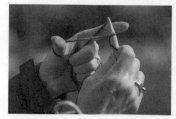 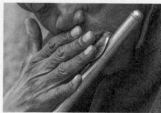 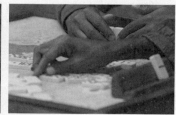

Fundamentals *of* Hand Therapy

Clinical Reasoning and Treatment Guidelines for Common Diagnoses of the Upper Extremity

Second Edition

Edited by

Cynthia Cooper, MFA, MA, OTR/L, CHT
Owner, Cooper Hand Therapy
Scottsdale, AZ
Adjunct Faculty
Occupational Therapy
A.T. Still University
Mesa, AZ

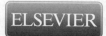

ELSEVIER
MOSBY

3251 Riverport Lane
St. Louis, Missouri 63043

Notice

Knowledge and best practice in this field are constantly changing. As new research and experience broaden our understanding, changes in research methods, professional practices, or medical treatment may become necessary.

Practitioners and researchers must always rely on their own experience and knowledge in evaluating and using any information, methods, compounds, or experiments described herein. In using such information or methods they should be mindful of their own safety and the safety of others, including parties for whom they have a professional responsibility.

With respect to any drug or pharmaceutical products identified, readers are advised to check the most current information provided (i) on procedures featured or (ii) by the manufacturer of each product to be administered, to verify the recommended dose or formula, the method and duration of administration, and contraindications. It is the responsibility of practitioners, relying on their own experience and knowledge of their patients, to make diagnoses, to determine dosages and the best treatment for each individual patient, and to take all appropriate safety precautions.

To the fullest extent of the law, neither the Publisher nor the authors, contributors, or editors, assume any liability for any injury and/or damage to persons or property as a matter of products liability, negligence or otherwise, or from any use or operation of any methods, products, instructions, or ideas contained in the material herein.

ISBN: 978-0-323-09104-6

Cover and part opener art designed by John Evarts

Content Strategist: Jolynn Gower
Senior Content Development Specialist: Christie Hart
Publishing Services Manager: Julie Eddy
Senior Project Manager: Marquita Parker
Design Direction: Jessica Williams

Printed in the United States

Last digit is the print number: 9 8 7 6 5 4 3 2

Working together
to grow libraries in
developing countries

www.elsevier.com • www.bookaid.org

Contributors

Sandra M. Artzberger, MS, OTR, CHT, CLT
Lecturer, Consultant, Clinician
Pagosa Springs, CO
Certified Hand Therapist
Rocky Mountain PT and Sports Injury Center
Pagosa Springs, CO

Jeanine Beasley, EdD, OTR, CHT, FAOTA
Associate Professor
Occupational Therapy
Grand Valley State University
Grand Rapids, MI
Hand Therapist
East Paris Hand Therapy
Mary Free Bed Rehabilitation Hospital
Grand Rapids, MI

Mark W. Butler, PT, DPT, OCS, Cert. MDT
Adjunct Associate Professor
School of Health Related Professions
Rutgers University
Stratford, NJ
Center Manager
Novacare
Medford, NJ

Shrikant J. Chinchalkar, MThO, BScOT, OTR, CHT
Hand Therapist
Hand and Upper Limb Center
St. Joseph's Health Care
London, Ontario, Canada

Cynthia Cooper, MFA, MA, OTR/L, CHT
Owner, Cooper Hand Therapy
Scottsdale, AZ
Adjunct Faculty
Occupational Therapy
A.T. Still University
Mesa, AZ

Jeffrey Cowdry, BS, OT, CHT
Hand Therapist
Hand Rehabilitation
Advanced Training and Rehab
St. Louis, MO

Lori DeMott, BS, OTR, CHT
Hand Therapy Manager
Therapy Services
Orthopedic One
Columbus, OH

Lisa Deshaies, BS, OTR/L, CHT
Clinical Specialist
Outpatient Therapy Services
Rancho Los Amigos National Rehabilitation Center
Downey, CA
Adjunct Clinical Faculty
Division of Occupational Science and Occupational Therapy
University of Southern California
Los Angeles, CA

Kelly Droege, MOTR/L
Occupational Therapist
Milliken Hand Rehabilitation Center
Healthsouth Corporation
St. Louis, MO

Lori Falkel, PT, MOMT, CHT, DPT, PT, CHT
Clinical Coordinator
Outpatient Therapies
Peace Health Saint John Medical Center
Longview, WA

Elaine Ewing Fess, MS, OTR, FAOTA, CHT
Adjunct Assistant Professor
Department of Occupational Therapy, SHRS
Indiana University
Indianapolis, IN

Sharon R. Flinn, PhD, OTR/L, CHT
Associate Professor
Division of Occupational Therapy
The Ohio State University Wexner Medical Center
Columbus, OH

Louann Gulick Gaub, MSA, OTR/L, CHT
Hand Therapist
Orthopedic One
Columbus, OH

William S. Graff, EdD
Licensed Psychologist
William S. Graff, EdD, PC
Phoenix, AZ

Vincent Hentz, MD
Emeritus Professor of Surgery and Orthopedic Surgery
Robert A. Chase Center for Hand and Upper Limb Surgery
Stanford University
Stanford, CA

Linda J. Klein, OTR, CHT
Hand Therapy Supervisor
Therapy Department
Hand Surgery, Ltd.
Milwaukee, WI

Paige E. Kurtz, MS, OTR/L, CHT
Hand Therapy Manager
Advanced Orthopedics
Richmond, VA
Adjunct Faculty
School of Physical Therapy
Old Dominion University
Norfolk, VA

Corey Weston McGee, PhD(c), MS, OTR/L, CHT
Assistant Professor
Program in Occupational Therapy
The University of Minnesota
Rochester, MN

Joel Moorhead, MD, PhD
Adjunct Assistant Professor
Environmental Health
Rollins School of Public Health/Emory University
Atlanta, GA
Clinical Director
FairCode Associates
Marco Island, GA

Patricia M. Moorhead, MHCA, OTR/L
Executive Director of Professional Services
WellStar Cobb Hospital
Austell, GA

Ryan Morgan, MS, OTR/L
Senior-Level Occupational Therapist
Occupational Therapy/Hand Therapy
Kentucky Hand & Physical Therapy
Lexington, KY

Anne M.B. Moscony, MA, OTR/L, CHT
Certified Hand Therapist
Occupational Therapy
Rothman Institute
Egg Harbor Township, NJ
Adjunct Faculty
Occupational Therapy - Graduate School
Philadelphia University
Philadelphia, PA

Brenda Nealy, PTA, BA
Certified Pilates Instructor, Master Pilates Certification
Strength-n-Length Pilates
Scottsdale, AZ

Carol Page, PT, DPT, CHT
Program Director, Hand Therapy Fellowship
Rehabilitation
Hospital for Special Surgery
New York, NY
Manager, Strategic Improvement
Rehabilitation
Hospital for Special Surgery
New York, NY

Julie Pal, OTR/L, CHT
Dept. of Occupational Therapy/Outpatient Rehabilitation
Saint Lukes Hospital
Kansas City, MO

Teri Britt Pipe, PhD, RN
Dean
College of Nursing and Health Innovation
Arizona State University
Phoenix, AZ

Joey G. Pipicelli, MScOT
Occupational Therapist, Certified Hand Therapist
Division of Hand Therapy
Hand and Upper Limb Centre, St. Joseph's Health Care
London, Ontario, Canada
Lecturer
School of Occupational Therapy, Faculty of Health Sciences
Western University
London, Ontario, Canada

Karen Donahue Pitbladdo, MS, OTR/L, CHT
Senior Occupational Therapist
Rehabilitation
San Francisco General Hospital
San Francisco, CA

Donald Greg Pitts, MS, OTR/L CHT
Clinical Specialist
Hand Therapy
Kentucky Hand and Physical Therapy
Lexington, KY
Faculty
Occupational Medicine
University of Kentucky
Lexington, KY

Gillian Porter, MA, MOT, OTR/L
Occupational Therapist
SWAN Rehab
Phoenix, AZ

Deborah A. Schwartz, OTD, OTR/L, CHT
Product and Educational Specialist
Physical Rehabilitation
Orfit Industries America
Leonia, NJ

Tracy M. Shank, MS, OTR/L, CHT
Hand Therapist
Nemours/A.I. duPont Hospital for Children
Wilmington, DE

Gary Solomon, MBA, MS, OTR/L, CHT
Director
Chicago Metro Hand Therapy, LLC
Arlington Heights, IL

Lara Taggart, MS, OTR/L
Faculty
Occupational Therapy Assistant Program
Brown Mackie College
Phoenix, AZ
Occupational Therapist
St. Joseph's Hospital
Phoenix, AZ

Marietta Tartaglia, MS, OTR/L
Occupational Therapist
Independent Contractor
Phoenix, AZ

Matthew J. Taylor, PT, PhD, ERYT-500
Director
Dynamic Systems Rehabilitation Clinic
Scottsdale, AZ

Aaron C. Varney, BS, MOTR/L, CHT
Clinical Specialist, Occupational Therapist, Certified Hand Therapist
Outpatient Therapies
PeaceHealth St. John Medical Center
Longview, WA

Rebecca von der Heyde, PhD, OTR/L, CHT
Director of Occupational Therapy Department
Concordia University Wisconsin
Mequon, WI

Jackie Wallman, OTR/L, CHT
Manager
Rehabilitation Services Department
Saint Luke's Hospital
Kansas City, MO

Colleen West, MS, OTR/L
Occupational Therapist
Advanced Home Care
Phoenix, AZ
Adjunct Faculty
A.T. Still University
Mesa, AZ

Christine M. Wietlisbach, OTD, OTR/L, CHT, MPA
Certified Hand Therapist
Rinker Hand Center
Eisenhower Medical Center
Rancho Mirage, CA
Assistant Professor
Occupational Therapy Program
Rocky Mountain University of Health Professions
Provo, UT

Jason Willoughby, MHS, OTR/L, CHT
Clinical Specialist
Hand Therapy
Kentucky Hand and Physical Therapy
Lexington, KY

Ranay Yarian, MA, CCRC
Community Outreach Manager
Integrative Oncology & Cancer Prevention
Banner MD Anderson Cancer Center
Gilbert, AZ
Faculty Associate
School of Social Work
Arizona State University
Tempe, AZ

Foreword

Again, Cynthia Cooper has honored me with the space to write an introduction to the second edition of her text, *Fundamentals of Hand Therapy: Clinical Reasoning and Treatment Guidelines for Common Diagnoses of the Upper Extremity*. By initially reviewing the Contents, the reader can see that this new edition, again, offers a unique and needed view of the practice of hand therapy not often seen in one volume. Cynthia has compiled authors able to provide the basic understanding of the fundamentals needed for understanding the anatomy and basic fundamentals used for evaluation and treatment interventions in the first section, Part One, "Fundamentals." The chapters that were retained were updated to more current application related to functional assessment, combining the mechanistic and organistic concepts needed to treat the whole person. Additions to this section include chapters related to orthoses and additional considerations of clinical reasoning and problem solving so needed for the hand therapist to provide optimal care. The addition of the chapter by Cooper and West of "Hand Coordination" is filled with such relevant and useful examples illustrated so well by the extensive figures included.

Part Two is focused on "Pain and Integrative Strategies," which is the unique and much-valued view of hand therapy from a client-centered point of view. The section includes concepts that are now more included and accepted in hand therapy practice, with additional evidence to support inclusions of the practices discussed. The concepts included in this section have been the perspective that Cynthia Cooper has offered us over the past several years at various presentations and through publications. Cynthia Cooper has a unique manner of ensuring that the need for occupation is included in the science of hand therapy in the intervention planned individually for each client treated. The concept of mind-body is not unknown to us, but putting the ideas together in one text makes this an unusual and very relevant read for the new as well as older generation of hand therapists. The inclusion of chapters related to the client-therapist relationship, offering examples through narratives in hand therapy, and relating the personality type to how best to provide patient/client education is a unique ability of Cynthia Cooper to put into conceptual thinking. The additional chapters that incorporate dance and Pilates in hand therapy continues to confirm this mind-body thinking along with more specific consideration to incorporate Yoga as a regular practice. This whole section is vital to hand therapists to read and integrate into their clinical thinking.

Finally, Part Three, "Clinical Reasoning and Treatment Guidelines for Common Diagnoses of the Upper Extremity" provides the clinician with the updated information needed in multiple diagnostic conditions found so useful in the first edition. Cynthia Cooper has added chapters in this section that begins with much needed information consolidated for the hand professional about wound care and ends with the addition of a topic for "Chemotherapy-Induced Peripheral Neuropathy." The assistance through updated knowledge offered within this text has essential use to the hand professionals to gain and/or improve knowledge of clinical reasoning for the usual and unusual clinical conditions seen in the clinic. I heartily recommend this textbook to all hand professionals, and again, I am honored to have the chance to review and write this piece on behalf of Cynthia Cooper and her original work.

Donna Breger Stanton, OTD, OTR/L, CHT, FAOTA
Associate Professor, Academic Fieldwork Coordinator
Samuel Merritt University, OT Program
Oakland, CA

To my wonderful husband,
John L. Evarts
You taught me to spread my wings and allow myself to take chances.
Once again, you have provided continuous emotional support,
artistic direction and insight, and valuable technical help.
You are an amazing person, a magnificent husband,
and will always be the love of my life.

Preface

Changes in reimbursements are affecting health care delivery and restricting clients' access to specialists. Even if their health plans support specialty care, they may have high co-pays or may live in remote locations where there are no hand therapy specialists. Therapists who are not familiar with the body of knowledge in hand therapy may inadvertently do more harm than good. Therapists who are unaware of tissue tolerances or who do not know about tissue timelines following injury or surgery can unintentionally injure clients, sometimes irrevocably.

The purpose of this book is to educate non-specialist therapists, hand therapists in training, and occupational and physical therapy students about the fundamentals of hand therapy, using didactic materials and case examples. It is also a recommended resource for therapists who are studying for the hand therapy certification examination. This textbook teaches reader's how to apply sound clinical reasoning to determine the needs of their clients with upper extremity problems. In addition, it provides clear treatment guidelines for common upper extremity diagnoses with content that is valuable, even for experienced hand therapists.

Good clinical reasoning skills are required in order for therapists to move beyond therapy protocols, to think critically about their clients' needs, and to provide safe and creative treatment. The content of this book enables therapists to treat their clients as unique people with individual needs, while applying appropriate and safe treatment.

The scope of this book is broad, with content that includes those diagnoses most typically referred to hand therapy. The book is organized into three parts. Part One lays the foundation and identifies fundamentals of hand therapy treatment. In this second edition, Part One has added new chapters on problem solving to prevent pitfalls, orthoses, and hand coordination. Part Two has been renamed "Pain and Integrative Strategies." In this edition, Part Two has new chapters on how therapists' words affect the therapeutic relationship, narratives in hand therapy, personality type and patient education in hand therapy, using dance in hand therapy, applying Pilates concepts to hand therapy by connecting through the hand, and Yoga therapeutics. Part Three covers "Clinical Reasoning and Treatment Guidelines for Common Diagnoses of the Upper Extremity." In this second edition, Part Three has new chapters on wound care, wrist instabilities, separate chapters on wrist fractures and hand fractures, the neurological hand, and hand therapy for chemotherapy-induced peripheral neuropathy.

The chapters in Part Three provide diagnosis-specific information. Although the reader should spend time with the entire book, the chapters in Part Three are useful as an easily accessed resource for common diagnoses of the hand and upper extremity. Most of the Part Three chapters use a similar organizational format that serves as a unifying framework:

- Anatomy
- Diagnosis/pathology

- Timelines and healing
- Nonoperative treatment
- Operative treatment
- Questions to discuss with the physician
- What to say to clients
- Evaluation tips
- Diagnosis-specific information that affects clinical reasoning
- Tips from the field
- Precautions and concerns
- Case examples

In addition, clinical pearls and precautions are highlighted throughout each chapter

This book is unique in that it explicitly aims to teach clinical reasoning in hand therapy. The special features in Part Three— questions to discuss with the physician, what to say to clients, tips from the field, precautions and concerns—can be used as mental prompts by therapists when treating their clients. Doing this will help them find their own clinical voices and will strengthen their clinical reasoning skills.

The case examples, many of which are not simple, serve two purposes. First, they demonstrate the use of clinical reasoning in treating the client. Second, they highlight the humanistic side of each client encounter. In reality, even a seemingly straightforward clinical case has its special challenges and intriguing moments. The cases were selected to remind the reader of the human side and humane concerns in caring for a hand therapy client.

I am hopeful that this book will spark therapists' passion for hand therapy and will teach them gentle ways of touching their clients' hands and lives.

Acknowledgments

I would like to acknowledge my mother, Delma P. Cooper, and my twin sister, Jan Carroll, for their interest in and enthusiasm for my work. I am extremely grateful to Kathy Falk, Executive Content Strategist, for her support and creativity in the development of the first edition of this book; to Jolynn Gower, Content Strategist, and to Christie Hart, Senior Content Development Specialist, for her guidance, vision, support, and expertise. I would also like to recognize Marquita Parker, who was the Senior Project Manager on this book. Thanks as well to Marietta Tartaglia, MS, OTR/L, for feedback and review of portions of the first and second editions; and to Sarah Arnold, OTS, Siaw Chui Chai, PhD., OT, and J. Robin Janson, MS, OTR, CHT, for reviewing some chapter proofs on a tight timeline. I am very grateful to Marcia McMurtrey, ACSW, LCSW, for helping me create opportunities to grow. Lastly, I wish to acknowledge the memories of my sister, Linda Cooper McGarry; my father, Herschel A. Cooper; and my friend, Gerald W. Sharrott. I know how pleased they would be for me to have this wonderful opportunity.

Contents

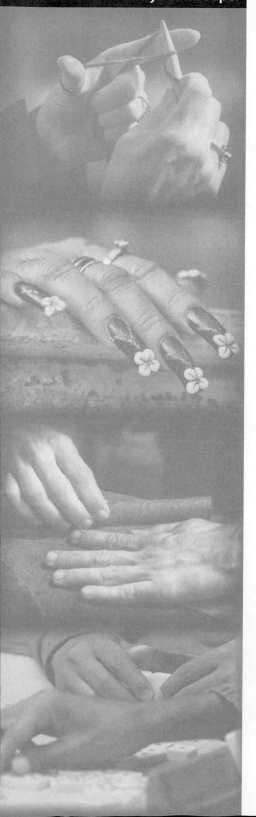

1

Fundamentals: Hand Therapy Concepts and Treatment Techniques

Cynthia Cooper

The more you know about something in detail, the less you know about it in general.

—From *The Child in Time* by Ian McEwan, Anchor Books, 1987

Hands are visible, expressive, and vulnerable. When clients use their hands to get dressed, eat, touch, gesture, or communicate, they are performing exquisite and complex movements. Limitations of motion or even a small scar can affect a person's life in profound ways.[1] When we touch our clients' hands, we touch their lives. Although it is very important to be knowledgeable about the details of hand anatomy and to be structure specific in our treatment, it is equally important not to lose sight of the whole person whose extremity we are treating. We must continuously encourage clients to tell us about themselves and their needs so that their therapy can be relevant and successful. While getting to know the person we are treating, we can explain how our interventions and the client's home programs will be helpful. As a rule, I find that if I listen well, clients frequently tell me in lay terms or even show me exactly what motion or function is missing. The challenge is to identify and treat clients' specific tissues effectively while not losing sight of them as people.

Hand Therapy Concepts

The anatomy of the hand is complex. Many structures are **multiarticulate** (that is, they cross multiple joints), and little room is available for scar tissue or edema to develop without affecting function. Injury in one area of the hand can result in stiffness in other, uninjured parts. A good demonstration of this is the **quadriga effect,** which illustrates the interconnectedness of the digits. If you passively hold your ring finger extended with your other hand and then try to make a fist, you will notice how limited the whole hand can feel when just one finger is held stiff. In this example, the flexor digitorum profundus (FDP) tendons to multiple digits have a shared muscle belly. Restricting movement at one finger restricts the other fingers when they try to flex. This example reminds us that clients can be limited in motion in areas not originally injured. Therefore the therapist needs to evaluate beyond the isolated area of injury when treating clients with hand problems.

To be competent in hand therapy, therapists must be able to do more than just note decreased range of motion (ROM). They must be able to figure out what structures are restricted and how these restrictions affect function (for example, the client has decreased digital flexion due to FDP adherence, preventing him from holding the steering wheel); they then must be able to target treatment to those particular tissues. These three elements are part of all the decisions we make as hand therapists. As treatment continues, re-evaluation reveals new findings with different tissues to target, and appropriate modifications and upgrades are made. This chapter addresses treatment concepts and techniques of hand therapy and concludes with some provocative thoughts to stimulate clinical reasoning.

Timelines and Healing

Tissues heal in predictable phases. However, the length of these phases varies depending on client variables, such as age and health. The three phases of healing are inflammation, fibroplasia, and maturation (also called *remodeling*). In the **inflammation phase,** vasoconstriction occurs, followed by vasodilation, with migration of white blood cells to promote **phagocytosis** in preparation for further healing. In this stage, which lasts a few days, immobilization often is advised, depending on the specifics of the diagnosis.[2] If wound contamination or delayed healing is a factor, this phase can last longer.[3]

The **fibroplasia phase** begins about 4 days after injury and lasts 2 to 6 weeks. In this phase, fibroblasts begin the formation of scar tissue. The fibroblasts lay down new collagen, on which capillary buds grow, leading to a gradual increase in the tissue's tensile strength. In this stage, active range of motion (AROM) and orthotics typically are used to promote balance in the hand and to protect the healing structures.[2]

The timeline for the **maturation (remodeling) phase** varies; this phase may even last years. In the maturation phase, the tissue's architecture changes, reflecting improved organization of the collagen fibers and a further increase in tensile strength. The tissue is more *responsive* (that is, reorganizes better) if appropriate therapy is started sooner rather than later. In this stage, gentle resistive exercises may be appropriate, and the client should be monitored for any inflammatory responses (also known as a *flare response*). Dynamic or static orthoses may also be helpful.[2]

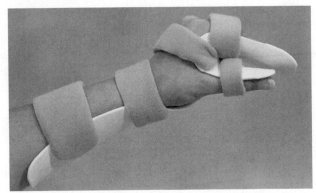

FIGURE 1-1 Antideformity (intrinsic-plus) orthotic position. (From Coppard BM, Lohman H, editors: *Introduction to splinting: a clinical-reasoning and problem-solving approach,* ed 2, St Louis, 2001, Mosby.)

Positioning to Counteract Deforming Forces

Predictable deforming forces act on an injured upper extremity (UE). **Edema** (swelling) routinely occurs after injury, creating tension on the tissues. The resulting predictable deformity posture is one of wrist flexion, metacarpophalangeal (MP) hyperextension, proximal interphalangeal (PIP) and distal interphalangeal (DIP) flexion, and thumb adduction.[4] This deformity position occurs as a result of tension on the extrinsic muscles caused by dorsal edema.

Use of the **antideformity (intrinsic-plus) position** is recommended after injury unless it is contraindicated by the diagnosis (for example, it is not used after flexor tendon repair). The antideformity position consists of the wrist in neutral position or extension, the MPs in flexion, the IPs in extension (*IPs* refers to the PIP and DIP joints collectively), and the thumb in abduction with opposition (Fig. 1-1). The antideformity position maintains length in the collateral ligaments, which are vulnerable to shortening, and counteracts deforming forces.

Joint and Musculotendinous Tightness

Joint tightness is confirmed if the passive range of motion (PROM) of a joint does not change despite repositioning of proximal or distal joints. **Musculotendinous tightness** is confirmed if the PROM of a joint changes with repositioning of adjacent joints that are crossed by that particular muscle-tendon (musculotendinous) unit.[5]

Joint tightness and musculotendinous tightness can be treated with serial casting, dynamic orthoses static progressive orthoses or serial static orthoses (see Chapter 7 and also the "Orthotics" section later in this chapter). With joint tightness, splinting can focus on the stiff joint, and less consideration is needed for the position of proximal or distal joints. With musculotendinous tightness, because the tightness occurs in a structure that crosses multiple joints, the orthotic must carefully control the position of proximal (and possibly distal) joints to remodel tightness effectively along that musculotendinous unit.

The client in Fig. 1-2, *A*, had an infected PIP joint in the index finger. He was treated with hospitalization, intravenous administration of antibiotics, and joint debridement. He arrived for therapy 2 weeks later than his physician had ordered; he had no orthotic, significant edema, and a severe flexion contracture of

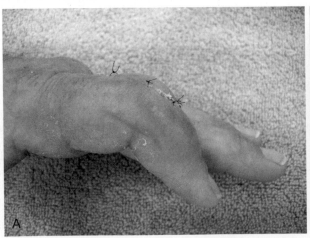
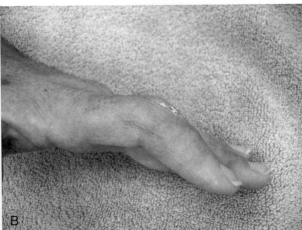

FIGURE 1-2 A, Unsplinted, infected index finger after surgery. **B,** Improvement in edema and improved extension range of motion (ROM) after 2 weeks.

the PIP joint. Because the stiffness was localized to the PIP joint, he needed only a digit-based extension orthosis for that joint. Fig. 1-2, *B*, shows his progress after 2 weeks of edema control and serial static digit-based orthoses.

Musculotendinous tightness can be a cause of joint tightness. Clients with tightness of the extrinsic flexors (that is, lacking passive composite digital extension with the wrist extended) are at risk of developing IP flexion contractures. Instruct these clients to passively place the MP in flexion and then to gently, passively extend the IPs to maintain PIP and DIP joint motion. In these cases, although you should consider night orthoses in composite extension to lengthen the extrinsic flexors, the better course may be to splint in a modified intrinsic-plus position with the MPs flexed as needed to support the IPs in full extension. This helps prevent IP flexion contractures.

Intrinsic or Extrinsic Extensor Muscle Tightness

Intrinsic muscles are the small muscles in the hand. **Extrinsic muscles** are longer musculotendinous units that originate proximal to the hand. Intrinsic tightness and extrinsic extensor tightness are tested by putting these muscles on stretch. This is accomplished by comparing the PROM of digital PIP and DIP flexion when the MP joint is passively extended and then passively flexed. With **interosseous muscle tightness,** passive PIP and DIP flexion is limited when the MP joint is passively extended or hyperextended (Fig. 1-3). With **extrinsic extensor tightness,** PIP and DIP flexion is limited when the MP joint is passively flexed (Fig. 1-4).[5]

To treat intrinsic tightness, perform PIP and DIP flexion with MP hyperextension. Functional orthotics are very helpful for isolating specific exercise to restore length to the intrinsics while performing daily activities (see the "Orthotics" section). To treat extrinsic extensor tightness, promote **composite motions** (that is, combined flexion motions of the wrist, MPs and IPs) with orthotics, gentle stretch, and exercise. Instruct the client that performing these exercises with the wrist in a variety of positions is helpful.

Extrinsic Extensor or Flexor Tightness

Extrinsic tightness can involve the flexors or the extensors. To test for tightness, put the structure on stretch by positioning the proximal joint crossed by that structure. With extrinsic extensor tightness, passive composite digital flexion is more limited with the wrist flexed than with the wrist extended. With extrinsic flexor tightness, passive composite digital extension is more limited with the wrist extended than with the wrist flexed.[5]

Lag or Contracture

> ◎ *Clinical Pearl*
>
> When PROM is greater than AROM at a joint, the active limitation is called lag.

A client with a PIP extensor lag is unable to actively extend the PIP joint as far as is possible passively (which may not necessarily be full extension). **Lags** may be caused by adhesions, disruption of the musculotendinous unit, or weakness.

> ◎ *Clinical Pearl*
>
> When passive limitation of joint motion exists, that limitation is called a *joint contracture.*

Joint contractures can be caused by collateral ligament tightness, adhesions, or a mechanical block. A *joint flexion contracture* is characterized by a stiff joint in a flexed position that lacks active and passive extension. A person with a joint flexion contracture whose passive extension improves may progress from having a flexion contracture to having an extensor lag. In your treatment communications and documentation, it is important to identify such changes, to use these terms correctly, and to be joint specific and motion specific. For example, you should note, "The client has full PIP passive extension but demonstrates a 30-degree PIP extensor lag."

When a lag is present (PROM exceeds AROM), treatment should focus on promoting active movement. Blocking exercises (Fig. 1-5), differential tendon gliding exercises (see Fig. 1-18), place and hold exercises (see Fig. 1-19), and dynamic or static functional orthotics can be helpful (Fig. 1-6). If a contracture is present, promote both PROM and AROM with the same exercises and with corrective orthoses, which may be the dynamic, static progressive, serial static, or casting type.

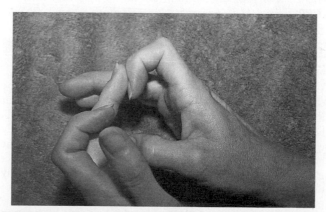

FIGURE 1-3 Interosseous muscle tightness. Proximal interphalangeal (PIP) and distal interphalangeal (DIP) flexion is passively limited when the metacarpophalangeal (MP) joint is passively extended or hyperextended.

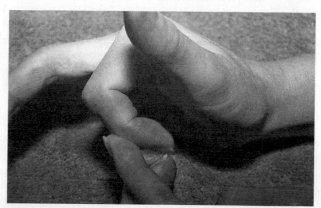

FIGURE 1-4 Extrinsic extensor tightness. PIP and DIP flexion is passively limited when the MP joint is passively flexed.

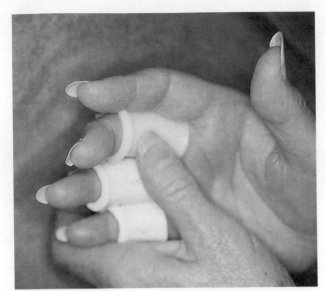

FIGURE 1-5 DIP blocking exercises with the MP in various positions.

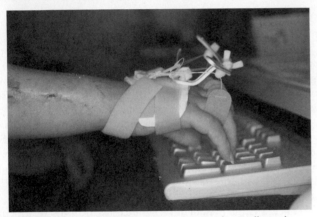

FIGURE 1-6 A dynamic MP extension assist orthosis allows the client to perform keyboard activities at the computer.

Joint End-Feel

A joint with a **soft end-feel** has a spongy quality at the end-range. This is a favorable quality that indicates a potential for remodeling. Orthoses for soft end-feel may be the static type or the low-load, long duration type (see the "Orthotic" section and Chapter 7).

A joint with a **hard end-feel** has an unyielding quality at end-range. This is a stiffer joint, and correcting it may require serial casting or static progressive orthoses with longer periods of splint wear.[2] Documenting the end-feel and explaining the implications of your findings to the client are very important.

Nociceptive Pain versus Neuropathic Pain[6]

Not all pain is the same physiologically or symptomatically. **Nociceptive pain** is caused by structural dysfunction, such as an arthritic wrist. Providing an orthotic to support the involved structures reduces the pain. **Neuropathic pain** is caused by some form of peripheral nerve dysfunction and is typically a sensory pain that is difficult for patients to describe in words. It may be burning or electrical. Providing sensory protection and minimizing peripheral nerve irritation reduces this type of pain.

Hand therapy patients may have nociceptive pain or neuropathic pain or a combination of the two. It is important to address this with patients so that your treatment targets their unique pain quality and can be most successful.

Preventing Pain

Precaution. *Pain with therapy is a signal that injury is occurring. Irreversible damage can result when clients or their families or, worse, therapists injure tissue by using painful force and PROM. Avoid pain in your hand therapy treatment. Being overzealous and ignoring objective signs of tissue intolerance is inexcusable.*

Teaching clients and their families that painful therapy is counterproductive can be a challenge. Often clients come to therapy with a "no pain, no gain" mentality. To make matters worse, this philosophy frequently is reinforced by their physicians and friends. Therapists have a duty to explain to their clients that imposing, prolonging, or aggravating pain slows the healing process, fosters more scarring and stiffness, and delays or eliminates opportunities to upgrade therapy.

> ### ⊚ *Clinical Pearl*
>
> Never tell your clients, "Exercise to pain tolerance" or "Go to pain." Instead say, "Avoid pain when you exercise. It's okay to feel a stretch that isn't painful, but it's not okay to feel pain when you exercise."

Taking Care with Passive Range of Motion

PROM of the hand should be performed gently and with care.

Precaution. *PROM can injure swollen and inflamed joints and tissues.* Colditz[5] cautions that the only joints for which manual PROM is safe are joints with a soft end-feel. Nevertheless, clients may request more aggressive therapy. They may even be passively stressing their swollen, stiff hands at home. It is very important that the therapist inquire about this and put a stop to it. Explain to your client how injurious and counterproductive it is, emphasizing that delicate hand tissues are all too easily injured (see Chapter 12).

Precaution. *PROM can trigger inflammatory responses, causing additional scar production, pain, and stiffness. PROM used inappropriately or painfully can incite complex regional pain syndrome (CRPS), which is also known as reflex sympathetic dystrophy (RSD).*

> ### 〔〕 *What to Say to Clients*
>
> #### If the Doctor Orders "Aggressive Therapy"

When a physician orders aggressive therapy for a client, I tell the client, "Your doctor wants you to make excellent progress. But the reality is that tissues in the hand are delicate and can easily be injured by too much force or pressure. We will promptly correct the restricted or injured tissues, and you will make the best progress by providing controlled stress to the proper structures. Painful, injurious treatment or exercise will only delay or even derail your progress. What we will do aggressively is to upgrade your program and encourage maximum results."

Hopefully, physicians soon will realize the wisdom of replacing the term *aggressive* with *progressive*. Until that happens, explain to your clients that pain-free, controlled stretching and remodeling have proved to be the best course of treatment for the fragile hand tissues.

Quality of Movement and Dyscoordinate Co-Contraction

Dyscoordinate co-contraction is a poor quality of movement that can result from co-contraction of antagonist muscles. Clients may demonstrate dyscoordinate co-contraction when they use excessive effort with exercise or when they fear pain with exercise or PROM, or it may be habitual. The resulting motion looks unpleasant and awkward. For example, you may feel the extensors contract as the client tries to activate the flexors. It is important not to ignore dyscoordinate co-contraction. Instead, teach the client pain-free, smooth movements that feel pleasant to perform. Replace isolated exercises with purposeful or functional activities and try proximal oscillations (small, gentle, rhythmic motions) to facilitate a more effective quality of movement. Biofeedback or electrical stimulation may also be helpful. Imagery offers additional possibilities (for example, ask your client to pretend to move the extremity through gelatin or water).[7] Do not bark at the client to "Relax!" Instead, be gentle with your voice and your verbal cues.

Adjunct Treatments

Superficial heating agents can have beneficial effects on analgesic, vascular, metabolic, and connective tissue responses. Analgesic effects are seen in diminished pain and elevated pain tolerance. Vascular effects are evidenced by reduced muscle spasms and improved pain relief. Metabolic effects are related to an increased flow of blood and oxygen to the tissues with improved provision of nutrients and removal of byproducts associated with inflammation. Connective tissue effects include reduced stiffness with improved extensibility of tissues.[8]

Many clients feel that heat helps prepare the tissue for exercise and activity. The safest way to warm the tissues of hand therapy clients is aerobic exercise, unless this is contraindicated for medical reasons. Tai chi, for example, provides multijoint ROM, relaxation, and cardiac effects.

Application of external heat (for example, hot packs) is a popular method in many clinics. Although the use of heat is fine if it is not contraindicated, be mindful that heat increases edema, which acts like glue, and this may contribute to stiffness. Heat can degrade collagen and may contribute to microscopic tears in soft tissue.[9] For these reasons, be very gentle and cautious if you perform PROM after heat application. Monitor the situation to make sure that the overall benefits of heat outweigh any possible negative responses. Measuring edema is a good way to objectify these responses.

Cold therapy (also called *cryotherapy*) traditionally has been used to relieve pain and to reduce inflammation and edema after injury (and sometimes after overly aggressive therapy). Cryotherapy typically is used after acute injury to reduce bleeding by means of vasoconstriction. Cold therapy reduces postinjury edema and inflammation and raises the pain threshold. However, remember: *cold therapy can be harmful to tissues; be cautious with this modality.*

Precaution. *Do not use cryotherapy on clients with nerve injury or repair, sensory impairment, peripheral vascular disease, Raynaud's phenomenon, lupus, leukemia, multiple myeloma, neuropathy, other rheumatic disease, or cold intolerance.*

Other modalities used in hand therapy include therapeutic ultrasound, electrical stimulation, and iontophoresis (provision of an agent such as an anti-inflammatory medication into tissue through use of low-voltage direct current). Therapists should study these topics further. However, they also must abide by their practice acts and the regulations of their state licensing agencies regarding the use of modalities. Never use a modality for which you cannot demonstrate proper education and training.

Scar Management

Scars can take many months to heal fully. Treat scar sensitivity with desensitization. If the sensitivity causes functional limitations, provide protection, such as padding or silicone gel. Scars are mature when they are pale, supple, flatter, and no longer sensitive. Scar maturation can be facilitated by light compression (for example, with Coban, Tubigrip [an elastic support sleeve], or edema gloves).

Precaution. *Always check to make sure the compression on the scar is not excessive (that is, the wrap, sleeve, or glove is not too tight).*

Inserts made of padded materials or silicone gel pads also help facilitate scar maturation.[10] This padding is thought to promote neutral warmth of the area and may decrease oxygen to the collagen, thus promoting collagen maturation. Another alternative for scar management is to use micropore paper tape applied longitudinally along the incision line once epithelialization has occurred.[11] I have found this to be very effective and cost-saving for patients. In addition, paper tape helps reduce neuropathic pain (see Chapter 41).

Instruct your clients to avoid sun exposure while the scar is still immature (that is, pink or red, thick, itchy, or sensitive). Sunlight can burn the fragile scar and darken its color, affecting the cosmetic result when the scar is mature. Frequent use of sunscreen is highly recommended (see Chapter 34). Although scar massage is often performed, it is important to monitor the client's tissue response.

Precaution. *If scar massage is too aggressive, it may cause inflammation and contribute to more extensive development or thickening of scar tissue.*

Do not encourage aggressive massage; instead, teach the client to perform gentler massage that does not cause a flare of tissues. Further research on this topic is needed.

Treatment Techniques

Orthoses

Orthotic Fabrication is a mainstay of therapy for UE problems. Orthotics can provide immobilization or selective mobilization. They can be used with exercise or to promote function. The topic of orthoses exceeds the scope of this chapter (see Chapter 7). I strongly advise readers to study more comprehensive resources on this subject.[2,12] In addition to learning about orthotic fabrication, readers should learn about strap placement for mechanical advantage and comfort.

Static orthotics are used to immobilize tissues, to prevent deformity, to prevent contracture of soft tissue, and to provide substitution for lost motor function. **Serial static orthoses** position the tissue for lengthening and are remolded at intervals. Static orthotics contribute to disuse, stiffness, and atrophy; therefore they should not be used more than necessary. **Static progressive orthoses** (also called *inelastic mobilization orthotics*) apply mobilizing force using nonmoving parts such as monofilament, Velcro, or screws. **Dynamic orthotics** (also called **mobilization orthotics**

or **elastic mobilization orthotics**) use moving parts, such as rubber bands or spring wires, to apply a gentle force. These orthotics are used to correct deformity, to substitute for absent or impaired motor function, to provide controlled movement, and to promote wound healing or help with alignment of fractures.[12,13]

Forearm-based orthotics should cover approximately two-thirds of the forearm. Have the client bend the arm at the elbow, and note the place where the forearm meets the biceps muscle. The proximal edge of the orthotic should be ¼-inch distal to this so that the orthotic is not pushed distally when the client flexes the elbow. Flaring the proximal edges of the orthotic is also important to ensure that the orthotic stays in place on the arm.[14] Clearing the distal palmar crease is extremely important. If the orthotic crosses this crease, MP flexion will be impeded. When you construct a dorsal forearm-based orthotic or a forearm-based ulnar gutter, pad the area of the ulnar head, because this bony prominence can become a pressure area. Always incorporate the padding into the molding of the orthotic; do not place it inside afterward as an addition. With mobilization orthotics, the best approach is to provide an orthotic your client can tolerate for long periods.

> ◎ **Clinical Pearl**
>
> Applying low tension that is tolerable and constant over prolonged periods is much more effective than applying strong forces over shorter periods.

The amount of safe force for the hand is 100 to 300 g.[15] Clients often ask that more force be used in their orthotics. These clients need repeated education that low load over a long duration is the safest and most effective way to remodel tissues and make clinical progress.

Precaution. *Painful splinting can be harmful.*

Skin blanching is a sign of high tension or incorrect orthotic mechanics.[3] The line of pull on the part being mobilized in a static progressive or dynamic orthotic must be a 90-degree angle from the **outrigger** (the structure from which the forces are directed). An outrigger can be high profile or low profile (Fig. 1-7). High-profile outriggers have certain mechanical and adjustment advantages but are bulkier and less attractive.[16]

Orthotics Used with Exercise

A dorsal dropout orthotic can be used to correct digital flexion or extrinsic extensor tightness. Mold the orthosis in a position of comfortable stretch. Use strapping as needed to keep it in place. The client should try to gently flex the digits away from the orthotic as able (Fig. 1-8). Having an object to reach for, such as a dowel in the palm, can be helpful.

Orthoses can be used to achieve various differential MP positions. The differential MP orthotic in Fig. 1-9 positions the long finger MP in greater flexion than the index and ring fingers. In this orthotic, active MP flexion of the index and ring fingers facilitates long finger flexion. Fig. 1-10 shows the opposite differential MP orthotic with the long finger MP more extended than the adjacent fingers. A differential MP orthotic with the small finger MP more flexed than the ring finger might be useful for a small finger metacarpal fracture with limited MP flexion. Active PIP flexion and extension within this type of orthotic at various MP positions also promotes PIP joint ROM and tendon gliding. This orthotic can be used during a progressive gripping activity (for

example, gripping a handful of dried beans, squeezing some out of the hand, and then gripping further).

A scrap of thermoplastic material can be used to create a cylinder to fit the client's available limited fist position. Sustained gripping of or holding onto this cylinder and "pumping" to flex and extend the digits around the cylinder may enhance composite digital flexion.

Chip Bags

Chip bags can be incorporated into orthotic regimens to maximize lymphatic flow and minimize the stiffness and adherence that otherwise would worsen as a result of the edema. A **chip bag** is a cotton stockinette bag filled with small foam pieces of various densities (Fig. 1-11). The foam can be cut from a variety of sources, including foam exercise blocks, padding, and soft Velcro materials. Chip bags traditionally have been used in the treatment of lymphedema; they are positioned over indurated areas of edema within external compressive garments or multilayered stretch bandages. Chip bags provide light traction on the skin, facilitate lymphatic stimulation, and promote neutral warmth. All these effects help reduce edema. The increased body heat under the chip bag and the light pressure exerted by the bag help soften thickened or fibrotic tissue.

In some cases, chip bags can be used alone without an accompanying orthotic. In such cases, they can be held in place with stockinette or a soft Velcro strap that is not applied tightly. Sometimes a less technical approach, such as using chip bags with orthotics, is a very effective option. Chip bags also can be positioned inside or in conjunction with orthotics to maximize edema control and reduce scar adherence. Clients find chip bags very comfortable. Some refer to the chip bag as their "pillow," which probably conveys the comfort they experience with it.

Soft Four-Finger Buddy Strap

A soft four-finger buddy strap can be made from Softstrap Velcro loop to provide transverse support that promotes more efficient primary function of the extrinsic flexors and extensors (see Fig. 1-20, *A-D,* on the Evolve website). This strap facilitates AROM for composite flexion and extension and for isolated extensor digitorum communis (EDC) and FDP tendon glide. It also stimulates lymphatic flow over the volar proximal phalanges, similar to chip bags. The soft four-finger buddy strap can relieve pain and promote AROM when hand stiffness is present. It also is helpful for symptom management in clients with lateral epicondylitis (tennis elbow) who have EDC involvement and pain on fisting.[17]

CASE STUDIES

CASE STUDY 1-1 ■

A client was in an altercation with a family member, and her hand was closed in a door during the argument. She was seen for malunion of a right distal radius fracture with right ulnar joint dislocation and extensor pollicis longus (EPL) rupture. She underwent open carpal tunnel release, corrective osteotomy of the distal radius fracture with internal fixation and bone grafting, and intercalary tendon grafting of the EPL tendon using the extensor indicis proprius (EIP). When

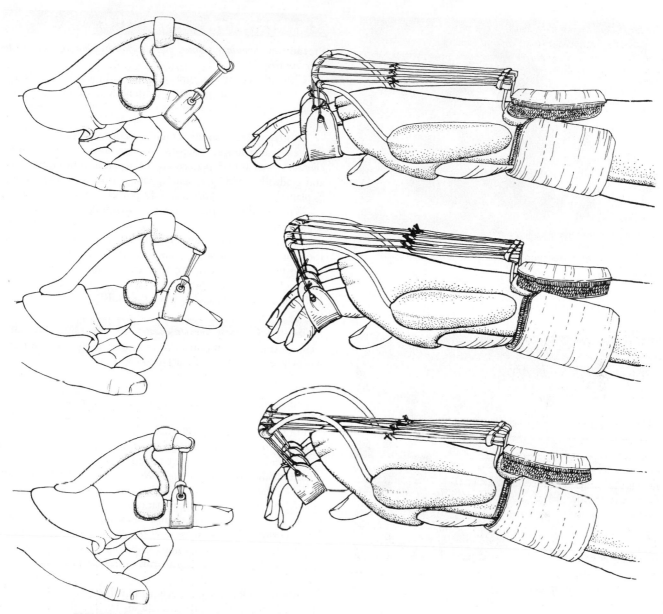

FIGURE 1-7 Examples of the 90-degree angle of pull with high-profile and low-profile outriggers. (From Fess EE: Principles and methods of splinting for mobilization of joints. In Mackin EJ, Callahan AD, Skirven TM et al, editors: *Rehabilitation of the hand and upper extremity,* ed 5, St Louis, 2002, Mosby.)

the client was seen in occupational therapy, her hand was extremely swollen and stiff, and she had severe extrinsic extensor tightness that limited full fisting. She developed CRPS and was treated successfully for this with a combination of stellate ganglion blocks and hand therapy. Note the dorsal scars and edema (Fig. 1-12, *A*). The style of chip bag incorporated into her volar wrist orthosis is shown in Fig. 1-12, *B*. This woman was a highly motivated client. At the time her therapy was discontinued, she had regained very good hand function.

CASE STUDY 1-2 ■

A client who underwent surgery for release of a Dupuytren's contracture developed a flare reaction. Note the incisional scar and fullness of the ulnar hand (Fig. 1-13, *A*), as well as the limitation in composite digital flexion (Fig. 1-13, *B*). This client used a chip bag inside an exercise orthotic designed to block the MPs and promote PIP and DIP

flexion exercise; the goals were to resolve intrinsic muscle tightness and promote composite digital flexion. Within 2 weeks, the client had made very good gains (Fig. 1-13, *C*).

CASE STUDY 1-3 ■

A woman who fell while hiking sustained a displaced distal radius fracture that required external fixation and percutaneous pin fixation. More than a week passed after her fall before she went to her physician. The woman explained this by noting that she has attention deficit disorder. She came to therapy 1 day after applying an elastic bandage tightly and irregularly around her external fixator. Note the indentations left on her skin by the wrap (Fig. 1-14, *A*). Chip bags were incorporated into the dressings and orthotics used in this case (Fig. 1-14, *B*), and the client progressed very well in therapy. She had good composite digital extension and flexion at the time of discharge (Fig. 1-14, *C* and *D*).

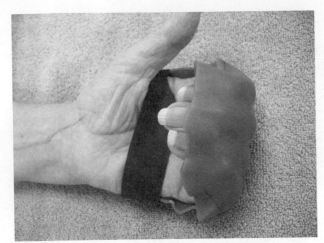

FIGURE 1-8 Client performing active digital flexion in a dorsal dropout orthosis.

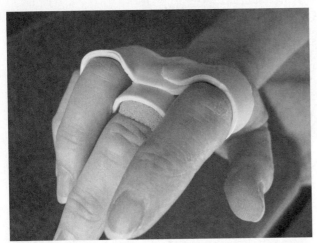

FIGURE 1-9 Differential MP positioning orthosis with long finger MP more flexed than adjacent fingers.

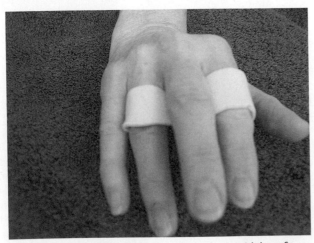

FIGURE 1-10 Differential MP positioning orthosis with long finger MP more extended than adjacent fingers.

Exercises for Upper Extremity Therapy

Precaution. *Shoulder stiffness can develop insidiously and can be very limiting.*

Check the client's posture and proximal motion initially and then at intervals. Incorporate proximal AROM into all home exercise programs even if this is only a preventive measure (see Chapter 22).

Shorter, milder sessions of exercise performed more frequently are better than longer, intensive sessions done less often. Some clients do well at first, performing five repetitions five times a day and gradually building to ten repetitions hourly during the day. Explain that exercises work well if the process is brief and frequent.

When working on isolated wrist extension, be sure to isolate the extensor carpi radialis brevis (ECRB), and teach clients how to extend the wrist with a soft fist that includes MP flexion. Have them hold an object so that the MPs are flexed. It is critical to retrain the ECRB to perform wrist extension. Without this isolation of motion, the client may learn to extend the wrist with EDC substitution instead of using the ECRB.

Clinical Pearl

Once established, the habit of extending the wrist with EDC substitution can be very hard to break.

To work on wrist active/active assistive range of motion (A/AAROM), put a towel on the table, and then place a coffee can (no bigger than the 3-lb size) on its side on the towel. Teach the client to place the involved hand on the can and to use the other hand to hold the involved hand flat on the can. The client then rolls the can using A/AAROM forward and backward. Clients like the feeling of this exercise, which also promotes proximal ROM and stimulates lymphatic flow.

In contrast to this, if extrinsic flexor tightness is a problem, the client would perform exercises involving wrist extension with simultaneous digital extension. Otherwise, exercises for wrist extension should be done primarily with a fist that includes MP flexion.

Always look at the client's wrist position when exercising the digits. Do not exercise or coax the digits into flexion with the wrist flexed unless you are deliberately trying to stretch the extrinsic extensors. It is biomechanically easier to achieve digital flexion with the wrist in extension, to achieve PIP joint flexion with the MP extended, and to achieve PIP joint extension with the MP flexed. If the client cannot sustain a position of wrist neutral or extension, use an orthosis or have the client self-support the wrist using the other hand when digital exercises are performed.

Instruct clients always to keep the upper arm locked at the side of the body when performing forearm rotation exercises.

Clinical Pearl

Do not perform forearm rotation exercises with the elbow on a table or even on a pillow; this prevents isolated forearm rotation and allows for substitution with humeral motions.

Teach the client that one way to do this is to keep a towel roll pressed to the side of the body with the arm used to perform forearm rotation exercises, because this requires that the elbow be kept close to the body.

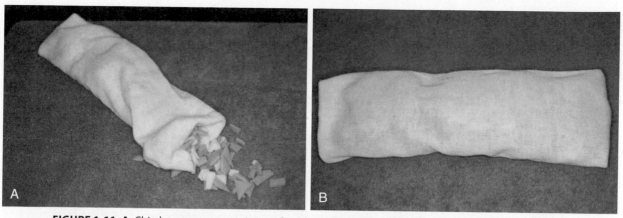

FIGURE 1-11 A, Chip bag contents consisting of small pieces of foam placed in a cotton stockinette. **B,** Ends of chip bag can be folded over and taped closed.

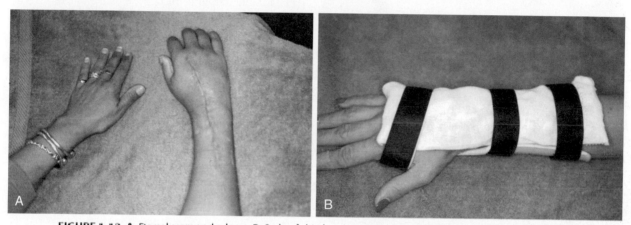

FIGURE 1-12 A, Dorsal scars and edema. **B,** Style of chip bag incorporated into the client's volar wrist orthosis.

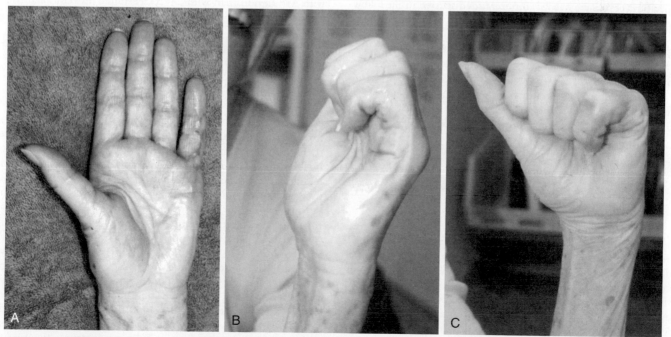

FIGURE 1-13 A, Flared incisional scar that developed after Dupuytren's release surgery. **B,** Limited active composite flexion. **C,** Full active composite flexion 2 weeks later.

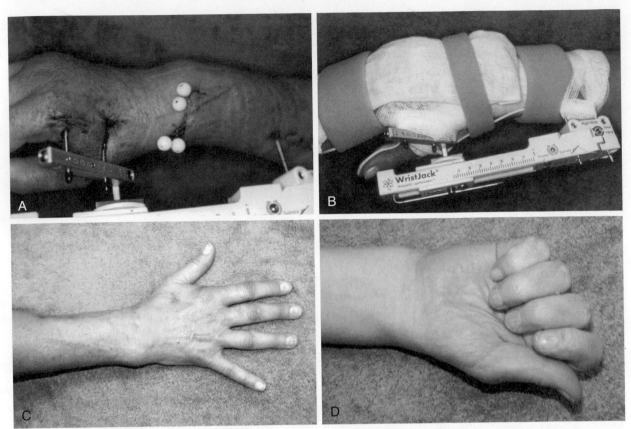

FIGURE 1-14 A, Indentations made by a tight elastic bandage applied by the client. **B,** Chip bags incorporated into dressings and orthosis with external fixator and pins. **C** and **D,** Resolution of edema and active digital extension and flexion at discharge.

In some cases, AROM through functional activity and exercise may be all that is needed to enable the client to recover full UE flexibility and function. When more isolated and structure-specific exercises are needed, the exercises discussed in the following sections may be helpful.

Blocking Exercises

Blocking exercises are exercises in which proximal support is provided to promote isolated motion at a particular site. They are helpful for clients with limitation of either AROM or PROM or both. Blocking exercises exert more force than nonblocking exercises.

> ### ◎ Clinical Pearl
>
> With blocking exercises, instruct the client to hold the position at comfortable end-range for 3 to 5 seconds; this allows remodeling of the tissues.

Blocking exercises can be accomplished in a variety of ways. You can use either commercially available devices or individual devices made from scraps of orthotic materials. Digital gutters or cylinders that cross the IPs help isolate MP flexion and extension. If the cylinder is shortened to free the DIP, then DIP blocking exercises can be performed. These exercises can be done with the MP in extension or in varying degrees of flexion. Often a client exerts too strong a contraction, and the PIP tries to flex within the blocking splint. Explain to the client that isolating motion

to only the DIP requires a soft quality of contraction so that the effort is not overridden by other structures. The biomechanical challenge to the FDP is greater when DIP flexion is performed with MP flexion than with MP extension. This positional progression can be used to upgrade the exercises.

> ### ◎ Clinical Pearl
>
> When a digital PIP block is used to promote MP flexion of the small finger, it is very helpful to stabilize the small finger metacarpal.

The ring and small finger metacarpals are more mobile at their carpometacarpal (CMC) joints than are the index and long finger metacarpals. If the metacarpal is supported by your hand or the client's other hand, more effective isolated motion can occur at the MP joint. This isolation and proximal support can be very helpful for clients trying to recover MP flexion after a small finger metacarpal fracture.

A blocking splint with the MPs flexed helps isolate active PIP extension (Fig. 1-15). Extending the PIP is easier biomechanically when the MP is flexed, because this position promotes central slip function. This same blocking splint also promotes composite flexion exercise and can be helpful for normalizing extrinsic extensor tightness. Conversely, a blocking splint with the MPs extended (Fig. 1-16) helps to isolate active IP flexion and FDP excursion and to resolve intrinsic tightness. These types of orthotics can be used with function, or they may be used only for exercise.

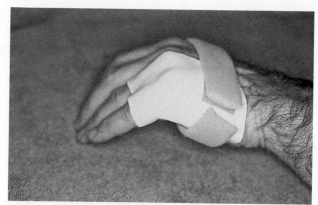

FIGURE 1-15 Blocking orthosis with the MP flexed helps isolate PIP extension and promotes extrinsic extensor stretch.

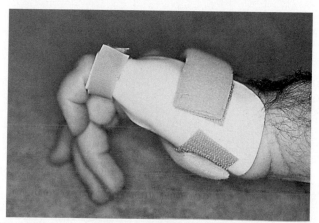

FIGURE 1-16 Blocking orthosis with the MP extended helps isolate active PIP flexion and flexor digitorum profundus (FDP) excursion and also helps resolve intrinsic tightness.

A DIP cap or flexion block diverts FDP excursion to the PIP and thus promotes isolated exercise of the FDS muscle with MP and PIP flexion and DIP extension. This blocking device may also help the client exercise the flexor digitorum superficialis (FDS) fist position more easily (see the following section).

Differential Tendon Gliding Exercises

Differential tendon gliding exercises are a mainstay of most home programs because they are easy to perform and they promote motion very effectively (Fig. 1-17).[18] They are a standard exercise for conservative management of carpal tunnel syndrome and are also used after carpal tunnel release. These exercises are an important option for all clients with hand or wrist stiffness. Rolling a thick highlighting pen up and down in the palm is an effective way to perform FDP gliding.

Place and Hold Exercises

Place and hold exercises can be helpful when PROM is greater than AROM (Fig. 1-18). Gently perform AAROM to position the finger (for example, in composite flexion). Then ask the client to sustain that position comfortably while releasing the assisting hand. The assisting hand may be yours or the client's other hand. Watch for co-contraction or force that is too strenuous as the client tries to sustain the exercise position. A combination of blocking exercises and place and hold exercises can be very productive. Also, you can try doing place and hold exercises with a blocking orthosis in place.

When the client releases the sustained contraction, pain sometimes may be felt in the area of a stiff joint. For instance, if the client performs place and hold exercises for composite fisting and then has PIP joint discomfort when releasing the fist, have the client relax the muscle contraction but stay in the same fisted position. While the client stays in that position, gradually provide assistance to gently begin extending the digit or digits (minimal joint distraction mobilization also can be helpful if not contraindicated). Next, ask the client to slowly actively extend the digits the rest of the way. This technique can be helpful for eliminating pain associated with end-ranges and AAROM.

Resistive Exercises

After clients have been medically cleared for them, resistive exercises are used for strengthening and to improve excursion of adherent tissue. Sometimes clients want to use a greater load than is safe for them. Teach clients that, for isolating wrist curls, they should not use as heavy a weight as they would for biceps curls.

Precaution. *Think carefully and critically about the status of your client's wrist if the person is recovering from a fracture, has had tendonitis, or is at risk for degenerative joint changes. Be very careful with wrist radial and ulnar deviation strengthening exercises, because these may provoke tendonitis.*

Generally speaking, the safest course in performing resistive exercises is to use more repetitions with a lower load. This approach promotes endurance. (A more detailed discussion of resistive exercise is presented in Chapter 4.)

Resistive exercise can take many forms, including progressive resistive exercises (PREs) and exercises performed with graded grippers, rubber bands, squeeze balls, graded clothespins, and putty. For example, marbles or other objects can be embedded in putty, requiring pinch and dexterity to remove them.

Functional Activity

It is essential that the client incorporate the gains made from exercising into functional UE use at home and at work. Practicing or simulating relevant activities in the clinic can reinforce this. Examples of such activities may include tying shoes, folding clothes, manipulating coins, writing with an adapted pen, using the involved hand for handshakes, hammering, using screwdrivers, or lifting. Putty can be used to simulate activities, such as turning keys. Adding visualization to the simulation enhances the treatment. The scope of practice for either occupational therapy or physical therapy dictates some of these choices.

Ball rolling can be used for wrist AROM, composite stretching, weight bearing, and closed chain exercise. The ball can be dribbled or thrown for strengthening or sports simulation. Balloons can also be thrown or batted with the hand.

Dried beans can be used for grip and release, for progressive gripping, and for fishing other objects (for example., marbles) out of the beans. Instruct the client to grip the beans and then to release them with full digital extension. Wrist motions can be varied, and tenodesis can be incorporated. You also can have the client use opposition of the thumb to each finger to pick up one bean and then release it with full digital extension.

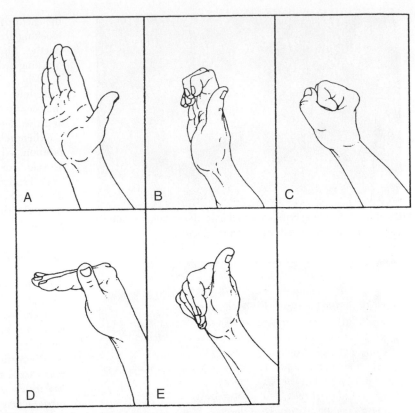

FIGURE 1-17 Differential tendon gliding exercises. A, Straight digits. **B,** Hook fist. **C,** Composite fist. **D,** Tabletop. **E,** Straight (flexor digitorum superficialis [FDS]) fist. (From Rozmaryn LM, Dovelle S, Rothman ER et al: Nerve and tendon gliding exercises and the conservative management of carpal tunnel syndrome, *Journal of Hand Therapy* 11:171-179, 1998.)

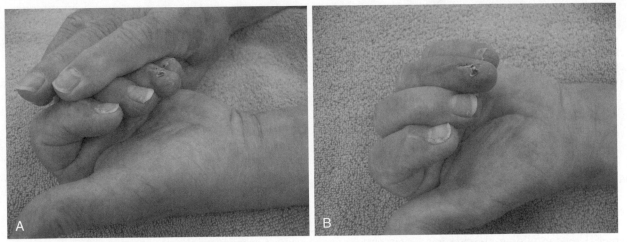

FIGURE 1-18 A, Place exercises for digital flexion. **B,** Hold exercises for digital flexion.

Pegs of varying sizes promote tendon gliding, sensory stimulation, and joint ROM. Fine motor activities (for example, threading beads, in-hand manipulation of marbles, and stacking blocks) can be modified with blocking orthoses to promote isolated ROM or tendon glide.

♡ Tips from the Field

- Look at all your clients and their hands with interest and curiosity. For example, what do you see in Fig. 1-19?
- Be tender when you touch your clients. If your hands are cold, try to warm them up a bit before you touch the person.

- Remember that you do not have to evaluate and treat everything on the first visit.
- Never yell at or order a client to "Relax!" Instead, encourage relaxation with a calm, slow voice.
- Working on one area of stiffness sometimes can also resolve stiffness in another area.
- *Example:* A client who sustained a distal radius fracture had limited AROM and PROM in wrist flexion and extension and decreased ECRB excursion (that is, passive wrist extension exceeded active wrist extension). Stretching led to improved wrist flexion. It also helped reduce ECRB adherence, which resulted in improved wrist extension.
- *Example:* A client had extrinsic flexor tightness after a distal radius fracture with edema and decreased wrist and hand

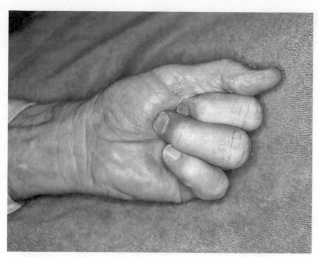

FIGURE 1-19 What do you see wrong with this client's hand?

AROM. As her extrinsic flexor tightness resolved (she recovered full passive composite extension), the active digital flexion also resolved because she had better mechanical function of the lengthened digital flexors.

- Keep the timeline open for more progress by not performing painful therapy and by avoiding a flare reaction.
- As a hand therapist, you won't be able to resolve every problem in every case. If prolonged, established stiffness is present, if the client has highly fibrotic tissue responses, or if client follow-through has been poor, residual limitations may exist that are beyond our ability to correct.
- Document explicitly if poor client follow-through is a factor. For example, a client was carrying a glass table that broke; the client received a laceration to his right-dominant forearm. Several flexor tendons and the median and ulnar nerves also were lacerated. The client missed many therapy visits and did not perform his Duran home program (see Chapter 30). The client returned to therapy with very poor passive digital flexion, severe edema, and skin maceration. In this case, documentation would include the following: "The patient had been instructed to perform hourly protected passive digital flexion within his orthotic, but he reports that he did not do so. He states that he understands the need to exercise as instructed. He also states that he understands that if he does not gain passive digital flexion soon, he may lose the opportunity to make maximum clinical gains." If appropriate, the progress note to this client's physician should report that the patient now agrees to increase the frequency of home exercise program (HEP) exercises, as he was previously instructed to do.
- If a client is not following through as instructed, it is important to investigate why this is happening and to work with the client to correct the situation. Clients can have a number of reasons for failing to follow their regimen. They may be uninformed about the importance of the HEP; they may think they can catch up and make progress later; they may have a secondary agenda, such as avoiding a return to work; they may be depressed; or they may need help to assimilate the HEP into their daily routine successfully. (See Chapter 15 for more information on functional somatic syndromes and challenging behaviors.)

- Help clients learn to be patient. Encourage them to continue with their home program and to celebrate small improvements. Assist them in finding meaningful ways to use their time (for example, find new interests and hobbies) if participation in an enjoyable activity has been temporarily disrupted.
- Replenish your own reserves so that you have the resources needed for complicated clinical situations (see Chapter 13). Give yourself a few moments to take some deep breaths and focus on the client as a person. Try to sense what it must be like for the client to have this injury. Carefully check for extensor habitus, which is habitual posturing in digital extension. The index finger is particularly prone to this response. Extensor habitus can occur after an injury as simple as a paper cut. It is important to identify this phenomenon and to correct it as soon as possible so that it does not become permanent and so that joint stiffness does not occur. Buddy straps and orthotics may be helpful.
- Take one day at a time with the therapy. Do not presume that you will pick up where your last session left off. Look at your clients with fresh eyes at each visit. Ask them what is better, what they are noticing about their hands, what they are able to do functionally now, and what they are still unable to accomplish functionally.

Thinking Outside the (Treatment) Box

When to Mix and Match

Mix and match your treatment repertoire. After reading the rest of this book, try to think outside the treatment box. Be creative, and have some fun. For example, why not perform early protective motions (for example, place and hold tenodesis motions described in Chapter 37) with most of your patients?

When Less Is More

Teaching your client the benefits of a "less is more" approach to UE exercises is very important. For example, a 12-year-old girl underwent flexor tendon grafting. In therapy, when trying to isolate FDP motion at the DIP with the PIP blocked, she was co-contracting and eliciting PIP flexion instead. The therapist taught her to contract more softly so as to isolate the FDP more effectively. The therapist used some helpful verbal cues, such as "Don't try so hard," "Stop trying altogether," and "Stop thinking." The therapist gave these cues in a soft, gentle voice and made sure to compliment the girl and smile when her isolated motion was of better quality. This activity was followed by place and hold exercises, which progressed successfully. Even though this client was very young, she learned the quality of isolated motion well, recognizing that "less is more." She also could see the improvement in her capabilities.

When to Stop Exercising for a Few Days

Another important lesson to teach clients is when to stop exercising for a short time. For example, a 53-year-old, right-dominant woman sustained a distal radius fracture when she fell while shopping. She developed significant, diffuse edema and stiffness of the shoulder, elbow, forearm, and hand. This client demonstrated objective signs of a flare response after efforts were made to upgrade her exercises gradually. She was at risk for IP flexion contractures of all digits. Her sisters came to visit her, and they all went to a spa for 4 days. During this time, the client stopped performing her assigned UE exercises while she pampered herself at the spa. When she came back to therapy, she had diminished flare responses, decreased edema, and improved ROM throughout the upper extremity. It helped her immensely to stop trying so hard. She was then able to resume "trying," but with a better sense of her tissue tolerances.

When to Accept a Stiff Hand and Get On with Life

Unfortunately, hand therapists cannot fix everything. In some cases, the client's injuries may be too severe to permit a full recovery. In other cases, a family crisis may prevent therapy from continuing in a timely manner. Under circumstances such as these, the client's best course of action is to accept the residual stiffness or limitations and to resume otherwise normal living. In such cases, therapists can perform the important role of identifying and teaching compensatory techniques to maximize the client's function.[19] Also, sometimes the therapist has the responsibility to identify a clinical plateau and to help clients realize that they may have achieved all that is possible at that time.

Summary

This chapter has identified fundamental hand therapy concepts that foster clinical reasoning. It also has highlighted treatment techniques and provided guidelines to promote interventions that are safe and appropriate. Most treatment techniques are not diagnosis specific, but rather can be applied to a variety of diagnoses. As a hand therapist, the challenge you face is to be tissue specific, to be aware of clinical precautions, and to adapt the appropriate treatment from your toolbox of techniques to a given diagnosis. As you continue with this book, I encourage you to ask yourself what interventions would be most appropriate and why. I also recommend that you return to this chapter and reread it after you have read the rest of the book. Rereading this chapter at that time will help you appreciate what you have learned; that, hopefully, will be how to apply clinical reasoning in selecting safe treatment choices for clients with many different diagnoses.

Acknowledgments to Chapter 1 in the First Edition

I wish to thank Sandra M. Artzberger, MS, OTR, CHT, CLT, for reviewing this chapter and for providing me the impetus to explore chip bags in conjunction with upper extremity orthotics; Patricia Zarbock Fantauzzo, COTA/L, for her creative ideas for using chip bags on clients with upper extremity problems; and Joel Moorhead, MD, MPH, John L. Evarts, BS, Lisa Deshaies OTR, CHT, and Sharon Flinn, PhD, OTR/L, CHT, CVE, for reading and critiquing this chapter.

References

1. Tubiana R, Thomine J-M, Mackin EJ, editors: *Examination of the hand and wrist*, ed 2, London, 1996, Martin Dunitz.
2. Fess EE, Gettle KS, Philips CA, et al, editors: *Hand and upper extremity splinting: principles and methods*, ed 3, St Louis, 2005, Elsevier.
3. Strickland JW: Biologic basis for hand and upper extremity splinting. In Fess EE, Gettle KS, Philips CA, et al: *Hand and upper extremity splinting: principles and methods*, ed 3, St Louis, 2005, Elsevier.
4. Pettengill KS: Therapist's management of the complex injury. In Skirven TM, Osterman AL, Fedorczyk JM, et al, editors: *Rehabilitation of the hand and upper extremity*, ed 6, Philadelphia, 2011, Elsevier.
5. Colditz C: Therapist's management of the stiff hand. In Mackin EJ, Callinan N, Skirven TM, et al, editors: *Rehabilitation of the hand and upper extremity*, ed 6, St Louis, 2011, Elsevier.
6. Gutierrez-Gutierrez G, Sereno M, Miralles A, et al: Chemotherapy-induced peripheral neuropathy: clinical features, diagnosis, prevention and treatment strategies, *Clin Transl Oncol* 12:81–91, 2010.
7. Cooper C, Liskin J, Moorhead JF: Dyscoordinate contraction: impaired quality of movement in patients with hand disorders, *OT Practice* 4:40–45, 1999.
8. Bracciano AG: Physical agent modalities. In Radomski MV, Latham C, editors: *Occupational therapy for physical dysfunction*, ed 6, Baltimore, 2008, Lippincott Williams & Wilkins.
9. Chen J-J, Jin P-S, Zhao S, et al: Effect of heat shock protein 47 on collagen synthesis of keloid in vivo, *ANZ J Surg* 81:425–430, 2011.
10. Anzarut A, Olson J, Singh P, et al: The effectiveness of pressure garment therapy for the prevention of abnormal scarring after burn injury: a meta-analysis, *J Plast Reconstr Aesthet Surg* 62:77–84, 2009.
11. von der Heyde RL, Evans RB: Wound classification and management. In Skirven TM, Osterman AL, Fedorczyk JM, et al, editors: *Rehabilitation of the hand and upper extremity*, ed 6, Philadelphia, 2011, Elsevier.
12. Coppard BM, Lohman H: *Introduction to splinting: a clinical reasoning and problem-solving approach*, ed 3, St Louis, 2008, Mosby.
13. Deshaies LD: Upper extremity orthoses. In Radomski MV, Latham C, editors: *Occupational therapy for physical dysfunction*, ed 6, Baltimore, 2008, Lippincott Williams & Wilkins.
14. Lashgari D, Yasuda L: Orthotics. In Pendleton HM, Schultz-Krohn W, editors: *Pedretti's occupational therapy practice skills for physical dysfunction*, ed 7, St Louis, 2013, Mosby.
15. Krotoski JAB, Breger-Stanton D: The forces of dynamic orthotic positioning: ten questions to ask before applying a dynamic orthosis to the hand. In Skirven TM, Osterman AL, Fedorczyk JM, et al, editors: *Rehabilitation of the hand and upper extremity*, ed 6, Philadelphia, 2011, Elsevier.
16. Fess EE: Orthoses for mobilization of joints: principles and methods. In Skirven TM, Osterman AL, Fedorczyk JM, et al, editors: *Rehabilitation of the hand and upper extremity*, ed 6, Philadelphia, 2011, Elsevier.
17. Cooper C, Meland NB: *Clinical implications of transverse forces on extrinsic flexors and extensors in the hand*, Unpublished paper presented at the annual meeting of the American Society of Hand Therapists, Seattle, Oct. 5-8, 2000.
18. Bardak AN, Alp M, Erhan B, et al: Evaluation of the clinical efficacy of conservative treatment in the management of carpal tunnel syndrome, *Adv Ther* 26:107–116, 2009.
19. Merritt WH: Written on behalf of the stiff finger, *J Hand Ther* 11:74–79, 1998.

2 Functional Anatomy

Sharon R. Flinn and Lori DeMott

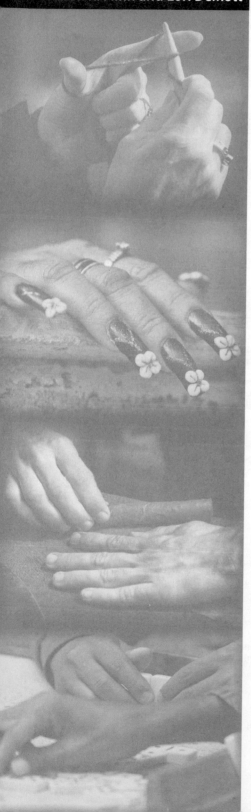

Introduction

Anatomy is the study of the physical structures within the human body. The skeleton provides the foundation for the body; muscles attach by way of bony origins and insertions. Knowledge of the nervous system provides us with a practical understanding of muscle action, tendon excursion, and joint motion. Therefore, the assessment of key postural markers throughout the upper extremity provides an understanding of proper skeletal alignment and balance in the neuromusculoskeletal system as well as a basis for comparing the normal default of **body conformation** to that of abnormal alignment.

As hand therapy professionals, we rely on the functional anatomy of the upper extremity as the main determinant in grading the success of our client's task performance. We can correlate abnormal postures to a client's functional complaints. Fundamentally and simplistically, the observation and assessment of the body's alignment is a measure of how the neuromusculoskeletal system is performing. The concept of balance and movement can provide a greater understanding of human anatomy and direct us to the contributions of soft tissue impairment. The important issue for us is that a postural assessment gives us the ability to evaluate the overall muscle balance and the response of the body as a whole to disease and trauma.

During purposeful activity, a client thinks more about *what* they want to do and less about *how* they do it. Frequently, unguarded movements lead to stressing joints and overloading muscles without knowing the consequences of their effects on healing tissues. When symptoms and functional limitations appear, pain is the body's response to injury. As the first line of defense, movement is altered unconsciously to reduce pain. Whether the complaints are global and diffuse or pinpoint and local, we cannot be fooled into narrowly interpreting the origin of their symptoms as the source of pathology to a specific body structure. Altered body movements and imbalances in resting neuro-muscular-skeletal alignment can cause mechanical pathology and can be the secondary complications that result in the client's chief complaint that is it "hurts."

Due to a fixed time period allotted for our evaluation, it is imperative that we observe our client's static body postures and movement patterns to understand the etiology of their physical impairment. Our efficiency and skill in evaluation is imperative to control health care dollars and, above all, to direct treatments to the best outcomes for each of our clients. During the initial interview of chief complaints and general medical history, you can simultaneously perform an assessment of posture. Observations can be done in static, resting positions while the client is sitting, standing, and lying down as well as during spontaneous, dynamic movements when the client first shakes your hand, takes off his/her coat, walks, sits down, or completes paperwork. These observations are the first quick functional anatomy screen of how the body is aligned, possible altered responses proximally and distally, and observations of the sites related to the client's physical complaints.

Resting and dynamic postural assessments assist us in developing a plan of care that provides a clear relationship between the desired improvements of the neuro-muscular-skeletal balances and functional tasks. Self-reports are obtained every visit on the client's satisfaction and ease of performance in doing purposeful daily activities. For example, the ability to wash hair will improve more efficiently and safely when scapular muscle stabilizers are strengthened and able to support free movement at the glenohumeral joint. Balanced **scapulo-thoracic rhythm** occurs at the normal starting position of retracted, downward rotation. This allows normal gliding of the rotator cuff tendons without impingement at the acromioclavicular joint and reduces subsequent pain. A systematic approach to screening the functional anatomy of the core and distal joints of the body combines the knowledge of kinematic chains, tissue imbalances, and compensatory movements in the recovery of the upper extremity from disease and trauma.

To enhance your clinical reasoning skills, this chapter will review anatomy and neurophysiology principles beyond the rote memorization of origins, insertions, nerves, and actions. Instead, the reader will be introduced to normal postural mechanics and the characteristics associated with healthy bones, joints, ligaments, muscles, tendons, and the neurovascular system of the upper extremity. Then, common clinical scenarios will illustrate abnormal deviations or faults in postural mechanics resulting from tissue imbalance and will provide suggestions for quick screens of the functional anatomy. An extensive review of anatomic features such as joint function, the lymphatic system, dermatome levels, sensory distributions, and pulleys for flexor tendons, are provided in other chapters of the book.

Normal Postural Mechanics

There are observable muscle behaviors that influence our posture and purposeful movements, also termed as our functional anatomy. Important distinctions should be made between anatomic characteristic of body positions, both at the initial static position of a kinematic event and then the return to our neuro-muscular-skeletal equilibrium of balance.[1] **Static posture** is the stationary position held against gravity, whereas **dynamic posture** refers to a series of positions that constantly change during movement and function. Both postures require equilibrium of the muscle system and are observed during relaxation, standing, sitting, or lying down.[1]

The neutral resting balance of our anatomy is the state of default or the **zero position** of the body.[2] The zero position is different from the anatomical position of the body. It represents the **normal resting balance** position where the upper extremities align themselves in space against gravity and where movement ceases and loads are removed. In zero position, the upper extremities are positioned in the midrange of glenohumeral and forearm rotation, the wrist is positioned in approximately ten degrees of extension, and the finger joints are positioned in approximately 45 degrees of flexion. Abnormal changes in functional anatomy cannot be understood without knowledge of the normal resting balance position. Fig. 2-1 illustrates zero position.

The upper extremities return to this default resting position, or *zero position,* in most static body postures. It is an assumed position of joint alignment where the tone of muscle activity is minimal, where the origins and insertions are in a "resting" tone, and where the tension of the joint is in a relaxed, balanced position. **Tone** is defined as the continuous and passive-partial contraction of the muscle or the muscle's resistance to passive stretch during the resting state.[3]

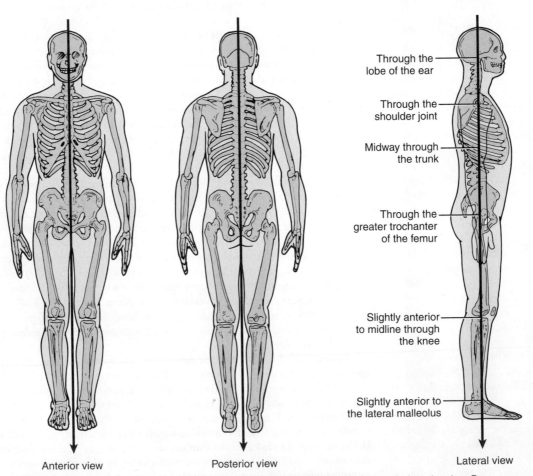

Anterior view   Posterior view   Lateral view

Through the lobe of the ear

Through the shoulder joint

Midway through the trunk

Through the greater trochanter of the femur

Slightly anterior to midline through the knee

Slightly anterior to the lateral malleolus

FIGURE 2-1 **The zero position of the body from the sagittal and coronal planes. A,** Anterior view. **B,** Posterior view. **C,** Lateral view. (Modified from Cameron MH, Monroe LG: *Physical rehabilitation: evidence-based examination, evaluation, and intervention,* St Louis, 2007, Saunders Elsevier.)

Functional anatomy, defined by postural kinematic expressions, is fundamentally based on a predictable design. Skeletal conformation is observed and analyzed by envisioning the underlying bone positions. By knowing the preset configuration, or default design, you can visually construct the muscle anatomy and its contribution to posture. The gross structure, knowledge of fiber alignment, location, and the origins and insertions from your human anatomy references will assist you in understanding the natural tone and potential force of a specific muscle. The angles and lines that are produced as well as the conformation of our body are indications as to how synergistic muscles and peripheral nerves are performing. Typically, the points of reference are anatomical landmarks and are observed in two body planes. The **coronal plane** is vertical and divides the body into anterior and posterior halves.[2] From the coronal plane, we draw a linear line, or plumb line, that forms an **axis of reference.** From the lateral view of the client, the alignment of the ear, shoulder, lateral elbow, posterior hip, anterior knee, and lateral malleolus are body landmarks that are located close to, if not directly within, the axis of reference. From the axis, you can observe the flexion, extension, anterior, and posterior adaptations of the body. Similarly, the **sagittal plane** is vertical and divides the body into right and left right halves.[2] Postures viewed from all sides include obvious body markers, such as head position, shoulder height and glenoid orientation, clavicle angle, scapular position, antecubital fossa (carry angle), hand orientation, and hip height. Fig. 2-1, *A* and *B*, illustrates the body in the sagittal plane and provides the anterior and posterior views of the body. Fig. 2-1, *C*, illustrates the body in the coronal plane and provides a lateral view of the body with a clear view of the arm position.

A functional anatomy screen is performed by envisioning the points at the joints, the anatomic landmarks, and the bone segments as they create altered angles in contrast to those described in the zero position. The differences in these angles or projections are used to hypothesize the influence of the associated muscle function. To understand postural forces of human anatomy and to utilize these concepts in practice, we need to apply the normal orientation of the ideal balance for the skeleton and muscles at rest and during movement throughout the entire kinematic chain. These "normal" default postures can then be compared to the patient who has compensatory adaptation and restrictions in his/her anatomical structures.

Mapping is a technique of drawing using the design and angles of the body that create a picture of alignment. Positions of mapping are in movement planes. The body's coronal and sagittal planes produce the lines of reference in static and dynamic body postures. The front and back views of the body allow the best view of symmetry. **Landmarks** are structures that identify a feature other than a joint. Examples of landmarks are the ear, forehead creases, palm and nail positions, the carry angle space, web spaces, and skin folds in the back and digital creases. Once the position of the joint articulation and landmarks are identified, the **segments** are drawn. The design is then analyzed using the expected functional anatomy as the reference point for identifying imbalances that can contribute to pain, weakness, and restrictions in movement.

The use of the two anatomic planes, axes of reference, and mapping techniques serve as a functional anatomy screening tool that allows the hand therapy professional to compare the ideal postural alignment to that of the assumed posture of the client. The deviation from the ideal can range from slight to severe and will guide the evaluator in understanding the problems associated with joint and muscle functions. Next, a review of the anatomical systems will be discussed in further detail including the characteristics associated with bones, joints, ligaments, muscles, tendons, and the neurovascular systems of the upper extremity and their the contribution to normal postural mechanics.

Bones, Ligaments, and Joints

Bones are responsible for the rigidity and structure of the entire foundation. The joint anatomy is designed to allow transmission of muscle force, at rest and during motion. Understanding the joint structure contributes to the overall whole of functional anatomy and posture configuration. The bone-to-bone connection meets to create the joint. The bone segments within the joint move in relation to each other. The configuration of the bony surfaces dictates the degree of freedom of a joint and creates a type of movement hinge.

The joint allows freedom of movement from one to three planes. Two bony segments move in relationship to each other. Usually one segment is stable while the other moves in relation to the base. At the joint there can be more than one articulation. For example, the glenohumeral joint has scapulo-humeral, sterno-humeral, and clavico-humeral articulations.[2] The control and stability of the joint's axis of rotation directly relates to the articular orientation of the bones. Without rules of engagement for the joint, the simplest movement can become weakened by loss of mechanical advantage. This is seen in joint dislocation and a segmental bone fracture, whereby the movement is not guided and irregular angulations are observed. Conversely, if the segments of bone are not congruent and there is altered space that changes the axis of movement, the normal extrinsic muscle pull can be offset and the movement will present with distorted mechanics that are less than desired.

Throughout the body, there are many axes of rotation. In the upper extremity there are flexion-extension, abduction-adduction, internal-external, radial-ulnar, and pronation-supination axes. The wrist has two, the elbow joint has one at the ulnohumeral joint axis, and the glenohumeral joint is a ball and socket joint with three axes of rotation. The relationships of joint axes have a normal presentation of balance that is predictable and can be assessed at rest and during movement.

The normal skeletal system of the upper extremity can be mapped to determine the **normal default state** of zero position. An imaginary overlay of the skeleton on the conformation of the body creates the approximate location of the joints and bone segments. These structures assist you in recognizing important landmarks. An example of important landmarks from Fig. 2-1 is the space between the arm and body. Fig. 2-2 identifies the mapping specific to the hand. Important landmarks for the hand are nail positions, the space between the index and thumb, the cascading flexion of the fingers, the mass of the thenar eminence, and the prominence of the ulnar head.

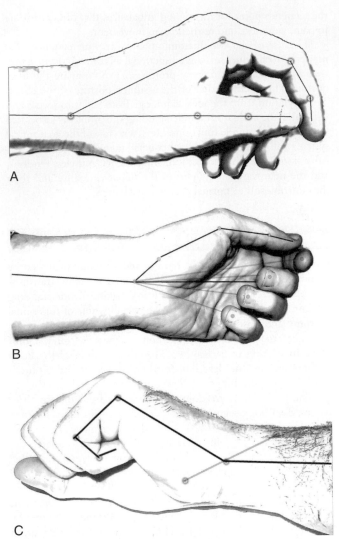

A

B

C

FIGURE 2-2 Mapping of the hand at rest in a pronated **(A)**, supinated **(B)**, and neutral forearm position. (From Donatelli RA: *Orthopaedic physical therapy*, ed 4, St Louis, 2010, Churchill Livingstone Elsevier.)

◎ **Clinical Pearl**

An understanding of normal anatomy and the ideal positions of balance is essential to recognize the imbalances in your client's neuromusculoskeletal anatomy.

Altered configuration of the joint's soft tissue matrix or bony constructs lead to the joint's failure to glide and can result in various types of joint collapses and deformities.[3] With joint laxity, the axis shifts into the direction of the weakened, degraded tissue integrity. Frequently, this is seen with attritional changes of the glenohumeral joint where the anterior capsulo-ligaments are weakened and attenuated. A shift in the joint axis results in changes in the anterior and posterior capsule and in the formation of adhesions.

Another example is seen with metacarpophalangeal (MP) joint subluxation and swan neck deformities in the hands of persons with rheumatoid arthritis. A common joint change is when the proximal phalanx segment shifts palmary toward the volar plate, descending and subluxing. What is observed at rest is

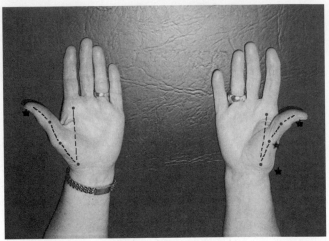

FIGURE 2-3 Mapping of a normal and pathological carpometacarpal (CMC) joint of the thumb. (Photo by Lori DeMott.)

the prominent head of the metacarpal. The forces from muscle contractions are transmitted through the altered axis and with changes in the moment arm of the tendon, the extensor becomes a flexor of the finger MP joint. The change in the axis of rotation alters not only the forces applied to the MP joint but also the kinematic chain of all joints that the muscle tendon unit controls. The shortening or lengthening of the long tendon, in conjunction with significant joint changes, presents with a zigzag of the fingers in proximal interphalangeal (PIP) hyperextension and distal interphalangeal (DIP) flexion joint postures.

Similar attritional changes often are observed with joint dysfunction to the carpometacarpal (CMC) joint of the thumb. Synovitis of the joint causes bone surface erosions and ligament laxity. Laxity of the stabilizing deep anterior oblique ligament (DAOL), called *the beak ligament,* causes the joint to sublux in a radial and palmar direction. Over time, the degenerative thumb CMC joint exhibits changes in appearance as seen with a prominent ledge that extends from the radial side of the base of the thumb. The loss of joint stability changes the characteristic of the surrounding muscular anatomy. The abductor pollicis brevis weakens and the adductor pollicis muscle contracts, unopposed. The thumb CMC joint is drawn into adduction and rotational supination. The imbalance of the thumb intrinsics change the axis of rotation, decrease the transmission of flexion forces across the metacarpal joint, and move the resting position of the MP joint from a flexed posture to extension. Over time, the metacarpal joint hyperextends as the mechanical advantage from the extensor pollicis brevis (EPB) muscle further aggravates the adductor pull on the CMC joint and the increasing severity of the contracture. The interphalangeal (IP) joint compensates for loss of metacarpal joint flexion and overly flexes to produce a functional tip pinch. The cascading events are self-perpetuating as the normal joint forces become pathologic. The anatomy of the arthritic thumb presents with imbalances, principally at the CMC joint level, with bone erosions and capsular instability that contribute to the distal joint changes at rest and during dynamic loads. Fig. 2-3 illustrates mapping of a normal and pathological CMC joint. The *dots* estimate the joint location, the *stars* are the landmarks, and the *dashes* are the bone segments. The disparities between the two thumbs are clear. Compared to the normal thumb, imbalances in the pathological thumb are identified by three visible landmarks; increased nail rotation, MP joint hyper-extension, and a protuberance at the CMC joint caused by the subluxing metacarpal.

◎ Clinical Pearl

The **kinematic chain** of mobility is controlled and primarily influenced proximally.

Mapping the skeletal alignment within the body conformation is a screening tool that you can utilize to assist with evaluation of the functional anatomy. The technique can be drawn on the client and, with practice, will be visualized as part of your observations during the functional anatomy screen.

Muscles and Tendons

Muscles work in groups and patterns of movement. Individual muscles have lengthening, contractile, excitable, and recoil characteristics. Contractility allows a muscle to shorten with force, to lengthen passively, and to move. **Excitability** allows a muscle to respond to a stimulus and to maintain chemical potentials across its cell membranes. **Extensibility** allows a muscle to be stretched, repeatedly and considerably, as needed, without being damaged. **Elasticity** allows a muscle to return to its normal length after being stretched or shortened. The end result is a force application. For example, a coordinated neuromuscular event occurs during the conscious decision to make a fist. The wrist extensors stabilize the wrist in approximately 35 degrees of extension, the extrinsic extensor digitorum communis (EDC) elongates into a full extensible position as the antagonist muscle, and simultaneously the extrinsic flexor digitorum profundus (FDP) and flexor digitorum superficialis (FDS) contract in their role as agonist muscles. The coordinated muscle contractions differentiate the glide that allows terminal distal joint flexion. Simultaneously, contraction of the intrinsic lumbrical and interossei muscles increase metacarpal joint flexion, stabilize and control the joint, and allow the digits to converge into a tucked position within the palm. The characteristics of the musculotendinous structures that contribute to muscle balance are located in Box 2-1.[3]

Nervous System

The peripheral, central, and autonomic nervous systems all combine to form one internal communication system for sensing and responding to internal and external stimuli.[4] The motor and sensory functions for the forearm, wrist, and hand are provided by the peripheral nervous system; consisting of the median, ulnar, and radial nerves. Each nerve has efferent motor and afferent sensory fibers arranged in bundles of axons. The axons are protected by layers of dense connective tissues called the epineurium, perineurium, and endoneurium. Each layer has a unique role to support the innermost structures of the nerve, modulate compressive and tensile forces, and allow gliding between nerve fascicles and the surrounding anatomical structures.[5] Electrical impulses are rapidly conducted via the nodes of Ranvier along a neural pathway, which originates at the spinal cord and brainstem and terminates in the fingers and toes. Due to the continuous nature and physiology of the peripheral nervous system, motions at a distal

---

BOX 2-1   Musculotendinous Characteristics that Contribute to Balance

1. The resting length of a muscle is the relationship and proportional stretch to the fully contracted muscle fiber.
2. At rest and even during sleep, there is a tendency of the muscle to contract and resist lengthening. This principle is influenced by the central nervous system and the intrinsic muscle structure and by definition is our muscle tone.
3. Ordinary normal range of motion at rest or during movement is influenced by the variability of length and pull of all of our contributing anatomy due to antagonist lengthening as well as synergistic coordination.
4. Gravity and the need for skeletal stability will change the resting muscle tone and therefore change distal joint position.
5. Length and cross-section of a muscle leads to predictable excursion and levels of muscle elasticity.
6. A muscle crossing multiple joints will provide a composite excursion; a proximal joint stability is necessary for increased distal joint mobility.
7. Passive joint mobility is without influence of soft tissue elastic characteristics.
8. Muscle balance is involuntary, and over time the resting length can change or be changed by an altered axis. As the joint moves, these altered forces create imbalances and lead to deformity.

---

site, such as the wrist joint, increase the strain at the cord level of the brachial plexus. Similarly, contralateral flexion of the cervical spine increases the strain in the cords of the brachial plexus and three major nerves in the arm.[4] Under tension, the neural tissue may have difficulty conducting electrical impulses, assuring adequate blood supply, and providing adequate axonal transport especially during movement.[5]

Several biomechanical properties are necessary to protect the nerve from tensile, shear, and compressive forces that occur across multiple joints in various postures and dynamic movements of the upper extremity during everyday activities.[5] The properties of the nerve protect it from the forces generated from whole body movements resulting from everyday activities. These protections are due to the nerve's capacity to change its length during movement, slide or glide relative to the surrounding interfacing tissue during movement, and tolerate increases in pressure or compression from the surrounding interfacing tissue.[5] When the nerve does not tolerate normal stresses, a "sensitized" protective state may result as the upper extremity joints usually adjust by flexion or extension to limit the nerve excursion. Symptoms can include increased pain or aberrant movements in the absence of altered nerve conduction.[4,5]

Observations of static and dynamic postures are essential to evaluate the neurodynamics of the peripheral nervous system in its entirety and the changes which can result from limited excursion or traumatized segment(s) of the nerve.[4] As simply observed in an acute nerve injury, the upper arm is held tightly in shoulder adduction, internal rotation, and elbow flexion. In the presence of long-standing trauma to the nerve, imbalances in motor function can be observed. For example, hyperextension of the thumb MP joint during resistive lateral pinch can be observed in persons

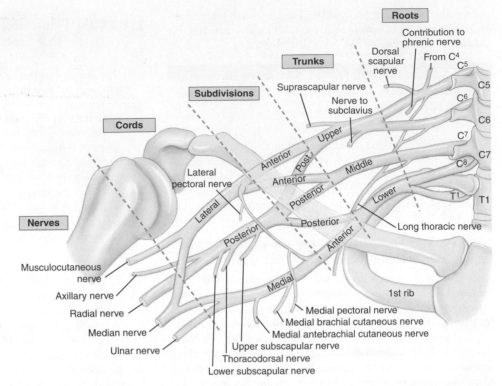

FIGURE 2-4 Diagram of the brachial plexus. (From Neuman D: *Kinesiology of the musculoskeletal system: foundations for rehabilitation*, ed 2, St Louis, 2010, Mosby.)

with ulnar nerve palsy. A zigzag deformity is observed as a result of absent function of the adductor pollicis muscle and imbalances created from a weakened intrinsic extensor mechanism and overpowering extrinsic long flexor.

A neuromusculoskeletal screen of the upper extremity is critical to understanding the changes that impact functional anatomy. Several observations of normal postures can be made. At rest, clients with neural tension postures will limit movement that places the nerve in full excursion. The elbow joint has a high degree of contribution to nerve glide. In resting postures the elbow will flex, and the head will laterally tilt to the affected side. During movement, the head may increase the degree of tilt or the elbow joint increase its flexed position to offset the increased demand at adjacent joints.

Now that you have a better understanding of normal postural mechanics and the neuromusculoskeletal systems, common clinical scenarios are provided to illustrate abnormal deviations, or defaults, in the postural mechanics that result from tissue imbalances. Quick screens will also be provided in each scenario to assist you in applying the principles of balance.

Scenario 1

How does proper cervical alignment facilitate normal functioning of blood vessels and nerve roots?

Proper cervical alignment is necessary for sound neurological and vascular function in the shoulder, arm, and hand. The normal relationships of bone, ligaments, disks, vasculature, and nerves provide the cervical spine with valuable mobility that other segments of the spinal column do not possess. The cervical spine supports motions of the head which consist of rotation from

side-to-side, flexion and extension, lateral flexion to each side, and all the motions in between. While the locations of the structures are designed to provide increased mobility at the cervical level, they are also vulnerable to injuries as a result of these anatomical relationships.

Proper cervical alignment of vertebrae, muscle, and soft tissue facilitates normal conduction and excursion of nervous tissue in nerves C1 to C8. In addition, alignment of these structures also provides for normal blood flow within the vertebral artery and the vertebral and deep cervical veins, insuring adequate blood flow and drainage for the cervical structures related to upper extremity function. Fig. 2-4 illustrates the anterior rami of nerves C5 to T1, which form the brachial plexus and innervate the entire upper extremity.

Symptoms of cervical misalignment may appear distal to the primary injury site and present as sensory, motor, or autonomic dysfunction. For example, forward head posture can be the cause of head, neck, shoulder, or mid and lower back pain as well as distal paresthesias. When the head moves forward, the axis of reference shifts, the cervical spine is pushed into compensatory extension, and the neck extensors shorten. Another **postural fault** is observed with the rounded shoulder posture found in many clients while sitting at their computers or while texting on a cell phone screen. An elevated, abducted, and upwardly rotated scapula influences the axis of the glenohumeral joint by changing the balance of the rotator cuff muscles. The orientation of the glenoid fossa is altered, leaving the humerus in more forward and internally rotated position. In time, a cascading event of changes occurs; the pectoralis minor, serratus anterior, and upper trapezius muscles shorten. The extrinsic muscle origins on the thoracic vertebrae, ribs, and scapula also contribute toward an elevated and upward scapular position. This adaptive shortening of soft tissue has been associated with nerve compression as the nerve plexus exits the thoracic outlet and influences the

TABLE 2-1 Common Cervical Injuries and Disorders and Resulting Impairment

Anatomic Structure	Injury or Disorder	Symptoms
Vertebrae	Subluxation, instability, fracture; abnormal bone development; arthritis; displacement; degenerative changes; stenosis; bony spurs	Disruption of sensory, motor, or vascular function throughout the UE
Muscle	Weakness; tightness; imbalance; hypertonicity or hypotonicity; spasm; overstretching; sprain or strain	Compression of nervous tissue characteristically results in numbness, pain, paralysis, and loss of function; vascular compression characteristically results in moderate pain and swelling[3]
Soft tissue	Disk protrusion, lax ligament; ligament avulsion; degeneration or thickening of dura; adhesions	***
Vasculature	Compression; constriction; mechanical irritation; congestion; reflex response; hemorrhage; stretching	Sympathetic symptoms associated with circulation can manifest in UE; decreased blood flow to UE tissues; temperature changes; pain; edema; decreased healing time
Nerve root and nerves	Decreased movement and elasticity; compression; strain, irritation, axonotmesis, severance	Pain at point of entrapment or along distal distribution in UE; decrease in or loss of sensation, motor control, or strength in UE; decreased UE deep tendon reflexes; decreased UE muscle tone; trophic changes in UE; sensation of deep pain; pain that radiates over shoulders and arms

UE, Upper extremity.

extremity, contributing to sensory disturbances distally. Further postural changes ensue within the pelvic and abdominal cores and are associated with the musculoskeletal changes of the low flat-back posture (posterior tilt), elongated and weaken hip flexors, and shortened hip extensors and anterior abdominals. Table 2-1 describes other disorders that result from misalignment of the cervical spine and can result in conditions that impair upper extremity function.

> **◎ Clinical Pearl**
>
> It is important to appreciate the upper extremity as multiple parts of a complex system; the client's complaints of pain or weakness may not be the source of the pathology.

Observations of static postures provide valuable information of the body's resting tone and default. A quick screen of functional anatomy can be done from the sagittal and coronal planes. From the anterior view, are the eyes, ears, and shoulders symmetrical? From the posterior view, does the position of the head or shoulders deviate laterally from the imaginary plumb line? From the lateral view, does the lobe of the ear align with the imaginary plumb line and the anterior one-third of the humerus? Fig. 2-5 identifies the mapping specific to normal and forward head positions. Disparities exist between the two head positions. Compared to the normal head position, imbalances in the pathological head position are identified by three visible landmarks; the position of the chin, ear, and scapula.

In addition to observations of static posture, active movements of the upper extremity are needed due to the additional tension created on the neurovascular bundle in the upper quadrant of the body. Common symptoms of the sensory, motor, or vascular systems are localized burning, cramping, or cooler temperature changes of the hand are common. When these movements are repeated over time, the temporary symptoms caused by the compression of the neurovascular bundle can become frequent or constant and somewhat unrelenting. Fig. 2-6 shows

common claviculocostal sites where increased neurovascular pressure occurs with upper body movement. The symptoms that occur at these sites are often referred to as *thoracic outlet syndrome.*

> **◎ Clinical Pearl**
>
> Joint pathologies can be observed, and should be palpated, at rest and during movements.

As a hand therapy professional, it is important for you to remember that increased neurovascular tension over time can lead to compression. Tension will occur with normal upper body movement. If the movement becomes repetitive over time, more long-standing compression will occur. Table 2-2 describes what occurs to the neurovascular structures with upper body movement. Many other upper extremity sites are prone to neurovascular compression as the result of poor posture, injury, and/or muscle imbalance due to weakness or malnutrition. A thorough understanding of the workings of the cervical spine is necessary to identify the source of injury for some patients having symptoms along the upper extremity. As part of effective intervention, educating the patient in appropriate cervical posture patterns will improve the kinematic chain of the upper extremity and potential rehabilitation outcomes.

Scenario 2

What is the relationship of the rotator cuff muscles to the glenohumeral joint that is intact and mobile?

The glenohumeral joint depends on the rotator cuff muscles for support, rather than from the bones or ligaments. Fig. 2-7 shows the relationship of the rotator cuff muscles, which include the subscapularis, the supraspinatus, the infraspinatus, and the teres minor. The glenohumeral joint is a ball-and-socket synovial joint that moves in multiple axes. The motion

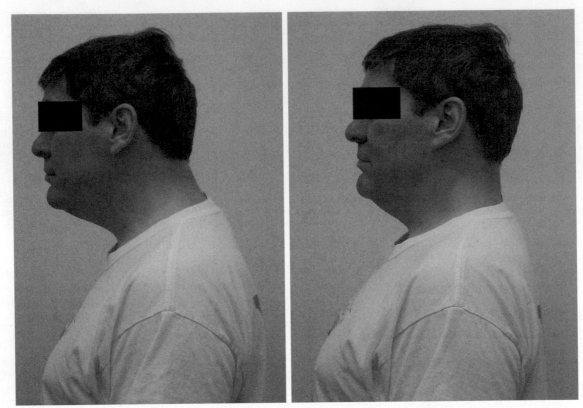

FIGURE 2-5 Mapping of normal and forward head positions. (From Sahrmann SA: *Movement system impairment syndromes of the extremities, cervical and thoracic spines: considerations for acute and long-term management*, St Louis, 2011, Elsevier Mosby.)

of the glenohumeral joint, provided by the rotator cuff muscles, is related to the angle of pull for each muscle. A quick screen of normal functional anatomy in a standing resting posture is the parallel orientation of the hand and scapula. The hand position changes with the scapular position. If the hand position is pronated, an abducted scapular position is assumed. Consequently, the abducted scapula has a direct effect upon the origin and insertion of the rotator cuff muscle actions and shortening or lengthening of these structures can be postulated. Table 2-3 identifies the locations of and motions provided by the rotator cuff muscles.[2]

> ### ◎ *Clinical Pearl*
>
> The position of the hand in relation to the zero position tells you about the functional anatomy of the scapula and suggests the orientation of the scapula and its relative position on the thorax.

In addition to the primary motions that the rotator cuff muscles have on the glenohumeral joint, they act as part of a force couple. Force couples are responsible for stabilizing joints through muscle co-contractions. The forces are parallel and equal in magnitude but opposite in direction.[6] For instance, the deltoid and supraspinatus muscles work as a **force couple** to produce glenohumeral abduction or flexion. The deltoid and teres minor work as a force couple to produce depression and stabilization of the humeral head. Another force couple is the deltoid muscle and the rotator cuff muscles for depression of the humeral head and flexion of the humerus.[6]

You also need to keep in mind the impact of forces and how they change with different positions and/or postures. For instance, painting a ceiling requires glenohumeral stabilization and flexion proximally. But how do the forces change when the position is held for an extended period of time and with the cervical spine extended? This could result in a variety of possible symptoms, such as dizziness, core lumbar pain, impingement of the rotator cuff muscles, triceps weakness, or sensory changes in the thumb side of the hand. Therefore, when treating clients with rotator cuff injuries, you need to consider the entire kinematic chain, all the forces applied to the upper quadrant, and the context of movement, not just the isolated motion of shoulder flexion.

A common example of a proximal upper extremity imbalance is seen with a client who demonstrates rounded shoulders with a forward head (RSFH) position. A functional anatomy screen of the upper quarter can be observed while the client is sitting at a table and reaching for a drinking cup. The upper arm movements of a client with normal balanced shoulder position consists of scapular abduction and depression while the kinematic expression of the arm reach is observed in neutral glenohumeral rotation, **forward elevation,** forearm in mid position and wrist extension. In contrast, scapular adduction, glenohumeral internal rotation and flexion, forearm pronation, and wrist flexion occurs in an over-the-top hand orientation to grasp. Fig. 2-8 shows the difference between the reaching patterns of an individual with normal balance and imbalance in the glenohumeral joint. There are clear differences in the amounts of internal rotation, forearm pronation, and wrist flexion required for the default position.

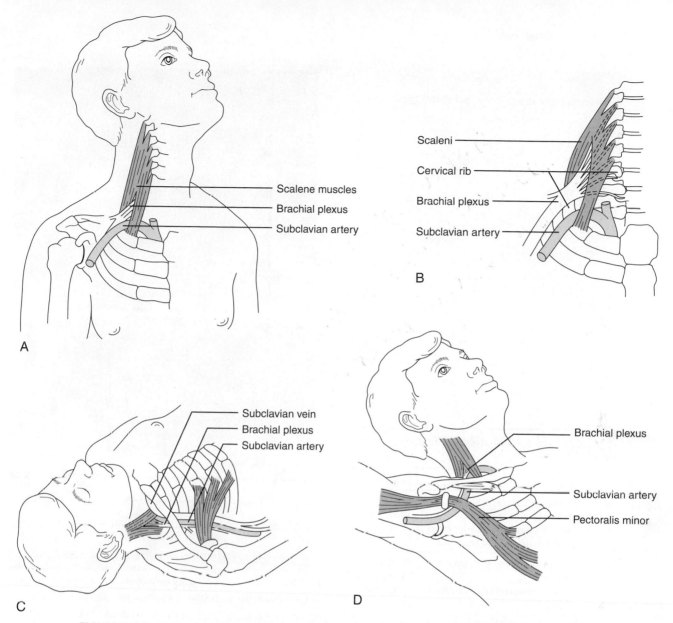

FIGURE 2-6 Common claviculocostal sites where increased neurovascular pressure occurs. **A,** Scalenus anterior syndrome. **B,** Cervical rib syndrome. **C,** Costoclavicular syndrome. **D,** Hyperabduction syndrome. (From Cummings NH, Stanley-Green S, Higgs P: *Perspectives in athletic training,* St Louis, 2009, Mosby.)

TABLE 2-2		Neurovascular Symptoms Associated with Upper Body Movement	
Body Part	**Motion**	**Result**	**Symptoms**
Shoulder	Depression	*Peripheral nerve:* Stretching of upper and middle trunks of brachial plexus over scalene muscle; pulling of lower trunks into angle formed by first rib and scalene tendon	Numbness and pain, particularly over ulnar distribution; pain worse at night because of positioning; intensity fluctuates throughout the day; arm fatigue, weakness, finger cramps, tingling, numbness, cold hand, areas of hyperesthesia, atrophy, tremor, and/or discoloration of hand
		Blood vessel: No compression of subclavian artery	
	Retraction	*Peripheral nerve:* No compression	
		Blood vessel: Compression of subclavian vein by tendon of subclavian muscle, *not* by clavicle	
	Abduction and retraction	*Peripheral nerve:* Clavicular compression on brachial plexus	
		Blood vessel: Clavicular compression of subclavian artery against scalene muscle	
Scapula	Retraction	*Peripheral nerve:* Compression of brachial plexus at point where it passes between clavicle and first rib	
		Blood vessel: Compression of subclavian artery at point where it passes between clavicle and first rib	

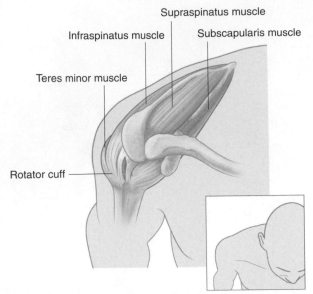

FIGURE 2-7 Tendons of the rotator cuff muscles. (From Cummings NH, Stanley-Green S, Higgs P: *Perspectives in athletic training*, St Louis, 2009, Mosby.)

TABLE 2-3 Location and Motion of Rotator Cuff Muscles

Muscle	Location	Motion
Supraspinatus	*Proximal attachment:* Supraspinous fossa of scapula *Distal attachment:* Superior facet of greater tubercle of humerus	Abduction and rotation
Subscapularis	*Proximal attachment:* Subscapular fossa *Distal attachment:* Lesser tubercle of humerus	Medial rotation and adduction
Infraspinatus	*Proximal attachment:* Infraspinous fossa of scapula *Distal attachment:* Middle facet of greater tubercle of humerus	Lateral rotation
Teres minor	*Proximal attachment:* Superior part of lateral border of scapula *Distal attachment:* Inferior facet of greater tubercle of humerus	Lateral rotation

Scenario 3

How do the ligamentous structures of the wrist and hand provide stability and assist with balanced movement during normal function? How do these structures change with different positions of movement? Are there postural deviations from the normal resting balance of wrist extension and digit flexion that contribute to the strength and movement of the hand?

The function of the collateral ligaments in the human body is to provide joint stability while functional activities occur within multiple planes of movement. Fig. 2-9 provides the ligamentous

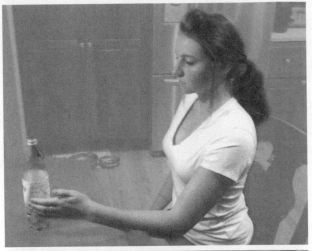

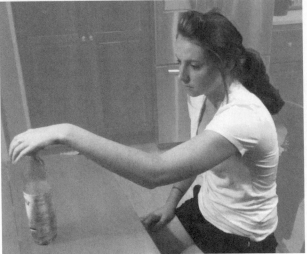

FIGURE 2-8 Reaching capacity expected for a client with and without balance in the glenohumeral joint. (Photo by Lori DeMott.)

system of the wrist. The palmar wrist ligaments provide support between the carpal bones. The dorsal wrist ligaments provide support between the carpal bones and the radius. The palmar radioscaphoid lunate ligament provides support for the radius, the scaphoid, and the lunate. The triangular fibrocartilage complex (TFCC) provides support between the carpal bones, the ulna, and the distal radial-ulnar joint. Each of the supporting structures is important in stabilizing the wrist in extreme ranges of wrist extension, flexion, radial deviation, and ulnar deviation.[7] Not only does stability of the joint affect mobility, but without adequate support on the ulnar border of the wrist, the amount of pinch strength on the contralateral side can be diminished.

Several imbalances of the wrist can occur from pathology. In the case of a displaced and angulated metacarpal fracture, the skeletal length changes and the shortened foundations can limit the ability of the extensor tendon to bring the MP joints into a complete end range of extension. This is an important function in initiating grasp for large objects, placing the hand into pockets, and for the fine manipulation of using a keyboard. Injuries to the wrist ligaments themselves have stabilizing effects that redirect the pull and balance of the long extrinsic tendons. This is seen in clients with distal radioulnar joint (DRUJ) instability. During forearm pronation, the ulna migrates dorsally and a prominent

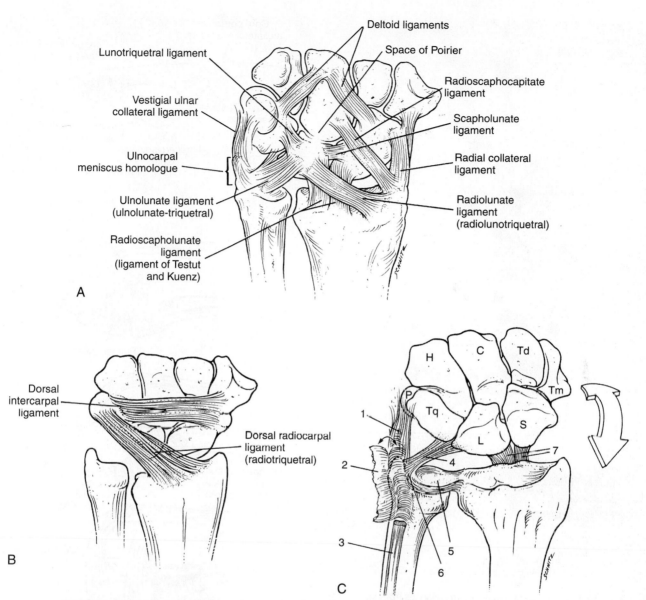

FIGURE 2-9 Ligamentous anatomy of the wrist. A, Palmar wrist ligaments. **B,** Dorsal wrist ligaments. **C,** Dorsal view of the flexed wrist, including the triangular fibrocartilage. *1,* Ulnar collateral ligament; *2,* retinacular sheath; *3,* tendon of extensor carpi ulnaris; *4,* ulnolunate ligament; *5,* triangular fibrocartilage, *6,* ulnocarpal meniscus homologue; *7,* palmar radioscaphoid lunate ligament; *P,* pisiform; *H,* hamate; *C,* capitate; *Td,* trapezoid; *Tm,* trapezium; *L,* lunate; *S,* scaphoid. (From Fess EE, Gettle K, Phillips C, et al: *Hand and upper extremity splinting: principles and methods,* ed 3, St Louis, 2005, Mosby.)

ulnar styloid is observed. The CMC joint of the small finger demonstrates mild changes but an obvious collapse proximally creates a visual fovea, or depression. The extensor carpi ulnaris (ECU) tendon that inserts onto the fifth metacarpal becomes inefficient and loses its ability to stabilize the metacarpal into extension during active grasp. The hand changes its appearance as the arch of the small metacarpal joint ascends and over time the entire hand radially deviates during grasp and pinch tasks. The ligaments by virtue of disease and overload from an altered axis will eventually cascade into instability and joint collapse. Fig. 2-10 maps the expected imbalances from the same client with ligamentous instability associated with a classical malunion of a distal radius fracture. In Fig. 2-10, *A,* shortening of the radius and carpal collapse demonstrates the radial bias of the wrist. Landmarks can be

observed with increased prominence of the ulnar styloid. In Fig. 2-10, *B,* the proximal elevation of the fifth metacarpal can be seen as a result of ulnocarpal ligament laxity. This instability results in the disruption of the distal transverse arch. Also, you will see an atrophied hypothenar eminence and a pronounced the extensor digitorum minimi, which assists with wrist extension. Other landmarks can be observed with abnormal depression from the metacarpal angle and prominence of the ulnar styloid; both are indicative of possible subluxation of the wrist carpus and DRUJ imbalance.

The ligamentous structures in the fingers differ considerably from those of the wrist. Fig. 2-11 reviews the supporting structures of the finger MP and PIP joints. The design of the collateral ligament is to ensure lateral support. When the joint is flexed,

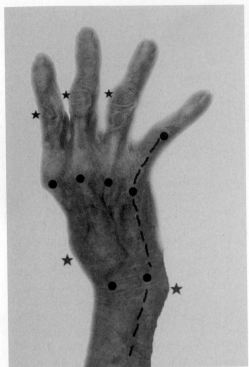

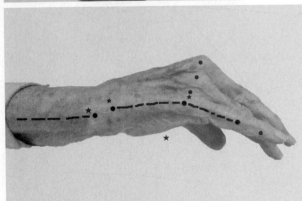

FIGURE 2-10 Mapping of the expected imbalances from ligamentous instability of the distal radial ulnar joint. (Photo by Lori DeMott.)

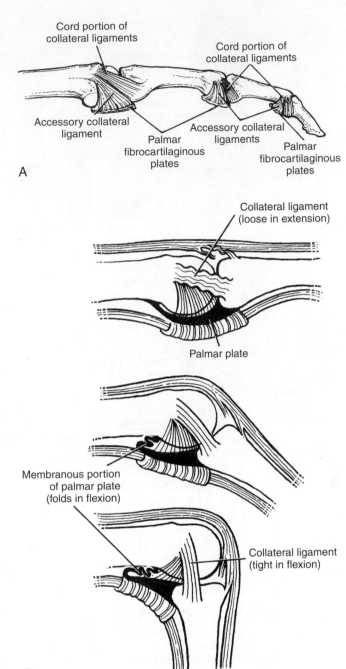

FIGURE 2-11 A, Ligamentous structures of the digital joints. **B,** At the metacarpal joint level, the collateral ligaments are loose in exertion but tighten in flexion. (**A,** From Fess EE, Gettle K, Phillips C, et al: *Hand and upper extremity splinting: principles and methods*, ed 3, St Louis, 2005, Mosby; **B,** Modified from Wynn-Parry CB: *Rehabilitation of the hand.* In Fess EE, Gettle K, Phillips C, et al: *Hand and upper extremity splinting: principles and methods*, ed 3, St Louis, 2005, Mosby.)

the collateral ligament lengthens to accommodate the movement and becomes slack when the joint is in an extended position. In addition to the lateral support of a joint, volar reinforcement is provided through strong membranous connections with the collateral ligament. The palmer (also called *volar*) plates are slack in flexion but become taut when the joint is extended, thus protecting the joint from hyperextension stresses or dislocations. Common postural changes for ligamentous instability of the fingers may include swan neck deformity of the digits. In the static and dynamic postures of the PIP joint, the palmar support attenuates over time and the lateral bands slide anterior to the joint axis into this new postural orientation.

As expected, the thumb has ligamentous supports at the IP joint, the MP joint, and the CMC joint. Of particular interest is the radial and ulnar collateral ligaments (RCLs/UCLs) of the MP joint. Fig. 2-12 illustrates the importance of this strong band of tissue in supporting pinch, especially for tip and lateral pinches. Common postural imbalances can be seen with ligamentous

instability when loading the joint through tip pinch. Observational mapping of unstable bilateral RCLs at rest shows increased angulation of the MP joints of the thumb, supination of the thumb nail, and loss of muscle mass in the thenar eminences (Fig. 2-12, *A*). Similar changes can be seen with observational mapping of an unstable UCL with pinch to include radial deviation of the MP joint and rotation of the thumb nail.

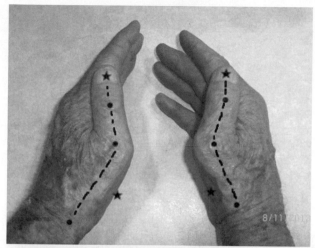

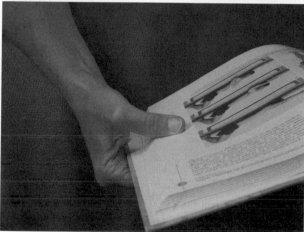

FIGURE 2-12 Diagram of unstable thumb MP joint collateral ligaments in static and dynamic postures. **A,** Bilateral radial collateral ligaments at rest and **B,** ulnar collateral ligament with movement (©Martin Dunitz Ltd., 2001.)

Scenario 4

If you were to identify the muscles that originate from the lateral and medial epicondyles, which muscles would they be? Why would it be useful to evaluate these muscles by this grouping?

Proper balance of the musculotendinous structures that originate from the lateral and medial epicondyles is necessary for positioning the hand in tasks away from the body. Actions of elbow extension and flexion, forearm rotation, wrist extension and flexion are controlled by these musculotendinous structures. Due to the length of these tissues, their actions cross as many as five joints and can influence reaching and positioning of the hand. Static or dynamic muscle imbalances can lead to pathologic joint stresses, muscle weakness, and ultimately with limitations in functional reach and grasp patterns.

Clinical Pearl

Shortened muscles are not stronger muscles.

Even though all of the muscles that originate from the lateral epicondyle are innervated by the radial nerve, a different picture

of function can be obtained when observing their influence on multi-joint, simultaneous movements. Table 2-4 provides a listing of the eight muscles, their origin, and their action.[2] It is easy to recognize that many of these muscles cross the elbow, the forearm, the wrist, and in some cases the fingers. In order to ensure full joint motion, pliability of the muscles and connective tissues, and strength testing individual or groups of muscles that originate from the lateral epicondyle can be useful. When testing range of motion of the wrist and hand, the position of the elbow and the forearm should be considered. For example, full passive stretch of the longest musculoskeletal structure originating on the lateral epicondyle, the EDC muscle, is obtained with elbow extension, forearm pronation, wrist flexion, and full finger flexion.

In discussing the muscles that originate from the medial epicondyle, a similar picture of function also can be obtained. Table 2-5 provides a listing of the five muscles, their origin, and their action.[2] In this case, all of the muscles are innervated by the median nerve with the exception of one, the flexor carpi ulnaris, which is supplied by the ulnar nerve. In spite of the differences in nerve innervations, the same principles for extensibility of these muscles can apply as was suggested for the muscles originating from the lateral epicondyle. For example, full passive stretch of the longest musculoskeletal structure originating on the medial epicondyle, the FDS muscle, is obtained with elbow extension, forearm supination, wrist extension, and full finger extension.

A functional anatomy screen of the muscles that originate from the lateral and medial epicondyles is essential to determine deviations from normal posture of the wrist and hand. At rest, imbalances cause unopposed muscles from the lateral epicondyle to change the positions of the upper arm joints. In a standing or sitting positions the client will present with subtle increases in the **carrying angle of the elbow,** the palm of the hand facing forward, the wrist in radial deviation, and the MP joints of the fingers in slight hyperextension. Similarly, the extrinsic flexor bias of the muscles from the medial epicondyle at rest can be observed with the back of the hand more prominent and the wrist in ulnar deviation. During movement, the client may have difficulty reaching in every plane of movement and may present with a more pronounced posture defect when carrying increased loads. Exaggerated movements of trunk flexion and glenohumeral rotation compensate for limitations in extensibility of the elbow extensors and wrist deviators.

As part of effective intervention for the musculoskeletal structures originating from the lateral and medial epicondyles, full extensibility is necessary to obtain multi-joint flexibility, balanced strength both proximally and distally, and full function in everyday life activities.

Scenario 5

If you were to complete a manual muscle test by nerve function, which muscles would be evaluated for the median, the ulnar, and the radial nerve distributions? What is the advantage of doing strength testing by nerve distribution?

Functional anatomy screening can be utilized to assess muscle adaptations that occur with acute and chronic nerve injury. Changes in muscle balance, and ultimately postures at rest and

TABLE 2-4   Muscles Originating from the Lateral Epicondyle

Muscle	Origin	Action	Position for Full Musculotendinous Flexibility
Anconeus	Lateral and posterior surfaces of proximal half of body of humerus and lateral intermuscular septum	Extends the elbow	Elbow flexion, forearm pronation
Brachioradialis	Proximal two thirds of lateral supracondylar ridge of humerus and lateral intermuscular septum	Flexes the elbow, assists with pronating and supinating the forearm	Elbow extension, forearm pronation or supination
Supinator	Lateral epicondyle of humerus, RCL of elbow joint, annular ligament of radius, and supinator crest of ulna	Supinates the forearm	Elbow extension, forearm pronation
Extensor carpi radialis longus	Distal one third of lateral supracondylar ridge of humerus and lateral intermuscular septum	Extends the wrist in a radial direction, assists with elbow flexion	Elbow extension, forearm pronation, wrist flexion in an ulnar direction
Extensor carpi radialis brevis	Lateral epicondyle of humerus, RCL of elbow, and deep antebrachial fossa	Extends the wrist, assists with wrist radial deviation	Elbow extension, forearm pronation, wrist flexion
Extensor carpi ulnaris	Lateral epicondyle of humerus, aponeurosis from posterior border of ulna, and deep antebrachial fossa	Extends the wrist in an ulnar direction	Elbow extension, forearm pronation, wrist flexion in a radial direction
Extensor digitorum communis	Lateral epicondyle of humerus and deep antebrachial fossa	Extends the MP joints of the second through fifth digits; in conjunction with the lumbricals and interossei, extends the PIP joints of the second through fifth digits; assists with abduction of the index, ring, and little fingers; and assists with extension of the wrist in a radial direction	Elbow extension; forearm pronation; wrist flexion; and MP, PIP, and DIP flexion of the fingers
Extensor digitorum minimi	Lateral epicondyles of humerus and deep antebrachial fossa	Extends the MP joint of the fifth digit; in conjunction with the lumbricals and interossei, extends the PIP joints of the fifth digit; assists with abduction of the fifth finger	Elbow extension; forearm pronation; wrist flexion; and MP, PIP, and DIP flexion of the little finger

DIP, Distal interphalangeal; *MP,* metacarpophalangeal; *PIP,* proximal interphalangeal; *RCL,* radial collateral ligament.

TABLE 2-5   Muscles Originating from the Medial Epicondyle

Muscle	Origin	Action	Position for Full Musculotendinous Flexibility
Pronator teres	Medial epicondyle of humerus, common flexor tendon, and deep antebrachial fascia	Pronates the forearm, assists with elbow flexion	Elbow extension, forearm supination
Flexor carpi radialis	Common flexor tendon of medial epicondyle of humerus and deep antebrachial fascia	Flexes the wrist in a radial direction; may assist with pronation of the forearm and elbow flexion	Elbow extension, forearm supination, wrist extension in an ulnar direction
Flexor carpi ulnaris	Common flexor tendon of medial epicondyle of humerus	Flexes the wrist in an ulnar direction; may assist with elbow flexion	Elbow extension, forearm supination, wrist extension in a radial direction
Palmaris longus	Common flexor tendon of medial epicondyle of humerus and deep antebrachial fascia	Tenses the palmar fascia, flexes the wrist, and may assist with elbow flexion	Elbow extension, forearm supination, wrist extension
Flexor digitorum superficialis	Common flexor tendon of medial epicondyle of humerus, UCL of elbow, and deep antebrachial fascia	Flexes the PIP joints of the second through fifth digits; assists with MP and wrist flexion	Elbow extension; forearm supination; wrist extension; and MP, PIP, and DIP extension of the fingers

DIP, Distal interphalangeal; *MP,* metacarpophalangeal; *PIP,* proximal interphalangeal; *UCL,* ulnar collateral ligament.

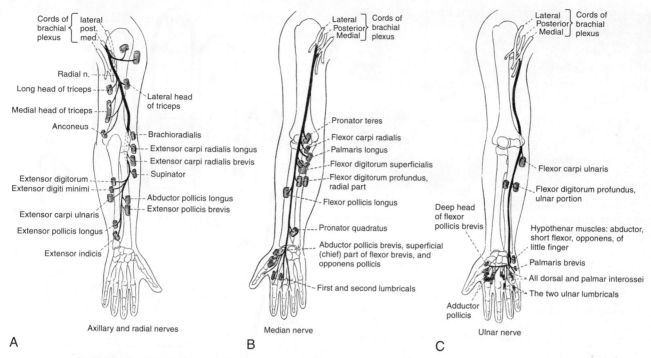

FIGURE 2-13 A, Axillary and radial nerves. **B,** Median nerve. **C,** Ulnar nerve. (From Jenkins DB: *Hollinshead's functional anatomy of the limbs and back*, ed 6, Philadelphia, 1991, WB Saunders.)

during movement, develop in response to pain. Symptoms of nerve pain can be reported within the cutaneous distribution or throughout the entire peripheral distribution from an injury to the nerve root. Unconsciously the nerve response to injury is to limit the stretch and excursion that occurs with joint movement. The muscles of the upper extremity limit the arc of motion by contracting the corresponding joint. An example can be seen in clients with an ulnar nerve injury. The shoulder, elbow, and wrist joints will limit tension and stress to that nerve. Neural tension increases with elbow flexion greater than 90 degrees and intrafascicular pressure intensifies with shoulder abduction, forearm supination and wrist extension. The neuromuscular system will prevent this undesirable painful posture by controlling joint motion in a cohesive manner. A functional anatomy screen for the composite joints of the upper extremity will find the arm bias of elbow flexion is short of 90 degrees, forearm movements range from neutral to pronation, and the wrist is flexed. If additional tension occurs, as when the client's head laterally flexes to the opposite side, the shoulder girdle and elbow may change position to accommodate proximal nerve glide without increasing neural tension. Measures are needed to decrease the pain and the neuromuscular response during intervention. Immobilization may be necessary, but overlooking the effects of pain reduction through postural modifications may lead to an undesirable response of joint and muscle adaptation.

In nerve injuries with a severe degree of conduction loss of both sensory and motor fascicles, a functional anatomy screening uses a more conventional assessment of imbalance. Frequently, manual muscle tests are performed by evaluating synergistic action of muscle groups, such as wrist extensors or finger flexors as a group. In reality, manual muscle testing can be a valuable tool in viewing muscle balance from other perspectives. Unrecognized impairments of the upper extremity can be discovered due to imbalances created from a diagnosis, such as peripheral neuropathy.

The findings of a manual muscle test can be more sensitive when selecting muscles innervated by various nerve distributions. For example, Fig. 2-13, *A*, provides the distribution of the muscles associated with the radial nerve. It is important to note that more than finger and wrist extension can be involved, especially with trauma to the nerve proximal to the elbow in the mid-humeral or brachial plexus regions. The selection of muscles to be evaluated should include wrist and finger extensors as well as those muscles that are responsible primarily for elbow extension, elbow flexion with the forearm in neutral position, supination, and thumb extension. In addition to wrist drop, common postural changes for radial nerve injuries at rest may be increased forearm pronation and thumb adduction.

When identifying the muscles that are innervated by the median nerve, the same approach could be used. Fig. 2-13, *B*, provides a visual representation of the muscles innervated by the median nerve. You may notice that several **extrinsic muscles,** those muscles which originate outside of the hand, are innervated by the median nerve. In some cases, the musculotendinous system can cross the elbow, the wrist, the fingers, and the thumb. In addition, there are several **intrinsic muscles,** those muscles that originate in the hand, which are innervated by the median nerve and provide movements to the thumb, the index, and the middle fingers. In a median nerve injury at the wrist, the motor loss to the abductor pollicis brevis, opponens pollicis, and a portion of the flexor pollicis brevis presents with loss of bulk to the thenar eminence. The loss of muscle tone from the median nerve innervated muscles increases the dominance of the ulnar nerve innervated muscles. The thumb is drawn into CMC adduction at rest, a posture called the *ape hand position.* The orientation of the thumb CMC joint changes to a flat posture, the flexor pollicis longus is without balance at the MP joint. With this

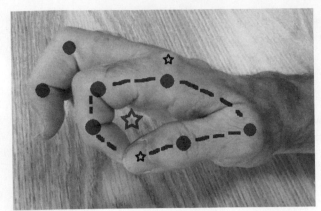

FIGURE 2-14 Mapping of a hand with limited median and ulnar nerve function. (Photo from Lori DeMott.)

loss of intrinsic abductor tension, the IP joint of the thumb is then persuaded into flexion. Weakened tip and chuck pinch may be present. Fig. 2-14 illustrates the mapping of postural imbalances created from the absence of the median nerve at the wrist. Important landmarks are changes in the orientation of the nail, the prominent head of the index MP joint, and the flat space between the index and thumb.

The muscles innervated by the ulnar nerve are identified in Fig. 2-13, *C.* Motor function is supplied to a wrist flexor, finger flexors to the ring and little fingers, and to many intrinsic muscles of the fingers and thumb. Compression of the ulnar nerve at the elbow can result in reduced grip from weakened FDP of the ring and little fingers and lateral pinch from weakened adductor pollicis. Recognizing patterns of muscle imbalance based on the nerve distribution provides a picture of function very different from that picture obtained from a generalized manual muscle test.

Scenario 6

If you were to check the excursion of the extensor and flexor tendons to the fingers, how do the location and the type of these structures affect movement?

The default position of the hand and wrist at rest is described as the "normal resting hand position." In this posture, the wrist is positioned in approximately 30 degrees of extension, the MP and IP joints of the fingers are in approximately 45 degrees of flexion, and the fingers abduct and converge towards the radius. At rest, the posture of the thumb joints is CMC abduction, MP flexion, and IP extension. The balanced relationship between the wrist, fingers, and thumb demonstrates the principle of **tenodesis.** That is, the **length-tension** of the musculotendinous structures and the ability of the extrinsic tendons to freely glide within their sheaths create movements at distal joints as a result of passive wrist repositioning. In the absence of active muscular contraction, flexion of the fingers and thumb occurs with wrist extension *and* extension of the fingers and thumb occurs with wrist flexion. A wrist-produced tenodesis can be beneficial in providing gross grasp, prehension, and release for individuals who lack C7 innervation, amplitude, and tensile strength from tendon transfers.[7] However, subtle limitations in tenodesis can result from joint and soft tissue problems, such as

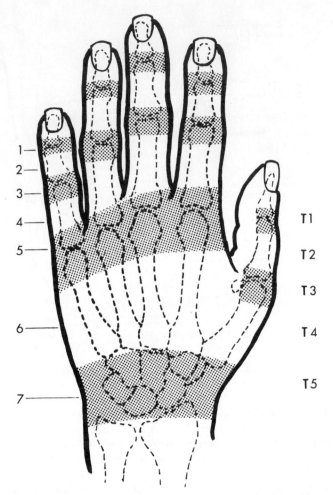

FIGURE 2-15 Extensor tendon zones as defined by the Committee on Tendon Injuries for the International Federation of the Society for Surgery of the Hand. (From Fess EE, Gettle K, Phillips C, et al: *Hand and upper extremity splinting: principles and methods,* ed 3, St Louis, 2005, Mosby.)

musculotendinous shortening, poor wrist patterns, and extrinsic tendon adhesions.[7] In the event where normal joint range of motion and length-tension of the musculoskeletal structures are present, the focus of the functional anatomy screen should be on the quality of **tendon gliding** through sheaths and the expectation of fluid distal joint flexion and extension. Different scenarios occur when adhesions are present at different locations in the arm and hand.

> **◎ Clinical Pearl**
>
> The wrist position is the key to changing the tension placed on the extrinsic fingers and thumb musculotendinous units.

You have learned that a muscle such as the EDC crosses the elbow, the forearm, the wrist, and the fingers. In addition to considering the length of a musculotendinous unit, the location of the extensor tendons is useful to appreciate the role of other structures which can impact tenodesis and tendon gliding.[7] Fig. 2-15 identifies the six locations, or zones, of the extensor tendons. Within an area at the wrist known as *Zone VI,* another important

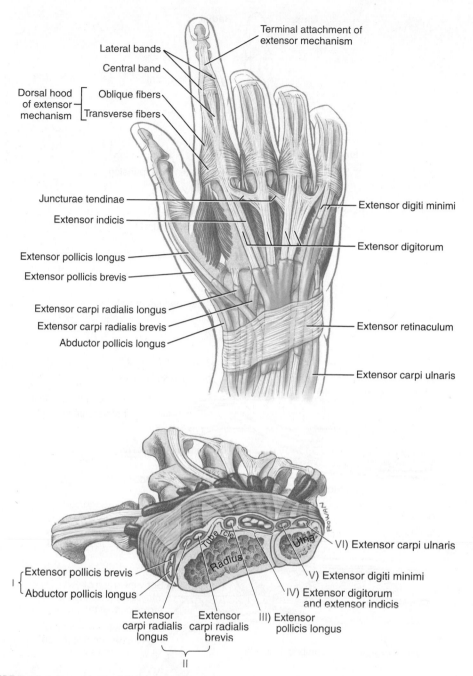

Terminal attachment of
extensor mechanism

Lateral bands

Central band

Dorsal hood
of extensor
mechanism

Oblique fibers

Transverse fibers

Juncturae tendinae

Extensor indicis

Extensor pollicis longus

Extensor pollicis brevis

Extensor carpi radialis longus

Extensor carpi radialis brevis

Abductor pollicis longus

Extensor digiti minimi

Extensor digitorum

Extensor retinaculum

Extensor carpi ulnaris

Extensor pollicis brevis

Abductor pollicis longus

Extensor
carpi radialis
longus

Extensor
carpi radialis
brevis

Radius

Ulna

VI) Extensor carpi ulnaris

V) Extensor digiti minimi

IV) Extensor digitorum
and extensor indicis

III) Extensor
pollicis longus

FIGURE 2-16 Arrangement of the extensor tendons in the compartments of the wrist. (From Neuman D: *Kinesiology of the musculoskeletal system: foundations for rehabilitation*, ed 2, St Louis, 2010, Mosby.)

contribution to the function of extensor tendon gliding is the presence of six compartments created by the deep layers of the dorsal fascia. Fig. 2-16 shows the tendons that are located in each of the numbered dorsal compartments of the wrist. Testing the independent movement of each extensor tendon by compartment provides a clearer picture of the effectiveness of tendon excursion through the dorsal pulley system and can supplement the findings of a more generic range of motion or manual muscle test. A functional anatomy screen at Zone VI for the extensor tendons may show changes at rest for the MP joints of the fingers with increased extension. With movement, passive and active limitations of wrist flexion and exaggerated finger extension can be observed.

Similarly, an appreciation of the extensor tendons to the fingers in Zones II-IV provides a different perspective of how location impacts tendon gliding. In Fig. 2-17, the extensor mechanism of a finger PIP joint is presented in a dorsal and lateral view with digital MP flexion and extension. One can see the balance that must occur between the intrinsic and extrinsic muscle groups so that full extension of a digit can occur. To assess the contribution of the extrinsic musculature with PIP extension, the wrist and the MP joints can be stabilized in extension. In this position, the power of the intrinsic muscles is minimized. When the PIP joint is held in extension and the DIP joint is actively flexed, a passive stretch to the lateral bands are completed that

Ulnar   Radial

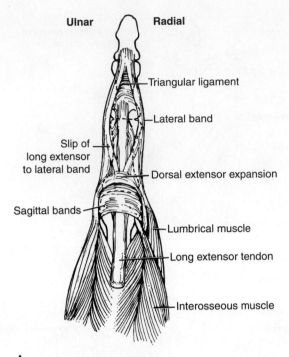

Triangular ligament

Lateral band

Slip of
long extensor
to lateral band

Dorsal extensor expansion

Sagittal bands

Lumbrical muscle

Long extensor tendon

Interosseous muscle

A

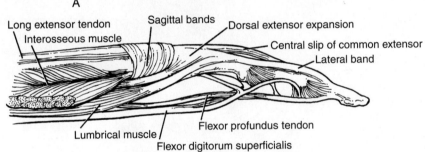

Long extensor tendon   Sagittal bands   Dorsal extensor expansion
Interosseous muscle   Central slip of common extensor
                                                       Lateral band

Lumbrical muscle
                              Flexor profundus tendon
          Flexor digitorum superficialis

B

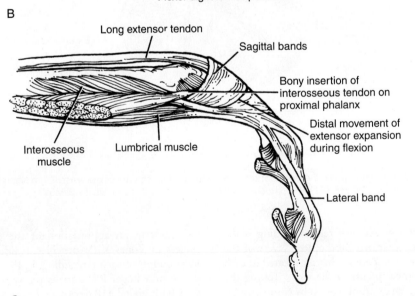

Long extensor tendon

Sagittal bands

Bony insertion of
interosseous tendon on
proximal phalanx

Distal movement of
extensor expansion
during flexion

Interosseous
muscle   Lumbrical muscle

Lateral band

C

FIGURE 2-17 Extensor mechanism of the digits. The figure shows distal movement of the extensor expansion with metacarpophalangeal (MP) joint flexion. (From Fess EE, Gettle K, Phillips C, et al: *Hand and upper extremity splinting: principles and methods*, ed 3, St Louis, 2005, Mosby.)

ultimately facilitates balanced extension between the PIP and the DIP joints. Knowledge of the extensor tendon anatomy, location by zone, and presence of surrounding structures is an important consideration in your assessment of the hand.

At rest, a functional anatomy screen for the extensor tendons in Zone II-IV can present with imbalances in PIP and DIP extension. An injury to the palmar plate at the PIP joint results in loosening of the volar supporting structures resulting in unchecked pull of the extensor tendon, increased dorsal orientation of the lateral bands, and hyperextension of the PIP joint. This imbalance results in a change of the PIP joint axis, loss of mechanical advantage, and flexion bias of the distal phalanx. At rest, the digit is observed in PIP joint extension and DIP joint flexion. The normal resting balance of flexion cascade in the MP, PIP, and DIP joints is also lost.

The finger flexors have similarities and contrasting differences from the extensor tendons. Fig. 2-18 illustrates the five flexor tendon zones to the fingers and three flexor tendon zones to the thumb. Zone IV contains the structures within the carpal tunnel, and Fig. 2-19 provides a cross-sectional view of their anatomy. When examining the excursion of the flexor tendons at this level, an assessment of the structures can be performed starting with the superficial tendons and progressing to the tendons in the deeper compartments of the carpal tunnel. The FDS to the middle and ring fingers would be the most superficial structure, followed by the FDS to the index and little fingers, and finally the FDP to all of the fingers. Two other structures are contained within the carpal tunnel, the flexor pollicis longus and the median nerve, as well as the synovium, which encases and lubricates the flexor tendons. Overall, it can be useful to isolate the excursion of these tendons by compartments as injuries that are more superficial, such as burns, which may have more effect on the FDS compared to injuries that are deeper—as is the case with fractures to the distal one-third of the radius. A functional anatomy screen for the flexor tendons in Zone IV can be exaggerated tenodesis or increased finger flexion with increased wrist extension.

Further considerations become evident in flexor tendon Zones I-II. At this level the relationship between the FDP and the FDS changes. Prior to entering Zone II, the FDP is deep to the FDS. In Zone II, the FDP passes through the decussation of the FDS, which can be visualized in Fig. 2-20. It becomes very

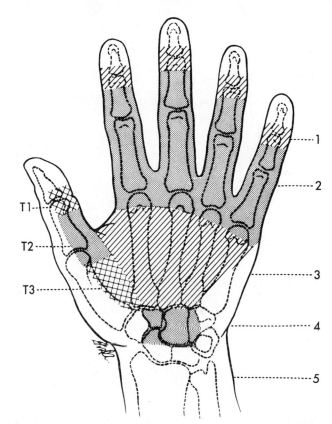

FIGURE 2-18 Flexor tendon zones of the hand. (From Kleinert HE, Schepel S, Gill T: Flexor tendon injuries, *Surg Clin North Am* 61(2): 267-286, 1981.)

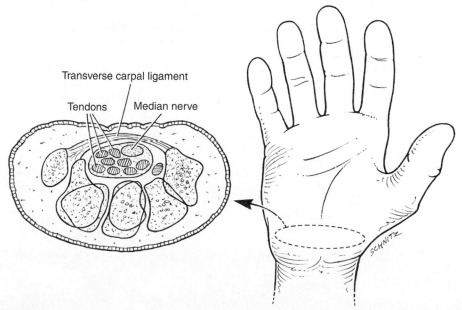

FIGURE 2-19 Cross-sectional view of the carpal tunnel anatomy. (From Fess EE, Gettle K, Phillips C, et al: *Hand and upper extremity splinting: principles and methods*, ed 3, St Louis, 2005, Mosby.)

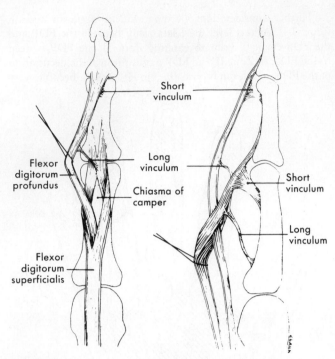

FIGURE 2-20 The flexor digitorum superficialis (FDS) lies volar to the flexor digitorum profundus (FDP) as the tendons enter the sheath. (From Schneider LH: *Flexor tendon injuries*, Boston, 1985, Little Brown.)

important to isolate each tendon when assessing its excursion. When testing the FDS, the effects of the FDP must be eliminated by the examiner holding the DIPs of the non-tested fingers in extension and allowing each individual finger to actively flex at only the PIP joint. When testing the FDP, the PIP joint can be supported in extension to allow only DIP flexion. In this way, isolated range of motion exercises can facilitate the independent function of these two important flexor tendons to the hand. A functional anatomy screen for the flexor tendons in Zones I-II can reveal imbalances, such as insufficient flexion of the DIP joint with full fisting of the hand.

Summary

It is critical that hand therapy professionals understand the role *and* interrelationships of joints, ligaments, muscles, tendons, and nerves in order to appreciate normal postural mechanisms that occur. Continued study and observations of normal anatomy during static and dynamic movements of the upper extremity are vital to recognizing the abnormal deviations, or defaults in posture resulting from tissue imbalance. The addition of a functional anatomy screen during the evaluation process will enhance the level of rehabilitation expertise needed to recognize the source of pathology and the influence of the kinematic chain at rest and during movements. Understanding these principles, along with continued study of human anatomy, will enable you to develop therapeutic interventions that address the imbalances of the upper extremity in order to help your clients recover from the devastating effects of injury, disease, and aging.

References

1. Donatelli RA, Wooden MJ: *Orthopedic physical therapy*, ed 4, St Louis, 2010, Churchill Livingston Elsevier.
2. Kendall FP, McCreary EK, Provance PG, et al: *Muscles: testing and function, with posture and pain*, ed 5, Baltimore, 2005, Lippincott Williams & Wilkins.
3. Brand PW, Hollister AM: *Clinical mechanics of the hand*, ed 3, St Louis, 1999, Mosby.
4. Walsh MT: Interventions in the disturbances in the motor and sensory environment, *J Hand Ther* 25:202–218, 2012.
5. Topp KS, Boyd BS: Peripheral nerve: from the microscopic functional unit of the axon to the biomechanically loaded macroscopic structure, *J Hand Ther* 25:142–151, 2012.
6. Rybski M: *Kinesiology for occupational therapy*, ed 2, Thorofare, NJ, 2011, Slack Incorporated.
7. Fess EE, Gettle K, Phillips C, et al: *Hand and upper extremity splinting: principles and methods*, ed 3, St Louis, 2005, Mosby.

3

Edema Reduction Techniques: A Biologic Rationale for Selection

Sandra M Artzberger

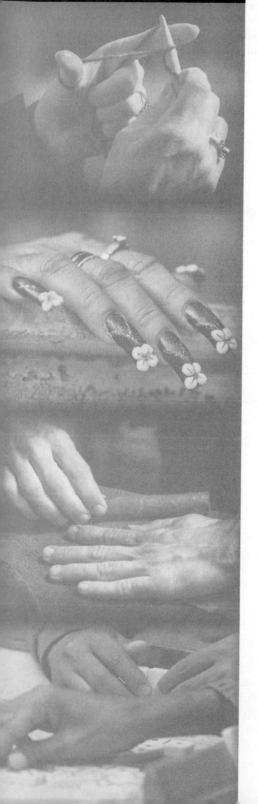

U nlike in the past, the treatment of hand edema no longer needs to be partly a guessing game. Modern treatment selections are more firmly grounded in anatomic and biologic principles and therefore are more successful. To treat edema effectively, the therapist must know the difference between the lymphatic and venous systems, including the role these systems play in edema reduction. It also is essential that the therapist understand the different types of edema. This chapter describes acute, subacute, and chronic edema. It reviews vascular and lymphatic anatomy and biology, and it describes appropriate interventions for edema, including the technique of **manual edema mobilization (MEM).** Special emphasis is placed on the clinical reasoning involved in selecting the appropriate treatment.

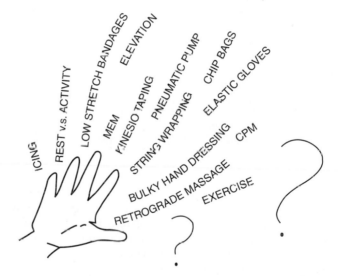

Overview of Lymphatic Anatomy Related to Edema Reduction

An overview of the capillary vascular structures and their relationship to each other is a prerequisite for a more detailed discussion of these systems. The vascular structures include the interstitium, the arteriole, and the venule. The **interstitium** is the space between cells. It contains both the smallest arterial vessel, called an **arteriole,** and the smallest venous structure, called a **venule.**[1, 2] Both the arteriole and the venule terminate in capillaries, which are joined histologically (Fig. 3-1). The heart is responsible for pumping blood through these structures.

Editor's Note: Before the importance of Sandra Artzberger's work on the treatment of edema was recognized, the edema techniques that hand therapists were taught were not specific to the lymphatic system and sometimes even damaged this delicate and amazing part of the body. Artzberger has done much to delineate the anatomy and physiology of post traumatic edema. She has changed our thinking and has overhauled the treatment repertoire, creating an approach that is based on science. Her technique of manual edema mobilization has resulted in much-improved management of edema in clients with upper extremity injuries.

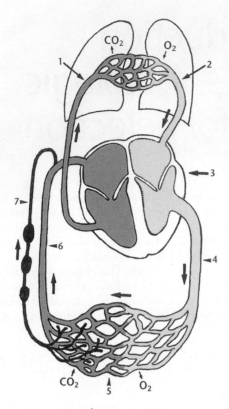

1 Pulmonary artery ⎫ pulmonary circulation
2 Pulmonary veins ⎭
3 Heart
4 Aorta – arterial system ⎫
5 Capillaries   ⎬ systemic circulation
6 Venous system   ⎭
7 Lymph vessels and lymph nodes

FIGURE 3-1 Blood and lymph circulatory systems. (From Foldi M, Foldi E, Kubik S: *Textbook of lymphology for physicians and lymphedema therapists,* Munich, 2003, Urban & Fischer Verlag.)

The lymphatic system originates in the interstitium with the smallest of the lymphatic vessels, called the **initial lymphatic** or **lymphatic capillary,** and culminates in the largest lymphatic structure, called the **thoracic duct.**[2] The venous system has a continuous-loop pump system based on the heart pumping oxygenated blood to the arteries, arterioles, venules, veins and back to the lungs and heart. However, the lymphatic system does not have this continuous central pump system (see Fig. 3-1).[3] Also, unlike with venous capillaries in the interstitium, molecules do not diffuse into the lymphatic capillary. Therefore the lymphatic system must be stimulated to activate a force pump, (external and internal vacuum stimulation that moves lymph), creating a vacuum and drawing the lymph proximally.[3] Initial lymphatics, which are larger than venules, are finger-shaped tubes that are closed on the distal end and lined with overlapping, oak leaf–shaped endothelial cells. Anchor filaments extend from the endothelial cells to the connective tissue (Fig. 3-2). Movement of the connective tissue pulls on the anchor filaments. This, in turn, pulls on the overlapping flaps (junctions) of the endothelial cells, and water and large molecules are admitted into the initial lymphatic.[1,2,4] Large molecules also enter the initial lymphatic when a change in the interstitial pressure causes the junctions of the endothelial cells

to spread apart. The initial lymphatic connection forms a net-like structure.[1,3]

The balance between fluid moving into and out of the vascular vessels on a cellular level, which was first described by Ernest Starling in the early 1900s, is called **Starling's equilibrium.**[1,2] This balanced movement of fluid functions as a gradient system from high to low pressure. On the capillary level, **arteriole hydrostatic pressure** (the pressure of the blood fluid exerted on the arteriole vessel wall) is 30 to 40 mm Hg, which is enough pressure to cause filtration of electrolytes, fluid, a few small plasma proteins, and other nutrients into the interstitium.[1,2] The colloid **osmotic pressure** (also called the **oncotic pressure**) in the interstitium is determined by the concentration of proteins in this intercellular space; this pressure is approximately 25 mm Hg.[2] Tissue cells in the interstitium absorb the nutrients, electrolytes, and other substances filtered out of the arteriole. Of the remaining substances, 90% diffuse by osmosis into the venous system.[1-3] The residual 10% of leftover substances are large molecules, which are absorbed by the lymphatic system.[1-3] These large molecules consist of plasma proteins, minerals, ions, hormone cells, bacteria, fat cells, and fluid.[1-5] Once the cells enter the initial lymphatic, they make up a substance called **lymph.**[2]

As lymph enters the initial lymphatic, it causes pressure changes that open the valve connected to the next lymphatic vessels, the three-celled **collector lymphatics** (Fig. 3-3). Clinically, the most important features of the tube-like collector lymphatics are a middle layer of muscle cell and the presence of valves every 6 to 8 mm along the tube.[1,3] The chamber between two valves is called a **lymphangion.**[3] As a bolus of lymph enters a lymphangion, the single layer muscle cell contracts against the expanding lymphangion and pushes the bolus proximally into the next lymphangion (see Fig. 3-3). This process continues until the bolus reaches the afferent lymphatic pathways of the lymph node.

◎ **Clinical Pearl**

Exercise moves lymph ten to thirty times faster through the collector lymphatics and increases the rate of lymphatic uptake from the interstitium.[1]

The pumping movement of the lymphangions resembles the peristaltic movement of the small intestine. The lymphangions pump at a rate of 10 to 20 times per minute,[3] and exercise can increase this pumping motion by 10 to 30 times.[1] Recent theories hold that peristalsis also creates a negative pressure that opens the junctions of the endothelial cells, enabling large-molecule substances to move from the interstitium into the initial lymphatic.[3]

Eventually the bolus of lymph moves into the afferent lymphatic pathways of the lymph nodes. **Lymph nodes,** which perform several immunologic functions, are composed of a series of complex sinuses and therefore often are considered "dams" or "kinks in the hose" in the movement of lymph. Excessive swelling distal to the lymph nodes does not increase their rate of filtration, but rather causes further congestion distally.[4] Venous vessels do not connect to lymph nodes and therefore do not reflect this slowing of fluid movement. Also, venous vessels do not carry bacteria or tissue waste products and therefore do not pass these

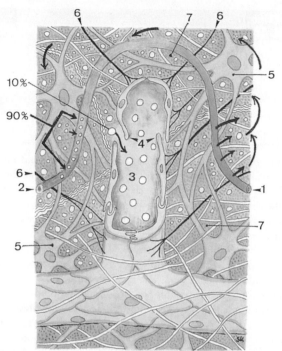

FIGURE 3-2 Incorporation of the lymph capillary into the interstitium. *1,* Arterial section of the blood capillary; *2,* venous section of the blood capillary; *3,* lymph capillary; *4,* open intercellular groove-swinging tip; *5,* fibrocyte; *6,* anchor filaments; *7,* intercellular space. *Small arrows* indicate the direction of blood flow; *large arrows* indicate the direction of intercellular fluid flow. (From Foldi M, Foldi E, Kubik S: *Textbook of lymphology for physicians and lymphedema therapists,* Munich, 2003, Urban & Fischer Verlag.)

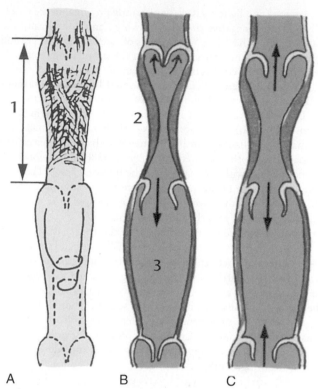

FIGURE 3-3 Structure and function of the valve segments in the collector lymphatics. A, Arrangement of the musculature. **B,** Normal function. **C,** Dilated lymph vessel with valvular insufficiency and reflux. (From Foldi M, Foldi E, Kubik S: *Textbook of lymphology for physicians and lymphedema therapists,* Munich, 2003, Urban & Fischer Verlag.)

substances through the lymph nodes for cleansing. Lymph nodes present significant resistance to the flow of lymph and must be massaged to facilitate a faster flow of the distal congested lymph.[4] The MEM method of massaging healthy and uninfected nodes uses *MEM pump point stimulation,* which is a method of simultaneously massaging two groups of nodes, bundles of lymphatic vessels, or **watershed areas** (anatomical drainage dividing areas), which theoretically speeds up the movement of lymph through the nodes.

From the nodes, lymph can enter the venous system directly, through **lymphovenous anastomoses** (areas where the small vessels of the lymphatic and venous systems join), or it can continue on in the lymphatic vessels and empty into either the right lymphatic duct or the largest lymphatic vessel, the thoracic duct. The thoracic duct lies anterior to and parallel with the spinal cord from approximately L2 and empties into the left subclavian vein.[2,3] The right lymphatic duct terminates in the right subclavian vein.

The movement of lymph in the thoracic duct is affected by changes in thoracic pressure. **Diaphragmatic breathing** expands the abdomen, causing changes in thoracic pressure that move the contents of the thoracic duct more proximally.[1,3] This action creates a vacuum, drawing lymph from the more distal vessels toward the thoracic duct.[1,3] Treatments such as MEM, therefore, begin with diaphragmatic breathing and trunk exercise. This is analogous to removing the plug from a drain or a clog from a backed-up sink. The clog must be removed before the water can flow out. In terms of clinical application, the vacuum created by

diaphragmatic breathing moves lymph more proximal in the thoracic duct, creating a space into which the more distal peripheral edema can move.

> **◎ Clinical Pearl**
>
> The key to successful edema reduction is to "remove the plug" by starting proximally at the trunk with diaphragmatic breathing and proximal exercise.

Before they reach the thoracic duct, the deep lymphatic trunks share a common vascular sheath with the venous and arterial structures.[3] Therefore exercise increases the rate of arterial flow and passively stimulates the lymphatic vessels, increasing the rate of lymph flow. Also, at least 200 lymph nodes are located centrally and around deep venous and arterial structures. Exercise of the abdominal muscles increases the pumping of blood, which stimulates the lymph nodes, moving lymph through them more rapidly—a force pump action.

"Exercise is key to lymphatic activation" is a frequently heard statement. Yet therapists know that in most cases, simply exercising the edematous hand or arm in the subacute phase does not significantly or permanently reduce edema. Lymphatic structures can exceed 30 times their normal capacity before edema becomes visible;[1] this means that proximal to the visible edema is the beginning of non-visible edematous congestion.

Exercise and light massage significantly proximal to the visible edema create a negative pressure, drawing lymph proximally and thus removing the "clog." The results of research by Pecking and colleagues[6] present a strong argument for stimulating lymphatic absorption and conduction significantly proximal to visible edema. In these researchers' study, **manual lymphatic drainage (MLD)** (the manual decongesting of lymph through activating the lymph uptake through massage, low-stretch bandaging programs, and so on) was performed exclusively to the contralateral, normal upper quadrant on 108 women with lymphedema caused by mastectomy; this resulted in a 12% to 38% lymph uptake in the hand, even without massage of the involved area.[6] The contralateral massage created a negative pressure (vacuum), drawing the lymph from the involved to the uninvolved area, where it could be absorbed into the normal system.

If we synthesize these findings with the theory that changes in thoracic pressure move lymph proximally, and add the knowledge that muscle contraction stimulates lymphatic uptake on many levels, we arrive at a very strong rationale for beginning edema reduction at the trunk even if edema is visible only in the hand. Clinically, this means that therapists should not begin edema reduction treatment where edema is visible; rather, they must begin in a normal, uninvolved area significantly proximal to the visible edema. Appropriate treatments include diaphragmatic breathing, trunk stretching and muscle contraction exercises and activities, and MEM massage that begins in the area of the uninvolved axilla. (MEM is discussed in more detail later in the chapter.)

Acute Edema Related to the Vascular Anatomy

The venous and lymphatic systems have many pump-like structures that help propel the blood back to the heart. Because of the descending gradient of hydrostatic pressures from the arteriole capillary to the venule capillary, small-molecule substances diffuse easily and are reabsorbed into the venous capillary through its thin wall.[2] Active muscle contraction acts as a pump as it compresses and empties the large deep venous vessels. As this blood is propelled proximally toward the heart, a negative pressure is created, which draws blood from the periphery into the deep veins.

Edema develops when the descending gradient of Starling's forces are disrupted by an interruption and an imbalance. The cascade of events that occurs after tissue laceration is a good example. Initially, an outflow of water and electrolytes (**transudate edema**) into the wound occurs. The mast cells then release histamines, which greatly increase capillary permeability, and plasma proteins, phagocytic cells, and other substances leak into the area. Plasma protein fibrinogen is converted to fibrin, which plugs the endothelial cells lining the lymphatics.[7] This prevents the lymphatics from temporarily removing the large molecules as the various **phagocyte cells** perform their "cleanup" function.[7] Edema results when excess fluid and plasma proteins are trapped in the interstitium. Starling's equilibrium is disrupted, because the trapping of excess proteins in the interstitium increases the colloid osmotic pressure.

The immediate goal of treatment by physicians and therapists is to limit the amount of outflow into the wound bed, thereby preventing excessive swelling, accumulation of blood, and further tissue damage. After 2 to 5 days, the swelling begins to subside as the surrounding intact venous capillaries start to absorb the transudate and the lymphatic vessels absorb the large-molecule plasma proteins not phagocytized by the **macrophages.**

> ◎ **Clinical Pearl**
>
> The anatomic differences between the lymphatic and venous systems determine the anatomically-based treatment of edema.

Reduction Techniques for Acute Edema

Bulky Dressing

Several techniques can be used to reduce excessive fluid outflow (edema). For example, a bulky hand dressing applied at the time of surgery gives counterforce to the outflow (filtration) by changing the tissue pressure. It is composed of appropriate wound care dressing, fluffy gauze sponges, and rolled-on gauze. After soft tissue trauma, immobilization for up to a week in a bulky dressing or plaster splint facilitates healing of involved structures by preventing stress on fragile tissue, which could cause microscopic rupture of vessels with resulting edema. The therapist should check the dressing or splint to make sure it is not too tight and should contact the physician immediately if this is a possibility. A bulky dressing that is too tight causes vascular changes, temperature changes, increased edema, or severe, painful compression of the fingers and can lead to tissue breakdown. The capillary refill test can be used to check vascular status (see Chapter 5). The therapist also must teach the client that any vascular changes (that is, changes in tissue color) or sensory changes must be reported immediately to the physician. Procedures, such as tenolysis and flexor tendon repair, involve minimal or no immobilization in a bulky dressing. However, even with these diagnoses, limited motion can increase edema, therefore early motion must be balanced with rest to prevent this.

High Voltage Pulsed Current

In animal studies, high-voltage pulse current (HVPC) used on very acute edema was reported to retard the high capillary permeability outflow [8,9] but has not been replicated in human subjects. Clinically, it is a frequently used modality to reduce acute edema.

Elevation

Elevation of the hand above the heart, if not contraindicated, also reduces outflow because it reduces the arterial hydrostatic pressure.[10] Elevation in the acute stage facilitates lymphatic flow because hydrostatic gradient pressure is increased along the lymphatic trunks.[4] Ideally, the involved extremity is elevated in a plus 45-degree "ski hill" position; this means that pillows are placed so that the elbow is above the shoulder, and the hand is above the elbow and wrist.

Keeping the arm elevated while sleeping can be difficult. Often clients use pillows on either side of them. A belt can be fastened around the pillows to keep them together. Also, the bed can be moved against the wall so that one set of pillows is pushed up against the wall, preventing them from falling. For clients with finger replantation, elevation no higher than the heart is recommended to avoid compromising arterial blood flow.[11]

Precaution. *Extreme elevation of the right arm must be avoided in stroke clients with right-sided heart weakness. Extreme upper extremity elevation may cause fluid to flow too quickly into the right side of the heart, because the right upper quadrant is drained by the right lymphatic duct that empties into the right subclavian vein.*

Cold Packs

Cold packs, if not contraindicated for vascular and tissue ischemia reasons or diseases such as Raynauld's, cause vasoconstriction and thus reduce the outflow of fluid in the acute stage. However, the temperature of the cold pack is a consideration. Research shows that when the temperature is lower than 59° F (15° C), proteins leak into the interstitium from lymphatic structures.[12] Excess proteins in the interstitium cause edema.

Precaution. *To prevent "ice burn" to tissue, always place a dry towel between the skin and the cold pack. Cold packs should not be used on a client with a replanted hand or digit because of the effect of vascular compromise on tissue viability.[13] A nerve repair may be injured by cold postoperatively. Clients should get explicit care instructions from their physicians, including precautions on the use of cold packs.*

Retrograde Massage

Light retrograde massage with elevation facilitates diffusion of small molecules into the venous system. The elevation reduces capillary filtration (outflow) pressure, and the light pressure from the retrograde massage aids in venous absorption of the small molecules (not large plasma proteins).

Precaution. *The pressure is kept light to avoid damaging the single-cell initial lymphatic structures in the dermal layer of the skin.*

Compression

Light compression, such as from an elastic glove, Coban (or similar type material) lightly spiral layered on a digit, or low-stretch finger bandage wraps (see video/slides on the Evolve website), facilitates small molecule absorption by the venous system and absorption of large and small molecules by the lymphatic system. A loose but compressive elastic glove generally is one in which the glove material can be pulled away from the hand and simultaneously on each side of finger at least ⅛ inch.

In the early post stroke stages, hand and arm edema is a transudate swelling because fluid leaks into the interstitium as a result of lack of muscle pumping activity on the vascular vessels. Elevation, light retrograde massage, and light compression from an elastic glove or elasticized arm stockinette are effective treatments that promote diffusion of leaked electrolytes and water back into the venous system.

Precaution. *When using an elasticized garment, observe two important precautions: (1) make sure it is not too tight (that is, it does not cause color or temperature changes in the hand or digit) and (2) with elasticized stockinette, make sure it cannot roll down, causing swelling distally.*

A body garment glue can be used to prevent the elastic stockinette from rolling down on itself, which can cause distal swelling. Keep in mind that some body garment glues are latex based; therefore always make sure your client does not have a latex allergy before using this type of glue.

Precaution. *An elastic glove should be fitted to give some compression but should feel loose on the hand and fingers. If the compression is too tight, fluid flow is restricted, which increases edema.*

Elastic Taping

Elastic taping is becoming the common generic term used to designate a variety of tapes similar to the original Kinesio Tex tape developed by a Japanese-born chiropractor, Dr. Kenso Kase, in the 1970s.[14] The cloth-like tape has acrylic glue applied to one side in a wave-like pattern, such as a finger print swirl. When the tape is applied in a specific manner it is theorized that the edema reduces because patient movement pulls the skin in the opposite direction from where the tape was applied. This movement puts a stretch on the initial lymphatic structures facilitating congested lymphatic absorption.[15] Increasing this space, creates a pull on the connective tissue anchor filaments attached to the endothelial cells of the initial lymphatics; this separates the planted endothelial junctions, thereby increasing lymph and fluid flow.

Indications for Manual Edema Mobilization in the Acute Stage

Many wonder why MEM is not started in the acute stage. In 1989, Hutzschenreuter and Brummer[16] did a research study on this point using sheep. They compared the results in two groups, one in which MLD was performed and one in which it was not over a defined period (that is, immediate postoperative to 3 weeks postoperative). They found that both groups showed minimal fluid reduction during the first week after surgery. However, after the first week, the MLD group had a significantly greater increase in fluid movement and edema reduction than the control group.[16] These results are not surprising because initially, acute edema is transudate that is changing to **exudate edema** as the plasma proteins invade and are contained. Only the lymphatic vessels can remove excess proteins from the interstitium.[1,2] MEM and **manual lymphatic treatment**[*] (MLT) programs are designed to activate lymphatic vessels.

Exercise

Some physicians prescribe proximal active motion of an extremity or gliding of the involved structures, or both, during the acute stage of wound healing. Proximal trunk and shoulder motion is excellent. It decongests the lymphatic vessels and removes tissue waste products, resulting in better oxygenation to tissue and faster wound healing. However, movement must be balanced with rest of involved structures. This is done by progressively grading the exercise so as not to increase hand inflammation, pain, and swelling. Always respect the fragility of healing tissue and vascular structures. When moving the involved structures, start with limited movement and check for signs of increased pain, swelling, or redness. If edema increases, rest the involved hand for a day (consider applying a static orthosis). Resume activity, but do less than previously and gradually increase the exercise over the next treatment sessions. I usually begin with the rule of three or five: three (or five) repetitions of an exercise three (or five) times a day. If this does not increase swelling, gradually increase repetitions or frequency, or both. Remember, edema and pain limit motion and retard progress.

> **◎ Clinical Pearl**
>
> Reducing edema is almost always the first priority; do this, and the client will gain motion.

---

[*]*Manual lymphatic treatment is the generic term used to describe the massage principles common to all schools of lymphatic drainage.[15]*

Summary of Reduction Treatment for Acute Edema

- Bulky hand dressing (usually applied by the surgeon postoperatively)
- High-voltage pulse current (HVPC) (used only for very acute edema; benefit in humans not yet proven)
- Elevation
  - Lesser degree of elevation is needed for replanted digits and/or hands.
  - Extreme elevation is contraindicated if right-sided heart weakness is present (that is, post stroke client).
- Cold packs (used in the first 24 to 48 hours only as directed by physician)
  - Cold packs should not be used for replants because cold causes vasoconstriction.
  - Precautions should be clarified with physician if a nerve is involved.
- Light retrograde massage
- Loose elastic glove or elastic stockinette
- Coban or similar self-adherent material (loosely placed on digit in spiral, distal-to-proximal pattern)
- Finger bandage wraps
- Limited active motion of uninvolved areas (excessive trunk/shoulder motion increases edema)
- Balance of activity and rest for all structures to prevent inflammation or increase in edema
- Elastic taping (that is, Kinesio taping)

Reduction Techniques for Subacute and Chronic Edema Based on the Lymphatic Anatomy

To review, the lymphatic system is an independent pump system that works on a negative pressure gradient. When lymph vessels fill (high pressure is created), lymph moves to an area of lower pressure.[1-4]

Clinical Pearl

The sooner lymphatic decongestion occurs, beginning at 1 week post-injury even with non-visible edema, the less the chances of developing tissue and scar thickening, fibrosis, and contractures.

The two keys to activating the lymphatic system are as follows:
- Key 1—Proximal, uninvolved lymphatic structures must be stimulated (massaged), creating a lower negative pressure to draw the most proximal edema out of the involved area.
- Key 2—Molecules are absorbed into the lymphatics from the interstitium because only changes in the interstitial fluid pressure (low to high) cause the endothelial cells lining the lymphatics to open.

Key 1 is based on the theory that negative pressure causes a suction effect that moves the more distal lymph proximally in the trunk and extremities.[1,3] Appropriate treatments to achieve this include MEM massage that starts at the uninvolved axilla, diaphragmatic breathing, trunk exercise, trunk exercise combined with breathing, proprioceptive neuromuscular facilitation (PNF) techniques combined with exhaling and inhaling, and easy yoga trunk stretching exercises. These are considered methods of internal stimulation of the deep lymphatics.

Key 2 involves external stimulation of the lymphatics to facilitate the uptake of lymph from the interstitium by creating changes in the interstitial pressure; by causing stretching of the anchor filaments attached to connective tissue; and by creating negative pressure, which causes the opening of lymphatics through lymphangion pumping. Appropriate treatments to achieve this include MEM, elastic taping, gentle myofascial release (MFR), bombardment of tissue with fluidotherapy particles at a machine temperature no higher than 98° F (36.7° C), active and passive exercise and the light compression provided by elastic gloves, chip bags, and low-stretch bandaging.

Contrast Baths

Some therapists use contrast baths to reduce edema, although currently no research is available that supports this practice.[17] If contrast baths are to be used, research findings on temperature need to be considered. Kurz[18] states that lymph flows best at temperatures between 71.6° F (22° C) and 105.8° F (41° C).[18] For therapy purposes, the hot temperature should not exceed 98° F (36.6° C) to avoid increasing capillary permeability (which is enhanced by heat) and thus edema. With regard to the cold temperature, as mentioned earlier, research has shown that the initial lymphatics actually leak protein into the interstitium at temperatures below 59° F (15° C).[12] Therefore, to avoid the leakage of more plasma proteins into the interstitium (potentially increasing edema), the cold temperature should not be lower than 59° F (15° C).

Precaution. *To avoid worsening the edema, set the temperatures for contrast baths between 71.6° F (22° C) and 98.6° F (37° C).*

Therapy with contrast baths commonly is performed by having the client immerse the hand in warm water for 3 minutes and then in cold water for 1 minute. This sequence is repeated four times, ending on cold.

Electrical Modalities

Published research regarding the use of electrical modalities, such as transcutaneous electrical nerve stimulation (TENS), Low Intensity Laser Therapy (LILT), and non-thermal therapeutic ultrasound, to reduce peripheral subacute edema is inconsistent. Resende, et al.[19] found that TENS did not reduce edema. For over 30 years, literature has been published regarding the multiple applications for LILT. However because of the variety of parameters used with LILT, comparing outcomes is difficult. Studies showing the use of LILT for edema control of ankle sprains were not positive.[20,21] In 2004, a post flexor tendon repair study using gallium arsenide (GaAs) laser therapy found edema reduced immediately and at 12 weeks post repair.[22] Clinically non-thermal therapeutic ultrasound is often implemented to reduce upper extremity edema, yet a peer-reviewed literature search did not find any supporting evidence.

HVPC has been shown to reduce acute edema in the animal model.[8,9,23] It has also been a consideration for subacute and chronic edema. For instance, Griffin and colleagues[24] found that HVPC did not reduce pre-existing edema.[24] However, a subsequent study by Stralka and coworkers[25] on employees with cumulative trauma disorders who wore an orthosis that incorporated HVPC while working showed a reduction in edema. This raises the question of whether the HVPC was reducing the acute edema occurring while working, or reducing a combination of acute and subacute edema. Further study is needed.

Thermal Modalities

Often with subacute edema the therapist additionally has to address joint and tissue stiffness and decreased range of motion (ROM). Heat will increase tissue elasticity. Heat between 71.6° F (21.9° C) and 105.8° F (41° C) will increase lymph flow[18] and soften tissue due to decongestion of the lymph. However, too much heat will increase capillary permeability, increasing the swelling. Therefore, therapists are recommended to keep heat to tissue at body temperature or just slightly above.

Clinically, the author has been able to use well-padded hot packs for 12 minutes on the edematous **indurated** (dense thickened) tissue area, gain tissue elasticity, and soften this edematous indurated tissue without increasing edema. This has been accomplished by doing a proximal MEM routine while the hot packs are on the extremity, followed by proximal to distal exercise after removal of the hot packs. Doing the MEM stimulates and decongests the proximal lymphatic system, creating the negative pressure vacuum to absorb and move the lymph from the area (see Case Study 3-1). A Fluidotherapy machine set at 98° F (36.6° C) to 100° F (37.7° C) will accomplish the same benefit.

Pneumatic Pump

Pneumatic pumps are rarely used by hand therapists. A combination of MEM, compression bandaging, elastic tapping on induration areas, and exercise will usually reduce the congested lymph. However, there might be rare instances where usage is needed, such as a temporary case of dependent edema from a neurological motor impairment, or extensive damage to the initial lymphatics, such as a massive crush injury to the entire arm. This edema will not stay reduced unless a low-stretch bandaging or garment system is applied to the extremity after using the pneumatic pump. Description of this type of a bandaging or garment program is beyond the scope of this chapter.

When using the pneumatic pump for post trauma/surgery chronic edema, the chamber pressures should never be greater than 40 mm Hg because of the potential to collapse the initial lymphatics where absorption occurs "having a tourniquet effect"[26] and because of potential calibration errors.[4,27] A pneumatic pump system was developed by Flexitouch in 2006, and research has shown it facilitates lymphatic uptake and moves lymphatic fluid.[28] This system mimics MLD by first decongesting trunk edema and then proceeding to the extremity(ies) with the sequence, a rolling light chamber pressure, and the timing used with MLD. The therapist must follow usage guidelines and precautions for all pump usage.

Elastic Taping

Clinically I have found elastic tape to be an excellent adjunct to MEM to soften tissue and to keep the lymphatics stimulated for absorbing lymph throughout the day and night. There are many applications for taping, and formal course completion is recommended. See the Reduction Techniques for Acute Edema section for a complete description

Myofascial Release

MFR is a manual technique that entails sustaining a very light gentle pressure on soft tissue that in turn impacts the fascial system directly below the therapist's hands and throughout other parts of the body. The result is elongation or softening of the fascia and its ground substances. Clinically, I frequently use one of several MFR techniques on a specific muscle area to reduce the fascial restriction, and then I get a better lymphatic flow and edema reduction. Here, also, formal coursework is needed before doing the technique.

Exercise

Exercise should start at the trunk to facilitate the lymphatic pump. Even low-level aerobic exercise causes thoracic pressure changes on the thoracic duct. The pressure changes move the lymph proximally into the venous system at the subclavian veins creating a vacuum drawing the lymph proximal from the periphery.[3] Shoulder and elbow exercise, if not contraindicated, should be done next in the sequence. This draws and moves edema proximal toward the thoracic duct, creating a space for the more distal edema to move proximally. Next, exercise is completed at the wrist and then at the hand/fingers.

> **Clinical Pearl**
>
> Do not begin exercises at, or just, proximal to the edema because it has to have a proximal space (decongested area) for the fluid to move within the lymph system.

> **Clinical Pearl**
>
> When MEM is contraindicated (such as, for cardiac, pulmonary, kidney disease reasons), some edema will be reduced by doing diaphragmatic breathing. Then begin exercise at the trunk and proceed proximal to the edema and potentially add an elastic stockinette to the edematous area.

Low-Stretch Bandages, Gloves, Massage, and Chip Bags

Massage or compression on tissue must be light to avoid collapsing the single-celled initial lymphatics in the dermal layer. Miller and Scale[30] reported that the initial lymphatics began to collapse at a pressure of 60 mm Hg and that they closed completely at 70 mm Hg when tested on a flat surface. Eliska and Eliskova[31] found that a 3 minute friction massage on edematous tissue at 75 to 100 mm Hg caused temporary damage to the endothelial linings of both the initial lymphatics and the collector lymphatics. Thus string wrapping should be avoided in all stages of edema because of the potential to damage fragile lymphatic structures and because fluid cannot be "pushed" into the lymphatic structures, but rather it has to be absorbed due to pressure changes. Applying this same information to the application of elastic gloves, finger and forearm wrapping, or massage means that the compression has to be light to cause interstitial pressure changes and lymphatic absorption. The movement and slight compression of a loose elastic glove or elastic stockinette causes interstitial pressure changes and lymphatic absorption. Clinically I have found that fingers of elastic gloves are most effective when they can be stretched simultaneously ⅛ of an inch on either side of the digit. An elastic stockinette must allow me to place my two hands on either side of the forearm when the patient is wearing it; otherwise it is too tight. MEM massage pressure is one half the weight of the hand, _block

---

...er than required to feel tissue moving over muscle. (See ...n Techniques for Chronic Edema and the Evolve website ...ailed description of bandaging and chip bags.)

Manual Edema Mobilization

As mentioned in treatment for acute edema, MEM is used to reduce persistent subacute edema where proteins are congested and trapped in the interstitium because of extensive tissue damage to lymphatic structures, fibrotic scarring, and so on. The technique reduces both visible and not yet visible edema when there is congestion of a normal, intact, but overloaded, lymphatic system.

MEM is a modification of MLT techniques used for lymphadenectomy and/or lymph node irradiation, primary (congenital) lymphedema, and lymphedema arising from filariasis. For those types of edemas, MLT very appropriately involves extensive rerouting of lymph flow around missing or permanently damaged nodes and lymphatic vessel areas.

I developed MEM after I became certified in lymphedema treatment and learned about the anatomic functioning of the lymphatic system. As I studied lymphatic anatomy and physiology, I realized that the traditional treatments for upper extremity edema could be improved if they were based on this knowledge. Specifically, I realized that the subacute edema that I struggled to reduce in my surgical, trauma, and stroke clients with hand edema was a lymphatic overloaded edema. In these cases, because the lymphatic system, although overloaded, was still intact, extensive rerouting wasn't necessary, just decongestion, starting at the trunk.

I first taught MEM in 1995, and it continues to evolve. Since then, three peer-reviewed studies (one case study, a single-subject design study, and a randomized controlled study)[32,33,34] have been published establishing the validity and showing outcomes of use of the MEM technique. There are no research-based articles for a "simple lymphatic" massage for subacute and chronic hand edema reduction. In other words, only MEM has been validated, and randomly modifying MLD has not been validated.

MEM is a significant modification of MLT in several ways: (1) it involves only one or two trunk rerouting techniques; (2) it requires exercise after each segment is massaged; (3) it has its own light hand massage patterns; (4) it includes scar rerouting patterns; (5) it relies heavily on client follow-through with a self-management program; and (6) it incorporates pump point stimulation, which is unique to MEM.

The full MEM program takes 30 minutes. The short version, consisting of trunk rerouting and pump point stimulation, takes 15 minutes. MEM can be combined with other edema reduction techniques, but it should be done before those techniques are performed. The reason for this is simple: MEM decongests the most proximal edema and moves that edema proximally, creating a space into which the more distal edema can move by means of a proximal negative pressure vacuum. The more traditional edema reduction techniques will be more effective after MEM, because then there is a space cleared to which the edema can be moved proximally.

Principles and Concepts

MEM is grounded in the following principles and concepts:[35]
1. Light massage is provided, ranging from 10 to 20 mm Hg, to prevent collapse of the lymphatic pathways and arterial capillary reflux.

2. When protocol allows, exercises are performed before and after the MEM session; these exercises are done in a specific sequence, starting proximal to the edematous area or in the contralateral quadrant if possible.
3. Massage is performed in segments, proximal to distal, then distal to proximal. Massage ends in a proximal direction (that is, toward the trunk).
4. When possible, the technique includes exercise of the muscles in the segment just massaged.
5. Massage follows the flow of lymphatic pathways.
6. Massage reroutes around scar areas.
7. The method of massage and the types of exercise do not cause further inflammation of the involved tissue.
8. A client home self-massage program is devised that is specific to the pathologic condition of the hand.
9. MEM can be adapted to various diagnoses and stages of high plasma protein edema.
10. Guidelines are included for incorporating traditional edema control, soft tissue mobilization, and strengthening exercises without increasing edema.
11. Specific precautions are observed.
12. When necessary, low-stretch compression bandaging or other compression techniques are used.
13. Pump point stimulation is used extensively.
14. MEM is beneficial in clients whose lymphatic vessels are intact but overloaded from congestion.

Contraindications

The precautions and contraindications for MEM include those that are common to most massage programs and others that are specific to the movement of a large volume of fluid through the system. Always consult a physician if you are concerned about the client's current or past cardiac and/or pulmonary status. For instance, if an 80 mL volumetric difference exists between the client's two extremities, inform the physician that with MEM, that much fluid may be moved through the heart and lungs. Ask whether this would compromise the client's cardiac status.

Therapists should not use MEM in the following circumstances:
- If infection is present, because the infection may be spread by the technique.
- Over areas of inflammation, because inflammation and pain may be increased; MEM should be performed proximal to the inflammation to reduce the amount of congested fluid.
- If a hematoma or blood clot is present in the area, because the clot may be activated (that is, it may move).
- If active cancer is present. A controversial theory notes the potential for spreading cancerous cells. MEM should absolutely never be done if the cancer is not being medically treated. The therapist should always seek the physician's advice.
- If the client has congestive heart failure, severe cardiac problems, or pulmonary problems, because the cardiac and pulmonary systems may be overloaded.
- In the inflammatory (acute) stage of acute wound healing (rationale explained previously).
- If the client has renal failure or severe kidney disease, because the edema in these cases is a low-protein edema, and the renal system may be overloaded and/or the fluid may be moved to some other undesirable site.

- If the client has primary lymphedema or lymphedema arising from a mastectomy. Successful treatment of this condition requires knowledge of ways to reroute lymph to other parts of the body, as well as specific techniques beyond the scope of this chapter.

Manual Edema Mobilization Massage, Drainage, and Definitions

U's Hand Movement Pattern

U's are a pattern of hand movement that involves placing a flat, but relaxed, hand lightly on the skin. The hand gently tractions (pulls) the skin slightly distal and then circles back up and around, ending in the direction of the lymph flow pattern. The movement is consistently a clockwise or counterclockwise motion in a U, or teardrop configuration. Very light pressure (10 mm Hg or less) is used to move just the skin, thereby stimulating the initial lymphatics. Clinically, this is taught by having the therapist first place the full weight of the hand on the client's arm; then, while the entire palm and the digits remain in contact with the client's skin, the hand is partly lifted so that only half of its weight rests on the arm. MEM massage proceeds at this very light pressure, moving in a U while tractioning (pulling), not sliding, the skin. This is a "skin" massage—just enough pressure to feel the skin move over muscles.

Clearing U's Skin Tractioning Pattern

Clearing U's is a pattern of skin tractioning (pulling) performed in segments. It starts proximally and moves to the designated distal part of the trunk or arm segment (that is, upper arm, forearm, or hand). A minimum of five U's are done in three sections for each segment. The purpose is to create interstitial pressure changes that cause the initial lymphatics to take up lymph.

Flowing U's Lymph Movement Pattern

Flowing U's is a pattern of sequential U's that starts in the distal part of the segment being treated and moves proximally past the nearest set of lymph nodes. This could be described as "waltzing" up the arm. The process of moving one U after another from distal to beyond the proximal node is repeated five times. After the final repetition is completed, the flowing U motion is performed all the way to the contralateral upper quadrant. The purpose is to move the softened lymph out of the entire segment and facilitate its eventual return to the venous system and the heart (Fig. 3-4). In other words, the direction of "flow" follows the lymphatic pathways toward the heart (that is, flowing proximally, not distally). If not contraindicated by the diagnostic protocol, active muscle contraction is done in each segment after "flow." This increases the rate of lymphangion contraction, which moves the lymph out of the area more quickly.

Pump Point Stimulation

Pump point stimulation involves simultaneous, synchronous movement of the therapist's two hands in a U pattern over areas of **lymphatic bundles** (groups of initial and collector lymphatics), watershed areas, and/or lymph nodes.[35] Because nodes pose resistance to the flow of lymph, pressure from the full weight of

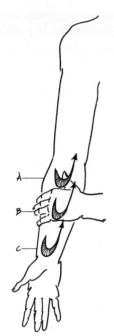

FIGURE 3-4 Forearm: Clear A, B, C. Flow C, B, A. (From Mackin EJ, et al, editors: *Rehabilitation of the hand and upper extremity*, ed 5, St Louis, 2002, Mosby.)

Summary of Reduction Treatment for Subacute Edema

- Start proximally with diaphragmatic breathing, trunk stretches, trunk exercises, easy (appropriate) yoga trunk stretches
- MEM
- Elastic taping
- Gentle myofascial release (MFR)
- Fluidotherapy machine (set at 98° F [36.6° C] or lower)
- Active and passive exercise (avoid excessive exercise, which can cause re-inflammation of tissue)
- Loose elastic glove; loose elastic stockinette; cotton finger wrap bandages; Coban wraps
- Pneumatic pump to soften lymph (set at 40 mm Hg or less)
- Low-stretch bandages, gloves, massage, chip bags

the hand is used. Typically the therapist does 20 to 30 Us in one area before proceeding to the next area of pump points. After pump point stimulation is performed in an area, MEM flow is done followed by exercise either in that area or proximal to it (see the Evolve website)

Therapists should not attempt MEM unless they have been trained in the technique. One- and two-day courses are available and required for any therapist who would like to use MEM as a treatment.

Clinical Pearl

Starting proximal at the trunk is the key to lymphatic decongestion; this is the first technique that must be done so that the other edema reduction techniques are effective.

Reduction Techniques for Chronic Edema

Chronic edema is persistent edema that lasts longer than 3 months and is indurated (hard) and difficult to pit.[35] As a result of the long-term entrapment of plasma proteins in the interstitium, the tissue becomes fibrotic. In part, treatment is the same as for subacute edema, but it includes softening of the fibrotic tissue to facilitate uptake by the initial lymphatics. Softening of indurated tissue can be accomplished with low-stretch bandaging, chip bags (convoluted foam pieces of different densities placed in a stockinette bag), foam-lined orthoses, silicone gel sheets, and elastomer pads (see the Evolve website). Neutral warmth builds up under these inserts, causing an enzymatic reaction that softens the indurated tissue. The varying densities of the foam chips in a chip bag can result in tissue pressure differentiation, stimulating protein uptake.

Low-Stretch Bandaging

Low-stretch bandages are cotton, nonelastic bandages that have a 20% stretch because of the weave of the bandage. These bandages are rolled on rather than stretched on. When a muscle contracts, it bulks up under the bandages. Because the bandages stretch only 20%, they provide a light counterforce, which is not enough to collapse the initial lymphatics. When the muscle relaxes, the bandages only collapse 20%, again not enough to collapse the initial lymphatics. Thus variation in tissue pressure facilitates lymphatic uptake and prevents refilling of stretched tissue. Research has shown that use of a combination of low-stretch and foam bandages on the forearm, along with exercise, increases protein uptake.[36] (See the Evolve website for more information on low-stretch bandaging.)

Low-stretch finger wraps also soften lymph and facilitate lymphatic absorption (see the Evolve website). These are often used when a client's hand is so edematous that it does not fit into an elastic glove. Low-stretch finger wraps are not used to squeeze the edema out, because that would collapse the delicate lymphatic structures. The distal-to-proximal spiral pattern in which the wraps are applied, the neutral warmth maintained by the finger bandages, and the effect of finger movement all soften the indurated tissue, improving lymphatic flow and edema reduction.

Chip Bags

Chip bags vary in size, depending on the area they are to cover. They consist of stockinette bags filled with various densities and sizes of foam. The ends of the bag are either taped or sewn closed. Chip bags can be worn under low-stretch bandages, loose elastic gloves, or orthoses (see the Evolve website). Various types of commercially-fabricated chip bags made of foam or wheat hulls are also available for purchase.

Self-Adherent Wrap

Coban or similar self-adherent wrap material is used by many therapists on edematous fingers. When placed on the finger or digit circumferentially, it creates a squeezing effect, pushing fluid distal or proximal, or both. Lightly overlapping spirals of self-adherent wrap distal to proximal down a digit facilitates the absorption and movement of fluid proximally (see the Evolve website). This wrap also creates a buildup of neutral warmth.

A small stockinette or powder can be put on the wrap once it is on the finger so that the wrapped fingers do not stick together.

> ◎ *Clinical Pearl*
>
> For chip bags, self-adherent wrap, or low-stretch bandaging to be successful, proximal MEM, or at least pump point stimulation (discussed earlier in the chapter), must be done first to decongest the lymph ("pull the drain plug") and move it proximal.

Summary of Reduction Treatment for Chronic Edema

- All techniques listed for treatment of subacute edema
- Methods to soften indurated tissue (that is, tissue that is hardening or already hard), including chip bags, convoluted foam in stockinette, elastomer and elastomer-type products, silicone gel sheets, foam-lined orthoses low-stretch bandages, cotton finger wraps, and loose elastic stockinette and/or gloves (see the Evolve website).

Other Types of Edema and Appropriate Treatment

Lymphedema

Lymphedema is a chronic, high-protein edema that results when a permanent mechanical obstruction of the lymphatic system creates a lymphatic overload.[37] Permanent obstruction can be caused by surgical removal of the lymph nodes, irradiation of the nodes or skin, **filariasis** (an infestation of worms that destroys the lymph nodes), or a congenital deficit of the lymph nodes and lymphatic vessels. Clients with lymphedema must be treated with a full MLT program performed by a trained and credentialed therapist. Treatment includes multiple rerouting of lymphatic flow patterns around deficit areas. MEM is not appropriate for these clients.

Precaution. *MEM is a treatment for clients with an overloaded but intact lymphatic system.*

Therapists working with hand clients may see a permanent deficit of the lymphatic system, resulting in persistent, sustained swelling. This is seen with circumferential scars, as with a replanted digit. It may also occur with circumferential skin grafting. Primary (congenital) or secondary lymphedema (for example, from the removal of diseased nodes) causes lymphatic congestion (slow outflow of lymph) in the subcutaneous, epifascial tissue space[38] which means that only the superficial lymphatic vessels are affected. Therefore a client whose fingers are edematous as a result of this type of lymphedema does not develop joint contractures (Fig. 3-5). If surgical or traumatic invasion (that is, laceration) into the deeper lymphatic structures around joints has occurred, joint contractures may develop. Soft tissue contractures are caused by laceration of superficial and deep lymphatic capillaries, high capillary permeability that causes leakage of plasma proteins, and prolonged congestion of plasma proteins around these joint and tendon structures leading to fibrosis.

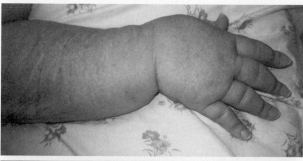
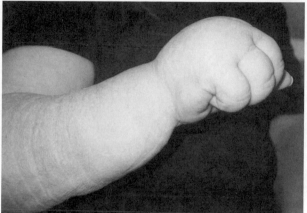

FIGURE 3-5 Lymphedema of the hand with no loss of mobility.

Complex or Combined Edema

Complex or combined edema is initially a transudate edema, such as acute flaccid stroke hand edema. With flaccidity, no muscle pump facilitates vascular flow, and water and electrolytes leak into the interstitium, resulting in a transudate edema. The treatment is the same as for acute edema. During this phase, night orthoses might be considered to prevent shortening of the extensor tendons. Three months later, the edema may have a viscous feel, but it is relatively fast to rebound, and it does not significantly or permanently reduce with elevation and/or the use of an elastic glove. The edema now has an exudate component. At this point, the lymphatic system, which initially was aiding in the removal of the excess fluid (transudate edema), has reached its maximum capacity. The lymphatic system is overloaded and has slowed down, resulting in lymphatic congestion. The congested plasma protein content of the fluid makes the edema feel viscous. The treatment is the same as for subacute and chronic edema. Often an orthotic program is needed to prevent or overcome joint contractures.

Precaution. *Overexercising or forcing joints in a flaccid or hemiparetic hand can cause microscopic rupture of tissue, resulting in inflammation and increased hand edema. Therefore a balance must be attained between gentle, progressive motion and rest of structures.*

Cardiac Edema

Cardiac edema occurs with a decline in the heart's ability to pump blood completely through the circulatory system. As a result, fluid accumulates in the extremities, especially around the ankles. Often cardiac edema manifests as bilateral ankle swelling with a slight pinkish tone to the tissue. Hand therapists treating older adults need to look for this type of edema.

Precaution. *MEM and many of the edema-reduction techniques are contraindicated for clients with cardiac edema, because movement of more fluid can further overload the already compromised cardiac system.*

Low-Protein Edema

Low-protein edema can manifest as extremity swelling caused by liver disease, malnutrition, or kidney failure (for example, nephrotic syndrome).[1,5] Edema results because too few plasma proteins are present in the interstitium to bond with the water molecule and bring fluid back into the vascular systems.

Precaution. *Low-protein edema has a systemic cause and must be treated with medication. MEM and many of the edema reduction techniques are contraindicated because they may overload the kidneys or liver. Also, even if these edema control techniques are used, this type of edema will return because of its systemic cause.*

Evaluation of Edematous Tissue

Edema reduces ROM both actively and passively because it increases the size of the fingers or hand. This, in turn, can reduce functional use and coordination of the hand. Once the edema has been reduced, if decreased ROM persists, the therapist can effectively evaluate and treat joint and/or soft tissue limitations. The sooner the edema is reduced, the less the buildup of plasma proteins in soft tissue, the less the fibrosis of the tissue, and the less the thickening of scar tissue.

Precaution. *Reducing edema does not reverse existing joint contractures.*

By taking circumferential measurements, the therapist can determine where on the hand specifically the edema is prevalent. For consistency, always use the same measuring device; also, take measurements at the same time of day and after the same amount of hand activity.

Edema rebound tests (see Chapter 5) can help determine whether treatment has reduced some of the viscous congested edema. For instance, if the edema rebound time was 65 seconds before treatment and 40 seconds after treatment, this indicates that lymph was moved out. To make this subjective test more consistent, devise a protocol for how much pressure is used and for how long it is applied.

Volumeters have been shown to provide reliable, valid edema measurements.[39] These measurements indicate whether volume reduction has occurred; they do not specify the location of the reduction.

The criteria for tissue quality assessment, another evaluation method, are as follows:

- *Acute edema:* Tissue pits deeply, rebounds rather quickly, and can be easily moved around.
- *Subacute edema or early stage chronic edema:* Tissue pits, is very slow to rebound, and has a viscous quality.
- *Chronic edema:* Tissue pits minimally and has a hard feeling.
- *Severe edema:* Tissue has no elasticity and is shiny, taut, and cannot be lifted.
- **Lymphorrhea:** Weeping of tissue occurs with an extremely congested edematous hand or arm. Lymph, a clear, yellowish fluid, escapes from the interstitium to the outside of the skin. Technically, weeping tissue is considered an open wound and must be treated as such. MEM techniques can rapidly decongest the lymph and stop the lymphorrhea.

Note: Always perform the capillary refill test if the client's hand has a bulky dressing or if the client is wearing finger bandages.

Precaution. *Color, temperature, and sensory changes may be signs of a problem. A purple color often indicates pooling of venous blood, and a whitish color means that arterial blood flow to the tissue is compromised. Immediately notify the physician of these signs.*

◎ Clinical Pearl

Macrophages are less effective in edematous tissue because it has less oxygen; phagocytic activity therefore is diminished.[4]

The therapist must be able to distinguish between congestion and infection. With an open wound, the classic signs of infection are redness, warmth, pain to the touch, odor, and/or cloudy drainage. With a closed wound, the signs of a subclinical infection are a pinkish red color and slight warmth; also, the wound may be painful to the touch and the tissue may be hard.[40] This is often seen with a very edematous extremity or hand if the first course of antibiotics hasn't fully resolved the infection. Extremely edematous hands often need a second course of antibiotics as determined by the treating physician.

Precaution. *If infection is suspected, MEM should not be started before a full course of antibiotics has been completed and the physician has assessed the status of the infection.*

The signs of congestion frequently are the same as those of a subclinical infection. The client's history can help determine whether the condition is congestion or infection (or both). Often congestion (and, possibly, infection) can be prevented if the therapist begins treatment of an uninfected extremity early, before visible edema is present, with the short version of MEM. Prolonged tissue congestion can lead to infection because congestion reduces oxygen delivery to tissue, diminishing the effectiveness of the phagocytic cells.

Both old and new scars can create a barrier to lymph flow. Check for proximal scars (for example, on the shoulder, back, or axilla). Soften both old and new scars with gentle MFR techniques, silicone gel sheets, paper tape, and/or elastic taping. Instruct the client in MEM techniques to reroute edema around scars and to soften scars.

Sensory testing is very important for an edematous extremity because edema often reduces sensation. As edema is reduced, the degree of sensation usually improves. Sensory testing, therefore, becomes an objective test that shows limitations and improvements that can be related to function.

Coordination often is diminished by edema in the hand. A nine-hole peg test can become a repeated, scheduled test for assessing hand function. Reducing hand edema should improve coordination, unless an underlying problem exists.

Pain assessment is very important. As edema declines, pain usually diminishes. Clinically, pain reduction often is noticed before ROM shows improvement. Keep in mind that pain can have many sources. For example, in a client with a Colles fracture, edema reduction can relieve the pain caused by the pressure of edema on the nerve receptors; however, the client still may have chronic pain specifically related to the fracture site. Therefore other, appropriate methods must be used to reduce that pain, which differs from edema-related pain. Even during treatment for a different cause of pain, the client should follow a MEM home program twice daily to eliminate any new, not yet visible congested edema.

CASE STUDY

CASE STUDY 3-1 ■

Marlene is a 58-year-old white woman from Texas who sustained a right complex distal radius fracture, abrasions and facial fractures, plus bruising to her right shoulder when she slipped off a chair hitting her granite countertop as she climbed down from cleaning overhead light fixtures. An orthopedic surgeon and plastic surgeon saw her in the emergency room and appropriate surgery was performed on all fractures during the next week. The complex distal radius fracture was treated with open reduction and internal fixation (ORIF), casting for 4 weeks, and then a soft wrist brace for 2 weeks.

At 6 weeks, Marlene saw a hand therapist for the first time. The therapist gave her the standard forearm, wrist, and hand active range of motion (AROM) exercises plus an elastic edema glove. Marlene explained they were leaving for Colorado for the summer in 2 days and would continue hand therapy there. It was another week before Marlene saw me for treatment in Colorado. An assessment revealed in part: significant decreased and painful shoulder ROM; forearm supination of 40 degrees and pronation 50 degrees; both wrist flexion and extension 20 degrees; radial deviation 10 degrees and ulnar deviation 5 degrees; active composite finger/thumb ROM was 25% of normal range and passive 50% of normal range. Forearm through fingers were extremely edematous with a total of 3½ inches greater than the circumference of the uninvolved left forearm/fingers. Sensation was impaired one grade overall in all fingers. The patient was extremely anxious about moving her dominant right upper extremity and guarded it.

Problem: I had only three visits that week to treat Marlene before going away for a week.

Thus treatment priorities had to be determined for hand therapy including that the patient needed to be competent with a home edema reduction and exercise program, patient psychological fears needed to be addressed, and she needed to be beginning to functionally use her right upper extremity. I requested physical therapy (PT) for shoulder issues so that I had adequate time to address the hand deficit areas.

After the evaluation, she was shown how to apply heat packs to her shoulder and perform traditional Codman's shoulder exercises to do until her PT visit. Knowing protein-rich, subacute edema is "glue" causing pain and decreased ROM, my first priority became to reduce the edema. I did the basic short MEM home program (Fig 3-6). Note that MEM and exercises are begun at the trunk and shoulder to reduce hand edema. For Marlene if MEM was just started at the elbow, the distal edema would have had no proximal lymphatic space for congested forearm edema to move into and out of the area. Also, the shoulder exercises as part of the MEM treatment facilitate proximal muscle pumping of the lymphatic system. I chose to do the MEM home program on the patient rather than a full therapist treatment, because I could teach the patient her home program while I was doing it. It was imperative for her to follow through three to five times a day. This also got her used to using and touching the right upper extremity. The AROM program previously given to Marlene was reviewed and incorporated into her daily routine. I loaned Marlene a 3½ inch ball to use for wrist/arm ROM exercises (see the Evolve website).

During the first treatment visit, we reviewed her MEM program that she had done two of the five recommended times a day. I took 30 minutes and did the entire therapist version of MEM to her right upper extremity and reduced the hand edema by 50%. Marlene was excited to see the edema reduction, plus her pain reduced from 6/10 at rest to 3/10 at rest. She also had a slight increase in active and passive ROM. During the last 15 minutes of the MEM treatment, I placed her forearm/hand between two hot packs in an effort to facilitate induration softening and elongation of tissue to increase ROM. I added a 6 oz weight hammer for supination/pronation exercises and wrist flexion/extension to her home program. She was also given sponges to carry around to do finger/wrist exercises multiple times a day. The use of a heat pack for 10 minutes four times a day was encouraged along with continuing the ball exercises, which she like to do because "it makes my wrist and arm feel good."

During the second treatment visit, Marlene was in full compliance with her home program because she experienced decreased pain and had started to use her hand for assistive light tasks, such as folding clothes and dusting. MEM was again 30 minutes as noted above with the hot pack placed 15 minutes on hand/forearm indurated tissue. Edema was reduced about 15% further. This was followed up by forearm/wrist MFR, grade one wrist joint mobilization, and instruction in scar massage. The forearm and wrist were elastic taped for edema reduction. Marlene loved to do color pencil sketching. She was asked to bring her tools to the next session.

During the third treatment visit, Marlene continued to be compliant with MEM and the exercise part of her home program, but she still was apprehensive about using her right upper extremity for routine light activities of daily living (ADLs), and so on. Between visits, the patient's hand edema had reduced another 10%. MEM with the usage of the hot pack was only 15 minutes during this treatment

session with a slight edema reduction noted. I performed MFR and joint mobilization. This session began with the use of mirror therapy to improve her hand/wrist ROM exercises and improve patterns of composite and spontaneous movement. Marlene was instructed in a simple mirror therapy home program to do two times daily. Her colored pencils were also built up for easier gripping, and I encouraged her to do sketching activities.

While I was on vacation, Marlene continued her home program but apprehension on her and her husband's part limited the frequency. There was neither further loss nor gain in edema. The remaining 25% of the increased edematous girth compared to the uninvolved extremity was reduced by my treatment in two subsequent 15 minute MEM sessions. More vigorous progressive strengthening exercises were started after the edema reduced (If started too soon and vigorously, this will cause an inflammatory response and increased edema.) and her upper extremity ROM started to significantly increase. It took a few more sessions for Marlene to lose her apprehension of using the right hand, and then she began again doing and enjoying her volunteer activity at a thrift store sorting and marking. She also felt she could safely enjoy long mountain hikes again.

Post note: Ideally I would have preferred seeing Marlene for treatment the first week post casting for a shoulder ROM program and an edema or preventative edema reduction program. If there were no complications (such as, blood clots or other MEM contraindications), then I would have begun shoulder/elbow ROM, dealt with patient psychological apprehension and ADL issues, and started a MEM home program addressing trunk to cast.

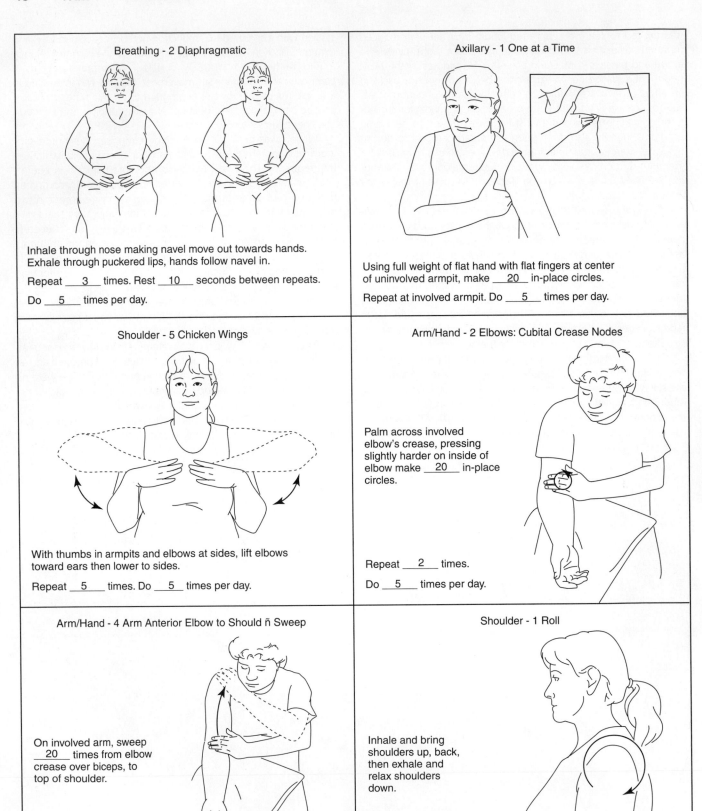

Breathing - 2 Diaphragmatic

Inhale through nose making navel move out towards hands. Exhale through puckered lips, hands follow navel in.

Repeat ___3___ times. Rest ___10___ seconds between repeats.

Do ___5___ times per day.

Axillary - 1 One at a Time

Using full weight of flat hand with flat fingers at center of uninvolved armpit, make ___20___ in-place circles.

Repeat at involved armpit. Do ___5___ times per day.

Shoulder - 5 Chicken Wings

With thumbs in armpits and elbows at sides, lift elbows toward ears then lower to sides.

Repeat ___5___ times. Do ___5___ times per day.

Arm/Hand - 2 Elbows: Cubital Crease Nodes

Palm across involved elbow's crease, pressing slightly harder on inside of elbow make ___20___ in-place circles.

Repeat ___2___ times.

Do ___5___ times per day.

Arm/Hand - 4 Arm Anterior Elbow to Should ñ Sweep

On involved arm, sweep ___20___ times from elbow crease over biceps, to top of shoulder.

Do ___5___ times per day.

Shoulder - 1 Roll

Inhale and bring shoulders up, back, then exhale and relax shoulders down.

Repeat ___5___ times.

Do ___5___ times per day.

FIGURE 3-6 Marlene's manual edema mobilization (MEM) home program. (From Visual Health Information (VHI) kits, used with permission.)

Arm/Hand - 6 Arm: Volar Elbow to Wrist ñ Clear

Involved hand palm side up, make __10__ in-place circles at elbow crease proceeding in sections to wrist.

Repeat __2__ times.

Do __5__ times per day.

Arm/Hand - 7 Arm: Volnar Wrist to Elbow ñ Sweep

Sweep __20__ times from involved arm wrist crease to elbow crease.

Do __5__ times per day

Wrist/Finger - 3 Wrist: Curl to Shoulder

Palm side of arm up, bend wrist toward elbow, bend elbow so hand rest on shoulder.

Repeat __5__ times. Do __5__ times per day.

Arm/Hand - 3 Hand: Dorsum of Hand to Axilla Sweep

Involved palm down, fingers in web spaces, sweep __10__ times over top of hand and forearm, back of upper arm, shoulder, chest front to uninvolved armpit.

Do __5__ times per day.

Arm/Elbow - 1 Upper Arm: Make Fist Overhead

With involved arm above head and straight, open and close hand __5__ times.

Repeat __2__ times.

Do __5__ times per day.

FIGURE 3-6, cont'd

References

1. Guyton A, Hall J: *Textbook of medical physiology*, ed 9, Philadelphia, 1996, WB Saunders.

2. Hole JW: *Human anatomy and physiology*, ed 4, Dubuque, IA, 1987, William C Brown.

3. Kubik S: Anatomy of the lymphatic system. In Foldi M, Foldi E, Kubik S, editors: *Textbook of lymphology for physicians and lymphedema therapists*, Munich, 2003, Urban & Fischer Verlag.

4. Casley-Smith JR: *Modern treatment for lymphedema*, ed 5, Adelaide, 1997, The Lymphoedema Association of Australia.

5. Chikly B: *Silent waves: theory and practice of lymph drainage therapy with applications for lymphedema, chronic pain, and inflammation*, Scottsdale, AZ, 2001, International Health & Healing Publishing.

6. Pecking A, et al: Indirect lymphoscintigraphy in patients with limb edema: progress in lymphology, *Proceedings of the Ninth International Congress of Lymphology*201–296, 1985.

7. Bryant WM: Wound healing, *Clin Symp* 29(3):1–36, 1977.

8. Reed BV: Effect of high voltage pulsed electrical stimulation on microvascular permeability to plasma proteins, *Phys Ther* 68(4):491–496, 1988.

9. Snyder AR, Perotti AL, Lam KC, et al: The influence of high voltage electrical stimulation on edema formation after acute injury: a systematic review,, *J Sport Rehabil* 19:436–451, 2010.

10. Vasudevan SV, Melvin JL: Upper extremity edema control: rationale of treatment techniques, *Am J Occup Ther* 33(8):520–523, 1979.

11. Buncke HJ, et al: Surgical and rehabilitative aspects of replantation and revascularization of the hand. In Hunter JM, Schneider LH, Mackin EJ, et al: *Rehabilitation of the hand: surgery and therapy*, ed 4, St Louis, 1995, Mosby.

12. Lievens P, Leduc A: Cryotherapy and sports, *Int J Sports Med* 5(Supplement):37–39, 1984.

13. Villeco JP, Mackin EJ, Hunter JM: Edema: therapist's management. In Mackin EJ, et al: *Rehabilitation of the hand and upper extremity*, ed 5, St Louis, 2002, Mosby.

14. Kase K, Stockheimer KR: *Kinesio taping for lymphoedema and chronic swelling*, Albuquerque, NM, 2006, Kinesio USA.

15. Kase K, Wallis J, Kase T: *Clinical therapeutic applications of the Kinesio taping method*, Toyko, 2003, Ken Ikai.

16. Hutzschenreuter P, Brummer H: [Experimental and clinical studies of the mechanism of effect of manual lymph drainage therapy], [Article in German], *Z Lymphol* 13(1):62–64, 1989.

17. Breger-Stanton D, Lazaro R, MacDermid J: A systematic review of the effectiveness of contrast baths,, *J Hand Ther* 22:57–70, 2009.

18. Kurz I: *Textbook of Dr. Vodder's manual lymph drainage*, ed 4, Heidelberg, 1997, Haug.

19. Resends MA, et al: Local transcutaneous electrical stimulation (TENS) effects in experimental inflammatory edema and pain, *Eur J Pharmacol* 504:217–222, 2004.

20. Michlovitz SL, Nolan TP Jr: *Modalities for therapeutic intervention*, ed 4, Philadelphia, 2005, FA Davis.

21. De Bie RA, et al: Low level laser therapy in ankle sprains: a randomized clinical trial, *Arch Phys Med Rehabil* 79:1415–1420, 1998.

22. Ozkan N, et al: Investigation of the supplementary effect of GaAs laser therapy on the rehabilitation of human digital flexor tendons, *J Clin Laser Med Surg* 22:105–110, 2004.

23. Snyder AR, et al: The influence of high voltage electrical stimulation on edema formation after acute injury: a systematic review, *J Sport Rehabil* 19:436–451, 2010.

24. Griffin JW, Newsome LS, Stralka SW, et al: Reduction of chronic post-traumatic hand edema: a comparison of high voltage pulsed current, intermittent pneumatic compression and placebo treatments, *Phys Ther* 70(5):279–286, 1990.

25. Stralka S, Jackson J, Lewis A: Treatment of hand and wrist pain, *AAOHN J* 46(5):233–236, 1998.

26. Grieveson S: Intermittent pneumatic compression pump settings for the optimum reduction of oedema, *J Tissue Viability* 13(3):98–100, 2003.

27. Segers P, et al: Excessive pressure in multichambered cuffs used for sequential compression therapy, *Phys Ther* 82:1000–1008, 2002.

28. Adams K, et al: Direct evidence of lymphatic function improvement after advanced pneumatic compression device treatment of lymphedema, *Biomed Opt Express* 1:114–125, 2010.

29. Giudice M: Effects of continuous passive motion and elevation on hand edema, *Am J Occup Ther* 44:10, 1990.

30. Miller GE, Seale J: Lymphatic clearance during compressive loading, *Lymphology* 14(4):161–166, 1981.

31. Eliska O, Eliskova M: Are peripheral lymphatics damaged by high pressure manual massage? *Lymphology* 28(1):21–30, 1995.

32. Roenhoej KK, Maribo T: A randomized clinical controlled study comparing the effect of modified manual edema mobilization treatment with traditional edema technique in patients with a fracture of the distal radius, *J Hand Ther* 24:184–193, 2011.

33. Priganc V, Ito M: Changes in edema, pain, or range of motion following manual edema mobilization: a single-case design study, *J Hand Ther* 21:326–333, 2008.

34. Howard SB, Krishnagiri S: The use of manual edema mobilization for the reduction of persistent edema in the upper limb, *J Hand Ther* 14:291–301, 2001.

35. Artzberger S, Priganc V: Manual edema mobilization: an edema reduction technique for the orthopedic patient. In Skirven T, et al: *Rehabilitation of the hand and upper extremity*, ed 6, St Louis, 2011, Elsevier Mosby.

36. Leduc O, et al: Bandages: scintigraphic demonstration of its efficacy on colloidal protein reabsorption during muscle activity, *Progress in Lymphology XII* 887:421, 1990.

37. Casley-Smith JR: Modern treatment of lymphedema, *Australas J Dermatol* 33(2):61–74, 1992.

38. Szuba A, Rockson S: Lymphedema: classifications, diagnosis and therapy, *Vasc Med* 3(2):145–156, 1998.

39. Waylett-Rendall J, Seibly D: A study of the accuracy of a commercially available volumeter, *J Hand Ther* 4:10, 1991.

40. Marcks P: Lymphedema pathogenesis, prevention, and treatment, *Cancer Pract* 5:32–38, 1997.

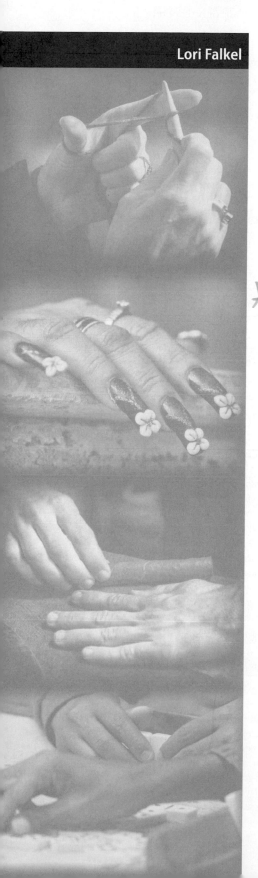

4 Tissue-Specific Exercises for the Upper Extremity

Lori Falkel

Tissue-specific exercise progressions can be thought of as the science of prescribing an accurate dosage of exercise. Tissue-specific exercise allows us to use our knowledge of exercise physiology to address the specific pathologic tissue conditions. When physicians prescribe medicine, they do not arbitrarily select a medication from the pharmacy and administer it. They prescribe medicine based on the pathologic condition.

With proper knowledge, exercise is the therapist's area of expertise. For optimal outcomes, exercise dosage must not be assigned arbitrarily; it should be dosed accurately according to the physiology of the tissue(s) involved. When designing an exercise program effectively to promote the recovery of the target tissue, the therapist needs to consider multiple variables. Some of these variables are the appropriate resistance; the repetitions and sets that will promote the desired response; the speed, frequency, breaks, and duration of exercise; the appropriate positioning of the limb and/or client; and the precise range of motion. Proper exercise equipment, to provide support, can be critical for restoration of physiologic motion. The types of muscle work (for example, concentric, eccentric, and isometric) are also important considerations.

The Ola Grimsby Institute developed Scientific Therapeutic Exercise Progressions (STEP), which is a concept of dosing exercises according to the specific pathologic condition and tissue tolerance of each client. STEP is based on principles of medical exercise therapy. It was developed in Norway and has been practiced throughout Europe for many years with excellent results. STEP addresses musculoskeletal dysfunctions with respect to their histologic, biomechanical, and neurophysiologic significance.*

Joint Dysfunction

Joint dysfunction occurs because of a compromise in connective tissue integrity. This may result from capsular, ligamentous, or cartilaginous causes. In cartilage, symptoms of joint dysfunction present as an inability to withstand compressive forces. If the joint dysfunction is capsular, joint swelling will be present. A ligamentous injury has point tenderness. The end result is altered mobility. Joint dysfunction can be labeled as a **hypomobility**, a **hypermobility**, or an **instability**. A joint is considered to be hypomobile when movement takes place about a physiologic axis but is less than normal. A hypermobile joint has greater than normal motion around a physiologic axis. Joint instability is motion around a nonphysiologic axis.[1] All synovial joints can be categorized by a joint mobility grading system[1] (Table 4-1).

Musculoskeletal Dysfunctions

The two main *causes* of musculoskeletal dysfunctions are acute trauma and cumulative trauma. Acute trauma is associated with an excessive contraction (muscle strain) or an externally applied force. Chronic overload, or cumulative trauma, is associated with prolonged static work, stress, and often reduced aerobic activity.

◎ Clinical Pearl

A large percentage of clients who have cumulative trauma injuries are deconditioned because of a fairly sedentary job or lifestyle.

---

*The Ola Grimsby Institute offers courses on a range of subjects pertaining to exercise and physical therapy if more information is needed.

TABLE 4-1 Joint Mobility Grading Scale

Grade	Joint Mobility	Treatment
0	Ankylosed	Surgery/no mobilization treatment
1	Considerable limitation	Articulation/ avoid exercise and manipulation
2	Slight limitation	Joint mobilization/self-mobilization
3	Normal	No treatment needed
4	Slight increase	Postural correction/ADLs and ANLs/check for hypomobility/taping/self-stabilization
5	Considerable increase	Postural correction/bracing/taping/self-stabilization/ADL and NDL/check for hypomobility/dry needling/sclerosing injections
6	Pathologically unstable	Surgery/no mobilization treatment

ADLs, Activities of daily living

Comorbidities Associated with Increased Prevalence of Musculoskeletal Dysfunction

The vast majority of clients who present for treatment in a hand clinic do not have only a hand injury. The therapist must be aware of the client's comorbidities and provide comprehensive treatment that addresses the client as a whole, rather than just an extremity. Some of the more common diseases that are associated with lowered tolerance of the musculoskeletal system are diabetes, hypothyroidism/hyperthyroidism, gastric ulcer, chronic/recurrent infections, colitis, and cardiovascular and respiratory diseases.

Diabetes causes the production and use of insulin in the body to be impaired. This results in an abundance of sugar in the bloodstream. With diabetes, the pancreas secretes little or no insulin (type I diabetes) or the body becomes resistant to the action of insulin (type II diabetes). If the disease is not treated, the level of sugar in the bloodstream builds up and leads to diabetic complications.

The thyroid gland affects all aspects of metabolism. The thyroid releases hormones that regulate heart rate, the strength of bones, how quickly calories are burned, and sensitivity to heat/cold. If the thyroid gland is underactive or overactive (hypothyroidism/hyperthyroidism), medical treatment is necessary to avoid complications.[2]

A gastric ulcer is an open sore that develops in the lining of the stomach. The ulcer may result from diet, stress, medication, or bacterial infection.

Infections can occur when the immune system is suppressed or comes in contact with an organism to which it does not have resistance. Bones and joints become susceptible to chronic infections that originate elsewhere in the body and are passed to them via the bloodstream.[3]

Colitis is a painful and debilitating chronic inflammation of the digestive tract.[4] Symptoms include bloating, cramping, abdominal pain, and loss of appetite. Cardiovascular and respiratory disease includes any of a multitude of problems involving the heart, lungs, and blood vessels. Some of these disease processes are preventable and are acquired over a lifetime; others are congenital. Cardiovascular disease is more prevalent than all of the previously mentioned diseases combined.[5,6]

BOX 4-1 Traits That Have Been Shown to Increase Risk for Fractures

Slender build
Fair skin
Family history of osteoporosis or osteoporotic fracture
Small muscle mass
Sedentary lifestyle
Small peak adult bone mass (approximately age 35)
Low calcium intake
Cigarette smoking
Excessive consumption of protein, sodium, and alcohol
One or more osteoporotic fracture(s)
A situation that increases the likelihood of falling (that is, wet floor, throw rugs, or small pets)

BOX 4-2 Common Age-Related Changes Affecting Bone Loss

Gradual increase in parathyroid hormone secretion as a result of chronic calcium deficiency
Decreased intestinal absorption of elemental calcium
Lower circulating calcitonin
Decreased sunlight exposure and dietary vitamin D intake
Decreased ovarian function causing altered estrogen balance

Exercise Considerations

Always use caution and discretion when prescribing the intensity of exercise. A thorough evaluation provides the necessary information regarding cardiovascular compromise or risk factors, pulmonary disease, diabetes mellitus, hypertension, obesity, peripheral vascular disease, arthritis, and renal disease.[5]

Precaution. *An exercise program may not be recommended for uncontrolled diabetes. A rigorous strengthening or aerobic exercise program, in this case, may cause a hyperglycemic effect because cellular absorption of glucose is restricted. Insulin-dependent diabetic clients may need to decrease insulin or increase carbohydrate intake when exercising. They should monitor their glucose more frequently when starting an exercise program. For this client population, the exercise should be dosed at a lower level of intensity and duration initially and should progress at a much slower rate.*[2]

Osteoporosis

An estimated 30 million Americans have osteoporosis. This disease is responsible for 1.5 million individuals sustaining bone fractures per year (200,000 wrist fractures, 300,000 hip fractures, and 300,000 non-wrist extremity fractures). Osteoporosis costs more than $18 billion per year in health care expenses and lost productivity. Bone mass attains a peak in males and females at approximately 30 to 35 years of age, with total bone mass beginning to decline 5 to 10 years later. Boxes 4-1 and 4-2 list traits and age-related changes associated with osteoporosis.[7,8]

BOX 4-3 Some Considerations for Exercise Selection

- Weight-bearing activities and strength training are ideal for bone stimulation.
- Increased strength improves balance and decreases the risk of falls.
- Walking is ideal because it is weight bearing, dynamic, and repetitive.
- Swimming or cycling use less weight-bearing forces and are less effective than walking.
- Nonimpact loading may cause damage to weakened bone.

BOX 4-4 Contraindicated Exercises for Advanced Osteoporosis

Vigorous aerobic workout
Exercises that require twisting or bending
Abdominal machines
Biceps-curl machines
Rowing machines
Tennis
Golf
Bowling

Males are less affected by osteoporosis than females. Males usually ingest more calcium and have higher levels of calcitonin. They also produce testosterone into the seventh and eighth decades of life as opposed to the decline in hormone production that females experience with menopause in the fourth or fifth decade. The increased calcium and hormone levels reduce the loss of bone mass, which in turn reduces the potential for development of osteoporosis.

Several factors can affect bone resorption levels. A lack of weight bearing and of activity in antigravity muscles changes the resorption rate, as does excessive thyroid and parathyroid hormones. Corticosteroids also have an impact.

Determinants of bone mass and loss are genetic, mechanical, or hormonal. Genetics can cause large-boned individuals to gain a relative immunity to osteoporotic fractures. The mechanics of bone density can aid in the prevention of fractures, but they also can be a possible cause. Increasing loading yields lead to increased bone mass, and decreased loading yields lead to decreased bone mass.

Exercise for Prevention/Treatment of Osteoporosis

Exercise can help prevent or slow down bone loss, improve posture, and increase overall fitness. For clients who are at risk of osteoporosis, a bone density test before beginning an exercise program is recommended. Box 4-3 lists factors to consider when selecting an exercise.[7]

Although walking is the best of all of the options listed in Box 4-3, those clients who are unable to tolerate walking because of comorbidities or advanced osteoporosis have other options. These options provide benefit by generating muscle tension, which provides needed stress to bone. To prevent injury to those with advanced osteoporosis, clients absolutely should avoid the exercises listed in Box 4-4.

Client Education for Osteoporosis

Education of the client on what impact osteoporosis will have on his or her life and what the client can do to prevent fractures or falls is important. Teach clients about proper body mechanics by demonstrating proper posture. When teaching lifting and carrying techniques, show the client how to hold loads close to the body. Explain that strengthening exercises improve balance and decrease the risk of falling. Address fall prevention. Wearing of proper shoes, removal of throw rugs, sufficient lighting, and use of handrails decrease the risk of a fall or fracture.

Precaution. *Avoid forceful, unguarded motions, such as opening a stuck window or bending forward to lift a heavy object. Instead, teach clients how to squat when lifting.*

Histology of Collagen, Bone, and Cartilage

Collagen

Collagen is the fundamental component of the connective tissues of the body, including fascia, fibrous cartilage, tendons, ligaments, bones, joint capsules, blood vessels, adipose tissue, and dermis. Collagen is the most abundant protein in the human body. It accounts for approximately 30% of all protein. Before 1970, researchers believed that all collagen was identical. Now, nineteen types of collagen are known that are differentiated by their protein composition. Type I and type II together compose approximately 90% of human connective tissue. *Type III collagen* is produced first, in the initial reparative phase, before type I collagen. Type III collagen also is found in arteries, the liver, and the spleen.[8]

Type I collagen constitutes about 90% of total body collagen. Type I collagen is found in bone, tendon, fascia, fibrous cartilage, derma, and sclera. This collagen is synthesized by **fibroblasts, osteoblasts,** and **chondroblasts.** Its primary function is to resist tension.

Type II collagen is found in hyaline and elastic cartilage and intervertebral disks. Type II collagen is synthesized by chondroblasts. Its primary function is to resist intermittent pressure.

Fibroblasts produce type I collagen fibers that are found in tendons, ligaments, and joint capsules. **Procollagen,** the precursor of collagen, is produced in the endoplasmic reticulum and is made up of polypeptide chains of lysine, glycine, and proline. **Tropocollagen** is the basic molecular unit of collagen fibrils and is found in the interstitial spaces; this collagen is the building block of collagen. The bonds of procollagen and tropocollagen are weak and easily deformed or ruptured. One must understand that collagen bonds are remodeled from mobilization or exercise.

Fibroblasts also produce **glycosaminoglycans.** These are **proteoglycans,** the fundamental components of connective tissue, which make up the **extracellular matrix** of tendons, ligaments, and articular cartilage. **Imbibition** is the primary nutritional source for avascular tissues, such as tendons, ligaments, cartilage, and vertebral disks. When tension/pressure increase, fluid is forced out of tissue and the volume of the tissue decreases. This causes an increase in the concentration of proteoglycan substances and an increase in osmotic pressure, which in turn produces imbibition. Glycosaminoglycans provide the fibers with nutrition via imbibition and lubrication. They allow space for elastic deformity of the tissue.[8] The half-life of glycosaminoglycans is 1.7 to 7 days. Immobilization for more than 1.7 to 7 days causes a 50% decrease in glycosaminoglycans. Therefore lubrication is decreased and the elastic range of collagen is decreased. A decrease in glycosaminoglycans causes a decrease in nutrition, which damages the tissue.

Bone

Bone is the protective and supportive framework that has rigid and static, elastic and dynamic properties. The properties and geometry of bone can be altered in response to internal and external stress and also in response to mineral demands. Bone has plastic qualities; it absorbs and stores compressional forces and transmits tensile forces. Bone also has elastic qualities. Long bone can deform up to 5%. The ability of bone to deform decreases with age.

Bone is composed of approximately 5% water and approximately 70% minerals (calcium hydroxyapatite, phosphate, magnesium, sodium, potassium, and fluoride carbonate); approximately 20% organic compounds, mostly type I collagen; and approximately 5% noncollagenous proteins. Osteoblasts are the functional building blocks of the **osteoid matrix;** they are located only at the surface of bone tissue. **Osteocytes** are mature osteoblasts. **Osteoclasts** are responsible for bone dissolution and absorption. Bone homeostasis balances synthesis, dissolution, and absorption with the forces that are applied on the skeleton.[9]

Cartilage

Cartilage is a semirigid connective tissue that is less dense and more elastic than bone. The functional unit of cartilage is the chondrocyte. Chondroblasts are immature **chondrocytes,** and they produce the **ground substance** or extracellular matrix of cartilage. This extracellular matrix consists of glycosaminoglycans and type II collagen. Water composes 65% to 80% of articular cartilage. Like fibroblasts, chondroblasts synthesize collagen and glycosaminoglycans when stimulated by mechanical tension. Mature cartilage is avascular and lacks nerve supply. Cartilage gets nutrition through imbibition. The mechanical forces of motion stimulate imbibition and removal of waste products.

The three types of cartilage are the following:

1. *Hyaline cartilage:* The most common and found on articular surfaces of peripheral joints, sternal ends of the ribs, nasal septum, larynx, and tracheal rings
2. *Elastic cartilage:* Found in the epiglottis, laryngeal cartilage, walls of eustachian tubes, external ear, and auditory canal
3. *Fibrocartilage:* Found in intervertebral disks, some articular cartilage, the pubic symphysis, dense connective tissue in joint capsules, ligaments, and the union of tendons to bone

The two primary functions of articular cartilage are to promote motion between two opposing bones with minimal friction and wear and to distribute the load applied to the joint surfaces over as great an area as possible.[10]

Optimal Stimulus for Regeneration of Collagen, Bone, and Cartilage

Collagen

The optimal stimulus for fibroblastic function in the regeneration of collagen is modified tension along the line of stress. This modified tension is not to exceed the level of tension that the newly formed polar bonds of tropocollagen can withstand. The tropocollagen is an immature precursor to the stronger, more resilient collagen. Once a certain level of tension is exceeded, tissue breakdown will occur instead of proliferation.

Precaution. *If tension exceeds this critical level, the signs and symptoms will be pain, inflammatory reaction, muscle guarding, decreased range of motion or loss of flexibility, and secondary scarring.*[8]

Bone

The optimal stimulus for osteoblastic production in the regeneration of bone is modified compression in the line of stress. Wolff's law states that bone will change its internal architecture according to the forces placed upon it.

Precaution. *Abnormal shear force may cause a pseudarthrosis.*

Pseudarthrosis or "false joint" occurs at the site of nonunion. **Osteophytes** are bony outgrowths that develop as the body attempts to provide stability or to repair itself. Shearing force stimulates undifferentiated mesenchymal cells to produce cartilage, and a false joint may be created at the fracture site.[9]

Cartilage

The optimal stimulus in the regeneration of cartilage is intermittent compression/decompression with glide. Joint movement (shear) is necessary to distribute synovial fluid over the cartilaginous surface and provide oxygen and other necessary nutrients. Intermittent compression forces the extracellular fluid within the joint to be compressed into the cartilage matrix. With joint immobilization, an alteration in joint mechanics and a decrease in the normal contact areas of cartilage occur. This eventually leads to joint dysfunction, hypomobility or hypermobility, and muscle guarding.

Precaution. *The body responds to the stresses placed upon it. With abnormal stresses, there will be dysfunctional remodeling. This manifests as joint degeneration, osteophytes, bone spurs, or pseudarthrosis.*[9]

Effects of Immobilization versus Early Mobilization

◎ *Clinical Pearl*

Early mobilization within a pain-free range of motion promotes faster healing of connective tissue, stronger collagen bonds, reduced scar tissue adhesions, and improved collagen fiber orientation.

After 9 weeks of immobilization, there is 14% loss of total collagen, and by 12 weeks there is a 28% loss. The half-life of

BOX 4-5 Home Exercise Program

The home exercise program should do the following:
1. Provide modified tension in the line of stress. Initially, this will be accomplished by performing light muscle contractions to move the joint through the full available pain-free range of motion.
2. Avoid re-injury. *Any exercise or activity that causes pain is an indication of tissue trauma.*
3. Provide the proper dosage. Give specific instructions about the number of repetitions, sets, breaks, positioning, and speed of exercises.
4. Indicate the frequency of exercise. This depends on healing time frames, intensity, volume, comorbidities, and the tolerance to stress of the tissue. Be clear in the instructions to the client about the frequency of exercise. Initially this may be three or more times per day, but with increased exercise stress, there will be a decrease in frequency.
5. Supply adequate nutritional support. Explain the importance of eating a balanced diet and drinking a sufficient amount of water to stay hydrated. A well-balanced diet combined with exercise promotes healthy tissue.

glycosaminoglycans is 1.7 to 7 days. The half-life of collagen is 300 to 500 days. For this reason, under normal physiologic conditions, it takes between 1 to 2 years for full healing to occur. Immobilization of cartilage causes a decrease in thickness and number of collagen bundles, a decrease in proteoglycan content, an increase in water content, a decrease in load-bearing capacity, softening of the articular surface, decrease in tensile strength of cartilage, and a decrease in oxygen content. To decrease these adverse effects of immobilization, one should institute an exercise model of high repetitions with low to no resistance. This model increases the oxygen content within the tissues by improving blood flow and imbibition. For maximal benefit, mobilization exercises should be performed several times a day.[8] A home exercise program helps accomplish these goals. Box 4-5 lists the qualities of a good home exercise program.

Neurophysiology

Muscle Spindles

Muscle spindles are proprioceptors that consist of intrafusal muscle fibers enclosed in a sheath (spindle). They run parallel to the extrafusal muscle fibers and act as receptors that provide information on muscle length and the rate of change in muscle length. The spindles are stretched when the muscle lengthens. This stretch causes the sensory neuron in the spindle to transmit an impulse to the spinal cord, where it synapses with alpha motor neurons. This causes activation of motor neurons that innervate the muscle. The muscle spindles determine the amount of contraction necessary to overcome a given resistance. When the resistance increases, the muscle is stretched further, and this causes spindle fibers to activate a greater muscle contraction.[11]

Golgi Tendon Organs

Golgi tendon organs (GTOs) are proprioceptors that are located in the tendon adjacent to the myotendinous junction. They are arranged in series with the extrafusal muscle fibers. They are sensitive to stretch but are activated most efficiently when the muscle shortens. The GTO transmits information regarding muscle tension as opposed to length. Neural input from the GTO causes an inhibition of muscle activation. This provides a protective mechanism to avoid development of excessive tension.[11]

Joint Mechanoreceptors

Four types of **mechanoreceptors** are found in the synovial joint capsules. Mechanoreceptors have a significant effect on muscle tone and pain sensation locally and distally along segmental innervations. The number of mechanoreceptors decreases with age. By age 70 the total number of receptors has decreased by about 50%, depending on factors such as genetics and activity level.[12]

Type I mechanoreceptors are found in the superficial layers of the joint capsule between the collagen fibers. A large percentage of the type I mechanoreceptors is found in the joints of the neck, hip, and shoulder. They have a great effect on the coordination of the tonic muscle fibers. They are slow-adapting and inhibit pain. They fire during movement and for about 1 minute after movement stops. They provide postural and kinesthetic awareness (awareness of the position of the body or body part in space). They are active in the beginning and end-range of collagen tension.

Type II mechanoreceptors are found in deep layers of joint capsules. A high concentration of the type II mechanoreceptors is found in the joints of the lumbar spine, hand, foot, and temporomandibular joint. They are fast adapting and pain inhibiting. They fire during movement and continue to fire until about ½ second after movement stops. They do not respond to stretch but are activated in beginning and midrange of collagen tension. They have more effect on the phasic muscle fibers and **kinesthesia.**

Type III mechanoreceptors are located in the deep and superficial layers of the joint capsules and ligaments. They are slow adapting and inhibit muscle tone in response to stretch at the extreme end-range of tension. They provide kinesthetic information, but their role is less understood than the type I and II mechanoreceptors.

Type IV mechanoreceptors are located in joint capsules, blood vessels, articular fat pads, anterior dura mater, ligaments of the spine, and connective tissue. They are not found in muscle. They fire when excessive levels of tension are reached in the collagen, and they warn of tissue trauma. They function as pain-provoking, nonadapting, high-threshold receptors. They fire continuously until the injurious stimulus is removed. They are provoked by excessive stretch, inflammation, high temperature (38° C to 42° C or 100.4° F to 107.6° F), or respiratory and cardiovascular distress.[12]

Pain has been defined by the International Association for the Study of Pain as an unpleasant emotional disorder evoked by sufficient activity in the **nociceptive** system and associated with real or potential tissue damage.[13] The irritation causing the pain may be due to immobilization, physical trauma, infection, or emotional tension.

Precaution. *Pain is a protective mechanism. Pain is not a warning that something is about to go wrong; it has already gone wrong! Pain is the way the body alerts the brain that an irritation to the tissue has occurred. For this reason, one must remember to exercise within a pain-free range of motion. In this case, feeling bad is a good thing because it is how your body communicates. Listen to the body.*

Traumatology

The response of the body to trauma is predictable and consistent, regardless of the tissue involved or the mechanism of injury. Trauma sets off a highly organized response involving chemical, metabolic, permeability, and vascular changes at a cellular level in preparation for tissue repair.

Phases and Time Frames of Healing

The initial response to a traumatic event is irritation. This lasts for 5 to 6 hours. Vasomotor constriction occurs in the first few seconds. An immediate release of chemical vasodilators occurs. These dilators are also transmitters for the nociceptive (pain) system. The vasodilation increases the hydrostatic pressure because of increased capillary permeability. Clinicians rarely can influence this phase because of its immediate occurrence.

The next stage of healing is the acute stage, which lasts for 1 to 3 days depending on the vascularity of the tissue. During this time frame, a migration of the larger cell bodies through the wall of the vessel occurs. Subsequently, blood flow increases to the area, increasing hydrostatic pressure and increasing bleeding. The large proteins leak out of the capillary, causing a shift in osmotic pressure with resultant pulling of fluid out of the capillary. Venous stasis occurs distal to the traumatized area, and edema results (see Chapter 3).

The third stage of healing is the subacute stage. The subacute stage begins with the settled stage, where muscle spasming occurs over the next 3 to 5 days. Bleeding is no longer present. Oxygen and macrophages are present. Walling off of the capillary occurs, which makes waste removal difficult. This leads to secondary healing or scarring. Externally applied heat in the settled stage promotes stasis and inflammatory exudates. The preferred method of heating tissue is internally. Initiating movement with low resistance exercise produces friction and naturally generates heat. This promotes increased blood flow.

The final stage is the chronic stage. Tissue becomes strongly chemical bonded (**covalent bonds**) and mature at 9 to 12 months. At this stage the tissue becomes nonelastic and cannot be deformed. Mature scar tissue may cause pain. Clinically, concentrate on increasing the tolerance of the tissue to tension about the scar by use of controlled stress through properly dosed exercises.

Tissue-specific exercise in the subacute stage provides the optimal stimulus for the removal of **metabolites,** which are products of metabolism, from the tissue. Muscle contraction is necessary to transport metabolites from the cell and provide oxygen/nutrition to the area. Increased vascularization accomplishes this goal. This is achieved through many repetitions of properly dosed exercise with minimal resistance while avoiding excessive tissue tension. In other words, the muscle contractions with proper exercise facilitate formation of capillaries, blood flow, and removal of metabolites.

Stages of Repair

The stages of repair can be categorized into three phases: inflammation, repair, and remodeling. During the inflammatory phase, the white blood cells/macrophages destroy cellular debris, synthesize fibronectin, and produce protein and fiber. During the repair stage, collagen is produced, and during the remodeling stage, the fibroblasts orient longitudinally within 28 days and repair is complete between 128 to 135 days. **Myofibroblasts** (involved in tissue reconstruction) are active from 5 to 21 days after trauma to up to 9 months. During the initial remodeling, a random configuration of collagen fibrils occurs. This arrangement provides minimal strength. During the maturation phase, the mechanical strength increases with remodeling and organization of fibers with modified tension in the line of stress.[8]

Muscle Physiology

> ◎ *Clinical Pearl*
>
> Strength is related to fiber diameter, not fiber type.

Type I muscle fibers are smaller in diameter than type II muscle fibers. Muscle recruitment progresses from smaller to larger diameter. **Tonic muscles** fire first because they are the primary dynamic joint stabilizers. Their nutrition mainly comes from the delivery of oxygen. They are predominantly type I or slow-twitch muscles and are responsible for sustaining proper joint **arthrokinematics** over time.[14]

Tonic versus Phasic Muscles

Tonic muscles initiate the easy work; they are better adapted for endurance exercise than **phasic muscles** because they have more capillaries, mitochondria, and metabolic enzymes (Table 4-2). With long-distance running the tonic muscles are primarily responsible for work because they are adapted for aerobic activity. The phasic muscles are recruited to participate if the load is too great or if it is increasing. They are better suited for short-duration activities that are of higher intensity. They also begin to participate if the light work has lasted for 2 to 3 hours, as seen with marathon runners who sprint when approaching the finish line. Phasic muscles are anaerobic and contract at a higher speed

TABLE 4-2	Comparison of Tonic and Phasic Muscle Fibers
Tonic	**Phasic**
Red: High myoglobin concentration	White: Lower myoglobin concentration
Slow twitch: 10 to 20 impulses per second	Fast twitch: 30 to 50 impulses per second
Type I	Type II
Arthrokinematic	Osteokinematic
Bipenate	Fusiform
Antigravity	—

and with greater force of contraction; they fatigue more quickly than tonic muscles.

The tonic muscle fibers atrophy almost immediately when immobilized after injury because they depend primarily on oxygen for metabolism. Therefore exercise to improve vascularization provides the oxygen necessary to nourish the tonic system.

Habitually overloading a system will cause it to respond and adapt. The rate of protein synthesis in a muscle is related directly to the rate of amino acid transportation into the cell. Amino acids transported into the muscle are influenced by the intensity and the duration of the muscle tension. Conversely, muscle atrophies as a result of disuse, immobilization, guarding associated with pain, or starvation.[14,17]

Types of Muscle Work and Training Effects

Isometric muscle contraction is the production of muscle tension without a change in muscle length or joint angle. The tension in the **cross-bridges** (the portion of myosin filament that pulls the actin filaments toward the center of the sarcomere during muscle contraction) is equal to the resistive force, thereby maintaining constant muscle length.

Concentric muscle contraction is muscle shortening as the muscle produces tension while the insertion moves toward the origin. Movement occurs in the same direction as the tension and joint motion because the contractile force is greater than the resistive force. Based on the **sliding filament theory,** the cross-bridges on the myosin filament attach to the active site on the actin filament. When all of the cross-bridges in a muscle shorten in a single cycle, the muscle shortens by approximately 1%. Muscles have the capacity to shorten up to 60% of their resting length; therefore the contraction cycle must be repeated multiple times.[15]

Eccentric muscle contraction is muscle lengthening as the muscle produces tension and the insertion moves away from the origin. The net muscle movement is in the opposite direction of the force of the muscle because the contractile force is less than the resistive force. Eccentric contractions require less energy than concentric contractions and are thought to be responsible for some aspect of postexercise muscle soreness. The cross-bridges of myosin stay attached to the active sites while the resistance is lowered. It may be the actual "tearing" away of the cross-bridges while resisting the lowering of a heavy resistance that results in the delayed-onset muscle soreness.[15,16]

Exercise

Functional Qualities of Exercise

Coordination refers to quality of motion. With atrophy of the tonic system, coordination is the first functional quality to be lost because the tonic muscles are the primary dynamic stabilizers of the joints. Therefore coordination must be the first functional quality to be restored. With an increase in speed or an increase in resistance comes a need for increased coordination. Normalization of a **reflex disturbance,** which is abnormal action of the cell, tissue, organ, or organism caused by overstimulation or understimulation, requires 5000 to 6000 repetitions. The repetitions are necessary to regain optimal coordination of movements about a physiologic axis.[17]

Endurance is the capacity to maintain an intensity of exercise for a prolonged period. Endurance requires continuous restoration of energy sources. Tonic muscles primarily require oxygen from the vascular system for their nutrition. Phasic muscles require glucose and body fat for their nutrition. Because the tonic system is the first to atrophy, because of muscle guarding and decreased motor recruitment, endurance is the quality that will increase nutrition through vascularization. Endurance exercise also promotes removal of waste products and prevents continued firing of the type IV mechanoreceptors caused by an abnormal chemical environment. Exercise dosage for endurance and vascularization requires many repetitions (three sets of 24) with low resistance.[17]

Speed is the time it takes to cover a fixed distance. Speed equals distance divided by time. With an increase in speed of movement is an increase in inertia, and overcoming this inertia requires a higher level of coordination. Speed of movement ultimately must be functional. During the initial phases of healing, coordination is not sufficient to exercise safely at a fast/functional speed.[18]

Volume refers to the total amount of weight lifted in a workout. The weight per repetition determines the appropriate volume per set. Heavy weights cannot be lifted for many repetitions in a set. Volume can be determined by multiplying the number of repetitions by the number of sets times the weight lifted per repetition. Three sets of 25 repetitions with 5 pounds would be calculated as $3 \times 25 \times 5$ lbs = 375 lbs of volume. If other sets also are performed with different amounts of weight, the volumes per set are calculated and then all are added together to obtain the total workout volume.[19]

Strength is the maximal force that a muscle or group of muscles can generate against a resistance at a given speed. Strength can be tested as a measure of **1 RM (resistance maximal;** see the following discussion for more on this topic). Strength training is performed at a percentage of 1 RM. For strength training, the number of repetitions decreases as the resistance increases. Increased resistance produces an increase in tissue tension and a decrease in blood flow to the capillaries during the muscle contraction, as well as an increase in blood flow when the exercise is over. Therefore only a few repetitions are performed. For pure strength gains, 85% of 1 RM (three sets of six) are performed. However, when there is muscle atrophy, after immobilization, strength gains are realized at 30% to 40% of 1 RM.[18-21]

Power is the ability to overcome resistance over a specific distance in a fixed time frame. Work equals force multiplied by distance. Power equals work divided by time. Power lifting is generally not a functional requirement for clients. However, increased power is necessary to perform a task at a faster rate. Power is therefore a critical component of exercise for clients.[22]

Dosing

Exercise initially is dosed based on the physiology of the type I muscle fibers and their depletion of nutrients in a state of guarding.

> ◎ *Clinical Pearl*
>
> Clinically, the first goal of dosing exercise is to deliver oxygen to the muscles, elicit no pain, and perform many repetitions.

Initially, focus on sustaining slow, coordinated movement around a physiologic axis. Ultimately, progress toward a fast/

functional speed while maintaining coordination and providing optimal stimulus for regeneration of the specific tissue(s) in lesion.[17] Resistance should be objective and measurable, physiologic, and adjusted to the tissues participating. (See later in the chapter for explanations of these concepts.) Training with free weights or a pulley system is easier to quantify and provides a more specific resistance throughout the entire range of motion than elastic bands.

Starting Positions

Determining a starting position depends on tolerance of the specific tissues to stress. Gravity assists, resists, or is eliminated, depending on what the tissue can tolerate while working in a pain-free synergy about a physiologic axis.

Precaution. *If there is pain while exercising against the force of gravity, position the limb in a posture that eliminates the effects of gravity.*[17]

If necessary, to complete a pain free arc of motion, the limb can be positioned so that the motion to be performed is assisted by gravity. This way, the **antagonists,** muscles that work in opposition to the prime movers, generate motion instead of the painful **agonists,** or prime movers.

Range of Motion

Initially, localize motion to a specific joint in a specific direction with controlled range of motion maintained throughout the arc. Monitor the tension on noncontractile tissues. Watch for controlled, normal physiologic motion, and educate the client to avoid compensatory motion while exercising. Adjust the resistance to allow for acceleration toward maximal length-tension range and deceleration away from it. Quality of motion, while avoiding pain-provoking end-ranges, dictates quantity.[18]

Work Capacity/Effects of Aging

An individual's sustainable work capacity is approximately 30% of that person's available energy. The remaining 70% of the stored energy in the body is needed for protein synthesis and maintenance of tissue (Fig. 4-1). The amount of energy available for maintenance, repair, and regeneration of tissue decreases with age. With age, it takes less activity to dip into the 70% of

energy reserve that is so necessary for tissue synthesis and repair (Fig. 4-2).

Precaution. *With an older client population, take care not to overexercise, or the risk for breakdown of collagen tissue and problems, such as tendonitis, will increase.*[17]

Calculating Dosage

In 1948, DeLorme defined the term *resistance maximal (RM).* This is the resistance that a group of muscles can overcome once. RM was used as a measure of strength. In the 1950s the Norwegian, Oddvar Holten, developed a curve that estimated guidelines for dosing repetitions/resistance for concentric work (Fig. 4-3).[17,23]

Calculating Resistance by Percentage of 1 RM

Repetitions of Exercise

Because 1 RM is the maximum resistance that can be overcome once, this resistance has a high risk of causing further injury to the already compromised tissue. When dosing an exercise program initially, the first functional qualities desired are to promote vascularization and endurance while maintaining coordination. For this to be accomplished, according to the Holten diagram, the exercise should be dosed at 30 repetitions (Fig. 4-4).[17,23]

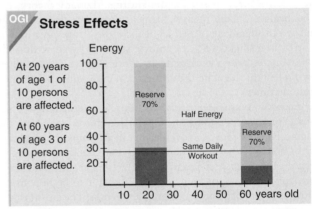

FIGURE 4-2 Effects of age on energy requirements. (Used with permission from the Ola Grimsby Institute.)

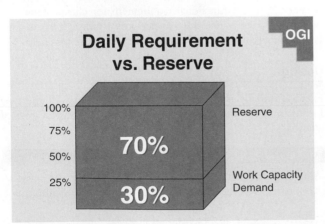

FIGURE 4-1 Total daily energy requirements. (Used with permission from the Ola Grimsby Institute.)

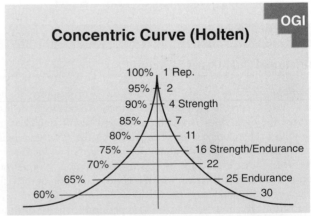

FIGURE 4-3 Holten diagram. (Used with permission from the Ola Grimsby Institute.)

The client is given a weight that the therapist predicts will cause fatigue in less than 30 repetitions. The client then performs as many repetitions as possible before the onset of fatigue, pain, or loss of coordination. As an example, the client is provided with a 3-pound weight and is able to perform 16 repetitions with this weight before becoming fatigued or experiencing pain (16 repetitions correlates to 75% of 1 RM according to the Holten diagram).

Therefore

$$\frac{x}{60} = \frac{3}{75}$$

$$x = \frac{180}{75}$$

$$x = 2.4 \text{ lb}$$

This client should be able to perform 30 repetitions with 2.4 pounds.

Speed of Exercise

Speed of exercise is another component that may change the dosage. Increased speed causes an increase in inertia and requires more coordination to execute. Oxygen debt is also important to avoid during exercising so as to provide the type I muscle fibers with nutrition while they are in a state of guarding.

Precaution. *If the client's respiratory rate is increasing during the exercise, then the speed of exercise must be decreased or there must be a longer break between sets or both.*

To increase the total number of repetitions while maintaining an accurate dose, increase the number of sets. It has been determined that to go from one set to three sets without changing the resistance, the number of repetitions must be decreased by 15% to 20%. By doing this, one set of 30 repetitions now becomes three sets of 24 to 25 repetitions. The amount of time between sets is determined by how long it takes the client to return to a **steady state respiratory rate** (equilibrium of the respiratory system). This is necessary to avoid oxygen debt.

When using pulleys to exercise the upper extremity, if the weight of the limb alone exceeds 60% of 1 RM, then a counterweight may be used to de-weight the arm. Other ways to decrease the weight of the limb for proper dosage are to position it in a gravity-eliminated position or even a gravity-assisted position.[17,23]

Length-Tension Relationship and Implications to Exercise

Blyx,[24] a Swedish physiologist, defined **muscle fiber length equilibrium** as the length the muscle will maintain when it is unaffected by outside forces. Muscle force production varies depending on the angle of the muscle in the arc of motion. The length/tension curve identifies the length at which a muscle generates the most contractile tension (Fig. 4-5). This length is influenced by histologic, biomechanical, and neurophysiologic factors. Histologically, the overlap of actin and myosin filaments is most extensive toward the midrange of motion. Biomechanically, the angle of the tendon insertion into the bone dictates where the greatest tensile strength will occur. The greatest amount of force is achieved when the moment arm for a muscular force is perpendicular to the lever arm. Neurophysiologically,

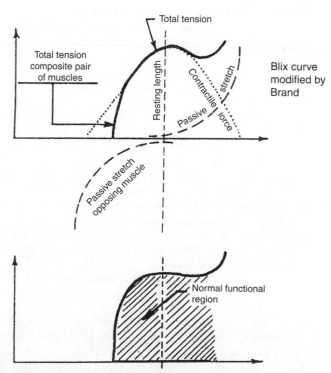

FIGURE 4-5 Length-tension curve. (From Brand PW, Hollister A: *Clinical mechanics of the hand*, St Louis, 1993, Mosby. In Trumble, *Principles of hand surgery and therapy*, St Louis, 2000, Philadelphia.)

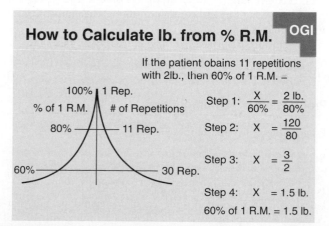

FIGURE 4-4 Example for calculating exercise dose. (Used with permission from the Ola Grimsby Institute.)

the joint mechanoreceptors influence muscle facilitation around the joint. Type I and type II mechanoreceptors fire at the beginning of range. Type II alone fires at midrange, and type I fires at the end-range of capsular tension.[12]

The clinical importance of the length/tension concept can be discussed in terms of concentric and eccentric aspects.

Concentric Aspects

When working concentrically with pulleys, set the rope perpendicular to the lever arm at 20% into the lengthened range of the muscle that is going to do the work. If using free weights, position the limb where it is perpendicular to the force of gravity, when the lever arm is at 20% into the lengthened range of motion.

Eccentric Aspects

When working eccentrically, have the maximal resistance set perpendicular to the lever arm at 20% to 30% into the shortened range of the muscle that is going to do the eccentric work. The length/tension concept reveals that muscle produces the least amount of power at the beginning and end-ranges. When activated, the muscle contraction accelerates toward the midrange and decelerates away from it. The variability of speed is an important component of all activities of daily living. Because activity is task specific, the variables of speed and resistance throughout the range of a contraction are important for fiber recruitment and physiologic coordination.[25,26]

Formulation and Progression of an Exercise Program

When formulating an exercise program for treatment of hypomobility or hypermobility, you should start by identifying the specific problems that exist. Examples of these problems are the following:
- The complaint of pain
- Muscle guarding of the tonics (rotator cuff)
- Decreased endurance, and limited range of motion (external rotation [ER] > abduction [ABD] > internal rotation [IR])
- Articular compression
- Decreased synovium/decreased articular cartilage nutrition
- Decreased mechanoreceptor input in the capsule
- Compensatory motion

Once an examination has been completed, establish functional or measurable goals that address the identified problems. The following suggestions are several possible goals for the client:
- Decrease pain with arm elevation (1 to 10 scale)
- Increase endurance with exercise (time and repetitions) and with functional work/avocation activities (time)
- Increase range of motion (specific planes of motion and to accomplish functional activities)
- Educate/improve posture to promote proximal stability and improved arthrokinematics of the glenohumeral joint (at work, with activities, time frames)
- Identify treatment approaches to resolve the goals:
  - *Decrease pain and guarding:* Distraction of the joint to fire type I mechanoreceptors
  - *Increase joint mobility:* Compression/decompression with gliding for cartilage, modified tension in the line of stress for joint capsule
  - *Hydrate/lubricate cartilage:* Compression/decompression with glide
  - *Increase proprioception:* Modified tension in the line of stress

---

BOX 4-6   Considerations for Exercise Program

Equipment: Consider using pulleys, benches, bolsters, and wedges for positioning; straps, free weights, and de-weighting devices.

Ropes: Consider the range of motion, and set the rope perpendicular to the lever arm and parallel to the muscle fiber.

Pulley: Should be single, double, concentric, or eccentric.

Starting positions: Consider recommending supine, prone, side-lying, sitting, standing, non–weight bearing, weight bearing, arm supported, or unsupported.

Movement range: Consider recommending full range of motion; inner, outer, or mid range of motion.

Weight: Consider the functional quality that is desired and what percentage of 1 RM is needed to accomplish that. (In this case, the functional qualities most likely would be endurance and vascularization.) Also take into account the body/limb position, gravity, and quality of motion when determining weight.

Dosage: The number of repetitions and sets is determined by the desired functional qualities. These include coordination, vascularization, endurance, strength, and power.[7,23]

Speed: This will vary, but early in the rehabilitation, when working on vascularization and endurance, it is important to follow respiratory rate at steady state to avoid oxygen debt. Speed should increase as coordination and function increase.

Rest: Breaks between sets are determined by respiratory rate. As the client starts to increase strength (x resistance + x repetitions), the rest breaks will increase. As resistance increases, the frequency of exercise decreases as well (three times per week).

Education: Instructions to the client must be specific. Demonstration of the exercise first or even guiding the client's limb through the arc of motion that is desired is often helpful. Use verbal, visual, and tactile cues as necessary.

Consider client and equipment needs before starting exercises. Box 4-6 outlines different aspects of an exercise program. Consider precautions and contraindications when implementing an exercise program.

Precaution. *Comorbidities (such as, cardiac or pulmonary disease, specific physician protocol, and other medical/surgical considerations) must dictate exercise decisions.*

Progressions of Hypomobilities

Progressions of hypomobilities has four stages (Table 4-3).

Stage I

Stage I begins with many repetitions to address coordination. Following the Holten diagram, 60% of 1 RM promotes vascularization. This is dosed at three sets of 25 repetitions. Fifty percent of 1 RM helps decrease joint edema. Beginning with 40% of 1 RM may be necessary when the amount of muscle fiber atrophy present is significant. Start at a slow speed with minimal

TABLE 4-3	Progression of Hypomobilities Stages I to IV	
Stage	Procedures	Goals
Stage 1	Many repetitions	Increase endurance
	Low speed	Increase circulation
	Minimal resistance	Increase exercise ability
	Outer range of motion	Avoid overexertion
Stage II	Increase repetitions	Increase endurance
	Increase speed	Increase fast coordination
	Do not increase resistance	
Stage III	Stabilizing exercise in the gained range of motion	Increase strength in the gained range of motion
	Concentric and eccentric	
Stage IV	Coordinate tonic and phasic function throughout physiologic range of motion	Functional stability

TABLE 4-4	Progression of Hypermobilities Stages I to IV	
Stages	Procedures	Goals
Stage I	Many repetitions	Increase endurance
	Low speed	Increase circulation
	Minimal resistance	Increase exercise ability
	Beginning or midrange of motion	Avoid overexertion
Stage II	Increase repetitions	Increase strength
	Include isometric contractions in inner range of motion	Increase sensitivity to stretch
Stage III	Submaximal (80% RM) resistance concentrically and eccentrically	Increase dynamic stability in the gained range of motion
	Include isometric contractions in the full range of motion (except the outer range)	
Stage IV	Coordinate tonic and phasic function throughout physiologic range of motion	Functional stability

RM, Resistance maximal.

resistance to maintain coordinated movement and help decrease inflammation. Work into the outer, pain-free range of motion to promote stimulation of fibroblasts and production of glycosaminoglycans. This stage of exercises stimulates joint mechanoreceptors and GTOs to inhibit pain and guarding. Begin with the joint in a resting position and provide support of bolsters or other equipment as needed to promote quality of motion around a physiologic axis. Start with concentric contractions initially to increase vascularity.[25]

Stage II

Have the client progress to stage II when the functional quality of coordination and vascularization is achieved. Signs for progressing to this stage are a decrease in complaint of pain, increased range of motion, increased speed of exercise, decreased muscle guarding, and less fatigue experienced by the client.

The goal of stage II is to increase endurance and speed. This is accomplished by increasing the number of sets and the number of exercises. With increased coordination, increase the speed of exercise. Do not increase resistance. At this point, remove the supportive bolsters so that the client can begin stabilizing proximally while improving the mobility of the hypomobile joint. Histologic changes that take place in stage II are improved nutrition to the joint cartilage through decreased viscosity of synovial fluid associated with the increase in speed.[25]

Stage III

Have the client progress to stage III when pain has resolved, full range of motion is regained, and when speed and coordination have increased. For the newly gained range of motion, there must be dynamic stability. This means that the musculotendinous units are strong enough to maintain controlled, physiologic mobility. Concentric and eccentric contractions in the newly gained range of motion promote functional stability. In stage III the resistance is increased to 60% to 80%, and the repetitions are decreased to 10 to 15 repetitions to promote strength/endurance. Begin triplanar motions by exercising in proprioceptive neuromuscular

facilitation patterns. Add isometric contractions in the newly gained end-range of motion to promote strength.

Stage IV

Have the client progress to stage IV when the client is able to increase the speed of exercise and still maintain coordination. Absence of delayed-onset muscle soreness is also an indication that it is time to progress to the next level. Stage IV emphasizes functional exercises and retraining for activities of daily living, essential job functions, and sport-specific activities. Exercises are performed through a full range of motion at up to 80% to 90% of 1 RM at a functional speed in order to achieve the functional quality of power.[18]

Progressions of Hypermobilities

Exercise progressions for hypermobilities have four stages (Table 4-4).

Stage I

Stage I for hypermobilities is identical to stage I for hypomobilities with one major exception. With a hypomobility the exercises are dosed to promote increased mobility, whereas with a hypermobility the goal is to increase stability. Therefore exercises for hypermobility are performed in the beginning and midrange of motion so that coordination can be maintained while developing stability.

Stage II

In stage II, increase repetitions, number of sets, and number of exercises. Add closed kinetic chain and slow plyometric exercises to increase sensitivity to stretch. Continue to perform exercise in a single plane of motion, and increase speed as coordination permits.

Stage III

In stage III, increase resistance to 80% of 1 RM and decrease the number of repetitions to promote strength. Perform concentric and eccentric contractions for increased stability in the physiologic range of motion. Add a set of one isometric contraction at 75% to 85% of **1 IM** (**isometric maximum**). This contraction should be held for 15 seconds. Fast **plyometrics** (when an eccentric contraction is immediately followed by a concentric contraction) for recruitment of the muscle spindle helps increase sensitivity to stretch and aids in stability. Triplanar motion can start in stage III for promotion of functional stability.

Stage IV

Hypermobility progression in stage IV is equivalent to that for hypomobilities. The exercises become more functional, and you should focus more on retraining for a job, activities of daily living, and sport. Increase the resistance to improve the qualities of power and speed.[18]

Monitoring of Vital Signs

Monitoring of vital signs is a reliable, valid, and meaningful way of measuring clients' response to exercise. It takes practice to become accurate with monitoring vital signs and to understand the significance of these values. Taking a resting heart rate, blood pressure, respiratory rate, and oxygen saturation (SpO_2) only measures the body systems at rest. To get baseline measurements, take vital signs before, during, and after exercise. Doing this provides critical information about how the body is responding to the exercise loads placed upon it, as well as how well it recovers from the stress of exercise.

Precaution. *Proper dosing of exercise can improve the efficiency of the cardiovascular system, whereas overdosing may cause irreversible damage.*

Heart rate/pulse may be altered by many medications and diseases. When this is the case, as in clients who are taking betablockers or are in congestive heart failure, monitoring of the heart rate in response to exercise may provide inaccurate or misleading information. In such cases, one must use other forms of measuring the response of the body to exercise.[5,6]

Rate of Perceived Exertion

Gunner Borg established the Borg scale (rate of perceived exertion, or RPE) in 1962. The RPE is a subjective measurement of how hard clients think they are exercising. The RPE has been proved to be a valid and reliable way of measuring exertion during exercise and functional activities. The original scale was based on numeric values that ranged from 6 to 20, with 6 being a perception of minimal effort, as in relaxing in a chair, and with 20 describing maximal effort, as in running up a steep hill. Target RPE is between 11 and 13 (fairly light to somewhat hard). This is a pace that could be maintained for at least a 15-minute workout. Breathing would be labored; one could carry on a conversation but likely would prefer not to do so. In more recent years, a modified RPE scale has become popular. This newer version is based on a 0 to 10 value system. Zero is equivalent to work at rest, and 10 is maximal exertion. Some find this modified scale easier to use. Table 4-5 gives the Borg RPE scales.[5]

TABLE 4-5   Borg Rate of Perceived Exertion Scales

Borg Scale	Newer Scale
6	0 Nothing at all
7 Very, very light	0.5 Very, very weak
8	1 Very weak
9 Very light	2 Weak
10	3 Moderate
11 Fairly light	4 Somewhat strong
12	5 Strong
13 Somewhat hard	6
14	7 Very strong
15 Hard	8
16	9
17 Very hard	10 Maximal
18	
19 Very, very hard	
20	

Training Modes

Cardiovascular warm-up not only gets the heart and lungs prepared for exercise, but it also is the healthy, natural way of preparing tissue for more vigorous, tissue-specific exercise. The warm-up may consist of 5 to 15 minutes of walking on the treadmill or riding on a stationary bike or upper body ergometer. This type of warm-up increases blood flow, heart rate, deep muscle/tissue temperature, and respiratory rate and decreases joint synovial fluid. This means of increasing circulation may be the wise choice as opposed to the passive hot pack application for tissue warming.

Core/proximal stabilization exercises are essential components of all phases of exercise and activities of daily living. For normal physiologic movement to take place, there must be distal mobility on proximal stability.

Precaution. *Increased mobility at the expense of proximal stability equates to compensatory or nonphysiologic movement.*

Therefore proper posturing and core stabilization exercises are an appropriate component of the hand therapist's repertoire.

Concentric exercise requires three times as much energy as does eccentric exercise. Most of the energy of the body is stored in muscle mass. Seventy percent of the stored energy is used to maintain all vital organ function. Thirty percent of the stored energy is used to carry out functional daily activities. If a person regularly exceeds the 30% of energy reserved for activities of daily living and dips into the 70% reserved for vital organs, pathologic conditions of the collagen will result. This may be manifested as a tendonitis, for example. To promote healing, when dosing initially for concentric exercise, it is best to require many repetitions with light resistance. Doing so will increase oxygen to the injured tissue by increasing its blood flow (Fig. 4-6).[14]

Isometric exercise occurs when a muscle contracts without joint motion. A strengthening effect for the muscle occurs at the

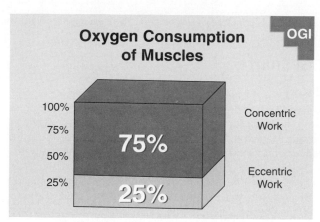

FIGURE 4-6 Oxygen consumption of muscles.

angle the joint assumes during the contraction and at 20 degrees on either side of that angle. For example, if the biceps are isometrically contracted with the elbow at 90 degrees, a strengthening effect will result from 70 to 110 degrees. This is a safe way to begin strengthening after an injury if the isometric exercises are performed in a pain-free range. Isometric exercises can be performed at varying angles and can be dosed at different intensities. The amount of force that can be maintained by an isometric contraction for 1 second is 1 IM. In rehabilitation, therapists dose isometric contractions at a percentage of 1 IM. Percentage of isometric resistance is dosed in relation to holding time. For example, 60% of 1 IM can be held from 50 to 60 seconds; 80% of 1 IM for 20-30 seconds; 90% of 1 IM can be maintained for 10 seconds.[14]

Open and closed kinetic chain exercises play an important role in rehabilitation of the upper extremity. Most functional activities of the upper extremity are **open chain.** Movement occurs from muscle origin to insertion, and the terminal joint is free. With **closed chain** exercises, movement occurs from muscle insertion to origin, and the terminal joint is constrained in a fixed position.[27]

Client Education

To increase compliance with exercise programs, it is essential to educate clients on why they are doing each component of the exercise program and what is being accomplished.

> ### ◎ *Clinical Pearl*
>
> Explain that the exercises that are dosed at high repetitions are to improve vascularization and endurance.

Movement is life, and conversely lack of movement will lead to tissue destruction. Many repetitions in a pain-free range of motion help to increase blood flow, which in turn brings more oxygen to the injured tissue. The body gets nutrition through the oxygen in the blood.

Precaution. *Avoid pain because pain indicates that the tissue is being irritated. With tissue irritation there will be more pain, which leads to muscle guarding, inflammation, and a decrease of blood flow/nutrition to the area.*

Emphasize quality of motion. The body responds to the stress placed upon it. Maintaining proper posture and body mechanics

during exercises and throughout the day and night will result in optimal health. Encourage clients to keep a journal of their activities and home exercise program. This is often helpful for accountability and guidance for upgrades.

CASE STUDIES OF EXERCISE PROGRESSIONS

CASE STUDY 4-1 ▪

History

TP is a 36-year-old left-hand dominant female secretary who spends 8 hours a day working on the computer and talking on the telephone. She also is attending night school and studying nursing. Because of limited free time, she reports that she has not been participating in any regular exercise program. She admits that she has gained quite a bit of weight over the last year. TP often studies in bed at night, propped up by pillows, until she falls asleep. She presents to therapy reporting that her right lateral elbow has been painful for approximately 3 months. She does not recall sustaining any injury. She notes that the pain in her elbow becomes more intense over the course of the workday. Upon questioning, she does recall that she often awakens during the night with numbness and tingling into the "whole hand."

Clinical Evaluation Findings

TP reports frustration because she has had 1 month of therapy for her elbow, and she feels that it has not improved but rather has gotten worse. She states that her therapy has consisted of hot packs, ultrasound, and stretching exercises. She also was provided with a wrist orthosis and tennis elbow strap.

Her evaluation was remarkable for rounded shoulder with a forward head (RSFH) posture, sixth cervical vertebra–facilitated segment (causing increased tone along the C6 distribution), pain to palpation at the origin of the extensor carpi radialis brevis, pain at end-range elbow extension, decreased grip on the right (because of pain), and pain with resisted wrist extension. After explaining the findings and outlining the treatment plan, the therapist established goals for therapy with TP, and she agreed to comply.

An ergonomic evaluation of the workstation was performed. Recommendations for computer monitor, keyboard height, and chair adjustments were made. New mouse placement and style were reviewed. A phone headset was ordered.

TP was instructed in some postural exercises, including pectoralis stretches, chin tucks, neck stretches, and gentle brachial plexus/peripheral nerve glides. The postural strengthening exercises included wall letters and scapular retraction and depression exercises. TP agreed to perform these exercises during breaks at work and at home.

TP agreed to start walking daily, beginning with 15 minutes a day at a comfortable pace while maintaining good posture. Duration of the walks is to increase by 2 minutes a week over the next 2 months, as she is able. Speed of gait is also to increase as TP becomes more comfortable and acclimated to her walking program.

The first therapy treatment was spent evaluating TP, and educating her on the different components of her present complaints. Explanations were provided on how posture, work, and exercise habits contributed to the elbow pain and how she could address this responsibly. She was provided with the foregoing home exercise program and was dosed for her clinical elbow exercise program.

The first stage of exercise was dosed with the physiology of the tonic muscle fiber of the elbow in mind. Three months of muscle guarding resulted in some tonic muscle atrophy, degeneration of collagen, and alteration in joint mechanics leading to a decrease in normal contact areas of cartilage. The optimal stimulus for regeneration of collagen is modified tension in the line of stress, and the optimal stimulus for regeneration of cartilage is compression/decompression with glide. Following the stage I protocol for hypomobility, it was determined that TP could tolerate 21 repetitions of concentric wrist extension against gravity before pain set in.

On the second visit, treatment commenced. All exercises were dosed at three sets of 25 repetitions to promote vascularization and endurance while maintaining coordinated movement around a physiologic axis throughout a full pain-free arc of motion. TP warmed up on the upper body ergometer for 12 minutes at 120 rpm, forward and backward to avoid fatigue. Please refer to the Evolve website for illustrations of the following exercises:

1. Concentric wrist flexion, with forearm supported on a table (see Evolve for Fig. 4-7, *A*)
2. Concentric wrist extension, with forearm supported on a table (see Evolve for Fig. 4-7, *B*)
3. Pronation, with forearm supported on a table (see Evolve for Fig. 4-8, *A*)
4. Supination, with forearm supported on a table (see Evolve for Fig. 4-8, *B*)
5. Elbow flexion/extension, with forearm supported on a table (see Evolve for Fig. 4-9)

After finishing the foregoing 375 repetitions, the home exercise program was reviewed to ensure that the exercises were being performed correctly. Treatment concluded with an ice massage. TP reported fatigue but no pain.

TP returned to therapy 2 days later reporting that she had been compliant with her home exercises, walking program, and working on proper posture throughout the day/night. Her complaint of pain had decreased approximately 25%, and the "numbness and tingling" in the hand had resolved. TP went through the foregoing exercise program again and then was scheduled for one visit per week in therapy to make upgrades in the program as necessary. She also agreed to add the dosed exercises to her current home exercise program.

One week later, she returned to the clinic and reported compliance and denied any problems with her exercises. She stated that the exercises were taking much less time now than they were originally. TP described minimal complaint of elbow pain during the workday and no more symptoms at night. The exercises were upgraded because she now could tolerate 30 repetitions. Please refer to the Evolve website for illustrations of the following exercises:

1. Wrist extension against gravity (see Evolve for Fig. 4-10)
2. Wrist flexion against gravity (see Evolve for Fig. 4-11)
3. Pronation with 1 lb (see Evolve for Fig. 4-12, *A*)
4. Supination with 1 lb (see Evolve for Fig. 4-12, *B*)
5. Elbow flexion—recumbent seated position flexion with 2 lbs (see Evolve for Fig. 4-13)
6. Elbow extension in prone with 2 lbs (see Evolve for Fig. 4-14)

TP agreed to continue with her home exercise program, adding the new upgrades with the three sets of 25 each.

Result of Care

On the following week, TP called to cancel her future therapy appointments. She reported that she had not had any elbow pain in the previous 4 days and that because of time constraints she felt that she could continue with her independent exercise program and make upgrades appropriately.

CASE STUDY 4-2 ■

History

RJ is a 42-year-old right-hand dominant male carpenter who sustained an injury to his left shoulder 3 weeks before presenting for therapy. He reports that when unloading his truck at the job site early one morning, he lost his footing and started to fall backward off the truck. At the time, he was holding his toolbox in his right hand. As he was falling, he reached out with the left hand and grabbed on to a long 4×4 that was sticking out of the bed of the truck. He reports that "it happened so fast," but he is sure that he did not actually fall onto the shoulder or bump it on anything. Over the next 2 hours, he found it difficult to do his job because of left lateral and posterior shoulder pain. He decided to go to the nearby urgent care facility when the pain did not resolve over the course of the day. X-ray films were taken, and no fracture was noted. Over the next 2 weeks, RJ tried to persevere at work and apply ice to the shoulder whenever he could. He returned to the physician because his shoulder "just wasn't getting any better."

Clinical Evaluation Findings

Magnetic resonance imaging confirmed a near full-thickness tear of the supraspinatus and partial tear of the infraspinatus. Therapy evaluation ruled out any cervical spine involvement. Manual muscle testing of the left shoulder revealed 3/5 grade strength of the supraspinatus and 4/5 grade strength of the infraspinatus. There was a positive sulcus test at zero degrees, positive Hawkins-Kennedy sign, and positive external rotation lag sign with the supraspinatus at greater than 10 degrees and with the infraspinatus at less than 10 degrees. The evaluation confirmed the magnetic resonance imaging findings, and it was determined that RJ had a right shoulder impingement with an underlying hypermobility because of the rotator cuff tear.

Goals of Therapy

The goals of therapy were as follows:
1. Decrease pain.
2. Resolve muscle guarding.
3. Restore functional range of motion around a physiologic axis.
4. Increase endurance/strength of the rotator cuff.

Initial Treatment

Exercises were selected for stage I hypermobilities:
1. Start with a warm-up exercise, such as the upper body ergometer for 10 minutes at 120 rpm.
2. Dose with many repetitions initially to increase endurance and circulation to the type I muscle fibers of the rotator cuff (three sets of 25).
3. Begin with slow speed to promote coordinated movement about a physiologic axis.
4. Choose starting positions that are in the inner range of motion to maintain stability from inner to mid range of motion.
5. Support the limb with equipment, as necessary, to aid with preserving proper joint arthrokinematics.

The following exercises were selected for Robert's shoulder rehabilitation. Please refer to the Evolve website for illustrations of the following exercises:
1. Scapular retraction (see Evolve for Fig. 4-15)
2. Internal rotation (see Evolve for Fig. 4-16)

3. External rotation (see Evolve for Fig. 4-17)
4. Abduction (see Evolve for Fig. 4-18)
5. Lateral pull downs (see Evolve for Fig. 4-19)
6. Triceps (see Evolve for Fig. 4-20)
7. Biceps (see Evolve for Fig. 4-21)

RJ's first treatment was spent evaluating and testing to determine the appropriate resistance to achieve the functional qualities of vascularization and endurance while maintaining coordination and quality of motion without eliciting pain. The outer range of motion initially was avoided because of instability. On return visits, he performed three sets of 25 repetitions for all of the foregoing exercises. He took rest breaks between sets. For each exercise the pulley rope was set perpendicular to the lever arm at 20% into the lengthened range of motion and parallel to the muscle fiber. Concentric contractions were performed initially, and between each repetition, the weight stack was let down to remove tension.

Continuing Care

RJ was scheduled for therapy three times per week for 4 weeks. On his third treatment, he was noted to be moving through his exercise program more quickly, maintaining coordination, and reporting no pain with exercise and decreased pain overall. He then was dosed for four more exercises. Please refer to the Evolve website for illustrations of the following exercises:

1. Horizontal adduction (see Evolve for Fig. 4-22)
2. Horizontal abduction (see Evolve for Fig. 4-23)
3. Extension (see Evolve for Fig. 4-24)
4. Flexion (see Evolve for Fig. 4-25)

On the fifth visit, RJ began stage II for hypermobility. Slow plyometrics were added with a 1-pound ball tossed against a wall, catching it with the left hand. Closed chain exercises were initiated by performing wall pushups. He started to perform (two sets of 25) concentric contractions and one set of isometric contractions in the inner to mid range of motion. The isometric contractions were dosed at 60% to 70% of 1 IM, which is a 40- to 60-second hold.

By the eighth visit, RJ was able to progress to stage III. Exercises were upgraded to include concentric contractions at 80% of 1 RM for two sets of ten repetitions and one set of isometric contractions in the mid to outer (stable) range at 85% of 1 IM for a 10- to 15-second hold. Fast plyometrics were performed to recruit the muscle spindle. He started to incorporate diagonal (proprioceptive neuromuscular facilitation) patterns into his exercise routine as well.

Result of Care

In the fourth week, Robert's rehabilitation introduced some retraining of some of his essential job functions. At that time, he was released back to full duty and was discharged from therapy. He decided to join a local gym and continue with his established exercise routine.

Acknowledgments

I would like to give special thanks to Ola Grimsby and the Ola Grimsby Institute for the invaluable education I received from them and the permission to share this knowledge with other clinicians.

References

1. Grimsby O, Rivard J, Kring R: Models of pathology in orthopaedic manual therapy. In Grimsby O, Rivard J, editors: *Science, theory and clinical application in orthopaedic manual physical therapy: applied science and theory*, Vol 1, Taylorsville, UT, 2008, The Academy of Graduate Physical Therapy, Inc., pp 161–224.
2. Goodman CC, Snyder TE: Screening for endocrine and metabolic disease. *Differential diagnosis for physical therapists: screening for referral*, ed 4, St Louis, 2007, Saunders Elsevier.
3. Goodman CC, Snyder TE: Screening for immunologic disease. *Differential diagnosis for physical therapists: screening for referral*, ed 4, St Louis, 2007, Saunders Elsevier.
4. Goodman CC, Snyder TE: Screening for gastrointestinal disease. *Differential diagnosis for physical therapists: screening for referral*, ed 4, St Louis, 2007, Saunders Elsevier.
5. ACSM: *American College of Sports Medicine: guidelines for exercise testing and prescription*, ed 8, Philadelphia, 2009, Lippincott Williams & Wilkins.
6. Goodman CC, Snyder TE: Screening for cardiovascular disease. *Differential diagnosis for physical therapists: screening for referral*, ed 4, St Louis, 2007, Saunders Elsevier.
7. Carmona RH, Beato C, Lawrence A: *Bone health and osteoporosis: a report of the surgeon general*, Rockville, Md, 2004, Department of Health and Human Services.
8. Grimsby O, Rivard J, Kring R: Exercise for collagen repair. In Grimsby O, Rivard J, editors: *Science, theory and clinical application in orthopaedic manual physical therapy: applied science and theory*, Vol 1, Taylorsville, UT, 2008, The Academy of Graduate Physical Therapy, Inc., pp 33–65.
9. Grimsby O, Rivard J: Exercise for bone repair. In Grimsby O, Rivard J, editors: *Science, theory and clinical application in orthopaedic manual physical therapy: applied science and theory*, Vol 1, Taylorsville, UT, 2008, The Academy of Graduate Physical Therapy, Inc., pp 19–31.
10. Grimsby O, Rivard J: Properties of cartilage. In Grimsby O, Rivard J, editors: *Science, theory and clinical application in orthopaedic manual physical therapy: applied science and theory*, Vol 1, Taylorsville, UT, 2008, The Academy of Graduate Physical Therapy, Inc., pp 67–82.
11. Hunter GR, Harris RT: Structure and function of the muscular, neuromuscular, cardiovascular and respiratory systems. In Baechle TR, Earle RW, editors: *Essentials of strength training and conditioning*, ed 3, Omaha, 2008, Human Kinetics, pp 3–12.
12. Grimsby O, Rivard J: Clinical neurophysiology. In Grimsby O, Rivard J, editors: *Science, theory and clinical application in orthopaedic manual physical therapy: applied science and theory*, Vol 1, Taylorsville, UT, 2008, The Academy of Graduate Physical Therapy, Inc., pp 137–158.
13. *Classification of chronic pain*, Seattle, 1994, IASP Press.
14. Grimsby O, Rivard J, Kring R: Muscle physiology. In Grimsby O, Rivard J, editors: *Science, theory and clinical application in orthopaedic manual physical therapy: applied science and theory*, Vol 1, Taylorsville, UT, 2008, The Academy of Graduate Physical Therapy, Inc., pp 107–135.
15. Cipriani DJ, Falkel JE: Physiological principles of resistance training and functional integration for the injured and disabled. In Lee AC, Quillen WS, Magee DJ, et al: *Scientific foundations and principles of practice in musculoskeletal rehabilitation*, St Louis, 2007, Saunders Elsevier.
16. Cheung K, Hume P, Maxwell L: Delayed onset muscle soreness: treatment strategies and performance factors, *Sports Med* 33:145–164, 2003.
17. Grimsby O, Rivard J, Kring R: Exercise prescription. In Grimsby O, Rivard J, editors: *Science, theory and clinical application in orthopaedic manual physical therapy: applied science and theory*, Vol 1, Taylorsville, UT, 2008, The Academy of Graduate Physical Therapy, Inc., pp 347–392.

18. Grimsby O, Rivard J, Kring R: Functional qualities and exercise dosage. In Grimsby O, Rivard J, editors: *Science, theory and clinical application in orthopaedic manual physical therapy: applied science and theory*, Vol 1, Taylorsville, UT, 2008, The Academy of Graduate Physical Therapy, Inc., pp 325–344.

19. Baechle TR, Earle RW, Wathen D: Resistance training. In Baechle TR, Earle RW, editors: *Essentials of strength training and conditioning*, ed 3, Omaha, 2008, Human Kinetics, pp 405–407.

20. Peterson MD, Rhea MR, Alvar BA: Maximizing strength development in athletes: a meta-analysis to determine the dose-response relationship, *J Strength Cond Res* 18:377–382, 2004.

21. Wolfe BL, LeMura LM, Cole PJ: Quantitative analysis of single vs multiple set programs in resistance training, *J Strength Cond Res* 18:35–47, 2004.

22. Harman E: The biomechanics of resistance exercise. In Baechle TR, Earle RW, editors: *Essentials of strength training and conditioning*, ed 3, Omaha, 2008, Human Kinetics, pp 73–78.

23. *Medical exercise therapy*, Oslo, 1996, Norwegian MET Institute.

24. Blyx M: Blyx curve, *Scand Arch Physiol*, 93–94, 1892.

25. Grimsby O, Rivard J, Kring R: Exercise progression. In Grimsby O, Rivard J, editors: *Science, theory and clinical application in orthopaedic manual physical therapy: applied science and theory*, Vol 1, Taylorsville, UT, 2008, The Academy of Graduate Physical Therapy, Inc., pp 431–472.

26. Ratamess NA, et al: Progression models in resistance training for healthy adults, *Med Sci Sports Exerc*, 687–708, 2009.

27. Brumitt J: Scapular-stabilization exercises: early-intervention prescription, *Athletic Therapy Today* 11(5):15–18, 2006.

5 | Evaluation of the Hand and Upper Extremity

Linda J. Klein

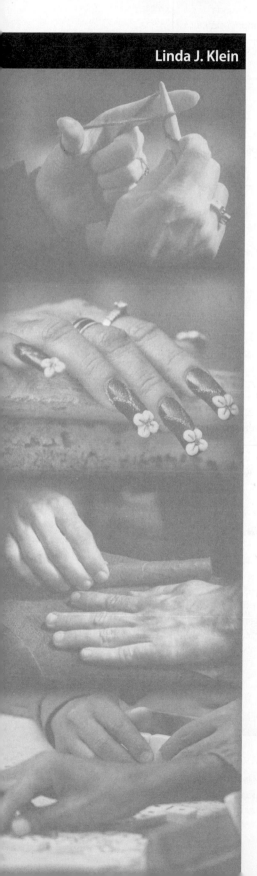

The client's initial evaluation sets the stage for successful rehabilitation. Evaluation establishes rapport, determines areas of functional deficit, and serves as the foundation for treatment and recovery. Only with an accurate assessment can the therapist determine the best course of treatment for the client's condition. A number of assessment processes and clinical assessment skills are needed to perform a thorough evaluation (Fig. 5-1). The main areas of assessment for the injured hand include pain, wound and scar status, vascular status, range of motion (ROM), swelling, sensation, strength, current and previous use of orthotics, and functional limitations. A screening of proximal motion, strength and posture are important to have a full understanding of deficits in the distal upper extremity. Periodic re-evaluations are necessary to show progress, identify new or remaining problems, and redirect goals.

Using an evaluation summary form is helpful (see Appendix 5-1). The form will guide you through each step of the assessment, ensuring that you do not forget any areas. Defer areas of an evaluation when it is not appropriate to perform them at a certain time in the tissue healing process or if the client simply cannot tolerate these procedures. Sometimes an additional specific form is needed for an assessment. For example, the evaluation summary form should have an area listed as sensation even though a separate form is used for sensory tests, including the Semmes-Weinstein monofilament test or two-point discrimination test. On the evaluation summary form, give a brief description that indicates where the client perceives altered sensation, including numbness, tingling, burning, or hypersensitivity. Then use the Semmes-Weinstein monofilament, two-point discrimination, or other sensation forms for more specific and objective information.

The evaluation summary form promotes clinical reasoning and assists the therapist's organization of thoughts and communication with a thorough and logical progression of categories.

Initial Interview

Obtaining a History

Before assessing the function of the client's hand, obtaining a history of the injury or symptoms that bring the client to the therapy clinic is essential. Understanding the onset of symptoms (for example, trauma versus gradual) is essential. Next, ask about any prior medical intervention. Has there been surgery? An injection? X-ray, magnetic resonance imaging, or computed tomography scan? Nerve study? Cast immobilization? Use of orthotics? Medication? Manual tests by the physician? Or has there been no intervention by the physician except to send the client to therapy for the therapist's expertise in evaluation and treatment? Understanding previous care that the client has experienced helps in a number of ways. It gives the client confidence that you understand what has been done, and it builds trust because in many cases you can explain what the physician was attempting to determine with various tests. Having clients develop trust in you leads to gaining their full cooperation and participation in the evaluation and rehabilitation process. In addition to the history of the injury or condition, you must understand the individual's pertinent medical history, because many medical conditions, such as diabetes or peripheral vascular disease, affect the healing process.

Observation

During the initial process of meeting new clients and discussing their history and symptoms, use your observation skills. Observe the client's nonverbal communication, including

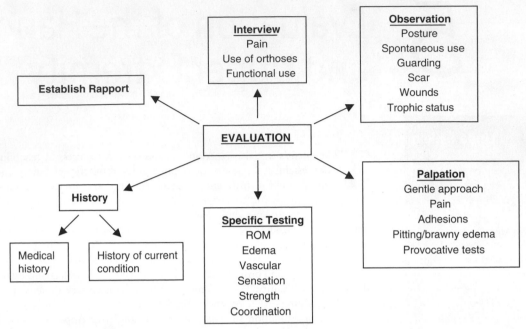

FIGURE 5-1 Summary of the evaluation process. *ROM,* Range of motion.

facial expressions and body language, as well as how the client holds and uses the injured extremity and trunk. The client often guards the injured extremity at the time of initial evaluation, possibly as a subconscious protection from pain. I also have seen situations in which the client guards the extremity or exaggerates limitations, such as strength or motion, during the evaluation to be sure that the therapist recognizes and appreciates the extent of deficit. In these cases, it is sometimes possible to observe them function better during a spontaneous situation than during the formal assessment. For example, a client with an elbow injury who lacks 40 degrees of elbow extension during formal assessment may be seen extending the elbow significantly further while removing or putting on his or her coat. Another example is the client who guards the hand by holding it close to the body during the assessment but uses the hand more freely with gestures during informal discussion.

Observe differences in posture and use of the upper extremity in spontaneous situations compared with formal assessment. This gives clues regarding the client's comfort with the extremity. Use different approaches to elicit the best response from clients who are not comfortable moving freely (see Chapter 15). In my experience, most clients with abnormal posturing (guarding) are unaware of their upper extremity positioning and are eager to change. In contrast, facilitation of positive involvement by clients who may be consciously controlling their responses in therapy is more challenging. I have had some success by reminding these clients that continued therapy is contingent on their showing progress. I have found that use of a nonjudgmental approach, pointing out inconsistencies between formal testing and observation is the most effective approach in this situation. Reinforcing that your goal is to work with the client toward recovery will maximize the client's positive involvement in the rehabilitation process.

In discussing each section of the evaluation, I will describe the tools and process of the evaluation, followed by inconsistencies and difficulties to be aware of, and when that portion of the evaluation should be deferred.

BOX 5-1   Pain Scales

- *Numeric analog scales:* A line with equal markings from 0 to 5, 0 to 10, or 0 to 20 is used to indicate the perceived level of pain at the initial evaluation compared with periodic re-evaluations.
- *Visual analog scale:* Provide the client with a 10-cm line drawn vertically on paper with one end labeled "no pain" and the other end labeled "pain as bad as it could be." The client marks the location and level of pain, and the examiner later divides the line into twenty equal portions to determine the distance from zero to the client's pain mark.
- *Verbal rating scale:* Client describes their pain with four to five descriptive words (for example, mild, moderate, or severe).
- *Graphic representation:* The client marks his or her pain location and type on a body chart.
- *Pain questionnaire:* Written pain questionnaires are available that obtain more information about the client's pain, such as the McGill Pain Questionnaire.[2] These questionnaires are probably used most in specialty centers dealing with management of pain, but the knowledge of the content of specific questionnaires may be helpful to develop your skills in discussing pain during an evaluation.

Assessment of Pain

Equipment

No equipment is necessary, but you may choose to use a pain scale during initial evaluation to summarize the client's overall perception of pain. Numerous pain scales are available (Box 5-1).[1]

Methods

Obtain a verbal or written description by the client regarding the level of pain, location, type of pain, frequency or cause, and duration of pain. Also document when pain occurs during other parts of the evaluation, such as with active range of motion (AROM) or passive range of motion (PROM), strength testing, or palpation:

- *Level of pain:* Using a pain scale, have the client describe the pain at its worst on the scale and then at its best, and also obtain an average pain level. Most often, I use the 0-to-10 pain scale or the verbal rating scale of mild, moderate, or severe. Documentation can then be done accordingly; for instance, "Pain is described as varying from mild at best to severe at worst."
- *Location of pain:* Have the client point to the area(s) of pain. For clients with a more diffuse pain that may involve more of the upper extremity, I use a body chart on which the client can circle the areas that hurt and rate each area if desired. When a client has **referred pain**—for instance, when palpation of one area results in pain in another area—this is best documented on a body chart as well. Referred pain can occur for a number of reasons, such as following a nerve injury where pain may be felt proximal or distal to the site of injury of the nerve.
- *Type of pain:* Ask the client to describe the pain as throbbing, aching, sharp, stabbing, shooting, burning, or hypersensitive to light touch.
- *Frequency or cause of pain:* Determine whether the pain is constant or intermittent. Have the client describe when the pain occurs and what seems to cause the pain. This information is helpful in determining a diagnosis if the physician has not provided a firm diagnosis.
- *Duration of pain:* Determine how long the pain has been present.

◎ Clinical Pearl

Pain in an area for longer than 6 months often is classified as chronic pain, as opposed to acute pain experienced following a recent injury.

- *Chronic pain:* Chronic pain often is associated with depression, anxiety, and other psychological involvement and may be helped best by a team approach with specialists in the area of chronic pain management.
- *Pain levels:* Note pain levels that occur during the evaluation, such as pain during AROM, PROM or strength testing. For instance, my evaluation might state, "Strength: Grip strength right hand 100#, left hand 50# with moderate pain identified in left volar wrist with grip." I may have a goal to reflect this in my initial evaluation note, such as "Increase left hand grip strength to 75# without pain." Tendonitis is more often associated with pain on AROM than PROM in the direction of motion of the involved muscle/tendon. Thus distinctions about pain during evaluation become part of the clinical reasoning and treatment process.

Discussion

I usually begin my assessment of a new client's injury by discussing the client's pain and reassuring the client that the evaluation is not intended to worsen the pain. As soon as the client has the opportunity to tell me about his or her pain, I see a level of relief develop. Many clients are apprehensive about attending therapy, concerned that the therapist may perform painful, provocative tests, might touch or grasp a sensitive or tender area or move the extremity beyond comfort. Knowing that the therapist is aware of the pain helps the client relax and participate in the rest of the evaluation process.

Clinical Problem Solving

At times, the therapist is not given a firm diagnosis by the referring physician and may be instructed to evaluate and treat for hand, wrist, elbow, or shoulder pain. The location of pain and whether pain occurs with active or passive motion can give the therapist clues as to the cause of the pain. Use provocative testing for specific conditions with the goal of reproducing the pain complaint for nerve compressions and tendonitis or tendinopathy (see Chapters 24 and 28).

Consider the following:

- Pain with AROM that is not present with PROM most likely is caused by a problem with the muscle or tendon.
- Pain with PROM is more likely due to a joint problem, such as tightness of the joint structures, ligament injury, cartilage injury, or inflammation (pain may be present equally with AROM in these situations).
- When a joint is limited in motion because of pain, and pain is present with distraction of the joint but not compression of the joint, pain is most likely due to a ligament or joint capsule being stretched with distraction and relieved with compression.
- If pain is present with compression of the joint but is relieved with distraction, pain is more likely due to a problem at the joint surface, such as thinning or loss of cartilage, inflammation within the joint or other abnormality, such as a bone spur.

Precaution. Aggressive clinical problem-solving methods can be used safely only when the physician has allowed AROM and PROM as part of treatment. These methods are not appropriate in the acute phase following a tendon, nerve, or ligament repair or tendon transfer.

Wound Assessment

Open wounds can be intimidating. Breaking the assessment down to wound size, depth, color, drainage, and odor is helpful (see Chapter 21). When wounds are closed, it is appropriate to skip this section and go on to scar assessment.

Consider the following:

- *Size:* Measure length and width with a ruler. Make a tracing of the wound for future comparison, or use transparent calibrated grids. Do not touch the wound with the ruler or other measuring device unless the item is sterile.
- *Depth:* Wound depth may be measured with a sterile cotton swab if the client and therapist are comfortable with this procedure.
- *Color:* Open wounds are referred to as red, yellow, or black.[3,4] Many wounds have a combination of these colors, and wounds progress through stages of these colors.
  - *Red wound:* Wound may be a superficial wound, second-degree burn, acute fresh wound, surgical wound, or a wound left open to heal by **secondary intention,** which is the process by which an open wound heals with granulation and new blood vessel formation.

- *Yellow wound:* Semiliquid to liquid slough (**exudate**) is present. Color ranges from cream to yellow. Pink or red **granulation tissue** usually is seen at the edges of or under the yellow tissue. Yellow tissue may facilitate infection. Yellow wounds are often in the late **inflammatory phase** or early **fibroplasia phase** and include exudates.
- *Black wound:* Wound characterized by necrotic black, brown, or gray tissue or thick **eschar** (layer of necrotic collagen over a wound). Pus may form at the edges because of **macrophage** (cell that assists in cleaning the wound of necrotic tissue and debris) activity. New granulation tissue forms under the eschar. If bacterial infection forms under the eschar, the wound edges can become red, painful, and swollen. The wound may be in all stages of wound repair, with inflammation present while macrophages remove necrotic debris, fibroblasts lay down new collagen under the eschar, **angiogenesis** (new vessels in the tissue of a healing open wound) begins to occur, and the wound tries to contract despite being blocked by eschar.

> ### ◎ Clinical Pearl
> Wounds almost always have more than one color present at one time. Treat the worst stage first; that is, progress from treatment of black to yellow and then yellow to red.

- *Drainage:* Attempt to quantify the amount of drainage (mild, moderate, heavy) and color of drainage. Clear, pink, or white drainage does not indicate presence of infection. Exudate may have a yellow color and may or may not indicate infection.

> ### ◎ Clinical Pearl
> If there is any question of the possibility of infection, have the drainage examined by a physician.

- *Odor:* Odors often indicate infection. Note any odor emanating from the wound, and have the wound assessed by a physician for potential infection.
- *Temperature:* Surface thermometers or temperature tapes can be used to compare temperature of an area near the wound with an unaffected area.

Scar Assessment

The characteristics to assess for scar status include color, size, whether it is flattened or raised, and the presence of **adhesion** (attachment) to underlying or surrounding tissue.

Consider the following:
- *Color:* Scars usually begin as deep red and gradually become lighter as time progresses.
- *Size:* Use a ruler to measure the length and width of the scar.
- *Flat/raised:* Use observation and palpation to assess how far the scar is raised above the skin level, and describe it using terms like *mild* or *moderate.* Sometimes the superficial scar may be flat, but there may be a lump under the skin. This happens most commonly on the dorsum of the hand or wrist with a lump under the surface scar that is a thickening composed of a combination of scar and fluid. This lump of scar and fluid can be described by size and height (for example, dorsal incisional scar is 3 cm in length

along the third metacarpal, with a thickened area under the skin of 3 mm in height and 2 to 3 mm in width surrounding the scar).
- *Adhesions:* Assessment of adhesions of surface scars to underlying tissue is done by observation and palpation. Some adhesions can be seen during active motion. When the adhesion is on the dorsal hand or wrist or the volar wrist/forearm, the scar is often seen to dip deeper, or dimple, when active motion is attempted because of adhesions from the superficial scar to underlying fascia and tendons. Also assess adhesions of skin to underlying tissue by palpation. Attempt to slide or lift the scar tissue in a manner similar to the surrounding uninjured tissue, and describe the level of adhesion as mild, moderate, or severely adherent.

Precaution. *Respect the level of healing of a new scar and the tissue to which it may adhere. Avoid aggressively attempting to move scar tissue within the first week following suture removal or when a portion of the wound is still open. Doing so may cause damage to fragile, healing tissue or possibly may reopen the wound. Avoid strong scar manipulation during assessment or treatment over a tendon in the early phase of healing.*

Vascular Status Assessment

A basic vascular evaluation of the hand can be done by observation (color or **trophic** changes, pain level), palpation (pulse, capillary refill assessment, modified Allen's test), and temperature assessment. Blood flow to the hand can be affected by proximal injury or diagnoses, such as thoracic outlet syndrome, injury to the hand itself, or conditions like Raynaud's phenomenon. Proximal conditions, such as thoracic outlet syndrome, are discussed in the Chapter 22.

Observation

Observation includes assessment of color and trophic changes in the hand. Increased levels of white (**pallor**), blue (**cyanosis**), or red (**erythema**) coloration of the skin are the most common changes noted.

> ### ◎ Clinical Pearl
> Arterial interruption usually produces a white or grayish discoloration of the affected area (pallor), whereas venous blockage produces a congested, purple-blue color.[5] Dusky blue may indicate chronic venous insufficiency. Redness may indicate loss of outflow of blood from the hand or a venous problem, but it also may be an indication of a normal inflammatory phase of wound healing or the presence of infection.

Trophic changes refer to the texture of the skin and nail. Changes in the trophic status can occur from sympathetic nerve or vascular changes. Note the presence of increased dryness or moisture of the skin of the involved hand and the presence of open wounds or necrotic tissue at the initial evaluation. Reevaluate these items frequently for improvement.

Pain is present in two-thirds of clients with upper extremity vascular disease.[6] Pain may be described as aching, cramping, tightness, or cold intolerance. Pain may be associated with activity that includes exposure to vibration, cold, or repetition.

Precaution. *Close monitoring of color and temperature change is important, and communication with the referring physician is* *recommended if abnormalities are worsening or not improving. Causes of vascular abnormalities are numerous, and in-depth evaluation and testing by the physician may be indicated.*

Palpation Tests of Vascular Status

Capillary Refill Test

To perform the capillary refill test, place pressure on the distal portion of the volar finger or over the fingernail of the digit until tissue turns white.[5,6] Capillary refill time is the number of seconds it takes for the color to return to normal after the pressure is released. Normal capillary refill time is less than 2 seconds, and the time can be compared with the same digit on the opposite hand or with uninjured digits.

Peripheral Pulse Palpation

Place light pressure over the radial artery or ulnar artery just proximal to the wrist crease to gain information about the strength of the pulse or blood flow to the hand.[7] If the pulse is weaker in one wrist than the other, there may be a potential problem with blood flow proximal to the wrist. Palpation of peripheral pulse is used frequently for assessing proximal vascular diagnoses, such as thoracic outlet syndrome. Check the pulse before and after exercise in certain positions to determine whether position or exercise diminish blood flow to the distal upper extremity. Refer to Chapter 22 for more information on specialized testing.

Modified Allen's Test

The modified Allen's test assesses the status of the blood supply within the hand through the ulnar and radial arteries of the wrist.[5,8] To perform the test, place firm pressure over the radial and ulnar arteries just proximal to the wrist crease. Instruct the client to make a tight fist and then open the fingers repeatedly until the palm turns white. Then instruct the client to relax the fingers to a partially opened position. Release the pressure from one side of the wrist, allowing blood flow through one of the arteries. Record the time it takes for the color to return to normal in the hand. Repeat the process, releasing pressure from the artery on the opposite side of the wrist. Record the time it takes for the color to return to normal in the hand. A normal response is 5 seconds or less and can be compared to the opposite extremity to confirm a normal response time for that individual.

Surface Temperature Assessment

Surface thermometers can be used to compare forearm temperature to fingertip temperature. If the forearm is at least 4° C (39° F) warmer than the fingertip surface, it may indicate vascular compromise. Assess Raynaud's phenomenon with a temperature assessment that measures the temperature of the involved fingertip(s) after being in a warm room (24° C [75° F]) for 30 minutes and then after being immersed in ice water for 20 seconds. Record the time it takes to return to the baseline temperature. The normal time for return to body temperature is within 10 minutes, but clients with Raynaud's phenomenon may take 20 to 45 minutes.[7]

Range of Motion Assessment

Assessment of ROM in this chapter is limited to the forearm, wrist, fingers, and thumb. A variety of ways to assess ROM are available and have resulted in the effort by the American Society of Hand Therapists to standardize this process.[9] This method is discussed later in this chapter; however, variations exist that are acceptable, and we should refer to recognized ROM references[10,11] when becoming familiar with ROM testing. All ROM of the forearm, wrist, and hand is performed with the client in the seated position. Clinical problem solving that interprets the cause of the limited ROM (for example, joint stiffness, **intrinsic tightness** which limits simultaneous MP extension and IP flexion, and **extrinsic tendon tightness** which limits composite wrist and digit motion in the same direction) is important for determining the most appropriate treatment.

Methods

Passive Range of Motion

PROM is the ability of a joint to be moved through its normal arc of motion while relaxed, with motion being performed by an outside source, such as the therapist's hand, the client's opposite hand, or gravity. Limitations in PROM indicate a problem within the joint (for example, stiffness caused by capsular or ligamentous tightness, decreased joint space, or bone spur). PROM also may be limited by tightness of the muscle/tendon group opposing the passive motion (for example, a tight or adherent extensor muscle/tendon will prevent full passive or active flexion).

    Precaution. *Traumatic injuries to the bone or joint in the acute phase of healing, or as determined by the physician, are limited to AROM, with no PROM allowed. PROM by an outside source may be performed too strongly, reinjuring the healing bone or ligament. Following a tendon repair in the early phase of tendon healing, PROM in the direction that would stretch the tendon is not allowed.*

Active Range of Motion

AROM is motion of a joint caused by musculotendinous contraction, most often from a voluntary muscle contraction. Limitations in AROM can result from a number of causes. Some of these causes include weakness of the muscle, loss of tendon continuity, adhesions of the tendon preventing its motion, inflammation or constriction of the tendon, decreased tendon mechanical efficiency because of loss of pulley (bowstringing), and disrupted nerve supply to the muscle.

    Precaution. *AROM using a repaired tendon (that is, contracting a repaired muscle/tendon) is not allowed following some tendon repairs or tendon transfers in the acute phase of tendon healing. This restriction lasts for approximately the first 4 weeks after the repair unless the type of repair performed by the surgeon allows use of an immediate active-motion protocol. Please refer to Chapters 30 and 31.*

    You must recognize that AROM or PROM also may be limited by pain. If the client describes pain during ROM testing, note this on the evaluation form.

    When there is no medical limitation regarding use of AROM and PROM, it is important to do the following:

- Measure passive and active motion for information that helps determine the cause of limitation.
- Compare ROM to the other hand to learn what is normal for that individual.
- Measure ROM at a consistent time or sequence in the treatment session (for example, before or after exercise) for a more accurate reading of improvement.

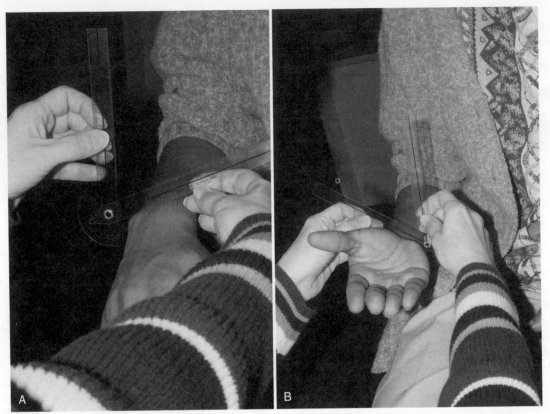

FIGURE 5-2 A, Pronation as measured with a standard 6-inch goniometer, demonstrating axis of motion on the dorsal distal ulna. **B,** Supination as measured with a standard 6-inch goniometer, demonstrating axis of motion on the volar distal ulna.

• Be consistent in position of hand and proximal joints. For instance, it is more difficult to perform finger flexion when the wrist is flexed compared with when the wrist is extended. When the extensors are adherent, each individual digital joint measured alone or independently will flex further than when all three finger joints are flexed at the same time.

Total Active Motion

Total active motion (TAM) is used to describe the full arc of active motion of the digit(s). TAM is measured as the total flexion of all three finger joints, subtracting any loss of full extension at all finger joints:

(MP + PIP + DIP flexion) - (MP + PIP + DIP extension loss) = TAM

where *MP* is metacarpophalangeal, *PIP* is proximal interphalangeal, and *DIP* is distal interphalangeal.

> ### ◎ *Clinical Pearl*
> Use TAM when reporting ROM in situations where tendon adhesions limit motion and composite motion is more limited than individual joint motion.

Total Passive Motion

Total passive motion (TPM) is the same process as TAM but is measured passively. This can be helpful to document the presence of adhesions.

> ### ◎ *Clinical Pearl*
> When flexor tendon gliding is limited by adhesions, TPM will be better than TAM.

Standard plastic goniometers work well for measurement. Large goniometers (12¼ inches) are recommended for the larger elbow and shoulder joints. Standard goniometers (6 to 7 inches) are used for measuring the forearm and wrist (Figs. 5-2 and 5-3). They can be cut down in length to measure finger ROM (Fig. 5-4). Metal finger goniometers are available at a higher cost and do not have the benefit of transparency when lateral placement is needed. Electronic and computer system goniometers are available at a much higher cost. For the wrist, I prefer the 6-inch goniometer with rounded ends because it allows dorsal placement on the wrist for flexion and extension (Fig. 5-5).

Hyperextension of the fingers is recorded with a plus sign (+), loss of full extension with a minus sign (−). When standard placement of the goniometer is not used because of scar, swelling, or wound, document the modified placement of the goniometer for future reference to allow for accurate comparative measurements.

Forearm Range of Motion

Consider the following for forearm ROM:
• Motions of the forearm are pronation and supination.
• Starting position is with the arm adducted at the side, elbow flexed to 90 degrees, forearm and wrist neutral.

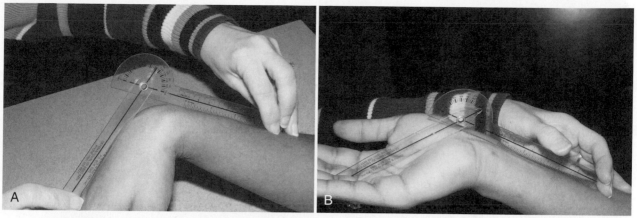

FIGURE 5-3 A, Wrist flexion measured dorsally over the central wrist with a standard 6-inch goniometer. **B,** Wrist extension measured along the volar surface over the central wrist with a standard 6-inch goniometer.

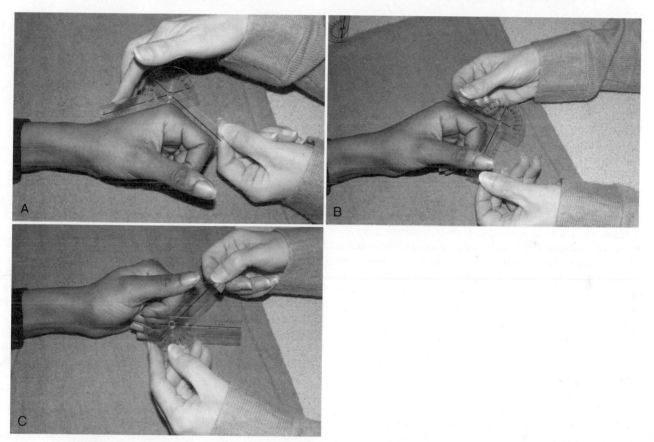

FIGURE 5-4 Finger flexion measured dorsally with a standard 6-inch goniometer that has been cut down in length. **A,** Demonstrates metacarpophalangeal (MP) flexion; **B,** demonstrates proximal interphalangeal (PIP) flexion; and **C,** demonstrates distal interphalangeal (DIP) flexion. Note the placement of the goniometer arms to allow DIP flexion to be measured in a composite flexion position.

- Axis of motion is the ulnar edge of the forearm, dorsally for pronation, and along the volar surface for supination.
- Placement of the goniometer is with both arms of the goniometer across the distal forearm, dorsally with axis placed at the lateral edge of the dorsal ulna for pronation, and along the volar surface of the distal forearm, with axis placed at the lateral edge of the volar ulna for supination.
- To measure pronation, one arm of the goniometer stays in place in the starting position (straight up), while the other

arm of the goniometer stays in contact with the dorsal distal forearm as it moves into pronation. The stationary arm of the goniometer, which stays in the starting position, is now straight up and should be aligned with the humerus if the client has maintained the correct starting position of the trunk and arm. The moving arm of the goniometer is to stay flat on the dorsum of the distal forearm, flush with the center of the distal forearm, between the ulna and radius (see Fig. 5-2, *A*).

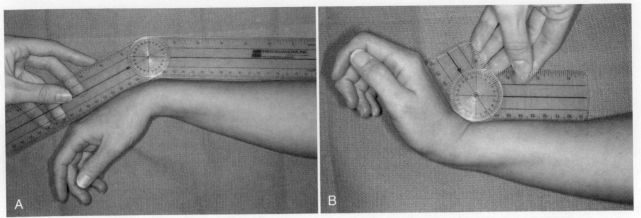

FIGURE 5-5 A, Alternate goniometer for wrist flexion, measured dorsally over the central wrist. **B,** Alternate goniometer with rounded ends used for wrist extension measured dorsally over the central wrist.

- To measure supination, one arm of the goniometer stays in place in the starting position (straight up), while the other arm stays in contact with the volar distal forearm as it moves into supination. The stationary arm of the goniometer, which stays in the starting position is now straight up and should be aligned with the humerus if the client has maintained the correct starting position of the trunk and arm. The moving arm of the goniometer is flush on the center of the volar forearm on the flattest portion of the midvolar forearm (see Fig. 5-2, *B*).

- If the humerus is not straight up and down due to body composition, I prefer to align the stationary arm of the goniometer with the humerus. This will provide an accurate measurement of forearm motion in relation to the humerus. It is important to perform the test in the same manner on retest.

- Frequent errors are made when measuring pronation and supination by allowing the goniometer to overturn and measure more along the distal radius or under-turn and measure more along the distal ulna, rather than correctly on the middle section of the distal forearm. Other common errors are to allow the client to lean or move the arm away from the starting position of humeral adduction against the side of the body. Feedback from an experienced therapist is helpful when learning to measure forearm motion.

Wrist Range of Motion

Consider the following for wrist ROM:
- Motions of the wrist are flexion, extension, radial deviation, and ulnar deviation.
- Starting position is with wrist neutral.
- Axis of motion is the center of the wrist.
- Placement of the goniometer according to American Society of Hand Therapists recommendations are along the volar surface for extension, dorsally for flexion, and dorsally for radial deviation and ulnar deviation. Lateral placement is appropriate when scar or swelling make dorsal or volar placements inaccurate.
- To measure flexion, place one arm of the goniometer along the dorsum of the forearm and the other arm along the third metacarpal on the dorsum of the hand (see Fig. 5-3, *A*).
- To measure extension, place one arm of the goniometer along the volar forearm and the other arm along the third metacarpal on the palmar side of the hand (see Fig. 5-3, *B*).

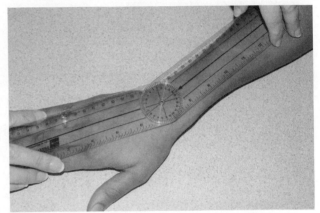

FIGURE 5-6 Wrist ulnar deviation measured dorsally.

- To measure radial and ulnar deviation, with hand flat on a table surface, place the goniometer flat on its side, one arm of the goniometer on the dorsum of the forearm, axis at the center of the wrist, and the other arm of the goniometer along the third metacarpal (Fig. 5-6).

Volar placement of the goniometer on the palm to measure wrist extension may be difficult because the goniometer does not lay flat on the many curves in the palm. A goniometer with rounded ends (see Fig. 5-5), which is available in many therapy supply catalogs, allows dorsal placement of the goniometer to measure flexion and extension of the wrist.

Digital Range of Motion

The MP, PIP joints, DIP joints of the fingers, and MP and interphalangeal (IP) joints of the thumb are measured with the same procedure and are described together next:
- Motions of the finger and thumb MP and IP joints are flexion and extension. The MP joints of the fingers also perform abduction and adduction, and although this can be assessed with goniometric measurements,[11] a tracing of the hand with the fingers fully abducted is also an effective way to show change over time.
- Starting position for measuring flexion and extension of the digit is extension. Neutral wrist is recommended for consistency in procedure.

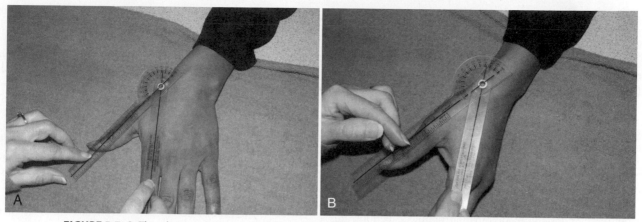

FIGURE 5-7 A, Thumb carpometacarpal (CMC) radial abduction measured dorsally with a standard 6-inch goniometer. **B,** Thumb CMC palmar abduction measured radially with a standard 6-inch goniometer.

- Axis of motion is centrally over the dorsum of the joint being measured.
- Placement of the goniometer for all finger measurements is on the dorsal surface. The MP joint is measured with one arm of the goniometer along the metacarpal, and the other arm of the goniometer along the proximal phalanx, with the axis at the dorsal MP (see Fig. 5-4, *A*). Placement of the goniometer for the PIP joint is with one arm of the goniometer on the proximal phalanx and the other arm on the middle phalanx (see Fig. 5-4, *B*). Placement for the DIP joints is with one arm of the goniometer on the middle phalanx and the other arm on the distal phalanx (see Fig. 5-4, *C*). Alternate placement of the goniometer is laterally along the finger if there is a lump or other abnormality preventing dorsal placement.
- To measure motion, note the maximal extension at each joint, and when moving into flexion, move the distal arm of the goniometer to maintain its position on the dorsum of the finger section noted before. Note the degree of flexion attained. If loss of full extension is present, record it with a minus sign (−); for example, −25 to 50 degrees MP motion means there was a loss of 25 degrees of extension and the joint was able to flex to 50 degrees of flexion. For hyperextension, use a plus sign (+): +25 to 50 degrees MP motion means there is 25 degrees of hyperextension at the MP joint and the joint was able to flex to 50 degrees of flexion.

Hyperextension is difficult to measure with the standard 6-inch goniometer or 6-inch goniometer cut down in length, and lateral placement is necessary for this measurement. The goniometer style with rounded ends described in the discussion section of wrist ROM (see Fig. 5-5) can be used to measure hyperextension of the digit joints with dorsal placement.

> ### ◎ *Clinical Pearl*
>
> Measurement of each digit in composite flexion and extension (TAM) is important during the initial evaluation.

Each joint may be near normal if measured in isolation, but significant limitation in ROM may be evident when total active flexion and extension are measured, due to tendon gliding or scar tissue limitations. The TAM of the digit measured in composite flexion and extension indicates the functional limitations of motion. Functional limitations of motion also can be demonstrated by measuring the distance, during a composite fist, from the fingertip pulp to the distal palmar crease of the hand.

Thumb Carpometacarpal Joint

Consider the following:
- Motions include palmar abduction, radial abduction, adduction, and opposition.
- Axis of motion is the intersection of lines extending down the first and second metacarpals on the dorsal radial aspect of the hand.
- Starting position is with the forearm pronated with hand flat on table for radial abduction or with the ulnar side of the hand on the table, forearm neutral for palmar abduction or opposition. The thumb is adducted to be flat along the side of the index finger.
- Placement of the goniometer is with one arm placed along the second metacarpal and the other arm placed along the first metacarpal, dorsally for radial abduction and radially for palmar abduction. The axis of the goniometer will be located at the first carpometacarpal (CMC) joint, where the first metacarpal articulates with the trapezium and trapezoid.
- To measure radial abduction, the goniometer arm placed over the second metacarpal is stationary, and the goniometer arm placed over the first metacarpal moves, staying in alignment over the first metacarpal as the thumb moves into radial abduction (Fig. 5-7, *A*).
- To measure palmar abduction, the goniometer arm placed on the radial side of the second metacarpal is stationary, and the goniometer arm placed on the dorsal first metacarpal moves, staying in alignment over the first metacarpal as the thumb moves into palmar abduction (see Fig. 5-7, *B*).
- Opposition can be assessed in a number of ways. One source recommends using a ruler to measure the distance from the volar IP joint of the thumb to the third metacarpal with the nail parallel to the plane of the palm when the thumb is in opposition.[9] Other sources suggest measuring opposition as the distance between the thumb tip and the base of the small finger.[10] Still others suggest having the patient touch the tip of the small finger with the thumb and assessing whether the nail of the thumb is perpendicular to the nail of the small finger and parallel to the plane of the metacarpals.[11] This is the method that I prefer to use. Because there are a number of

different ways to assess opposition, it is important to define the method used in the documentation and be consistent when retesting.

Thumb CMC joint ROM testing is difficult to perform consistently because placement of both arms of the goniometer is done using visual judgment of the therapist. Placing the goniometer arms correctly over the first and second metacarpal with the axis at the CMC joint can be difficult, and practice with an experienced therapist is recommended.

Clinical Problem Solving

When ROM of the digits is limited, it is important to determine whether the limited ROM is due to joint stiffness, extrinsic tendon tightness or adhesions, or intrinsic tightness. Perform this type of assessment as soon as active and passive motion is allowed because it dictates the most appropriate type of treatment by determining the limiting structure(s).

Follow these steps:

- *Step 1:* Measure and record composite flexion and composite extension of the digits with the wrist in neutral to slight extension.
- *Step 2:* Compare composite flexion and extension of the fingers with the wrist fully extended and fully flexed (to determine whether extrinsic tendon tightness or adhesions are present).
- *Step 3:* Screen ROM of each finger joint separately with the proximal joints supported in neutral (to determine whether limited motion is isolated to the joint, regardless of the position of the proximal joints).
- *Step 4:* Perform passive motion of the digits. Comparison of passive motion to active motion provides information regarding tendon adhesions that may be limiting active motion.

The following is a description of the causes of finger joint motion limitations in each of the screened positions:

- If AROM of a joint is the same as PROM, and the motion is the same regardless of the position of proximal joints, the limitation is due to joint stiffness.
- If passive flexion is better than active flexion, the limited active flexion is due to weak or paralyzed flexor muscles, or flexor tendon adhesion or rupture.
- If passive extension is better than active extension, the limited active extension is due to weak or paralyzed extensor muscles, or extensor tendon adhesion or rupture.
- If active and passive flexion are equal, and flexion is better with the proximal joint(s) in extension than with the proximal joint(s) in flexion, the limited flexion is due to extrinsic extensor tendon tightness or adhesions.
- If active and passive extension is equal and extension is better with the proximal joint(s) in flexion than extension, the limited extension is due to extrinsic flexor tendon tightness or adhesions.
- If the IP joints of the finger can be flexed passively further with the MPl joint flexed than when the MP joint is extended, the limitation is due to intrinsic tightness.

Treatment choices can be made accordingly. For example, when limited flexion is due to tight or adherent extensor tendons, treatment should address the extensor tendon length and ability to glide, not the motion at individual joints. This type of situation occurs frequently following an open reduction and internal fixation of a metacarpal fracture with scar tissue adhesions to underlying extensor tendons. My treatment choice would include applying heat over the hand that is placed in a composite flexion position with a wrap that supports the flexed fingers in a comfortable stretch. Following the heat treatment with the tissue in its lengthened position, manual techniques would include massage to the dorsal scar that is adherent to the extensor tendons and ROM exercises emphasizing composite flexion of the fingers distal to the site of adhesion. I would not choose to do joint mobilization or individual joint stretches, ultrasound, or heat to an individual joint. However, if the assessment shows individual joint stiffness, my treatment choice would include joint mobilization (when passive motion is allowed), modalities to the limiting joint structures, as well as AROM and PROM of the individual joint and composite motion to encourage functional use of the injured hand.

Swelling

Swelling of the hand occurs after every surgery or injury to some extent and is the normal response of the body to injury, bringing cells that are important for healing to the injured area. Normal reduction of swelling begins within 2 weeks of the injury or surgery but may take a number of months to complete. Excessive edema or edema that is not decreasing gradually but instead remains in an area longer than 2 weeks can become problematic because it becomes more like gel, interfering with joint and tendon motion and functional use of the hand.

Precaution. *Awareness of edema and assessment of the amount and characteristics of edema present are critical.*

As discussed in Chapter 3, numerous types of swelling occur in the extremity. Inflammatory edema that occurs after injury, surgery, or other insult is initially fluid but over time may become spongy and eventually fibrotic and thus more resistant to methods aimed at reducing the swelling.

Amount of Swelling

The amount of swelling in the hand and wrist is assessed most often using circumferential and volumetric measurements. The characteristics of edema typically are evaluated by observation and palpation.

Volumetric Displacement

Equipment
The volumeter kit available in supply catalogues includes the volumeter tank, a collection beaker, and graduated cylinder for measuring the displaced water. A hand volumeter and arm volumeter are available.

Method
Always use the same level surface for each test. The client's hand must be free of jewelry or other objects. If jewelry cannot be removed, document such.

Follow these steps:[12]

Step 1: Fill the volumeter with room temperature water to the point of overflow, to allow an accurate starting point. Allow excess water to flow out into a beaker, and then empty the beaker.

Step 2: Position the hand so that the palm faces the client and the thumb faces the spout of the volumeter. Keep the hand as vertical as possible; avoid contact with sides of volumeter

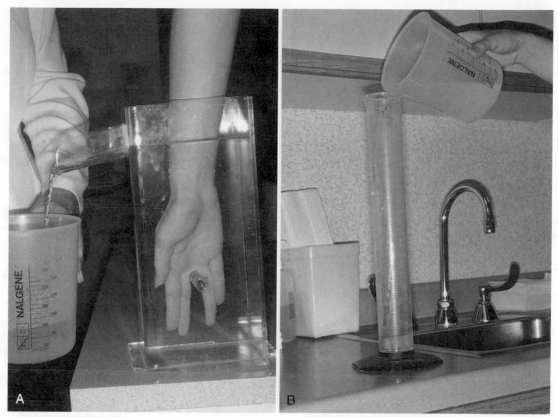

FIGURE 5-8 A, Edema measurement using the volumeter. The water that is displaced by immersion of the hand and distal forearm into the volumeter overflows into a collection beaker. **B,** Volumeter measurement is completed when the water from the collection beaker is poured into a graduated cylinder for accurate reading.

(surfaces that are too high prevent the client from placing the arm straight down into the volumeter).

Step 3: Lower the hand slowly into the volumeter until the dowel in the volumeter is firmly seated between the middle and ring fingers. Collect the displaced water in the beaker. Hold the hand still in the volumeter until water stops dripping into the collection beaker (Fig. 5-8, *A*).

Step 4: Pour the displaced water from the beaker into the graduated cylinder for final measurement (see Fig. 5-8, *B*).

Step 5: Repeat the previous steps if you would like to average results for increased accuracy.

Step 6: Compare the volume to the other hand to determine a relative normal for the individual and to determine whether a systemic increase in volume is occurring. The difference between the two extremities is the most valuable information because there is a normal daily variance in volume, even in uninjured extremities. This test has been determined to be accurate to 5 mL, or 1% of the volume of the hand. Therefore a 10-mL difference is considered a significant change from one measurement to the next.[13]

Precaution. *Volumetric measurement should not be performed with open wounds, with an unstable vascular status, casts, external fixators, percutaneous pins, or other nonremovable supports or attachments to the extremity.*

Discussion

To increase reliability with volumetric testing, it has been helpful in my experience to use a waterproof marker to mark the spot on the forearm at the edge of the water when it is lowered into the water on the first trial. When swelling is reduced, it is possible for the hand and forearm to be lowered further into the volumeter because the web space between the fingers that is used as a stopping point against the dowel may deepen as swelling reduces. Thus there are times when I see a significant decrease in edema of the hand; however, because the forearm is lowering deeper into the volumeter, there is little if any change in the volumeter reading. Ensuring that the hand and forearm are lowered to the same depth on each repeat test minimizes this variable.

Circumferential Measurement

Equipment

Tape measure or tape measure/loop for finger circumference is available in catalogs. When measuring circumference, identify the area being measured in relation to anatomic landmarks, and use the same amount of tension on the tape measure for each test.

Method

Follow these steps:

Step 1: Apply tape measure around area to be measured.

Step 2: Tighten lightly (Fig. 5-9).

Step 3: Record the circumference. Be sure to note exactly where tape was placed; for example, 4 cm proximal to radial styloid, around radial styloid and distal ulna, proximal phalanx, or PIP joint. Note positioning, such as elbow flexed or extended, wrist neutral, or fingers relaxed or extended.

Discussion

Consistency of repeat measurements with a tape measure is difficult because the tightness with which the tape measure is applied can vary with each application. Having the same therapist perform repeat measurements can help decrease variability of tightness.

Characteristics of Edema

Observation

The skin becomes shiny and more taut with loss of wrinkles or joint creases when there is an increase in swelling. A description of the appearance of the skin may be documented. The evaluation form may have a checklist to choose from a variety of options, such as shiny, dry, and partial or full loss of joint creases. The color of the skin is also helpful to document and can be described as having increased redness (erythema), bluish tinge (cyanosis), or pallor (loss of normal color).

Palpation

Pressure with the examiner's finger into the swollen area may allow an indent into the swelling and may provide feedback as to the firmness of the swelling. If the examiner's finger is able to push into a soft edema fairly quickly, it is characterized as **pitting edema,** which is made up of large amounts of free fluid in the

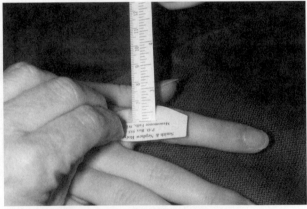

FIGURE 5-9 Edema measured using circumferential finger tape available in therapy supply catalogs.

tissue that can be displaced by pressure, leaving a pit that slowly fills back up when the pressure is removed[14] (Fig. 5-10).

As the edema becomes more spongy and gel-like, it will refill more slowly than fluid edema. As time goes on, if the edema becomes very firm, it will decrease the ability of the fluid to move out of the way with pressure and no longer will be pitting. The more firm edema is characterized as **brawny edema** and usually is caused by the interstitial fluid becoming clogged, preventing it from moving easily.[12] The terms *mild, moderate,* and *severe* can be used to quantify the extent of the pitting or brawny characteristic; however, this is a subjective observation made by the examiner.

Sensation

Static Two-Point Discrimination

The static two-point discrimination test measures **innervation density** (the number of nerve endings present in the area tested). Flexor zones I and II are tested (the area between the distal palmar crease and the fingertips). Two-point discrimination determines the ability to discern the difference between one and two points and relates to clients' ability to determine not only *if* they can feel something but also *what* they are feeling.

Equipment

The device used for this test is the Disk-Criminator, also known as the Boley gauge, and is available in therapy supply catalogs.

Method

Follow these steps:[15,16]

Step 1: Instruct the client to respond to each touch, with vision occluded, by saying "one point" or "two points."

Step 2: Support the client's hand to avoid movement of fingers when touched by the point(s). Putty commonly is used as a support for the fingers.

Step 3: Occlude the client's vision. Begin at 5 mm. Touch the client's fingertip with one or two points, randomly applied (Fig. 5-11).

Step 4: The force of the touch pressure is just to the point of blanching, in a longitudinal direction to avoid crossing digital nerve innervation in the finger, perpendicular to the skin.

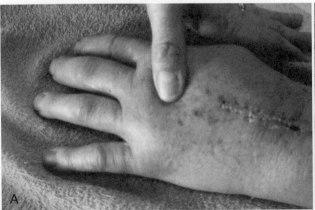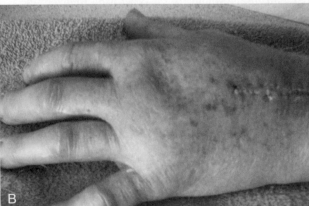

FIGURE 5-10 A and **B,** Pitting edema is seen when pressure from the examiner's finger leaves an indent, or "pit," when removed.

Step 5: Increase or decrease the distance between the two points. If the client is unable to discriminate two points correctly at 5 mm, increase the distance between the points. If the client is able to discriminate two points correctly at 5 mm, decrease the distance, and continue until you have determined the smallest distance the client can discriminate as two points.

Step 6: Begin distally and work proximally from fingertips to distal palmar crease.

Discussion

Seven out of ten correct responses in one area are required for a correct response. Box 5-2 describes two-point discrimination scoring.

Moving Two-Point Discrimination

According to Dellon,[17] moving two-point discrimination always returns earlier than static two-point discrimination after nerve laceration, and it approaches normal 2 to 6 months before static two-point discrimination. This test is used to determine progress in return of sensation following nerve injury.

Equipment

The device used for this test is the Disk-Criminator, or Boley gauge.

Method

Follow these steps:[17]

Step 1: Describe the test to the client.

Step 2: Fully support the client's hand.

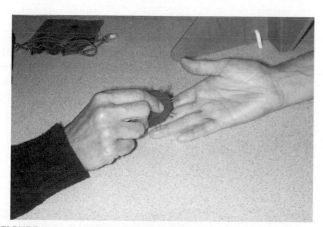

FIGURE 5-11 Two-point discrimination test is performed with the points placed longitudinally onto the skin of the fingertips with pressure just to the point of blanching.

BOX 5-2   **Static Two-Point Discrimination Scoring[15,16]**

1-5 mm = Normal
6-10 mm = Fair
11-15 mm = Poor
One point perceived = Protective sensation only
No points perceived = Anesthetic

Step 3: Occlude the client's vision.

Step 4: Instruct the client to respond with either "one" or "two" to the stimulus provided.

Step 5: Application is from proximal to distal on the volar distal phalanx of the fingertip. The points are longitudinal to the axis of the finger and are placed perpendicular to the skin. Move the points along the fingertip only, from proximal to distal. Speed has not been addressed.

Step 6: Begin with a distance of 5 to 8 mm, and increase or decrease as needed.

Step 7: Lift the points off the tip of the finger. Do not allow the points to come off the tip of the finger separately because this gives the client information that it was two points.

Discussion

Seven of ten correct responses are needed for an accurate response. Two millimeters is considered normal moving two-point discrimination. A common error is to press too hard during the testing process, and inconsistency in amount of pressure placed on the device and skin is the main problem with reliability of this test.

Touch/Pressure Threshold Test (Semmes-Weinstein Monofilament Test)

This test determines light touch thresholds. The test is effective in identifying impairments in nerve compression injuries.

Equipment

The Semmes-Weinstein Pressure Aesthesiometer Kit is available in catalogs with 5 or 20 monofilaments. The monofilaments are color coded with green monofilaments indicating light touch within normal limits, blue monofilaments indicating diminished light touch, purple monofilaments indicating diminished protective sensation, and red monofilaments indicating loss of protective sensation. If only the largest monofilament is felt, it indicates deep pressure sensation only; and if the largest monofilament is not felt, it indicates that light touch sensation is "untestable" (Table 5-1).[15] The 5-monofilament screening kit contains the largest monofilament in the categories of normal, diminished light touch, diminished protective sensation, and the smallest and largest monofilament in the loss of protective sensation category.

TABLE 5-1	**Semmes-Weinstein Monofilament Categories/Scoring[15]**	
Color Code	**Definition**	**Monofilament Size Range**
Green	Normal light touch threshold	1.65 to 2.83
Blue	Diminished light touch	3.22 to 3.61
Purple	Diminished protective sensation	3.84 to 4.31
Red	Loss of protective sensation	4.56 to 6.65
Untestable	Unable to feel largest monofilament	—

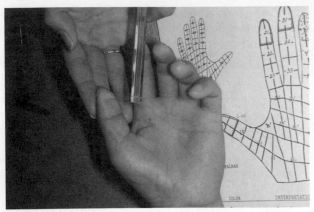

FIGURE 5-12 Semmes-Weinstein monofilament test measures touch force threshold.

Method

Follow these steps:[15]

Step 1: Describe the test to the client.

Step 2: Support the client's hand on a rolled towel to prevent the fingers from moving with the touch.

Step 3: Occlude the client's vision with a screen or folder.

Step 4: Instruct the client to respond with "touch" each time a touch is felt.

Step 5: Begin with the largest monofilament in the normal category (2.83). Proceed to larger monofilaments if there is no response.

Step 6: For the smaller monofilaments, sizes 1.65 to 4.08 (green and blue categories), the filament needs to be applied for three trials. One correct response to the three trials is considered a correct response. All larger monofilaments are applied only one time for each trial.

Step 7: Begin testing distally and move proximally.

Step 8: Apply the monofilament perpendicular to the skin until the monofilament bends. Apply it slowly (1 to 1½ seconds) to the skin, hold for 1 to 1½ seconds, and then lift slowly (1 to 1½ seconds) (Fig. 5-12).

Step 9: Record on a hand map the monofilament size that the client correctly perceives.

Localization of Light Touch

The localization of light touch test is used to determine functional ability to locate touch on the hand.[15] The ability to localize light touch returns after light touch threshold and can cause significant problems following a nerve repair.

Equipment

The equipment needed is the Semmes-Weinstein monofilament (the smallest monofilament to be determined intact on threshold testing described previously). If monofilaments are not available, a cotton ball or pencil eraser has been used. It is important to use the same item for retests.

Method

Follow these steps:

Step 1: Describe the test to the client. The client is to open his or her eyes and point to the location the touch was felt after the stimulus is given.

Step 2: Provide a light touch stimulus to an area. Place a dot on the hand map where the stimulus was placed.

Step 3: Following the client's response, if touch is felt in another place than given, draw an arrow pointing to the location the client felt touch from the location given. If the client did feel touch where given, draw the dot alone.

Additional Tests

Additional tests for assessing sensation are the following:[15]

- *Ninhydrin test:* Used to evaluate sudomotor or sympathetic nervous system function. It does not require a voluntary response from the client and therefore can be used for children or individuals with cognitive impairments. Ninhydrin spray is a clear agent that turns purple when it reacts with a small concentration of sweat. The individual's hand is cleansed and air dried for at least 5 minutes. The fingertips are then placed on bond paper for 15 seconds, and traced. The paper is sprayed with the ninydrin spray reagent and dried according to directions. The prints are then sprayed with the ninhydrin fixer reagent, and areas where sweat is present will appear as dots. The test identifies areas of distribution of sweat secretion after recent, complete peripheral nerve lesions. No sweat will be present in a particular nerve's innervation area after a complete nerve laceration.

- *O'Riain wrinkle test:* Used to evaluate sympathetic nervous system function or recovery following a complete nerve lesion. Denervated palmar skin does not wrinkle when soaked in 42° C (108° F) water for 20 to 30 minutes, as normal skin will.

- *Vibration:* Used to determine frequency response of mechanoreceptor end organs. Tuning forks of 30 and 256 cps are most frequently used. It has been noted that there is currently no equipment that controls for force and technique at this time.[15]

- *Moberg's pick-up test:* Used to determine tactile gnosis, or functional discrimination. Using specific small objects, the client picks the objects up with each hand and is timed, with vision and without vision. The time to place the objects in the box with and without vision is recorded, and the quality of movement and use or disuse of specific digits is observed.

Discussion

Although it is helpful to be aware of the battery of sensory evaluations described, a standard screening of sensation is limited to one or two assessments. I recommend use of the Semmes-Weinstein monofilaments for nerve compressions (such as, carpal tunnel or cubital tunnel syndrome), and monofilaments, two-point discrimination testing, and functional test (such as, Moberg pickup test) following a nerve injury or laceration. Following a nerve laceration, touch threshold (Semmes-Weinstein monofilaments) will show an improvement before the ability to discriminate touch (two-point discrimination).

Coordination

Coordination is the ability to manipulate items in the environment. This ranges from gross coordination to fine coordination tasks. A large number of standardized coordination tests are available with methodology available for each test. Standardized coordination tests include O'Connor Dexterity Test, Nine-Hole

Peg Test, Jebsen-Taylor Hand Function Test, Minnesota Rate of Manipulation Test, Crawford Small Parts Dexterity Test, and the Purdue Pegboard Test.[18] A simple test for a quick screening of coordination is the Nine-Hole Peg Test.[18,19] This test is standardized yet allows use of a low-cost homemade board and pegs. The Jebsen-Taylor Hand Function Test assesses functional tasks, such as writing, as well as the ability to manipulate large and small items.[18,20] The methodology is available with each test and will not be specified in this chapter because of the number of tests available. Use of a standardized test is helpful particularly for clients whose injuries might affect their coordination.

Strength Testing

Grip and Pinch Strength Testing

Grip and pinch strength testing is the standard method used for decades to determine functional grasp and pinch strength. The tests are used initially and in periodic retests to demonstrate improvement in the strength available to grasp or pinch. Contraindications are noted in the following discussion.

Contraindications

Do not perform these tests when resistance has not yet been approved by the referring physician. Grip and pinch strength testing are maximally resistive tests. Testing is contraindicated before full healing following a fracture, ligament repair, tendon laceration, or tendon transfer of the forearm, wrist, or hand, or as determined by the referring physician.

Precaution. *An acute joint, ligament, or tendon injury or sprain of a digital joint or wrist are contraindications for maximal grip or pinch strength testing until resistive exercises are appropriate.*

For any traumatic injury, I defer testing of grip or pinch strength until resistive exercises or strengthening have been approved by the referring physician. For a gradual-onset condition or injury (such as, tendinopathy or carpal tunnel syndrome), I will test strength at the time of initial evaluation, even though my initial treatment plan may not include strengthening until the level of pain decreases. At the time of initial evaluation for this type of condition, I modify the instructions and tell the client to stop grasping when mild pain occurs to prevent an increase in pain following use of the test, and I document when pain does occur with the test. Determination of initial grip and pinch strength for tendinopathy or nerve compressions is important to determine future progress.

> ◎ **Clinical Pearl**
>
> The question to always ask yourself before performing strength testing is whether there are any healing tissues that can be damaged by this test.

Grip Strength Test

Equipment

To assess grip strength, the Jamar dynamometer is recommended by the American Society for Surgery of the Hand and the American Society of Hand Therapists.[18,21] The test has been determined to be accurate and reliable. Annual calibration is recommended and should be done more often in high-use settings. Do not ignore calibration. Pinchmeters are commercially available; however, no one specific type is endorsed by the aforementioned associations.

Method

The client is seated with shoulder adducted, elbow flexed to 90 degrees, and forearm and wrist neutral. The therapist places the dynamometer in the client's hand while gently supporting the base of the dynamometer, and he/she instructs the client to squeeze as hard as possible. Grip force should be applied smoothly, without rapid jerking motion. Allow the wrist to extend during the grip.[18,21]

Consider the following:

- *Standard grip test:* Three trials on the second handle-width setting.
- *Five-level grip test:* One trial on each of the five handle-width settings. This test is used to determine a bell curve when graphed. The strongest grip is almost always on the second or third handle-width setting. The weakest grips normally occur at the most narrow and widest settings with scores on the middle three handle settings falling between the strongest and weakest scores, assimilating a bell curve. Lack of maximal effort may be a possibility when the five handle setting scores show a flat line when graphed, where readings at all handle settings are almost the same, or when there is an up/down-up/down type of curve.
- *Rapid exchange grip test:* The examiner rapidly moves the dynamometer, alternating from the client's right to left hands, for ten trials to each hand. This test had been thought to prevent voluntary control of grip strength by the client, making it more difficult for a client to self-limit the grip response or provide less than maximal effort.[22] More recently, Schectman and colleagues[23-25] have articulated well-founded concerns about the methods with which clinicians interpret sincerity of effort of grip tests. Their work provides some thought-provoking findings on the topic.

Discussion

Normative data exists for grip and pinch strength testing.[26] In addition, the American Society of Hand Therapists recommends that you compare readings with the client's opposite extremity if it is uninjured.

Pinch Strength Test

Equipment

The device used is the pinchmeter (styles vary).

Method

With the client seated, elbow flexed to 90 degrees with arm adducted at side, and forearm neutral, proceed as follows:[18]

- *Lateral pinch (key pinch):* Place the pinchmeter between the radial side of index finger and thumb, and instruct the client to pinch as hard as possible.
- *Three-point pinch (three jaw chuck pinch):* Place the pinchmeter between the pulp of the thumb and pulp of the index and middle fingers. Instruct the client to pinch as hard as possible.
- *Two-point pinch (tip to tip pinch):* Place the pinchmeter between the tip of the thumb and tip of the index finger, and instruct the client to pinch as hard as possible.

Discussion

Repeat each test three times and calculate an average. Calibrate equipment at least annually.

Manual Muscle Test

Manual muscle strength is essential to test and document for improvement when there is weakness related to a nerve injury or compression. Identifying the strength of various muscles along a specific nerve distribution helps determine the level of nerve injury and improvement over time. Measurement of manual muscle strength also is helpful in order to document improvement when weakness is present because of disuse, such as after prolonged immobilization.

Equipment

Manual muscle testing is a form of strength testing that measures the client's ability to move the body part being tested against gravity and, if able to move fully against gravity, to maintain the position against the examiner's resistance. Thus the only equipment needed is a reference book and a form on which to record the results.

Method

Manual muscle testing is performed according to methods documented in numerous sources. Strength is graded according to normal, good, fair, poor, and trace strength definitions—with fair strength defined as the ability to move the body part through its full available range against gravity, although not able to tolerate any additional resistance. Also acceptable is a number grading system where 5 corresponds to normal, 4 to good, 3 to fair, 2 to poor and 1 to trace strength. Description of the method of applying resistance to each muscle of the hand, wrist, and forearm is beyond the scope of this chapter. An excellent reference for specific testing procedures for each muscle is found in *Muscles: Testing and Function* by Peterson Kendall, et al.[27] I recommend use of a form designed for manual muscle testing with the muscles listed in relation to their nerve innervation, as described in this reference.

Discussion

Manual muscle testing is contraindicated in the same situations as for grip and pinch strength testing, or when pain prevents full effort by the client. Because manual muscle testing is a maximally resistive test, any injury with healing tissues (bone, ligament, and tendon) that could be reinjured should not be tested until determined to be safe by the referring physician or the appropriate time after surgery allows resistance.

Precaution. *Finger or thumb tendon repairs are not sufficiently strong to test until 14 weeks after surgery.*

Use of Orthotics

Many clients have obtained their own orthotic or have been given a prefabricated orthotic by their primary or referring physicians. Determine the use of any orthotics and the amount of time and activities during which they are worn. This information is helpful in determining the client's functional limitations and allows you to offer insight into the appropriate use of orthotics for the client's condition (see Chapter 7).

Functional Use

Functional use is an area that should be assessed as part of every evaluation. This portion of the evaluation is important to determine functional goals with the client and to document them for the insurance company. Determining difficulty in daily activities helps you set goals in conjunction with the clients' perception of their needs. This area often is forgotten or bypassed in a busy clinic situation. Discussing functional limitations and goals helps clients recognize that the therapist is aware of the ways that their injury affects their life and gives them confidence that they are working together toward common and meaningful goals.

Equipment

A checklist to help the client think of areas in which they are successful or in which they have difficulty may be helpful. Categories such as self-care skills, home management (outdoor and indoor), and vocational tasks can be included. The evaluation summary form (see Appendix 5-1) may include a list of common tasks, such as opening containers or performing fasteners. Some therapists prefer to take notes about specific functional tasks that the client describes as difficult. Please see Chapter 8 for more about functional assessments.

Method

Functional use is assessed through discussion with the client or simulation of activities. The extremity may be completely nonfunctional because of the presence of a cast and/or limitations due to the injury, such as a flexor tendon repair in the early stage of healing, a complex injury, inability to move the digits to grasp an object, loss of muscle innervation, or loss of sensation. In these cases, to list all the functional tasks that are limited is impossible, and it may be more appropriate to state the limitations such as, "Unable to use the right upper extremity for any functional tasks other than support of a light object using the forearm, as the hand is unable to grasp." At the other extreme may be a client with a single digit injured with hypersensitivity that limits fine coordination. In this case, it may be possible to list specific task limitations. I prefer to include the category of functional use as the last section of the evaluation documentation. Following documentation of the status of pain, wounds/scars, ROM, sensation, and strength, the functional use statement becomes a reflection of the way that the previously noted deficits affect the client's daily life.

In some situations, time limitations may preclude an in-depth assessment of all areas of the upper extremity in one session. A screening of some sections may be done with a full assessment deferred to the next session. For instance, I may screen the area of sensation by asking about the client's sensation and may defer monofilament or two-point discrimination testing to the next visit.

Summary

Awareness of the areas to include in a thorough evaluation is enhanced by use of an evaluation summary form (see Appendix 5-1), which facilitates the logical progression through the steps of the evaluation.

Precaution. *Awareness of situations in which it is unsafe to perform certain assessments is essential.*

Much evaluation is done by observation. Effectiveness as a therapist is enhanced when the therapist takes the time to communicate well with a new client during the evaluation. This occurs not only by describing the process of the assessments but also by listening as the client attempts to communicate verbally and nonverbally. The information gained during the assessment process is the foundation upon which treatment choices rest, and the connection the therapist makes with each new client is the foundation upon which the client's confidence in the treatment rests. Both are equally important.

References

1. Fedorczyk JM: Pain management: principles of therapist's intervention. In Skirven TM, Osterman AL, Fedorczyk JM, et al, editors: *Rehabilitation of the hand and upper extremity*, ed 6, Philadelphia, 2011, Elsevier Mosby, pp 1461–1470.
2. Melzack R: The short-form McGill pain questionnaire, *Pain* 30: 191–197, 1987.
3. Cuzzell JZ: The new red yellow black color code, *Am J Nurs* 88(10):1342–1346, 1988.
4. von der Heyde RL, Evans RB: Wound classification and management. In Skirven TM, Osterman AL, Fedorczyk JM, et al, editors: *Rehabilitation of the hand and upper extremity*, ed 6, Philadelphia, 2011, Elsevier Mosby, pp 219–232.
5. Seiler JG III: Physical examination of the hand. *Essentials of hand surgery*, Philadelphia, 2002, Lippincott Williams & Wilkins, pp 23–48.
6. Taras JS, Lemel MS, Nathan R: Vascular disorders of the upper extremity. In Mackin EJ, Callahan AD, Skirven TM, et al, editors: *Rehabilitation of the hand and upper extremity*, ed 5, St Louis, 2002, Mosby, pp 879–898.
7. de Herder E: Vascular assessment. *Clinical assessment recommendations*, ed 2, Chicago, 1992, American Association of Hand Therapists, pp 29–39.
8. Hay D, Taras JS, Yao J: Vascular disorders of the upper extremity. In Skirven TM, Osterman AL, Fedorczyk JM, et al, editors: *Rehabilitation of the hand and upper extremity*, ed 6, Philadelphia, 2011, Elsevier Mosby, pp 825–844.
9. Adams LS, Greene LW, Topoozian E: Range of motion. *Clinical assessment recommendations*, ed 2, Chicago, 1992, American Association of Hand Therapists, pp 55–70.
10. Seftchick JL, Detullio LM, Fedorczyk JM, et al, editors: Clinical examination of the hand. In Skirven TM, Osterman AL, Fedorczyk JM, et al, editors: *Rehabilitation of the hand and upper extremity*, ed 6, Philadelphia, 2011, Elsevier Mosby, pp 55–71.
11. Reese NB, Bandy WD: *Joint range of motion and muscle length testing*, ed 2, St Louis, 2010, Saunders.
12. Villeco JP: Edema: therapist's management. In Skirven TM, Osterman AL, Fedorczyk JM, et al, editors: *Rehabilitation of the hand and upper extremity*, ed 6, Philadelphia, 2011, Elsevier Mosby, pp 845–857.
13. Waylett-Rendall J, Seibly D: A study of the accuracy of a commercially available volumeter, *J Hand Ther* 4(1):10–13, 1991.
14. Colditz JC: Therapist's management of the stiff hand. In Skirven TM, Osterman AL, Fedorczyk JM, et al, editors: *Rehabilitation of the hand and upper extremity*, ed 6, Philadelphia, 2011, Elsevier Mosby.
15. Bell Krotoski JA: Sensibility testing: history, instrumentation, and clinical procedures. In Skirven TM, Osterman AL, Fedorczyk JM, et al, editors: *Rehabilitation of the hand and upper extremity*, ed 6, Philadelphia, 2011, Elsevier Mosby, pp 894–921.
16. Dellon AL, Mackinnon SE, Crosby PM: Reliability of two-point discrimination measurements, *J Hand Surg Am* 12(5 Pt 1):693–696, 1987.
17. Dellon AL: The moving two-point discrimination test: clinical evaluation of the quickly adapting fiber/receptor system, *J Hand Surg* 3:474–481, 1978.
18. Fess EE: Functional tests. In Skirven TM, Osterman AL, Fedorczyk JM, et al, editors: *Rehabilitation of the hand and upper extremity*, ed 6, Philadelphia, 2011, Elsevier Mosby.
19. Mathiowetz V, Volland G, Kashman N, et al: Adult norms for the nine-hole peg test of finger dexterity, *Am J Occup Ther* 39(6):386–391, 1985.
20. Jebsen RH, Taylor N, Trieschmann RB, et al: An objective and standardized test of hand function, *Arch Phys Med Rehabil* 50(6):311–319, 1969.
21. Fess EE: Grip strength. *Clinical assessment recommendations*, ed 2, Chicago, 1992, American Association of Hand Therapists, pp 41–45.
22. Hildreth DH, Breidenbach WC, Lister GD, et al: Detection of submaximal effort by use of the rapid exchange grip, *J Hand Surg Am* 14(4): 742–745, 1989.
23. Shechtman O: Using the coefficient of variation to detect sincerity of effort of grip strength: a literature review, *J Hand Ther* 13:25–32, 2000.
24. Taylor C, Shechtman O: The use of rapid exchange grip test in detecting sincerity of effort, Part I: administration of the test, *J Hand Ther* 13(3):195–202, 2000.
25. Shechtman O, Taylor C: The use of rapid exchange grip test in detecting sincerity of effort, Part II: validity of the test, *J Hand Ther* 13(3): 202–210, 2000.
26. Mathiowetz V, Kashman N, Volland G, et al, editors: Grip and pinch strength: normative data for adults, *Arch Phys Med Rehabil* 66(2):69–74, 1985.
27. Kendall FP, McCreary EK, Provance PG, et al: *Muscles testing and function with posture and pain*, ed 5, Baltimore, 2005, Lippincott Williams & Wilkins.

Evaluation Summary Form

History of Injury/Condition _____

_____

Pertinent Medical History: _____

Pain Level   0 – 1 – 2 – 3 – 4 – 5 – 6 – 7 – 8 – 9 – 10   At best_____Worst_____
                  (mild)   (intolerable)

Description (Circle all that apply):
    Sore   Aching   Throbbing   Burning   Sharp   Stabbing   Radiating

Location: _____

Frequency: Intermittent (Occasional   Frequent) / Constant
             At rest   With use   With exercise   Other_____

Scar   Location:_____
           Raised/Flattened   Color:_____

Adhesions (circle one):   Adherent   Partially adherent   Non-adherent

Wound (circle one):   Closed   Eschar   Sutured   Open

Wound color: Red   Yellow   Black   Combination   Size:_____

Location: _____

Drainage Amount and Color: _____

Vascular Status   Color (circle one):   Normal/Pink/Red/Blue/White/Mottled

Trophic: Normal   Dry/Moist   Shiny/Dull   Location: _____

Peripheral Pulse Strength/Quality: Right _____   Left _____

Capillary Refill Time: _____   Location: _____

Allen'sTest: _____

Surface Temperature: Location/Degrees _____

Fingertip Pulp Changes: Narrowing/Thickened/Other: _____

Fixation Devices   Pins (Internal/Protrude through skin) _____

Screw(s) _____   Plate _____

External Fixation _____   Other _____

Use of Orthotics (Describe Orthotic and Times of Use) _____

Swelling	Visual Inspection (circle one)	Volumetric Measurements
	Not significant	Injured hand: _____ mL
	Mild	Noninjured hand: _____ mL
	Moderate	Difference: _____ mL
	Moderate +	
	Severe	Pitting/Brawny Location: _____

Circumferential Measurements (cm)

	Right	Left
Forearm (Location_____)		
Hand (MCP)		
Wrist		
Digit (Circle)	Thumb IF MF RF SF	Thumb IF MF RF SF
Proximal Phalanx		
PIP joint		
Middle Phalanx		
DIP joint		

Range of Motion (endRange) A= Actn P= Passv.

		Right	Left			Right	Left
Shoulder	Flexion			**Index Finger**	MP		
	Extension				PIP		
	Ext Rot				DIP		
	Int Rot			**Middle Finger**	MP		
Elbow	Flexion				PIP		
	Extension				DIP		
Forearm	Supination			**Ring Finger**	MP		
	Pronation				PIP		
Wrist	Extension				DIP		
	Flexion			**Small Finger**	MP		
	Radial Dev				PIP		
	Ulnar Dev				DIP		
Thumb MP				**Thumb CMC**	Radial Abd		
Thumb IP					Palmar Abd		

Sensation

Circle One: Intact Hypersensitive Tingling Numb Frequency: Intermittent/Constant

Occurrences: With use / At rest / Prolonged position / Repetitive use / At night

Semmes-Weinstein monofilament / Two-point discrimination / Other (see separate forms)

STRENGTH	Right	Left
Grip		
Lateral pinch		
2 point pinch		
3 point pinch		

Five-level or rapid exchange grip if indicated—see separate form

Manual muscle test if indicated—see separate form

Coordination

Observation: _____

Test Results (see separate form)

Functional Use Patient has difficulty with the following (circle all that apply):

Self-Care	*Home Management*
Dressing	Washing dishes
Fasteners	Mealpreparation
Eating	Laundry
Bathing	Openingcontainers
Hygiene	Cleaning—light
Hair care	Cleaning—heavy (floors, tub)
Other	Lawn/outdoor maintenance
Driving/starting vehicle	Grocery shopping
Opening doors	Computer use
Writing	

Vocational (Describe)

Computer use, assembly, heavy lifting

Other_____

Avocational (Describe)

Hobbies, gardening

Other_____

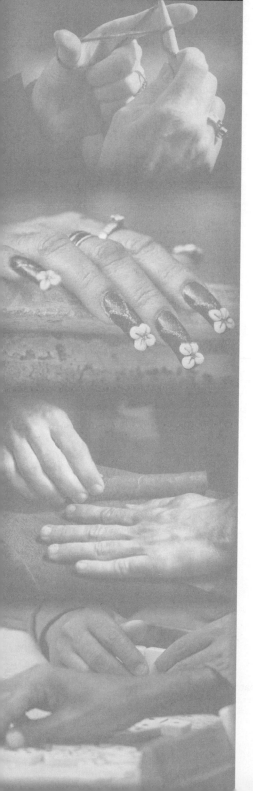

6

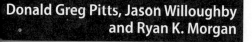

Donald Greg Pitts, Jason Willoughby and Ryan K. Morgan

Clinical Reasoning and Problem Solving to Prevent Pitfalls in Hand Injuries

Introduction and Clinical Reasoning

Identification and evaluation of pitfalls are paramount in the management of hand injuries. A pitfall is an unexpected problem or difficulty that limits the potential to maximize function. Therapists must anticipate pitfalls and prioritize in treatment plans of injured hand patients. Treatment plans should reflect pitfalls in the short and long term goals as cornerstones to good functional outcomes. The healing hand is multi-factorial with therapists constantly providing clinical reasoning and problem solving based upon the application of specific healing rates in different tissues. Primary skills that are needed for treating upper extremities include the understanding of the pathological conditions, surgical repairs, and the healing rates of loose and dense connective tissues. These clinical reasoning and problem-solving skills empower clinicians to design specific and custom personal rehabilitation plans for each patient. The ability to identify current and future pitfalls directly impacts the design and application of an orthotics and activity of daily living (ADL) participation plan maximizing occupational performance. The most common pitfalls seen in upper extremity patients include edema, scar adhesions, maladaptive pain reflex, abnormal neural-tension, adaptive shortening of contractile and non-contractile tissues, and scapular dyskinesia. If biomechanical derangement exists from these pitfalls, the therapist must anticipate the potential problems and develop a proactive rehabilitation program maximizing patients' outcomes. Therapists should constantly question what is missing in the evaluation process to ensure good functional outcomes.

Human Factors

Human factors that a therapist should consider when evaluating pitfalls in patients with upper extremity injuries are intrinsic values, interests, and work habits. The perceptions of function by the patient are critical to establishing functional baselines to determine the clinical effectiveness of the treatment plan. The Quick Disabilities of the Arm, Shoulder, and Hand (DASH) is an eleven-item questionnaire providing subjective data on ADL capacity. The Quick DASH is clinically efficient if used once every 2 weeks as a gauge for the effectiveness of a treatment plan. The patient's positive perception of treatment improves follow through of home exercise programs and active clinical treatment. The focus on patient-centered functional goals with return to the physical demands of past occupations helps establish short- and long-term goals.

Systemic Factors

The medical records of patients assist therapists in yielding detailed data on systemic diseases that impact healing processes and treatment plans. The more common confounding medical problems include diabetes, thyroid dysfunction, pulmonary and heart diseases, congenital abnormalities, and rheumatoid arthritis or osteoarthritis. The clinician's understanding of diseases ensures appropriate goals for the patient's education and custom rehabilitation processes.

Stages of Wound Healing

The stages of wound healing are commonly placed into three basic categories: inflammatory, proliferation, and maturation (Fig. 6-1).[1-4] Therapists should strive be competent in their understanding of the stages of wound healing and how each type of tissue heals at a different rates.[1]

The therapist must place healing timelines on the patient's pathology based upon classifying healing tissues into either loose or dense connective tissue categories (Fig. 6-2). Loose connective tissues include skin, blood vessels, and muscle.[5-7] The normal healing rates for loose connective tissues in the inflammatory phase is between 1 to 3 days, the proliferation phase is between 3 to 10 days, and the maturation phase is from 11 to 21 days. Dense connective tissues include bone, joint capsule, ligament, tendon, and fascia.[1,8,9] The approximate healing timeline for dense connective tissues in the inflammatory phase is from 1 to 4 weeks, the proliferation phase is from 4 to 8 weeks, and the maturation phase is from 8 to 12 weeks.

Fig. 6-3 is an example of a clinical-level system for communicating with therapists about therapeutic exercises for use throughout a common pathology of the hand and upper extremity.[10]

The evaluation processes by the clinician identifies the healing rates of repaired or injured tissues and anticipates the potential pitfalls prioritizing treatment plan options. The consideration of wound healing ensures that the patient receives maximum functional outcomes with minimal chance for long-term disabilities.

Therapists should consider the occupational environments of the patient at home, work, and play. Clinical education programs provide patients with a clear understanding of tissue healing rates, pathophysiology of injuries, and the expected timelines of functional recovery. Occupational goals and wound healing education are reinforced daily. This promotes intrinsic buy-in throughout the rehabilitation processes, which is vital to facilitating therapist-patient relationships.[4,11]

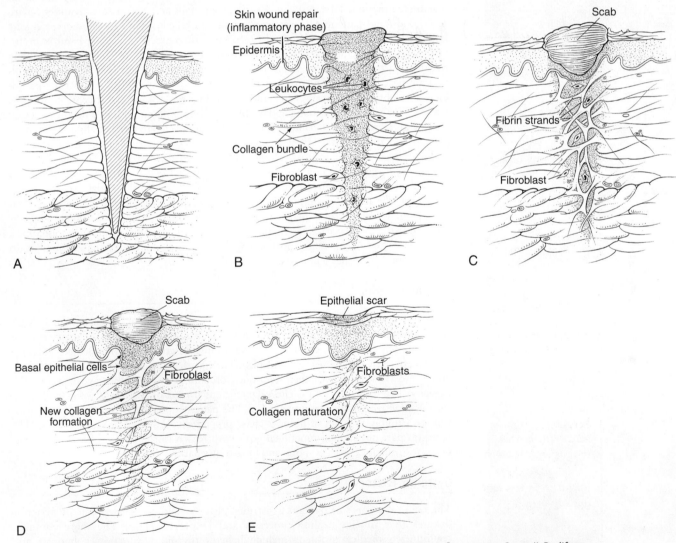

FIGURE 6-1 The basic stages of the wound-healing process with Stage I, Inflammatory; Stage II, Proliferation; and Stage III, Maturation. The therapist's understanding of loose versus dense connective tissue healing rates allows safe, proper, and graded progression of treatment. (From Fess EE, Gettle KS, et al: Hand and upper extremity splinting: principles & methods, 3e, St. Louis, 2005, Mosby, Inc.)

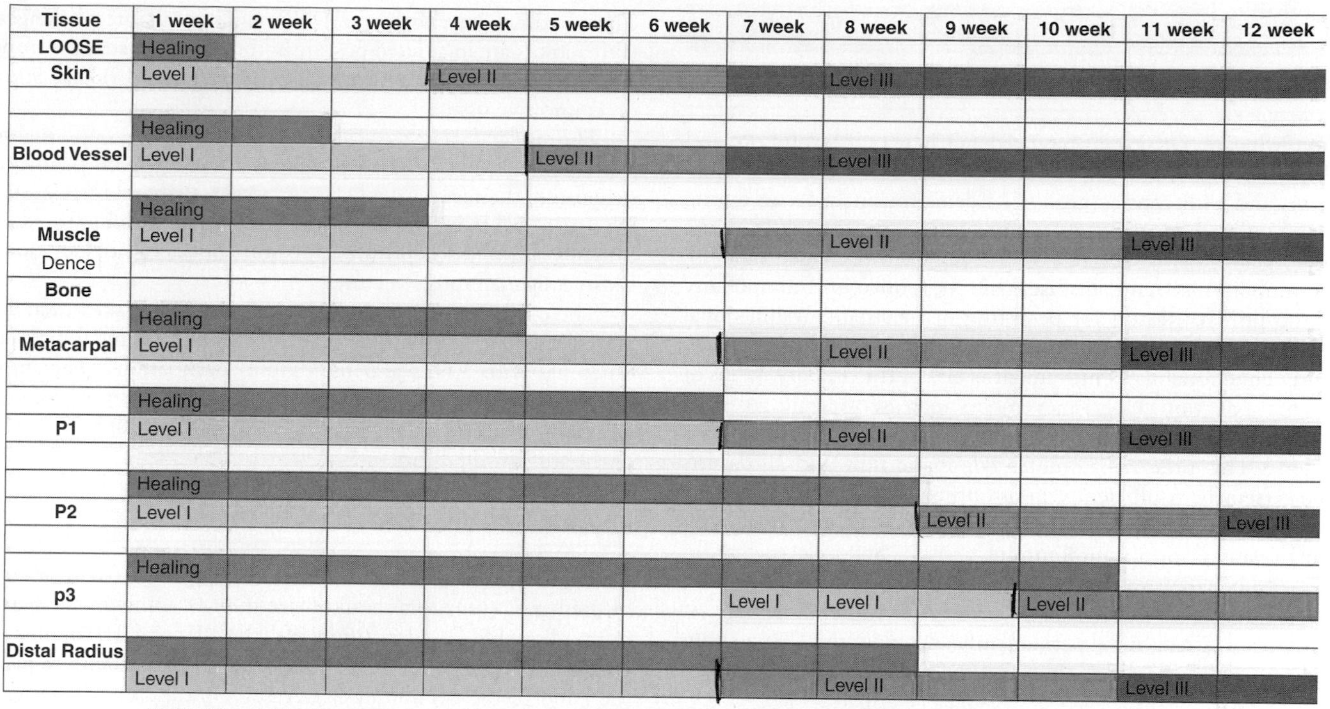

Tissue	1 week	2 week	3 week	4 week	5 week	6 week	7 week	8 week	9 week	10 week	11 week	12 week
LOOSE	Healing											
Skin	Level I			Level II				Level III				
		Healing										
Blood Vessel	Level I				Level II			Level III				
		Healing										
Muscle	Level I							Level II			Level III	
Dence												
Bone												
		Healing										
Metacarpal	Level I							Level II			Level III	
		Healing										
P1	Level I							Level II			Level III	
		Healing										
P2	Level I								Level II			Level III
		Healing										
p3							Level I	Level I		Level II		
Distal Radius												
	Level I							Level II			Level III	

FIGURE 6-2 Healing rates and stages of common tissues seen in the upper extremity treatment clinical setting. (Data from Pitts G, Willoughby J: Rehabilitation of wrist and hand injuries. In Andrews J, Harrelson G, Wilk K: *Physical rehabilitation of the injured athlete*, ed 4, Philadelphia, 2012, Saunders.)

Level I	Level II	Level III
Inflammatory/healing Wound care	**Maturation/ Load Rehabilitation**	**Maturation Rehabilitation**
Dressing Changes	Joint Mobilization Grade III	Overhead tasks
Debridement	Increase Load	Torque tasks
Edema control	Strengthening	Ulnar and Radial Deviation
Coban /compression wrap	Isometric/ isotomic	Pronation and Supination
Scar Management	No overhead tasks	**Sequnce of Risk Factor Exposure**
Elastomere/ silicon	Stress Loading	A. Exposure to Torque Motion
Scar massage/ vibration	Weight bearing	B. Motion plus load
Orthoses	Lifting carry tasks	C. Pace
Protec healing tissue, Reduce pain reflex and decrease inflammation	*Focus on LADL tasks	Time all tasks / stop with pain
	Scapular stabilization	Starloadphase only if motion phase is completed (5 min exposure at a rate of 1 rep per second)
Rehabilitation	Open and closed kinetic chain exercises	Start pace phase only if 80% of load and torque goals are completed
Joint Mobs Grade I–II		Torque simulation should match essential job or recreational tasks
Muscle balancing	**Orthoses**	Scapular stabilization with load to simulate work or recreation
Nerve glides	Corrective Splints	
Tendon glides	**Avoid**	**Goals**
Scapular stabilization	Pronation/supination & ulnar / radial deviation with force	Independence in Essential Job Tasks
ADL/LADL modification	PDL to Med according to the dictonary of occupational titles	
*Focus on ADL Skills	Start Level III once the patient reaches 80% ofload goals	
Goals	**Goals**	
Independence with self-care tasks	Independence IADL tasks	

FIGURE 6-3 The clinical-level system of functional return. An explanation of the appropriate rehabilitation techniques for various phases of the wound-healing process.

Edema

Pathophysiology

According to Dr. Paul Brand, edema is scar in evolution, and if it is left untreated, it will result in adaptive shortening, adhesions, and joint contractures.[12-15] Edema routinely occurs during acute inflammatory processes from infections, traumatic injury, or surgery. Edema can also be present from decreased mobility (immobility), systemic diseases, and local infections. Immobility is the primary reason for persisting or persistent dysfunctional edema of the hand from a traumatic injury or post-surgical procedure. Functional hand movement is one of the primary means of edema reduction. Hand movements increase pressure gradients on the arteriole and venous systems creating fluid shifts of pooled edema. This pressure promotes lymphatic flow and also assists the extremely insufficient venous outflow system of the hand.

Systemic edema can result from a non-functional lymphatic system or an autoimmune disease. Systemic edema can be extremely detrimental to hand function due to the prolonged stress on the musculoskeletal system, joints, and nerves.[14-16] Prolonged stress may permanently derange the ligamentous structures that stabilize joints and tendon systems that produce functional dexterity [17]

Infection

In 1904, Dr. Kanavel first described the identification and evaluation of infectious edema. He described the four cardinal signs of infection as symmetrical edema, flexed digital posture, pain with extension of digit, and pain with palpation along the tendon sheath (Fig. 6-4). The clinician should document the patient's pain levels on a scale of 0 to 10 at rest and with ADL tasks and note the number of Kanavel signs present. This documentation will allow the therapist to evaluate progression or regression.

Evaluation

Edema may be on the dorsum of the patient's hands due to the limited lymphatic drainage. Patients displaying persistent edema often develop the classic stiff hand posture. When the hand is subjected to pitting edema, the position of least resistance is often referred to as the *loose pack position* (Fig. 6-5).[7,18] Edema diminishes the capacity for functional tendon excursions by a phenomenon known as *fabric bias*.[15,18]

The stiff hand (open pack) posture presents with the metacarpal joints in extension due to edema pooling in the dorsum of the hand and stress applied to the extrinsic extensor mechanism.[15,19,20]

The proximal interphalangeal (PIP) and distal interphalangeal (DIP) joints are in a flexed posture with the edema stress creating a tenodesis effect on the extrinsic flexors from the fabric bias stress on connective tissue.[21]

The stiff hand posture can be extremely problematic due to the open-pack non-stressed position of the collateral ligaments supporting the metacarpophalangeal (MP), PIP, and DIP joints.[7] This may lead to insufficient glides of contractile tissues (tendon, muscle) and stress deprivation of non-contractile tissues (joint capsule, ligamentous structures).[15,18,22]

These pitfalls may result in joint contractures, tendon adhesions, and long-lasting pain reflexes inhibiting functional outcomes with ADLs and meaningful occupations. Therapists must evaluate the effects of the edema and adjust the patient's treatment plans on a daily basis in order to diminish the chances of the stiff hand posture pitfalls.[2,8]

Physical Examination

When assessing the effects of edema on ligamentous structures of the hand, evaluators should place the MP joints in the maximum allowable flexed position and the PIP and DIP joints in maximum extension.[14,15,18,22] Therapists should attempt to place the hand in the commonly referred safe position for long-term functional outcomes.

The standard edema evaluations for hand injuries are volumetric and active range of motion (AROM) (Fig. 6-6). According to Waylett-Rendall and Seibly, volumetric testing has been found to have a high level of inter-/intra-rater reliability and repeatability.[23] Often volumetric devices are not feasible due to open wounds from injury or surgery. Therapists should consider AROM and passive range of motion (PROM) of the digits with the evaluations of fingertips to distal palmar crease (DPC) and palmar digital crease (PDC) (Fig. 6-7). These evaluations allow therapists a fast and reliable way to determine the negative impact edema has on functional movement.

Dr. Brand describes a clinical evaluation of edema based upon the viscoelastic properties of loose and dense connective tissues. He describes the application of graded force to joints over a set time. He recommends recording torque range of motion (TQROM) obtained with a force gauge and plotted on a graph.[12,24,25] The type of tissue and edema involved is based on the shape of the plotted TQROM timed stress strain curve

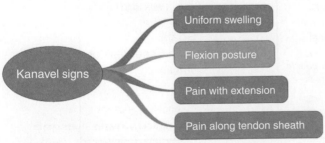

FIGURE 6-4 The four cardinal signs of infection described by Dr. Kanavel.

- Kanavel signs
  - Uniform swelling
  - Flexion posture
  - Pain with extension
  - Pain along tendon sheath

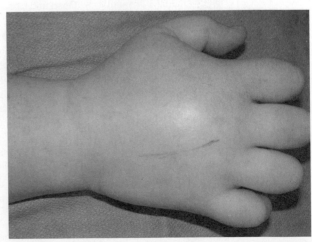

FIGURE 6-5 Extremely swollen hand in a loose pack position.

(Fig. 6-8 and Fig. 6-9). A long shallow curve with a gradual peak at the end range will indicate a loose connective tissue problem (soft-end feel). This is demonstrated with an end range can be reached at a fast rate, the edema is fluid in nature and may respond to mobility and compression. A steep curve with an often painful hard end range reached at a slow sluggish rate indicates the edema is mature and protein-filled with great potential for stiffness.[14,15,18]

Scarring

Scarring is the natural process by which the body heals. It is imperative that therapists use clinical reasoning and manual skills to evaluate effects of scar synthesis-lysis on contractile and non-contractile tissue. *Synthesis-lysis* is a term used to describe the metabolism of scar production and absorption rates that determine the integrity, type, and amount of scar produced post injury or surgery.

Clinical Pearl

Individuals produce scar tissue at varying rates with some producing only a small amount of scar tissue, whereas others produce a large amount.

Scar tissue can alter tendon glide and change joint function (see Fig. 6-10).[26-28] If the scar is not stressed appropriately in

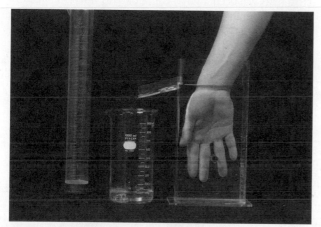

FIGURE 6-6 Volumetric test. A volumeter is used to measure edema in the hand by comparing the amount of water displacement by the affected to the unaffected extremity. (From Fess EE, Gettle KS, et al: *Hand and upper extremity splinting: principles & methods*, 3e, St. Louis, 2005, Mosby, Inc.)

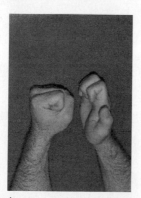

FIGURE 6-7 Distal palmar crease (DPC) *(left)* is a measurement that hand therapists utilize to assess the client's ability to make a "fist" for functional activity. Palmar digital crease (PDC) *(right)* is a measurement utilized to assess for tightness of intrinsic muscles and the ability of clients to make a "hook" with their hand. (From Pitts G, Willoughby J: *Rehabilitation of wrist and hand injuries*. In Andrews J, Harrelson G, Wilk K: *Physical rehabilitation of the injured athlete*, ed 4, Philadelphia, 2012, Elsevier Saunders.)

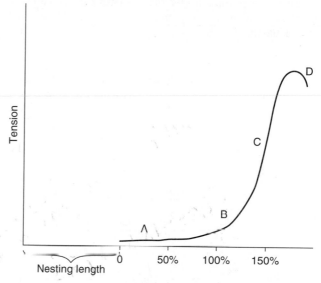

FIGURE 6-8 Diagram of loose connective tissue stress strain curve. The diagram demonstrates a gradual stress strain curve with a slow slope to peak, which is characteristic of loose connective tissue with a soft-end feel of resistance.

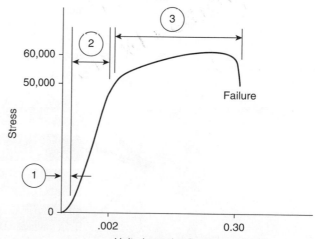

FIGURE 6-9 Diagram of dense connective tissue stress strain curve. The diagram demonstrates a steep stress strain curve with and immediate peak, which is characteristic of a dense connective tissue with a hard-end feel.

the early phase (inflammatory) of rehabilitation process, non-functional adhesions and joint contracture can result limiting function.[14,15, 29,30] Scar tissue will respond to gentle graded stresses at the early stages of the rehab process. Stress application to a mature scar will take longer and be less predictive to realize effective change. Rehabilitation programs with aggressive stress can keep the tissue in an inflamed state longer or create an inflammatory state in mature tissue thus creating excessive scar tissue.

> ### ◎ *Clinical Pearl*
>
> Active range of motion (AROM) evaluates contractile tissue function. Passive range of motion (PROM) evaluates non-contractile tissue.[14,15]

The evaluating therapists must understand that the position of the proximal joints directly impacts length-tension relationship of the extrinsic muscles affecting joint positions.[22] As an example, if positioning the MP joint in extension limits flexion of

PIP but if MP flexion yields increase in PIP flexion, this indicates intrinsic tightness. If movement of a distal joint is not altered by proximal joint position, then adhesions in the joint structures is probable. [14,15]

Dr. Brand pioneered the evaluation techniques necessary to implement a treatment plan to target specific altered tissue types with the application of progressive stress (Fig. 6-11). The controlled application of stress plotted on a stress strain curve can clearly identify the maturation of the scar, tissue type, and rehabilitation approach needed to avoid a pitfall.[14,15] If the curve plotted is long with a gradual slope and a soft-end feel, then the problem is mechanical stiffness. If the curve plotted is shallow with a steep slope and a hard-end feel, then the problem is biological stiffness.[31-35]

> ### ◎ *Clinical Pearl*
>
> If excessive manual stress is applied to mature scar tissues, micro tears will occur in the scar beds. This will result in additional scar formation, stiffness, and a harmful pain reflex.

Stress application measured with a Haldex gauge and a goniometer allows therapists to plot changes in joint motion with the application of progressive measured force (Fig. 6-12).

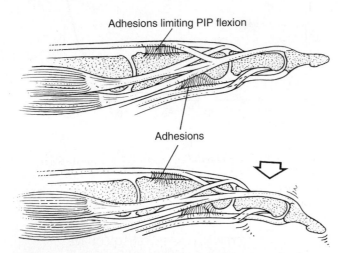

FIGURE 6-10 Scar adhesion of extensor and flexor mechanism. This picture demonstrates how adhesions form surrounding a proximal interphalangeal (PIP) restricting gliding structures of both extensor and flexor mechanisms. (From Fess EE, Gettle KS, et al: *Hand and upper extremity splinting: principles & methods*, ed 3, St. Louis, 2005, Mosby, Inc.)

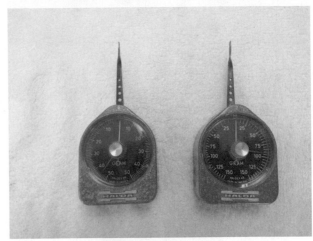

FIGURE 6-12 Haldex gauge. Force application is effective in addressing joint stiffness and controlled safe tissue elongation.

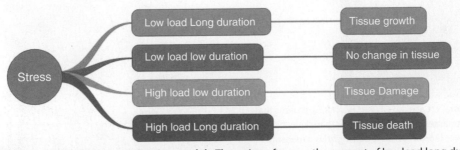

FIGURE 6-11 Rules for stress application model. Therapists often use the concept of low load long duration *(green)* to facilitate a change in tissue length and tissue growth. The use of low load low duration will result in no change in tissue growth or length *(blue)*. The use of high load low duration can result in tissue damage *(yellow)*. If the stress is too aggressive and or long duration, this can lead to tissue death *(red)*. (From Pitts G, Willoughby J: Rehabilitation of wrist and hand injuries. In Andrews J, Harrelson G, Wilk K: *Physical rehabilitation of the injured athlete*, ed 4, Philadelphia, 2012, Saunders.)

The data plotted will allow the treating therapist to determine if the lack of functional motion is due to loose or dense connective tissue. This allows proper selection and type of force when fabricating dynamic and static progressive orthoses (Fig. 6-13).[10,18]

Scar tissue can have direct negative impact on tendons with attempted functional movement. These types of pitfalls include gliding structures through scar, scar in gliding structures, and nerve glide through scar. Examples of gliding structures through scar include flexor and extensor tendon adhesions. Examples of scar in gliding structures include de Quervain tenovaginitis and trigger finger tendonitis.[15,36]

Examples of nervous tissue gliding through scar include digital nerve repairs, carpal tunnel syndrome, and cubital tunnel syndrome. This simple classification of scars when applied can assist therapists in the selection of proper treatment approaches to avoid functional impairments that limit social roles.[37]

Joint Dysfunction

Joint dysfunction can create many occupational performance limitations if not identified and corrected prior to permanent impairment.[38] The joint is a biodynamic system that moves with exact precision producing virtually no friction or drag.[19,20,39]

An articulating joint is made up of congruent joint surfaces with a basic shape of concave or convex. The knowledge of the joint shape allows the clinician to understand the direction the articulating bone moves during a functional task. The basic convex-concave rule exists to explain joint kinematics and the identification of joint.[7,14,16,39]

If the distal joint is concave and the proximal joint is convex, the distal joint will move in the same direction with functional motion. If the distal joint is convex and the proximal joint is concave, the distal joint will move in the opposite direction with functional motion. This allows the clinician to evaluate normal kinematics of joint roll and glide. If an injury occurs to the joint system, a change in the ratio of roll and glide can occur resulting in extreme pain and a change in motor control. There are intrinsic and extrinsic joint structures that can impede joint motion (Fig. 6-14). The intrinsic structures include the joint capsule, volar plate, and the collateral and accessory ligaments.[15,22]

The evaluation of an injured joint should start with the therapist placing the affected joint in a position that eliminates the drag of extrinsic muscles an open pack joint posture. Application of distraction to the joint is applied by the therapist allowing evaluation of joint glide, roll and stability. The manual skills of the therapist in the detection of abnormal kinematics are acquired through seeking mentorship, practice, and clinical experience.[39]

Therefore, it is imperative that therapists have sound clinical knowledge of joint kinematics and how a dysfunctional joint can impede performance. Joint dysfunction left undetected leads to early arthritis, heightened pain reflexes, and diminished motor control skills. If missed early in the rehabilitation phase, this pitfall may negatively affect the functional outcomes of the clients by prolonging therapeutic interventions and lengthening the return to independence (Fig. 6-15).

Intrinsic Tightness

The intrinsic and extrinsic muscles work in harmony to allow the hand to smoothly transition from dexterity to power tasks.[40,41] If patients are suffering from intrinsic tightness, they will experience difficulty in making both a hook fist to PDC (palmar digital crease) and a full fist to DPC (distal palmar crease) (Fig 6-16).

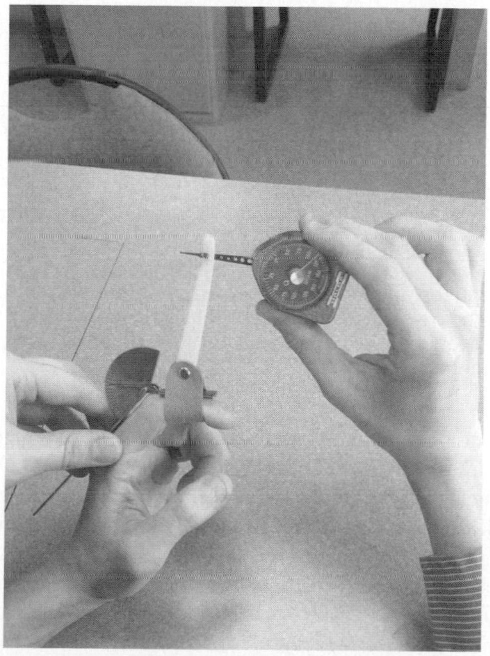

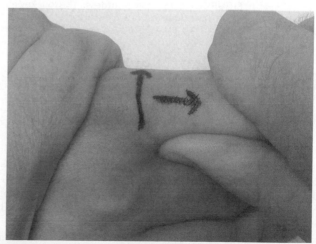

FIGURE 6-13 Stress application measured with a Haldex gauge and a goniometer allows therapists to plot changes in joint motion with the application of progressive measured force. The data plotted will allow the treating therapist to determine if the lack of functional motion is due to loose or dense connective tissue. This allows proper selection and type of force when fabricating dynamic and static progressive orthosis.

FIGURE 6-14 The MP joint is in an open pack extended posture allowing joint mobilization *(left)*. The MP joint is being distracted to allow joint glide with joint mobilization *(right)*.

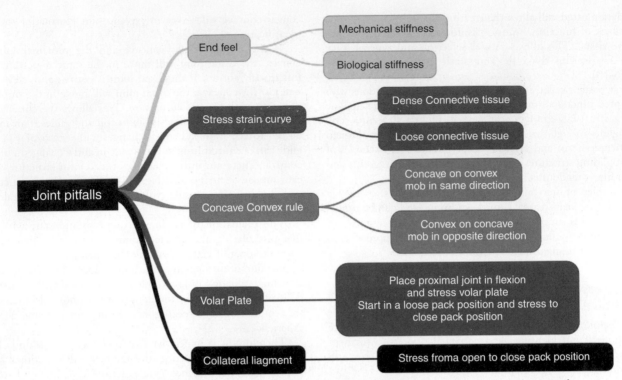

FIGURE 6-15 Joint pitfalls. A variety of assessments utilized by hand therapists when assessing the type of lesions or impairments clients need to address throughout rehabilitation. (From Pitts G, Willoughby J: Rehabilitation of wrist and hand injuries. In Andrews J, Harrelson G, Wilk K: *Physical rehabilitation of the injured athlete*, ed 4, Philadelphia, 2012, Elsevier Saunders.)

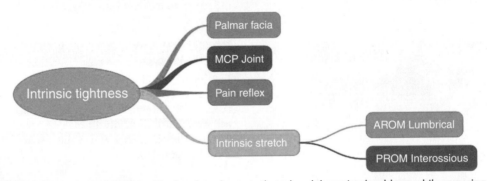

FIGURE 6-16 Intrinsic tightness. The four key elements that a hand therapist should use while assessing for intrinsic tightness of a client are: (1) the palmar fascia should be addressed, (2) followed by the ligamentous and capsular tightness of the MP joint, (3) the therapist should consider the pain reflexivity of the client, and (4) check both active and passive palmar digital crease (PDC) measurements.

◎ *Clinical Pearl*

The most important clinical evaluations that a therapist can master are the skills of assessing intrinsic tightness.

Intrinsic tightness, at the basic level, is a clinical description of the muscles in the palm of the hand (lumbrical and interossei) that become tight as a result of stress deprivation. Intrinsic lumbrical tightness limits force production due to the origin on the flexor digitorum profundus (FDP) (the powerhouse of hand) and insertion on the lateral bands.[12,16,36,42] This muscle imbalance changes the reciprocal inhibition reflex between the intrinsic lumbrical and extrinsic muscles. This tightness will create a gross weakness with functional grasp and limit fine motor dexterity, which are both vital to performing meaningful occupations.

To assess intrinsic tightness, the MP joint of the finger being assessed must be placed into supple hyperextension. Once the joint is held in supple hyperextension by the evaluator, you must then ask the client to "flex the tip" of the distal phalanx down toward the PDC.[43-45] The distance will then be measured in centimeters (cm) from the tip of the distal phalanx to the PDC. The MP joints are placed in slight flexion, and again ask the client to pull the distal phalanx toward the PDC.

The evaluator records this measurement and assesses the difference between the first and second measurement. If measurements of the distal phalanx to PDC is greater with the MP joint hyperextended versus flexed, the patient has intrinsic tightness. This measurement procedure should be repeated with PROM (Fig. 6-17). If PROM of the PIP joint will not change with position of the MP, then PIP joint derangement and extensor

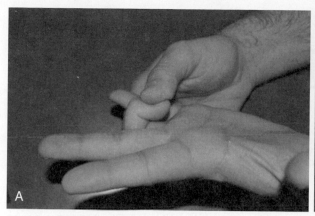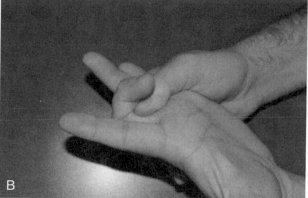

FIGURE 6-17 A, Passive range of motion (PROM) of the intrinsic muscle functions. **B,** Active range of motion (AROM) of the intrinsic muscle functions. Therapists should evaluate both active and passive intrinsic function holding the MP in hyperextension. This ensures full stress on the intrinsic muscles and accurate assessment the tightness.

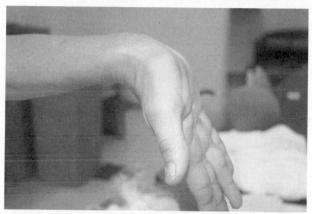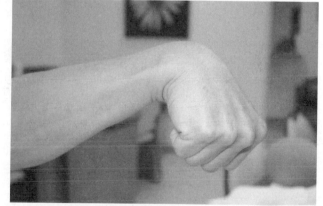

FIGURE 6-18 Volar compartment (VC). A measurement of the extrinsic flexors in the forearm is shown here by having the patient fully extend and supinate the forearm while extending the wrist and digits.

FIGURE 6-19 Dorsal compartment (DC). A measurement of the extrinsic extensors in the forearm is shown here by having the patient fully extend and pronate the forearm and fully flex the wrist while maintaining a fist posture.

adhesions must be ruled out. Intrinsic tightness is one of the largest pitfalls found in the treatment of hand injured patients.

Extrinsic Tightness

Often in upper extremity practice, patients experience a phenomenon where the muscles that originate in the forearm develop adaptive shortening resulting in extrinsic tightness.[12,16,36,42] This can result from sprains, strains, or traumatic events that lead to post-operative procedures with the patient to succumb to a state of immobility. This immobility forces the muscles in the forearm to adaptive shortening.[15,16]

The therapist can assess the difference between the extrinsic flexor length and extrinsic extensor length by comparing two measurements: one that assesses joint mobility, and one that assesses muscle length. This is commonly found in a patients' sustaining distal radius fractures, but it is an extremely important and valid assessment to use in many hand pathologies.[46]

The therapist should first assess the joint mobility of the wrist by taking measurements of volar flexion and dorsal flexion (extension). Therapists should ask the patient to "relax the fingers"

and bring the wrist forward "as much as possible" and record the measurement. The same is true for dorsal flexion, except that the patient will then extend their wrist as much as possible while keeping the fingers in a relaxed position, eliminating the pull of the superficial and deep extrinsic flexors.

To measure the length of the muscle, the therapist will record a volar compartment (VC) and dorsal compartment (DC) measurement. To assess VC length, patients will be asked to bring their arm into supination and full elbow extension. Then patients will be asked to keep their fingers straight and extend their wrist. Therapists should measure the length of the VC at the axis of the carpus. To assess DC length, patients will be asked to bring their arm into full pronation with the elbow fully extended. Patients should then be asked to make a fist and flex their wrist to maximum flexion. The therapist measures this at the level of the axis of the carpus. These compartment lengths can be measured both actively and passively.

To accurately evaluate the extrinsic tightness the therapists should now compare the VC measurement to the dorsal flexion measurement, and then compare the DC measurement to a volar flexion measurement (Fig. 6-18 and Fig. 6-19). If there is a difference in the two, then the patient is experiencing a phenomenon

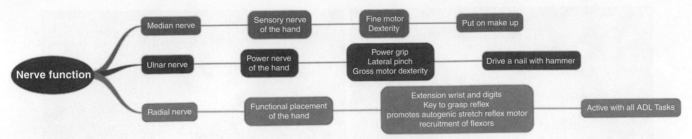

FIGURE 6-20 Nerve pathways/functional implications for each nerve. This map shows each of the three main nerves of the hand/upper extremity and what each of the functional implications are for each one individually.

called *extrinsic tightness.* If there is a difference in the VC and DC measurements, then the patient is said to have a muscle imbalance. Muscle imbalance of the extrinsic musculature can limit power potential and change the kinematics of the entire kinetic chain when attempting large reach tasks. This would prompt the therapist to implement compartment stress through a variety of techniques both manual (passive) and non-manual (active).

Nerve Function and Pitfalls

There are three basic nerves that innervate the hand in upper extremity practice. These include the median, ulnar, and radial nerve distributions. Each nerve has its own unique behavior, nerve pattern, and/or distribution and can be exposed to traction or compression through awkward postures within the human body. It is important for the treating therapist to understand the difference in evaluation of the dermatomes and myotomes when assessing a patient that is experiencing nerve symptoms. Additionally, it is important to learn how to "map" a neurological lesion in the upper extremity of the patient. If missed, this can lead to frustration in the treatment approach of the therapist and frustration and irritability on the part of the patient who is experiencing neurological discomfort.

In the evaluation of pitfalls for nerve injuries, the therapist should consider the severity, location, and functional neuropathies of the peripheral nerves (Fig. 6-20). This will allow the therapist to identify the loss of function and predict recovery based upon the location, severity, and age of the patient.[47-49] Therapists mastering upper extremity function based upon neuropaths and nerve lesions will gain insight into problem solving for many clinical pathologies.

The severity of nerve injuries is classified into three basic categories.[49] These categories are neuropraxia, axonotmesis, and neurotmesis. Neuropraxia lesions are the result of the loss of myelin along the sheath of the affected nerve.[47] This will diminish nerve conduction and create symptoms of numbness and motor control with ADL tasks.[47] Functional return for this lesion is 90% spontaneous recovery within 2 to 4 months.

Axonotmesis lesions are the result of the loss of axons within nerve fascicle bundles resulting in loss of motor output (efferent) or sensory input (afferent).[47] This will diminish motor control and create weakness due to muscle atrophy and decrease force output of the muscle group involved. Functional return for this lesion is 50% to 70% spontaneous recovery with treatment in 6 to 10 months.

Neurotmesis lesions are the result of a complete laceration of all the axons of the nerve resulting in loss of sensory input and motor output.[47] This will create complete paralysis with resulting muscle atrophy, loss of force output, and no sensory input to the

brain. Functional return for this lesion is 0% recovery without a primary nerve repair, with no predictable return of sensory or motor skills.[50] The location of the nerve lesion is of great concern, because this will impact the functional outcome. Lesions located above the elbow have a decreased chance of recovery due to an increase in complexity of the nervous system.[47,51]

The sensory and motor fibers are mixed together in a complex matrix that makes repair of an axonotmesis or neurotmesis injury very unpredictable with recovery taking many months to years. Nerve recovery post-repair of a complete nerve laceration (neurotmesis) is a slow process with the first month consisting of Wallerian degeneration followed by a regeneration rate of a one millimeter a day or an inch a month in healthy individuals. This basic healing concept assists the therapist in determining the rate of functional return.

This knowledge allows the therapist to provide custom treatment, prevention and patient education to diminish the patient's fear, anxiety, and depression, and improve the understanding of expected sensory and motor return. The treating therapist can start sensory motor reeducation and ADL tasks graded to precisely challenge the patient's level of functional return and prevent frustration by limiting exposure to tasks that exceed current sensory motor skill levels.

The median nerve is made up of the lateral and medial cord at the brachial plexus level. The median nerve courses downward along the medial boarder of the upper arm and crosses anterior at the level of the elbow. The median nerve then courses down the forearm and into the wrist via the carpal tunnel.[52]

The afferent sensory input of the median nerve includes the volar portion of the thumb, index, middle, and half of the ring fingers.[45] The efferent motor output from proximal to distal include pronator teres (PT), flexor carpi radialis (FCR), palmaris longus (PL), index and middle finger flexor digitorum profundus (FDP), flexor pollicis longus (FPL), pronator quadratus (PQ), abductor pollicis brevis (APB), opponens pollicis (OP), flexor pollicis brevis (FPB), and lumbricals 1 and 2 .

◎ *Clinical Pearl*

The median nerve is the sensory nerve of the hand, producing fine-motor dexterity output. This nerve applies makeup, completes sewing tasks, and interfaces with technology devices (such as, using your iPad). Paralysis of this nerve results in a hand deformity with loss of intrinsic fine-motor ADLs dexterity and the inability to manipulate small objects.

The ulnar nerve is made up of the medial cord at the brachial plexus level. The ulnar nerve courses downward the medial border

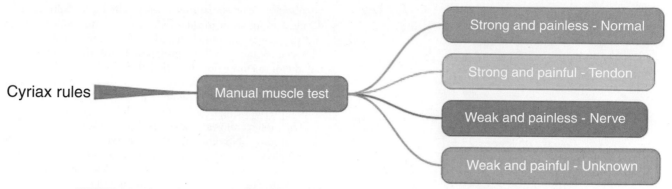

FIGURE 6-21 Cyriax's rules of orthopaedic evaluation. The mind map displays the four possible results in assessing symptoms or impairments through the art of manual muscle testing.

of the upper arm and crosses at the elbow level on the posterior side of the medial epicondyle through the cubital tunnel and then courses down the forearm and into the wrist through the Guyon canal.

The afferent sensory input of the ulnar nerve includes the volar ulnar portion of the ring finger and the small finger. The dorsum branch arises 5 cm proximal to the ulna styloid and enters the dorsum of the hand from wrist to the tips of ring and small fingers (dorsal cutaneous branch of the ulnar nerve). The efferent motor output from proximal to distal include flexor carpi ulnaris (FCU), FDP for the middle, ring, and small fingers, opponens digiti minimi (ODM), flexor digiti minimi (FDM), abductor digiti minimi (ADM), lumbrical 3 and 4, dorsal interosseous, palmar interosseous, and the adductor pollicis.

> ### Clinical Pearl
>
> The ulnar nerve is the power nerve of the hand, producing primarily grip strength, lateral pinch, and wrist ulnar deviation with force. This is the nerve that drives nails, turns car keys, and opens jars. Paralysis of this nerve results in the claw hand deformity and the loss of power grasp and lateral pinch.

The radial nerve is made up of the posterior cord at the brachial plexus level. The radial nerve courses downward the upper arm posteriorly and around the humerus crossing at the lateral elbow level, coursing through the extensor muscles of the forearm and into the wrist.

The afferent sensory input of the radial nerve is the dorsum of the hand from the wrist to the tip of the thumb, index finger, and middle fingers. The efferent motor output from proximal to distal include brachioradialis (BR), extensor carpi radialis longus (ECRL), extensor carpi radialis brevis (ECRB), extensor digitorum communis (EDC), extensor carpi ulnaris (ECU), extensor pollicis longus (EPL), abductor pollicis longus (APL), extensor pollicis brevis (EPB), extensor digiti minimi (EDM), and extensor indicis proprius (EIP).

> ### Clinical Pearl
>
> The radial nerve is the functional positioning nerve that fires with every functional task to enhance dexterity and strength. This is the nerve that allows the hand to produce graded functional motor control tasks. Paralysis of this nerve results in the inability to conduct basic self-care ADL tasks and the inability to extend the wrist or digits.

If left untreated, the patient will have extreme depression with no use of their affected hand. Impairments include elongation of the extensor mechanism, adaptive shortening of the flexor tendons, and joint contractures of the MP and PIP joints.

If treating therapists understand the significance of the severity index, location, and function of nerves, they can foresee future functional pitfalls and understand the duration of dysfunction and the expected level of functional return. This is invaluable in the management of pitfalls for establishing treatment goals, the application of orthoses and patient education on return to function.

Muscle Weakness

The evaluation of muscle is a very valuable skill that is needed to determine focal weakness of a patient and also to determine the lesion location and type.[47,53] Therapists should utilize Cyriax's rules of orthopaedic evaluation (Fig. 6-21). Cyriax's rules have been utilized by physicians and therapists providing detailed diagnostics that far exceed a simple manual muscle score (that is, 4/5).

> ### Clinical Pearl
>
> Manual testing of specific muscles or muscle groups with strong and painless results indicates normal tissue with no lesions. If the muscle is strong and painful, then a tendon lesion at the location of pain is probable. If the muscle is weak and painless, this suggests a lesion of neurological origin. If the muscle is weak and painful, this suggests a lesion of mixed origin that could include a joint, a muscle-tendon, a nerve, or a mixture of all three.

The MicroFET is an available tool that allows treating therapists to measure exact amounts of force output thereby eliminating the subjective evaluation of a clinician, and allowing a more objective and comparative numerical value to the unaffected extremity (Fig. 6-22).

Pitfalls with Pain Reflexes

Often upper extremity rehabilitation programs providing PROM result in patients experiencing excruciating pain reflexes. This is

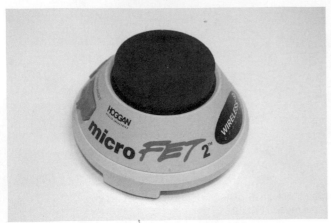

FIGURE 6-22 MicroFET. This tool is often used in assessing the strength or power of a muscle in the hand and upper extremity. Although the microFET has a myriad of functions, it is most easily used in looking at the pound/kilogram of force that a specific muscle or group of muscles exerts, each one individually. (From HOOGAN Health Industries, Salt Lake City, UT, http://hogganhealth.net/welcome/microfet2.php).

why therapists treating upper extremity injuries need to understand the basic science of reflexes.[48,54,55]

The pain reflex can initiate a heavy muscle co-contraction of the agonistic and antagonistic muscle simultaneously to stop external painful applied stress . If painful stimuli occurs for a long period of time, the patient can develop a cortical representation of pain.

This will, in turn, increase muscle tension and diminish functional movement. The pain reflex response speed is between 25 to 50 ms, and it will fire fast-twitch muscle fibers prior to slow-twitch muscle fibers. Pain reflexes are activated when excessive stress is applied to an imbalanced muscle system or adhesion formation altering normal tendon glide. A patient will display extreme pain with AROM prior to the tissue completing normal excursion. The pain reflex can present in injured or deranged joint systems creating an intense response prior to PROM end range. These pain reflexes can coexist and require daily evaluation.

Motor Reflexes

When evaluating occupational performance and functional tasks, it is important for therapists to view muscles as a sensory organ. When muscles are stressed, the muscle spindle apparatus, which is located in the muscle belly, is distorted, and a sensory impulse travels to the central nervous system (CNS) in the form of a stretch reflex. The sensory input travels up the afferent nerve fibers into the spinal cord and synapses with the alpha-motor neurons. This stress on the muscle spindle results in a gain in contraction potential of the particular muscle that has been stressed. This is known

as an *autogenic* or *muscle stretch reflex.* The muscle spindle relays detailed information to the CNS in regards to motion velocity and the amount of muscle length with all functional tasks.[54,55] This sensory motor reflex loop repeated over time creates essential motor memory for dexterity, force regulation, and power production with ADL tasks. Muscle spindles are under constant tension, even while the muscle is in a shortened position with constant monitoring by the gamma reflex.

This reflex allows a continuous sensory feedback loop between the CNS and peripheral nervous system with the muscle physically engaged in all forms of functional tasks. Therapists should evaluate functional activities and occupational performance to assess the motor patterns and maladaptive motor patterns of patients with upper extremity injuries. This allows the therapist to understand the motor coping mechanism and change the patient's motor patterns to restore appropriate motor control.

Functional goals and directed ADL tasks have the highest values of motor control. These tasks are learned motor patterns over many years of imprinting into the motor memory of the CNS. Functional tasks graded to the patient's functioning level allows the recruitment of the appropriate motor sequences with the proper type of motor fibers with the exact number of motor units at a subconscious level. Occupational tasks restore force regulation and efficient occupational performance motor output.

Therapists need to establish batteries of fine and gross motor ADL tasks coupled with standardized functional motor tests to evaluate normal and compensatory patterns of movement. Task analysis performed by therapists should focus upon grasp patterns, delivery of hand to task, placement of the hand for static tasks, quality of movement, speed of motion, and core stability with proper shoulder scapular motor control. These are critical evaluation skills based upon the intrinsic values of the patients, the science of human physiology, and the pathophysiology of injuries or surgery. This is the starting point for all motor control graded functional tasks.

Upper Limb Tension Testing

There are a set of examinations described by Butler[56] called *upper limb tension tests (ULTTs)* that help therapists to better understand the origin of a nerve lesion. There are three basic ULTTs with a multitude of variability in how to perform these assessments. However, the most basic assessment will be discussed in this text.

Upper Limb Tension Test for the Median Nerve

To perform the ULTT for the median nerve, (C5-7) the examiner will first place the patient in a supine position on a plinth in the anatomical position (Fig. 6-23). The patient will then be asked to first abduct his/her arm of the affected extremity to a 90-degree posture. Then, the clinician will ask the client to fully extend the wrist to supple end-range. While depressing the clavicle and first rib and controlling for excessive scapular winging, the clinician will ask the client to rotate his/her neck away from the abducted arm and hold this position for a maximum of 60 seconds. This test is considered positive if the client experiences an increase in neurological symptoms (that is, numbness/tingling).

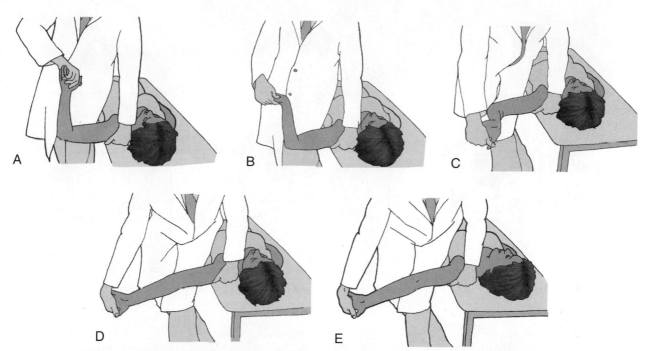

FIGURE 6-23 ULTT median nerve. Upper limb tension test 1 (ULTT1): Median nerve dominant utilizing shoulder abduction. A, Position the patient with the shoulder abducted to 90 degrees and in neutral rotation, the elbow flexed to 90 degrees, and the wrist in neutral. Then extend the shoulder to neutral. B, Extend the wrist and fingers. C, Externally rotate the shoulder. D, Extend the elbow. E, Side bend the neck away from the side being tested. *Adapted from Butler DS:* Mobilisation of the Nervous System, *Edinburgh, 1991, Churchill Livingstone.* (From Cameron M: *Physical Rehabilitation,* St. Louis, 2007, Saunders).

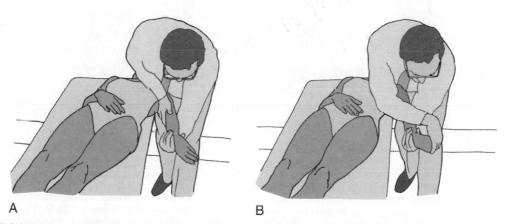

FIGURE 6-24 ULTT radial nerve. Upper limb tension test 2b (ULTT2b), radial nerve dominant utilizing shoulder girdle depression plus internal rotation of the shoulder. A, Position the patient as in ULTT2a and extend the elbow. Then medially rotate the shoulder and pronate the forearm. B, Flex the wrist, fingers, and thumb. *Adapted from Butler DS:* Mobilisation of the Nervous System, *Edinburgh, 1991, Churchill Livingstone.* (From Cameron M: *Physical Rehabilitation,* St. Louis, 2007, Saunders)

Upper Limb Tension Test for the Radial Nerve

For the ULTT that specifically addresses the radial nerve distribution (C5 to T1), place the patient in a supine position on a plinth in the anatomical position (Fig. 6-24). This test can be performed while sitting or standing as well. Have the patient extend his/her shoulder to supple end-range and then bring their wrist into volar flexion. While depressing the clavicle and first rib and controlling for excessive scapular winging, have the patient laterally flex their cervical spine away from the extended shoulder. Hold this position for a maximum of 60 seconds or until the patient complains of heightened neurological symptoms. This test is positive if the patient is experiencing an increase in neurological symptoms.

Upper Limb Tension Test for the Ulnar Nerve

The final ULTT assesses the neurological irritation of the ulnar nerve distribution (C8 to T1) (Fig. 6-25). Start by placing the patient in a supine position on a plinth in the anatomical position. Have the patient abduct their shoulder to a 90-degree position. Next, have the patient fully flex their elbow and extend their wrist. While depressing the clavicle and the first rib, have the patient laterally flex their cervical spine away from the side

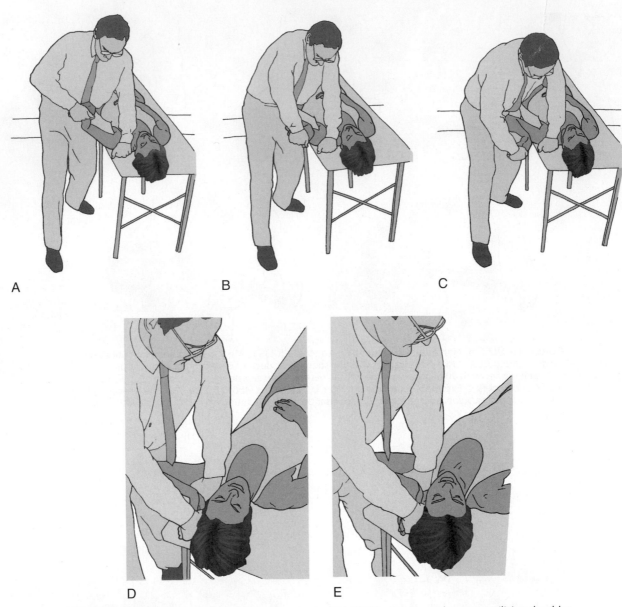

FIGURE 6-25 ULTT ulnar nerve. Upper limb tension test 3 (ULTT3), ulnar nerve dominant utilizing shoulder abduction and elbow flexion. A, Position the patient as for ULTT1. Then extend the wrist and supinate the forearm. B, Fully flex the elbow. C, Depress the shoulder girdle and externally rotate the shoulder. D, Abduct the shoulder. E, Side bend the neck away from the side being tested. *Adapted from Butler DS:* Mobilisation of the Nervous System, *Edinburgh, 1991, Churchill Livingstone.* (From Cameron M: Physical Rehabilitation, St. Louis, 2007, Saunders)

being examined. Hold this position for a maximum of 60 seconds or until the patient complains of heightened neurological symptoms. This test is considered positive if the patient is experiencing an increase in neurological symptoms.

These tests are best utilized when there is an expectation by the treating therapists that the nerve symptoms that the patient is experiencing are from a more proximal origin versus a distal origin. They are often used when a patient is experiencing bilateral symptoms distally in the hand secondary to a proximal nerve compression.

For example, if you have a patient who has undergone a carpal tunnel release surgery, has attended hand therapy sessions from the initial 3 day post-operative evaluation through 8 weeks of active therapy, and is still experiencing numbness and tingling in the median nerve distribution, then a "red flag" should go off in the therapist's mind suggesting that there could be a neuropraxic compression that has origins proximal to zone 4 of the hand. This could lead to the therapist utilizing the ULTT for the median nerve distribution to rule out upper plexus compression or potential cervical radiculopathy. Through using the ULTT, the therapist might find a positive result and recommend a more proximal treatment approach in addressing the neurological lesion.

Although there are a myriad of tests that can help "map" out a neurological lesion, one of the biggest pitfalls in hand therapy practice is a failure to address proximal muscle balance or imbalance of a patient through upper limb tension testing. Finally, it is vital for the therapist not only to assess where the nerve lesion is but to adapt the treatment plan through clinical reasoning to address the specific neurological problem.

The pitfalls of edema, scar adhesions, joint derangement, muscle imbalances, muscle weakness, upper plexus irritation and pain reflexes directly impact the expedient return to social role independence. If therapists miss these pitfalls early, they will manifest into long-standing functional impairments. Proactive awareness of pitfalls can diminish rehabilitation timelines and financial burden of return to function. Additionally, it is important to consider what is meaningful to the patient. Taking this into account will aid in the motivation to return to meaningful occupational performance, thereby increasing the volition to participate in motor-control activities that the patient feels are most important to them.

References

1. Madden JW: Wound healing: the biological basis of hand surgery, *Clin Plast Surg* 3(1):3–11, 1976.
2. Madden JW, Peacock EE Jr: Studies on the biology of collagen during wound healing: dynamic metabolism of scar collagen and remodeling of dermal wounds, *Ann Surg* 174(3):511–520, 1971.
3. Arem AJ, Madden JW: Is there a Wolff's law for connective tissue? *Surg Forum* 25(0):512–514, 1974.
4. Arem AJ, Madden JW: Effects of stress on healing wounds: I. intermittent noncyclical tension, *J Surg Res* 20(2):93–102, 1976.
5. Baker S, Swanson N: Rapid intraoperative tissue expansion in reconstruction of the head and neck, *Arch Otolaryngol Head Neck Surg* 116:1431–1434, 1990.
6. Beauchene J: Biochemical, biomechanical, and physical changes in the skin in an experimental animal model of therapeutic tissue expansion, *J Surg Res* 47:507, 1989.
7. Hertling D, Kessler R: *Management of common musculoskeletal disorders:physical therapy principles and methods*, 1996, Lippincott Williams & Wilkins.
8. Madden J. Wound healing: biologic and clinical features. In Sabiston J, Davis-Christopher, editors: *Sabiston textbook of surgery*, ed 12, Philadelphia, 1981, Saunders.
9. Weeks PM, Wray RC, editors: *The management of acute hand injuries: a biological approach*, St. Louis, 1973, Mosby.
10. Pitts G, Willoughby J: Rehabilitation of wrist and hand injuries. In Andrews J, Harrelson G, Wilk K, editors: *Physical rehabilitation of the injured athlete*, ed 4, Philadelphia, 2012, Elsevier Saunders.
11. Mason ML, Allen HS: The rate of healing of tendons: an experimental study of tensile strength, *Ann Surg* 113(3):424–459, 1941.
12. Brand PW, Hollister AM: *Clinical mechanics of the hand*, ed 2, St Louis, 1993, Mosby Yearbook.
13. Brand PW, editor: *Clinical mechanics of the hand*, St. Louis, 1985, Mosby.
14. Brand PW: Mechanical factors in joint stiffness and tissue growth, *J Hand Ther* 8(2):91–96, 1995.
15. Brand PW, Hollister AM: *Clinical mechanics of the hand*, ed 3, St Louis, 1999, Mosby.
16. Brand PW: Hand rehabilitation: management by objectives. Brand PW: The forces of dynamic splinting: ten questions before applying a dynamic splint to the hand. In Hunter JM, Schneider, Mackin, et al, *Rehabilitation of the hand: surgery and therapy*, ed 3, St Louis, 1989, Mosby.
17. Bell-Krotoski J: Biomechanics and evaluation of the hand. In Hunter JM, Mackin, Callahan, et al, editors: *Rehabilitation of the hand and upper extremity*, ed 5, St Louis, 2002, Mosby.
18. Brand PW: Hand rehabilitation: management by objectives. In Hunter JM, Schneider LC, Mackin E, editors: *Rehabilitation of the hand*, ed 2, St. Louis, 1984, Mosby.
19. Kaltenborn FM: *Manual mobilization of the joints*, ed 7, Minneapolis, 2011, Orthopedic Physical Therapy Products.
20. Kapandji AI: *The physiology of the joints*, ed 6, Philadelphia, 2007, Churchill Livingstone Elsevier.
21. McKee P, Hannah S, Priganc VW: Orthotic considerations for dense connective tissue and articular cartilage—the need for optimal movement and stress, *J Hand Ther* 25(2):233–243, 2012.
22. Riordan DC: A walk through the anatomy of the hand and forearm, *J Hand Ther* 8(2):68–78, 1995.
23. Waylett-Rendall J, Seibly D: A study of the accuracy of a commercially available volumeter, *J Hand Ther* 4:10–13, 1991.
24. Breger-Lee DE, J. B.-K.: Torque range of motion in the hand clinic, *J Hand Ther* ***:7–13, 1990.
25. Breger-Lee D, Voelker ET, Giurintano D, et al: Reliability of torque range of motion: a preliminary study, *J Hand Ther* 6(1):29–34, 1993.
26. Gelberman RH, Manske PR: Factors influencing flexor tendon adhesions, *Hand Clin* 1(1):35–42, 1985.
27. Micks JE, Reswick JB: Confirmation of differential loading of lateral and central fibers of the extensor tendon, *J Hand Surg Am* 6(5):462–467, 1981.
28. Garcia-Elias M, An KN, Berglund L, et al: Extensor mechanism of the fingers. I. A quantitative geometric study, *J Hand Surg Am* 16(6):1130–1136, 1991.
29. Strickland JW, Gettle K: Flexor tendon repair: the Indianapolis method. In Hunter J, Schneider L, Mackin E, editors: *Tendon and nerve surgery in the hand—a third decade*, St. Louis, 1997, Mosby.
30. Manske PR, Gelberman RH, Lesker PA: Flexor tendon healing, *Hand Clin* 1(1):25, 1985.
31. Duran R, et al: Management of flexor tendon lacerations in zone 2 using controlled passive motion postoperatively. In Hunter JM, editor: *Tendon surgery in the hand*, St Louis, 1987, Mosby.
32. Evans R: Immediate active short arc motion following tendon repair. In Hunter JM, Mackin EJ, Schneider LH, editors: *Tendon and nerve surgery in the hand: a third decade*, ed 1, St Louis, 1997, Mosby.
33. Gelberman RH, Manske PR: Factors influencing flexor tendon adhesions, *Hand Clin* 1(1):35–42, 1985.
34. Kleinert HE, et al: Primary repair of flexor tendons in no-man's land, *J Bone Joint Surg* 49A:577, 1967.
35. Hunter JM, Mackin EJ, Schneider LH: *Tendon and nerve surgery in the hand: a third decade*, ed 1, St Louis, 1997, Mosby.
36. Brand PW, Beach RB, Thompson DE: Relative tension and potential excursion of muscles in the forearm and hand, *J Hand Surg Am* 6(3):209–219, 1981.
37. (Mark Linsay personal communication 1994)
38. Bell-Krotoski JA, Fess EE: Biomechanics: the forces of change and the basis for all that we do, *J Hand Ther* 8(2):63–67, 1995.
39. Mennell J: *Science and art of joint manipulation*, Vol 2, London, 1952, Churchill.
40. Tubiana R, Thomine JM, Mackin E: *Examination of the hand and wrist*, Philadelphia, 1996, WB Saunders Company.
41. ***
42. Brand PW, Hollister A, Thompson D: Mechanical resistance. In Brand PW, Hollister A, editors: *Clinical mechanics of the hand*, ed 3, St. Louis, 1999, Mosby.
43. Smith P: *Lister's The Hand*, ed 4, Livingstone, 2001, Churchill.
44. Roberson L, Giurintano DJ: Objective measures of joint stiffness, *J Hand Ther* 8(2):163–166, 1995.
45. Hoppenfeld S: *Physical examination of the spine & extremities*, East Norwalk, CT, 1976, Appleton-Century-Crofts (Prentice-Hall).
46. Elfman H: Biomechanics of muscle, *J Bone Joint Surg [Am]* 48A:363–377, 1966.
47. Smith P: *Lister's the hand: diagnosis and indications*, ed 4, Philadelphia, 2002, Churchill Livingstone.
48. Covington TJ: Evaluation and treatment of pain: aspects for nerve injury and rehabilitation, *J Hand Ther* 6(2):161–169, 1993.

49. Dahlin L: The biology of nerve injury and repair, *J Hand Surg Am* 143–155, 2004.
50. Topp KS, Boyd BS: Peripheral nerve: from the microscopic functional unit of the axon to the biomechanically loaded macroscopic structure, *J Hand Ther* 25(2):142–152, 2012.
51. Novak CB, Mackinnon SE: Repetitive use and static postures: a source of nerve compression and pain, *J Hand Ther* 10(2):151–159, 1997.
52. Walsh MT: Interventions in the disturbances in the motor and sensory environment, *J Hand Ther* 25(2):202–219, 2012.
53. Kendall FP, Provance P, McCreary EK: *Muscles testing and function: with posture and pain*, ed 4, Baltimore, 1993, Lippincott Williams & Wilkins.
54. (Mayer, 1997)
55. Carr J, Shepherd R: *Neurological Rehabilitation: Optimizing motor performance*, ed 2, Livingston, 2010, Churchhill.
56. Butler DS: *The sensitive nervous system*, ed 1, Minneapolis, 2006, Orthopedic Physical Therapy Products.

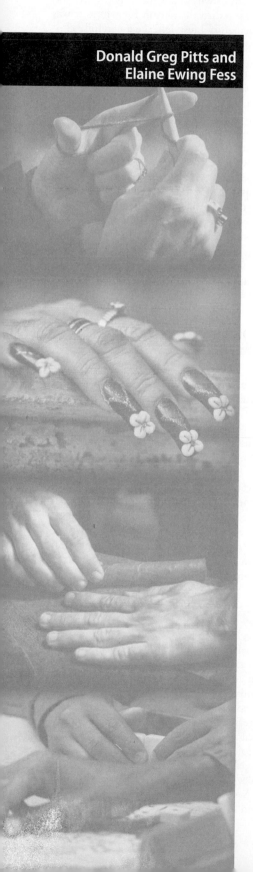

7

Orthoses: Essential Concepts

**Donald Greg Pitts and
Elaine Ewing Fess**

Written for therapists with novice to intermediate level experience, this chapter is not intended to provide comprehensive information for therapists with extensive experience in the field of hand/upper extremity rehabilitation. Instead, this chapter provides straightforward answers to the following basic questions relating to orthotic theory and clinical practice:

- Getting started
- What is the historical perspective for orthotic intervention provided by therapists?
- Who makes orthoses?
- Why are orthoses applied?
- What factors guide orthotic design?
- What tools and materials are used to fabricate orthoses?
- How do orthoses work?
- How do wound healing stages guide orthotic intervention?
- What is tissue remodeling?
- How are orthoses named/classified?
- What are the most commonly fabricated orthoses?

Getting Started

Perusing published literature regarding orthotic theory and application can be daunting, especially for therapists who are inexperienced in fabricating orthoses. However, it is important to remember that each "experienced" therapist had to begin by making his/her first orthosis. Orthotic fabrication is a skill that is developed through experience and over time. It is not an inherited trait. Practice is imperative. Being familiar with materials and understanding basic anatomy, kinesiology, and biomechanical concepts are the keys to success. As with all new skills, orthotic proficiency involves a crucial learning curve. Those who do not take the time to prepare, never learn. Conversely, those who persevere in developing their skills through practice and application, become increasingly adept. Upgrading skills and knowledge is also important as new materials and concepts are introduced.

Historical Perspective[1]

Application of orthoses is not a contemporary concept. Leaves, reeds, bamboo, and bark with linen padding were used to immobilize fractures in early antiquity. By the 1500s, copper orthoses augmented treatment of individuals with burn injuries; and Hippocrates applied orthoses to either immobilize or distract fractures (460-377 BC). Created by armor-makers, turn-buckle orthoses were used to correct joint contractures by 1517; and surgeons worked with "appliance-makers" to create custom orthoses from the 1750s to the 1850s. Plaster of Paris became a popular orthotic material in the mid-1850s; and the first book dedicated to describing orthoses was published in 1888. The era of surgeon-fabricated orthoses began in the late 1800s, continuing well into the 20th century. From early to late 20th century, eight major factors influenced orthotic practice, including (1) disease; (2) political conflict/war; (3) surgical advances; (4) commercial products; (5) basic science advances; (6) governmental agency support; (7) creation of specialized hand centers; (8) knowledge dissemination and organizational leadership. The consequences of epidemiologic disease (for example, infection, polio) and war injuries provided momentum to surgical and basic science advances (for example, anatomy, wound healing, tissue remodeling), eventually resulting in governmental support of early specialized hand/upper extremity, hospital-based treatment venues. Government agencies also supported dissemination of evolving knowledge through workshops and publications focused on teaching therapists about hand/upper extremity orthotic concepts and techniques. Concomitantly, material innovations facilitated orthotic fabrication, starting with aluminum (1920s) and moving through the "plastics revolution" (1930s to present). The race for space during the Cold War introduced even more sophisticated materials that were adapted by commercial entities for orthotic application. Based on Dr. Paul Band's rehabilitation center in India, the first hand center in the United States (US) was established in 1961 in Chapel Hill, North Carolina. The 1970s were expansion years for hand surgeons and therapists. Surgeons began relying exclusively on therapists to provide orthoses and treatment for individuals in their care who had sustained upper extremity injuries; and cutting-edge specialty centers dedicated solely to treating upper extremity problems were established across the US. Professional hand specialty organizations for surgeons (American Society for Surgery of the Hand [ASSH], American Association for Hand Surgery [AAHS]) and therapists (American Society of Hand Therapists [ASHT], American Hand Therapy Foundation [AHTF], Hand Therapy Certification Commission [HTCC]) provided and continue to provide educational and research forums relating to orthotic intervention for the upper extremity; and the *Journal of Hand Surgery* and the *Journal of Hand Therapy* disseminate up-to-the-minute orthotic concepts. While books and manuals relating to upper extremity orthoses reached their pinnacle in the 1980s, production of orthotic-specific publications continue to the present.

Makers of Orthoses

Although their respective areas of expertise differ, currently, both therapists (occupational therapists and physical therapists) and orthotists create and apply orthotic devices. Traditionally, therapists work closely with hand/upper extremity surgeons to fabricate orthotic devices that most often require application during early- to mid-treatment intervention. These orthoses routinely necessitate frequent adjustments and alterations in order to keep up with clients' changing medical requirements; and are usually constructed from less durable materials, such as thermoplastics, or even plaster of Paris. In contrast, orthotists traditionally work with orthotic materials that are more durable in order to achieve the requisites of clients that are well past their immediate remedial needs.

Rationale for Orthotic Application

Reasons for orthotic intervention directly correlate with injury-specific and/or disease-specific patient diagnoses. In a review of published literature spanning over a fifty-year time frame, twenty-seven different rationales for orthotic intervention were identified; with the six most frequently cited reasons, listed in rank-order, including to (1) increase function; (2) prevent deformity; (3) correct deformity; (4) protect healing structures; (5) restrict motion; and (6) allow tissue growth/remodeling.[1]

Design

Although orthotic devices often are crucial "door-openers" for subsequent referrals, they are never regarded as stand-alone interventions. Instead, each orthosis is created to reflect individual contextual conditions of why the orthosis is needed and how it will be used to help return the person for whom it was created to an active participatory lifestyle. Like a carefully choreographed dance, the tempo of which is dictated by wound healing status, therapists create and modify orthoses in accordance with a multitude of client variables including, but not limited to, diagnosis, wound status, concomitant exercise programs, physical and mental status, age, motivation, intelligence, activities of daily living (ADLs), instrumental activities of daily living (IADL), work, family support, distance from the clinic, etc. Unfortunately, client third-party payer status sometimes must also be part of these considered factors. Meeting individual needs requires therapist creativity and understanding of the ramifications of design options. Even if two clients have similar diagnoses, their resulting orthoses may differ due to their respective individual circumstances.

In addition to satisfying client-specific requisites, orthoses absolutely must function properly. In other words, they must accomplish, in the most efficacious manner possible, the purposes for which they are applied. Otherwise, they limit the rehabilitation potential of those who wear them.

Materials and Equipment

As noted in the "Historical Perspective" section, orthotic materials evolve as technology becomes more sophisticated. Chemical composition differentiates physical properties of thermoplastic materials. Both high and low temperature thermoplastics become malleable through heat application. Most thermoplastics used in clinical situations are low temperature materials; although some high temperature thermoplastics are used for outrigger components or as reinforcement for weaker materials. While more uniform levels of heat transfer are achieved via wet heat, the majority of thermoplastic materials currently available to therapists may be warmed using either wet or dry heat. Thermoplastic materials are often described by their "draping" capacity. Some materials require a given amount of finger pressure to mold them to an extremity, while others simply drape or "flow" themselves onto and into extremity contours. Each material has advantages and disadvantages. Astute therapists coordinate material physical properties to meet the needs of their individual clients.

Companies that supply orthotic materials encourage therapists to familiarize themselves with a wide range of orthotic products by making available at no cost or minimal cost, "sample kits" of orthotic materials. In addition to thermoplastic materials, do not dismiss the conforming advantages of plaster of Paris. This material continues to hold a special place in orthotic fabrication, especially for orthoses created to mobilize joints via application of orthoses that are changed serially.

Basic equipment for fabricating orthoses includes, but is not limited to, a water heat pan, several pairs of sharp scissors, a heat gun, a rotary hole-punch, box cutter, wire cutters, an awl, and a goniometer (Fig. 7-2). Scissors that are used for cutting Velcro should be segregated and used only for this task since they tend

> **◎ Clinical Pearl**
>
> Limiting oneself to just one thermoplastic material considerably narrows ones' ability to provide optimal therapeutic intervention for clients. Practicing with new materials as they are introduced to the market is essential for both novice and experienced therapists (Fig. 7-1).

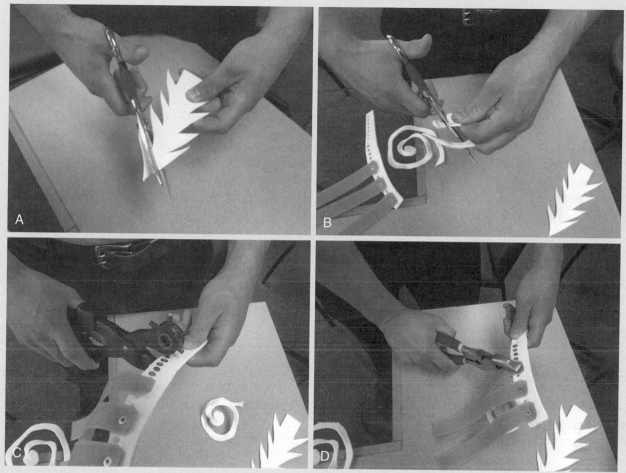

FIGURE 7-1 Using scrap orthotic materials, practice cutting various shapes **(A, B)** and setting rivets **(C, D)** improves novice skill sets; and familiarizes experienced therapists with properties of new materials.

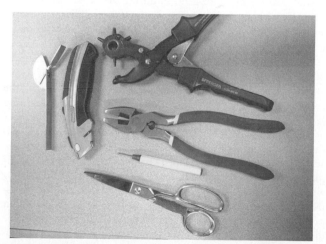

FIGURE 7-2 Basic tools used to fabricate orthoses may be found in most hardware stores.

to become "gummy" from the Velcro adhesive, making them unsuitable for cutting heated thermoplastic materials.

Ergonomic use of tools and equipment is essential to producing orthoses that are professionally assembled and finished. Simple practices, like rounding orthotic corners and strap-end eliminates uncomfortable pointed ends and edges (Fig. 7-3).

> **◎ Clinical Pearl**
>
> Not fully closing scissor blades when cutting warm thermoplastic materials, produces smooth cut edges. This is in contrast to the regular-occurring-sharp-points along cut heated material edges when scissor blades are closed completely.

Additionally, improper use of equipment may injure the hands of those who fabricate orthoses. When cutting materials, therapists should keep their hands and wrists in neutral postures and bring materials to the scissors to avoid "chasing"

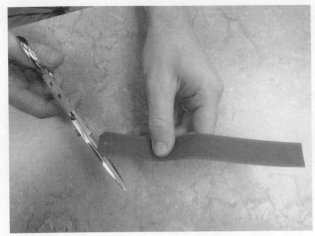

FIGURE 7-3 Rounding strap corners increases orthosis cosmesis and eliminates pointed ends that can cause skin irritation.

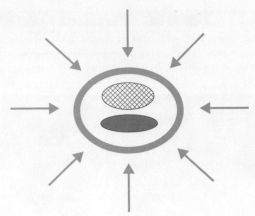

FIGURE 7-5 With circumferential configurations, coadaptation orthoses do not have a middle reciprocal force. (From Fess EE: Splints: mechanics versus convention, *J Hand Ther* 8(2):124-130, 1995.)

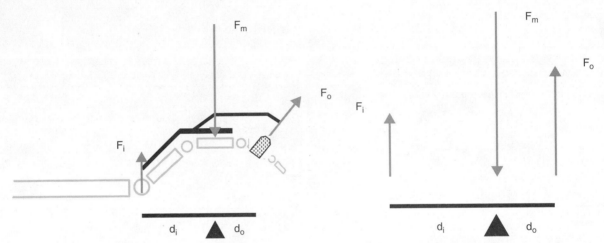

FIGURE 7-4 Orthoses with three-point pressure systems have a middle reciprocal force, the magnitude *(Fm)* of which is the sum of the opposing proximal *(Fi)* and distal *(Fo)* forces. *di,* input distance; *do,* output distance. (From Fess EE, Gettle K, Philips C, et al: *Hand and upper extremity splinting: principles and methods,* ed 3, St Louis, 2004, Mosby Elsevier.)

the material, which increases exposure to risk factors associated with awkward postures. Over time, therapists who ignore ergonomic concepts while fabricating orthoses tend to develop finger and thumb joint pain from stress and overuse injuries. For example, commonly seen thumb carpometacarpal (CMC) and/or metacarpophalangeal (MP) joint pain often stems from the chronic practice of cutting under-heated thermoplastic materials.

Factors That Allow Orthoses to Work Effectively

In mechanical terms, orthoses function either as lever systems that apply *three-point pressures* in reciprocal patterns (Fig. 7-4); or they apply *two-point pressures* in opposing patterns (Fig. 7-5). The vast majority of orthotic designs utilize *three-point pressures.* Although less frequently used, the most common reasons for applying two-point pressure orthoses are to support stable fractures (for example, humerus; metacarpals) or to support healing/repaired pulleys of digital flexor tendons.

See Table 7-1 for mechanical principles for creating effective orthoses.[2]

Wound Healing Stages

Orthotic intervention directly correlates with tissue-specific wound healing stages. In general, during the acute *inflammatory stage (0 to 2 weeks),* tissues are rested via immobilization orthoses; or for some tendon repairs, orthoses that apply minimal stress may be applied under very specific conditions in order to minimize/control scar tissue development and to increase tensile strength of repairs. Note that early passive and early active motion programs for tendon repairs are undertaken only with the consent of the referring physicians. During the *fibroplasia stage (2 to 4 weeks),* wound tensile strength increases and the focus of orthotic intervention is protection of soft tissue structures and their associated repairs while initiating minimal to moderate active motion without resistance. Orthoses used during the fibroplasia stage often restrict joint motion in specific directions while allowing motion in other directions. For example, minimal resistance may be allowed with the direction of repaired structures but prohibited in directions against the repairs. These orthoses are diagnosis-specific and vary widely in design. During the *maturation phase (more than 4 weeks),* graded resistance against the direction of repairs may be initiated. Maturation phase orthotic

TABLE 7-1 Mechanical Principles of Orthotic Fabrication and Fit

Principle	Implication
1. Understanding force systems	Know when to use three-point pressure orthotic designs and when to use two-point pressure orthotic designs.
2. Increase the area of force application	Wider orthotic components decrease pressure and increase comfort.
3. Increase mechanical advantage	Longer orthotic components decrease pressure and increase comfort.
4. Use optimum rotational force	Application of corrective force is most efficient at a 90-degree angle.
5. Consider torque effect	The further away from the main focus joint a force is applied, the greater the torque on that joint will be. Be careful to not exceed tissue and/or pain thresholds.
6. Control reaction at secondary joints	Prevent subluxation of joints proximal and/or distal to primary focus joints within longitudinal rays.
7. Consider reciprocal parallel force effect	• Middle reciprocal pressure in a three-point pressure orthosis equals the sum of proximal and distal forces. • Monitor the area under middle-reciprocal-pressure components carefully for soft tissue breakdown.
8. Use appropriate outrigger systems	• Outriggers must be of sufficient strength to support pull from traction devices (for example, rubber bands). • As joint motion changes, alter outrigger length to maintain a 90-degree angle of pull.
9. Incorporate articulated components appropriately	Carefully align orthosis joints/hinges with corresponding anatomical joints.
10. Increase material strength through contour	Contoured material provides strength to orthotic components.
11. Eliminate friction	• Eliminate orthosis slippage or "pistoning" on the extremity as clients move. • Design orthoses according to key skin creases to ensure that orthotic material does not impede desired joint motion.
12. Avoid high shear stress	• High shear stress causes soft tissue breakdown. • Monitor extremity for pressure from orthosis edges. • When possible, widen narrow components that contact the extremity. • Monitor soft tissue beneath narrow orthotic components.

intervention frequently deals with, but is not limited to, problems relating to limitations in joint motion. It is important to remember that wound healing stages progress at different rates depending on the types of tissues involved. Normal healing time is delayed with contaminated wounds, wounds that are overly stressed or traumatized, with specific metabolic conditions, with patients taking certain pharmacologic drugs, and with chronic smokers. Additionally, orthotic intervention is influenced by types of repairs and patient-specific variables, such as age, intelligence, motivation, and so on.[2]

Soft Tissue Remodeling Concepts

Cells strive for equilibrium by compensating biologically via a process known as *remodeling*. When under greater than normal tension, the number of cells increases through mitosis; and when tension is less than normal, cells are absorbed so that normal cell equilibrium is reestablished[3] (Fig.7-6). Understanding and effectively utilizing soft tissue remodeling is fundamental to successful orthotic intervention.[2,4,5]

Clinical Pearl

Application of too much tension tears soft tissue, exacerbating the inflammatory process and creating more scar; while too little tension results in delayed minimal to no tissue remodeling.

The key to success is knowing how much tension to apply and when to do so. Orthoses designed to correct digital joint contractures apply between 100 to 300 grams of traction.[2] Larger joints require somewhat greater forces. Inexperienced therapists tend to use too much corrective traction on joints with range of motion (ROM) limitations.[2]

Naming and Classifying Orthoses

Similar to animal and plant taxonomic names, orthoses have multiple designations, including colloquial names, L-Code classifications, and scientific nomenclature. Utilization of these respective identifications is situation-dependent. For example, colloquial labels are more frequently utilized in informal settings; L-Codes are the foundation for billing; and scientific terminology is employed when very precise connotations are required.

The ability to express information clearly and distinctly, without confusion, directly reflects the level of sophistication of populations and the professions within those populations. How orthoses are named and classified is critical to the development, recognition, and credibility of the occupational and physical therapy professions.

Colloquial names, like street jargon, reflect regional geographic locales. These names often make little sense to outsiders but within regional groups they carry distinct meaning. Unfortunately, these local dialects inhibit professional

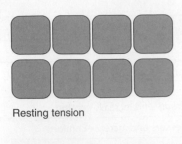

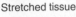
Resting tension

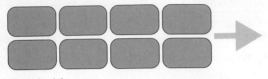
Stretched tissue

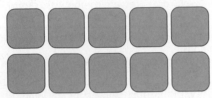
Growth restores resting tension

FIGURE 7-6 Mechanical stress-tension initiates tissue remodeling. (From De Filippo RE, Atala A: Stretch and growth: the molecular and physiologic influences of tissue expansion, *Plast Reconstr Surg* 109(7):2450-2462, 2002; adapted from www.plasticsurgery.org.)

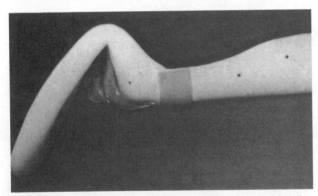

FIGURE 7-7 *Index-small finger MP flexion and IP extension, thumb CMC radial abduction* and *MP-IP extension mobilization orthosis, type 1 (16)* MP flexion, IP extension of the digits, with thumb radial abduction and extension mobilization orthoses are frequently used during the early stages of burn, crush, or frostbite injuries. Orthotic intervention is critical to prevent unwanted deformity. (From Fess EE, Gettle K, Philips C, et al: *Hand and upper extremity splinting: principles and methods*, ed 3, St Louis, 2004, Mosby Elsevier.)

communication across geographic boundaries. For example, this orthosis (Fig. 7-7) has multiple colloquial names including, but not limited to, "resting pan," platform," "night splint," "resting platform," "functional position splint," "burn orthosis," and "clam-digger." In reality, none of these names adequately describes the pictured orthosis.

L-Codes were developed in the late 1970s by orthotists in order to standardize billing for orthoses and prostheses. In 2006 and 2007, as a result of Centers for Medicare and Medicaid

Services (CMS) collaborating with the American Occupational Therapy Association (AOTA), the American Physical Therapy Association (APTA), and the ASHT L-Code Task Force, twenty-four new L-Codes that better reflect the orthoses that therapists create were added to existing codes.[6] In addition to L-Code terminology that describes anatomical segments influenced by orthoses (for example, finger, hand, wrist, elbow, shoulder and combinations thereof), L-Code descriptions also define whether or not orthoses include articulations, and whether they are custom-made or prefabricated. Describing form rather than function, the L-Code system results in simplistic descriptive phrases that define letter/number codes. For example, L3808 is a *Wrist hand finger orthosis, rigid without joints, may include soft interface material; straps, custom fabricated, includes fitting and adjustment.*

While L-Codes are a major improvement over colloquial names, relying on L-Codes as a means to classify orthoses precisely and in a scientific manner is fraught with limitations, the greatest of which is that the codes group all sorts of unrelated orthoses together. The only commonality is that group members have similar configurations. Because of this shortcoming, it is difficult, if not impossible, to correlate L-Codes with International Classification of Diseases (ICD)-9/10 diagnostic codes.[7] Further, L-Codes are not reflective of the high functioning level at which hand/upper extremity specialist therapists operate. Language-wise, L-Codes are analogous to, "Me Tarzan, you Jane."

Scientific nomenclature systems that successfully and accurately sort items often utilize organizational structures that progressively move from comprehensive to fine detail. The scientific classification that groups living biological entities into eight hierarchal taxonomic ranks (life, domain, kingdom, phylum, class, order, family, genus, and species) is an excellent example of this type of ranked classification system.

Orthosis Classification System and Expanded Orthosis Classification System[1]

In 1992, the ASHT published a theoretical foundation for an important scientific system of classifying splints/orthoses that is based on function rather than form called the Orthosis Classification System* (OCS);[8] and in 2004, Elaine Ewing Fess, Karan Gettle, Cynthia Philips, and Robin Janson expanded this system to include, in addition to the original orthoses group, an additional purpose; and two new major device groups, splint-prostheses and prostheses called the Expanded Orthosis Classification System (EOCS). Nearly 1,200 orthotic and prosthetic devices are scientifically classified in the third edition of their book,[2] a feat that was not possible previously.

Learning the OCS/EOCS

Is relatively simple. Orthoses are first divided according to whether or not they influence articular structures. *Nonarticular* orthoses do not influence joint action. When named, these orthoses always carry the "nonarticular" designation in their respective scientific names. Nonarticular orthoses are further subdivided according to the anatomical segment to which they are fitted (Table 7-2).

---

*The terms, splint and orthosis, are used interchangeably in the OCS and EOCS. Orthosis is the New Latin form of the word, orthotic. Orthoses is the plural of orthosis.

TABLE 7-2	EOCS Nonarticular Orthosis Nomenclature
NONARTICULAR ORTHOSES	
Anatomical segment	For example, humerus; metacarpal; forearm, proximal phalanx, and so on
Example	*Nonarticular proximal forearm orthosis*
Photo	(Fig. 7-8)

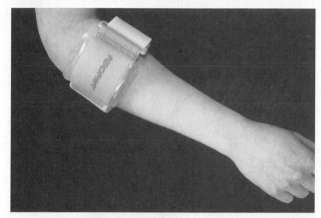

FIGURE 7-8 Nonarticular proximal forearm orthosis. This nonarticular forearm orthosis design may reduce pain during activities that induce lateral epicondylitis. A variety of nonarticular forearm orthosis design options are available. (Courtesy of Aircast, Summit, NJ.)

In contrast, *articular* orthoses affect joint motion. Because the vast majority of orthoses are articular, for convenience, the designation "articular" is dropped from these scientific names. Articular orthoses are further ranked according to five hierarchical sub classifications (Table 7-3).

The OCS and EOCS identify four purposes for orthotic application:[2,8]

1. *Immobilization* orthoses stop motion at main/primary joints via external forces.
2. *Mobilization* orthoses increase motion at main/primary joints via external forces.
3. *Restriction* orthoses limit normal arc of motion of main/primary joints via external forces.
4. *Torque transmission* orthoses redirect internal forces to main/primary joints.

It is important to understand that these four purposes describe orthosis function rather than orthosis form. In contrast, the terms, "static," "dynamic," and "static-progressive" are archaic descriptors of orthosis form/configuration, and they have no place in the OCS/EOCS scientific classification system.

With the exception of the Type category, the subclassifications associated with articular orthoses are intuitive. Type describes the less important joints that are included in an orthosis to stabilize the orthosis on the extremity and/or to enhance its mechanical performance. In contrast to the main/primary joints that are named, Type joints' names are not included in the scientific designation. Instead, Type joints are counted according to their transverse alignment levels. For example, the MPs are counted as only one (1) level regardless of how many MP joints are included in an orthosis. Potentially, there are ten upper extremity levels, shoulder, elbow, forearm, wrist, finger MP, finger proximal interphalangeal (PIP), finger distal

TABLE 7-3	EOCS Articular Orthosis Nomenclature
ARTICULAR ORTHOSES	
Primary anatomical joint(s)	These are the very specific joints upon which the orthosis is designed to act. These joints are named in the scientific designation (for example, shoulder, elbow, finger MP, and so on); and they are further described by direction and purpose categorizations.
Direction	Extension, flexion, radial deviation, ulnar deviation, circumduction, abduction, adduction, and so on
Purpose	Immobilization, mobilization, restriction, torque transmission
Type	Count of secondary joint *levels;* these joint levels are *not* specifically named in the scientific designation; only their number of levels are counted. Secondary joints are included to stabilize the orthosis on the extremity. They are "anchor" joints, "holding on" joints, or "positioning" joints. There is no direction or purpose associated with these joints. These joints are included in the orthosis to improve its function mechanically.
Total joint(s)	Count of all joints included in the orthosis
Example	*Small finger MP flexion mobilization orthosis, type 0 (1)*
Photo	(Fig. 7-9)

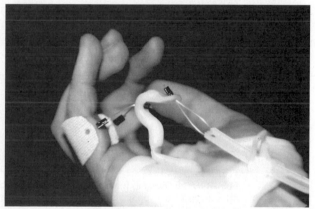

FIGURE 7-9 Small finger MP flexion mobilization orthosis, type 0 (1). This specialized outrigger maintains a 90-degree angle to the proximal phalanx as MP joint motion changes, and the unique inelastic mobilization assist facilitates tension adjustments. (Courtesy of Nelson Vazquez, OTR, CHT, Miami, FL, and Damon Kirk, WFR Corporation, Wyckoff, NJ.)

interphalangeal (DIP), thumb CMC, thumb MP, and thumb interphalangeal (IP). Type classification ranges from 0 (no secondary joint levels included) to 9 (nine secondary joint levels included).[2,8]

Applying the OCS/EOCS

As noted earlier, the OCS and EOCS describe orthoses according to function. This means that some orthoses with identical configurations can have different functions. For example, the ubiquitous "wrist cock-up" orthosis (Fig. 7-10) may be fitted for the following reasons, each with a different ICD-9 code (see Table 7-4).

In comparison, because L-Code designations are based on form rather than function, the L-Codes for three of the above four scenarios are identical: L3906—*Wrist hand orthosis, without joints, may include soft interface, straps, custom fabricated, includes fitting and adjustment.*[9] Significantly, there is no L-Code designation for "static" orthoses that are designed to mobilize joints (increase joint motion) via serial changes. While acceptable for billing purposes, L-Codes are woefully inadequate in terms of being an efficacious scientific language.

A summary example of the power of the OCS/EOCS involves an orthosis that often is used to correct boutonniere deformity at the PIP joint (Fig. 7-11). This small orthosis includes three purposes in its EOCS designation, each correlated with correcting a specific anatomical problem within the boutonniere deformity. The EOCS designation for this orthosis is: *Long finger PIP extension mobilization / DIP extension restriction / DIP flexion torque transmission orthosis, type 0 (2).* The orthosis simultaneously remodels the PIP flexion contracture via serially applied inelastic extension traction; stops DIP hyperextension via a dorsal block; and remodels the shortened oblique retinacular ligaments via active torque transmission forces. The ICD-9 code is 842.13.[7] Colloquially,

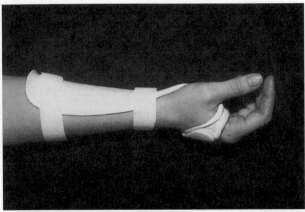
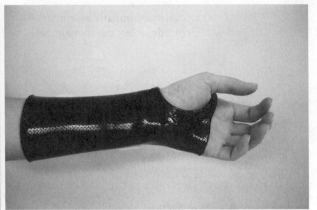
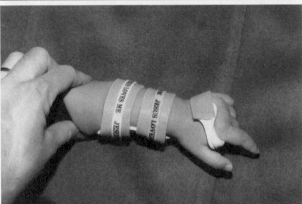

FIGURE 7-10 Wrist extension mobilization orthosis, type 0 (1). Type 0 wrist mobilization orthoses may be fitted to provide mobilization forces to stiff, weakened, or paralytic joints. When used to increase passive joint range of motion (ROM), they may be serially adjusted allowing continuous application of mobilization forces until the desired goal is achieved. (From Fess EE, Gettle K, Philips C, et al: *Hand and upper extremity splinting: principles and methods,* ed 3, St Louis, 2004, Mosby Elsevier.)

TABLE 7-4	EOCS Correlation with ICD-9 Codes	
Purpose	**EOCS Name**	**ICD-9 Code[7]**
To stop wrist motion	*Wrist neutral immobilization orthosis, type 0 (1)*	354.0— Nerve entrapment, median nerve, carpal tunnel syndrome
To increase wrist motion (via orthosis serial changes)	*Wrist extension mobilization orthosis, type 0 (1)*	944.07—Burn, wrist
To restrict wrist motion	*Wrist flexion restriction orthosis, type 0 (1)*	881.2— Laceration, tendon
To improve active finger flexion and extension (extrinsic muscle-tendon excursion)	*Index-small finger extension and flexion torque transmission orthosis, type 1 (13)*	927.3— Crush, fingers

EOCS, Expanded Orthosis Classification System; *ICD,* International Classification of Diseases.

this orthosis is called a *serial cast;* and, like the second example in Table 7-4, there is no L-Code for a "static" orthosis that mobilizes joints through serial changes. Yet, its EOCS designation is elegantly and comprehensively descriptive. Anyone reading the EOCS designation for this orthosis would know immediately why it was applied even without being given the associated diagnosis.

In the future, EOCS designations will be linked to their corresponding ICD-9 (10) codes via extensive databases. Orthoses will have to match their ICD-9 (10) codes in order for reimbursement to occur. Slipshod and inappropriate application of orthoses will be quickly and easily identified; and those who take advantage of the system by overcharging their patients will be indisputably labeled and dealt with accordingly. Additionally, clinicians and researchers finally will be able to compare different configuration orthoses that function similarly on clients with same ICD-9 (10) codes, thereby advancing the therapy profession considerably.

Four Commonly Fabricated Orthoses

Expertise in fabricating a few basic orthoses serves as a foundation from which to make more complicated orthoses. Novice therapists often find an easy initial orthosis upon which to practice is a simple "hand-based thumb spica" or *Thumb CMC palmar abduction immobilization orthosis, type 1 (2)*. This orthosis incorporates only one main/primary joint (thumb CMC) that is positioned in palmar abduction. The thumb MP joint is a Type joint level, adding mechanical advantage and stability to the orthosis. Creating a pattern from paper towel is an inexpensive way to check accuracy of fit prior to cutting thermoplastic material. Selecting a material that has some "draping" properties eases fitting (Fig. 7-12). This orthosis is routinely used for CMC arthritis and MP collateral ligament injuries. The application of an outrigger to this orthosis to correct IP and MP joint contractures converts its purpose to that of mobilization.

A "forearm thumb spica" or *Thumb CMC palmar abduction immobilization orthosis, type 2 (3)* is simply an elongated version of its hand-based counterpart. This orthosis has two Type levels, the thumb MP and the wrist. As with the shorter hand-based orthosis, inclusion of the thumb MP as a Type level increases mechanical advantage on the CMC joint and improves overall orthosis stability on the extremity. Although the normal wrist is included to control tenodesis effect of the long extrinsic finger extensors and flexor muscles, the wrist is not a main/primary joint (Fig. 7-13). This orthosis is commonly used for de Quervain's tenosynovitis, scaphoid fractures, thumb fractures,

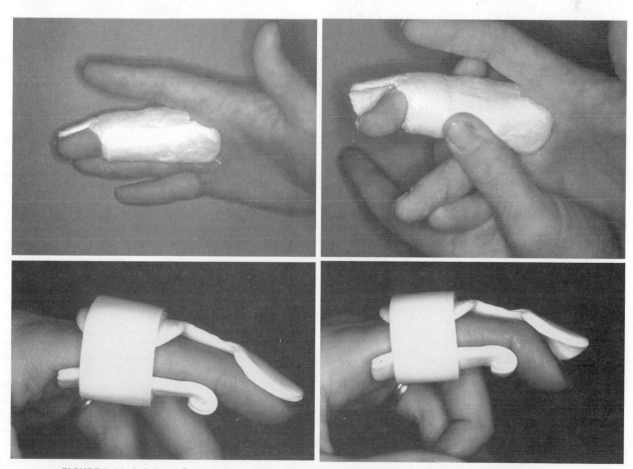

FIGURE 7-11 **A, B, Long finger PIP extension mobilization/DIP extension restriction/DIP flexion torque transmission orthosis, type 0 (2).** This orthosis involves sophisticated understanding of PIP and DIP joint biomechanics. It uses torque transmission to actively move the DIP joint and over time to remodel shortened oblique retinacular ligaments. Concomitantly, through serial adjustments, it uses inelastic traction to remodel PIP soft tissues and increase PIP joint extension. (Courtesy of Christopher Bochenek, OTR/L, CHT, Cincinnati, OH.)

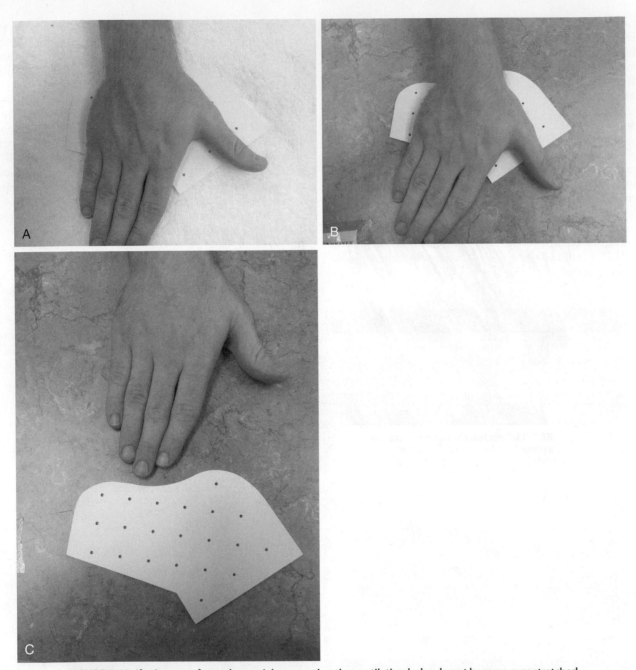

FIGURE 7-12 If using a perforated material, ensure that the ventilation holes do not become over stretched and enlarged. **A,** Drawing pattern; **B,** hand with cut-out material; **C,** cut-out material prior to fitting.

arthritis, arthroplasties, and tendon lacerations of the thumb flexors and extensors.

The EOCS designation for a "wrist cock-up" or "wrist gauntlet" orthosis is a *Wrist extension immobilization orthosis, type 0 (1)*. This orthosis has no Type level and only one main/ primary joint is included, making it an ideal "starting" orthosis upon which to learn. Again, a paper pattern helps ensure that the final orthosis will allow full thumb and finger motion while at the same time immobilizing the wrist (Fig. 7-14). This orthosis is the workhorse of the hand rehabilitation world. The *Wrist extension immobilization orthosis, type 0 (1)* is by far the most common orthosis and is used to treat wrist; fractures, instability, arthritis and cumulative trauma disorders. Dorsal applied

dynamic outriggers can protect repaired extensor tendons and volar static progressive digital straps with a 90-degree angle of applied force can correct difficult MP joint contractures.

An *Index-small finger MP flexion and IP extension, thumb CMC radial abduction and MP-IP extension mobilization orthosis, type 1 (16)*, commonly referred to as a *safe position* or *resting hand orthosis*, is the most complicated of the four orthoses discussed in this section (Fig. 7-15). This orthosis includes all digital joints as main/primary joints; with the wrist being the only Type level joint. An important mainstay design, this orthosis is associated with two different diagnostic groups that are differentiated by how the digital joints are positioned in the orthosis:

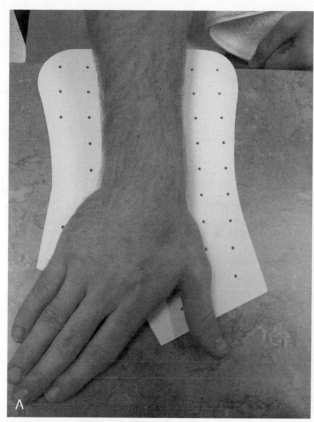

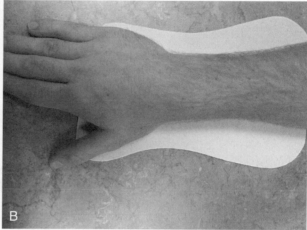

FIGURE 7-13 First learning to fabricate the shorter, hand-based version of this CMC immobilization ortho-sis is a prelude to becoming proficient in creating and fitting this elongated orthosis that incorporates one more joint, the wrist. Different material properties result in slightly differing patterns. **A,** Less stretchy material; **B,** stretchy material.

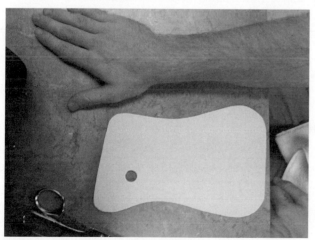

FIGURE 7-14 Selecting a material that will stretch and contour easily as the thumb and its thenar eminence are pulled through the thumbhole in the thermoplastic, facilitates fitting this wrist immobilization orthosis.

1. *Safe position:* If the finger MP joints are held in 70 to 90 degrees of flexion, the IP joints are in extension and the thumb CMC joint is in palmar or radial abduction, then the ortho-sis is probably made for a person who has sustained either a burn or crush injury to the hand. The primary function of this orthosis is to maintain collateral ligament length at the finger and thumb joints.

2. *Functional position:* If the finger MP and IP joints are in 30 to 40 degrees of flexion and the thumb CMC joint is in palmar abduction, then the orthosis may be applied to "rest" digital joints affected by arthritis or to position digits incapacitated by a stroke.

   It is important to understand that the latter described orthosis does not maintain finger collateral ligament length at the MP and IP joints. These orthoses are commonly used to treat joint contractures of burned hands and control edema of traumatic hand injuries.

Summary

Integral components to the rehabilitation process, orthoses must be carefully synchronized with diagnostic-specific, wound healing-specific, and client-specific factors in order for patients to achieve their maximum rehabilitation potential. "One-design-fits-all" and "one-size-fits-all" approaches are indicative of igno-rance, demonstrating serious lack of knowledge. Conversely, learning to fabricate a wide variety of orthoses is both fun and challenging. More importantly, knowing that you have mastered an important skill that helps direct and speed the rehabilitative process along is invaluable!

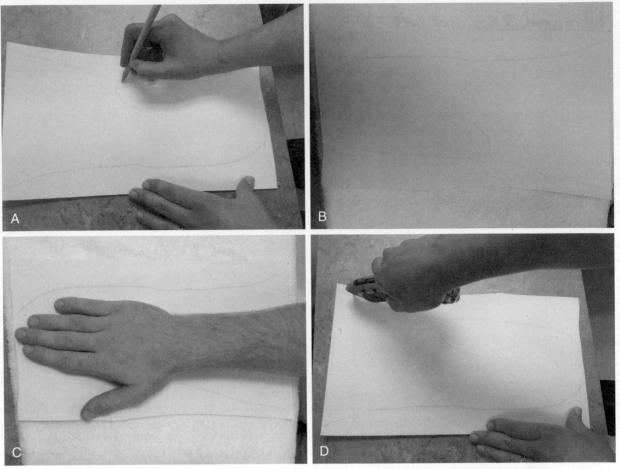

FIGURE 7-15 Because multiple surface planes are involved, pre-fitting a paper pattern is helpful to both novice and experienced therapists. **A,** Drawing pattern; **B,** pattern transferred to orthotic material; **C,** accuracy check with hand before cutting material; **D,** cutting material.

References

1. Fess EE: A history of splinting: to understand the present, view the past, *J Hand Ther* 15:97–132, 2002.
2. Fess EE, Gettle K, Philips C, et al: *Hand and upper extremity splinting: principles and methods*, ed 3, St Louis, 2004, Mosby Elsevier.
3. De Filippo RE, Atala A: Stretch and growth: the molecular and physiologic influences of tissue expansion, *Plast Reconstr Surg* 109(7):2450–2462, 2002.
4. Brand PW, Hollister AM: *Clinical mechanics of the hand*, ed 3, St Louis, 1999, Mosby.
5. Fess EE: Orthoses for mobilization of joints. In Skirven TM, Osterman AL, Fedorczyk JM, et al, editors: *Rehabilitation of the hand and upper extremity*, ed 6, Philadelphia, 2011, Elsevier Mosby, pp 1588–1598.
6. Blake C, et al: *American society of hand therapists, L-Codes task force*, Chicago, 2006-2007, The Society.
7. PMIC: *ICD-9-CM, international classification of diseases, 9th revision, clinical modification*, ed 6, 2012, Practice Management Information Corporation.
8. Bailey J, et al: *American society of hand therapists, splint classification system*, Chicago, 1992, The Society.
9. * Alkaline Software: *The web's free 2013 medical coding reference: 2012 HCPCS L3906* (website): http://www.icd9data.com/HCPCS/2012/L/L3906.htm. Accessed April 8, 2013.

8 Assessment of Functional Outcomes

Rebecca von der Heyde
and Kelly Droege

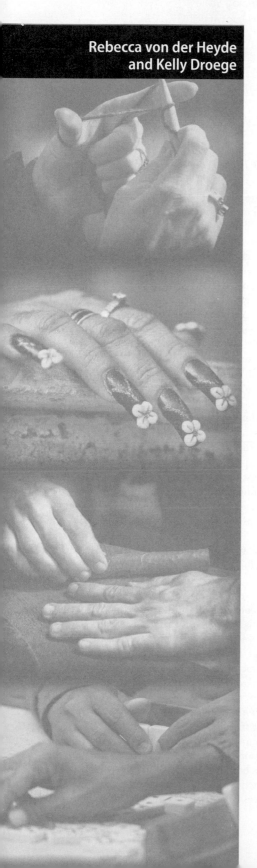

Client-centered care is a high priority in the health professions. The commonly used subjective, objective, assessment, and plan (SOAP) note method of documentation denotes the client's subjective discussion of recovery as our first priority. The problem, however, is the effective intake of the client's point of view and the consideration of this information from a quantitative and qualitative perspective. **Quantitative** aspects of evaluation and treatment include those variables that are measured in a standardized fashion and result in numeric data.[1] Typical quantitative tools include goniometric measurement, manual muscle testing, and sensory evaluations. These tests often are referred to using terms such as *objective* or *performance-based*.[2,3] **Qualitative** information, in comparison, is subjective and often consists of client narratives[1] (Box 8-1). Symptoms, abilities, and participation in daily activities are typical examples of *subjective* information. For client-centered care providers, the challenge lies in attempting to measure and interpret qualitative information as a means of directing evaluation and treatment. Subjective information is considered to play a crucial role in maximizing therapeutic outcomes, and much research has been dedicated to this topic.

Literature pertaining to client outcomes is littered with terms such as *quality of life, emotional function, disability,* and *health status*.[4,5] Many researchers are pursuing measurement of these complex components in the form of **client self-report outcome measures.** These measures most often are found in questionnaire form using the **visual analog scale (VAS)** or **Likert scale** (Box 8-2). The development of these tools can be considered a conduit toward incorporating subjective data into evaluation and treatment planning and a means for analyzing and adding to the current evaluative repertoire.

As therapists, our goal is to evaluate our clients accurately and consistently with tools that are designed to detect changes in clinical status. Research terms for these expectations include validity, reliability, and responsiveness. As a group, these variables are known as **psychometric properties. Validity** is the degree to which an instrument measures what it is intended to measure.[1] An outcome measure can be defined specifically as having construct, criterion, and/or content (face) validity. **Construct validity** refers to a comparison between a new measure and an associated measure, **criterion validity** compares a new measure with a gold standard, and **content validity** considers accurate measurement of a specific domain.[6] **Reliability** is the degree of consistency with which an instrument or rater measures a variable, and responsiveness is the ability of a test to demonstrate change.[1] **Responsiveness** often is referred to as *sensitivity to (clinical) change* and is established if change in scores accurately represents change in clinical status.[7] Similarities between measurement of responsiveness and validity have been addressed recently by researchers who question whether the two are distinct psychometric properties.[8]

Normative data, minimal detectable change, and **minimally clinically important difference (MCID)** are terms used to define analysis of client scores. Normative data can be considered as average scores for large groups of clients with similar diagnoses and abilities. As clinicians, we are familiar with norms in objective measures, such as grip and pinch strength. Normative values are helpful in providing a framework with which to compare client scores. With therapeutic progress or decline, we should expect to see a change in client-rated scores. The minimal detectable change is defined as a valid change in score that is not due to chance. MCID, in comparison, goes beyond valid change to assess meaningful difference in client function.[9]

The assessment of clinical outcomes from a qualitative and quantitative perspective is strongly encouraged in response to research findings.[10] Clinical evaluation tools, such as range of motion, have been shown to demonstrate poor reliability[11] and decreased responsiveness when compared with client self-report measures.[12-14] Research also has shown a suboptimal relationship between client self-report of quality of life and ratings from health care providers.[15]

BOX 8-1   Quantitative and Qualitative Aspects of Client Evaluation

Quantitative
Variables that are measured in a standardized fashion and result in numeric data[1]
Examples: Goniometric measurement, manual muscle testing, and sensory evaluations

Qualitative
Client narratives, self-report of symptoms or recovery, and subjective opinions
Examples: Subjective section of a SOAP note and personal communication with therapist

---

◎ ***Clinical Pearl***

Client perception of ability has been suggested as being more valuable than the therapeutic evaluation of independent function.[16]

In addition, it is recommended that the client is the one who ultimately should assess the importance of change in health status.[17] Despite these findings, incorporation of standardized, self-report outcome measures in treatment and/or clinical research is currently inconsistent.[18]

Over the past 25 years, client self-report outcome measures have been researched extensively and are readily available for use in clinical practice. These measures can be categorized as generic, regional, or disease-specific. **Generic measures** can be used to compare health conditions and therefore can assist in the analysis of policies and funds distribution. **Regional measures** are designed to demonstrate changes at the systems level, whereas **disease-specific measures** are intended to be highly responsive for individual diagnoses.[13] The purpose of this chapter is to introduce standardized, self-report outcome measures in the regional and disease-specific categories as a means of facilitating their incorporation into upper extremity evaluation and intervention.

Regional Measures

Disabilities of the Arm, Shoulder, and Hand Index

The Disabilities of the Arm, Shoulder, and Hand (DASH) index was a joint effort of the American Academy of Orthopaedic Surgeons (AAOS), American Society for Surgery of the Hand (ASSH), American Association for Hand Surgery (AAHS), the Council of Musculoskeletal Specialty Societies (COMSS), and the Institute for Work and Health (IWH).[19] The DASH was conceptualized as a tool that would facilitate comparison of conditions throughout the upper extremity while considering it a single functional unit. Careful development of this tool, including an extensive literature review[19,20] and consideration of questions and attribution,[21] have made it a well-recognized and popular tool in upper extremity research and clinical practice.

Thirteen existing outcome measures were reviewed to create a pool of more than 800 possible items. These items were reduced to 30 through a process of expert opinion and group

---

BOX 8-2   Visual Analog and Likert Scales

Visual Analog Scale
How much pain do you have at night?
No pain   Extreme pain

Ten-Interval Visual Analog Scale
How much pain do you have at night?
0   1   2   3   4   5   6   7   8   9   10
No pain   Extreme pain

Likert Scale
How much pain do you have at night?
?   ?   ?   ?   ?
No pain   Mild   Moderate   Severe   Extreme pain
           pain   pain   pain

---

selection.[19,20] Two concepts of symptoms (9 items) and functional status (21 items) are addressed in the DASH with functional status being classified further into domains of physical, social, and psychological status. A Likert scale format is used for assessment; options range from 1 (no difficulty, symptoms, or limitations) to 5 (unable to complete activities and extreme symptomatology). The DASH is scored when at least 27 items have been completed using a simple equation offered by the authors.[22] This equation anchors the score to a zero base; resultant scores range from 0 (no disability) to 100 (completely disabled). The DASH also includes optional work and sports/performing arts modules (4 items each).[10] The DASH has been shown to correlate with both general health measures and joint-specific measures.[23] A systematic review has been published stating that the DASH remains reliable and valid when translated into Armenian, Russian, Chinese, French, German, Swedish, Italian, Portuguese, and Greek.[24] **Normative data,** including mean scores and standard deviations, have been published by the AAOS.[25]

Psychometric properties of the DASH have been researched thoroughly. Studies in upper extremity clinics including a variety of diagnoses have demonstrated validity, excellent reliability, and responsiveness to clinical change.[22,26-29] The DASH also has been established as possessing the following attributes: content validity for clients with psoriatic arthritis;[30] construct validity for clients with ulnar wrist disorders,[31] carpal tunnel syndrome, and subacromial impingement;[32] reliability for clients with pathologic conditions of the elbow[18,33] and musculoskeletal complaints from textile workers;[34] convergent and divergent validity for clients following arthroplasty of the CMC joint;[35] and test-retest reliability, concurrent, convergent, and face validity for patients with rheumatoid arthritis.[36] Responsiveness/sensitivity to clinical change has been recognized for the DASH when used with clients following carpal tunnel release,[37-39] distal radius fracture,[40,41] wrist pain,[39] humeral fractures,[42] rotator cuff repairs,[43,44] shoulder instability,[45] rheumatoid arthritis,[46,47] and various shoulder pathology.[48] In addition, the DASH has been used to determine outcomes for clients with distal humeral fractures,[49,50] radial nerve palsy,[51] and acute traumatic hand injuries.[52]

The DASH was found to be the best instrument for evaluating patients with disorders involving multiple joints in the upper limb[53,54] and has been suggested as the most widely tested instrument.[55] The content of the DASH has been found to link well with the International Classification of the Functioning,

Disability, and Health (ICF) framework[56,57] and has been reported as a potential patient-centered tool to aid in comprehensive care.[58,59] On the other hand, the DASH has been demonstrated to be comparable to, but slightly less responsive than, the Canadian Occupational Performance Measure (COPM),[26] the Patient-Rated Wrist/Hand Evaluation (PRWHE),[28] the Boston Questionnaire,[37,38] the Western Ontario Shoulder Instability Index (WOSI),[45,60] and the Shoulder Pain and Disability Index (SPADI).[61] The DASH was found to be less sensitive to differences in functional outcomes between clients with hand injuries[62] and clients following wrist arthroplasty or arthrodesis.[63] In addition, a Rasch analysis questioned the validity of the DASH when utilized for patients with multiple sclerosis.[64]

QuickDASH

The QuickDASH was developed by Dr. Borcas Beaton and colleagues at the IWH in 2005. The purpose of creating the QuickDASH was to provide a valid and reliable shortened version of the full DASH that would be easier to use in a clinical context for both the patient and clinician/researcher.[65] The full DASH consists of 16 domains, but for the purposes of the QuickDASH, only 11 domains were utilized; therefore reducing the number of items for the assessment to 11. Three item-reduction techniques were utilized to analyze the 30 item full DASH to determine which 11 items would be clinically sensible to include in the QuickDASH.[65]

The QuickDASH consists of 11 items addressing the symptoms and functionality of people with any or multiple disorders of the upper extremity. The QuickDASH is similarly formatted to the full DASH using a Likert scale with the options ranging from 1 (no difficulty, symptoms, or limitations) to 5 (unable to complete activities and extreme symptomatology). The QuickDASH can be scored when 10 of the 11 items have been completed; allowing only one "missed" item. The scoring equation used to calculate the full DASH is also used to score the QuickDASH with scores ranging from 0 (no disability) to 100 (completely disabled).[65] The QuickDASH has been translated into the Turkish language and deemed as reliable and valid as the original tool for patients with carpal tunnel syndrome.[66]

The QuickDASH was originally found to have reliability, construct validity, and responsiveness to clinical change when used with 200 patients with either proximal or distal disorders of the upper extremity.[65] The QuickDASH and full DASH were found to have similar responsiveness to clinical change for patients with hand trauma and degenerative hand conditions.[67] The QuickDASH was significantly correlated with changes of ROM and can be utilized to detect clinical change in children with supracondylar humeral fractures.[68] The QuickDASH is an adequate tool for a summary assessment of symptoms and functionality, but the full DASH should is suggested for differentiating assessment of symptoms and function for patients following shoulder and carpometacarpal arthroplasty.[69] The cross-sectional and test-retest reliability of the full DASH and the QuickDASH are similar, insinuating that the QuickDASH can be used in clinical practice instead of the full-length DASH.[70]

Michigan Hand Outcomes Questionnaire

The Michigan Hand Outcomes Questionnaire (MHQ) was developed by Dr. Kevin Chung and colleagues[71] at the University of Michigan in 1998. The MHQ is defined as a hand-specific questionnaire; the authors specifically address function of each upper extremity separately as a means of analyzing independent use, hand dominance, and bilateral involvement.[10] Previously established tools and client input were used to create the MHQ.[71]

The MHQ consists of 67 questions including six domains, demographics, and work history. Domains of overall hand function, physical function with activities of daily living tasks, esthetics, and satisfaction with hand function are answered specific to each hand. Responses in the domains of pain and work performance are given regarding both hands. All domain items are formatted in Likert scales ranging from 1 to 5 with lower scores indicating higher function in all domains except pain. If less than 50% of a scale is complete, the scale is not scored, and if more than two scales are incomplete, a final score cannot be calculated. Raw scores are summed for each hand; bilateral scores are calculated by averaging scores from both hands. Summed and averaged scores are normalized from 0 to 100 according to the scoring algorithm as found in the original publication.[71] Scores closer to 100 on all scales indicate increased function and decreased pain. The MCIDs for the MHQ have been published specifically for patients with carpal tunnel syndrome (pain: 23, function: 13, work: 8) and rheumatoid arthritis (pain: 11, function: 13).[72]

The MHQ was originally found to be reliable and valid in a study including 200 clients with various upper extremity diagnoses.[71] Responsiveness as a function of significant clinical change was noted in a similar, diverse client group.[7] In addition, the MHQ has been found to be sensitive to clinical change for patients with carpal tunnel syndrome,[39,55] carpal tunnel release,[73-76] distal radius fractures,[77] wrist pain, and finger contracture.[39] The MHQ has been established as valid and reliable for clients with rheumatoid arthritis,[78,79] osteoarthritis,[80] and diabetes.[81] The MHQ has been suggested to be reliable and valid for patients with finger and wrist disorders but less so for nerve disorders.[82] Multiple sources have disputed which functional outcome assessment, MHQ or DASH, is considered to be most responsive to clinical change.[62,83,84] The MHQ has been correlated to grip strength[85] and a standardized test of activities of daily living function,[86] and it was reported to be sensitive to change in a long-term follow-up study of clients with metacarpophalangeal joint arthroplasties.[87] Most recently, a brief, 12-item version of the MHQ has been created and was reported to maintain the same psychometric properties as the original MHQ.[88]

Patient Evaluation Measure

The Patient Evaluation Measure (PEM) was introduced by Macey and Burke[89] in 1995. Developed in the United Kingdom, the PEM is novel in that it addresses client satisfaction as a primary component of outcome measurement.

The original PEM included three parts: treatment (5 items), "how your hand is now" (10 items), and overall assessment (3 items). A second version was published in 2001 that titled the second section as the Hand Health Questionnaire and added a question to this section addressing duration of pain. The PEM is presented in a seven-interval VAS with lower scores indicating increased satisfaction and function. Parts two and three are summed and calculated as a percentage of the possible score. Part one is not included in the scoring process, and the authors suggest that clients should be given their previous answers when repeating this measure.[90] A cultural difference in language is noted in the use of the activity example "fiddly things," which is clarified as fine dextrous tasks.[91]

The PEM was found to be reliable, highly valid, and highly responsive in patients with carpal tunnel syndrome[76] and a study of 80 clients with scaphoid fractures.[90] Research including 35 clients with multiple diagnoses demonstrated very good reliability and validity as correlated with grip strength.[91] The PEM was also used for outcomes measurement in a follow-up study of clients with palmar wrist ganglia[92] and found to be valid when assessing the outcomes of patients with distal radius fractures.[93] The PEM was compared to the DASH and MHQ and found to be the easiest to use according to 100 randomly selected patients with varying hand and wrist disorders.[82,94] In addition, the PEM was found to be more responsive to change than the DASH when used as an outcome measure for patients with carpal tunnel syndrome.[94]

Patient-Rated Evaluation Methods

Dr. Joy MacDermid and colleagues in Ontario, Canada, have carefully researched and developed four client-rated tools for outcome evaluation: the Patient-Rated Wrist Evaluation (PRWE), the Patient-Rated Tennis Elbow Evaluation (PRTEE), the Patient-Rated Elbow Evaluation (PREE), and the Patient-Rated Wrist/Hand Evaluation (PRWHE). The PRWE was the first measure of the four to be developed; the process included a survey of the International Wrist Investigators for content and format. The goal in creating the PRWE was to capture client-rated measurement of impairment, disability, and handicap that could be used in clinical and research settings.[3] The three remaining tools were published as adaptations to the PRWE that more specifically could address measurement of outcomes for clients with lateral epicondylitis (PRTEE), pathologic conditions of the elbow (PREE), and hand injuries (PRWHE).

All four tools include two scales of pain and function. The pain scales include 5 to 6 items that address magnitude and frequency of pain. Activities that might precipitate pain are specific to each tool. Function scales are divided further to specific and usual activities. Usual activities are identical for each tool and include personal care, household management, work, and recreation. Specific activities on PRWE, PRWHE, and PRTEE consist of 10 items that pertain to the anatomic area under consideration. In comparison, the PREE lists 15 specific activities. Responses are marked on a scale ranging from 0 (no pain/difficulty) to 10 (worst pain imaginable/unable to do) as perceived over the past week. The authors present multiple scoring options; scales can be summed individually or combined with simple calculations to yield a total score of up to 100 points.[3,18] Higher scores on all scales indicate increased pain and decreased function.

The PRWE was published in 1996.[3] Reliability and content, construct, and criterion validity have been established for this tool.[3,95] These properties were reinforced in clients with distal radius and scaphoid fractures, and the PRWE total score was found to demonstrate greater reliability than individual subscale scores.[96,97] Responsiveness of the PRWE was determined in a prospective study of 275 clients with distal radius fractures; this publication also offers means and standard deviations for the tool.[98] The PRWE was more responsive than the DASH and SF-36 for clients following distal radius fracture.[40,53,98] The PRWE was not sensitive to differences in outcomes between clients with wrist arthroplasty or arthrodesis[63] and was less sensitive than grip strength testing for clients with unstable wrist fractures.[99] The

PRWE was chosen as an outcome measure in a publication that advocates low-level heat wraps for wrist pain,[100] and translations into Japanese,[101] Hindi,[102] and Swedish languages[103,104] have been considered as valid and reliable as the original tool.

The PREE was introduced in 2001 in a study that articulated excellent reliability for the total score, high reliability for the pain subscale, and moderate to high reliability for the function subscale.[18] The PREE has successfully been translated in to a German version suggested to be as reliable and valid as the original tool.[105] The PRWHE differs from the PRWE only in introductory wording, changing "wrist" to "wrist/hand," and the addition of one appearance question. The PRWHE was found to be more responsive than the DASH in a study of 60 clients with a variety of hand injuries; however, the appearance question was less responsive than comparable scales.[28] Furthermore, according to a systematic review of functional outcome assessments, the PRWHE was found to have good construct validity and responsiveness for patients with varying wrist injuries, which was considered to be marginally superior than the DASH.[55] The PRWHE was also found to be a valid tool when assessing pain and/or disability following arthroplasty of the carpometacarpal joint in the osteoarthritic hand.[106]

American Shoulder and Elbow Surgeons Standardized Shoulder Assessment

The American Shoulder and Elbow Surgeons (ASES) Standardized Shoulder Assessment form was developed by the Research Committee for American Shoulder and Elbow Surgeons in 1993 and published in 1994.[107] A later publication excluded five questions and subsequent studies of psychometric properties are based off of this modified edition.[108]

The ASES was designed to be a baseline measurement of shoulder and elbow function that would be applicable to any diagnosis involving these anatomical structures.[107] The ASES consists of two sections: pain and activities of daily living (ADLs). The pain section is rated on a VAS ranging from 0 (no pain at all) to 10 (pain as bad as it can be).[107] The ADL section assesses ten ADLs on a four point ordinal scale ranging from 0 (unable to do the activity) to 3 (no difficulty). Each upper extremity is assessed separately and scored according to the equation provided by the authors.[107,108]

The ASES was found to have test-retest reliability; construct and discriminant validity; and responsiveness to clinical change for patients with various shoulder pathologies; and a MCID of 6.4.[108-111] It was suggested to demonstrate reliability and construct validity for patients following shoulder joint operations,[112] and reliability and responsiveness following shoulder surgery.[113,114] In addition, the ASES was found to have reliability; criterion and construct validity; and responsiveness to clinical change for 455 patients with shoulder instability, rotator cuff disease, and shoulder arthritis.[115]

The Shoulder Pain and Disability Index

The Shoulder Pain and Disability Index (SPADI) was designed as a regional measure aimed at capturing patient self-reported pain and disability about the shoulder. Originally presented as VAS,[116] the more commonly used second version includes a numerical rating scale for ease in administration and scoring.[117]

The SPADI includes two domains: a five-item pain subscale and an eight-item disability subscale. Patients are allowed to mark one item as not applicable that is then omitted from scoring. In cases with more than two not applicable prompts, no score is calculated. Summation and transformation of subscales yields a score out of 100; averaging the pain and disability scores then creates a final score. A higher score on the SPADI is indicative of higher perceived pain and/or disability. The MCID for this tool has been reported to range between 8 and 13 points.[61] The SPADI has been validated in Turkish,[118] German,[119] Portugese,[120,121] and Norwegian.[122]

Excellent reliability has been consistently reported for this tool[61,95] with high internal consistency suggested for the pain and disability subscales in patients with chronic shoulder symptoms.[123,124] The SPADI was found to be significantly more responsive than: the Western Ontario Rotator Cuff Index (WORC) and Oxford Shoulder Scale for patients with rotator cuff disease;[125] the Croft Index and DASH for patients with adhesive capsulitis;[126] the Sickness Impact Profile for patients with shoulder pain;[127] and the DASH for patients following total shoulder arthroplasties.[128]

Research suggests a strong negative correlation between the disability subscale scores and shoulder range of motion and a positive correlation between the disability subscale scores and age.[124] Higher pain and disability have also been correlated with passive or negative coping strategies.[123] Limitations of the SPADI include its identification as unidimensional for patients with adhesive capsulitis[129] and its limited attention to occupational/recreational disability.[127] Table 8-1 provides information on the aforementioned regional measures.

Disease-Specific Measures

Arthritis Impact Measurement Scales 2 Short Form

The Arthritis Impact Measurement Scales 2 Short Form (AIMS2-SF) was established by Guillemin et al.[130] in France in 1997. The original Arthritis Impact Measurement Scales (AIMS) and Arthritis Impact Measurement Scales 2 (AIMS2) were published in 1980 and 1992, respectively, to measure quality of life for clients with rheumatoid arthritis. The new, shorter form was developed to reduce completion time and client/therapist burden. Contributors to this process included expert and client panelists.

The AIMS2-SF includes questions in five domains: physical components (twelve questions), symptom components (three questions), affect components (five questions), social interaction components (four questions), and role components (two questions). These questions are answered on a Likert scale with options ranging from "all days" to "no days" in the past 4 weeks. Scores are summed and normalized when at least 50% of the domains have been completed; the role component is excluded for those clients who are unemployed, disabled, or retired. A composite score is given that ranges from 1 to 10 with a higher score indicating decreased status. This tool is available in English, Dutch, French, and Persian.[131]

With the exception of the social interaction domain, the remaining components of the AIMS2-SF demonstrate acceptable levels of reliability, validity, and sensitivity to change for clients with rheumatoid arthritis[130] and osteoarthritis.[132,133] The AIMS2-SF also was found to be in agreement with and demonstrate responsiveness comparable to the AIMS2.[134] An interesting note is that multiple authors have recommended changes in the questions originally chosen from the AIMS2 to increase reliability, validity, and sensitivity to change of the social interaction and symptom domains.[134-136] With these changes, the AIMS2-SF was found to be preferable to the modified Health Assessment Questionnaire (HAQ) for detecting clinical change in clients with rheumatoid arthritis.[136] For those patients with osteoarthritis, it was found to be less efficacious as compared to functional measures, including the Functional Index of Hand Osteoarthritis and the Moberg Pick-Up Test.[137]

Australian/Canadian Osteoarthritis Hand Index

Development of the Australian/Canadian (AUSCAN) Osteoarthritis Hand Index took place at two medical centers across the globe from one another: the University of Western Ontario in Canada and the University of Queensland in Australia. Dr. Nicholas Bellamy and colleagues[17] intended to create a disease-specific, self-report outcome measure for clients with osteoarthritis of the hand. Client interviews were used as an integral part of the development process.

The AUSCAN is a 15-item questionnaire that is available in Likert scale, VAS, or numeric rating scale response formats. The AUSCAN includes three subscales of pain (five items), stiffness (one item), and physical function (nine items). Clients consider items based on the past 4 weeks; Likert scale items include responses ranging from no days to all days. Scoring options include summation, normalization, pooling, or weighting as proposed in the user guide.[138] The Likert scale version of the AUSCAN results in a summed, total score ranging from 0 to 61. The VAS version ranges from 0 to 1500. A score of 0 on either version indicates that the client is asymptomatic. A lower score, therefore, indicates decreased pain and stiffness and increased physical function of the client with osteoarthritis of the hand. For the client who has not performed a task as listed on the AUSCAN, the authors recommend exchanging the item with a similar task.[78] This measure has been translated into more than 25 languages.

The AUSCAN demonstrates good construct validity,[78,139-141] criterion validity,[142] internal consistency,[140] and responsiveness to clinical change,[139] notably in the areas of pain, stiffness, and function.[140] Scale performance has been suggested to improve with removal of "pain at rest" from the pain scale and with division of physical function into high precision and grip strength tasks.[143] The AUSCAN has been noted as offering comparatively better data quality than the Functional Index for Hand Osteoarthritis[141,143] and the AIMS2.[143] The AUSCAN is promoted as relevant to clinical and research applications,[138] and age- and gender-specific normative values have been published for the physical function subscale.[144]

Boston Questionnaire

The Boston Questionnaire was developed by Levine et al.[145] at the Brigham and Women's Hospital as an assessment tool for clients with carpal tunnel syndrome. Consisting of an eleven-item Symptom Severity Scale and an eight-item Functional Status Scale, the tool was not given a formal name in the initial publication. This outcome measure therefore has been referred to by these individual scales and multiple other names in the literature, including the Brigham and Women's carpal tunnel questionnaire,[13,37] the Carpal Tunnel Syndrome Assessment Questionnaire,[146,147] the CTS instrument,[14] the Brigham (carpal tunnel) questionnaire,[22] and the Boston Carpal Tunnel Questionnaire.[148]

TABLE 8-1	Regional Measures			
Title	**Date and Location**	**Questions**	**Format**	**To Obtain**
DASH	1996, AAOS, ASSH, AASH, COMSS, and IWH	Symptoms: 9 Functional status: 21 **Total: 30** Optional—Work: 4 Sports/performing arts: 4	Likert scale	www.dash.iwh.on.ca
QuickDASH	2005, IWH	Symptoms: 3 Functional: 8 **Total: 11**	Likert scale	www.dash.iwh.on.ca/quickdash
MHQ	1998, University of Michigan	**Total: 67** Hand function, physical function with ADL, esthetics, satisfaction with hand function, demographics, and work history	Likert scale	www.med.umich.edu/surgery/plastic/research/department/studies/mi_hand_outcome.shtml
PEM	1995, United Kingdom	Treatment: 5 Hand Health Questionnaire: 11 Overall assessment: 3	7-interval VAS	Dias et al[90]
PRWE	1996, Ontario	Pain: 5 Function: 10 **Total: 15**	10-interval VAS	Dr. Joy MacDermid Hand and Upper Limb Centre St. Joseph's Health Centre 268 Grosvenor Street London, Ontario N6A 3AB
PREE	2001, Ontario	Pain: 5 Function: 15 **Total: 20**	10-interval VAS	Dr. Joy MacDermid Hand and Upper Limb Centre St. Joseph's Health Centre 268 Grosvenor Street London, Ontario N6A 3AB
PRWHE	2004, Ontario	Pain: 5 Function: 10 **Total: 15** Optional—Appearance: 1	10-interval VAS	Dr. Joy MacDermid Hand and Upper Limb Centre St. Joseph's Health Centre 268 Grosvenor Street London, Ontario N6A 3AB
ASES Standardized Shoulder Assessment Form	1993, Research Committee for American Shoulder and Elbow Surgeons	Pain: 1 Function: 10 **Total: 11**	Pain: VAS Function: Likert scale	Michener LA, McClure PW, Sennett BJ[108]
SPADI **Total: 13**	1991 Roach KE, Budiman-Mak E, Songsiridej N, et al[116] Williams JW Jr., Holleman DR Jr., Simel DL[117]	Pain: 5 Disability: 8	Likert scale	www.workcover.com/public/download.aspx?id=799

AAOS, American Academy of Orthopaedic Surgeons; *AASH,* American Association of Hand Surgery; *ADL,* activity of daily living; *ASES,* American Shoulder and Elbow Surgeons; *ASSH,* American Society for Surgery of the Hand; *COMSS,* Council of Musculoskeletal Specialty Societies; *DASH,* Disabilities of the Arm, Shoulder, and Hand, *IWH,* Institute for Work and Health; *MHQ,* Michigan Hand Outcomes Questionnaire; *PEM,* Patient Evaluation Measure; *PREE,* Patient-Rated Elbow Evaluation; *PRWE,* Patient-Rated Wrist Evaluation; *PRWHE,* Patient-Rated Wrist/Hand Evaluation; *SPADI,* Shoulder Pain and Disability Index; *VAS,* visual analog scale.

Despite the confusing nomenclature, these scales include a reasonable number of questions and scoring that benefit client and therapist. The Symptom Severity Scale addresses pain, numbness, weakness, tingling, and difficulty with fine motor tasks on a typical day in the past 2 weeks. The Functional Status Scale considers the relationship between symptoms and function, including activities, such as buttoning, writing, and ADL tasks. These tasks also are evaluated for a typical day in the past 2 weeks. Questions are answered on a Likert scale with a score of 1 indicating a low level of symptom/difficulty and 5 indicating highly symptomatic or unable to complete functional tasks. The answers are averaged with a higher score indicating decreased status, and questions that are not answered simply are not included in the scoring process.

The Boston Questionnaire has been demonstrated as reliable, valid, and sensitive to change in clients with carpal tunnel syndrome.[14,38,145,149-152] No differences in psychometric properties were noted when used with workers' compensation recipients, indicating its' utility for this patient population.[153] The Symptom Severity Scale has been found to be four times more sensitive to change and the Functional Status Scale has been found to be two times more sensitive to change than standard measures of strength and sensibility.[13] Current findings regarding relationships between the two scales and pre- and post-operative nerve conduction studies are conflicting.[154-157] The Symptom Severity Scale has been suggested as a means to triage patients; higher initial scores and/or failure to change in short-term were correlated with ultimate surgical release.[158] Overall, this measure has been reported to be more sensitive to change in carpal tunnel syndrome than generic[13,14,37,146] and regional[55] measures. Copies of the Symptom Severity Scale and Functional Status Scale, as well as mean scores, can be found in the original publication.[145]

Patient-Rated Tennis Elbow Evaluation

The Patient-Rated Tennis Elbow Evaluation (PRTEE) is the only disease-specific tool included in the patient-rated evaluation methods by Dr. Joy MacDermid and colleagues in Ontario, Canada (see the "Patient-Rated Evaluation Methods" section). An adaptation to the PRWE, the PRTEE was specifically designed to address pain and function in patients with lateral epicondylitis. Four out of the five pain scales and the usual activity subscale are identical to PRWE model with the addition of specific functional activities appropriate to tennis elbow (that is, "wring out a washcloth or wet towel").

The PRTEE was originally published as the Patient-Rated Forearm Evaluation Questionnaire[159] with a resultant name change and minor revisions in wording in 2005.[160] Translations of this tool have been psychometrically tested in Canadian French,[161] Swedish,[162] and Turkish,[163] and the MCID has been suggested to range from 7 to 11 points or 22% to 37%.[164]

Excellent test-retest reliability of the PRTEE and its subscales was reported by the original authors, although it was significantly lower for patients with work-related conditions.[159] Reliability, validity, and sensitivity of the tool have been confirmed in subsequent studies;[165,166] however, moderate test-retest reliability, low convergent validity, and questionable sensitivity to change were published in a recent study.[167]

Western Ontario Shoulder Instability Index

Dr. Alexandra Kirkley has worked with colleagues in Ontario, Canada, to research and develop client self-report outcome measures for evaluation of shoulder-specific diagnoses.[168] The first measure offered was the Western Ontario Shoulder Instability Index (WOSI).[45] This tool was designed to consider those clients with combinations of traumatic and atraumatic anterior, posterior, or multidirectional shoulder instability, and clients were consulted during development and research.

The WOSI consists of 21 items, each measured on a 100 mm VAS. Four domains of physical symptoms (ten questions), sports/recreation/work (four questions), lifestyle (four questions), and emotions (three questions) are framed to evaluate client perception during the past week. Clients are instructed clearly to make their "best guess" to questions that do not currently pertain to them. Raw scores range from 0 to 2100; scores closer to 0 indicate higher quality of life. Scores also can be converted quickly to percentage with 100% designating normal function. The MCID value for the WOSI has been calculated as 10%.[114,168] The questionnaire is offered in the form of a packet including directions and scoring. Psychometric properties of this tool have been validated for Swedish,[169] Japanese,[170] and German[171] translations.

Reliability of the WOSI was established with a group of 51 symptomatically stable clients.[49] In addition, this tool was found to be valid and responsive in two groups of clients with anterior instability. The WOSI also was indicated to be more responsive to clinical change than generic, regional, and clinical (range of motion) measures for these clients.[45,172] Finally, the WOSI was noted to be an internally consistent tool for use with patients following shoulder surgery.[113]

Western Ontario Rotator Cuff Index

The Western Ontario Rotator Cuff Index (WORC), also published by Dr. Alexandra Kirkley and colleagues, is targeted for use with clients diagnosed with rotator cuff disease, including tendonitis, tendinosis with no tear, partial-thickness tears, full-thickness tears, and rotator cuff arthropathy.[173] Consistent with previous methodology, the authors included clients in each step of the development process.

The WORC has 21 items in four domains, including physical symptoms (ten questions), sports/recreation/work (four questions), lifestyle (four questions) and emotions (three questions). Raw scores range from 0 to 2100 with a higher score indicating decreased quality of life due to pathological condition of the rotator cuff. Mathematic conversion yields a percentage score; higher percentages indicate proximity to normal function. The MCID value for the WORC is 275 points[125] or 12% to 13%.[114] The WORC has been psychometrically tested in multiple languages, including English, French, German, Portugese,[121] Turkish,[174] Norwegian,[122] and Persian.[175]

The WORC was suggested to be reliable and valid in a study that included 110 clients being treated with operative and non-operative interventions following rotator cuff injury.[173] This tool was found to be responsive to clinical change in a group of 30 clients following subacromial decompression[176] and demonstrated cross-sectional convergent validity and sensitivity to change in post-surgical shoulder patients.[177] In a sample of over 300 patients awaiting rotator cuff surgery, the five-domain model of the WORC was not supported.[178] It was found to be significantly more responsive than the Oxford Shoulder Scale but less responsive than the SPADI for patients receiving corticosteroid injections for rotator cuff disease.[125] Table 8-2 provides information on the aforementioned assessment instruments.

Incorporating Self-Report Measures into Clinical Practice

Choosing a Measure

With such a vast array of options for assessing functional outcomes, the task of choosing a measure for clinical practice or research may seem daunting. Dr. Peter Amadio,[179] who has extensive experience in the development and research of client self-report outcome measures, offers a simple solution. His advice is to "define the job, then pick the tools." For a research study including multiple upper extremity diagnoses, a foundational, generic measure could be used along with a regional measure and objective assessments. For a research study specific to a diagnostic group, a specific measure could be added. Choosing a measure to assess individual outcomes daily requires

TABLE 8-2	Disease-Specific Measures				
Title	**Date and Location**	**Diagnosis/ Population**	**Questions**	**Format**	**To Obtain**
AIMS2-SF	1997, France	Rheumatoid arthritis	Physical: 12 Symptom: 3 Affect: 5 Social interaction: 4 Role: 2 **Total: 26**	Likert scale	www.hopkins-arthritis. som.jhmi.edu/mngmnt/ forms/aims2-sf.pdf
AUSCAN Osteoarthritis Hand Index	2002, Australia and Canada	Primary hand osteoarthritis	Pain: 5 Stiffness: 1 Function: 9 **Total: 15**	Likert scale (LK3.0) VAS (VA3.0)	Professor Nicholas Bellamy nbellamy@medicine.uq.edu.au University of Queensland, Australia
Boston Questionnaire (Brigham & Women's Hospital; carpal tunnel syndrome assessment questionnaire)	1993, Boston	Carpal tunnel syndrome	Symptom Severity Scale: 11 Functional Status Scale: 8	Likert scale	Levine et al.[87]
PRTEE	1999, Ontario	Tennis elbow	Pain: 5 Function: 10 **Total: 15**	10-interval VAS	Dr. Joy MacDermid Hand and Upper Limb Centre St. Joseph's Health Centre 268 Grosvenor Street London, Ontario N6A 3AB
WOOS	2001, Canada	Osteoarthritis of the shoulder	Pain/physical symptoms: 6 Sports/recreation/ work: 5 Lifestyle: 5 Emotions: 3 **Total: 19**	100 mm VAS	Sharon Griffin stdshg@uwo.ca Fowler Kennedy Sports Medicine Clinic, London, Ontario
WORC	2003, Canada	Rotator cuff disease	Pain/physical symptoms: 10 Sports/recreation/ work: 4 Lifestyle: 4 Emotional: 3 **Total: 21**	100 mm VAS	Sharon Griffin stdshg@uwo.ca Fowler Kennedy Sports Medicine Clinic, London, Ontario
WOSI	1998, Canada	Shoulder instability	Pain/physical symptoms: 10 Sports/recreation/ work: 4 Lifestyle: 4 Emotional: 3 **Total: 21**	100 mm VAS	Sharon Griffin stdshg@uwo.ca Fowler Kennedy Sports Medicine Clinic, London, Ontario

AIMS2-SF, Arthritis Impact Measurement Scales 2 Short Form; *AUSCAN,* Australian/Canadian; *PRTEE,* Patient-Rated Tennis Elbow Evaluation; *VAS,* visual analog scale; *WOOS,* Western Ontario Osteoarthritis of the Shoulder Index; *WORC,* Western Ontario Rotator Cuff Index; *WOSI,* Western Ontario Shoulder Instability Index.

analysis of multiple factors, many of which are based on therapist and clinic preference.

Time

Time as a function of client self-report outcome measures can be considered in two separate ways. The first is time taken to administer and score a questionnaire. The obvious preference would be toward shorter and more efficient tools; however, minutes in the waiting room or on a modality could become productive and proactive. Correct scoring takes practice and attention to detail,

much like goniometric measurement, and becomes quicker over time. Simplicity of scoring systems leads to increased inter-rater reliability in the clinic. The second aspect of time is included in the instructions of each tool. A therapist must be confident that the client accurately can recall the past few days, the past week, or the past month.

Format

Format options include scale type, left-to-right organization and consistency, and question complexity. Likert scales and VASs are standard questionnaire formats (see Box 8-2). Likert scales have been discussed as difficult to construct in terms of meaning, consistency, and spacing, and comprehension of VAS has been found to be challenging, especially for elderly clients.[3] Few tools offer choice in this area.

The English language includes a standard left-to-right reading format. With this in mind, it seems logical that numbers would increase from left to right. The problem that arises is that while we want function to increase, we want symptoms to decrease. In other words, a score of 10/10 for function is good, but 10/10 for pain is bad. Some scales attempt consistency of left and right as positive or negative, whereas some maintain the standard left-to-right increase. Assessment of whether the client is confused by response options and intervention as necessary for clarification are important.

Complexity of questions also can lead to misinterpretation. Double-barreled questions ask clients to consider two variables at the same time, such as the effect of pain on function. Asking clients clearly to assess one variable facilitates reliability over time. It also has been suggested that the provision of previous answers decreases response variability,[180] but this was recommended only for one of the measures reviewed.[90]

Instructions

Questionnaire instructions should be clear and without room for error by the therapist or client. Individual clarifications and assumptions should be avoided because this decreases reliability in administration and completion. Instructions for scoring also should be used consistently and should be compared between clinicians.

Results and Goal Setting

Understanding what scores mean and how to interpret clinical change is a difficult yet necessary component of using self-report outcome measures as part of holistic therapeutic intervention. Simply writing down numbers in a chart would be comparable

to performing manual muscle tests and noting results without application to treatment planning or short-term goals.

Dr. Joy MacDermid, a clinical epidemiologist and physical therapist, has made a concerted effort to develop, research, and assist in the everyday understanding and use of outcome measures in therapy practice. She advocates practice and, therefore, experiential learning as the best way to become versed in the use of these tools.[9] Approximately half of the tools reviewed here were found to include normative values or discuss MCID in scoring. Dr. MacDermid clarifies equations that can assist with the calculation of MCID using data retrieved from the literature and advocates the use of MCID for short- and long-term goal setting.[9]

Clinic Outcomes and Marketing

Once a tool has been chosen and the therapy staff is comfortable with administration, scoring, and analysis of scores for intervention and goal setting, data can be compiled to consider larger issues pertaining to clinic management. Outcomes for client groups, individual therapists, and surgeons can be used to reflect on quality of client care and treatment strategies. Positive trends can be used as tools for marketing and year-end reports. Quality of life and overall outcomes can make a significant impact on the justification currently needed for reimbursement in health care settings.

Summary

Treatment of the client with a hand or upper extremity injury requires knowledge and attention to fine details. One of the most important details is the clients' perception of their abilities and health status. Current methods for client evaluation are moving toward a consistent and comprehensive assessment of quality of life and functional ability, and client self-report outcome measures have been developed and can be used clinically for this purpose. Consistent incorporation of these tools requires time for research, practice, and discussion, but ultimately results in a renewed focus on client-centered care and holistic evaluation.

References

1. Portney LG, Watkins MP: *Foundations of clinical research: applications to practice*, ed 2, Upper Saddle River, NJ, 2000, Prentice Hall Health.
2. Bindra RR, Dias JJ, Heras-Palau C, et al: Assessing outcome after hand surgery: the current state, *J Hand Surg* 28(4):289–294, 2003.
3. MacDermid JC: Development of a scale for client rating of wrist pain and disability, *J Hand Ther* 9:178–183, 1996.
4. Kirshner B, Guyatt G: A methodological framework for assessing health indices, *J Chronic Dis* 38(1):27–36, 1985.
5. Fienstein AR, Josephy BR, Wells CK: Scientific and clinical problems in indexes of functional disability, *Ann Intern Med* 105(3):413–420, 1986.
6. Salerno DF, Copley-Merriman C, Taylor TN, et al: A review of functional status measures for workers with upper extremity disorders, *Occup Environ Med* 59(10):664–670, 2002.
7. Chung KC, Hamill JB, Walters MR, et al: The Michigan Hand Outcomes Questionnaire (MHQ): assessment of responsiveness to clinical change, *Ann Plast Surg* 42(6):619–622, 1999.
8. Lindeboom R, Sprangers MA, Zwinderman AH: Responsiveness: a reinvention of the wheel? *Health Qual Life Outcomes* 3(1):8, 2005.
9. MacDermid JC, Stratford P: Applying evidence on outcome measures to hand therapy practice, *J Hand Ther* 17:165–173, 2004.
10. Amadio PC: Outcome assessment in hand surgery and hand therapy: an update, *J Hand Ther* 14(2):63–68, 2001.
11. Koran LM: The reliability of clinical methods, data and judgments, *N Engl J Med* 293:642–646, 1975.
12. Katz JN, Gelberman RH, Wright EA, et al: Responsiveness of self-reported and objective measures of disease severity in carpal tunnel syndrome, *Med Care* 32(11):1127–1133, 1994.
13. Amadio PC, Silverstein MD, Ilstrup DM, et al: Outcome assessment for carpal tunnel surgery: the relative responsiveness of generic, arthritis specific, disease-specific, and physical examination measures, *J Hand Surg Am* 21(3):338–346, 1996.
14. Atroshi I, Gummesson C, Johnsson R, et al: Symptoms, disability, and quality of life in patients with carpal tunnel syndrome, *J Hand Surg Am* 24(2):398–404, 1999.
15. Sprangers MAG, Aaronson NK: The role of health care providers and significant others in evaluating the quality of life of clients with chronic disease: a review, *J Clin Epidemiol* 45(7):743–760, 1992.
16. Ripat J, Etcheverry E, Cooper J, et al: A comparison of the Canadian Occupational Performance Measure and the Health Assessment Questionnaire, *Can J Occup Ther* 68(4):247–253, 2001.
17. Bellamy N, Campbell J, Haraoui B, et al: Dimensionality and clinical importance of pain and disability in hand osteoarthritis: development of the Australian/Canadian (AUSCAN) Osteoarthritis Hand Index, *Osteoarthritis Cartilage* 10(11):855–862, 2002.

18. MacDermid JC: Outcome evaluation in clients with elbow pathology: issues in instrument development and evaluation, *J Hand Ther* 14(2):105–114, 2001.

19. Hudak PL, Amadio PC, Bombardier C: Development of an upper extremity outcome measure: the DASH (disabilities of the arm, shoulder, and hand), *Am J Ind Med* 29(6):602–608, 1996.

20. Davis AM, Beaton DE, Hudak P, et al: Measuring disability of the upper extremity: a rationale supporting the use of a regional outcome measure, *J Hand Ther* 12(4):269–274, 1999.

21. Marx RG, Hogg-Johnson S, Hudak P, et al: A comparison of clients' responses about their disability with and without attribution to their affected area, *J Clin Epidemiol* 54(6):580–586, 2001.

22. Beaton DE, Katz JN, Fossel AH, et al: Measuring the whole or the parts? Validity, reliability, and responsiveness of the Disabilities of the Arm, Shoulder and Hand outcome measures in different regions of the upper extremity, *J Hand Ther* 14(2):128–146, 2001.

23. Smith MV, Calfee RP, Baumgarten KM, et al: Upper extremity-specific measures of disability and outcomes in orthopaedic surgery, *J Bone Joint Surg* 94:277–285, 2012.

24. Alotobaibi NM: The cross-cultural adaptation of the disability of arm, shoulder, and hand (DASH): A systematic review, *Occup Ther Int* 15(3):178–190, 2008.

25. Hunsaker FG, Cioffi DA, Amadio PC, et al: The American academy of orthopaedic surgeons outcomes instruments: normative values from the general population, *J Bone Joint Surg* 84-A(2):208–215, 2002.

26. Case-Smith J: Outcomes in hand rehabilitation using occupational therapy services, *Am J Occup Ther* 57:499–506, 2003.

27. SooHoo NF, McDonald AP, Seiler JG 3rd, et al: Evaluation of the construct validity of the DASH questionnaire by correlation to the SF-36, *J Hand Surg Am* 27(3):537–541, 2002.

28. MacDermid JC, Tottenham V: Responsiveness of the Disability of the Arm, Shoulder and Hand (DASH) and Patient-Rated Wrist/Hand Evaluation (PRWHE) in evaluating change after hand therapy, *J Hand Ther* 17:18–23, 2004.

29. Stiller J, Uhl TL: Outcomes measurement of upper extremity function, *Human Kinetics* 10(3):24–25, 2005.

30. Navsarikar A, Gladman DD, Husted JA, et al: Validity assessment of the Disabilities of Arm, Shoulder and Hand questionnaire (DASH) for clients with psoriatic arthritis, *J Rheumatol* 26(10):2191–2194, 1999.

31. Jain R, Hudak PL, Bowen CV: Validity of health status measures in clients with ulnar wrist disorders, *J Hand Ther* 14(2):147–153, 2001.

32. Gummesson C, Atroshi I, Ekdahl C: The disabilities of the arm, shoulder, and hand (DASH) outcome questionnaire: longitudinal construct validity and measuring self-rated health change after surgery, *BMC Musculoskelet Disord* 4:11, 2003.

33. Turchin DC, Beaton DE, Richards RR: Validity of observer-based aggregate scoring systems as descriptors of elbow pain, function, and disability, *J Bone Joint Surg Am* 80(2):154–162, 1998.

34. Kitis A, Celik E, Aslan UB, Zencir M: DASH questionnaire for the analysis of musculoskeletal symptoms in industry workers: A validity and reliability study, *Appl Ergon* 40:251–255, 2009.

35. MacDermid JC, Wessel J, Humphrey R, et al: Validity of self-report measures of pain and disability for persons who have undergone arthroplasty for osteoarthritis of the carpometacarpal joint of the hand, *Osteoarthritis Cartilage* 15(5):524–530, 2007.

36. Bilberg A, Bremell T, Mannerkorpi K: Disability of the arm, shoulder, and hand questionnaire in Swedish patients with rheumatoid arthritis: A validity study, *J Rehabil Med* 44:7–11, 2012.

37. Gay RE, Amadio PC, Johnson J: Comparative responsiveness of the disabilities of the arm, shoulder, and hand, the carpal tunnel questionnaire, and the SF-36 to clinical change after carpal tunnel release, *J Hand Surg Am* 28(2):250–254, 2003.

38. Greenslade JR, Metha RL, Belward P, et al: DASH and Boston questionnaire assessment of carpal tunnel syndrome outcome: what is the responsiveness of an outcome questionnaire? *J Hand Surg Br* 29(2):159–164, 2004.

39. McMillan CR, Binhammer PA: Which outcome measure is the best? Evaluating responsiveness of the disabilities of the arm, shoulder, and hand questionnaire, the Michigan hand questionnaire, and the patient-specific functional scale following hand and wrist surgery, *Hand* 4(3):311–318, 2009.

40. MacDermid JC, Richards RS, Donner A, et al: Responsiveness of the short form-36, disability of the arm, shoulder and hand questionnaire, patient-rated wrist evaluation and physical impairment measurements in evaluating recovery after a distal radius fracture, *J Hand Surg Am* 25(2):330–340, 2000.

41. Hwang JJ, Goldfarb CA, Gelberman RH, et al: The effect of dorsal carpal ganglion excision on the scaphoid shift test, *J Hand Surg Br* 24(1):106–108, 1999.

42. Ring D, Perey BH, Jupiter JB: The functional outcome of operative treatment of ununited fractures of the humeral diaphysis in older clients, *J Bone Joint Surg Am* 81(2):177–190, 1999.

43. Skutek M, Fremerey RW, Zeichen J, et al: Outcome analysis following open rotator cuff repair: early effectiveness validated using four different shoulder assessment scales, *Arch Orthop Trauma Surg* 120(7-8):432–436, 2000.

44. Getahun TY, Mac Dermid JC, Patterson SD: Concurrent validity of patient rating scales in assessment of outcomes after rotator cuff repair, *J Musculoskelet Res* 4(2):119–127, 2000.

45. Kirkley A, Griffin S, McLintock H, et al: The development and evaluation of a disease-specific quality of life measurement tool for shoulder instability: the Western Ontario Shoulder Instability Index (WOSI), *Am J Sports Med* 26(6):764–772, 1998.

46. Aktekin LA: Disability of arm shoulder and hand questionnaire in rheumatoid arthritis patients: relationship with disease activity, HAQ, SF-36, *Rheumatol Int* 31:823–826, 2011.

47. Ishikawa H, Murasawa A, Nakazono K, et al: The patient-based outcome of upper-extremity surgeries using the DASH questionnaire and the effect of disease activity of the patients with rheumatoid arthritis, *Clin Rheumatol* 27:967–973, 2008.

48. Slobogean GP, Slobogean BL: Measuring shoulder injury function: common scales and checklists, *Injury* 42:248–252, 2011.

49. McKee MD, Wilson TL, Winston L, et al: Functional outcome following surgical treatment of intra-articular distal humeral fractures through a posterior approach, *J Bone Joint Surg Am* 82-A(12):1701–1707, 2000.

50. McKee MD, Kim J, Kebaish K, et al: Functional outcome after open supracondylar fractures of the humerus; the effect of the surgical approach, *J Bone Joint Surg Br* 82(5):646–651, 2000.

51. Hannah SD, Hudak PL: Splinting and radial nerve palsy: a single-subject experiment, *J Hand Ther* 14(3):195–201, 2001.

52. Wong JYP, Fung BKK, Chu MML, et al: The use of Disabilities of the Arm, Shoulder, and Hand Questionnaire in rehabilitation after acute traumatic hand injuries, *J Hand Ther* 20:49–56, 2007.

53. Changulani M, Okonkwo U, Keswani T, et al: Outcome evaluation measure for wrist and hand—which one to choose? *Int Orthop* 32:1–6, 2008.

54. Stiller J, Uhl TL: Outcomes measurement of upper extremity function, *Athl Ther Today* 10(3):34–36, 2005.

55. Hoang-Kim A, Pegreffi F, Moroni A, et al: Measuring wrist and hand function: common scales and checklists, *Injury* 42:253–258, 2011.

56. Drummond AS, Sampaio RF, Macini MC, et al: Linking the disability of the arm, shoulder, and hand to the international classification of functioning, disability, and health, *J Hand Ther* 20:336–344, 2007.

57. Dixon D, Johnston M, McQueen M, et al: The disability of the arm, shoulder, and hand questionnaire (DASH) can measure the impairments, activity limitations, and participation restriction constructs from the international classification of functioning, disability, and health (ICF), *BMC Musculoskelet Disord* 9:114, 2008.

58. Jester A, Harth A, Wind G, et al: Disabilities of the arm, shoulder, and hand (DASH) questionnaire: determining functional activity profiles in patients with upper extremity disorders, *J Hand Surg Br* 30(1):23–28, 2005.

59. John R, Verma CV: Changes in the health status and functional outcomes in acute traumatic hand injury patients, during physical therapy treatment, *Indian J Plast Surg* 44(2):362–367, 2011.

60. Lopes AD, Villar e Furtado R, Augusto da Silva C, et al: Comparison of self-report and interview administration methods based on the Brazilian versions of the western Ontario rotator cuff index and disabilities of the arm, shoulder, and hand questionnaire in patients with rotator cuff disorders, *Clinics* 64(2):121–125, 2009.

61. Roy JS, MacDermid JC, Woodhouse LJ: Measuring shoulder function: A systematic review of four questionnaires, *Arthritis Rheum* 61(5):623–632, 2009.

62. Horng YS, Lin MC, Feng CT, et al: Responsiveness of the Michigan Hand Outcomes Questionnaire and the Disabilities of the Arm, Shoulder, and Hand questionnaire in patients with hand injury, *J Hand Surg Am* 35(3):430–436, 2010.

63. Murphy DM, Khoury JG, Imbriglia JE, et al: Comparison of arthroplasty and arthrodesis for the rheumatoid wrist, *J Hand Surg Am* 28(4):570–576, 2003.

64. Cano SJ, Barrett LE, Zajicek JP, et al: Beyond the reach of traditional analyses: using the Rasch to evaluate the DASH in people with multiple sclerosis, *Mult Scler* 17(2):214–222, 2011.
65. Beaton DE, Wright JG, Katz JN, et al: Development of the Quick-DASH: comparison of three item-reduction approaches, *J Bone Joint Surg Am* 87(5):1038–1046, 2005.
66. Dogan SK, Ay S, Evcik D, et al: Adaptation of Turkish version of the questionnaire Quick Disability of the Shoulder, Arm and Hand (QuickDASH) in patients with carpal tunnel syndrome, *Clin Rheumatol* 30:185–191, 2011.
67. Whalley K, Adams J: The longitudinal validity of the quick and full version of the Disability of the Arm, Shoulder, and Hand questionnaire in musculoskeletal hand outpatients, *Hand Ther* 14:22–25, 2009.
68. Colovic H, Stankovic I, Dimitrijevic L, et al: The value of modified DASH questionnaire for evaluation of function after supracondylar fractures in children, *Vojnosanit Pregl* 65(1):27–32, 2008.
69. Angst F, Goldhahn J, Drerup S, et al: How sharp is the short Quick-DASH? A refined content and validity analysis of the short form of the disabilities of the shoulder, arm and hand questionnaire in the strata of symptoms and function and specific joint condition, *Qual Life Res* 18:1043–1051, 2009.
70. Gummesson C, Ward MM, Atroshi I: The shortened disabilities of the arm, shoulder and hand questionnaire (QuickDASH): validity and reliability based on responses within the full-length DASH, *BMC Musculoskelet Disord* 7:44, 2006.
71. Chung KC, Pillsbury MS, Walters MR, et al: Reliability and validity testing of the Michigan Hand Outcomes Questionnaire, *J Hand Surg Am* 23(4):575–587, 1998.
72. Shauver MJ, Chung KC: The minimal clinically important difference of the Michigan Hand Outcome Questionnaire, *J Hand Surg Am* 34(3):509–514, 2009.
73. Klein RD, Kotsis SV, Chung KC: Open carpal tunnel release using a 1 centimeter incision: technique and outcomes for 104 clients, *Plast Reconstr Surg* 3(5):1616, 2003.
74. Chatterjee JS, Price PE: Comparative responsiveness of the Michigan Hand Outcomes Questionnaire and the Carpal Tunnel Questionnaire after carpal tunnel release, *J Hand Surg Am* 34(2):273–280, 2009.
75. Kotsis SV, Chung KC: Responsiveness of the Michigan Hand Outcomes Questionnaire and the Disabilities of the Arm, Shoulder and Hand questionnaire in carpal tunnel surgery, *J Hand Surg Am* 30(1):81–86, 2005.
76. Sambandam SN, Priyanka P, Gul A, et al: Critical analysis of outcome measures used in the assessment of carpal tunnel syndrome, *Int Orthop* 32:497–504, 2008.
77. Kotsis SV, Lau FH, Chung KC: Responsiveness of the Michigan Hand Outcomes Questionnaire and physical measurements in outcome studies of distal radius fracture treatment, *J Hand Surg Am* 32(1):84–90, 2007.
78. Massy-Westropp N, Krishnan J, Ahern M: Comparing the AUSCAN osteoarthritis hand index, Michigan Hand Outcomes Questionnaire, and Sequential Occupational Dexterity Assessment for clients with rheumatoid arthritis, *J Rheumatol* 31(10):1996–2001, 2004.
79. Waljee JF, Chung KC, Kim HM, et al: Validity and responsiveness of the Michigan Hand Questionnaire in patients with rheumatoid arthritis: a multicenter, international study, *Arthritis Care Res* 62(11):1569–1577, 2010.
80. Poole JL, Lucero SL, Mynatt R: Self-reports and performance-based tests of hand function in persons with osteoarthritis, *Phys Occup Ther in Geriatr* 28(3):249–258, 2010.
81. Poole JL, Gonzoles I, Tedesco T: Self-reports of hand function in persons with diabetes, *Occup Ther Healthc* 24(3):239–248, 2010.
82. Dias JJ, Rajan A, Thompson JR: Which questionnaire is best? The reliability, validity and ease of use of the patient evaluation measure, the disabilities of the arm, shoulder, and hand and the michigan hand outcome questionnaire, *J Hand Surg Eur Vol* 33(1):9–17, 2008.
83. Adams J, Mullee M, Burridge J, et al: Responsiveness of self-report and therapist-rated upper extremity structural impairment and functional outcome measures in early rheumatoid arthritis, *Arthritis Care Res* 62(2):274–278, 2010.
84. Schoneveld K, Wittink H, Takken T: Clinimetric evaluation of measurement tools used in hand therapy to assess activity and participation, *J Hand Ther* 22:221–236, 2009.
85. Michener SK, Olson AL, Humphrey BA, et al: Relationship among grip strength, functional outcomes, and work performance following hand trauma, *Work* 16(3):209–217, 2001.
86. Umraw N, Chan Y, Gomez M, et al: Effective hand function assessment after burn injuries, *J Burn Care Rehabil* 25(1):134–139, 2004.
87. Goldfarb CA, Stern PJ: Metacarpophalangeal joint arthroplasty in rheumatoid arthritis: a long term assessment, *J Bone Joint Surg Am* 85(10):1869–1878, 2003.
88. Waljee JF, Kim HM, Burns PB, et al: Development of a brief, 12-item version of the Michigan Hand Questionnaire, *Plastic Reconstructive Surg* 128(1):208–220, 2011.
89. Macey AC, Burke FD: Outcomes of hand surgery, *J Hand Surg Br* 20(6):841–855, 1995.
90. Dias JJ, Bhowal B, Wildin CJ, et al: Assessing the outcome of disorders of the hand: is the client evaluation measure reliable, valid, responsive, and without bias? *J Bone Joint Surg Br* 83(2):235–240, 2001.
91. Sharma R, Dias JJ: Validity and reliability of three generic outcome measures for hand disorders, *J Hand Surg Br* 25(6):593–600, 2000.
92. Dias J, Buch K: Palmar wrist ganglion: does intervention improve outcome? A prospective study of the natural history and client-reported treatment outcomes, *J Hand Surg Br* 28(2):172–176, 2003.
93. Forward DP, Sithole JS, Davis TR: The internal consistency and validity of the Patient Evaluation Measure for outcomes assessment in distal radius fractures, *J Hand Surg Eur Vol* 32(3):262–267, 2007.
94. Hobby JL, Watts C, Elliot D: Validity and responsiveness of the patient evaluation measure as an outcome measure for carpal tunnel syndrome, *J Hand Surg Br* 30(4):350–354, 2005.
95. Simmen BR, Angst F, Schwyzer HK, et al: A concept for comprehensively measuring health, function, and quality of life following orthopaedic interventions of the upper extremity, *Arch Orthop Trauma Surg* 129:113–118, 2009.
96. MacDermid JC, Turgeon T, Richards RS, et al: Patient rating of wrist pain and disability: a reliable and valid measurement tool, *J Orthop Trauma* 12(8):577–586, 1998.
97. Hemelaers L, Angst F, Drerup S, et al: Reliability and validity of the German version of "the Patient-Rated Wrist Evaluation (PRWE)" as an outcome measure of wrist pain and disability in patients with acute distal radius fractures, *J Hand Ther* 21:336–376, 2008.
98. MacDermid JC, Richards RS, Roth JH: Distal radius fracture: a prospective outcome study of 275 clients, *J Hand Ther* 14(2):154–169, 2001.
99. Karnezis IA, Fragkiadakis EG: Association between objective clinical variables and client-rated disability of the wrist, *J Bone Joint Surg Br* 84(7):967–970, 2002.
100. Michlovitz S, Hun L, Erasala GN, et al: Continuous low-level heat wrap therapy is effective for treating wrist pain, *Arch Phys Med Rehabil* 85(9):1409–1416, 2004.
101. Imaeda T, Uchiyama S, Wada T, et al: Reliability, validity, and responsiveness of the Japanese version of the Patient-Rated Wrist Evaluation, *J Orthop Sci* 15(4):509–517, 2010.
102. Mehta SP, Mhatre B, MacDermid JC, et al: Cross-cultural adaptation and psychometric testing of the Hindi version of the Patient-Rated Wrist Evaluation, *J Hand Ther* 25:65–78, 2012.
103. Navarro CM, Ponzer S, Tornkvist H, et al: Measuring outcome after wrist injury: translation and validation of the Swedish version of the Patient-Rated Wrist Evaluation, *BMC Musculoskelet Disord* 12:171, 2001.
104. Wilcke MT, Abbaszadegan H, Adolphson PY: Evaluation of a Swedish version of the Patient-Rated Wrist Evaluation outcome questionnaire: food responsiveness, validity, and reliability in 99 patients recovering from a fracture of the distal radius, *Scand J Plast Reconstr Surg Hand Surg* 43:94–101, 2009.
105. John M, Angst F, Pap G, et al: Cross-cultural adaptation, reliability, and validity of the Patient rated Elbow Evaluation (PREE) for German-speaking patient, *Clin Exp Rheumatol* 25:195–205, 2007.
106. MacDermid JC, Wessel J, Humphrey R, et al: Validity of self-report measures of pain and disability for persons who have undergone arthroplasty for osteoarthritis of the carpometacarpal joint of the hand, *Osteoarthr Cartil* 15(5):524–530, 2007.
107. Richards RR, An KN, Bigliani LU, et al: A standardized method for the assessment of shoulder function, *J Shoulder Elbow Surg* 3(6):347–352, 1994.
108. Michener LA, McClure PW, Sennett BJ: American Shoulder and Elbow Surgeons standardized shoulder assessment for patient self-report section: reliability, validity and responsiveness, *J Shoulder Elbow Surg* 11:587–594, 2002.
109. McClure P, Michener L: Measures of adult shoulder function, *Arthritis Rheum* 49(5):50–58, 2003.

110. Dowrick AS, Gabbe BJ, Williamson OD, et al: Outcome instruments for the assessment of the upper extremity following trauma: a review, *Injury* 36:468–476, 2005.

111. Stiller J, Uhl TL: Outcomes measurement of upper extremity function, *Athl Ther Today* 10(3):34–36, 2005.

112. Simmen BR, Angst F, Schwyzer HK, et al: A concept for comprehensively measuring health, function, and quality of life following orthopaedic interventions of the upper extremity, *Arch Orthop Trauma Surg* 129:113–118, 2009.

113. Oh JH, Jo KH, Kim WS, et al: Comparative evaluation of the measurement properties of various shoulder outcome instruments, *Am J Sports Med* 37(6):1161–1168, 2009.

114. Roy JS, Esculier JF: Psychometric evidence for clinical outcome measures assessing shoulder disorders, *Phys Ther Rev* 16(5):331–346, 2011.

115. Kocher MS, Horan MP, Briggs KK, et al: Reliability, validity, and responsiveness of the American Shoulder and Elbow Surgeons subjective shoulder scale in patients with shoulder instability, rotator cuff disease, and glenohumeral arthritis, *J Bone Joint Surg Am* 87(9):2006–2011, 2005.

116. Roach KE, Budiman-Mak E, Songsiridej N, et al: Development of a shoulder pain and disability index, *Arthritr Care Res* 4:143–149, 1991.

117. Williams JW Jr, Holleman DR Jr, Simel DL: Measuring shoulder function with the Shoulder Pain and Disability Index, *J Rheumatol* 22(4):727–732, 1995.

118. Bumin G, Tüzün EH, Tonga E: The Shoulder Pain and Disability Index (SPADI): cross-cultural adaptation, reliability, and validity of the Turkish version, *J Back Musculoskel Rehabil* 21(1):57–62, 2008.

119. Goldhahn J, Mannion AF, Roach KE, et al: Cross-cultural adaptation, reliability and validity of the German Shoulder Pain and Disability Index (SPADI), *Rheumatol* 46(1):87–92, 2007.

120. Martins J, Napoles BV, Hoffman CB, et al: The Brazilian version of Shoulder Pain and Disability Index— translation, cultural adaptation and reliability, *Rev Bras Fisioter* 14(6):527–536, 2010.

121. Puga VOO, Lopes A, Costa LOP: Assessment of cross-cultural adaptations and measurement properties of self-report outcome measures relevant to shoulder disability in Portuguese: a systematic review, *Rev Bras Fisioter* 16(2):85–93, 2012.

122. Ekeberg OM, Bautz-Holter E, Tveitå EK, et al: Agreement, reliability and validity in 3 shoulder questionnaires in patients with rotator cuff disease, *BMC Musculoskelet Disord* 9:1–9, 2008.

123. MacDermid JC, Solomon P, Prkachin K: The Shoulder Pain and Disability Index demonstrates factor, construct and longitudinal validity, *BMC Musculoskelet Disord* 7:11–12, 2006.

124. Hill CL, Lester S, Taylor A, et al: Factor structure and validity of the shoulder pain and disability index in a population-based study of people with shoulder symptoms, *BMC Musculoskelet Disord* 12(1):1–6, 2011.

125. Ekeberg OM, Bautz-Holter E, Keller A, et al: A questionnaire found disease-specific WORC index is not more responsive than SPADI and OSS in rotator cuff disease, *J Clin Epidemiol* 63(5):575–584, 2010.

126. Staples MP, Forbes A, Green S, et al: Shoulder-specific disability measures showed acceptable construct validity and responsiveness, *J Clin Epidemiol* 63(2):163–170, 2010.

127. Heald S, Riddle DL: The shoulder pain and disability index: the construct validity and responsiveness of a region-specific disability measure, *Phys Ther* 77(10):1079–1090, 1997.

128. Angst F, Goldhahn J, Drerup S, et al: Responsiveness of six outcome assessment instruments in total shoulder arthroplasty, *Arthritis Rheum* 59(3):391–398, 2008.

129. Tveitå EK, Sandvik L, Ekeberg OM, et al: Factor structure of the Shoulder Pain and Disability Index in patients with adhesive capsuliti, *BMC Musculoskelet Disord* 9:1–7, 2008.

130. Guilleman F, Coste J, Pouchot J, et al: The AIMS2-SF: a short form of the Arthritis Impact Measurement Scales 2: French Quality of Life in Rheumatology Group, *Arthritis Rheum* 40(7):1267–1274, 1997.

131. Askary-Ashtiani AR, Mousavi SJ, Parnianpour M, et al: Translation and validation of the Persian version of the Arthritis Impact Measurement Scales 2-Short Form (AIMS2-SF) in patients with rheumatoid arthritis, *Clinical Rheumatol* 28:521–527, 2009.

132. Ren XS, Kazis L, Meenan RF: Short-form Arthritis Impact Measurement Scales 2: tests of reliability and validity among clients with osteoarthritis, *Arthritis Care Res* 12(3):163–171, 1999.

133. Taylor LF, Kee CC, King SV, et al: Evaluating the effects of an educational symposium on knowledge, impact, and self-management of older African Americans living with osteoarthritis, *J Community Health Nurs* 21(4):229–238, 2004.

134. Haavardsholm EA, Kvien TK, Uhlig T, et al: A comparison of agreement and sensitivity to change between AIMS2 and a short form of AIMS2 (AIMS2-SF) in more than 1,000 rheumatoid arthritis patients, *J Rheumatol* 27(12):2810–2816, 2000.

135. Taal E, Rasker JJ, Riemsma RP: Psychometric properties of a Dutch short form of the Arthritis Impact Measurement Scales 2 (Dutch-AIMS2-SF), *Rheumatology* 42:427–434, 2003.

136. Taal E, Rasker JJ, Riemsma RP: Sensitivity to change of AIMS2 and AIMS2-SF components in comparison to M-HAQ and VAS-pain, *Ann Rheum Dis* 63:1655–1658, 2004.

137. Stamm T, Mathis M, Aletaha D, Kloppenburg M, et al: Mapping hand functioning in hand osteoarthritis: comparing self-report instruments with a comprehensive hand function test, *Arthritis Rheum* 57(7):1230–1237, 2007.

138. Bellamy N: *AUSCAN Hand Osteoarthritis Index: user guide II*, Queensland, Australia, 2003, Centre of National Research on Disability and Rehabilitation Medicine.

139. Bellamy N, Campbell J, Haraoui B, et al: Clinimetric properties of the AUSCAN Osteoarthritis Hand Index: an evaluation of reliability, validity and responsiveness, *Osteoarthritis Cartilage* 10(11):863–869, 2002.

140. Allen KD, Jordan JM, Renner JB, et al: Validity, factor structure, and clinical relevance of the AUSCAN osteoarthritis hand index, *Arthritis Rheum* 54(2):551–556, 2006.

141. Moe RH, Garratt A, Slatkowsky-Christensen B, et al: Concurrent evaluation of data quality, reliability and validity of the Australian/Canadian Osteoarthritis Hand Index and the Functional Index for Hand Osteoarthritis, *Rheumatol* 49(12):2327–2336, 2010.

142. Jones G, Cooley HM, Bellamy N: A cross-sectional study of the association between Herberden's nodes, radiographic osteoarthritis of the hands, grip strength, disability, and pain, *Osteoarthritis Cartilage* 9(7):606–611, 2001.

143. Haugen IK, Moe RH, Slatkowsky-Christensen B, et al: The AUSCAN subscales, AIMS-2 hand/finger subscale, and FIHOA were not unidimensional scales, *J Clin Epidemiol* 64:1039–1046, 2011.

144. Bellamy N, Wilson C, Hendrikz J: Population-based normative values for the Western Ontario and McMaster (WOMAC®) osteoarthritis index and the Australian/Canadian (AUSCAN) hand osteoarthritis index functional subscales, *Inflammopharmacol* 18(1):1–8, 2010.

145. Levine DW, Simmons BP, Koris MJ, et al: A self-administered questionnaire for the assessment of severity of symptoms and functional status in carpal tunnel syndrome, *J Bone Joint Surg Am* 75(11):1585–1592, 1993.

146. Bessette L, Sangha O, Kuntz KM, et al: Comparative responsiveness of generic versus disease-specific and weighted versus unweighted health status measures in carpal tunnel syndrome, *Med Care* 36(4):491–502, 1998.

147. Bessette L, Keller RB, Lew RA, et al: Prognostic value of a hand symptom diagram in surgery for carpal tunnel syndrome, *J Rheumatol* 24(4):726–734, 1997.

148. Giannini F, Cioni R, Mondelli M, et al: A new clinical scale of carpal tunnel syndrome: validation of the measurement and clinical-neurophysiological assessment, *Clin Neurophysiol* 113(1):71–77, 2002.

149. Mondelli M, Reale F, Sicurelli F, et al: Relationship between the self-administered Boston Questionnaire and electrophysiological findings in follow-up of surgically treated carpal tunnel syndrome, *J Hand Surg Br* 25(2):128–134, 2000.

150. Heybeli N, Kutluhan S, Demirci S, et al: Assessment of outcome of carpal tunnel syndrome: a comparison of electrophysiological findings and a self-administered Boston Questionnaire, *J Hand Surg Br* 27(3):259–264, 2002.

151. Leite JC, Jerosch-Herold C, Song F: A systematic review of the psychometric properties of the Boston Carpal Tunnel Questionnaire, *BMC Musculoskelet Disord* 7:78, 2006.

152. Senthil NS, Priyanka P, Gul A, et al: Critical analysis of outcome measures used in the assessment of carpal tunnel syndrome, *Int Orthop* 32(4):497–504, 2008.

153. Katz JN, Punnett L, Simmons BP, et al: Workers' compensation recipients with carpal tunnel syndrome: the validity of self-reported health measures, *Am J Public Health* 86(1):52–56, 1996.

154. Kurt S, Cevik B, Kaplan Y, et al: The relationship between Boston Questionnaire and electrophysiological findings in carpal tunnel syndrome, *Arch Neuropsychiatr* 47(3):237–240, 2010.

155. Green TP, Tolonen EU, Clarke MRA, et al: The relationship of pre- and postoperative median and ulnar nerve conduction measures to a self-administered questionnaire in carpal tunnel syndrome, *Clin Neurophysiol* 42(4):231–239, 2012.

156. Cevik MU, Altun Y, Uzar E, et al: Diagnostic value of F-wave inversion in patients with early carpal tunnel syndrome, *Neurosci Letters* 508(2): 110–113, 2012.

157. Ortiz-Corredor F, Calambas N, Mendoza-Pulido C, et al: Factor analysis of Carpal Tunnel Syndrome Questionnaire in relation to nerve conduction studies, *Clin Neurophysiol* 122(10):2067–2070, 2011.

158. Boyd KU, Gan BS, Ross DC, et al: Outcomes in carpal tunnel syndrome: symptom severity, conservative management and progression to surgery, *Clin Invest Med* 28(5):254–260, 2005.

159. Overend TJ, Wouri-Fearn JL, Kramer JF, et al: Reliability of a Patient-Rated Forearm Evaluation Questionnaire for patients with lateral epicondylitis, *J Hand Ther* 12:31–37, 1999.

160. MacDermid JC: Update: the Patient-Rated Forearm Evaluation Questionnaire is now the Patient-Rated Tennis Elbow Evaluation, *J Hand Ther* 18:407–410, 2005.

161. Blanchette M-A, Normand MC: Cross-cultural adaptation of the Patient-Rated Tennis Elbow Evaluation to Canadian French, *J Hand Ther* 23:290–300, 2010.

162. Nilsson P, Baigi A, Marklund B, et al: Cross-cultural adaptation and determination of the reliability and validity of PRTEE-S (Patientskattad Utvärdering av Tennisarmbåge), a questionnaire for patients with lateral epicondylalgia, in a Swedish population, *BMC Musculoskelet Disord* 9:1–8, 2008.

163. Altan L: Ercan İ, Konur S: Reliability and validity of Turkish version of the patient rated tennis elbow evaluation, *Rheumatol Int* 30(8):1049–1054, 2010.

164. Poltawski L, Watson T: Measuring clinically important change with the Patient-Rated Tennis Elbow Evaluation, *Hand Ther* 16(3):52–57, 2011.

165. Newcomer KL, Martinez-Silvestrini JA, Schaefer MP, et al: Sensitivity of the Patient-Rated Forearm Evaluation Questionnaire in lateral epicondylitis, *J Hand Ther* 18:400–406, 2005.

166. Rompe JD, Overend TJ, MacDermid JC: Validation of the Patient-Rated Tennis Elbow Evaluation Questionnaire, *J Hand Ther* 20:3–11, 2007.

167. Chung B, Wiley JP: Validity, responsiveness, and reliability of the Patient-Rated Tennis Elbow Evaluation, *Hand Ther* 15(3):62–68, 2010.

168. Kirkley A, Griffin S, Dainty K: Scoring systems for the functional assessment of the shoulder, *Arthroscopy* 19(10):1109–1120, 2003.

169. Salomonsson B, Ahlström S, Dalén N, et al: The Western Ontario Shoulder Instability Index (WOSI): validity, reliability, and responsiveness retested with a Swedish translation, *Acta Orthop* 80(2):233–238, 2009.

170. Hatta T, Shinozaki N, Omi R, et al: Reliability and validity of the Western Ontario Shoulder Instability Index (WOSI) in the Japanese population, *J Orthop Sci* 16(6):732–736, 2011.

171. Hofstaetter JG, Hanslik-Schnabel B, Hofstaetter SG, et al: Cross-cultural adaptation and validation of the German version of the Western Ontario shoulder instability index, *Arch Orthop Trauma Surg* 130(6):787–796, 2010.

172. Kirkley A, Griffin S, Richards C, et al: Prospective randomized clinical trial comparing the effectiveness of immediate arthroscopic stabilization versus immobilization and rehabilitation in first traumatic anterior dislocation of the shoulder, *Arthroscopy* 15(5):507–514, 1999.

173. Kirkley A, Griffin S, Alvarez C: The development and evaluation of a disease-specific quality of life measurement tool for rotator cuff disease: the Western Ontario Rotator Cuff Index (WORC), *Clin J Sport Med* 13:84–92, 2003.

174. El O, Bircan C, Gulbahar S, et al: The reliability and validity of the Turkish version of the Western Ontario Rotator Cuff Index, *Rheumatol Int* 26(12):1101–1108, 2006.

175. Mousavi SJ, Hadian MR, Abedi M, et al: Translation and validation study of the Persian version of the Western Ontario Rotator Cuff Index, *Clin Rheumatol* 28(3):293–299, 2009.

176. Kirkley A, Litchfield RB, Jackowski DM, et al: The use of the impingement test as a predictor of outcome following subacromial decompression for rotator cuff tendinosis, *Arthroscopy* 18(1):8–15, 2002.

177. Razmjou H, Bean A, van Osnabrugge V, et al: Cross-sectional and longitudinal construct validity of two rotator cuff disease-specific outcome measures, *BMC Musculoskelet Disord* 7:26–27, 2006.

178. Wessel J, Razmjou H, Mewa Y, et al: The factor validity of the Western Ontario Rotator Cuff Index, *BMC Musculoskelet Disord* 6:22–27, 2005.

179. Amadio PC: *Outcomes measures: disease specific versus global instruments*, Fajardo, Puerto Rico, 2005, AAHS Hand Therapy Day.

180. Guyatt GH, Bombardier C, Tugwell PX: Measuring disease-specific quality of life in clinical trials, *CMAJ* 134:889–895, 1986.

9 Hand Coordination

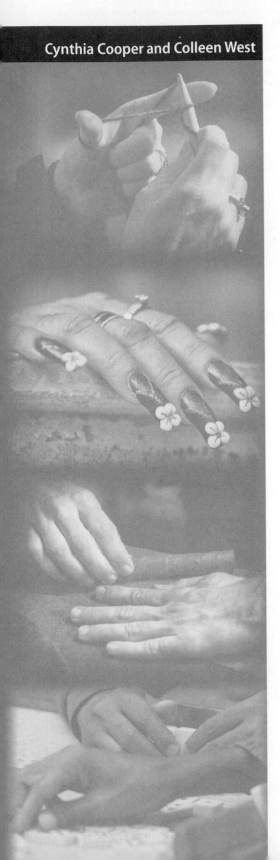

Cynthia Cooper and Colleen West

Background

The hand is a perceptual entity that has been described as an information-seeking organ. Its use provides patients with the ability to interpret and analyze tactile properties, such as shape, size, and texture. Hand use also enables patients to manipulate objects in order to identify and handle them effectively. Using coordinated hand function, we manually explore and recognize the relationship of objects to our bodies and to gravity.[1]

Hand skills require tactile-proprioceptive and visual information, but if the somatosensory functions are good, then visual feedback is not mandatory. Patterns of hand skills are reach, grasp, carry, voluntary release, in-hand manipulation, and bilateral hand use. The latter two patterns are considered to be more complex skills than the first four. The radial digits are considered to be the skill side (manipulative side) of the hand, while the ulnar digits are considered to be the stability side of the hand.

Definitions[2]

Reach is defined as moving and extending the arm for placing or grasping an object. **Grasp** is attaining an object with the hand. **Carry** is transporting an object in the hand to another place. **Voluntary release** is intentionally letting go of an object in the hand at a specific place and time. **In-hand manipulation** means adjusting an object in the hand after grasping it. **Bilateral hand use** means using two hands together in order to accomplish an activity and follows unilateral hand use developmentally. An example of bilateral hand use is steering a bicycle or throwing a large ball. **Bimanual hand use** means each hand does different things in the activity. An example of bimanual hand use is tying shoelaces or cutting with scissors.

Hand movements are classified as non-prehensile and prehensile. **Non-prehensile movements** use the fingers or the entire hand to lift or push an object. **Prehensile movements** incorporate grasping of an object and can be subdivided into two purposes, precision grasp and power grasp. **Precision grasp** uses opposition of the thumb to the fingertips. Power grasp uses the whole hand with thumb flexion or abduction according to the control needed for the task.

Another classification system differentiates patterns of grasp by the inclusion or exclusion of thumb opposition. Hook grasp, power grasp, and lateral pinch do not incorporate thumb opposition. **Hook grasp** is useful for sustaining a grip to carry objects. **Power grasp** is useful for controlling objects, such as tools. Using a hairbrush is an example of power grasp with oblique positioning of the object in the hand and more flexion of the ulnar digits than the radial digits. **Lateral pinch** is useful when one needs power to manipulate or hold a small object. Turning a key in the door is an example of lateral pinch.

Tip pinch and palmar grasp differ from hook grasp, power grasp, and lateral pinch because they do incorporate thumb opposition. **Tip pinch** is demonstrated by opposition of the tips of the thumb and index finger with all joints of the thumb and index finger being partially flexed, forming a circle. Patients with anterior interosseous nerve injury are unable to perform tip pinch because they lack the function of the flexor pollicis longus and the flexor digitorum profundus to the index finger.

Palmar grasp is further categorized into standard, cylindrical, disk, and spherical grasps. With **cylindrical grasp,** flattening of the transverse arch facilitates holding of the fingers against the object. In **disk grasp**, there is metacarpophalangeal (MP) hyperextension and finger abduction that is adjusted according to the object's size. When we open a jar, the hand stabilizing the jar demonstrates a cylindrical grasp, and the hand opening the lid uses a disk grasp. **Spherical grasp** occurs with wrist extension, digital abduction, and some MP and interphalangeal (IP) flexion, as in holding a tennis ball. This prehension pattern requires control and balance of the intrinsic and extrinsic muscles.

Pinches are classified according to the number of digits involved. **Two-point pinch,** also called **pad-to-pad pinch** or **pincer grasp,** occurs when the thumb opposes the index finger pad only. **Three-point pinch** or **three-jaw chuck** grasp occurs when the thumb opposes the index and middle finger pads simultaneously. This pinch provides better prehension stability than does two-point pinch.

Manipulation Skills

There are five pattern types of in-hand manipulation, and in order to perform them, the patient must be able to control the palmar arches. The pattern types are finger-to-palm translation, palm-to-finger translation, shift, simple rotation, and complex rotation. Varying definitions of finger-to-palm translation are offered in the literature. Exner[2] defines **finger-to-palm translation** as the grasping of an object with the thumb and finger pads and then moving the object into the palm. This is exemplified by the activity of picking up a button with the thumb and fingers and then moving the button into the palm. **Palm-to-finger translation** occurs in the opposite direction and is more difficult to do. This is performed when a person has coins in their palm, and they move one coin from the palm to the finger pads in preparation for inserting the coin in a slot. **Shift** is demonstrated when an object that is being held on the radial aspect of the hand is moved linearly on the finger surface in order to reposition it on the finger pads. Repositioning a pen after grasping it is an example of shift. **Simple rotation** occurs when an object is turned or rolled less than or equal to 90 degrees in the finger pads. Opening a small bottle cap is an example of simple rotation. **Complex rotation** is similar to simple rotation, but the object is rotated 180 to 360 degrees. Turning a pencil in order to use the eraser end is an example of complex rotation. **In-hand manipulation with stabilization** is defined as the performance of any in-hand manipulation skill while the person has other objects stabilized in the hand.

Using Hand Coordination Activities to Improve Hand Function

Having functional range of motion, sensation, and stength does not guarantee coordination abilities. Patients and therapists are often surprised at the challenge posed by tasks that look easy to perform. This is why it is so important to include coordination activities in hand therapy treatment.

> ◎ *Clinical Pearl*
>
> Having excellent range of motion (ROM) or good somatosensory function does not guarantee good coordination. For hand therapy patients, coordination activities that look easy may in fact be quite challenging, particularly for their non-dominant extremity.

> ◎ *Clinical Pearl*
>
> Fine motor skills result from combinations of various factors including excellent control of finger motions. But it is the impact of the central nervous system that truly provides the foundation for specialized hand use.[3]

Grading the Coordination Activities

> ◎ *Clinical Pearl*
>
> Developmentally, prehension precedes manipulation.

Coordination activities may be graded from gross motor control to fine motor control; from handling of rubbery or textured objects to use of smooth, slippery, or wet objects; from activities near the body to activities farther away from the body; from use of proximal support to no proximal support; from gravity-assisted to gravity-eliminated to anti-gravity positions; and from non-resistive to resistive.

Examples

See Figs. 9-1 through 9-20 for examples of coordination exercises.

Conclusion

Through complex sensorimotor capabilities of hand use, motion is transformed into function. Adding coordination activities to hand therapy treatment provides a way to transform objective clinical improvements, such as increased range of motion (ROM) into meaningful gains of hand function and use.[4]

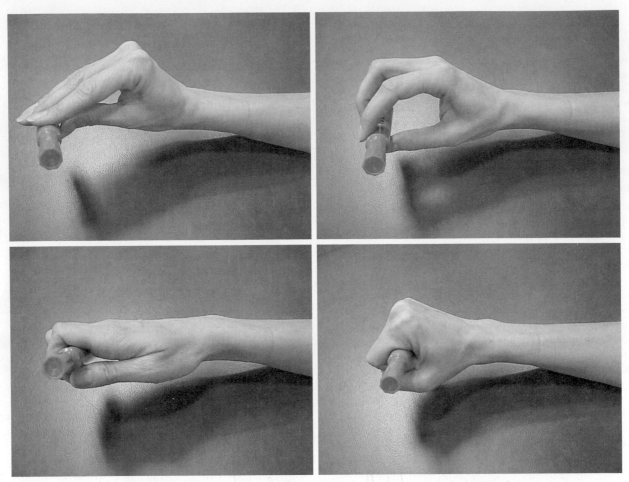

FIGURE 9-1 Finger-to-palm translation. (Copyright Cynthia Cooper and John Evarts.)

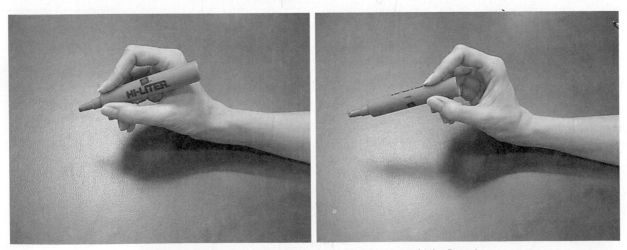

FIGURE 9-2 Shift or scoot. (Copyright Cynthia Cooper and John Evarts.)

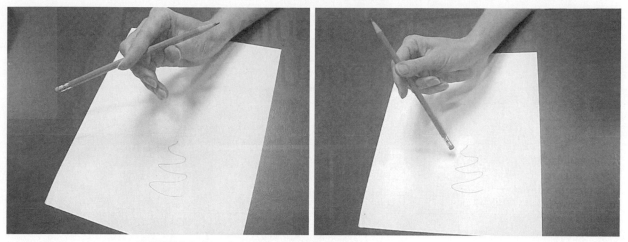

FIGURE 9-3 Complex rotation. (Copyright Cynthia Cooper and John Evarts.)

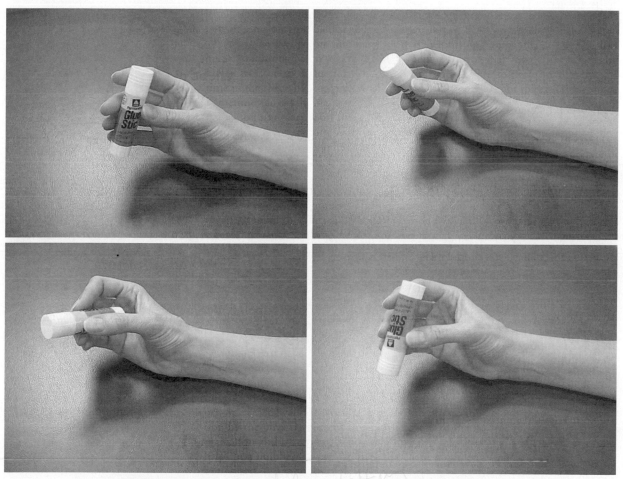

FIGURE 9-4 Complex rotation in steps. (Copyright Cynthia Cooper and John Evarts.)

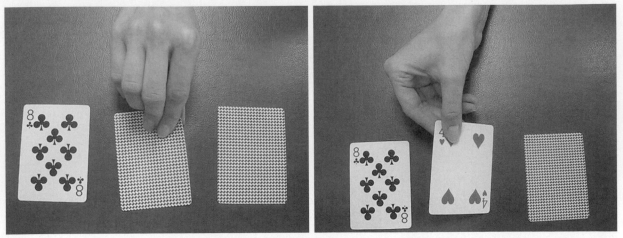

FIGURE 9-5 Card flip. (Copyright Cynthia Cooper and John Evarts.)

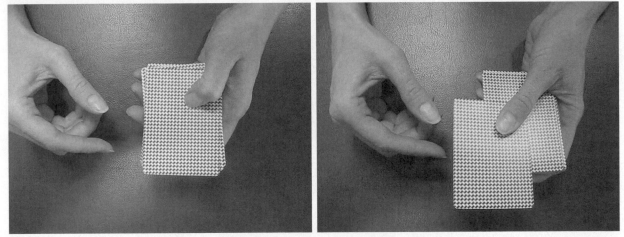

FIGURE 9-6 Dealing cards. (Copyright Cynthia Cooper and John Evarts.)

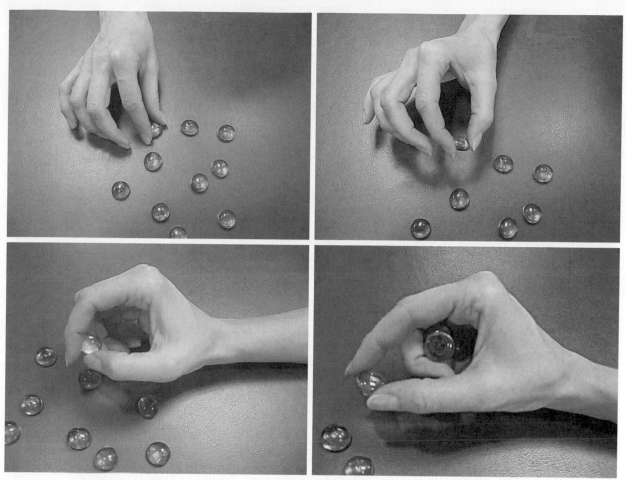

FIGURE 9-7 Finger-to-palm translation with stabilization. (Copyright Cynthia Cooper and John Evarts.)

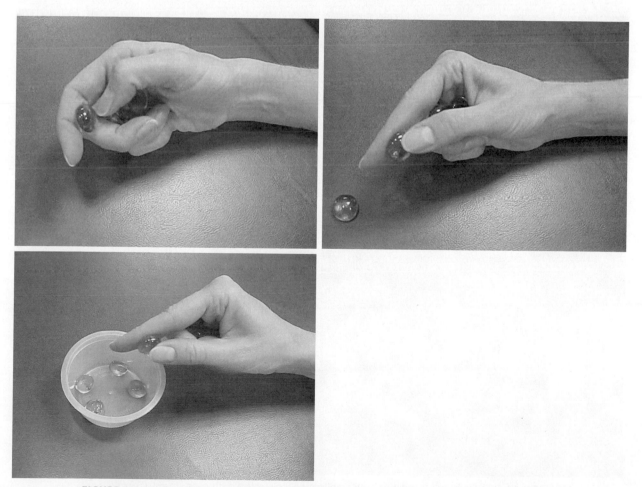

FIGURE 9-8 Palm-to-finger translation with stabilization. (Copyright Cynthia Cooper and John Evarts.)

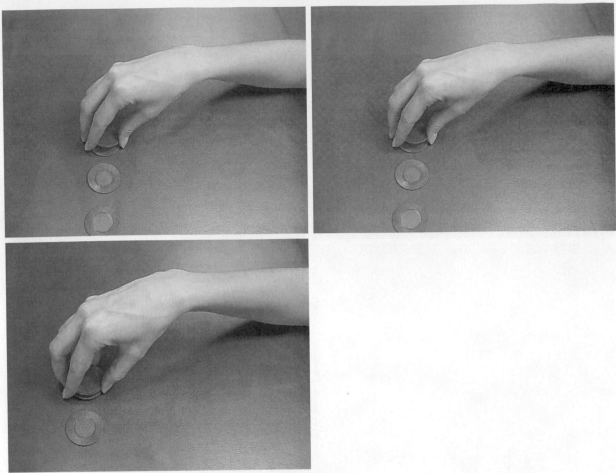

FIGURE 9-9 Stacking checkers and graded release. (Copyright Cynthia Cooper and John Evarts.)

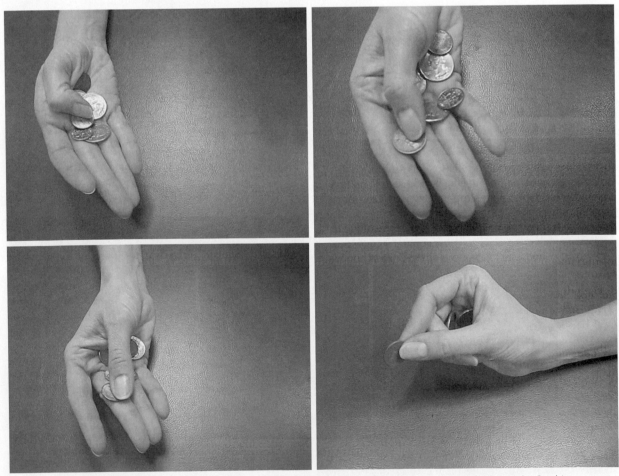

FIGURE 9-10 Palm-to-finger translation with stabilization, coin select with eyes closed. (Copyright Cynthia Cooper and John Evarts.)

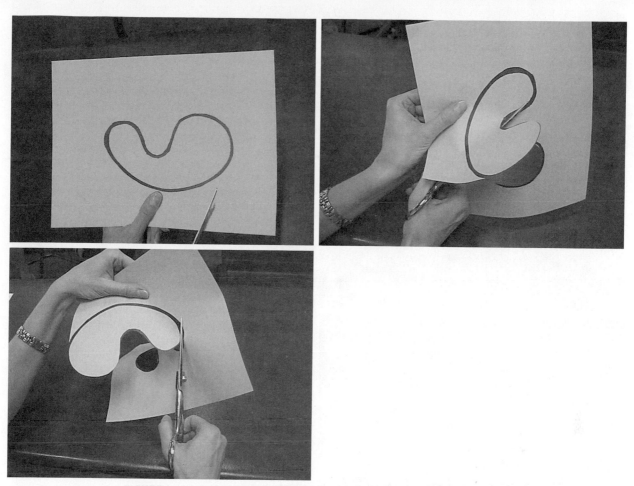

FIGURE 9-11 Bimanual task: scissors. (Copyright Cynthia Cooper and John Evarts.)

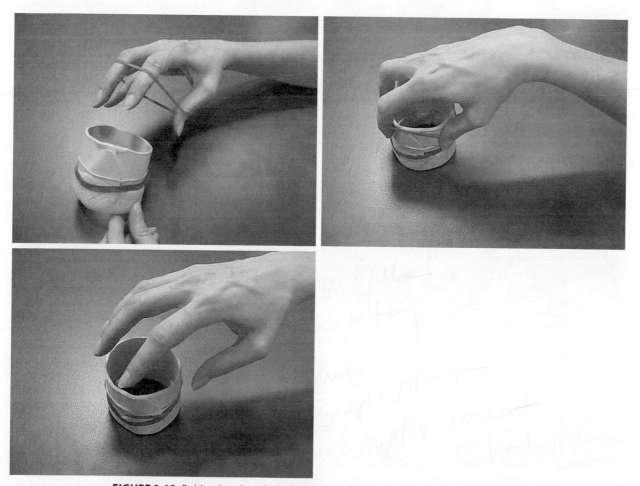

FIGURE 9-12 Rubber band graded release. (Copyright Cynthia Cooper and John Evarts.)

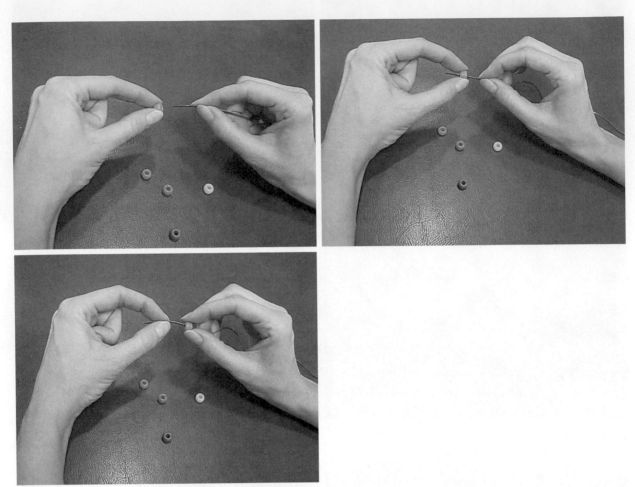

FIGURE 9-13 Stringing. (Copyright Cynthia Cooper and John Evarts.)

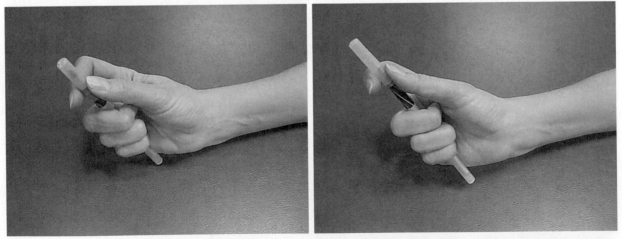

FIGURE 9-14 Pen cap removal with thumb and index fingers while holding pen in the hand. (Copyright Cynthia Cooper and John Evarts.)

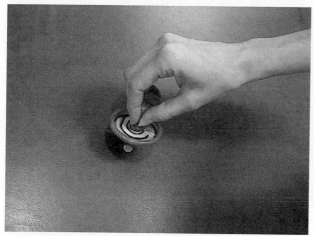

FIGURE 9-15 Lateral pinch to spin a top. (Copyright Cynthia Cooper and John Evarts.)

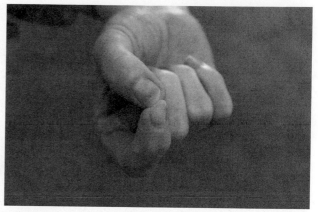

FIGURE 9-16 Flicking fingernails. (Copyright Cynthia Cooper and John Evarts.)

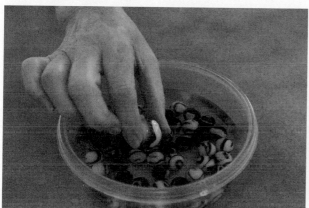

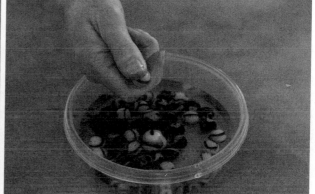

FIGURE 9-17 Finger-to-palm translation of slippery marbles in water. (Copyright Cynthia Cooper and John Evarts.)

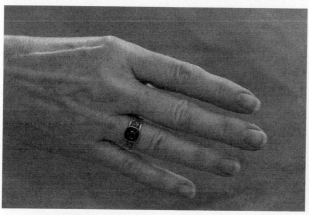

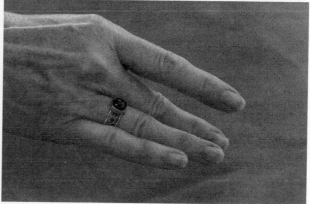

FIGURE 9-18 Rolling a ring around on the finger using the two adjacent fingers. (Copyright Cynthia Cooper and John Evarts.)

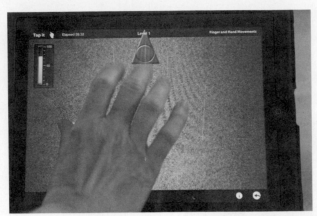

FIGURE 9-19 Dexteria application for iPad. (Copyright Cynthia Cooper and John Evarts.)

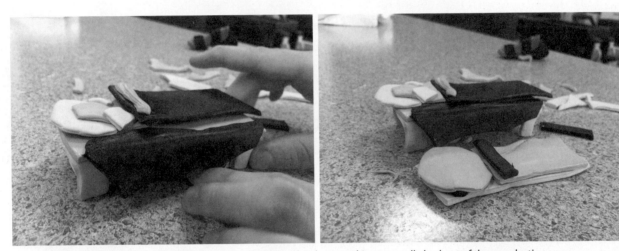

FIGURE 9-20 Young girl with juvenile rheumatoid arthritis making a trundle bed out of thermoplastic scraps. (Copyright Cynthia Cooper and John Evarts.)

References

1. Stilwell JM, Cermak SA: Perceptual functions of the hand. In Henderson A, Pehoski C, editors: *Hand function in the child: foundations for remediation*, St Louis, 1995, Mosby, pp 55–80.
2. Exner CE: Development of hand skills. In Case-Smith J, editor: *Occupational therapy for children*, ed 5, St Louis, 2005, Mosby, pp 304–355.
3. Exner CE, Henderson A: Cognition and motor skill. In Henderson A, Pehoski C, editors: *Hand function in the child: foundations for remediation*, St Louis, 1995, Mosby, pp 93–110.
4. Cooper C, West CG: *Coordination activities for hand therapy patients* Boston, 2008, (unpublished work, poster presented at the American Society of Hand Therapists Annual Meeting): http://evarts.net/ASHT-2008/ASHT_2008_Cooper_poster.pdf. Accessed April 16, 2013.

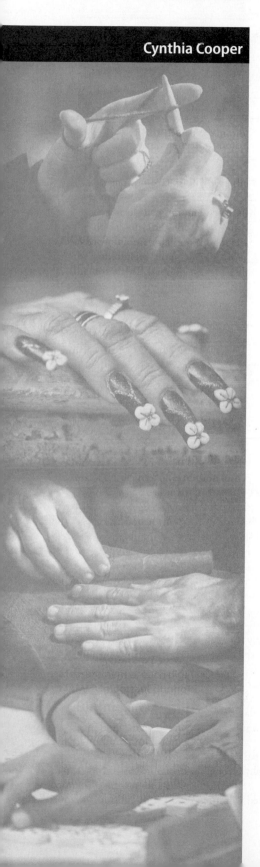

10

Roles of Therapy Assistants in Hand Therapy

Cynthia Cooper

The managed care system affects all health care fields, including hand therapy. One result of this change in the approach to health care is the increasing amount of treatment provided by occupational therapy assistants (OTAs) or physical therapy assistants (PTAs). This trend is likely to persist, and higher caseloads, shorter treatment times, and budget constraints will mean staffing patterns in which more assistants perform therapy. A knowledgeable, well-trained assistant can improve the care provided in a hand therapy program. This chapter discusses the roles of therapy assistants and suggests ways to develop and maximize an effective team. For clarity, the chapter uses the term *assistant* to mean an OTA or a PTA and the term *therapist* to mean an occupational therapist (OT) or a physical therapist (PT). It is understood that all are professionals who are therapy practitioners and that semantics vary.

In some states, therapy assistants need a license to practice. The fields of occupational therapy and physical therapy have separate practice acts and different licensing agencies, which can affect the staffing options of hand therapy programs. Typically, OTAs must work under the supervision of OTs and follow an occupational therapy plan of care,[1] and PTAs must work under the supervision of PTs and follow a physical therapy plan of care. A PTA with hand experience can be added to a hand therapy program only if the assistant reports to a PT. However, more OTs practice hand therapy than do PTs. These types of considerations affect staffing decisions.

The therapist sets the standard of care for the program. The assistant is responsible for adhering to these standards. Ideally, therapists and assistants work collaboratively. The term *collaboration* has more than one definition; in this sense, it means "working together, especially in a joint intellectual effort."[2] By definition, collaboration implies a hierarchy with the assistant reporting to the therapist. The hand therapist is responsible for the care that the client receives; the therapist also determines the level of supervision that an assistant requires. The assistant aids in the client's goal setting and contributes ideas for the client's program.[1] Assistants' responsibilities are increased as appropriate, depending on their clinical skills. All therapists and assistants are responsible for learning about and following their state laws concerning supervision and scope of practice.

Hand Therapy Experience Matrix

The hand therapy experience matrix (Fig. 10-1) is a model of collaborative roles for therapists and assistants.[3] The x axis represents the therapist's level of experience in hand therapy. The y axis represents the assistant's level of experience in hand therapy. The hand therapy team's goal is to move to a higher quadrant through supervision and training with competencies demonstrated in a manner consistent with state and facility guidelines.

In quadrant I, both the therapist and the assistant are inexperienced in hand therapy. In such cases, you (the therapist) should study as much as possible about the diagnosis and arrange for mentoring from and close communication with experienced hand therapists. If you have hand therapy colleagues in the area, phone calls may be helpful. Also, keep in close touch with the physician's office about the client's status. Be honest with the referring physician and communicate well; this style of interaction can build trust and lead to a close working relationship with a strong likelihood of future referrals.

In quadrant II, an inexperienced therapist is paired with an experienced assistant. The therapist must supervise the assistant but may not even know what is clinically wrong with the client. The assistant cannot fully evaluate the client and cannot and

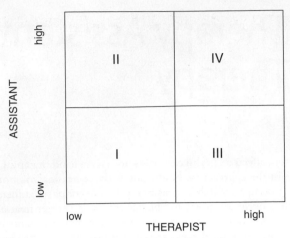

FIGURE 10-1 Hand therapy matrix.

should not supervise the therapist. In this case, the therapist and the assistant, working as a team, should pool their knowledge, read as much as possible about the diagnosis, and follow the suggestions for a quadrant I situation. Special care must be taken in these cases to avoid any role reversal of therapist and assistant.

In quadrant III, an experienced therapist is working with an inexperienced assistant. The therapist can help train the assistant, and competencies can be achieved in accordance with the facility's guidelines, maximizing the assistant's potential to broaden clinical skills. In this team, it is important for the therapist to supervise the assistant closely. The therapist should create a structured learning program with the assistant's assistance, identifying reading assignments, reviewing cases, and sharing resources from conferences and journals. This enrichment is more meaningful if it is shaped to match existing clients. For example, if a client has just been referred to you and your assistant for therapy after repair of the flexor pollicis longus, try to make that diagnosis your topic of study so that it is relevant to your case. If you have a client with adhesions, study scar management with your assistant and ask the OTA or PTA how the knowledge gained can be applied to the client's treatment. Box 10-1 presents a tool that can help assistants develop their clinical reasoning capabilities in reviewing hand therapy cases.

Quadrant IV is the best of both worlds. In this situation, both the therapist and the assistant are experienced in hand therapy. This team can continue to grow professionally and clinically by discussing cases, studying review articles, and keeping up with professional journals.

In all quadrants, it is very important that the assistant know when to ask the therapist for input about the client; this comes closest to a truly collaborative relationship.

An inexperienced therapist practicing hand therapy faces increased risk and a reduced likelihood of a favorable outcome. Inexperienced therapists should always use extra caution and should keep striving to learn. They should seek out all possible avenues for obtaining mentoring from other hand therapists and physicians. It strengthens, rather than weakens, your credibility and authority as a therapist if you are willing to ask questions and admit that you do not know something, rather than pretending to be more knowledgeable than you are. Most professionals will respect you more for this approach. Even the most experienced therapists do not know everything; there is always more to learn in hand therapy. The knowledge will come if you apply yourself, follow the suggestions made previously, and stay committed to reading and studying. The knowledge base for hand therapy is very broad; in fact, it can be overwhelming. It takes time to learn all this material and to see all these clients, who will continually teach you more. Pacing yourself through this learning process is far better than overdoing it, which can result in burn out.

Diagnoses that ideally should be referred to more experienced hand therapists include the following:

- Flexor tendon injury
- Extensor tendon injury
- Rheumatoid reconstruction
- Replantation/revascularization
- Complicated crush injury
- Nerve injury
- Complex regional pain syndrome (CRPS, also called reflex sympathetic dystrophy [RSD])
- Dupuytren's release
- Significant or infected wound

Developing a Respectful and Effective Team Relationship

Clients are sensitive to the subtleties of communication among coworkers, and they often comment on their perception of a team's work relationships. In a professional environment, the therapist explicitly shows respect for and appreciation of the assistant's work in front of clients. If the assistant reciprocates, this is all the better. Clients may remark on the friendly flow they notice among team members; this type of collaborative arrangement is very favorable to a successful clinical experience. Conversely, clients can tell if tension exists among coworkers; this situation affects the quality of care and reduces clients' comfort and satisfaction with the program.

Promoting a Learning Experience for Assistants

When all team members have a high level of clinical skills, the result is a better program. Supervising therapists should serve as role models and foster continual learning for the entire staff. For example, the staff could hold a journal club meeting once a month at lunch, sharing information from conferences that team members have attended and encouraging assistants to attend courses and read about hand therapy.

An awkward situation can arise if a team member feels that a therapist or an assistant is using outmoded treatment techniques. Some such techniques might include treating subacute hand edema with string wrap or retrograde massage instead of manual edema mobilization (MEM); failing to recognize or ignoring obvious and objective clinical signs of tissue intolerances (flare reaction); or performing hands-on treatment (for example, passive range of motion [PROM]) that is painful, aggressive, and/or injurious. In such cases it may help to challenge that practitioner to bring in evidence from the literature supporting that choice of treatment. At the same time, recommend and provide reading that supports MEM or explains flare reactions.

What to Say to Clients

Hand therapists and assistants should explain their roles when they introduce themselves to clients. This should be done in a way that conveys both the concept of teamwork and the fact that the assistant's contributions are a valued component of therapy. Team members must have a thorough understanding of their different roles if they are to explain them well to clients.

The hand therapist and OTA or PTA might introduce themselves to a client as follows:

Hand therapist: "Hello, my name is Jane. I will be your hand therapist, and today I will evaluate you. This is Sam, who is an [occupational or physical] therapy assistant. We will be your hand therapy team, and both of us will be working with you."

OTA or PTA: "Hello, my name is Sam. I will be working with you today. I am a(n) [occupational or physical] therapy assistant. Jane is your hand therapist. We are your hand therapy team, and we both will be involved with your care."

Tips from the Field

- When a physician calls about a client, the therapist should take the call if available. If the assistant handles the call, the assistant should inform the therapist. Also, if the therapist is not available and the assistant takes the call, the assistant should ask the physician if he or she would like to discuss the case further with the hand therapist. If so, this should be arranged.
- Therapists should show respect for assistants' knowledge and their desire to learn. Hand therapy assistants with good experience can be more knowledgeable in some areas than relatively new hand therapists. Assistants who have just attended a conference have educational material to share; they should be allowed to do so without awkwardness, because this will help to improve client care.
- Team members should have as much clinical and philosophic compatibility as possible.
- The therapist should know about tissue tolerances. If the assistant is being too aggressive on a client, this must be corrected with instruction and hands-on practice. Conversely, if a therapist is not well versed in tissue tolerances, the assistant should not be overly aggressive just because the therapist orders it.
- The therapist makes the final decisions about treatment, including modalities. The assistant can provide input and suggestions, but the therapist is responsible for the decision.
- The therapist and assistant should meet regularly to review their client cases, including cases in which the clinical needs seem to be minor. The therapist is responsible for ensuring that clients' therapy programs are appropriate and are upgraded regularly. For this and other reasons, the hand therapist should see each client approximately every third or fourth visit if possible. Some state licensing agencies stipulate how often the therapist must be directly involved with care that is provided by an assistant.
- Assistants should always feel that they can question or ask about the treatment a therapist prescribes. However, these discussions should take place in private.
- The therapist should try to avoid correcting or reprimanding an assistant in front of a client. Instead, the therapist and assistant should use an agreed-upon set of signals that convey specific messages that may mean, for example:
  - Stop doing that immediately. What you are doing is not safe or appropriate for the client.
  - We need to go down the hall immediately to discuss what you are doing before continuing treatment.
  - This client needs both of us now to reinforce an instruction or a precaution.
  - Please come help with this orthosis or dressing.

CASE STUDIES

CASE 10-1 ■

An assistant was trained by a relatively new, inexperienced hand therapist. The assistant was not taught to instruct clients with wrist fractures to isolate the wrist extensors when they performed wrist active range of motion (AROM) exercises during the home exercise program. The assistant had more years of experience than the new therapist had.

An experienced hand therapist subsequently was hired, and he identified wrist extensor isolation as an important clinical priority. This therapist began his discussion with the assistant by complimenting her for her hard work and acknowledging her clinical strengths. The therapist then said, "I know you have many years of clinical experience. As we develop our work relationship, I will be identifying things that I want us to do more similarly. Feel free to ask me more about these topics. I will be happy to recommend reading on these subjects. It is very important to teach clients how to isolate the wrist extensors when they are learning AROM after wrist fracture so that they do not substitute this motion using the extensor digitorum communis (EDC). Let's practice this together, and I will tell you what I like to say to clients so that they learn this motion well. Clients find it much harder to learn this motion if they have already learned to extend the wrist with the EDC; that is why I prioritize this technique and want you to practice it with clients quite a bit, so that they learn it thoroughly."

CASE 10-2 ■

An inexperienced hand therapist worked on a team with an experienced assistant who was excellent at making orthoses. The therapist acknowledged her need for more practice making orthoses. The assistant shared her expertise, and they practiced together. The assistant made it clear that she enjoyed orthotic fabrication and did not want to lose the opportunity to be involved in that work. The therapist improved her orthotic fabrication skills and made sure that the assistant continued to have rewarding opportunities to make orthoses.

Summary

Much of hand therapy probably falls into quadrants I and II of the hand therapy matrix. Be careful with this; *a well-intended but inexperienced therapist or assistant can do permanent harm to a hand client.* For this reason, it is critical that the hand therapy team recognize clinical limitations and improve competencies. Therapists and assistants who are inexperienced in hand therapy but are treating these clients should consult or network with more experienced hand therapists while advancing their clinical skills through reading, workshops and conferences, professional networks, and self-study. The rewards are well worth the effort. At the same time, therapists and assistants should work to maximize their team effectiveness, because this enhances personal satisfaction and improves client care.

References

1. Brayman SJ, Clark GF, DeLany JV, et al: Guidelines for supervision, roles, and responsibilities during the delivery of occupational therapy services, *Am J Occup Ther* 58:663–667, 2004.

2. American Heritage Dictionaries: *The American heritage dictionary of the English language*, ed 3, Boston, 1996, Houghton Mifflin.

3. Cooper C, Zarbock P, Zondlo JW: OTR and OTA collaboration in hand therapy, *AOTA Physical Disabilities Special Interest Section Quarterly* 23:2–4, 2000.

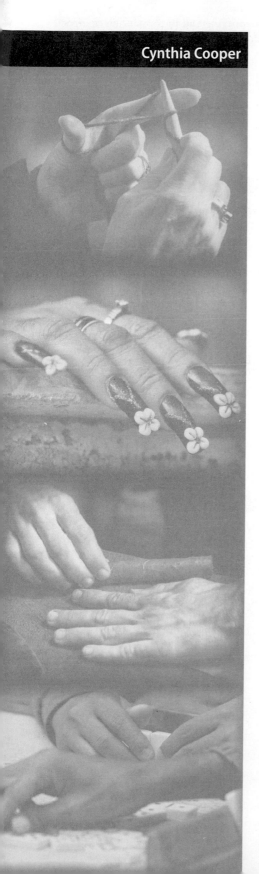

11

Some Thoughts on Professionalism

Cynthia Cooper

Sincerity is the most important thing... learn to fake that, and you've got it made.

—From *The Human Stain,* by Philip Roth, New York, 2000, Vintage International.

What Is Professionalism?

Professionalism is a combination of maturity and effectiveness. In the workplace, professional behavior is demonstrated by being the best you can be and doing the best you can, even if you are not in the mood to do so. Professionalism has been described as being a "class act" with emotionality being replaced by focus and responsibility. Instead of making decisions based on emotion, the professional relies on intellect and experience. Although professionalism implies treating others with respect, it does not imply elimination of empathy. While behaving professionally, we should still wonder what it is like to be in the client's shoes. In other words, we should try to understand our clients' subjective experiences.

Why Is Professionalism Important in Hand Therapy?

Lack of professionalism contributes to low morale, which reduces job satisfaction and also negatively affects our clients' experiences. Professional behaviors foster team work, which is advantageous for meeting clients' needs. Opportunities for advancement and success are associated with being perceived as a professional. Additional benefits of professional behavior include receiving the trust of clients and the admiration of colleagues and coworkers.

Communication Skills Related to Professionalism

Professionalism is exemplified by polite and respectful styles of communication, efficient use of time, punctuality, and integrity. These behaviors help convey the message that the client comes first. Minimizing interruptions, answering questions, smiling, having a friendly or open facial expression, and providing eye contact are examples of effective communication. Projecting a sense of confidence and staying calm during difficult situations are additional examples of professionalism.

Examples of Non-Professional Behavior

Example One

AA is an attractive female hand therapist who is single. She would like to meet a doctor at work. She wears low-cut tops and skimpy clothes to work, eliciting the attention of male clients and physicians. She has conversations in front of clients about her dates from previous nights. She is asked by doctors in front of clients if she would like to be fixed up with their single friends.

Questions: How does AA's behavior affect the professionalism of the clinic? What can be done to help correct this situation?

Example Two

BB is a hand therapist who feels she has excellent orthotic fabrication skills. When a coworker's client returns to clinic after not showing for appointments for 3 weeks, BB assesses the client's orthosis and notices that it no longer fits well due to clinical changes in the client's forearm and hand over the 3-week absence. BB states to the client, "This orthosis was made poorly and does not fit well. In fact, it is causing damage to your tissues. I will fix it for you and will make sure the other therapist is informed of the poor quality of her orthosis."

Question: How could she have worded this more professionally?

Example Three

DD is a therapist who believes that hand therapy should be painful. She imposes painful forces on delicate finger joints during passive range of motion (PROM) and tells clients that this will help them. Her clients frequently have flare responses with pain, edema, and stiffness. She yells at her clients to "Relax!" while she performs painful PROM on their digits.

Questions: Is this an issue of professionalism or is it a lack of clinical understanding? What type of communication skills would be more effective in helping a client relax? For example, before removing sutures, what could you say to your client, and how would you say it?

Example Four

EE is a hand therapist who is hoping to find a new career. She treats a client who is self-employed. She begins a business relationship with the client, exploring prospects to start a business together while still treating him. She uses the work computer on this project while her scheduled clients wait to be seen by her, which causes her appointments to run late.

Questions: What problems in professionalism do you see here? What solutions do you suggest?

Example Five

FF is an experienced hand therapist who has a very busy home life. She talks to her clients more about her own home life than about their lives or their hand therapy. She often receives presents from clients.

Question: What changes in behavior would improve FF's professionalism with her clients?

Characteristics of Professional Behavior

- Arrive at work on time, and start your first clients on time.
- Notify clients who are waiting if you are running late.
- Listen to your clients.
- Take pride in your work.
- Take initiative by identifying and implementing changes that improve efficiency and clinical care.
- Be open to constructive feedback.
- Ask for help if you need it.
- If you do not know something, admit it.
- Be trustworthy.
- Be pleasant.
- Be aware of your facility's policy about receiving gifts from clients.

♡ Tips from the Field

- Start the day with a pleasant expression on your face, even if you are not feeling that way. Doing so may actually make you feel better.
- Be hopeful with clients and pleasant with colleagues.
- Present a harmonious team front to clients, even if there are differences to be ironed out in private. Be as professional as possible.
- Do not discuss politics or religion with clients.
- Do not have any business activity with clients.
- Be open to suggestions from colleagues, and give positive feedback for good suggestions.
- Do not feel obliged to become friends with or socialize with team members. Prioritize a good working relationship that focuses on clients' needs. If your clients feel well-cared for, you will become close with your team members on a professional level.
- If the workload is skewed, try to help each other as is appropriate.

Summary

Our profession is hurt by therapists who are competent in hand therapy if they are incompetent in professionalism. We probably all recognize acquaintances or colleagues in the examples cited above. In truth, we may even recognize ourselves a little bit. These thoughts and case examples remind readers that therapists and clients alike can benefit from ongoing efforts to improve our professionalism.

12

Perspectives on Pain

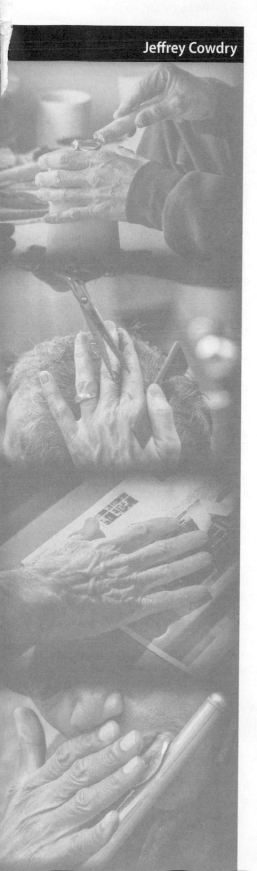

Jeffrey Cowdry

Pain is common to most of the patients that we treat. It is easy to develop a calloused attitude toward pain when you treat it every day. We may in fact laugh with our patients who, having progressed through a pain phase of their treatment, refer to us as their physical "torturer." But eventually we stop laughing. Either we experience pain ourselves or we treat an individual whose pain will not go away despite our best efforts to conquer it. Indeed, hand pain has been identified as "one of the most acutely stressful aspects of traumatic injuries and their treatment."[1]

Pain is one of the first things that we ask patients to rate or describe. We use pain to establish boundaries on exercises and stretches. Without pain to guide us, tendons would rupture, ligaments would tear, and wounds would not heal. Indeed, "pain protects us from destroying ourselves."[2] In his book, *Pain: The Gift Nobody Wants,* Dr. Paul Brand describes the fate of those with Hansen's disease (Leprosy) who, lacking the ability to feel pain, slowly lose fingers, toes, ears, their nose, and often go blind (forgetting to blink). I highly recommend this book to all therapists treating patients with pain. The book serves to stimulate both our scientific and our humanitarian natures. Several box inserts will be used as pearls throughout this chapter to highlight insights from Dr. Brand's book.[2]

◎ Clinical Pearl

"Touch…conveys to my patients a sense of personal concern that may help calm their fear and anxiety—and thus help reduce their pain"[2]

Finding the origin of pain can be difficult. For example, compare parts *A* and *B* in Fig. 12-1. Look at the thumb carpometacarpal (CMC) joints in these radiographs. It may seem clear that Fig. 12-1, *A,* is of a patient who has severe CMC pain and the patient in Fig. 12-1, *B,* is pain free. In reality the hand in Fig. 12-1, *A,* is that of a woman I know who has no thumb pain at all. Fig. 12-1, *B,* is my hand that from time to time gives me bouts of severe CMC pain.

Consider also a gentleman I treated for a crush injury to the hand. The initial surgical repairs included a carpal tunnel release. Long after the wounds healed and after many weeks of therapy this man had unrelenting pain and stiffness. The diagnosis was changed from crush injury to reflex sympathetic dystrophy (RSD). No treatment helped this man until a different doctor performed a revision carpal tunnel release. The surgeon's suspicion that an incomplete carpal tunnel release was the problem was correct. Once the nerve was completely decompressed the patient's pain went away immediately along with much of the stiffness.

Sometimes the origin of pain can be determined but not successfully treated. An extreme example of this is a patient who I saw for stump desensitization. He had an above the wrist amputation with a hypersensitive stump. His history included an original trigger finger release, neuromas, neuroma surgeries, and finally complex regional pain syndrome (RSD) of the hand. He told me that prior to the amputation, the hand pain was so intense he could not stand for even water to touch the hand. The hand eventually became filthy and then infected. The pain was so severe and the infection so bad that the man elected hand amputation. The sad ending to this story is that this patient eventually went on to have two more amputations (one below elbow and one above elbow). The last I heard about this patient was that he was suing his fourth surgeon who operated on his frozen shoulder, which made the pain worse.

Fortunately most of our patients respond well to over the counter or prescription analgesics to control pain. I find that hand patients who are on pain medication longer than two weeks are the exception. Many patients tell me that they only took their pain

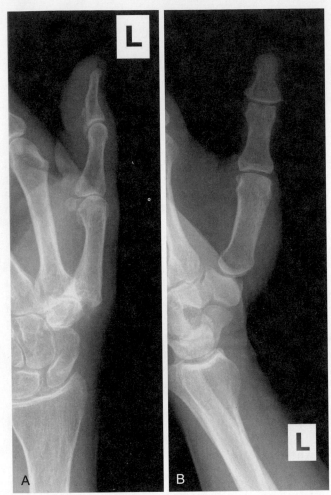

FIGURE 12-1 A, Patient with thumb CMC arthritis but no pain. **B,** Patient with painful thumb CMC but no significant radiological findings. (Courtesy of Jeffery Cowdry.)

(From Li Z, Smith BP, Smith TL, et al: Diagnosis and management of complex regional pain syndrome complicating upper extremity recovery, *J Hand Ther* 18(2):270-276, 2005.)

BOX 12-1   Definitions of Pain Terminology

Allodynia: Pain in a specific dermatomal or autonomous distribution associated with light touch to the skin; a stimulus that is not normally painful.

Analgesia: Absence of pain in response to an insult that should produce pain.

Hyperalgesia: Increased sensitivity to stimulation (includes allodynia and hyperesthesia).

Hyperesthesia: Increased sensitivity to stimulation (pain on response to a mild noxious stimulus).

Hyperpathia: Abnormally painful reaction to a stimulus (especially repetitive); often includes extended duration of pain, frequently with a delay.

Hypoesthesia: Decreased sensitivity to stimulation.

Nociception: Response to an unpleasant (noxious) stimulus that produces pain in human subjects under normal circumstances.

Pain: An unpleasant perception associated with actual or potential cellular damage.

Sympathetic pain: Pain in the presence of and/or associated with over-action of the sympathetic pain fibers; by definition the pain is relieved by sympatholytic interventions.

---

medication one or two nights to help them sleep after their operation. From a therapy standpoint some of the techniques used to control pain are: rest, immobilization, physical agent modalities, elevation, soft tissue massage, active range of motion (AROM), functional activities, joint protection education, adaptive equipment, and ergonomic education.

Although pain is a guide, in the United States we usually try to eliminate pain as fast as possible. If pain is not controlled quickly, patients will change doctors and therapists just as quickly. I learned this myself when treating my own tennis elbow (lateral epicondylalgia). When one treatment did not work, I would quickly try another. I tried many things, including joint taping, manual therapy, eccentric exercises, swimming, physical agent modalities, a cortisone injection, orthoses, and straps. I even tried a method that purposefully induces pain in order to stimulate the inflammatory process of the healing cycle. Just like my own patients, I shopped around and experimented until I found something to take away the pain.

Documenting baseline pain and performance is essential to helping patients get through their pain. Pain is a cardinal sign that is to be assessed by the therapist. Patients usually have poor recall about their initial pain. It is common after two or three weeks of therapy for them to say, "My pain is no better." It is helpful to show them how they initially rated their pain and its effects. The baseline evaluation includes:

- Swelling (using circumferential or volumetric measures)
- Observations of appearance (color, use, dryness, or sweating)
- Sensory testing (monofilaments or two point discrimination)
- Pain assessment (visual analogue scale, pain diagram, pain questionnaire)
- Range of motion, strength, and fine motor testing

For more information on baseline evaluation and rating pain, please see Chapter 5.

When documenting pain there are terms that are helpful to know. Pain from the periphery that alerts us to damage or potential damage of tissue is called **nociceptive pain,** carried by the nociceptive fibers of the sensory nerves. Pain originating from damage to the nerve itself is called **neuropathic pain. Allodynia** is pain that occurs after a stimulus that is normally not painful. Painful light touch following sunburn is an example of allodynia. **Hyperpathia** is pain that is more intense than normally expected and/or lasts longer than normally expected. Pain lasting for hours after gentle passive range of motion (PROM) is an example of hyperpathia. See Box 12-1 for a summary of pain terminology.

Complex Regional Pain Syndrome/Reflex Sympathetic Dystrophy

A day may come when you receive a referral diagnosing a patient with CRPS or RSD. CRPS/RSD has been described as "the most controversial and frustrating of all hand disorders."[3] It is a clinical syndrome in which there is extreme pain with allodynia

---

BOX 12-2   Different Names Used for CRPS/RSD

Acute atrophy of bone	Post-traumatic pain syndrome
Algodystrophy	Post-traumatic spreading neuralgia
Algoneurodystrophy	Post-traumatic sympathalgia
Babinski-Froment syndrome	Post-traumatic sympathetic dystrophy (disorder)
Causalgia	Pseudoneurological syndrome
Chronic segmental arteriospasm	Ravaut neurotrophic rheumatism
Chronic traumatic edema	Reflex atrophy
Complex Regional Pain syndrome (Types I and II)	Reflex hyperemic deossification
Drug-induced neurotrophic disorders	Reflex nerve atrophy
Erythralgia	Reflex nervous dystrophy
Erythromelalgia	Reflex neurovascular dystrophy
Idiopathic neurodystrophic disorders	Regional migratory transient osteoporosis
Leriche post-traumatic osteoporosis	Rheumatisme neurotrophique
Major causalgia	Shoulder-hand syndrome
Minor causalgia	Steinbrocker syndrome
Neurodystrophic syndromes	Sudeck atrophy (syndrome)
Neurotrophic rheumatism	Sudeck-Leriche syndrome
Osteoporose douloureuse traumatique	Sudeck osteoporosis
Painful osteoporosis	Sympathalgia
Peripheral neuralgia	Sympathetic dystrophy
Peripheral trophoneurosis	Sympathetic neurovascular dystrophy
Post-infarction sclerodactyly	Sympathetically maintained pain
Post-traumatic arterial spasm	Thalamic syndrome
Post-traumatic arthritis	Transient osteoporosis of the hip
Post-traumatic dystrophy	Traumatic angiospasm
Post-traumatic edema	Traumatic edema
Post-traumatic neurovascular pain syndrome	Traumatic reflex osteodystrophy
Post-traumatic osteoporosis	Traumatic vasospasm

(From: Merritt WH: *Reflex Sympathetic Dystrophy/Chronic Regional Pain Syndrome*, ed 2, vol 7, Philadelphia, 2006, Saunders/Elsevier.)

---

and hyperpathia. There is usually associated edema, stiffness, skin color and temperature change (often red and warm initially, changing to blue and cold over time), excessive sweating or dryness, excessive or diminished hair growth on the arm or hand, and changes in the nails/nail beds and pads of the fingers. It affects all ages, all races, both sexes, and can occur spontaneously or be caused by trauma, cerebrovascular accident (CVA) also known as stroke, heart attack, and shingles.[3] Because carpal tunnel syndrome and distal radius fractures are among the most common hand disorders, they are often cited as the event preceding the onset of CRPS/RSD.

The term RSD, coined in the 1940s, has been replaced by the term CRPS. RSD implies reflex to an injury causing a disease directly related to the sympathetic nervous system. CRPS conversely describes the complex nature of the disorder that attacks regionally (usually the arm or the leg), is severely painful, and is best thought of as a syndrome—not a disease. This is not the first time a new label has been used for this disorder. There are over 60 terms used to describe the condition (see Box 12-2). It is important to know that renaming RSD does not change the fact that there is no clear explanation, no precise way to diagnose, and no universally accepted treatment for this disorder.

CRPS has two divisions: Classic RSD is known as **CRPS Type I.** In this clinical condition (pain outside the boundaries of expectation, autonomic dysfunction, trophic changes, and functional impairment), there is no known nerve injury contributing to the problem.

Classic causalgia is known as **CRPS Type II.** This appears with the same signs and symptoms as Type I but is directly related to a nerve injury. *Causalgia* comes from the Greek words, *Kausis* (heat) and *algos* (pain). The term was coined during the American Civil War era to describe the intense burning pain soldiers felt from penetrating injuries.[3]

CRPS Type I and II may be further divided into categories based on response to blocked sympathetic nervous system function. When pain is improved by the use of sympathetic blocking treatments, such as oral antidepressants, anticonvulsants, or stellate ganglion blocks, the condition is called *sympathetically maintained pain (SMP)*. When sympathetic blocking treatments do not improve pain, the condition is called *sympathetically independent pain (SIP)*.

When communicating sympathetic changes that you observe in your patient, you will use specific terminology. Changes in color and temperature are due to **vasomotor** changes (*vas* is Latin for "vessel"). Changes in sweat are due to **sudomotor** changes (*sudor* is Latin for "sweat"). **Trophic** (*trophe* is Greek for "nourishment") changes affect nail and finger pad appearance, skin appearance, and even bone health. Nails may become talon-like, curled, or ridged. Finger pads may lose their bulk, and skin may become thin and shiny. **Pilomotor** (*pilus* is Latin for "hair") changes affect the goosebump flesh appearance of skin.

CRPS/RSD patients leave a lasting impression on you. They may initially refuse to be touched due to their pain intensity and often due to pain-producing prior therapy services. They may seem to act guarded toward you concerning their therapy, but this may be due to their frustration and fatigue of having relentless and high levels of pain. They desperately want someone to listen to them about their pain, but they also may be cautious. It may seem that they might be communicating hesitation in response to your attempts to work with them, but if they feel like you are listening to them, they will usually be receptive.

As mentioned earlier, you may rely heavily on baseline information from the initial evaluation to prove to the patient that positive changes are occurring. Showing patients improvement even in small amounts my help reduce pain. At night, resting orthoses can help prevent the pain of contracture, especially for proximal interphalangeal (PIP) flexion contractures or shortening of the muscle tendon unit to the digits.

> ◎ **Clinical Pearl**
>
> "The best rehabilitation takes place, I have found, if I can convince you of the truth that you are doing it all yourself"[2]

Although the patient may protest, one of the most important things to do to help the pain is to achieve movement of the arm.[4] Starting with the shoulder, it is imperative to get the patient to move the extremity. If they cannot tolerate motion of the involved upper extremity (UE), have them perform AROM of the uninvolved UE. Manual edema mobilization (MEM) is very helpful in reducing their pain (see Chapter 3).

> ◎ **Clinical Pearl**
>
> "You must prevent adhesive capsulitis or frozen shoulder from occurring"

Soon movements of the elbow, wrist, and hand will add to increasing amounts of pain-free range of motion. Get the patient to participate in self-care using the involved arm. The benefits of functional and occupational tasks are enormous for these patients. Focusing on and accomplishing a task helps toward pain reduction.

It is felt by some researchers that there is a central nervous system component that contributes to the cause and maintenance of CRPS/RSD.[3] Therefore, it behooves us to incorporate bilateral activity and functional activity into the exercise regimen. This may begin with self-care activities. Regarding exercises, I find that bilateral activities (such as twisting a flexible rubber bar, holding and catching a light ball, and mirror therapy) are good treatment techniques. I also find that exercise machines are useful in most phases of CRPS/RSD therapy. The latissimus pull down machine, the seated press up machine, the triceps extension machine, and the upper body ergometer all do well incorporating bilateral movements and include the shoulder.

Regarding the efficacy of exercise with CRPS/RSD, Sluka reports that "there is moderate evidence from control trials, both randomized and non-randomized, to support the use of exercise for the treatment of CRPS. There is good evidence to support the use of transcutaneous electrical nerve stimulation (TENS) and mirror image therapy for neuropathic pain and CRPS."[5]

The good news for hand therapists is that CRPS/RSD patients have a high response rate to placebo treatments.[3] Some studies show the response rate to be equal to stellate ganglion blocks. These patients are so desperate for relief that they respond well to the power of suggestion. The relief they get is from an expected good outcome, which may be due to physiological reasons such as the release of endorphins into the bloodstream. Therefore, have a positive approach to each treatment session. Show enthusiasm for any positive changes. Help the patient have faith in you and the treatment you select.

> ◎ **Clinical Pearl**
>
> "The essence of rehabilitation—indeed the essence of health—was to restore to my patients a sense of personal destiny over their bodies"[2]

CRPS/RSD is usually not the first diagnosis a patient receives. Their initial diagnosis may be the single working diagnosis for weeks or months. This is because patients may be dismissed as complainers or symptom magnifiers. Also, signs and symptoms do not always immediately develop into full blown CRPS/RSD. The clinical picture may begin with pain, stubborn edema, and stiffness while other signs and symptoms gradually develop.

It is common for RSD to be referred to in one of two stages: an early stage where the extremity is red, warm, and swollen and a later stage where the hand or extremity is blue, cold, sweaty, and atrophic. These phases of RSD can be confused with other disorders (see Box 12-3).

I have treated a number of patients diagnosed with RSD (CRPS Type I) who were in reality CRPS Type II. I reported earlier about a man diagnosed with RSD who was helped by revision carpal tunnel surgery. This taught me that one surgical nerve decompression does not always mean a nerve is fully decompressed. I will never forget the patient who I met at a surgeon's office waiving her arm in the air exclaiming, "I haven't been able to raise my arm for four years!" She had been unable

---

> **BOX 12-3** **Problems in the Differential Diagnosis of Complex Regional Pain Syndrome**
>
> A hot, red, painful swollen hand may be due to:
> - Septic arthritis
> - Acute trauma
> - Insect bite
> - Local allergy
> - CRPS/RSD
>
> A cold, blue, sweaty, atrophic painful extremity may be due to:
> - Chronic vascular insufficiency
> - Disuse (stroke, neural injury)
> - Immobilization
> - CRPS/RSD

to use her arm since an unsuccessful ulnar nerve transposition by another surgeon 4 years earlier. The first surgeon is an excellent nerve surgeon who teaches that the medial antebrachial cutaneous nerve (MACN) must be isolated and freed during ulnar nerve transposition. But following the original surgery this woman had intractable pain. She complained so much that she was eventually dropped by the first surgeon and was labeled "combative." The patient sought help for years and eventually was treated by the second surgeon. By carefully listening to the patient, the second surgeon was able to determine that the original postoperative pain began in a specific cutaneous nerve pattern, that of the MACN. He operated and found that the MACN was severely entrapped in scar. After releasing the MACN the patient's pain resolved, and with therapy her function returned.

> ◎ **Clinical Pearl**
>
> "…in pain management I have no choice but to work in partnership: pain occurs "inside" the patient, and the patient alone can guide me"[2]

As a final example of pain resolution, I will share the story of a patient who had denervation of the anterior shoulder capsule. Previously, the patient had four unsuccessful shoulder surgeries to reduce his shoulder pain. Pain prevented him from lifting his arm more than 25% toward his head. The surgeon removed the nerve supply to the anterior capsule, and the patient's pain resolved. He eventually had near complete, pain-free shoulder range of motion. Rehabilitation consisted primarily of strengthening the muscles that had weakened after years of disuse.

Concluding Thoughts

Most patients that we see have pain. While we respect pain, we do not let it rule us. We usually ask patients to find the boundary of their pain, and then we guide them to work toward their therapy goals while avoiding undue pain. We need to take a good history and determine, if possible, any cutaneous or dermatomal patterns that exist or that may have initially existed. We need to take good baseline measurements in order to encourage the patient about their progress. And we need to pay close attention to any patterns that look like emerging CRPS/RSD.

Research Considerations

The American Society of Hand Therapists (ASHT) members were surveyed, and a summary of their preferred research priorities was published.[6] RSD and pain were ranked nine and ten behind cumulative trauma disorder, flexor/extensor tendon, carpal tunnel syndrome, scar, tendinitis, edema, arthritis, and fracture. While ranked in the middle of all categories surveyed, pain nevertheless is a significant factor in most of the leading categories. As more and more financial burden is shifted from the payer to the patient, it is likely that pain and its effect on function will be a primary reason for seeking help from a therapist.

"A scientific revolution focusing on the phenomenon of pain has been occurring for three decades," therefore, the research-minded therapist is to be encouraged.[7] An area for research might include the functional effects of joint denervation. Intrigued by an article written by Elisabet Hagert, MD, PhD, on wrist proprioceptive reflexes,[8] I conducted my own experiment on the functional effects of wrist denervation. I asked Dr. Robert Hagan to block the primary nerves to my wrist joint, the anterior interosseous and the posterior interosseous nerves. Prior to the block, I timed and measured myself in six functional tasks. These tasks were starting a manual gyroscope, manipulating a bent-wire with ring dexterity device, gross grip strength testing, the Purdue Pegboard assembly subtest, manipulating Chinese balls, and typing for speed. Except for a slight increase in typing errors, there were only subtle differences in time, strength, and function after the wrist was temporarily blocked. I feel this was due to the fact that the sensory receptors of my skin and muscles were not interrupted, and they provided the necessary feedback to perform the functional tasks. Wrist proprioception should be studied carefully since Dr. Hagert's research shows the possibility of negative functional issues following denervation of the wrist.

Much more research needs to be done for lateral epicondylalgia. Two areas I looked at were electromyogram (EMG) activity during exercise and the effects of temporary lateral elbow denervation. Regarding exercise training, I looked at what activities elicited the greatest response of the extensor carpi radialis brevis (ECRB) muscle on EMG readings. I found that in my arm there is more ECRB motor recruitment during concentric contraction than eccentric and much more recruitment during elbow-flexed gripping than elbow-extended gripping. In my arm, the ECRB contracts little during resisted finger extension. The ECRB is less active during wrist extension while lifting a weighted ball (presumably due to the assistance of the finger extensors) than when lifting an equivalent weighted dumbbell. Further study in this area may help clarify best practice recommendations for lateral epicondylalgia exercise training.

While experiencing chronic lateral elbow pain, I tested my grip strength before and after a temporary nerve block to my lateral epicondyle. Following the block, my grip strengths improved significantly but not to normal. The pain in the lateral epicondyle region abated, but I still had lateral forearm muscular pain that lowered my grip strength. This led me to an experiment with one of my "tennis elbow" patients. I tested his grip in the normal way and got a reading of 10 pounds. I then applied a TENS unit to the radial nerve branch to the lateral elbow. The grip reading then was 80 pounds. However, when I removed the TENS unit, the patient had significant post-test pain. It would be interesting to rehabilitate an individual with tennis elbow using a portable TENS unit, attempting to block the pain while undergoing strength training.

In preparing a lecture on pain, I received communication from two hand therapists regarding research in the area of pain. Elaine Fess, MS, OTR, FAOTA, CHT, an enthusiastic advocate of evidence-based practice and statistics editor of the *Journal of Hand Therapy* between 1988 and 1998, writes "According to LeMotte, the continuum of sensibility testing includes the areas of sympathetic response, detection, discrimination, quantification, and identification. To date, none of these areas have been correlated with function and outcomes. Considerable research is needed before we truly understand the intricate and complex realm of sensibility."[9]

Judith Bell Krotoski, MA, OTR, CHT, FAOTA, a well-known therapist/researcher and colleague of Dr. Paul Brand writes, "If a test is not repeatable in force of application, then it follows that it is not a valid test, no matter how popular." She also says that, "You get farther with more success in touching a patient's heart before you touch their hand."[10]

As we think about pain, it is good to remember that pain is not necessarily an enemy. We need to learn from pain what the body is trying to tell us. We need to have compassion for those who suffer from it. We need to keep a calloused attitude in check. We need to carefully document our observations and relate them to function. We need to push our patients forward but always with concern for their discomfort. This is perhaps best summarized by Dr. Brand regarding his observation of leprosy patients trying to build a new life for themselves, "I began to see my chief contribution as one I had not studied in medical school: to join with my patients as a partner in the task of restoring dignity to a broken spirit. That is the true meaning of rehabilitation."[2]

References

1. Koestler AJ: Psychological perspective on hand injury and pain, *J Hand Ther* 23:199–211, 2010.
2. Brand P, Yancey P: *Pain, the gift nobody wants*, New York, 1993, Harper Collins. pp 57, 159, 219, 225, 242–243.
3. Merritt WH: *Reflex sympathetic dystrophy/chronic regional pain syndrome*, vol 7, ed 2, Philadelphia, 2006, Saunders. pp 823, 827, 828, 830, 843.
4. Kim DH, Midha R, Murovic JA, et al: *Kline & Hudson's nerve injuries*, ed 2, Philadelphia, 2008, Elsevier. pp 420.
5. Sluka KA, editor: *Mechanisms and management of pain for the physical therapist*, Seattle, 2009, ISAP Press, p 345.
6. MacDermid JC, Fess EE, Bell-Krotoski J, et al: A research agenda for hand therapy, *J Hand Ther* 15(1):3–15, 2002.
7. Gifford LS, Butler DS: The integration of pain sciences into clinical practice, *J Hand Ther* 10(2):86–95, 1997.
8. Hagert E: Proprioception of the wrist joint: a review of current concepts and possible implications on the rehabilitation of the wrist, *J Hand Ther* 23(1):2–16, 2010.
9. Fess E: Personal communication. 24 May 2010.
10. Krotoski JB: Personal communication. 21 June 2010.

13 Fundamentals of Client-Therapist Rapport

Teri Britt Pipe

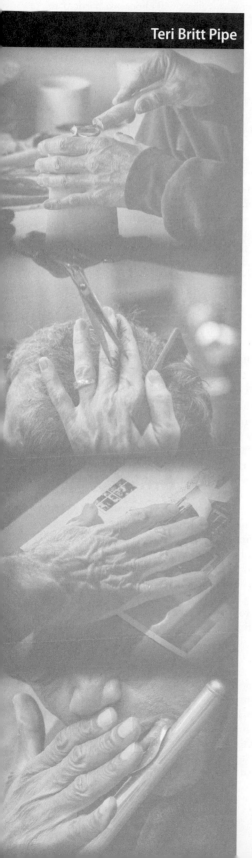

Importance of the Therapeutic Relationship

Holistic, client-focused care is a unifying goal among client care professionals. Holistic care involves viewing clients as complex, dynamic beings with evolving, developing personas, needs, and strengths. Developing and nurturing the therapeutic relationship are the keys to understanding clients from a holistic perspective. The client-therapist relationship then can serve as the foundation for assessment, prioritization, mutual goal setting, and shared decision making.

Creating and maintaining rapport are essential first steps in coming to know and understand the client. Much more than simply being nice or acting respectful, truly knowing the client is part of effective clinical care and has important implications for client outcomes. **Knowing the client** means comprehending the client's physical, emotional, cognitive, spiritual, and social sense of personhood and connecting to it as one human being to another within the boundaries of a professional therapeutic relationship.

Research and theory provide evidence that knowing the client is crucial to one of the most important yet basic aspects of clinical care: ensuring the client's safety. Learning more about clients, understanding their unique perspectives, listening to what is and is not said, and accurately reading behaviors to formulate a correct clinical impression are all vital steps in keeping clients aligned with their therapeutic program and keeping them from harm. For instance, research indicates that the clinical behaviors of knowing and connecting with clients provide protection against untoward events and promote early recognition of client problems.[1] Serving as a client advocate and guarding clients' best interests are professional responsibilities that are deeply rooted in the therapeutic relationship.

In addition to having implications for the client's safety and well-being, meaningful therapeutic relationships also have implications for professionals. At times therapists may not be fully aware of the impact on clients of "simple" interventions, such as listening, being present, and offering encouragement. Behaviors such as these lead to knowing the client. Perhaps if therapists understand the depth of caring that can be conveyed by a simple gesture or by listening to clients talk about their experiences, they can find renewal and healing in their practice.

Developing a Successful Therapeutic Relationship

Developing a therapeutic relationship is fundamental to working well with clients. The most effective approach is guided by a theoretical context so that thoughts and behaviors can be seen in a broader, systematic perspective of caring for the client as a comprehensive whole. A theoretical perspective helps the therapist perceive, recognize, and process clinical information in a systematic way and can help bring order out of chaotic clinical data. The theoretical perspective that provides a framework for this part of the chapter is Watson's theory of human caring.[2] This model is not simply "applied to" a situation; rather, it lends itself to being experienced so that the elements of the model come alive for the participants in caring relationships and encounters.

Watson's Theory of Human Caring

Watson's model has gained international recognition and has been used by a variety of disciplines since its origin in nursing. For the purposes of this chapter, the therapist is the "self," and the client is the "one being cared for." The theory of human caring is also sensitive to the changing realities of society and health care.[3] This chapter presents an overview of some of the theory's major concepts as well as examples based on clinical experience. The three major components used to frame the discussion are caritas, transpersonal caring healing relationships, and the caring moment.

Caritas

Caritas derives from the Greek word meaning "to cherish, appreciate, and give special attention, if not loving attention, to; it connotes that something is very fine, that indeed it is precious." Caritas characterizes how hand therapists may choose to approach their clients.

> ◎ *Clinical Pearl*
>
> A positive, respectful regard for the client is the very first step in the therapeutic relationship.

Whether they meet clients in the home, hospital room, office, or other setting, therapists' extension of a positive *caritas* regard for clients and their personal environment sets the stage for the development of therapeutic rapport. The ideal way to begin is to spend a moment or two mentally settling down and reaching a clear state of mind before meeting the client. This centering approach need not take a great deal of time; it requires merely the time it takes to inhale and intentionally clear one's focus in preparation for the client encounter. It is a way of cultivating mindfulness about one's practice.

Mindfulness is simple but not easy; it requires effort and discipline to "pay attention in a particular way: on purpose, in the present moment and nonjudgmentally."[4] The purposes of this centering moment are (1) to bring therapists awareness and understanding of their own minds; (2) to teach them how this can influence perceptions and actions; and (3) to show them how perceptions and actions influence the clinical environment, the client-therapist relationship, and the clinical encounter. The essence of mindfulness is to cultivate self-awareness through self-observation, self-inquiry, and mindful action. The overall attitude is one of gentleness, gratitude, and nurturing.[4] From this point of inward clarity, the therapist can progress to the therapeutic relationship with the client. Again, this practice of focused attention need not take a great deal of time; it can be done in a moment. Yet the effects can be quite powerful because of the intention and focus this approach brings to the clinical encounter.

Watson's theory of human caring delineated ten caritas processes,[2,5-9] which are used to explore the development of the therapeutic relationship. The discussion of each process includes common pitfalls and ways the therapist can avoid them.

Caritas Process 1: "Practice of Loving-Kindness and Equanimity within Context of a Caring Consciousness"

The word *practice* in the definition of Caritas Process 1 is a reminder that the attitude of loving-kindness and equanimity is not something that can be accomplished quickly or permanently; therapists practice it not with the goal of achievement, but rather with the objective of becoming more conscious of how they approach clients.[10] **Equanimity** is the quality of being calm and even tempered. It is an evenness of mind characterized by calm temper or firmness of mind, reflected as patience, composure,

and steadiness of mind under stress. For the hand therapist, cultivation of this mindful, caring approach to the therapist-client relationship translates into reflections such as, "Who is this person? Am I open to participating in his or her personal story? How ought I be in this situation? What are the client's priorities?" The client's response is also affected and may include the person's perceptions of how the interaction and relationship will be part of the healing process and how the client will choose to participate in the therapist-client relationship.

> ### Common Pitfalls and How to Avoid Them
>
> 1. Allowing yourself to be distracted: When you find yourself thinking about something other than the client in the present moment, gently refocus your attention. Try not to scold or reprimand yourself, because this is a fairly common occurrence, particularly early on in the development of a reflective practice.
> 2. Forgetting to take a moment to focus: Generally, once you notice how much more productive your focused encounters are, the reward will reinforce the practice of taking the small amount of time required.
> 3. Letting your mind say, "This client is just like that other client I had last week …": Remember that just as you are different from any other person and your reactions are unique, so is this client different from any other, and his or her reactions are unique.

Caritas Process 2: "Being Authentically Present and Enabling and Sustaining the Deep Belief System and Subjective Life World View of Self and One Being Cared for"

Authenticity requires that hand therapists know who they are and how they can contribute to their clients' care. Although authenticity sounds very simple, it can be counterintuitive in the context of modern standardized health care practice to remember that each therapist and each client brings something unique to the therapeutic relationship; unless therapists know their individual talents and gifts, those talents and gifts can't be shared. Discovering one's unique sense of authenticity involves taking the time to reflect on how experiences, clinical learning, personal knowledge, culture, belief system, aspects of personality, and a vast array of other factors unique to each individual can be cultivated to help in the current clinical situation. During this phase of the therapist-client relationship, the therapist is using his or her sense of self to be intentionally present with the client. This means being able to focus on only the client for this time. It means turning attention to what it is the client is experiencing in order to support the client in his or her belief system and discovering the things that will sustain and inspire hope or faith for that client.

In this phase of rapport building, helpful questions therapists might ask themselves include, "What information is needed to care for this person? Can I imagine what this experience is like for this client and what it means in his (or her) life?" Likewise, the client can contribute to the clinical relationship by sharing stories of his or her past as it relates to the person's current health status, exploring sources of strength and meaning that can be used in the work of hand therapy.

Common Pitfalls and How to Avoid Them

1. Thinking that a diagnosis (for example, a fractured wrist) has the same meaning to every client: Remember that this client will formulate a personal meaning from this condition and about the therapy.
2. Failing to assess or understand the client's sources of strength and meaning: It is refreshing for clients to be reminded that they have overcome challenges in the past and that they have a reservoir of strengths to use in the present and future.

◎ *Clinical Pearl*

Clients often are pleased and relieved to be asked about the strengths they bring to a situation, because health care providers generally ask instead about weaknesses or problems.

Caritas Process 3: "Cultivation of One's Own Spiritual Practices and Transpersonal Self, Going beyond Ego Self"

This element of caring requires a delicate balance. Caring involves tapping into one's own source of strength according to a personal belief system while taking care not to assume that the client shares those values. In order to use the **transpersonal self,** the therapist must sustain healthy personal boundaries and put aside personal concerns, worries, and needs to care for the client. This part of the rapport-building process involves supporting the client in his or her **spiritual** beliefs and source or sources of strength and meaning, even when those differ from the therapist's own beliefs. Going beyond the **ego self** means acknowledging the uniqueness of each individual while recognizing that the connections between individuals can be used for healing.

In this phase, the therapist may reflect on a question such as, "How am I attending to this person's spiritual needs and soul

Common Pitfalls and How to Avoid Them

1. Assuming the client shares the therapist's belief system: Ask the client; don't presume to know even if seemingly obvious signs are present (for example, religious symbols).
2. Failing to clarify and uphold professional boundaries: Clients can feel vulnerable and may say things to please the therapist. Always keep in mind the influence of the healer on the client, and use it responsibly.
3. Neglecting to call in resources: The trust between client and therapist is strengthened if limitations are communicated and arrangements or referrals are initiated for social workers, community providers, and other sources of help.
4. Neglecting to devote the time and energy to "feed one's own soul," leading to a professional sense of eroded spirit and diminished effectiveness: This is perhaps the most common pitfall among health care professionals. The remedy is to cultivate activities and recreational pursuits that strengthen the sense of self. Find a source of restoration and recreation that builds your self-confidence and self-respect. Your clients will benefit, because you will be much more effective in your professional role.

care?" The client can assist in building this part of the relationship by identifying the aspects of his or her life style that the client feels "feed my spirit."

Precaution. *Remember to use your own personal sources of strength but not to overstep professional standards regarding relationship boundaries.*

Caritas Process 4: "Developing and Sustaining a Helping-Trusting Authentic Relationship"

Participating with a client in a caring, healing relationship is a choice. The therapist can "go through the motions" and still deliver safe, effective care; however, a much higher standard is set when the therapist deliberately creates the potential for the development of a healing relationship. Within this framework, the professional must cultivate a caring consciousness that is integral to the healing process, requiring self-development and ongoing personal growth.

The therapist's thinking about the therapeutic relationship should include questions such as, "What significance does this illness or injury have for this client, and how can I honor that meaning? What are the specific forms of caring and hand therapy that will best acknowledge, affirm, and sustain this client?"

From the client's perspective, this phase of the relationship means choosing and showing a degree of trust and openness with the hand therapist. The client may show signs of willingness to relate to the therapist by sharing experiences and deeper meanings, past occurrences, and validating the therapist's understanding of concerns, needs, and priorities.

Common Pitfalls and How to Avoid Them

1. Getting caught in the routine and distracted by time constraints and schedules: Keep your attention and focus on what is happening with *this* client, in *this* moment. Verbally set realistic and positive expectations about time with your client by saying something such as, "Mr. Smith, we have 15 minutes together to accomplish our work. This will be ample time, so let's get started."
2. Rushing into a client's space before considering the best approach: Try to imagine what it would be like to have to ask for help from someone and then having that person disrespect your sense of privacy and your need for personal space.
3. Overlooking the significance that illness, injury, and therapy have for clients: The hand therapist represents a significant source of hope, repair, and return to function for the client.
4. Failing to recognize that trust is a changing characteristic: Be patient and allow the trusting relationship to develop. Once it does, diligently guard that trust.

Caritas Process 5: "Being Present to and Supportive of the Expression of Positive and Negative Feelings as a Connection with a Deeper Spirit of Self and the One Being Cared for"

The hand therapist recognizes that within a trusting relationship, the client will feel more comfortable if he or she can share negative as well as positive aspects and can voice disagreements and deeper feelings than might not otherwise be exchanged. The hand therapist's role is to listen to what is said and to understand what is left unsaid (that is, read between the lines). It is a good idea to confirm or validate verbally what you understand from the client's expression. This is crucial with expressions of pain or discomfort, which is highly subjective and open to interpretation.

What is perceived becomes reality. However, two realities, the client's and the therapist's, operate within the relationship. Clients may be trying to assimilate what their injury, disease, symptoms, diagnosis, or treatment means within their culture or personal relationships. Clients also are often trying to get a clear picture of what the current health situation means for their life and future.

◉ Clinical Pearl

Keep in mind that your time will be better spent if you slow down and focus.

Common Pitfalls and How to Avoid Them

1. Feeling offended when the client expresses negative emotions or behaviors: Remember that if the client didn't trust you, he or she would not reveal these feelings to you. Demonstrating that you accept the negative as well as the positive is one way of showing a caring attitude.
2. Forgetting to validate meanings: Verbally acknowledge the behavior or expression and verify the meaning of what you observed. For example, "You are crying and seem upset right now. I wonder if you are physically tired or maybe you are frustrated that you aren't completing this activity as well as you'd like, or maybe it is something else. Can you help me understand?"
3. Dismissing the client's stories as irrelevant to the current clinical situation: Remember that for the client, the story may be connected to the client's view of his or her health condition and therapy.

Caritas Process 6: "Creative Use of Self and All Ways of Knowing as Part of the Caring Process; to Engage in Artistry of Caring-Healing Practices"

In many cases, standardized methods of structuring client care serve as guidelines for a certain diagnosis or treatment approach. The art of caring involves a spirit of willingness to explore and discover other approaches to care that build on the unique aspects of the particular client and on situations that might lend themselves to creative or artistic healing methods.[11]

The hand therapist might choose to address the following reflections to support the artistry of caring: "What are the unique attributes of this client and this situation? How can I use the environment to support healing for this client?"

Clients' perspectives include determining the degree to which they feel comfortable disclosing their uniqueness as individuals and their ways of expressing themselves. Clients may also be coming to new levels of understanding about their pattern of response to the health situation, changes in roles and responsibilities, and how their lifestyle may change.

Creative innovations can be very simple, and many hand therapists incorporate artful insight into their practice with each client. Such innovation could involve simply finding out the kind of food the client likes to cook or eat and then facilitating some aspect of that food preparation as part of hand therapy, or finding out the kind of music the client enjoys and incorporating that into the practice environment. If the client enjoys writing, the hand therapist may ask the client to keep a journal of what the recovery process means to him or her, describing important milestones and setbacks along the way.

Common Pitfalls and How to Avoid Them

1. Failing to consult the client regarding preferences about artful ways of caring: Remember that some clients are more willing than others to incorporate nontraditional approaches. The client's comfort level is always the guide.
2. Becoming disappointed or discouraged if an artful approach does not work: Role model the qualities of persistence and optimism for the client.
3. Forgetting to ask about role changes and significant issues: Take the time to figure out what this illness or injury means to the client as you go about designing an artful approach. For example, if a pianist is working to recover from a hand injury, the significance of using music in the therapy will rest on whether the client finds this approach motivating or if it is a source of despair.
4. Moving too quickly into the artful approach without building a sense of rapport: Wait until you can gauge the types of approaches to which the client might respond, and then share the ideas with the client at the appropriate time.

Caritas Process 7: "Engaging in a Genuine Teaching-Learning Experience That Attends to Unity of Being and Meaning, Attempting to Stay within the Other's Frame of Reference"

Teaching and learning are key activities in the hand therapist-client relationship. The hand therapist's role is to create a teaching-learning environment that supports the client's progression through healing.

◉ Clinical Pearl

Although the primary outward activities of hand therapy involve the body, a significant part of treatment also involves the client's mind and spirit.

Teaching requires attending to the client's ways of learning and preferences for information exchange and decision making. The hand therapist may ask, "Is this person able to understand what he or she is experiencing? How can I share knowledge and expertise with this client in a way that is relevant and meaningful for facilitating self-healing?"

It is very important to ascertain the client's definition of health, healing, and wholeness so that the therapist can incorporate this into the teaching-learning plan. The hand therapist also must assess the client's understanding of self-care needs, limitations, resources, and strengths.

Common Pitfalls and How to Avoid Them

1. Focusing only on the physical aspects of treatment and overlooking the cognitive, emotional, and spiritual impact hand therapy can have: Bring an intentional awareness to how the treatment may be influenced by the client's thoughts, attitudes, beliefs, and experiences. It may be beneficial to ask the client to help you understand what questions or concerns he or she is having about therapy and what it means for the healing process.
2. Failing to use the client's strongest learning style: People usually find it easiest to teach in the style in which they learn best; take care that you don't always choose the teaching approach that best suits *you*. Some clients prefer multiple approaches (for example, visual, auditory, kinesthetic); therefore offer a variety of activities.

Caritas Process 8: "Creating a Healing Environment at All Levels, Physical as Well as Nonphysical, a Subtle Environment of Energy and Consciousness Whereby Wholeness, Beauty and Comfort, Dignity, and Peace Are Potentiated"

The hand therapist can work with the client to create the best environment, physical and nonphysical, to promote healing. Manipulation of the environment can range from basic methods to more complex approaches. The treatment environment should be well-lighted, ventilated, and clean. Beyond that, the hand therapist can incorporate elements of beauty, including sources of color, movement, texture, and form, to enhance the healing environment. When possible, a view of the outdoors, a change in surroundings, paintings, flowers, plants, and music can also be included. It is important to eliminate or reduce unnecessary noise, clutter, and other distractions from the environment during the clinical interaction.

The hand therapist can focus on questions such as, "What is important to this person to make his or her experience comfortable? How can healing art be incorporated into this space and time? How can I use creativity in managing institutional imperfections, constraints, contingencies, and scheduling issues while sustaining the context of a healing environment?" The client's role is to participate with the therapist in the creation of an environment that is most suitable. It is very important that the client is honest and forthcoming in discussions of how the environment can be adapted to be more pleasing to the senses.

> ◎ *Clinical Pearl*
>
> A positive attitude conveyed by the hand therapist can make a significant difference in the client's immediate surroundings.

Caritas Process 9: "Assisting with Basic Needs, with an Intentional Caring Consciousness, Administering Human Care Essentials That Potentiate Alignment of Mind/Body/Spirit Wholeness and Unity of Being in All Aspects of Care, Tending to Both Embodied Spirit and Evolving Spiritual Emergence"

It is essential to the building of a therapeutic relationship that the therapist take care to notice the client's very basic needs for safety, comfort, nutrition, clothing, cleanliness, privacy, and the need for relationships with others. Until these basic needs are attended to, the goals of hand therapy cannot be fully addressed. These facts seem self-evident, but many clients start hand therapy when they are hungry, weak, in pain, or not fully clothed (for example, hospital gowns), or they are experiencing alterations in their normal patterns of personal hygiene. All these factors can leave clients feeling eroded in spirit and "less" than they could be. By putting the client in the best condition possible for therapy and acknowledging the impact of basic human needs, the therapist can more effectively accomplish the goals of the therapeutic session, and the client probably will be more confident about trying new approaches. As a result, the client-therapist relationship operates on a higher level.

The hand therapist can reflect on questions such as, "Am I process focused or outcome focused? Can I let go of the need to fix things? Am I honoring this person in my actions? What is the practice I can use now that will honor caring as a moral ideal?" The client's role is to provide honest and timely information about his/her own experience of how well basic needs are met. For instance, the client can be as prepared as possible for the therapy experience by having toileting needs met prior to therapy, eating a small meal or snack prior to therapy as appropriate, and being open about telling the therapist when needs are unmet. Also, the client can share with the therapist the approaches that will help the client feel most cared for. The therapist can work to set this expectation with the client in the initial meeting.

Common Pitfalls and How to Avoid Them

1. Trying to do everything yourself: Hand therapists are probably more aware of the environmental aspect of care than many of their professional counterparts. Ask for help from the client or family in creating a healing environment, or talk with others on the health care team to share ideas and insights. This type of collaborative work will enhance the client-therapist relationship and can promote teamwork among members of the interdisciplinary team.
2. Neglecting the physical and psychologic environment: Remember that a link exists between the physical environment and how a person feels emotionally and physically. Change the physical environment as much as possible to support the healing process; when this is impossible, do your utmost to create a positive psychologic environment.

Common Pitfalls and How to Avoid Them

1. Overlooking basic needs: To the extent that you can, make sure the client comes to the clinical encounter with basic needs met.
2. Forgetting to honor the process: Remember that outcomes are very important, but the journey is too.
3. Focusing only on the "broken" body part: Remember and remind clients that they are more than this part of their body and that many aspects of the body and spirit remain strong, even in times of illness or injury. Avoid using terminology such as "the bad arm;" instead use "the affected arm." A small semantic difference may help the client reframe the injury and see the body as an integrated whole rather than made up of "good" and "bad" parts.

Caritas Process 10: "Opening and Attending to Spiritual-Mysterious and Existential Dimensions of One's Own Life-Death; Soul Care for Self and the One Being Cared for"

During times of illness or injury, clients often have questions about their future and what the health event means for them personally. At this juncture, clients often confront issues of loss and mortality, even if the injury or illness is not considered life-threatening. Clients may experience heightened emotions as they consider these existential questions.

> ◎ **Clinical Pearl**
>
> Bring honor to the process of your work with clients by developing an unhurried presence, one that reassures clients that their individual treatment journey is an essential part of arriving at the outcome.

In this phase, the hand therapist focuses on how the client views the future for himself or herself and others, how the client can find meaning in the current experience, and how he or she can make good decisions about life and death. Therapists may ask themselves, "What are the life lessons in this situation for the client and for me? What soul care is useful for this client at this time?"

The client can consider his or her openness to deeper self-exploration and soul care and what that means in relation to healing. Key existential questions may arise during this time of illness or injury. The hand therapist's role is not to provide answers to these questions, but rather to support clients as they ask the questions and then realize that they simply may have to live with uncertainties. Clients may be facing critical life decisions that require deep reflection, and this may affect their physical stamina and motivation.

> **Common Pitfalls and How to Avoid Them**
>
> 1. Feeling fearful or uncomfortable about bringing up difficult issues: Remember that your role is to walk along with this client through a difficult time in the person's life. Sometimes the most helpful thing you can do for clients is not to do anything, but simply to "be" (that is, be present with them, listen to them and, if they ask questions or express deep spiritual needs beyond your comfort level or professional preparation, ask them for permission to arrange a referral to others trained in these areas).
> 2. Failing to recognize the limitations of hand therapy: Work within the scope of professional practice, and consult others for assistance and referral as needed.

> ◎ **Clinical Pearl**
>
> You are not charged with meeting all the client's needs, but you can be instrumental in arranging the right combination of resources to do so.

Transpersonal Caring Healing Relationships

The second major element of Watson's theory of human caring is transpersonal caring healing relationships. Transpersonal caring "conveys a concern for the inner life world of another seeking to connect with and embrace the soul of the other through the processes of caring and healing and being in authentic relation, in the moment."[12] A **transpersonal caring relationship** connotes the sharing of authentic self between individuals and within groups in a reflective frame. All parties are changed within the relationship.

Care is founded on transpersonal caring relationships and is built on moral commitment, intentionality, and caritas consciousness. It is a vehicle for healing through the auspices of the relationship. The hand therapist recognizes and connects with the inner aspect of the other through presence, being centered in the caring moment, and through actions, words, intuition, body language, cognition, thoughts, senses, and other ways of interacting and connecting with others.[12]

An assumption of transpersonal relationships is that "ongoing personal and professional development, spiritual growth, and personal spiritual practice assist the [therapist] in entering into this deeper level of professional healing practice."[12] The hand therapist learns how to build and expand transpersonal caring relationships based on his or her own life history and previous experiences or conditions or by having imagined others' feelings in various circumstances.

The Caring Moment

The third component of Watson's theory of human caring is the caring moment or occasion. The **caring moment** happens when the therapist and the client come together with their unique life histories and enter into the human-to-human transaction in a given focal point in space and time.[12]

There is awareness that the moment in time is transient; one makes choices about how to spend the time, occasion, or opportunities that transcend the moment itself. If the caring moment is characterized by transpersonal relationship and caritas consciousness, a connection develops between the therapist and the client at a spiritual level, transcending time and space and creating the potential for healing and human unity at deeper levels.[12] On a more global plane, "We learn from one another how to be human by identifying ourselves with others, finding their dilemmas in ourselves. What we all learn from it is self-knowledge. The self we learn about ... is every self. It is universal—the human self. We learn to recognize ourselves in others, [it] keeps alive our common humanity and avoids reducing self or other to the moral status of object."[8]

Nonverbal Aspects of Communication

Personal Space, Body Language, and Gestures

The first impression a client gets is often the nonverbal communication that begins before the conversation ever starts. Hand therapists' posture and use of personal space often are clues to how they feel about themselves and their practice. *Personal space* can be thought of as an invisible bubble or zone that varies from person-to-person and depends on the circumstances. Studies of personal space generally describe four zones: *intimate distance,* for embracing or whispering (6 to 18 inches); *personal distance,* for conversations among good friends (1½ to 4 feet); *social distance,* for conversations among acquaintances (4 to 12 feet); and *public distance,* for public speaking (12 feet or more). With most clients, the personal zone becomes the territory of the health care team for the purposes of assessments, treatments, and therapies. However, by always maintaining an awareness of personal space and its influence on client comfort, therapists can more easily comply with the client's preferences and take care not to compromise communication by violating this space.

> ◎ **Clinical Pearl**
>
> A person's space becomes his or her safety zone, and people feel varying degrees of ownership and territoriality about their personal space.

The position and posture of clients (and of hand therapists, too) can convey relevant information about physical and emotional health, comfort with communication strategies, and general attitude. Clearly, nonverbal communication can be an important source of clinical information for the hand therapist, but it is a subjective means and can be misinterpreted. Therefore a very important part of therapy is validating the meanings of nonverbal communication with the client.

Therapists also must take special note of how they use space, body language, speech tone, and volume when engaging in activities with clients. Much of the work of hand therapy is performed within personal boundaries that would be considered socially uncomfortable in another context.

Studies of physician nonverbal behaviors have indicated that behaviors, such as increased facial expression, frequent eye contact, smiling, leaning forward, open body posture, and nodding correlate with client satisfaction in a variety of clinical scenarios.[13] Also, in the most favorably rated clinical encounters, the clinician's behaviors often mirror or are patterned after the client's behaviors. Two people in conversation usually tend toward this mutual behavior when they are on good terms and relating well. This is **interactional synchrony**, a term used to describe the extent to which behaviors in an interpersonal interaction are patterned or synchronized. The patterning can take place in the way movements and behaviors are timed or in the actual behaviors themselves, such as scratching one's nose or leaning forward.[14] This model of rapport includes three elements: mutual attentiveness, positivity, and coordination. Although the hand therapist may not consciously try to match the client's behavioral conversational responses, the natural unfolding of this mutual conversational pattern may positively affect the sense of rapport reported by the client.

Nonverbal communication can provide valuable clinical information and can serve as a tool for enhancing the therapeutic relationship. However, the therapist must always use caution in interpreting nonverbal cues. Culture, health issues, context, and the social situation are just a few of the many variables that can alter the meaning of nonverbal communication. Therapists should always confirm their understanding of nonverbal behaviors with the client.

Reading between the Lines

Sometimes the hand therapist must call attention to something that is not said or a gesture that is not made. At times the verbal message conflicts with the nonverbal message. Some clients are very reluctant to open up to the health care team, even about health-related issues, such as pain or functional status. Pain is one of the most difficult factors to assess because of its subjective nature; some people have a very high tolerance, whereas others have a very low threshold. An effective approach to dealing with this is to continue to ask verbal questions while assessing nonverbal cues until the client verifies that the therapist understands what the client means. For example, you might say, "You are rating your pain as a 3, yet we aren't seeing the movement in your finger that we did yesterday. Can you tell me more about your discomfort or stiffness so that I can understand it better?"

Empathy is a strong component of an ability to understand what might be missing from a conversation. By truly trying to put oneself in the client's place, the hand therapist may gain further insight into what is not part of the conversation. For example, if the hand therapist is working with a young farmer who recently had an upper extremity amputation, yet the subject of farming and role change has not yet been introduced, the hand therapist may surmise that the client might like to talk about this issue but does not know how to begin—it is the proverbial pink elephant in the middle of the room. Unspoken concerns, such as this one, require a sensitive approach because they usually represent very difficult issues. In most cases, giving the client the chance to express concerns opens up new possibilities. The energy that was spent worrying about the issue now can be spent addressing it.

The ability to figure out what is left unspoken or unexpressed is a high-level clinical skill that therapists develop after experiencing several similar client care scenarios. Patterns of expected behaviors and issues usually begin to make sense after the therapist sees clients in similar circumstances. Then, when a client's specific communication does not fit with the basic pattern, the therapist may conclude that something unspoken warrants attention.

Listening

In our fast-paced culture of information overload, people often are forced to triage information rather than truly listen. Paying attention can mean skimming through the bulk of the material present to pick out what is really useful. "Sound bites," text messaging, digital images, and executive summaries are the norm. Listening is more difficult and takes longer.

> ◎ **Clinical Pearl**
>
> Listening requires one to stop, put an end to personal internal chatter, and fully attend to what the other person is saying, how he or she is saying it, what the person's behavior shows, and what the environment is like.

Listening means perceiving the words and creating meanings or interpretations for them. Listening also means mentally capturing the concrete message the client is sending while at the same time exploring deeper meanings that might be part of the message. For example, if a client says, "My hand is killing me," it probably means the client is in physical pain. The deeper meaning may also be true; this statement may also send a message of loss and grief that would not be discerned if the listener only hears the text of the concrete message.

For therapists, listening requires more than sorting through information to decipher which data are clinically meaningful.

It means incorporating what the client is saying into the therapist's perception of that person as a whole. For instance, if a client starts talking about the quilt she hoped to make for her new grandson and this expression is dismissed as irrelevant to the clinical encounter, the hand therapist might miss an important opportunity, such as the chance to learn what is meaningful to the client and to work with the client on skills that would allow her to regain this function and restore her sense of role competency.

Listening takes time. Listening with the focused intention of caring and concern is a therapeutic technique in its own right. Often when clients are asked which interventions they find most meaningful, they report that when therapists listen to their concerns, they feel understood and cared for. Listening can be a means to the desired result of a productive therapist-client relationship, and it can also be an outcome in and of itself. Listening provides a chance to connect with the client in a meaningful way, and it also can be very rewarding for the therapist.

Even when the client cannot communicate verbally, listening is still an important skill. Listening can be accomplished with more than the ears and through means other than sound. Consider how attention might be turned to the client in a meaningful, silent way, supporting and accepting the person's sense of being without words.

Clinical Pearl

Some of the most stunning listening takes place in silence.

Hope

Hope is a positive attitude or orientation toward the future. It has cognitive aspects (such as when the client thinks about how treatment will affect outcomes) and affective components (such as the emotional excitement a client feels when thinking about regaining abilities). Scientists also are investigating the physiologic aspects of hope, such as how hope may affect neurologic and immunologic function.

Clinical Pearl

Hope can be present even in the most desperate circumstances.

Individuals can simultaneously feel hopeful about one thing and hopeless about another. Sometimes hope extends beyond the constraints of the physical world; that is, sometimes, in the face of impending death, clients express hope for a future beyond death or describe hope in the people or things they will leave behind. Hope can be vested not so much in extending the quantity of life, but rather the quality. Clients look for signs of hope in the faces of those who care for them. The simple words, "The body has an amazing capacity for healing," can provide clients with a foundation for believing hand therapy can and will work for them.

Clinical Pearl

Providing realistic hope is a crucial aspect of care.

BOX 13-1   Herth Hope Index

1. I have a positive outlook toward life.
2. I have short-range and/or long-range goals.
3. I feel all alone.
4. I can see possibilities in the midst of difficulties.
5. I have a faith that gives me comfort.
6. I feel scared about my future.
7. I can recall happy/joyful times.
8. I have deep inner strength.
9. I am able to give and receive caring and love.
10. I have a sense of direction for my life.
11. I believe that each day has potential.
12. I feel my life has value and worth.

(From Herth K: Abbreviated instrument to measure hope: development and psychometric evaluation—the Herth hope index, *J Adv Nurs* 70:1251-1259, 1992.)

Hope plays an important role in health and healing and in adjusting to serious injury, illness, and death. Taking away hope can have devastating effects. Hope can be viewed conceptually as requiring four critical attributes: a time-focused future orientation, energized action, the existence of a goal or desired outcome, and a feeling of uncertainty.[15] Hope is both a universally important construct and a very individualized experience.

Statements that clients can rate to indicate their level of hope are found in Herth's Hope Index,[16] an instrument used to measure hope in research settings (Box 13-1).

Hope is an attitude that can be affected by clinical interventions; to some degree, an outlook of hope can be taught. Important work is emerging that focuses on specific, scientifically based interventions designed to inspire hope[17] and to teach people thought patterns and behavioral competencies that enhance personal happiness and meaning.[18]

How should clinicians approach the issue of supporting realistic hope while not making unwarranted positive predictions or statements? In his book, *The Anatomy of Hope*, Jerome Groopman[19] addresses this question from the point of view of a medical oncologist caring for clients with life-threatening illness. He explores the dangers of taking away psychologic hope by providing only survival statistics and factual summaries, as well as the perils of giving too much hope or unrealistic hope. The approach he finds most therapeutic is to balance a straightforward appraisal of the worst-case scenario with realistic optimism. He finds that clients are very appreciative when practitioners show an awareness of their diagnosis and predicted course and that these clients make the most beneficial personal strides in building a sense of meaning and hope when they have a realistic picture combined with emotional support and reinforcement of hope.

The hand therapist can assume an important role in assessing hope and providing clients with realistic hope for the progress and outcomes of hand therapy. Hope can be conveyed in words, through encouraging remarks, or by reminding clients how far they have progressed. Helping clients to identify their individualized sources of support and to build on past successes are two approaches that go a long way in sustaining hope. Clients are much more likely to reach the physical and functional goals of hand therapy when they participate with a sense of hope intact.

Creating a Motivating Environment

One function of the therapeutic relationship is to create an environment in which the client can reach the very best possible clinical outcome. Motivation plays a key role in how much effort, dedication, and resilience a client will have in the therapeutic regimen. Naturally motivating factors and ways the therapist can enhance that motivation include the following:

1. Significant contributions: Identify the efforts clients are making; help them see the work they are accomplishing.
2. Goal participation: Take the time and effort to achieve mutual goal setting.
3. Positive dissatisfaction: When clients are not comfortable with their current status, help them use this dissatisfaction as a positive motivator for change.
4. Recognition: Create ways of acknowledging progress.
5. Clear expectations: Clarify reasonable goals, strategies, and regimens with the client; be a leader, encouraging and inspiring the client to reach beyond current abilities.

Clients often need help learning how to be successful in their treatment; they must realize that knowledge alone does not necessarily get them to the goal. The most effective rewards usually are those that are positive, valued by the individual client, and intermittent.

Clients become motivated when therapists help them find meaning in their therapeutic regimen. Point out the link between the activities or exercises and the way they will help the client go about daily life, especially the activities most important to the client. Share your observations with the client, such as, "Your range of motion is much better today." Even the simplest observation conveys to the client that you are paying attention to the person's progress (or lack thereof), and this feedback itself provides motivation. Also use any available nonverbal means of feedback (for example., chart, graph, or journal for keeping track of progress) for motivation.

Certain strategies do not work as motivational tools and can even set back motivational success. These include belittling clients, treating them in childlike ways, drawing attention to weaknesses or calling clients lazy, showing insensitivity to cultural or age-related norms, and in general behaving disrespectfully. Negative reinforcement should not be used. Sometimes confronting people about their negative behaviors or lack of focused effort is a reasonable tactic, but it should be done with care and respect.

◎ *Clinical Pearl*

Clients find it easier to be motivated if the hand therapist also is motivated or energized.

Clients are keenly aware of the authenticity of encouragement. Therefore the therapist must find ways to maintain a personal sense of energized optimism. Clearly this is tied to self-care strategies; for example, taking good care of your own health and well-being has some of its clearest implications for professional success when it comes to providing motivation. A tired, depleted, "burned out" hand therapist finds it very difficult to support clients in the motivational domain. Find and engage in personal strategies that provide opportunities for healthy growth and development so that these strengths can be shared with your clients.

Working with clients who have little motivation can be particularly frustrating for the therapist. Clients have differing levels of readiness for adopting the changes required by hand therapy. Patience, gentle persistence, and time generally are the most effective strategies for managing weak motivation.

A motivating hand therapist provides the client with clear direction about goals, how therapy will progress, what to expect along the way, how long it will take, and the results. Providing honest, constructive feedback during each session and about the whole course of therapy is the most effective way to maintain motivation for most clients. Reinforcing a client's "can do" spirit and conveying an attitude of "I knew you could do it" are excellent ways to boost motivation. Such encouragement leaves clients better prepared to draw from this motivation as a resource in the future when they are discharged from therapy. The hand therapist can make the impossible become possible and can give the client the courage to turn a possibility into a reality.

Terminating the Therapeutic Relationship

It is important that the therapist take the time and opportunity to acknowledge the end of the therapeutic relationship if at all possible. The client may be discharged from the hand therapy program for a variety of reasons. At this juncture, the therapist should note the progress that was made, not only in terms of functionality, but also in terms of the process of therapy. The therapist may want to share some thoughts with the client about the goals accomplished, the strengths or characteristics that most obviously helped on the journey, and any reflections about humorous, meaningful, or important moments the therapist and client shared.

Clients often feel a great deal of gratitude to the hand therapist for the work that has been accomplished, and they may have difficulty expressing this gratitude in a way that is fitting within the professional culture of the therapist. For instance, clients may offer gifts or tokens of appreciation. As a rule, it is best to thank the client and explain that you really can't accept personal gifts. Maintaining professional boundaries is very important, even as the therapist-client relationship is coming to a close.

Some of the most difficult good-byes can arise when a client enters a phase in treatment in which hand therapy is no longer relevant because of the client's declining condition or impending death. It is important not to ignore the transition. Instead, tell the client good-bye. You might take the chance to say how much you enjoyed working with the client and spending time together.

Other situations also can create difficulty in maintaining social and professional roles. For instance, in a large health care organization, some of the hand therapist's clients may be fellow employees. In rural settings, clients may also be neighbors. In these situations it is helpful to acknowledge that the professional therapeutic relationship is ending but that the social role will continue. If this transition in roles is acknowledged verbally, the former client is far less likely to ask a therapy question in the hospital elevator or request advice in the grocery store.

The end of the therapeutic relationship sometimes can cause emotions the client may be feeling about the hand therapist to bubble up. These can range from gratitude for reaching a therapy goal to frustration that goals were not accomplished. A client may even have just stopped therapy abruptly without giving notice. Most health care professionals develop a personal method of managing these thoughts and emotions, such as talking to colleagues, journaling (using no client names or identifiers), and finding ways to "let go" of clients when they leave. After you have been in practice for a while, you will have many client stories; some of them will be good memories, some not. Your expertise will be deepened by the complicated parade of clients that comprise an active clinical practice.

CASE STUDIES

CASE STUDY 13-1 ■

An 80-year-old, right-dominant woman arrives for hand therapy accompanied by her 54-year-old son, who recently lost his job and now lives with his mother, "working" as her caregiver. The client was referred with a diagnosis of stiff fingers of both hands secondary to disuse after right shoulder surgery to repair the rotator cuff. The physician's notes explicitly state that the son aggressively debated the issue of surgery with the physician and that he had been argumentative at office visits. He also had "pestered" the physician to the extent that the physician suggested that the client and son find another doctor with whom they might be happier. The client and son have decided to stay with this physician, but they make derogatory remarks about the doctor to the hand therapist. At the first hand therapy visit, the son challenges every recommendation the therapist makes and is reluctant to let his mother participate in the conversation. The son also makes numerous recommendations that are clinically contraindicated.

1. What is your first client/family relationship priority?
2. What is your clinical priority?
3. How do you plan the therapeutic interventions so that they will have the greatest effect?

Suggested Approach

The physician's notes make it clear that this will be a psychosocially complex case. The initial priority is to establish a trusting professional relationship with the client and her son. The clinical priority is safety for the client, followed by the formulation of clear working relationship roles and responsibilities that support the physical work of therapy.

Before initiating the client encounter, the hand therapist might take a moment to clear his or her mind of other distracting thoughts and to bring into focus a "fresh start" perspective for this client/family visit. A first step here might be to request and arrange for separate times with the client and the son and to arrange a physical setting that is conducive to privacy. Reassure both that they will have an adequate opportunity to voice concerns and questions. Recognizing that the son may have a lot of emotional investment in his caregiving role since he is otherwise unemployed, the therapist may find it beneficial to comment on his strengths in this area. It will be important to draw clear lines about how the hand therapist will treat the family as a unit, but the primary therapeutic recommendations and work will be focused on the client's priorities. Building a positive rapport with the son will facilitate the care of the client. The hand therapist might ask what the son's priorities are, if he feels that his priorities match the client's goals, and what the barriers have been up to this point. When talk turns to complaints about the physician,

the hand therapist could refocus the son, saying, "Let's focus on what we can accomplish for your mother here today." After rapport is established, it will be more feasible to discuss therapeutic recommendations with the son. If he continues to suggest things that are clinically contraindicated, the therapist can explain the reasons for the contraindication. If rapport is not well established, the son is likely to dismiss the therapist's recommendations.

In the client encounter, it is important for the therapist to notice nonverbal communication and to do an unobtrusive assessment for possible elder abuse. In scenarios in which the caregiver expresses a lot of anger and blame, the elderly individual sometimes is at risk for verbal, physical, or financial abuse. If signs of abuse are present and the client seems comfortable talking with the therapist, the therapist can assess the situation verbally to discern whether the client feels vulnerable. If so, a referral to social services and/or the elder abuse hotline is in order. If no signs of abuse are noted, the therapist proceeds with assessing the client's goals for therapy and her readiness to begin.

The private consultation with the client focuses on gaining trust, establishing priorities, and clarifying everyone's roles: client, son, hand therapist, and physician. Once the part each person plays in the client's therapy is clearly understood, realistic goals can be established. In this situation, establishing trust and rapport may take longer, but without these elements hand therapy probably will be unsuccessful. The time spent "up front" in establishing a positive working relationship will pay benefits by fostering a more productive therapeutic progression.

The hand therapist must be very careful to document the findings in this case thoroughly because of the son's issues with anger and hostility. It also is important for the therapist to have an opportunity to debrief and reflect about his or her time with this client and son. Progress probably will take time, and this case has the potential to be discouraging if the therapist focuses only on physical gains. The first major accomplishment in this case will be creating rapport with and establishing realistic expectations for all those involved; these outcomes are more difficult to see. After each visit, the therapist should take a few moments to reflect on the strategies that did and did not work in this particular situation and to envision how things might be more successful in future encounters.

CASE STUDY 13-2 ■

A precocious 9-year-old arrives for hand therapy with her mother, a pediatric nurse. The child has been referred with a diagnosis of bilateral wrist tendonitis. She is in gifted classes at school and is an avid reader. She is quite active and has trouble sitting in one place for longer than 5 minutes. She does not make eye contact with her mother or the therapist unless the mother specifically commands her to do so; she then makes eye contact for less than 30 seconds. Her hand therapy examination does not reveal any isolated structures that fit the criteria for tendonitis. She is hypermobile in numerous joints, including her wrists, and she has a habitual practice of forcefully passively stretching her wrists into extremes of flexion and extension. She does this often and states that it both "hurts and feels good." The mother is concerned that the physical problem causing the child's painful wrists has not been properly diagnosed, and she hopes that therapy will correct the condition.

1. How can rapport be gained?
2. What are the competing clinical priorities?
3. What referrals would be appropriate?

Suggested Approach

Presenting a focused, calm, accepting demeanor will be particularly helpful in this case; therefore the hand therapist might want to spend a few moments getting focused and clearing the mind of distractions before initiating this encounter. This client will be particularly sensitive to anxiety carried by the therapist. Maintaining a calm presence will be challenging, given the client's many movements and lack of eye contact, as well as the mother's presence. A very simple, yet effective, way therapists can remain focused and serene is to be aware of their own breathing, focusing on making the exhalation longer than the inhalation. This means of slowing down can have a positive effect on the client, who typically will slow her own breathing in response. Getting the client to slow down and focus is a critical first step in establishing rapport.

The hand therapist probably suspects that this child is experiencing anxiety or attention deficit characteristics. Further assessment of these suspicions warrants a complete history and may involve referrals to other professionals and perhaps school personnel. Competing clinical priorities include clarification of the behavioral issues that seem to be exacerbating the tendonitis, discerning medical versus psychologic etiologies for the behaviors, and identifying social or academic issues that might be compounding the condition. The fact that the child is academically precocious may mask her other developmental needs, which may be more in line with those of the average 9 year old. Although there may be interventions the hand therapist can recommend for the tendonitis, the picture is complicated by the child's repeated behaviors. Treating the underlying psychosocial conditions extends the effectiveness of hand therapy. Referrals to developmental specialists, social workers, psychologic and medical care providers, and the school counselor may also be appropriate. Again, the referral process can be facilitated if the therapist develops a sound, trusting relationship with the client and her mother, particularly if this is their first encounter with the health care system regarding this constellation of issues.

As in Case Study 13-1, the hand therapist should evaluate the client away from the mother's presence if at all possible. The mother's presence may be interfering with the daughter's ability to focus. Also, the girl may have goals for therapy that are different from those of her mother, which will be important to discern. The therapist can capitalize on the client's love of reading by giving her age-appropriate books or pamphlets about her tendonitis and its treatment. The therapist also should work with the client to identify ways of creating a soothing environment for her treatment, techniques that may extend to her living and academic activities. For example, the therapist might help the client identify music that she finds relaxing or activities that help her unwind before therapy.

The hand therapist must work to gain an understanding of the significance of the client's repeated flexion and extension of her wrists. Is this action symbolic of a desire for flexibility? Is the client's "hurts and feels good" statement symbolic of what it is like for her to be academically gifted, given the social realities of her school setting? These symbolic meanings can greatly influence the client's desire to quit the behaviors if the movements themselves are comforting psychologically.

Working separately with the mother, the hand therapist must first establish rapport and then gauge the mother's understanding of her daughter's underlying anxiety or attention-related condition. If no workup has been done on these issues, it is important that the therapist address the possibility of referrals. It is essential that the therapist make no assumptions about the mother's cognitive understanding of her daughter's condition; just because the mother is a pediatric nurse does not mean that she can objectively identify issues in her own family. The hand therapist must verify the mother's understanding and her concerns verbally, in addition to assessing her nonverbal communication. Working with the mother to identify priorities for diagnosis and treatment comes after this basic assessment of her understanding the larger picture of her daughter's condition. Supporting the mother and helping her accept the possible psychosocial diagnoses for her daughter also strengthens the therapeutic rapport and places the client in a better environment for improvement in overall well-being.

CASE STUDY 13-3 ■

A 61-year-old, right-dominant teacher is referred for hand therapy after repair of a fracture of the right distal radius with plating. The referral is for pain management, edema, and stiffness that limit functional use of her hand. She tells the therapist that she is an overachiever and is highly motivated to recover. The therapist provides the woman with written instructions for gentle exercises; she also instructs her to stop or modify the exercises if they cause pain or do not feel good. When the client arrives for the next therapy session, the pain, swelling, and stiffness are all worse. She states that she had tripled the recommended exercise regimen, although she realized immediately that it increased her pain, swelling, and stiffness. She explains that she did this because she was eager to recover. The client is developing a highly guarded posture of the painful right upper extremity that is contributing to the worsening of all symptoms, and she is at risk for complex regional pain syndrome (CRPS).

1. How can you sustain this client's high level of motivation, yet convince her that she has overdone her exercises?
2. How can you best approach this client about the worsening symptoms and pain?

Suggested Approach

The hand therapist can draw on the client's many strengths to optimize treatment. First, the woman is highly motivated to get better. Second, she clearly understands the link between treatment and outcomes. Third, she must have a high level of trust in the hand therapist, as evidenced by her wanting to follow the recommendations, if not the level of gentleness, recommended by the therapist.

The therapist's first step is to capitalize on the rapport already established. The therapist should acknowledge the client's hard work and then gently but firmly remind her that in her case, "less is more." The link between exercise and rest should be explained, as well as how pain affects mobility. The teacher is highly motivated to learn and likely will respond to logical, clear, and multifaceted explanations of why vigorous or repeated exercise is causing her pain. In this case it probably will be beneficial to give the physiologic explanations of overuse, edema, and pain. These explanations will appeal to the client's sense of reason, and this is likely to increase her motivation to be slower and gentler in her approach.

The hand therapist should not scold the client or trivialize the time and work she has already invested in her recovery. Shaming this client would be very detrimental to her overall well-being and to her progress in therapy. However, the hand therapist might want to gently inquire about other reasons the client overdid her therapy. Are there underlying reasons for her not to want to regain function, or was the overexertion truly related to wanting to get better faster? Such questions may help the client come to a better understanding of herself and her motives. If her sole motive is a speedy recovery, helping her discover that the most beneficial method is a gently paced approach that respects tissue tolerances may give her a deeper insight into other areas of her life.

References

1. Minick P: The power of human caring: early recognition of client problems, *Sch Inq Nurs Pract* 9:303–317, 1995.
2. Watson J: *Postmodern nursing and beyond*, Edinburgh, 1999, Churchill-Livingstone/Harcourt-Brace.
3. *** http://www2.uchsc.edu/son/caring/content/jwbio.asp.
4. Kabat-Zin J: *Wherever you go, there you are: mindfulness meditations in everyday life*, New York, 1994, Hyperion.
5. Watson J: Watson's philosophy and theory of human caring in nursing. In Riehl-Sisca J, editor: *Conceptual models for nursing practice*, ed 3, Norwalk, CT, 1989, Appleton & Lange.
6. Watson J: A meta-reflection on reflective practice and caring theory. In Johns C, Fleshwater D, editors: *Transforming nursing through reflective practice*, London, 1998, Blackwell Science.
7. Watson J: New dimensions of human caring theory, *Nurs Sci Q* 1:175–181, 1988.
8. Watson J: *Nursing: human science and human care*, New York, 1985, Appleton-Century.
9. Watson J: *Nursing: the philosophy and science of caring*, Boston, 1979, Little, Brown.
10. Pipe TB, Bortz JJ: Mindful leadership as healing practice: nurturing self to serve others, *International Journal for Human Caring* 13(2):34–38, 2009.
11. Pipe TB, Buchda VL, Launder S, et al: Building personal and professional resources of resilience and agility in the healthcare workplace, *Stress Health* 28(1):11–22, 2012.
12. *** http://www2.uchsc.edu/son/caring/content/transpersonal.asp.
13. Griffith C, Wilson J, Langer S, et al: House staff nonverbal communication skills and standardized client satisfaction, *J Gen Intern Med* 18:170–174, 2003.
14. Bernieri F, Rosenthal R: Interpersonal coordination: behavior matching and interactional synchrony. In Feldman R, Rime B, editors: *Fundamentals of nonverbal behavior*, London, 1991, Cambridge University Press.
15. Haase J, Britt T, Coward D, et al: Simultaneous concept analysis of spiritual perspective, hope, acceptance, and self-transcendence, *Image J Nurs Sch* 24:141–147, 1992.
16. Herth K: Abbreviated instrument to measure hope: development and psychometric evaluation—the Herth hope index, *J Adv Nurs* 70:1251–1259, 1992.
17. Herth K: Development and testing of a hope intervention program, *Oncol Nurs Forum* 28:1009–1016, 2001.
18. Foster R, Hicks G: *How we choose to be happy*, New York, 1999, Perigee Books.
19. Groopman J: *The anatomy of hope: how people prevail in the face of illness*, New York, 2004, Random House.

14

How Hand Therapists' Words Affect the Therapeutic Relationship

William S. Graff

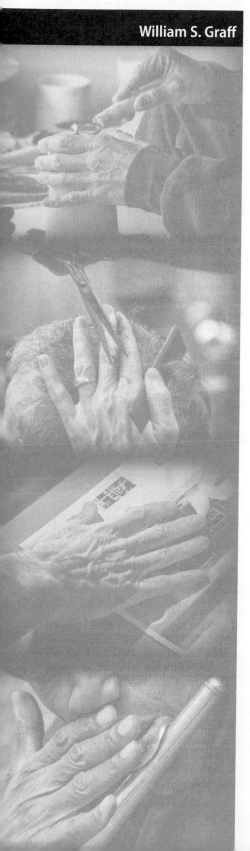

"Sticks and stones may break my bones, but words can never hurt me." Remember that little ditty from childhood? Let's examine it. Is it true, or is it false? The first part, of course, is true. Sticks and stones, in fact, are sometimes the cause of the injury you treat in your practice. But "words can never hurt me?" Abjectly false. Via both conscious and subconscious processes, words can have a devastating effect, not only on the human psyche, but on the human body as well. Conversely, words can have a profound healing effect on both the psyche and the physical body. Face-validity proof of the healing effect of words is revealed by the mere fact that the service of psychotherapy exists, and that it works to facilitate healing. The primary tool of psychotherapy is the spoken word. I'm not going to deal directly with psychotherapy in this chapter, but I would like to convince you that you are in a professional helping *relationship* with your patient.

◎ Clinical Pearl

Therefore the *words* you use as a hand therapist can have a profound healing effect on your patient, and I hope to contribute to your understanding of how to put healing words together in a sentence.

Pam Schindeler, OTR/L, CHT and Caroline W. Stegink-Jansen, PT, PhD, CHT wrote in the *Journal of Hand Therapy* that "[t]he empathy we share with our patients is the building block of trust and rapport, and the foundation for effective communication."[1] Indeed, yet how is empathy *created* from scratch?

Let's start with the difference between sympathy and empathy. Exaggeration is sometimes helpful in understanding abstract verbal concepts, so allow me to exaggerate the idea of sympathy. Extreme forms of sympathy often involve pity, condescension, and reinforcement of dependence. This is a harsh definition of a form of communication that can be simply supportive, yet you might see that sympathy has its risks when attempting to use it in healing.

◎ Clinical Pearl

Empathy is commonly more effective than sympathy.

Empathy can work both as a communication device and as a method of moving people toward health and self-sufficiency. The trouble with empathy is that it's harder to learn than sympathy and, probably for that reason, it's more rarely delivered. To put it another way, unfortunately, it takes more skill to deliver empathy than it does to deliver sympathy.

The all-time classic sympathy response is, "poor baby." Of course you would never say this sentence to a patient, but the "poor baby" meta-message may be implied in nearly any effort you put into sympathizing: "There's something wrong with you, so I feel bad for you." Via sympathy, you make a negative judgment about this other person, and then there's an "I" statement concerning what you are going to do about it for yourself (for example, "feel bad"). Sympathy can quickly turn into a bit of a problem.

The healing power of empathy, on the other hand, is subtle, almost translucent, because a transcribed helper empathy response doesn't look like much. In real time, in vivo, it doesn't sound like much, so bear with me while I explain the mysterious power of simple empathy.

Empathy

What *is* empathy? Let me define empathy in terms of its parts. Empathy has two parts. The first part is a perception. The second part is a delivery. Without both parts, there is no empathy.

Perception

Empathy requires accurate perception of the immediate emotional state of the patient. An example of one of these emotional states might be fear, so in this case the patient feels afraid. Well of course this patient might be afraid, you say to yourself. He hurt his hand moving a large landscape stone at work, and he is afraid he might lose his job because he's had anxiety for years; he thinks of the worst possibility first, and he's afraid of change in general. Still, this lifestyle fear, if you will, is one of this man's long-term traits, and it is not exactly immediate to the problem at hand. Let the psychologist use specialized empathy techniques to work on this long-term *trait* problem.

In your treatment setting, however, this man's immediate emotional *state* has more to do with fear of the environment, fearful skepticism concerning the rehabilitation process, fear of more pain right now, and even fear of you, the practitioner. So attempt to perceive the emotional state at the moment the patient is in front of you.

> ◎ **Clinical Pearl**
>
> *Look at state not trait.* Then come up with a word for the emotional state.

Now these emotional-state, or affective-condition, words can be harder to think of than you might suspect. ("Affect," pronounced similarly to "adjunct," is another word for emotion.) It takes effort to build a collection of these words into your professional, working vocabulary. Would it come to mind that, in addition to feeling fear, this injured worker is also feeling pride? After all, he was the only man on the work crew strong enough to move the landscape stone. But then, as this worker tells his story, can we stack embarrassment on top of pride and fear? Why yes we can. The man is embarrassed that he hurt himself. Can accurate empathic perception become complicated? Indeed we can perceive *layers* of state emotions, which is one of the reasons why empathy requires more skill than sympathy.

Yet to keep this empathy process reasonable, it's a good idea to focus on *one* of the patient's affective conditions at a time. So let's pick fear. At this point you *perceived* fear, along with a couple other immediate state emotions, and you *picked* fear.

Delivery

Now for the delivery. For empathy to occur, it's not enough that you know what this stone mover is experiencing emotionally; you must *prove* to him that you know. You must somehow deliver your perception to him.

But wait. Even though your perception of his very real fear is accurate, is the word "fear," or the word "afraid," going to be tolerated by the strongest man on the landscape-construction crew? Probably not. So even though, before your eyes, fear is exactly this man's emotional phenomenology, for you to reflect out loud that he feels afraid may not match his attempted opinion of himself. He may even take your comment as an insult. Now what?

In your mind, try to reduce the intensity of this word, "afraid." Let's see. "Anxious" is a bit clinical. "Nervous" may work. "Uncomfortable" could turn out to be too vague. Maybe "nervous" then—not just even though it undershoots the target of "afraid," but *because* it undershoots this target emotion. "Nervous" comes close, while allowing this fellow to save face. Okay, then, "nervous." Somehow you are going to *deliver* the word "nervous," as an aspect of your perception of his fear.

Delivery options at this juncture are endless. Most practitioners initially move toward asking questions. Now as simple as this sounds, questions end in question marks. Keep this in mind, because soon I will discriminate between delivery sentences that end in question marks and delivery sentences that end in periods. The difference between these two forms of delivery is significant. For now, though, let's ask this man a question. "Do you feel nervous?"

"No," he says.

Oops. What happened? What happened was that this question is a closed-ended, yes-or-no question. The patient not only decided on "no," but he also decided on denial. Let's open the question up a little and give the man some less-specific wiggle room. "Have you noticed that you've felt a little nervous around medical practitioners before?"

"A little," he says. Then he looks at you to see who you are again, because you just made *emotional* contact with this fellow. The *intellectual* contact was made when you heard about the three-dimensional physics of his injury story. Yet suddenly you used a different language to communicate with the emotional experience of his physical body at that moment in time. Initially it was information that passed between the two of you. Now it is almost as though something else, something invisible and something very important just passed between the two of you. Regardless, he now knows that *you* know about his affective condition in the present moment, because you just got done creating empathy.

During social and colloquial conversation, we usually assume that a question is a good way to start a conversation and a good way to keep a conversation going. However it is often a question that stops the conversation, which then requires another question to start the conversation up again, but which has the effect of bringing the conversation to a new halt. Person A asks person B a question, "How do you feel about hurting your hand?" Person B answers the question, and the conversation stops. "I feel stupid."

"Why do you feel stupid?"

"Because I hurt my hand."

The conversation has stopped twice now, each time that a question got answered. The question, a sentence that ends in a question mark, can be a somewhat difficult method to deliver empathy, or to create exploratory conversation. People who ask questions for a living typically hope for the conversation to stop after the question gets answered so that the answer can get noted and a new question can be quickly asked. In these scenarios, empathy communication is purposely shunned in favor of rapid information transfer. The comfort level of person B is not a concern, and tactics such as intimidation may be employed to push the information flow along. Communication situations such as these are commonly seen around medical emergencies, disaster-control efforts, interrogations, or cross-examinations.

You think you just asked a supportive, open-ended question, yet person B may feel interrogated and then respond in kind with a short, conversation-stopping answer. Interrogation and empathy may be on opposite poles of one aspect of communication. We'll look closer at similar conversational polarities later.

So what empathy-delivery form might we use besides a sentence that ends in a question mark?

◎ *Clinical Pearl*

An excellent empathy-delivery form is a sentence that ends in a period.

"Hey, you're probably feeling a little bit nervous about being here." Believe it or not, these empathy-delivery statements that do *not* end in a question mark, but that *do* end in a period, cause people to talk and talk and talk. I use the phrase "believe it or not," because most people, professional or otherwise, to whom I introduce this concept do *not* believe it. Regardless, empathy efforts via *question* can cause people to miss the empathy event and to reject the conversation. Empathy attempts via *statement* can cause people to self-disclose their phenomenological affective conditions concerning the immediacy of those agitating, distracting, and otherwise undesirable nemeses known clinically as Psychosocial Stressors. To put it another way, a non-question helper empathy statement causes a patient to talk about his or her immediate feelings regarding recent bad luck.

But we might back up a step in order to confirm the value of properly used questions. It is *essential* when performing a diagnostic or a history-taking interview that you ask specific questions, usually a *protocol* of *pointed* questions, and that you get *answers* to those questions. Please understand the difference between a question designed to obtain information, versus a question or a statement designed to enhance communication or, perhaps, healing. At the same time, however, while it is important to know the difference between practitioner verbalizations that either (1) serve to glean information or (2) serve to cause affective communication, keep in mind that it is not necessary to divide these two verbal methods into two separate events. The second category (affective communication) can be mixed among the first category (information gathering) to enhance the very act of gathering information. A patient who becomes guarded about your questions concerning the details that produced an impaired hand for example, may open up instantly if you make a statement that targets the emotional condition at the moment. "You feel unhappy about getting into the details."

Even if the patient agrees with you about this discomfort, then quits talking, you have proven your perception, and you have begun to build an emotional bridge across the divide in the direction of this patient, which may connect with the patient later. Often the information you seek will come out spontaneously after you render a couple more strategically spaced empathy reflections.

The historical healing use of empathy is lost in the shrouds of history, and probably dates back to shamans and to the wiser of our elders. The professional use of empathy was emphasized by psychologist Carl Rogers. If there was ever a stereotype picturing what Carl Rogers did for a living, it was that he rendered reflective empathy responses. Carl Rogers led the Client-Centered psychotherapy movement that, beyond empathy, called for a therapeutic relationship, practitioner genuineness, and unconditional positive regard for the patient. Rogers championed a form of psychotherapy in which empathy was a central component, and it became an uncanny yet undeniable fact that the heavy use of psychotherapist empathy is a powerful factor that can facilitate patient healing.

Rogers wrote that for healing to happen, the patient must perceive, "… to a minimal degree, the acceptance and empathy which the therapist experiences for him. Unless some communication of these attitudes has been achieved, then such attitudes do not exist in the relationship so far as the client is concerned…"[2]

"Since attitudes cannot be directly perceived, it might be somewhat more accurate to state that therapist behaviors and words are perceived by the client as meaning that to some degree the therapist accepts and understands him."[2]

Empathy is neither the territorial possession of Carl Rogers nor of psychotherapists. Empathy has never had a patent number or a copyright or a purchase price, and there are almost no warnings or restrictions when it comes to its use. You don't need to talk to your doctor before you attempt it. Empathy requires no specialized equipment. You can even try it at home. Some people, without any training whatsoever, become, simply by inclination and by experience, potent natural empathizers. Empathy is observed at picnics, at grocery stores, and on work crews. A few people are so good at empathy that they deliver their perceptions nonverbally with facial expressions alone. Empathy can be a natural act and, as such, is a simple human behavior that preceded the much more complicated professional behaviors required during the performance of psychotherapy. Once colloquial empathy became recognized for its power, however, it became incorporated into communication skills as a tactic, and it became included in psychotherapy as a core component, among others.

In 1969, Robert R. Carkhuff published the classic, *Helping and Human Relations*, which is still one of the most quoted works ever written on the components of psychotherapy. In this two-volume set, Carkhuff attempted to quantify some of these core psychotherapy components.[3] The art of using these components in a coordinated fashion during psychotherapy is complicated. Still, like empathy, these components did not come into existence *for* psychotherapy. They were in existence as part of language and communication well *prior* to psychotherapy, and they are available to hand therapists as techniques to improve contact with patients, and to thereby improve the overall potential for healing. Actually we have already casually looked at a few of these components, so I will introduce them formally here.

Specificity

Consider specificity. Back when we were trying to pick a word among the words "afraid," "anxious," "nervous," or "uncomfortable," one way to look at what we were really doing is that we were picking a point along a spectrum of specificity. If you examine the *order* in which these words appear above, they do seem to progress from more specific to less specific. I mentioned that the word "afraid" could be insulting. The reason for the insulting characteristic of this word is that it was *too* very true and *too* accurately specific, as it applied to the injured landscaper. The word "afraid" wasn't too true or too specific, as it applied to your perception or to an accurate description of the man's emotion, but it was too specific as it applied to the word's palatability. The word would have tasted bad, and this man would have refused to digest it.

I also mentioned that the word "uncomfortable" was too vague, and this brings up a more general concept around the nature of conversational specificity. It is nearly the average patient's "job" to refuse specificity and to fight in favor of the vague. It is nearly your job to refuse the vague and to fight in favor of the specific. Some people will present themselves as exceptions to this "rule," of course, but this specificity-versus-vagueness battle rages between practitioner and patient every day all over the world. This battle can almost be thought of as a standard aspect of the nature of practitioner/patient communication. So if the patient is predisposed in favor of the vague, we do *not* want to supply the patient with pro-vague words, such as "uncomfortable." Not only is this word too vague to be useful, but it allows the *structure* and *balance* of the conversation to tip in favor of any tendency the patient may have to retreat from the specifics required to bring about health. Even single words spoken by the practitioner can have a dynamic effect on the course and success of treatment, because "…words are not created equal and word choice matters," stated David Ring, MD, PhD, writing from Massachusetts General Hospital's Department of Orthopaedic Surgery.[4] Specificity is one of the core communication components that Carkhuff listed, and a hand therapist who can manage the specificity of words is a fluid practitioner indeed.

As you can see, by intentionally choosing a moderately nonspecific word like "nervous," it is not the practitioner's goal to win the battle of specificity. It is to the patient's advantage, though, if the practitioner can visualize words on a spectrum of specificity, and then use words accordingly to enhance a patient's approach to health at that immediate moment in time.

Immediacy

The phrase "immediate moment in time" refers to another core communication component studied by Carkhuff, that of immediacy. Again the standard battle. The patient wishes to deal with material that happened before, or that will happen later, none of which is occurring in the clinic, before your eyes, at that immediate moment in time. Both historical information and patient goals are exquisitely relevant to the patient's case, but after that information is established, the sparring begins. The patient, if you observe closely, will tend to deal with verbal material that is neither of the treatment setting nor in the now. The practitioner may decide to pull the patient into the present, regardless its inconveniences, or disagreeable qualities, or, for that matter, pain. Recognizing patient immediacy refusal is more difficult than it might appear. Humans in general tend to deny the immediate regardless, so the practitioner can get caught up in this human tendency, simply because the practitioner is human. A mutual comfort can develop between practitioner and patient when a nonverbal "agreement" is reached to avoid conversation concerning the treatment process, *now*. Immediacy appears achieved when the injured extremity is being treated, but what is the content of the conversation? Not as easy to do as it seems, it is important to constantly examine the *immediacy* content of the words in use.

One method of examination is to ask yourself whether patient references to people refer to people you don't know—outside relationships—or to you, the practitioner, and to the professional helping *relationship* the patient has with *you*.

Examine the question, "Have you noticed that you've felt a little nervous around medical practitioners before?" Can you identify what the practitioner did with immediacy, here? This wise practitioner purposely diluted immediacy so that the patient could stomach both the threatening situation and the threatening reference to it. The practitioner *created* a lack of immediacy to cook a somewhat sour soup, but one that could be swallowed. "Have you noticed that you've felt…". This is a reference to the *past*. Nobody is calling the patient nervous *now*. Oh, no. Nobody around *here* is nervous *at this moment*. Right? Maybe, though, at some distant point in the *past*, away from *here*, you *have felt* a little nervous. *Before*.

Not only did the practitioner dilute immediacy, but the practitioner pretended there was no immediate *here-and-now relationship* which, at that *moment*, was a relationship nearly defined by fear of the practitioner. Oh, no, again. Nobody around here is afraid of the practitioner at *this very moment*. But maybe, however, at some distant time in the *past*, away from *here*, "you've felt a little nervous around" not *me*, of course, but people *like* me.

The practitioner *gave* the patient a sample of his coveted immediacy refusal in order to begin serving this sour soup with stock made from fear. Eventually, if the practitioner wants to assist the patient in dropping this interfering fear, perhaps we keep the somewhat unspecific word "nervous," yet we assist this man in owning his fear at some point *now*, in *this* room, of *this* practitioner so that this fear can be identified and removed as a barrier to progress. This fear, obviously, might also be titrated nonverbally as a simple result of time spent with the therapist. Either way, the therapist is aware of the fear factor. Still, and most importantly, this practitioner intentionally gave immediacy away but, later, especially if this fear does not dissipate, it could become a good idea to take immediacy back.

As with the specificity battle, the immediacy battle does not have to be won, and sometimes it is important to lose the battle to win the healing. What is more important is that the practitioner keeps active track of the fluctuating position of immediacy during the treatment process and makes good *use* of it.

Carkhuff's core conditions are exceedingly helpful as a method for understanding not only what you say to patients, but why you say what you say. You do not, though, have to use the vocabulary of these core conditions; you can use your own experience, concepts, and language to comprehend the effects of your words. Still it does help to think of your concepts in terms of conversational polarities. Empathy versus interrogation is an arbitrarily fabricated construction, but this polarity does give a map for finding your last spoken sentence somewhere in verbal space. "You feel embarrassed" is one thing. "Why did you make that stupid move?" is another. How are these sentences alike? Why does it seem reasonable to place them on the same continuum? These sentences are conversationally polar and on the same spectrum because, albeit in different ways, they will yield the same information. The poles become more obvious when the first sentence also produces emotional affiliation, while the second sentence produces emotional distance. So it is possible to get two forms of communication out of the first sentence—informational and affective—but only one form of communication out of the second.

The other two conversational polarities that I covered here are specificity versus vagueness, and then immediacy versus spatial, temporal, and interpersonal distance. Should you become interested in additional core communication conditions elucidated by Carkhuff, I urge you to look at his system. Yet I will cover one more of these core conditions, but in a way which Carkhuff did not specify, and that is the core condition of confrontation.

Confrontation

We all know that when confrontation is improperly applied, it results in resistance. It can nearly be asserted, however, that without confrontation there is no learning, no change, no healing. Rehabilitation in any form is, by definition and in and of itself, a confrontation. We confront disabling conditions. We confront refusals. We confront restrictions. We confront barriers. We confront bad habits. We confront resistance. We confront entire lifestyles. And we confront people.

For now, however, let me talk about a more specific form of confrontation that revolves around words and that is brought to us by the development of cognitive-behavioral psychotherapy, a specialty that examines cognitions or thoughts. Then allow me to explain a small and focused aspect of cognitive psychotherapy, the irrational belief. And here we go again with which came first, the conversational tactic or the psychotherapy. I do this chicken-egg thing so you are sure in your mind that these techniques, as they stand alone, are not owned by psychotherapists, and you may use them ethically with the clear goal of producing the best upper extremity rehabilitation possible. Keeping in mind that full-on psychotherapy is maddeningly complex, it is not untrue that the older and wiser among us have always been able to identify and challenge what we today call irrational beliefs, and this human endeavor has been going on long before cognitive psychotherapy pulled itself together as a discernable, formatted structure and service.

There are many, many contributors to the field of cognitive psychotherapy, yet I would like to give credit to Albert Ellis since he was so fond of pointing out all the lives that have been reduced to rubble by chronic addictions to the toxic substance known as the word "should." Albert Ellis was the New York psychologist who created Rational Emotive Behavior Therapy, which is perhaps *the* cornerstone cognitive psychotherapy.

This word "should" has been written about so much that comprehension of the true problem with the word can be reduced to memorized, trite, and meaningless aphorisms. Let me attempt to refuse to contribute to this problem.

Ellis wrote that, "If you face yourself honestly, you can admit that when you view some loss or frustration as *awful,* you usually mean that, because it is quite disadvantageous; it *should* not, *must* not, *ought* not exist. You don't merely see it as undesirable but claim that the universe *shouldn't* foist it on you. Nor do you mean that because of its badness this event *preferably* should not exist. You mean that it *absolutely* should not! This kind of *should*-ing, *must*-ing, and *ought*-ing is unrealistic, illogical, and self-defeating..."[5]

"Should" is a disguised word for the idea of "need." Now relegate the definition of "need" to what you *need* for sheer, physical survival: air, water, food, clothing, shelter. You do not need to keep your job. You do not need love. The loss of either, or even both simultaneously, will not kill you. As stunning as this point of view can be to people who have not been exposed to it before, it is a healthy way to think. The moment the concept of *need* is bone-deep accepted in this way, life, and the universe along with it, greatly calms down and simplifies.

People use the word "should" to disguise misappropriated, irrational belief in so-called "needs" which are irrelevant to *survival.* You need your cell phone, now, don't you? Well maybe you don't, but your teenager does. "I should have a cell phone. I really should. What if there's an emergency?" That last sentence falls under the category of *evidence in favor of the irrational belief.*

"I should not have moved that stone, because I need this hand." This is not a reality-based statement and, as such, is an irrational belief. Actually this sentence holds *two* irrational beliefs. Notice the "should" word. The phrase, "I should not have moved that stone..." ignores reality, because this man already moved the stone. To actualize, "I should not have moved that stone..." requires either a time machine or magical powers. The stone-moving behavior is forever done now and is a part of recorded history.

Notice the "need" word. The phrase, "I need this hand," is not a reality-based statement and is also an irrational belief simply since not a few people with one hand are alive and are in no danger of dying. Other words interchangeable with "should," and that camouflage the misappropriation of the concept of *need* are "must," "ought to," and "have to." Also there is "should not," "ought not," and "must not," and you can see from the above example that the first of the two irrational beliefs is actually a "should not." I've seen it written that you should never use the word "should." Try not to think too hard about that sentence. Beyond that sentence's preposterous circularity, "should" is a perfectly fine word if used sanely. You *should,* for instance, breathe at least somewhat regularly. Breathing is a rational *need.* Whenever you get confused about foundational rational-versus-irrational beliefs, think in terms of lethality. Thwarting an irrational "need" or "should" will not kill you. Thwarting a rational *need* or *should* will.

Challenging an irrational belief is risky business because irrational beliefs are stacked one on top of another much like a huge cairn of rocks—remove one and there's another underneath—and people tend to guard these cairns with years of territorial and practiced "evidence" to support their irrational beliefs. I write about these irrational beliefs so that you might simply *hear* them in your patients, and then use the presence of these irrational beliefs to gauge the weight of any mental barriers to progress. There are a few of these irrational beliefs that you might add to your list of possible verbal confrontations, but only if you study your patient carefully, and only if you can estimate with confidence that your confrontation is feasible.

◎ Clinical Pearl

During any confrontation of even the most mild, irrational belief, you must know when to quit, and you must know when to sound a full retreat.

Remember trait versus state? If an irrational belief is a *trait* belief, stay away from it. "I *should* have this disease. I *shouldn't* be able to open my hand the whole way. I was terrible to my children when they were young." This form of irrational thinking may result from a long-term *trait* or personality-disorder condition, where confrontation will likely produce complications. Refer this cognitive, hand-health block to an experienced psychologist.

Conversely an irrational belief such as, "I *should* be healing up faster than this," which is a belief stemming from the *current state of affairs,* might be feasibly confronted with a simple supply of information. "No. I've seen and treated this diagnosis many times, and your rate of recovery is right out of the book." So far, so good. Then why not add an empathy statement? "I know you feel frustrated."

Here's a reassuring fact about empathy statements. It helps if your initial perception regarding the patient's immediate, state emotional experience isn't wrong most of the time. But the wonderful part about *genuinely attempted* empathy is that, if you're wrong now and then, *it doesn't matter.* A perceptual miss by the practitioner is taken by most patients instantaneously as a good try, and the patient will correct you without missing a beat and keep on talking. You lose no points at all.

So you say, "I know you feel frustrated."

Then the patient pounds the table with his good hand and says, "No, dammit. I *wish* I felt frustrated. I feel *angry. Really* angry. I could have paid my parents back by now, but I've lost so much money by not working that I'm just seething. I had this all figured out to pay them back and then buy them a vacation, and I could just spit. My dad's *never* gonna quit thinking I'm just lazy."

Did this patient clam up because you missed the perception? Not at all. The result is the same whether you perceived the correct emotional state or not. How can this be? This can be because the patient shifted over to rely on your genuineness rather than on your perception. Practitioner genuineness, by the way, was already mentioned here as one of the Rogerian core conditions, and it was also listed by Carkhuff. Genuineness, or congruence, is a *trait* condition of the *practitioner* that, hopefully, has been intact all along—something of a way of life—and which shows itself to the patient without much effort on the part of the practitioner.

There *is,* however, a problem with empathy. It almost doesn't matter in what setting or to whom empathy training is presented; trainee skepticism is the nearly standard response. A question seems more efficient, while a reflective empathy statement appears weak. Regardless, an examination of the ubiquitously stock social greeting may help clear up any confusion: "Hi. How ya doin'?"

"Fine."

Done. This question ends the conversation before it starts and often, perhaps usually, produces a lie. I am baffled by the use of this social habit in a clinical setting, yet it is used nearly as often in clinical situations as it is in social ones. Why ask this social question, collect a lie, and then ask the same question clinically a minute later and expect the truth? When greeting a current hand-therapy patient, it is more helpful to avoid this question altogether and then to either ask a direct question concerning hand functioning in the clinic, or to provide an empathy statement. "Good morning, Gwen. Come in. We're going in the second door on the right, there." Once the patient is seated, "Have you noticed any improvements?" Or, depending on your perception of the patient's emotional state, perhaps, "You seem, maybe, a little beside yourself."

The hand-function question will produce direct clinical information that could indirectly lead to a patient's latest relevant narrative story. Or the empathy statement can directly produce the life narrative. "Beside myself? Oh, I couldn't open a jar of peanut butter at home this morning, and how I'm supposed to keep running a restaurant, I'll never know."

You see, you couldn't have known to ask either about a peanut butter jar or about her restaurant anxiety, but you found out about both by *not asking a question.* And you already refused to ask the "How ya doin'?" question because both you and the patient know that the "fine" response is in direct contradiction to the presence of this patient at your facility.

If you already employ empathy responses in your hand-therapy work, you may be interested to know that there is no end to the ways by which these responses can be dressed up, modified, morphed, and developed. Should you be skeptical concerning the power of empathy, the best way to move beyond your reservations is to try empathy out.

Start by looking closer at the people, not just the patients, who pass within your visual range all day. Mentally choose an individual, and attempt to perceive that person's affective state. Then, silently in your mind, find the one word that identifies that state. Choose the person. Identify the state. Find the word.

I keep saying that aspects of these forms of communication can be more difficult than they appear at first. This is because aspects of these forms of communication can be more difficult than they appear at first, and I want you to know that any frustration you experience as you try to learn how to communicate in this manner is normal. Are you comfortable with words like "grumpy," "ecstatic," or "totaled?" Are such words even retrievable during the rigors of hand therapy work? Have you been contaminated by recent cultural refusals to use *any and all* affective identifiers? In the common vernacular, these words that name emotions have been dropped in favor of guttural sounds. Instead of saying, "You feel sickened by this," people now say, "Dude, you're, like, going *bluahh.*" Yes, the affective state in question is "like" the non-word grunt, yet this empathy attempt is a failed one for lack of specificity and, moreover, for lack of language. Find the *word.*

So you've chosen a person, and you've perceived the emotional condition. Now, silently, create a three-word sentence. "You feel _____" and fill in the blank. I know; this fill-in-the-blank technique appears canned and artificial. Nonetheless, for now, *try it.* Say the sentence to yourself mentally, "you feel sickened," "you feel cheated," or "you feel relieved." Consider the word that seems to fit.

The next step is to attempt these sentences out loud on people to see what happens. The worst-case scenario is the person who snaps, "Don't *you* tell *me* how *I* feel." This angry comeback is rare, and here we have, again, trends in the trait area of personality disorders. Back off—you didn't cause this trait condition— and try a "you-feel" sentence on somebody else. Most often, even the most basic "you-feel" effort on your part will cause speech to occur in this other individual. In fact, once you become comfortable with morphing "you-feel" statements into a less stark and smoother delivery, you will learn to look at the clock *prior* to providing empathy, because once you make the delivery, you will want to ensure that you have *time* to listen to all that follows. Otherwise you could produce *unethical* empathy, where you set the patient up to talk to you, and then you interrupt that expectation and send the patient out the door. Once you deliver empathy, you must be prepared to *listen,* and part of this preparation involves learning to value the art of listening and the *reason* for listening. In "Narratives in Hand Therapy," hand therapist Cynthia Cooper wrote that "...the listening skill can stimulate powers of self-healing for the patient." And, "It is amazing how effective it can be to just listen."[6]

What are some smoother forms of "you-feel?" Maybe, "just a bit jumpy, there," or "trapped like a bird in a cage." Or simply look the person in the eye, lower your head, raise your eyebrows, and say the single word, "pissed."

A word about television and movies. Hollywood seems to have trouble finding psychotherapy consultants to advise writers and actors who try to depict the roll of a psychotherapist. These uninformed actors, revealing no perception of the "patient's" emotional state, commonly say to the patient, "So, how does that make you feel?" In real life, this question negates the patient's state feeling at hand and causes a brand new feeling in response to the questioner. This brand-new patient feeling is typically, to say the least, not good. This actor question is a frequent media event, and yet it is almost completely irrelevant to professional healing efforts. Make it a point to avoid this hollow question. It has almost no therapeutic value at all. Rather perceive and identify the patient's emotional state. Find the word for that affective condition. Take a congruent, genuine dare at delivering the most accurate and feasible emotion word you can think of.

My goal is to convince you that properly chosen words can have a powerful therapeutic influence, and I hope that I have demonstrated some ways by which you may string words together to produce this healing effect during your hand therapy work. This healing-words process can become self-reinforcing, because once you see how well it works, you'll engage in increasing curiosity around its efficacy, and you'll want to do more of it.

Okay, so let me attempt an empathy statement on *you*. You feel mildly intrigued. As I already mentioned, you may feel skeptical, yet, admit it, a wee bit fascinated. This word thing could be *doable*. You are a healer—a very specific kind of healer with specific training and specific goals and specific parameters and limitations—but a healer. This vocational condition of yours, then, could very well have you chronically interested in this amazing process called *healing*. You may even wish to be good at what you do. Reasonable assumption? Likely. So within the ethical confines of your area of expertise, you hope to use all applicable tools, techniques, and creativity at your disposal to facilitate the fullest-functioning feasible result in the human beings who come to you for help. A portion of what you may ethically use to facilitate healing is called the *professional helping relationship* and much of that relationship is delivered using *words*. Therefore a portion of what you may ethically use to facilitate healing (and to stay, here, with the spirit of immediacy and specificity) is *you*.

References

1. Schindeler P, Stegink-Jansen CW: Introduction: psychosocial issues at hand, *J Hand Ther* 24(2):80–81, 2011.
2. Rogers CR: The necessary and sufficient conditions of therapeutic personality change, *Psychotherapy* 44(3):240–248, 2007.
3. Carkhuff RR: *Helping and human relations*, New York, 1969, Holt, Rinehart and Winston.
4. Ring D: The role of science and psychology in optimizing care of hand illness, *J Hand Ther* 24(2):82–83, 2011.
5. Ellis A, Harper RA: *A guide to rational living*, ed 3, Chatsworth, CA, 1997, Melvin Powers, Wilshire Book Company, pp 90–91.
6. Cooper C: Narratives in hand therapy, *J Hand Ther* 24(2):132–139, 2011.

15

Clients with Functional Somatic Syndromes or Challenging Behavior

Joel F. Moorhead and Cynthia Cooper

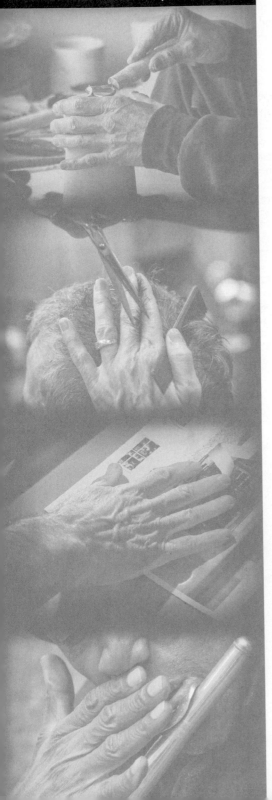

Clients with Functional Somatic Syndromes

A **functional somatic syndrome (FSS)** is defined as a physical illness that cannot be explained by an organic disease and that involves no demonstrable structural lesion or established biochemical change.[1] The distinction between *disease* and *illness* is particularly important. A **disease** is an anatomic or physiologic impairment of function in a structure or biochemical process. An **illness** is the client's personal experience of poor health. Clients frequently have illnesses that are not fully explained by available medical evidence of disease. FSSs can be classified as undifferentiated somatoform disorders, somatization disorders, factitious disorders, or malingering, depending on whether the client's actions are intentional or unintentional and whether motivation is conscious or subconscious.

The goal of giving clients satisfying and health-promoting rehabilitation care is particularly challenging for therapists treating clients with FSS. When the client's distress is disproportionate to the medical evidence of impairment, reducing the degree of impairment may not reduce the client's distress. The goal of this chapter is to help therapists become familiar with the types of FSS seen in clinical practice so that they can build a therapeutic relationship with even the most challenging client.

Undifferentiated Somatoform Disorders

Clients with symptoms that are out of proportion to impairments most often manifest one of the somatoform disorders, in which symptom magnification is subconscious and unintentional (Table 15-1).

Clients with **hypochondriasis** show excessive concern about minor health disturbances or intense worry over the possibility of future ill health. Clients with **body dysmorphic disorder** become preoccupied with imagined or innocent variations in appearance. Clients with **conversion disorder** have a bodily event (for example, paralysis or seizure) that is psychologic in origin. Clients with psychogenic pain and unspecified psychophysiologic dysfunction have persistent symptoms without apparent organic origin and without other distinctive classifying features. Clients with medically unexplained pain may have other diagnostic features as well, which could lead to a diagnosis of one of the somatization disorders below.

Somatization Disorders

More controversial are the **somatization disorders,** in which clients experience persistent or recurrent symptoms without objective or measurable medical evidence of impairment. Although these disorders occur frequently, general agreement is lacking on the cause and the treatment, and even on the status of some of them as legitimate diagnoses. However, questioning the validity of the diagnosis does little to help the client become more functional and may do irreparable harm to the therapeutic relationship. This chapter makes no judgment on the diagnostic legitimacy of the somatization disorders, but it recognizes the high level of distress in many clients diagnosed with these conditions.

Fibromyalgia

Fibromyalgia is perhaps the most common somatization disorder. The criteria for a diagnosis of fibromyalgia, established in 1990 by the American College of Rheumatology,

TABLE 15-1	Diagnostic Classification of Functional Somatic Syndromes	
Diagnosis	**ICD-9 Code**	**ICD-10 Code**
Undifferentiated somatoform disorders	300.82	F45.1
Hypochondriasis	300.7	F45.2
Body dysmorphic disorder	300.7	F45.1
Conversion disorder	300.11	F44.9
Psychogenic pain	307.8	F45.4
Unspecified psychophysiologic malfunction	306.9	F59
Somatization disorders	300.81	F45.0
Fibromyalgia	729.1	M79.0
Chronic fatigue syndrome	780.81	F48.8
Multiple chemical sensitivities	955.2	T88.7
Psychogenic tremor	306	F44.4
Factitious disorders	300.19	F68.1
Munchausen syndrome	301.51	F68.11
Clenched fist syndrome	300.19	F68.1
Secretan's syndrome	300.19	F68.1
Malingering	V65.2	Z76.5

ICD, International Classification of Diseases.

BOX 15-1   Criteria for Chronic Fatigue Syndrome

Major Criteria
- Fatigue is unexplained by other diagnoses.
- Fatigue has been present longer than 6 months.
- Fatigue has a definite time of onset.
- Fatigue has resulted in decreased activity level not due to ongoing exertion.
- Fatigue isn't substantially relieved by rest.

Minor Criteria
Four or more of the following symptoms are present:
- Impaired short-term memory or concentration
- Sore throat
- Tender lymph nodes
- Myalgias
- Arthralgias
- Headaches
- Nonrestorative sleep
- Postexertional malaise (lasting longer than 24 hours)

include pain on both sides of the body, above and below the waist, accompanied by tenderness at eleven or more of eighteen specific tender point sites.[2] Fibromyalgia affects approximately 2% of the population, although clients with fibromyalgia may account for 10% to 20% of visits to rheumatology clinics. The prevalence is inversely related to income and level of education, and females are affected more frequently than males at a ratio of up to 6:1. Fifty-nine percent of clients with a diagnosis of fibromyalgia rate their health as fair or poor.[3] Clients with this diagnosis commonly have other, associated symptoms, including nonrestorative sleep, fatigue, headaches, diarrhea or constipation, numbness, tingling, stiffness, a sensation of swelling, anxiety, and depression. Clients with rheumatoid arthritis and osteoarthritis report similar levels of distress, according to one measurement tool, the Rheumatology Distress Index;[4] however, clients with fibromyalgia report higher levels of distress in the areas of anxiety, depression, sleep disturbance, global severity, and fatigue.[4] Fatigue is also prominent in another disorder in this classification, chronic fatigue syndrome.

Chronic Fatigue Syndrome

The case definition of **chronic fatigue syndrome (CFS),** or **chronic fatigue and immune dysfunction syndrome (CFIDS),** includes several important criteria: (1) the fatigue cannot be explained by other diagnoses; (2) it must persist for longer than 6 months; (3) it must have a definite time of onset; (4) it must result in a decreased activity level but cannot be the result of ongoing exertion; and (5) it must not be substantially relieved by rest.[5]

This case definition, like that for fibromyalgia, was established primarily to identify subjects for clinical research. Salit[6] notes that these criteria "are not suitable for the determination of the presence and severity of illness, either in general medical settings or for medicolegal or insurance purposes" and that "clinical management should be based on an assessment of the client" (Box 15-1).

The case definitions for fibromyalgia and CFS overlap substantially. About 70% of clients with CFS meet the case definition for fibromyalgia, and 70% of clients with fibromyalgia meet the case definition for CFS.[7] Both disorders result in a high prevalence of work disability. Bombardier and Buchwald[8] found that 37% of clients with a diagnosis of CFS were unemployed. The prevalence of unemployment rose to 52% for clients diagnosed with CFS and fibromyalgia.[8]

Multiple Chemical Sensitivity Syndrome

A third somatization disorder that can affect perceived ability to work is **multiple chemical sensitivity (MCS) syndrome.** Clients with multiple chemical sensitivities, or **idiopathic environmental intolerance (IEI),** experience medically unexplained symptoms in response to low-level, identifiable environmental exposures.[9] Among the postulated mechanisms for MCS syndrome are **time-dependent sensitization (TDS)** and the development of **conditioned responses.** In TDS, repeated stressful episodes make an individual increasingly sensitive to low-level environmental stimuli.[10] With conditioned responses, cardiovascular, respiratory, gastrointestinal, or immunologic responses are triggered by heightened perception of environmental stimuli.[11]

Psychogenic Tremors

As with MCS syndrome, stress can be a factor in the development of **psychogenic tremors.** Psychogenic tremors of the hands and arms can manifest in unusual ways and have variable clinical characteristics. The severity of the tremor may be task specific, with the tremor often improving when the client is distracted.[12] Shaking of the limbs or body can appear exaggerated, whereas finger tremors often are absent. A twisting or ballistic component to the tremor can create the appearance of chorea.[13] Psychogenic tremor as a somatization disorder appears unintentionally and without conscious client awareness of motivation.

Factitious Disorders

Factitious disorders result from intentional client action, but without conscious client awareness of motivation. They more often arise from a psychologic need to be sick than from a conscious effort for material gain.[14] Clients with factitious disorders knowingly cause their own disease but are unaware of the underlying reason or reasons for their behavior. Several factitious disorders can affect clients' hands.

Munchausen's syndrome derives its name from Baron Karl Friedrich Hieronymous von Munchausen, an eighteenth century nobleman known for telling vivid but untrue stories. Clients with Munchausen's syndrome may cut, bruise, bite, or inject their hands and then give an untruthful history to the medical professionals who care for the resulting injuries.[15]

Clients with **clenched fist syndrome** have stiff, tightly curled fingers that resist extension.[15] The thumb and index fingers often are spared, enabling the client to maintain a level of function with the involved hand. Nerve block of the affected upper extremity or examination under anesthesia produces some relaxation of the hand, but often not full extension of the involved fingers. Some edema of the hand may be present, but it is not as great as in a hand that is repeatedly traumatized. (See Case Study 15-1.)

Clients who repeatedly strike their hands on a wall or other hard surface eventually develop chronic dorsal hand edema, a condition that has been called *secretan's syndrome*.[15] The fibrotic changes that develop in a repeatedly traumatized hand eventually create an appearance similar to the brawny edema that develops in the lower legs of clients with chronic vascular insufficiency.

Malingering

Malingering can be defined as the intentional presentation of false or misleading health information for personal gain. This personal gain is described as *secondary gain,* distinct from the primary gain of recovery from illness. Some malingering clients are seeking financial gain, whereas others are consciously seeking social or interpersonal benefits.[16] Although malingering generally is recognized as an uncommon condition (prevalence 5% or less), Mittenberg and colleagues[17] estimate that 29% of personal injury cases, 30% of disability cases, 19% of criminal cases, and 8% of medical cases probably involve malingering and symptom exaggeration.[17]

Evaluation Tips: Findings Suggestive of Simulated or Exaggerated Upper Extremity Deficits

Inconsistent Force Generation

Manual muscle testing provides information to the examiner in several ways. First, normal strength through a joint's functional range of motion (ROM) reassures the examiner that no abnormalities have been identified on this screening test. Second, examination of a client with organic weakness, such as that caused by neuropathy or myopathy, will disclose a smooth, consistent inability to resist the examiner's opposition. For example, the examiner will be able to flex the client's extended wrist smoothly despite the client's full effort to maintain wrist extension. An experienced examiner takes into account the client's age, muscle mass, and overall medical condition when assessing the significance of such a finding. Third, a client with disease or injury may be unable to maintain consistent force generation because of pain or structural instability. This results in a sudden release of resistance to the examiner's opposition. The client can be expected to describe the reason for this release of resistance clearly, providing information that is helpful for diagnosis and management. Fourth, the client may release resistance inconsistently, without other organic signs of impairment and without reporting incapacitating pain or instability. This *cogwheel,* or *give-way, weakness* is one of the physical signs reported by Waddell and colleagues[18] as suggestive of nonorganic pain.[18]

Nonphysiologic Pain and Movement Patterns

Clients with simulated or exaggerated upper extremity deficits may exhibit additional **Waddell's signs,** including extreme reaction to light touch (overreaction), tenderness that does not conform to established myotomal or segmental patterns, and sensory disturbances that do not conform to established dermatomal or segmental patterns.[18] Other similar and easily observed tests include Mannkopf's test and O'Donoghue's maneuver.

Mannkopf's test relies on the observation that the pulse rate rises when a client experiences acute pain. The absence of a rise in heart rate of at least 5% on palpation of a reportedly painful area suggests symptom magnification. **O'Donoghue's maneuver** relies on the observation that passive range of motion (PROM) generally is greater than active range of motion (AROM) when structures in and around a joint are painful. The possibility of symptom magnification is raised when AROM is greater than PROM.[19]

Associated Movements and Vicarious (Trick) Movements

Taking possibly simulated wrist extensor weakness as an example, several techniques can be used to assess the veracity of a client's complaints. A client simulating wrist extensor weakness may use the wrist normally when unaware that he or she is being observed. A client with a simulated wrist drop can be asked to make a fist while the examiner observes the actions of the wrist extensors. The wrist normally extends when a person makes a fist; only if the wrist extensors are truly paralyzed, as in a complete radial nerve injury, can the client make a strong fist without associated wrist extension.[16]

Even if the wrist extensors are truly paralyzed by radial nerve injury, a client with intact median innervation will be able to extend the interphalangeal joint of the thumb. This vicarious, or trick, movement is mediated by the abductor pollicis brevis and flexor pollicis brevis muscles, both of which insert onto the extensor expansion of the thumb.[20] Absence of this movement may be an indicator of symptom magnification.

Correct diagnosis of symptom magnification or an FSS is important for several reasons. First, an accurate anatomic or physiologic diagnosis for the client's complaints is an important step in determining what additional diagnostic tests, if any, are indicated. Second, the clinician becomes aware of the complexity of managing such a client and can plan to spend the needed additional time and mental energy to achieve a therapeutic alliance and a favorable outcome. Third, correct diagnosis is essential to designing a successful treatment plan.

♡ Tips from the Field

Treatment of Clients with Functional Somatic Syndromes

As mentioned previously, the distinction between disease and illness is very important in the treatment of clients with FSS. To recap, disease is a demonstrable alteration in anatomy or physiology with unfavorable consequences for the client; illness is the client's perception and experience of poor health. Both disease and illness are valid and important concerns for clients and the health care professionals who treat them.

◎ Clinical Pearl

Disease should be treated only when present; illness should always be treated.

Clients with a conversion disorder are unaware that their physical symptoms have a psychologic origin. Clients with somatization disorders feel unwell and can become truly convinced that they have a life-threatening or incapacitating disease or injury; this phenomenon has been called **dissimulation**.[16] Clients with factitious disorders have diseases or injuries that require treatment; in addition, to prevent future disease or injury, attention must be paid to the factors that caused these clients to harm themselves. As Hippocrates observed, "It is more important to know the person who has the disease, than the disease the person has."[21]

Clients with Challenging Behaviors

Reaching Agreement on a Treatment Plan at Every Stage of Treatment

Treatment of clients with FSS requires attention to the biologic, psychologic, and social factors that influence a client's illness (that is, a *biopsychosocial* approach).[22] Kleinman[23] observes that clinicians tend to evaluate treatment success by improvement in signs of disease, whereas clients view success as healing of illness. The five-step strategy recommended by Kleinman recognizes the importance of the clinician and client finding enough common ground to reach agreement on a treatment plan (Box 15-2).

Not every client requires or wants the type of negotiated understanding produced by this five-step process. This is fortunate for the busy clinician, because the discussion can take a bit longer than the 10 to 15 minutes estimated by Kleinman. This is especially true when the client's and the clinician's models for explaining illness have little in common. The therapist often has the luxury of being able to work through these five steps gradually over two or three therapy visits, taking advantage of the natural rhythm and growing trust that develop between client and therapist over time. The experienced clinician is alert for opportune moments to explore psychologic or social factors that may contribute to a client's illness.

Windows of Opportunity

In their study on client interaction with five experienced physicians, Branch and Malik[24] described "windows of opportunity" as unique moments in which clients briefly discuss personal, family, or emotional issues with clinicians. Based on the findings from

---

BOX 15-2 Five-Step Strategy for Reaching Agreement on a Treatment Plan

Step 1: The clinician develops an understanding of the client's explanatory model of his or her illness and the meaning of the illness to the client.

Step 2: The clinician presents his or her explanatory model for the client's illness in nontechnical terms.

Step 3: Clinician and client compare models.

Step 4: Clinician and client discuss illness problems.

Step 5: Clinician and client develop and agree upon specific interventions and elements of a plan for treating the client's illness.

From Kleinman A: Clinical relevance of anthropological and cross-cultural research: concepts and strategies, *Am J Psychiatry* 135:427-431, 1978.

---

their study, they suggested the following four ways clinicians can explore important issues efficiently:

- Listen attentively.
- Ask open-ended questions, such as, "Is there anything else I can do for you today?"
- Listen for and recognize changes in the client's emotions, appearance, posture, or voice. These windows of opportunity often occur in the middle of the visit. Ask a second question in a softer, gentler tone. Use silence, nods, and small comments to encourage the client to talk while you listen.
- Know when to end the conversation. Summarize the discussion and convey understanding and empathy.

Other authors have offered additional suggestions for establishing therapeutic relationships with challenging clients; these are presented in Box 15-3.

The health care professionals most likely to be sued are those whose clients feel that they were rushed, that they were not given enough information, and that their complaints were ignored.[25] Physician traits associated with malpractice suits include aloofness, lack of good communication with the patient, and too great a desire to accommodate or please the patient even if the request is not rational. It is very important to document when the client does not participate in his or her care. It also is important not to overly accommodate inappropriate requests (see Case Study 15-6).[26]

Participatory Decision Making

Clients who have been encouraged to participate in decision making demonstrate better follow through on their decisions than those who have not been encouraged to participate. Clients with the best health outcomes are those who express their opinions, who indicate their preferences about their treatment during appointments, and who ask questions. Physicians who regularly include their patients in treatment decisions are those who offer opinions and talk about the advantages and disadvantages of the options, who ask for input about patient preferences, and who pursue mutual agreement about treatment plans. These physicians demonstrate a *participatory* style. They elicit greater patient cooperation and better health outcomes than physicians who have more controlling styles of decision making.[27] This probably is also true for hand therapists.

BOX 15-3　Establishing Therapeutic Relationships with Challenging Clients

- Build trust. Positive client-therapist interactions require trust. Actions foster trust as much as words do. For example, return the client's phone calls and provide materials as promised.
- Provide good instructions. Focus on the client's agenda whenever possible. Clear instructions that fit with the client's agenda result in better client satisfaction and improved outcomes.
- Let the client talk without interruption at the beginning of the appointment. Identify which problems can be covered in the time available and which problems can be addressed at subsequent visits.
- Stay attuned to your sense of frustration, because this may be a sign that you find the client to be "difficult" (see Case Study 15-2).
- Be client centered. Use simple explanatory models that are easily understood. Avoid blaming the client; the therapeutic relationship can be harmed by the client's perception that he or she is being blamed (see Case Study 15-3).
- If a consensus cannot be reached with a challenging client despite compassionate listening, it may be best to refer the client elsewhere. Barriers to reaching a consensus include unexpected resistance from the client and communication mismatch. Noncompliance or the expression of opposition from a client is exemplified by denial of disease, conscious

- or unconscious sabotaging of the treatment, or a need to control every detail (see Case Study 15-4).
- Try to develop and convey unconditional positive regard for the client, family, and caregiver. Respect the client's autonomy and individuality and be willing to learn from clients' various backgrounds (see Case Study 15-5).
- Give your undivided attention to complaining clients. Dissatisfied clients tell twenty people, and satisfied clients tell three.
- Avoid dealing with difficult clients when you are too tired or busy.
- Don't downplay the client's perception of the seriousness of the complaints. Give each client time to describe his or her illness in its entirety. Listen responsively, but avoid interrupting.
- Make a statement that is empathetic. Work to establish a good rapport with the client, and do not be defensive. Convey that you are working with, not against, the client.
- Ask additional questions and take control of the situation. Ask what clients would like to be done or how they believe the problem can be solved. Create an action plan, and describe that plan in positive terms.
- Explain changes in treatment ahead of time. Fewer problems arise when there are fewer surprises.
- Follow up in a timely fashion and document the situation.

Modified from Levinson W, Stiles WB, Invi TS, et al: Physician frustration in communicating with patients, *Med Care* 31:285-295, 1993; Lin EHB, Katon W, Vo Korff M, et al: Frustrating patients: physician and patient perspectives among distressed high users of medical services, *J Gen Intern Med* 6:241-246, 1991; Lerner AM, Luby ED: Error of accommodation in the care of the difficult patient, *J Psychiatry Law* 20:191-206, 1992; Kaplan CB, Siegel B, Madill JM, et al: Communication and the medical interview: strategies for learning and teaching, *J Gen Intern Med* 12(suppl 2):S49-S55, 1997; and Baum NH: Twelve tips for dealing with difficult patients, *Geriatrics* 57:55-56, 2002.

Participatory decision making can be defined as the practice of offering clients choices among several treatment options and of giving them a sense of control and responsibility for their care.[27] Kaplan and colleagues[27] studied physicians' practice habits to determine the characteristics that promote participatory decision-making styles. They found that physicians who demonstrate participatory decision making are willing to spend extra time with patients and have lower volume practices.

Participatory physicians reported greater satisfaction with the autonomy they experienced in their personal lives. Short office visits in busier practices have demonstrated poorer outcomes. Medical office visits shorter than 18 minutes are associated with poor quality of information. Patients who had more time with their physicians rated the physicians more favorably. Physicians whose communication styles are less dominant receive higher satisfaction ratings than physicians who communicate in a more dominant manner.[27] In current practice, unfortunately, fiscal demands and business issues may challenge the ability of some physicians and hand therapists to provide participatory care.

Partnerships in Client Care

Quill[28] makes the following observations and recommendations:
- The relationship between the therapist and client is not obligatory, it is consensual. The therapist may speak with authority but should not be authoritarian. The client may ask questions, present alternatives, seek other opinions, or choose a different caregiver.

- The two parties must respect and trust each other.
- The client gets healed, cured, and/or relieved of pain. The provider derives enjoyment from being able to help, experiences personal or intellectual satisfaction from solving a problem, and receives financial compensation.
- The client's request may be incompatible with what the health care professional feels is the client's best interest, or it may conflict with the professional's personal beliefs. The caregiver should not compromise ethical, medical, or personal standards because of a client's request.
- Not all clients participate equally in their care. Caregivers may need to encourage clients to participate. It may be helpful, when appropriate, to request that clients participate more actively in their own treatment.

CASE STUDIES

CASE STUDY 15-1　■

A 58-year-old woman had tightly clenched long, ring, and small fingers on her nondominant left hand. This posture had persisted for 2 years and had been refractory to treatment by medications for dystonia and muscle relaxation. The client was able to use the thumb and index fingers to some degree. A diagnosis of clenched fist syndrome was made. Further discussion revealed that the condition began at the time of a stressful change at her workplace.

Treatment Approach

Make sure the client understands that she has a condition that requires treatment and that the likelihood of improvement with treatment is excellent. Perform an examination under regional anesthetic block, and fit the client for a custom wrist-hand orthotic while the arm is still under the effects of anesthesia. See the client daily for at least 2 weeks to reinforce wearing of the wrist-hand orthotic to preserve the ROM gained by the procedure. Perform and teach assertive passive, active-assisted, and active ROM exercises with the goal of restoring full ROM. Consider a custom dynamic wrist-hand orthotic to speed restoration of full ROM. Consider the timing of recommending psychologic counseling. Often the time to suggest counseling is when the client reports feeling sad or anxious, as many clients naturally will do as they become more comfortable with the therapist. Work closely with the referring physician to achieve the best outcome from a mental health referral.

CASE STUDY 15-2 ■

A female executive was seen after excision of a recurrent glomus tumor of the nondominant left small finger. She experienced a Code Blue that was narcotics induced. She stated at her next visit that her hand therapist had caused the code by upsetting her with a discussion of her therapy authorization status.

Treatment Approach

Validate the client's concerns. Tell her that you recognize that discussions about therapy authorization can be upsetting and that you are sorry she was upset. Ask how she would like to be kept informed about authorization status in the future. Recommend that the client discuss the factors that led up to the Code Blue with her physician. Call the physician so that he or she is prepared to discuss the Code Blue with the client. Coordinate all care as a medical team and document the situation carefully.

CASE STUDY 15-3 ■

A 60-year-old, right-dominant retired male executive suffered a radial collateral ligament injury to the small finger of his right hand while bicycling. He was shocked to learn that it would take longer than 2 weeks to recover from this injury. He could not accept this and demanded that he recover normal ROM and resolution of edema in 2 weeks' time.

Treatment Approach

Supervise the client's home program closely. Provide good explanations of the typical recovery timeline at every visit and include the physician in this explanation. Offer encouragement and enthusiasm for the client's progress, and explore ways he can pass the recovery time meaningfully.

CASE STUDY 15-4 ■

An elderly female underwent open reduction and internal fixation with volar plating for a left nondominant distal radius fracture. At follow-up, she had shoved long black strings from her holiday ham into her postoperative dressing; she claimed that these were her sutures, which had "fallen apart."

Treatment Approach

Make sure to notify the physician, who can explain to the client that the black threads are not her sutures. Also, document the situation carefully. Focus therapy on functional needs and positive aspects of the client's recovery.

CASE STUDY 15-5 ■

An elderly right-dominant female underwent excision for recurrent sarcoma of the right forearm, with radiation and multiple tendon transfers. She had had eleven previous surgeries on the involved extremity and was a well-informed client who had realistic expectations of her functional prospects. She followed her home program very well and often suggested appropriate upgrades. She and her therapist had a seemingly compatible and effective relationship. Near the end of one therapy session, she voiced an ethnic slur that was personally hurtful and offensive to the therapist.

Treatment Approach

Try to strike a balance between sincerity and professionalism. Focus on the client's clinical picture, and use the situation as an opportunity to practice professionalism.

CASE STUDY 15-6 ■

An operating room nurse was treated nonoperatively for a boutonniere deformity of the dominant long finger. She refused to make appointments and frequently arrived at hand therapy unscheduled. She was unwilling to wait to be seen even though she had no scheduled appointment. She called and interrupted the department director to complain, wrote letters of complaint, and also complained to the hand surgeon about being told she needed to make appointments to be seen in hand therapy.

Treatment Approach

Provide a nonemotional, factual explanation to the department director and the physician, and be consistent in requiring all clients to have appointments for therapy. Offer the client the option of seeking care elsewhere if she prefers to do that.

Summary

Ideally, the hand therapy client and the hand therapist will have similar goals. Also ideally, the client will attend therapy as scheduled, describe his or her illness honestly and accurately, make clinically appropriate requests, participate actively in treatment, and follow the treatment plan. When the therapist-client relationship does not benefit from these positive attributes, the relationship can deteriorate.

Through their recognition of the various patterns of FSS and the characteristics of challenging clients, hand therapists can more effectively shape rewarding therapeutic relationships. These positive relationships can favorably affect the clinical outcome for even the most challenging clients. Challenging client situations are opportunities for professional growth and can bring out the best care we have to offer.

References

1. Manu P: *Functional somatic syndromes*, Cambridge, 1998, Cambridge University Press.
2. Wolfe F, Smythe HA, Yunus MB, et al: The American College of Rheumatology 1990 criteria for the classification of fibromyalgia: report of the Multicenter Criteria Committee, *Arthritis & Rheumatism* 33:1863–1864, 1990.
3. Wolfe F, Anderson J, Harkness D, et al: Health status and disease severity in fibromyalgia: results of a six-center longitudinal study, *Arthritis & Rheumatism* 40:1571–1579, 1997.
4. Wolfe F, Skevington SM: Measuring the epidemiology of distress: the rheumatology distress index, *J Rheumatol* 27:2000–2009, 2000.
5. Fukuda K, Straus SE, Hickie I, et al: The chronic fatigue syndrome: a comprehensive approach to its definition and study, *Ann Intern Med* 121:953–959, 1994.
6. Salit IE: The chronic fatigue syndrome: a position paper, *J Rheumatol* 23:540–544, 1996.
7. Aaron LA, Buchwald D: A review of the evidence for overlap among unexplained clinical conditions, *Ann Intern Med* 134(9 pt 2):868–881, 2001.
8. Bombardier CH, Buchwald D: Chronic fatigue, chronic fatigue syndrome, and fibromyalgia: disability and health-care use, *Med Care* 34:924–930, 1996.
9. Cullen MR: The worker with multiple chemical sensitivities: an overview, *Occup Med* 2:655–661, 1987.
10. Sorg BA, Prasad BM: Potential role of stress and sensitization in the development and expression of multiple chemical sensitivity, *Environ Health Perspect* 105(suppl 2):467–471, 1997.
11. MacPhail RC: Evolving concepts of chemical sensitivity, *Environ Health Perspect* 105(suppl 2):455–456, 1997.
12. Koller W, Lang A, Vetere-Overfield B, et al: Psychogenic tremors, *Neurology* 39:1094–1099, 1989.
13. Deuschl G, Koster B, Lucking CH, et al: Diagnostic and pathophysiological aspects of psychogenic tremors, *Mov Disord* 13:294–302, 1998.
14. Iverson GL, Binder LM: Detecting exaggeration and malingering in neuropsychological assessment, *J Head Trauma Rehabil* 15(2):829–858, 2000.
15. Kasdan ML, Stutts JT: Factitious disorders of the upper extremity, *J Hand Surg Am* 20(3 Pt 2):S57–S60, 1994.
16. Green LN: Malingering, dissimulation, and conversion-hysteria, *Trauma* 6:3–21, 2002.
17. Mittenbert W, Patton C, Canyock EM, et al: Base rates of malingering and symptom exaggeration, *J Clin Exper Neuropsychol* 24(8):1094–1102, 2002.
18. Waddell G, McCulloch JA, Kummel E, et al: Nonorganic physical signs in low back pain, *Spine* 5:117–125, 1980.
19. Kiester PD, Duke AD: Is it malingering or is it real?: eight signs that point to nonorganic back pain, *Postgrad Med* 106:77–84, 1999.
20. Parry CBW: Trick movements, *Proc Royal Soc Med* 63:674–676, 1970.
21. Novack DM, Epstein RM, Paulsen RH: Toward creating physician-healers: fostering medical students' self-awareness, personal growth, and well-being, *Acad Med* 74(5):516–520, 1999.
22. Goldberg RJ, Novack DH, Gask L: The recognition and management of somatization: what is needed in primary care training, *Psychosomatics* 33:55–61, 1992.
23. Kleinman A: Clinical relevance of anthropological and cross-cultural research: concepts and strategies, *Am J Psychiatry* 135:427–431, 1978.
24. Branch WT, Malik TK: Using "windows of opportunity" in brief interviews to understand patients' concerns, *JAMA* 269:1667–1668, 1993.
25. Eisenberg L: Medicine: molecular, monetary, or more than both? *JAMA* 274:331–334, 1995.
26. Lerner AM, Luby ED: Error of accommodation in the care of the difficult patient, *J Psychiatry Law* 20:191–206, 1992.
27. Kaplan SH, Greenfield S, Gandek B, et al: Characteristics of physicians with participatory decision-making styles, *Ann Intern Med* 124:497–504, 1996.
28. Quill TE: Partnerships in patient care: a contractual approach, *Ann Intern Med* 124:228–234, 1983.

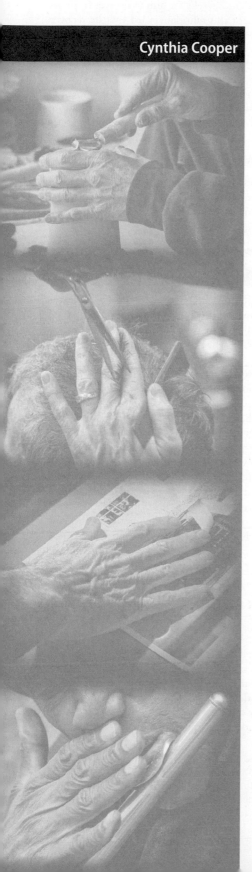

16 Narratives in Hand Therapy*

Cynthia Cooper

Statement of the Problem: The Illness Experience

Clinicians and patients do not always use the same end points to define the patient's recovery as a success. Clinicians may include in their definitions of success measures of reductions in disease and impairment, whereas patients tend to measure their success in terms of recovery of function.[1] Given the strong correlation between disability and mood, stress, and beliefs and the usually more limited correlation with disease or impairment,[2] a patient's physical problem, such as a hand injury, cannot be separated from the personal experiences that give the problem its meaning. The meaning a problem or injury embodies for a patient is idiosyncratic, circumstantial, and personal. The illness experience can help explain how a person's diagnosis affects his or her life.[3,4,5] Narrative medicine helps therapists treat the illness experience, not just the disease. This involves listening empathetically, trying to imagine how the situation feels to the patient and also how it changes the patient's life and story.[6]

Narrative Example of the Illness Experience

Martha's Story

An 80-year-old retired woman fell while walking and fractured her left dominant distal radius. She elected cast treatment and healed with some malalignment. She presented for hand therapy 3 months later with a stiff, edematous, dysesthetic hand and wrist. She relied on her right hand for self-care. She told the therapist that she loved to take walks but had not resumed this activity.

Therapist Reflection

Through conversation, Martha revealed that her morning walk was not just for exercise. She explained that it could take her more than 2 hours to walk around the block, because she paused and visited her friends and neighbors along the way. Walking was her social outlet, and her illness experience had disrupted it.

Solution

With further discussion, her hand therapist helped her explore ways to reestablish sufficient confidence to resume taking walks. She gradually incorporated arm exercises into her walking.

Narrative Message

The patient was very pleased to be able to resume walking. Recovering her social connection helped her reconnect with her pre-injury experiences and gave her a renewed sense of hopefulness about restoring her involvement in other activities as well.

Introduction to Narrative Medicine

Dr. Rita Charon's appreciation that a substantial portion of medicine involves the exchange of stories motivated her to earn a PhD studying narrative in English literature while she was active in her primary care practice. Finding that her improved understanding of narrative helped her better connect with her patients, she developed this aspect of her practice and coined the term "narrative medicine." Absorbing and interpreting the patient's story and being able to retell that story and give it form and meaning helped her

This chapter is a reprint of Cynthia Cooper's article for the Journal of Hand Therapy, Volume 24, Issue 2, Pages 132-139, April 2011.

and her patients realize the complexity of the illness experience, creating new possibilities for healing.[7] The narrative approach asks health providers to absorb, interpret, recognize, and be moved by patients' stories.

Operationally, narrative medicine looks like casual conversation between the provider and patient. The provider uses communication techniques that elicit personal and meaningful information from the patient. Both the patient and the provider are engaged in the exchange with the provider listening actively, reflecting, maintaining eye contact, avoiding interruptions, and asking open-ended questions.[8] Patients feel listened-to by being given opportunities to convey personal and emotional aspects of their illness.

When we listen to patients' stories, we collaborate with them and can empower them to create new life stories. In other words, providers who facilitate the unfolding of patients' stories[6] help them to become authors of their lives, which restores or enhances a sense of control.[9] To do this requires engagement with the patient. In other words, just listening is not enough; the therapist must also be engaged in the interaction.[10]

Another aspect of the practice of narrative medicine is the process of reflection. Charon[10] describes the "reflective space" that leads to a fresh or clearer version of the meaning of one's story. When therapists state the patients' narrative back to the patient, they show that they are listening and reflecting.

The **narrative fallacy** occurs when we create a story that confirms our flawed interpretation of a circumstance.[11] When patients' stories are reinforcing their illness, pain, or disability, therapists can help develop a more accurate, adaptive, and enabling story. For example, a patient who is having trouble performing range of motion soon after tenolysis for fear of hindering healing may do better when encouraged to adopt the more accurate and adaptive narrative of performing range of motion to remodel soft tissue and prevent adhesions.

Emotional Labor

Practicing narrative medicine is not easy. It requires emotional labor. Emotional labor occurs when clinicians regulate the emotions they display to convey a desired professional image.[12] Narrative medicine helps physicians (and therapists) become more supportive as colleagues, enhancing self-reflection that fosters greater sensitivity to the complexity of peoples' lives. In this way, narrative medicine promotes a sense of physician (and therapist) society, where individual patient stories matter.[10]

Regulating one's emotional display while looking sincere can be challenging at times, such as when a patient's ideas about the injury are very dissimilar to the clinicians. Understanding the importance and strength of one's intuition can help depersonalize these disagreements and keep the relationship from becoming adversarial. It is not that the patient lacks respect for your views as the expert, it is just that—right or wrong—they value and respect their own intuition and gut feelings more than your expert advice.

Narrative Example of Emotional Labor

Jack's Story

An active 60-year-old male executive sustained a radial collateral ligament injury to his right dominant small finger proximal interphalangeal joint while bicycling, which was one of his favorite activities.

Therapist Reflection

This patient loved to ride his bicycle. When discussing his progress and the typical timeline for recovery, he was shocked to learn that it could take longer than 2 weeks for him to recover from his injury. He could not accept this and demanded that he recover normal range of motion and resolution of all symptoms in 2 weeks' time.

Solution

The therapist helped him explore other activities to do temporarily while recovering, which helped him occupy his time more effectively, and the hand team provided enthusiasm and encouragement for his progress.

Narrative Message

This patient was used to being in charge in all aspects of his life, and he was going stir-crazy not being able to perform his usual high-demand athletic activities.

Procedural Reasoning versus Interactive Reasoning

Narrative medicine emphasizes interactive over procedural reasoning. **Procedural reasoning** is where an expert uses structured actions (procedural knowledge) to accomplish goals. Procedural reasoning is used to decide what treatment to use at what frequency or intensity.[13,14] There is a certain comfort in having procedures and rules for care but when providers use only procedural reasoning, evaluation and treatment may resemble a cookbook approach. By comparison, when providers collaborate with patients to understand their unique needs, it is called **interactive reasoning**.[13,15] Interactive reasoning looks like a social interaction but is actually a purposeful process that helps the therapist understand the patient while also building rapport.[13] Interactive reasoning uses the patient interaction to bring to light and amplify information that is relevant to recovery.[4] This is facilitated when the therapist elicits the patient's story and appreciates the patient's emotional tone and nonverbal communication.[6] By eliciting and restating the patient's narrative, both the patient and therapist come to a better understanding of how the patient makes sense of his or her illness experience.[14,16] This insight can create new opportunities for addressing the illness.

Narrative Example of Interactive Reasoning

Ms. Jones' Story

A young woman was experiencing nonspecific pain related to typing at work. She was taught postural exercises by a hand therapist as part of a program to help her be more comfortable at work. She returned to the therapist reporting that she had not performed her postural exercises as instructed, although she could demonstrate that she understood them.

Therapist Reflection

After confirming her desire for relief of symptoms, the patient noted that she was feeling self-conscious because she had been gaining weight, and she was concerned that practicing better posture would make her look heavier and "less attractive." The consequent discussion of weight management options was meaningful to the patient. Once she started participating in a program for weight reduction, she might be willing to practice better posture as well.

Solution

The patient's narrative helped the therapist understand the lack of follow-through. Elucidation of the patient's experience of the illness and suggested treatments improved the therapist's connection with the patient and led to useful support and guidance with participation in a weight reduction program.

Narrative Message

What looked like noncompliance was not straightforward refusal to follow suggestions. This patient was not able to practice better posture at work if it made her feel like she looked heavier.

Mechanistic Paradigm versus Phenomenological Paradigm

A study of clinical reasoning among occupational therapists identified two paradigms of treatment: the **mechanistic paradigm** and the **phenomenological paradigm**. The mechanistic or Newtonian paradigm assumes that humans work much like machines. This has also been referred to as the *biomedical model*. It is provider or expert centered and has an authoritarian nature with the provider telling the patient what to do. Objective measures and quantitative language typify this paradigm. The therapist focuses on measurable improvement in impairments rather than on the patient's quality of life and function/disability. In the mechanistic approach, the therapist is in control of the treatment process and the measures of success, and the patient is expected to comply with the therapist's instructions and derive satisfaction from improvements in the measures.

The phenomenological paradigm places emphasis on how things appear to be as being as important, or more important, than how things actually are. This paradigm centers on the patient's experience of their illness and promotes shared decision making. Subjective measures and qualitative language represent this paradigm.[17] This is also referred to as the *biopsychosocial* in contrast to the biomedical model of medicine.

In this model, the therapist sees the whole person, not just the injured part or the pathophysiology (disease). There is collaboration between patient and therapist, and the patients' interests, abilities, and motivation are considered when working together to make decisions about treatment.[18] The therapist understands the impact of the illness on the patient's life and addresses this while also performing the tissue-specific interventions of mechanistic care. The effort involved in this more holistic approach is well worth it—the patients' compliance is reported to be greater when they are encouraged to tell their stories.[19]

Narrative Example of Phenomenological Paradigm

Emily's Story

A female music professor found it difficult to play her instrument because of pain in her left wrist. Her pain increased after operative treatment of an ulnar styloid nonunion and triangular fibrocartilage complex defect.

Therapist Reflection

Emily told the hand therapist that music was her passion and "her life."

Solution

Working within this narrative, the therapist addressed the uniquely personal and symbolic (that is, phenomenological) aspects of her illness by suggesting that she bring her flute to hand therapy and by incorporating the functional demands of playing the flute in her hand therapy program.

Narrative Message

This patient found it very distressing that she could not even assemble, let alone play, her flute because of the pain in her wrist. She later told the therapist that bringing her flute to therapy was very important for her, because it was like bringing her best friend to therapy for support.

The Medical History Is Only Part of the Story

Patients' lives and experiences are complex and multifaceted. Time constraints may force therapists to focus on the medical history, but this should not preclude our efforts to learn more about the patient. The use of a narrative approach broadens awareness of our patients' illness experience. Hand therapists and other medical providers may feel required to focus on pathology. Clinical conversations tend to emphasize impairments and symptoms. Mattingly[6] refers to this as chart talk. An alternative is to place emphasis on the patient's story. The use of storytelling in narrative medicine leads to greater appreciation of the complexity of the illness experiences and promotes more patient-centered care.

Narrative Example of Learning More of the Story

Mrs. Smith's Story

A middle-aged woman with hearing impairment and cochlear implants was sent to hand therapy with a diagnosis of left hand numbness. Nerve conduction studies were normal. Her symptoms were vague, variable, and not characteristic of a specific disease. When the patient was encouraged to tell her story, she revealed that she had recently been to the emergency department with uncontrolled right hand and upper extremity spasms and had been told that her symptoms were "psychological." She expressed concern to her physicians that she wondered if she might have multiple sclerosis. She has been told by her doctors that because of her cochlear implants, she is not a candidate for a computed tomographic scan.

Therapist Reflection

During her visits to the hand therapist, the patient explained that she works two jobs, her son's friend recently committed suicide, and her daughter was missing the year in school because of illness. She also explained that her hearing diminished as a young girl at a time when her parents were divorcing and she was being taken care of by her older sister who "yelled all the time." The patient describes spontaneously losing her hearing, but after a few years she experienced some return of hearing. After seeing many experts, she was diagnosed with hearing impairment of psychological origin.

Solution

When therapists feel that patients' stories are difficult to relate to and hard to imagine, they should draw on their resources of professional behaviors and think of these differences as an opportunity to react sensitively and to be moved by the life challenges and adversities that are revealed in patients' stories. Doing so can clarify the differences between impairment and disability, disease and illness, increasing empathy and decreasing frustration. It can also help the therapist place realistic limits on their role without taking hope from the patient.

Narrative Message

The narrative approach requires therapists to try to understand what it must be like to be in the patient's situation.[20,21] It is easiest to experience empathy with patients who are similar to ourselves.[12]

Stories Are Not Trivial

What looks like idle chit chat in the clinic may in fact be essential for uncovering and incorporating narrative in hand therapy. A brief remark or detail from a patient may seem to be trivial from the mechanistic viewpoint but may be quite significant from the phenomenological viewpoint. Said more plainly, a detail that seems trivial from a physical point of view may actually be very important to that patient from a psychological point of view.[4]

Narrative Example of a Seemingly Small Detail

Rebecca's Story

A 64-year-old female sustained an embarrassing fall in public with resulting right dominant shoulder pain and rotator cuff tendinopathy. Her pain worsened during her initial therapy sessions. She changed providers and was diagnosed with complex regional pain syndrome. She received multiple stellate ganglion blocks, along with other medications and attended hand therapy after her blocks. She developed severe stiffness of her wrist and digits. Her hands were edematous and dysesthetic. In the patient's words, "I thought I would be cured after the first injection, even though I had been told otherwise, so it was disappointing when I was not dramatically better all of a sudden." She further commented, "It is exhausting to hurt all the time. And my pain affects my entire family. I have learned to appreciate those who have to live with constant pain."

Therapist Reflection

Before the fall, the patient had been very independent. She was widowed and had raised five children on her own. She told the therapist, "I was used to taking charge of things. It is very difficult to have to rely on others to help with driving, dressing, and personal care. This cannot be me."

Solution

The therapist provided extra time for conversation and discussion with Rebecca. She made good functional improvement over time and valued the opportunity to tell her story.

Narrative Message

Having to rely on others was extremely difficult for this patient who was proud of her independence and self-sufficiency. Talking helped her recognize this and led to her being able to receive help from friends temporarily. In her words, "I am the type of person who has to talk about things. Physicians typically do not have time to do that. It has made a big difference for me to be able to listen, learn, and talk in hand therapy."

Hand Therapy Can Help Even If It Cannot Cure

Hand therapists need to know their limitations, but even with limitations, the listening skill can stimulate powers of self-healing for the patient. Narrative medicine helps therapists have an impact on patients' well-being beyond the upper extremity. An underacknowledged but substantial part of hand therapy involves the mind and the spirit of the patient. Therapists who present a positive and respectful regard establish more of the rapport needed to elicit patients' stories.[22] Some patients' stories are so sad or complex that the hand therapist may feel overwhelmed. It will help to remember that therapists are not expected to solve all the patients' problems. It is amazing how effective it can be just to listen. Even in the most challenging of clinical cases, details will surface in patients' stories that open new avenues for problem solving leading to productive hand therapy interventions and experiences.

Narrative Example of Helping without Curing

Mrs. Miller's Story

An elderly patient was referred to hand therapy with bilateral wrist tendinitis and trapeziometacarpal arthrosis. She had a medical history including lung cancer, diabetes, balance disorders, and chronic pain. The hand therapist provided several interventions with minimal relief of pain.

Therapist Reflection

Mrs. Miller had weathered multiple illnesses in the past. She had surely developed strategies that helped her through these prior challenges.

Solution

Attention was focused on the patient's illness experience. The therapist encouraged her to describe the strengths she drew on in difficult times.

Narrative Message

This patient's stories led to an exploration of strategies for temporary pain relief. The patient acknowledged that hand therapy had not been able to cure her pain, but it had helped her to manage and live with her pain.

Patients as Actors in Their Real Worlds

A hand injury may disrupt an entire life. Therapists who appreciate this can help patients mend the disruption. By seeking information from the patient and then modifying therapy goals accordingly, a truly individualized treatment program is achieved.[4] Narrative medicine helps therapists create experiences for patients that give them identities other than that of an ill person, instead becoming actors in their real worlds.[6]

Narrative Example of Idiosyncratic and Personal Intervention

Jean's Story

A middle-aged woman fractured her distal radius in a fall while hiking. She did not go to a doctor until more than a week after the injury. The fracture was displaced and was treated with external fixation and percutaneous pin fixation. She told the hand therapist that she was bipolar and had attention-deficit disorder and other psychiatric diagnoses. During some of her therapy sessions, she was medicated and lethargic. It was frequently difficult for her to maintain her attention and focus at the hand therapy sessions.

Therapist Reflection

Jean required a unique and very nontraditional approach to hand therapy. She told the hand therapist that she loved to dance and that she would like to perform "theatrical dances" in hand therapy to express herself.

Solution

Jean performed dances in which she used her entire body, and she received the stretch and stimulation to the upper extremities that she needed.

Narrative Message

Traditional hand therapy did not fit this patient's narrative. Hand therapy by way of dancing allowed her to choreograph and accomplish her hand therapy in her own world and way.

Listening

Listening to a patient's story is one aspect of their healing.[23] When patients describe their stories, it is therapeutic because finding words helps contain the disorder and its associated worries, while also providing a sense of control over the chaos of illness or injury.[7] There are some situations where simply listening helps patients with their pain more successfully than the actual physical treatment.

Narrative Example of Listening

Patty's Story

A 30-year-old right dominant female dishwasher was referred to hand therapy with a diagnosis of right arm pain. She reported that an aggressive coworker who "had hurt other employees before" had maliciously shoved a crate of dishes forcefully into her, hitting her right forearm. X-rays and magnetic resonance imaging were normal.

Therapist Reflection

Sally presented with an intense expression of pain, wincing and moaning even when her arm was at rest. She told the therapist that she had been transferred by her employer from another state and had not been told that she would have a significant pay cut with the transfer. For this reason, she had to work 60 hours per week to make ends meet. She described a crowded and under-resourced living situation with family members and her children.

Solution

After having an opportunity to tell about herself, she stated that her pain was improved and that by listening, the hand therapist had helped her more than anyone else had.

Narrative Message

This patient had no one to confide in. Simply having an opportunity to express problems and frustrations and be listened to can help quiet an illness.

Enter the Patient's Subjective World

Narratives do not always have to reveal deeper psychological issues but may also assist the therapist in interventions, such as complicated ergonomic analysis. The art of hand therapy occurs when we allow patients to guide us to and through their problems.[24] To do this, our patients must have time to talk.[25] Yerxa[21] encourages us to enter the subjective world of our patients and to welcome the complexity of human nature.

Narrative Example of Entering the Patient's Subjective World

Mrs. Clark's Story

A 35-year-old woman who was wheelchair bound because of complications from surgery for a heart problem resulting in incomplete quadriplegia as a teenager, presented with nonspecific right dominant wrist and hand pain. She is a certified recreational therapist and an administrator at a center for independent living, where she also teaches independent living skills. There was no objective impairment, but 9/10 pain in response to palpation of the A-1 pulley of the right long finger. There was crepitus with composite digital flexion but no locking in composite flexion. She had no edema and no sensory complaint. She did demonstrate pain at the metacarpophalangeal (MP) joint of the right long finger, which was worse with passive MP hyperextension and hyperflexion, positions she used with transferring from wheelchair to bed and when crawling on the floor, which she did regularly at home. In addition, she had inconsistent vague pain at the ulnar right wrist that was worst when keying at the computer—a task that was necessary for work.

Therapist Reflection

When asked what she thought had caused or contributed to her right upper extremity pain, Mrs. Clark identified two factors: propelling her manual wheelchair and transferring from her wheelchair to her bed. When asked if she could perform transfers with more neutral MP joint positioning, she felt strongly that this would not be possible for various reasons. Splinting options were offered as part of a comprehensive treatment program, but she had particular needs and requests that were, frankly, contrary to the textbook solutions.

Solution

Ergonomic recommendations were made to accommodate the extremes of motion that Mrs. Clark used with propelling her wheelchair and transferring to her bed. In addition, nontraditional splints were made to help with soft tissue protection.

Narrative Message

Through narrative, patients may show us how to help them achieve their goals, sometimes in unconventional ways.

Conclusion

The practice of narrative medicine allows patients' stories to unfold so that their hand therapy care can be made personal and meaningful to them. This article applies the concepts of narrative medicine to hand therapy. The illness experience is explained, along with background on the development of narrative medicine. Obstacles to practicing narrative medicine, such as emotional labor, are addressed. Procedural reasoning is compared with interactive reasoning, and mechanistic versus phenomenological paradigms are discussed. Case examples based on the author's

clinical experience are provided to illustrate a narrative approach and methods of interaction that elicit self-healing powers among our hand therapy patients.

◎ Clinical Pearls

The recommendations below are based on the author's personal experience and on the literature:[26]
- Try to listen initially in the visit without interruption.
- Do not condescend or criticize patients when they express their views or beliefs.
- Ask patients and escorts open-ended questions about their view of the problem. For example, "Tell me more;" "Is there anything else?;" "This must be very difficult."
- Be yourself with the patient, and trust your feelings.

References

1. Kleinman A: Clinical relevance of anthropological and cross-cultural research: concepts and strategies, *Am J Psychiatry* 135:427–431, 1978.
2. Vranceanu A-M, Cooper C, Ring D: Integrating patient values into evidence-based practice: effective communication for shared decision-making, *Hand Clin* 25:83–96, 2009.
3. Mattingly C, Fleming MH: *Clinical reasoning*, Philadelphia, 1994, F.A. Davis.
4. Mattingly C: What is clinical reasoning? *Am J Occup Ther* 45:979–986, 1991.
5. Jackson J: Living a meaningful existence in old age. In Zemke R, Clark F, editors: *Occupational science: the evolving discipline*, Philadelphia, 1996, F.A. Davis, pp 339–361.
6. Mattingly C: The narrative nature of clinical reasoning, *Am J Occup Ther* 45:998–1005, 1991.
7. Charon R: Narrative medicine: a model for empathy, reflection, profession, and trust, *JAMA* 286:1897–1902, 2001.
8. Boyle D, Dwinnell B, Platt F: Invite, listen, and summarize: a patient-centered communication technique, *Acad Med* 80:29–32, 2005.
9. Frank G: Life histories in occupational therapy clinical practice, *Am J Occup Ther* 50:251–264, 1995.
10. Charon R: *Narrative medicine: honoring the stories of illness*, New York, 2006, Oxford University Press.
11. Taleb NN: *Nassim Nicholas Taleb, Wikipedia (website)*. http://en.wikipedia.org/wiki/Nassim_Taleb. Accessed March 21, 2009.
12. Larson EB, Yao X: Clinical empathy as emotional labor in the patient-physician relationship, *JAMA* 293:1100–1106, 2005.
13. Higgs J, Jones M: *Clinical reasoning in the health professions*, ed 2, Burlington, VT, 2000, Butterworth/Heinemann.
14. Schell BAB, Schell JW: *Clinical and professional reasoning in occupational therapy*, Baltimore, MD, 2008, Lippincott Williams & Wilkins.
15. Fleming MH: The therapist with the three-track mind, *Am J Occup Ther* 45:1007–1014, 1991.
16. Mallinson T, Kielhofner G, Mattingly C: Metaphor and meaning in a clinical interview, *Am J Occup Ther* 50:338–346, 1995.
17. Gillette NP, Mattingly C: Clinical reasoning in occupational therapy, *Am J Occup Ther* 41:399–400, 1987.
18. Brody H: The biopsychosocial model, patient-centered care, and culturally sensitive practice, *J Fam Pract* 45:585–587, 1999.
19. Barrier PA, James T-C, Jensen NM: Two words to improve physician-patient communication: what else? *Mayo Clin Proc* 78:211–214, 2003.
20. Yerxa EJ: Seeking a relevant, ethical, and realistic way of knowing for occupational therapy, *Am J Occup Ther* 45:199–204, 1991.
21. Yerxa EJ: Confessions of an occupational therapist who became a detective, *Br J Occup Ther* 63:192–199, 2000.
22. Pipe TB: Fundamentals of client-therapist rapport. In Cooper C, editor: *Fundamentals of hand therapy: clinical reasoning and treatment guidelines for common diagnoses of the upper extremity*, ed 1, St Louis, 2006, Mosby, pp 126–140.
23. Charon R: *Narrative medicine creates alliance with patients, Medscape Med Students (website)*. http://www.medscape.com/viewarticle/520704. Accessed May 20, 2010.
24. Morris MB, Morris B: *Personalized medicine and patient-centric learning: a core requirement for informed decision making, Medscape Per Med (website)*. http://www.medscape.com/viewarticle/576151. Accessed May 20, 2010.
25. Marvel MK: Soliciting the patient's agenda: have we improved? *JAMA* 281:283–287, 1999.
26. Branch WT, Malik TK: Using "windows of opportunities" in brief interviews to understand patients' concerns, *J Am Med Assoc* 269:1667–1668, 1993.

17

Personality Type and Patient Education in Hand Therapy*

Joel Moorhead, Cynthia Cooper and Patricia Moorhead

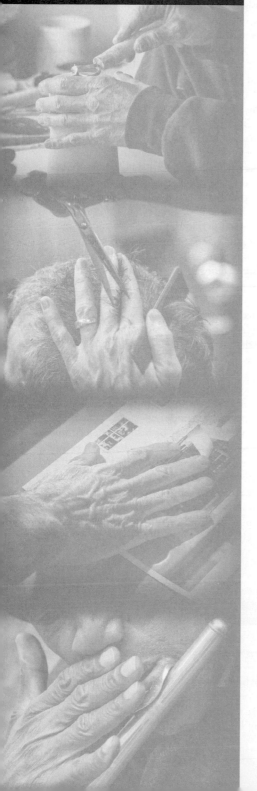

The MedlinePlus Medical Dictionary defines "personality" as "the complex of characteristics that distinguishes an individual, especially in relationships with others."[1] Personality theorists in the early 20th century began to challenge the assumption that people are inherently similar in character and temperament. In 1907, Adickes identified four basic ways of viewing the world, "dogmatic, agnostic, traditional, and innovative."[2] Kretschmer proposed different classifiers, "hyperesthetic, anesthetic, melancholic, and hypomanic."[2] The Myers–Briggs type indicator (MBTI) classification, developed in the 1950s, is based on the views of Carl Jung.[2] Personality classifications do not describe biological differences, such as being male or female; rather, such classifications provide a structure for appreciating the different ways in which people view the world and process information. For the sake of simplicity, this article will discuss aspects of personality as classified by the MBTI profiles.

Each patient who enters the hand therapist's office arrives with an upper extremity problem and a personality that can influence the therapist–patient relationship. The clinical setting for hand therapy encourages close therapeutic relationships. The therapist meets with the patient multiple times, face-to-face, helping the patient to reach goals that are of vital importance. The patient often enters the therapeutic relationship in a vulnerable state, feeling traumatized and unable to regain a high level of function without help. The personality characteristics of both the patient and the therapist can help build or can hinder this therapeutic relationship. A patient's personality characteristics may be an important aspect of his or her illness experience.

Injury is a universal human experience, more common in some people than in others. Factors associated with frequent accidents include emotional dissatisfaction, external locus of control, impulsiveness, hostility, and antisocial attitudes.[3] Marušič et al.[4] identified three personality factors that could identify injury-prone individuals. The first is "sensitization": the tendency to report more intense emotional reactions than those reported by other persons under similar circumstances. The second is an "avoidance coping style": the tendency to withdraw from sources of stress rather than to engage stressors directly. The third is a tendency toward extraversion, although this may be mitigated somewhat by a preference to cope with stress by direct engagement. Marušič et al.[4] suggested that the risk of injury may be increased in extraverts because of a tendency to become distracted and in persons whose intense emotional reactions prevent them from engaging situations directly.

The tendency to be competitive may increase injury risk when accompanied by personality factors, such as impatience, aggressiveness, and achievement drive.[5] Ekenman, et al.[6] found that runners scoring high on competitiveness and dependence on exercise for mood regulation were more likely to be diagnosed with a tibial stress fracture. Athletes with these personality traits may not reduce the frequency or intensity of their chosen sport in spite of symptoms, such as pain or swelling. This intensity of training can be adaptive, resilient, and healthy, but it can be taken too far in some circumstances.[6]

How can the knowledge that personality factors affect recovery from illness or injury increase the effectiveness of our patient education efforts? Do patients with different personality traits have distinctive learning styles based on their personality preferences? How can hand therapists recognize and apply this information in daily practice? This article will explore ways for therapists to transfer knowledge to patients most effectively

*This chapter is a reprint of the article by Joel Moorhead, Cynthia Cooper, and Patricia Moorhead for the Journal of Hand Therapy, Volume 24, Issue 2, Pages 147-154, April 2011.

by adjusting to differences in personality and learning style. The goals of this article are to present the MBTI profiles as a model for illustrating personality differences, to highlight the differences in learning styles that may be associated with personality preferences, and to provide examples of ways in which patient education can be tailored to each patient's learning style preferences.

Patient Narratives

Medical anthropologist Arthur Kleinman[7] described a five-step process to reach agreement on a treatment plan. The first of these five steps is to listen to the patient's explanatory model for his or her illness or injury.[7] The patient's explanatory model is the basis for achieving mutually accepted explanations of illness and plans for treatment. Hand therapists have the opportunity to learn from rich patient narratives, such as those discussed by Cooper in this issue, fostered by responsive listening over multiple patient visits. Empathy is demonstrated as the therapist understands in greater detail the meaning of the illness to the patient and the goals that the patient would like to achieve through treatment. To paraphrase a quote attributed to William Osler,[8] "Listen to the patient—he or she is telling you the treatment plan." Empathy flows more easily into a mutually accepted treatment plan if the patient and therapist share basic personality traits and preferences.[9]

One widely used model of basic personality traits and preferences is based on MBTI profiles. A discussion of the reliability and validity of the Myers–Briggs instrument is beyond the scope of this article but is available online.[10] The MBTI model will be used as a frame of reference for this discussion of personality types and patient education.

Myers–Briggs Type Indicator Profiles

The MBTI classifies personality types according to four pairs of personality preferences. People differ in fundamental ways on each of these dimensions,[2] briefly summarized by the following preference pairs:

Extraversion (E) versus Introversion (I)

- Extraverts are energized by contact with people.
- Introverts need more time alone to keep a high energy level.[2]

Intuition (N) versus Sensation (S)

- Persons with an intuition preference think conceptually and focus on future possibilities.
- Persons with a sensation preference want facts and focus on the present.[2]

Thinking (T) versus Feeling (F)

- Persons with a thinking preference tend to be analytical and objective. This is the only dimension with a strong gender association. Persons with a thinking preference are predominantly male.
- Persons with a feeling preference tend to consider situations in terms of how the situation personally affects themselves and others. Persons with a feeling preference are predominantly female.[11]

Judging (J) versus Perceiving (P)

- Persons with a judging preference like future events to be fixed and settled.
- People with a perceiving preference are more comfortable with having lots of options.[2]

The MBTI profiles are expressed as four letters, one from each preference pair, indicating the stronger characteristic within each preference pair. For example, an extravert with sensation, feeling, and judging preferences would be assigned MBTI type "ESFJ." An introvert with intuition, thinking, and perceiving preferences would be assigned MBTI type "INTP."

The words that patients choose as their narratives unfold can provide important clues to their preferences in each of the aforementioned dimensions. An extravert with a feeling preference may begin his or her narrative promptly with little coaching, talking about friends and family and how the injury has affected his or her own life and the lives of loved ones. In contrast, an introvert with a thinking preference may initially say very little, breaking silence to ask clinically oriented questions about his or her illness or about the natural history of recovery experienced by patients in general. A person with intuition and perceiving preferences may ask a number of "what if" questions about hypothetical future scenarios, whereas a person with sensation and judging preferences may ask for details of the therapist's current assessment and a treatment plan with specific dates and milestones.

Personality classifications, such as the MBTI, are nonspecific and are not intended to guide clinical treatment of psychological disorders. It is important to recognize that therapists will not be making a "personality diagnosis" based on the awareness of personality traits. Every patient will exhibit each preference to a different degree and may have an approximately equal balance of both dimensions of a preference. Preference terms like "extravert" are not intended to be labels or stereotypes. Preference terms describe relative tendencies, not a rigid or immutable state of being. Preference terms are concepts that can help the therapist to work effectively with each individual patient.

The purpose of developing a greater understanding of different personality preferences in the setting of clinical hand therapy is to communicate with the patient more effectively. The therapist's first efforts at communicating may be based on perceptions that are inaccurate. The patient's responses can give the therapist important clues about the effectiveness of the initial approach to patient education. If one approach is not effective, the flexible therapist can try another approach more tailored to the patient's personality characteristics. Packaging health care information in a form that is easily accepted by the patient may be more effective clinically and is ultimately most respectful to each patient as an individual.

Recommendations Based on Myers–Briggs Type Indicator Preferences and Learning Styles

Schedule extraverts with other patients or overlap their appointments. Schedule introverts with one-on-one time and no overlapping of appointments.

Extraverts may do best when a strong external motivator spurs them to learn. Extraverts may talk while they learn and do well if they can interact with others in a learning situation. In contrast, introverts may be motivated more by internal factors.

TABLE 17-1 Clinical Recommendations Based on the Myers–Brigg Type Indicator Preferences[12]

Preference Pair	Preference	Characteristics	Learning Style	Recommendation
E/I	Extraversion	Motivated by external factors	Talk while learning	Overlap appointments so that extraverts can interact
	Introversion	Motivated by internal factors	Need quiet time to process before talking	More one-on-one time with therapist
S/N	Sensing	Anchor learning on familiar facts	Linear thinkers; move from one concrete reality to the next	Few exercises; repetition; concrete facts
	Intuition	Focus on general concepts	Global thinkers; comfortable with complexity; "big picture" view	Original and imaginative exercises; let patient explore potential of equipment
T/F	Thinking	Analytical frame of reference	Challenge ideas based on thorough knowledge	Cite literature; be prepared for far-reaching analytical discussion
	Feeling	Personal frame of reference	Value approach based on caring and context of personal values	Create warm and caring professional relationship; context of patient's personal life
J/P	Judging	Value structure and schedule	Adhere to schedule with orderly progression	Create and follow written schedule of treatment with concrete milestones and goals
	Perceiving	Value choices and options	Explore options on choices at every step	Flexible treatment plan with goals and milestones that change as therapy progresses

Introverts may need time to think before they talk or act and may process an idea for an extended period of time before being ready to discuss it.[12]

Provide sensing patients with fewer exercises or activities that are graded in difficulty and spend more time on each. Provide intuiting patients with more variety of exercises or activities; allow them to explore the therapy equipment.

Persons with a sensing preference may anchor their learning on familiar facts. Sensing persons may relate well to concrete examples, moving in relatively linear fashion from one established reality to the next. Persons with a sensing preference are likely to be comfortable with repetition. In contrast, persons with an intuiting preference are more likely to focus on general concepts, as those concepts relate to the "big picture." Intuiting persons may respond well to creative and imaginative ideas that are complex, inventive, and original. Persons with an intuiting preference may be less comfortable with unvarying repetition, preferring frequent opportunities to look at situations from a different frame of reference.[12]

Talk about clinical evidence and evidence-based practice with thinking patients. Offer them references or articles. In contrast, express concern and caring messages to feeling patients.

Persons with a thinking preference are likely to question a statement if that statement is not supported by reasonable supporting analysis. Persons with a thinking preference may respond best when given the opportunity to challenge, explore, and analyze all aspects of a situation. In contrast, persons with a feeling preference may respond well to a warm professional relationship with the therapist. Persons with a feeling preference may make the best progress if they feel that the therapist cares about them personally and is working with them in the context of their own personal values.[12]

With judging patients, be on time, provide objective feedback regarding the clinical picture, and relate clinical findings to the status of goals. With perceiving patients, ask what they would like to start with or which activity or exercise feels most helpful to them.

Persons with a judging preference may respond best if they know exactly what is expected of them and when it is expected. Persons with a judging preference may value orderly, consistent adherence to schedule. In contrast, persons with a perceiving preference may respond more positively to choices and options at each step of the therapeutic process. Persons with a perceiving preference may value openness to new and changing circumstances and possibilities and may respond well to playful techniques that are educational as well.[12]

The clinical recommendations in this section are summarized in Table 17-1.

Examples of How Awareness of Personality Styles Can Improve Hand Therapy

A comparison between two opposite MBTI personality types may illustrate the very different ways in which each type adapts to the hand therapy experience and communicates within that experience.

The Extraversion Sensation Feeling Judging Patient

The ESFJ pattern of preferences is found in 13% of the population.[11] The ESFJ personality type may thrive on the social aspect of therapy and on developing a relationship with the therapist. She may want to know the therapist as a person and may ask questions about the therapist's family, education, or other topics that will help to strengthen the relationship. She may want the therapist to ask similar questions about her so that they can get to know each other. She may look forward to her therapy sessions if she enjoys the company of the therapist and may look forward to the social aspect of the session. This relationship-building helps to develop trust, which may serve both the patient and therapist well in therapy sessions.

The ESFJ patient may not question authority and may trust that the therapist is skilled and competent. She may be inquisitive and want to know why the therapist is using different modalities and treatments but may not question the rationale for the decisions. The ESFJ patient may want to know if the therapist has treated others with the same conditions—not to question the therapist's experience but to know that she has a connection with other patients like herself. She may even ask the therapist about the former patients.

The ESFJ patient may be goal oriented and organized and may approach her therapy in this manner. She may appreciate an organized and well-planned treatment session. She may become frustrated if the therapist does not have a plan before the session and appears unprepared. She may thrive on order and may expect structure in therapy sessions. She may do well with a written home program and can be relied on to carry out her home exercises with minimal encouragement.

The ESFJ personality may want to be liked by the therapist. It may be important to praise her for her progress from session to session, as she may need affirmation that she is doing well. She may especially like to hear that she is doing better than expected. This may encourage her to work even harder to please the therapist.

The ESFJ patient may be very conscious of her surroundings and may take note of things that others may not even notice. She may note the cleanliness of the treatment area, the organization of the splinting area, and the appearance of the therapist. She may form impressions about the clinic based on these observations. It may be important to pay attention to these details before the session by clearing a treatment space, straightening up the room, and acknowledging imperfections in the treatment area so that she knows you are aware of them. She may feel better knowing that the coffee stain on the therapist's shirt is because of a morning commute mishap and not because the therapist ran out of clean clothes.

The Introversion Intuition Thinking Perceiving Patient

The INTP pattern of preferences is found in only 1% of the population.[2] Let us say that this patient is a male. He may be an independent learner. He may read every reference that you provide as well as a few more. As he reads, he may instinctively look for associations with other facts and concepts. He may find those associations interesting, especially if they are surprising or unexpected. The INTP patient may want to discuss the concepts in these references with the therapist and may lose confidence in the therapist if he or she is not prepared for that discussion. The INTP patient may be disappointed if the therapist does not express interest in the concepts and creative associations that he believes make the treatment situation interesting. He may be particularly pleased if something that he reads results in a significant improvement in his condition or functional ability.

The INTP patient may not have a natural enjoyment of social interaction and may show little interest in the pleasant small talk that fills the air during treatment with other patients. However, he may have interests that he will discuss with great pleasure and animation. It may take the therapist some time to unearth these interests, because the INTP patient may not talk about them spontaneously. These interests may be difficult to predict. Asking if he has favorite TV shows, or if he likes going to the movies may be a start. Asking what magazines he reads may be an entry into his interests. The INTP patient may feel valued and understood as a person if the therapist can share those interests and chat a bit in those areas during the treatment session.

The INTP patient may not accept the therapist as an authority figure until the therapist demonstrates knowledge and expertise that he can verify independently, either by his own experience or by confirmation from reputable sources. He may not adhere to a treatment plan unless he understands the scientific foundations for that treatment plan in a depth, which approaches that of the therapist. Rigid treatment protocols may be a problem for the INTP patient. The INTP patient may believe that people and situations have a depth of complexity that is not appropriate for "cookie-cutter" treatment by rigid protocol. The INTP patient may be more comfortable if the therapist introduces a protocol as a "guideline," explaining in depth the reason for each aspect of the protocol and expressing openness to modify the schedule or content of the protocol as treatment progresses.

The INTP patient may be comfortable with silences, during which he may be processing something that the therapist has said. He may learn best if the therapist gives him a couple of minutes of quiet time after introducing a concept or change in the treatment plan. He may not appreciate feeling rushed through this processing time nor will he be likely to appreciate being expected to adhere to the therapist's guidance simply because he has been instructed to do so. The "P" (perceiving) aspect of the INTP profile indicates an enjoyment of processing information.[11] The INTP may benefit from thorough and ongoing discussion, in contrast to the preference for early closure that may be more pleasing to persons with a "J" (judging) preference.

The INTP patient may enjoy being given problems to solve as part of the patient education process—either conceptual problems or problems requiring manual activity—all the better if those activities are playful or help him to learn a new skill. Asking the patient with fine motor impairment to make a pipe cleaner animal is an example. The animal could be imaginary with the INTP patient having the opportunity to tell the therapist all about the previously nonexistent mythical creature that he has created.

What If the Treatment Plan Is Not Going Well?

Differences in personality style between patient and therapist can feel adversarial. Depending on how these feelings are handled, the therapist may decide that he or she does not "like" the patient. The patient may or may not be aware of the therapist's feelings.[13] The patient's "likeability" may affect the therapists' treatment decisions. One study using simulated patients found that "likeable–competent" patients were encouraged more often to telephone and return for follow-up visits than simulated patients considered unlikeable or incompetent. Unlikeable patients received more counseling on psychological aspects of care in this study than did simulated patients who were considered to be likeable.[14] The message here is that we may treat patients differently depending on whether we like them or not. Two aspects of this situation offer hope for successful treatment under these circumstances.

First, the subjective judgment of likeability can change over time. Some people are just easier to get to know than others.

Others will "grow on" us over time. Second, our difficulty working with patients who may seem unlikeable may be related to our relative inability to communicate with them. Appreciating and taking into account the differences between patients' communication styles can turn an "unlikeable" patient into a very "likeable" patient over time.

Patients with dependent personality characteristics may fall into the "unlikeable" category for some therapists. Dependent patients rely on other people for "support, direction, and nurturance."[15] Some therapists may prefer patients whom they view as taking more active responsibility for their own recovery. Therapists may work with such patients more effectively if they focus on the positive aspects of the dependent patient's personality in the treatment setting.

First, the dependent patient may report important physical symptoms promptly and accurately. Second, the inherently dependent role of being a patient may be instinctively comfortable for the dependent person. Third, dependent persons may instinctively have a more positive attitude toward health care professionals than nondependent persons. And fourth, dependent persons have been shown to adhere to treatment plans with greater frequency than patients with less dependent personality traits.[16] Appreciating these strengths may increase the therapist's enjoyment of treating the dependent person and the therapist's effectiveness in treating that person.

Even with the best possible therapeutic relationship, sometimes, the patient's impairments are so severe that he or she will fail to reach important treatment goals. Personality factors can determine how well the patient adapts to permanent impairment. One study on health education in diabetes found that personality characteristics, such as extraversion, agreeableness, and emotional stability, were associated with relatively positive perceptions of potentially adverse health care consequences. The strongest predictor of emotional response was "perception of the ways in which diabetes was explained to them"—in other words, communication style.[17] Considering patients' preferred communication styles can help therapists to discuss difficult topics with patients in a supportive and respectful way.

Lastly, some patients have dysfunctional personalities that are beyond normal variations in personality preference. In one study, 7 of 21 patients who were described as "difficult" by physicians had clinical personality disorders compared with only 1 of 22 control subjects.[18] Another study found personality disorders in 72% of the patients with somatization disorder, versus 36% in controls. Therapists may choose to consult mental health professionals for advice on improving communication with patients who have mental health disorders.[19] At a minimum, knowledge that some personalities are pathological will help frame the limits of what can be accomplished by working on awareness of personality styles and communication skills, which should help limit stress when things do not go as we wish.

Case Illustrations

Allen and Brock[11] provide tips for recognizing preference types and for maximizing patient follow through using the MBTI framework. They recommend that the therapist ask the following:

- Is the patient talking a lot (extraversion) or does the patient seem to be thinking a lot (introversion)?
- Does the patient seem focused on specifics (sensing) or the big picture (intuition)?
- Is the patient expressing logical implications (thinking) or the impact on others (feelings)?
- Does the patient appear more interested in closure (judging) or in processing (perceiving)?

The following case illustrations aim to demonstrate these tips:

- A 72-year-old semiretired man fell while exercising and underwent open reduction and internal fixation (ORIF) of his left nondominant olecranon with ulnar nerve transposition. He was quiet during the hand therapy evaluation and answered questions concisely after pausing to think about the questions. The therapist's initial efforts at friendly conversation elicited a cool response with only brief, terse answers. As the therapist recognized the introversion aspects of this patient's personality, she became more able to be quiet during longer intervals of his appointment time. When talking, she chose concrete clinical details for conversation, such as range of motion (ROM) gains. The patient gradually started to ask more questions in therapy, but the questions were mostly about the facts of his injury and timelines for recovery. The therapist communicated in these terms throughout the course of care. At this sensing patient's last visit, he stated that he had found the therapy helpful and educational.
- A 17-year-old learning-disabled woman was referred to hand therapy for bilateral upper extremity strengthening. She did not like typical hand therapy exercises and lost interest quickly but participated willingly in more creative activities, such as "sculpting" with putty. When a variety of exercise materials were placed in front of her, she spontaneously constructed mixed media creations with the therapy equipment using both hands (Fig. 17-1), and she did not want to stop at the end of these therapy sessions. By fitting the therapy to her intuitive style, she was able to build her upper extremity strength and enjoy the process.
- A 35-year-old nurse sustained a crush injury to her left index finger with resulting sensory loss. She had difficulty palpating

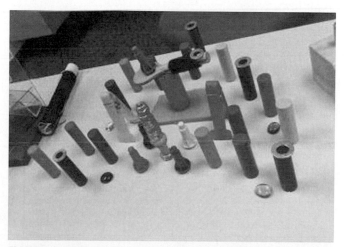

FIGURE 17-1 Free-form creation made by a patient with an intuitive learning preference, showing varied multimedia use of objects commonly available in a hand therapy department. (Courtesy of Cynthia Cooper.)

veins with the injured finger when initiating IVs. She had read articles about digital nerve injuries before initiating therapy. The therapist recognized the patient's thinking preference and provided additional references and spoke in clinical terminology. The patient read the articles, asked more questions, and made suggestions about her therapy treatments based on her readings. She especially appreciated learning that she was likely to continue to recover sensation and function over time. Having that knowledge enabled her to focus on compensatory functional strategies that she had been less receptive to initially.

Conclusion

Personality type may affect all aspects of clinical relationships between patients and hand therapists. Knowing what to do clinically may not be enough to guarantee good patient follow-through or a successful outcome. This may be particularly true when there is a mismatch between the therapist's and patient's personality types. Therapists who provide patient education that is tailored to each individual patient's personality and learning preferences can create therapeutic experiences that may be more rewarding for their patients and for themselves.

References

1. *MedlinePlus Medical Dictionary*. http://www.merriam-webster.com/medlineplus/personality. Accessed June 8, 2013.
2. Keirsey D, Bates M: *Please understand me: character and temperament types*, Del Mar, CA, 1984, Prometheus Nemesis Book Company.
3. Vavrik J: Accident prone, *Recovery* 9:2, 1999.
4. Marušič A, Musek J, Gudjonsson G: Injury proneness and personality, *Nord J Psychiatry* 55:157–161, 2001.
5. Costa PJ, Krantz D, Blumenthal J, et al: Task force 2: psychological risk factors in coronary artery disease, *Circulation* 76(Suppl 1):145–149, 1987.
6. Ekenman I, Hassmen P, Koivula N, et al: Stress fractures of the tibia: can personality traits help us detect the injury-prone athlete? *Scand J Med Sci Sports* 11:87–95, 2001.
7. Kleinman A: Clinical relevance of anthropological and cross-cultural research: concepts and strategies, *Am J Psychiatry* 135:427–431, 1978.
8. Pitkin R: A lasting influence: listen to the patient, *BMJ* 316:1252, 1998.
9. Larson E, Yao X: Clinical empathy as emotional labor in the patient-physician relationship, *JAMA* 293:1100–1106, 2005.
10. Schaubhut N, Herk N, Thompson R: *MBTI Form M manual supplement, CPP, Inc* (website). https://www.cpp.com/products/mbti/index.aspx. Accessed 2009.
11. Allen J, Brock J: *Health care communication using personality type*, New York, 2000, Taylor & Francis, Inc.
12. Lawrence G: *Looking at type and learning styles*, Gainesville, FL, 1997, Centre for Applications of Psychological Type, Inc.
13. Lieberman M, Rosenthal R: Why introverts can't always tell who likes them: multitasking and nonverbal decoding, *J Pers Soc Psychol* 80:294–310, 2001.
14. Gerbert B: Perceived likeability and competence of simulated patients: influence on physicians' management plans, *Soc Sci Med* 18:1053–1059, 1984.
15. Overholser J: The dependent personality and interpersonal problems, *J Nerv Ment Dis* 184:8–16, 1996.
16. Bornstein R: Depathologizing dependency, *J Nerv Ment Dis* 186:67–73, 1998.
17. Lawson V, Bundy C, Harvey J: The influence of health communication and personality traits on personal models of diabetes in newly diagnosed diabetic patients, *Diabet Med* 24:883–891, 2007.
18. Schafer S, Nowlis D: Personality disorders among difficult patients, *Arc Fam Med* 7:126–129, 1998.
19. Stern J, Murphy M, Bass C: Personality disorders in patients with somatisation disorder: a controlled study, *Br J Psychiatry* 163:785–789, 1993.

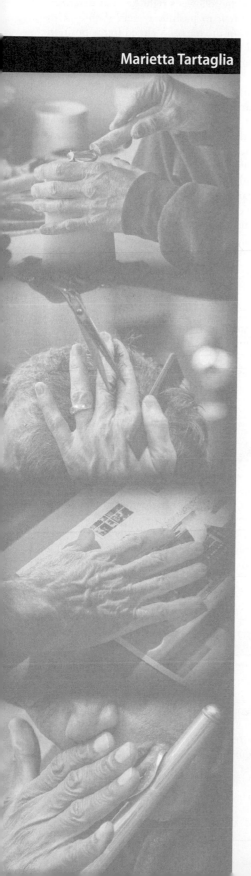

18 Using Dance in Hand Therapy

Marietta Tartaglia

Long before the dawn of history, long before man could sing or even speak, he danced. Moving to his own internal rhythms, the pounding to his heart, the beating of his pulse. Man danced. It is within us all... always.

—Gene Kelly, from the film, *That's Dancing!*, 1985

A Therapist's Occupations

"What's in your hand?" That is a question I once heard a prominent speaker ask when talking about the tools we have to engage in life successfully. It is a question all therapists should ask themselves when considering the best ways to interact with their patients. I am a ballroom dancer/instructor turned occupational therapist. In this chapter I hope to illustrate the unique partnership that is "the dance" of therapy. At the end of the chapter, I will describe how dance can be incorporated into hand therapy to promote upper extremity recovery.

The Basics of Ballroom Connection

Ballroom dancing is an umbrella term that encompasses a group of many partner dances. A few examples are waltz, tango, foxtrot, rumba, salsa, samba, and swing. While some of these dances draw from the more popular singular styles of ballet and jazz, they differ in one elemental way: ballroom dancing, like therapy, always requires a partner. In fact, it would not be considered ballroom dancing if there were not another person present, and the rules for engaging require the consideration and connection of the other person.

When a new student arrives to the studio for their first dance lesson, regardless of the dance they would like to learn, the very first thing I teach is connection. Whether they come in with a partner or by themselves, we practice moving as a unit. The basis of every lesson is learning not only how to move one's own body, but how to make two bodies cooperate as one unit. This connection requires a very special style of communication that occurs primarily through the hands. In ballroom dance, specifically in open position, the hands are an extension of the center and are extended outward from the body to connect in various ways to the partner's hands. Most of the information about body position, direction and intention communicated by both partners is coming through this hand connection and flowing in an open and dynamic fashion as an active channel.

In partner dancing, there is an active role and a passive role. Often the leader is in the active role, and the follower is in the passive role. The leader intends the movements and steps; the follower receives the information and responds to the intention. If the intention is not communicated clearly by the leader through the hands or is not received by the follower clearly through the hands, then the move will not be executed correctly, and the two partners lose their feeling of oneness. The range of motion, responsiveness, stability and sensitivity of the wrists, hands and fingers are requisite to making the dance beautiful and successful. This is what makes partner dancing a salient form of hand therapy.

In addition to thinking about connection while partner dancing, the student of dance must also learn a skeleton of standardized dance steps. It matters not whether the student is learning salsa or waltz; what is important is that the steps will become like second nature, as all of one's attention moves into the partner connection of providing or receiving direction.

Adding the Music and the Joy

Once the basic steps are learned and the connection is established, the appropriate music is played, and the student begins to perform these new movements to rhythm. This is where the moment of truth arrives. There is an exhilaration that is felt once the student begins to step in time with the music hand-to-hand and in unison with another person. This is the moment when if dance is going to have an analgesic effect, it will. As two move as one, distracted by the timeless feel of moving to rhythm and being in connection with another human being, the previous feelings of pain, incompetence, frustration, and inhibition that often accompany injury can seem to melt away. Dance becomes a beautiful method of shifting the focus from disablement to empowerment.

Incorporating Dance into Hand Therapy

It does not take years of experience to learn a few basic dance-related concepts to add into a therapy session. In the very advanced levels of professional dancing, both partners take on the leader and follower roles at different times during the dance. For the purpose of consistency I will give a description of the leader's role for use by the therapist, and the follower's role will be intended for the client. A video of these concepts is provided on the Evolve website.

From Therapist to Dance Leader

To create a social partnership frame in closed position, the dance leader will place the right hand onto the left scapula of the follower. The follower's left arm rests upon the strongly positioned right arm of the leader. The height of the leader's right elbow is dependent upon the height of the follower, but should rest in such a way that the follower's elbow rests below their own shoulder. If an outside pressure were to be applied downward on the leader's arm, the arm would not move. The right arm of the leader should maintain its position at all times. The left arm of the leader in closed position will extend outward in such a way that both elbows are in the same plane sagittally. The left arm of the leader connects to the right arm of the follower in a mirror-like fashion. This frame is extended outward and connects to the leader's center of gravity. When the torso moves, the frame moves as a function of the torso (see Video 18-1 on the website).

Open position is another very useful dance frame in which both of the leader's hands are held downward at the level where the forearms are parallel to the ground and the elbows are at approximately 90° of elbow flexion. In actuality, the follower's elbows should be in this position, and the leader will adapt their own arms so that the follower will maintain this relaxed position. The wrists will be held in neutral with slight wrist extension, the metacarpophalangeals in full flexion, and the fingers just shy of full extension. The leader is providing "handlebars" that the follower's hands will rest comfortably over. It is important not to involve the thumbs in the grip at all as gripping with the thumbs cuts off the available movement of the follower while performing turns (see Video 18-2 on the Evolve website).

From Client to Dance Follower

The leader will take a closed frame position with the right arm as described above. Instruct the client to place the left arm on yours but to hold it in such a way as to not weigh heavily on the frame of the leader. Connect to the follower's right hand as described above, and instruct the client to push away very slightly with both hands to create tone in the frame. A closed frame position for the follower is useful for creating shoulder stability, scapular depression, nerve gliding, elbow mobility, rhomboid strength, and overall posture.

To instruct the client into an open dance frame position, the leader will extend forth their hands as explained above and ask the follower to place their hands within. The follower will place their hands into those of the leader, holding their fingers in "hooks" over the "handlebars" of the leader's fingers. The weight of gravity will gently allow the wrists to fall into extension so that the leader's fingers make contact with the follower's palms. In this frame, a client is able to work on achieving wrist extension with composite digital flexion. The follower must allow gravity to naturally relax and extend the wrists into the hands of the leader, while gently maintaining composite digital flexion as a means to remain connected in the hands of the leader.

Dancing Together

Without learning any formal steps, there are many ways that both the open and closed dance frame may be used therapeutically. Any type of music can be played, and the closed frame can be employed to step side-to-side, forward and back, or even in a box step, moving as one unit in time with the music (see Videos 18-1 and 18-2 on the website).

Summary

Ballroom dance has, with growing popularity, found its place within many therapeutic contexts and among varying clinical populations. As I hope to have demonstrated, it also has its place within hand therapy as a means for promoting upper extremity motion and function. Not only is it a unique method for the therapist and client to work together, it is also a fun approach to incorporate posture, core, joint stability, range of motion, and coordination into the therapy experience.

CASE STUDY

CASE STUDY 18-1 ■

A female patient was attending hand therapy after sustaining a right distal radius fracture, status post open reduction and internal fixation (ORIF), with allodynia of her right wrist and hand radiating to the index finger where maximal hypersensitivity was experienced. She displayed proximal upper extremity guarding, holding her wrist in neutral and index finger extended. Wrist extension was painful, and tactile stimulation to her index finger was aversive. The patient often expressed that physical connection was important to her, and the hypersensitivity and pain associated with her injury prevented her from engaging in many of the activities she once enjoyed, especially horseback riding. Dance therapy was offered as a means to help recover wrist extension, desensitize the index finger, recondition the right upper extremity, and to give her a sense of the physical connection she felt she had been missing.

Dance sessions began with simple exercises to teach her how to find her center as well as to feel her weight distributed through her feet on the ground (see Fig. 18-1). In addition, a large emphasis was placed on creating a connection with her hands through her elbows and shoulders to her center as a means of directly communicating with both her partner and her own center. The patient's husband was present for the sessions and was able to assist her as well as discuss the similarities between dance and horseback riding (see Fig. 18-2).

Once the relevant dance frame and connection points had been established, a few basic dance steps were presented. As the patient learned to move her feet in time with the music and in connection with the signals provided through her hands from the leader, she became filled with joy and laughter. She began to lose the guarding behavior that she had previously demonstrated and began to flex, extend, and rotate her proximal upper extremity, elbow, forearm, and wrist. She tolerated tactile stimulation to her index finger without guarding while dancing with a partner to the music. This patient was now flourishing under the subtle guidance of human touch and interaction. Dance therapy was a safe, appropriate, and therapeutic substitute for the connection she felt she had been missing in her daily life after the onset of the injury.

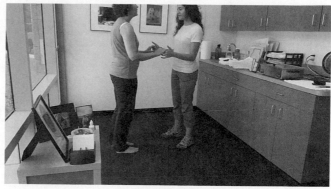

FIGURE 18-1 Patient and therapist in open dance frame with feet firmly planted and center engaged through upper extremity.

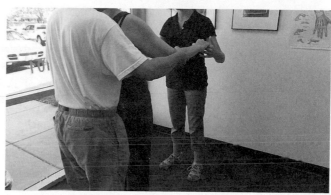

FIGURE 18-2 Patient and therapist in open dance frame with husband assisting from behind.

19

Applying Pilates Concepts to Hand Therapy: Connecting through the Hand*

Brenda Nealy and Cynthia Cooper

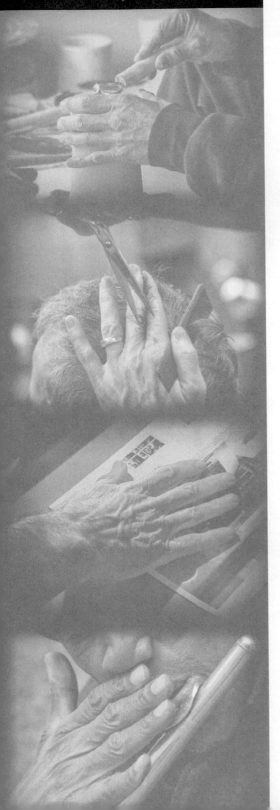

PILATES PRINCIPLES

A primary goal of the Pilates Method is to create a connection between the mind and the body so that without thinking, one would be able to stand, move and carry out daily activities with control and ease.

In the Pilates Method work, there are six basic principles.[1,2] The way in which the Pilates exercises are performed is based on these principles. Following these principles while performing the exercises will train the mind and body to connect, producing an attention-free movement. The way the exercises are performed is more important than the exercises themselves.

Concentration

To perform the exercises correctly, one needs to concentrate on the details of the positioning and placement of the whole body. The correct placement of the limbs will allow for a connection of the limbs into the core. In the Pilates Method, every position and movement of the body is interrelated and important.

Control

All exercises in the Pilates Method need to be performed with control. This is why one needs to concentrate on the details of every movement. There needs to be control not just of the large movements of the limbs but of the small movements as well. One needs to control the positions of the fingers and toes, rotation of the wrists and the curve of the spine. The awareness and control of these details will connect the mind and the body.

Centering

The center of the body is the focal point of the Pilates Method. This is often referred to as the "Powerhouse." It is the area that wraps around the entire torso from the bottom of the ribcage to the top of the hip bones. The goal while performing the Pilates exercises is to connect into the core muscles or the "Powerhouse."

Editor's Note: "Connecting through the Hand" is an original work in progress evolving from Cynthia Cooper's ongoing one-on-one Pilates sessions with Brenda Nealy.

Flow of Movement

The movement of each exercise should flow evenly and smoothly, Not too fast or too slow, Not too rigid or too loose. To keep the flow of the movement requires concentration and control from the center.

Precision

The whole focus is to do each movement with precision. It is better to do one repetition perfectly than it is to do many repetitions poorly.

Breathing

According to the Pilates Method, correct breathing is a vital part of the exercise program. Joseph Pilates, the founder of Pilates, wanted full inhalations and complete exhalations while performing the exercises. He felt this was a way of cleansing the body and getting rid of wastes. The inhalation should be on the point of effort and the exhalation should be on the return or relaxation. This will allow for a deeper abdominal connection. The breath is coordinated with the movements.

APPLICATION TO HAND THERAPY

A primary goal of Pilates is to achieve uniform development throughout the entire body obtaining a balanced muscular system. As we know, poor posture can have a significant impact on the upper extremity (UE), causing many UE dysfunctions. These muscular imbalances can increase the risk for nerve entrapment, fascial tightening, loss of musculotendinous length, and altered biomechanics of the UE. Posture plays a contributing role in many of the common diagnoses treated by hand therapists, including tendinopathies, overuse syndromes, and nerve entrapments, such as carpal tunnel syndrome. Poor posture may cause or contribute to the UE problem, or it may be caused by the impact of an UE injury, as is the case when a patient "carries" an injured arm by assuming a position of shoulder internal rotation and elbow flexion.

This protective position compromises shoulder mobility and scapular stability and promotes thoracic tightness. Whether the poor posture is the cause of the injury or is secondary to the injury, both dysfunctions need to be addressed from a whole body standpoint.

Where Does Proximal Stability Originate From?

Drawing on Joseph Pilates' classical school of thought, this section encourages hand therapists to rethink how to connect the UE into the body to allow the UE to function freely as an integrated part of the whole system. The idea that proximal stability facilitates distal function is a traditional concept in rehabilitation. Working from this concept, patients would first "correct" their posture and then work on their distal exercises or activities. We believe that stabilizing proximally in order to treat distally can often create an artificial stabilization, which is a held or locked

down position not allowing free movement throughout the system.

An alternate way of creating UE stability is to engage from the hand distally to facilitate a proximal stability. This concept of engaging the hand first elicits recruitment of the muscles distally to proximally, allowing the UE to move freely in a way that is connecting to the whole body. This is a natural stabilization. We propose that natural stabilization promotes a freedom of movement which improves range of motion (ROM) and enhances neuromuscular responses of the UE in hand therapy. In other words, we (the authors) recommend trying to connect distally from the palm through the arm into the whole body, and then proceeding with hand therapy interventions while sustaining the whole body connectedness. To better visualize this concept, think of a feedback-feedforward loop. Input from the hand connecting proximally (feedback loop) stimulates and elicits improved quality of motion distally (feedforward loop).

How to Connect From the Palm

To create a natural recruitment distally to proximally, the palm of the hand needs to be activated. It is easiest initially to activate the palm of the hand from a supine position. The therapist should first manually assist posterior shoulder connectedness by stabilizing the scapula, externally rotating the humerus, extending the elbow, pronating the forearm, and gently pressing the patient's neutral wrist into the treatment table surface with digits extended and relaxed (see Video 19-1 on the Evolve website). Note that the wrist is in neutral position in both of the planes of flexion/extension and radial/ulnar deviation. The middle finger should be aligned with the middle of the wrist. Our patients often report that this neutral position feels unfamiliar to them, and they perceive that their hand is ulnarly deviated when it is really in neutral alignment. Help the patient distribute weight equally at the heel of the hand (proximal palm) and the ball of the hand (distal palm) to create a doming or arching of the palm. When the palm is domed, the digits can move freely, because there is a reduced need to "grab" with the fingers (see Fig. 19-1 and Fig. 19-2).

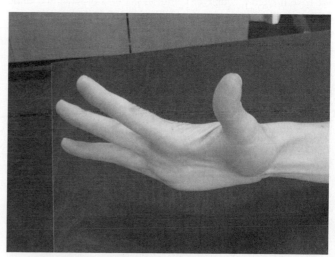

FIGURE 19-1 Domed palm. (Courtesy of Cynthia Cooper.)

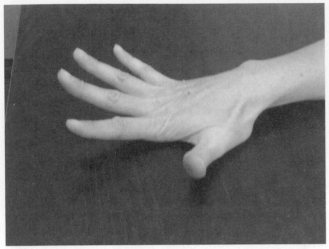

FIGURE 19-2 Domed palm on table. (Courtesy of Cynthia Cooper.)

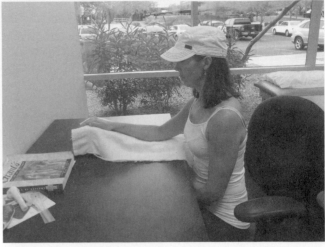

FIGURE 19-4 Good seated posture. (Courtesy of Cynthia Cooper.)

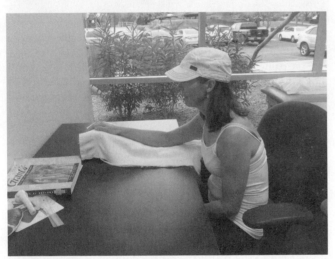

FIGURE 19-3 Poor seated posture. (Courtesy of Cynthia Cooper.)

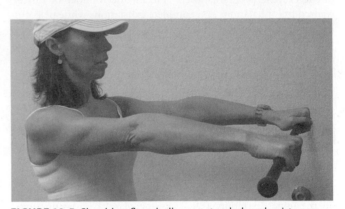

FIGURE 19-5 Shoulders flexed, elbows extended, and wrists neutral. (Courtesy of Cynthia Cooper.)

perspective, these patterns need to be corrected to allow for an UE connectedness promoting energy flow into the entire system.

Patterns of Upper Extremity Disconnectedness in Hand Therapy Patients

We have noticed a couple of common patterns of habit and comfort among hand therapy patients. One pattern includes slight wrist flexion with digital flexion with the patient grabbing with their fingers, thus overworking their digital flexors. This held pattern blocks energy flow and does not allow free movement (feedback) throughout the UE and instead creates a holding pattern with dominance of the extrinsic flexors. Patients with this tendency usually present with an overactive hand. Their forearms tend to be overworked, and they often hold their ribcage and thoracic region very rigidly. Habitual finger grabbing may contribute to fascial tightness of the hand and increased pressure on the median nerve at the wrist.

Another common pattern is resting in wrist extension with some radial deviation and digital flexion. This posture represents dominance of the wrist extensors. It promotes a "wimpy" hand and lacks connectedness throughout the UE. This position is associated with shoulder internal rotation, overuse of the wrist extensors, pectoral muscles, and the upper trapezius with a lack of shoulder stabilization, disconnecting the patient's hand and from the shoulder and interfering with proximal stability. From a classical Pilates

Treatment

For seated patients, they should be using good posture with both feet on the floor and the sitz bones (ischial tuberosities) back in the chair with the ribcage centered over the pelvis (see Fig. 19-3 and Fig. 19-4). The patient's hand should be placed on the table with the wrist in a neutral position in both flexion and extension as well as radial and ulnar planes. Then, have the patient gently apply equal weight through the heel and the ball of the hand to achieve a domed hand. Another approach is to have the patient hold a bar with shoulders flexed and arms extended in front, elbows extended, and wrists neutral (Fig. 19-5). Show the patient how to position the thumbs alongside the index finger instead of in opposition or palmar abduction (see Fig. 19-6). There is an energy line (or flow) of reaching through the middle finger. From this position and with neutral wrists, cue the patient to gently squeeze the small fingers. The triceps and posterior shoulder and inner arm will automatically activate (see Video 19-2 on the Evolve website). When patients truly connect through the hand, there is automatic contraction of posterior shoulder and inner arm muscles, connection into the shoulder girdle, and stabilizing

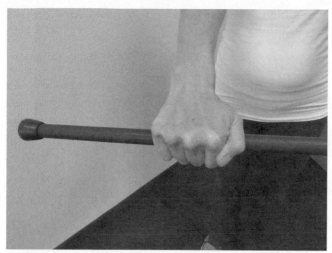

FIGURE 19-6 Thumb alongside the index finger. (Courtesy of Cynthia Cooper.)

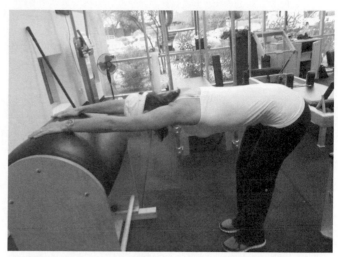

FIGURE 19-8 Thoracic stretch with arms extended. (Courtesy of Cynthia Cooper.)

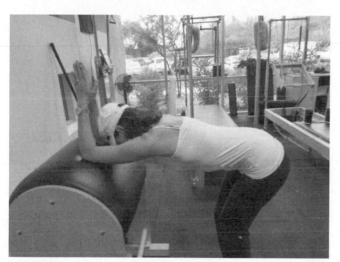

FIGURE 19-7 Thoracic stretch with elbows flexed. (Courtesy of Cynthia Cooper.)

onto the ribcage. This is the natural stabilization discussed earlier. From this position, depending on the person's posture, the upper chest usually needs to be lifted to connect the shoulder girdle and scapular stabilizers into the upper abdominal muscles. The image of "lifting your pretty necklace" facilitates the lift of the upper chest (see Video 19-3 on the Evolve website). Watch for a flaring of the ribcage or arching in the mid back. Patients tend to lift the entire ribcage/thoracic spine. This is often due to thoracic tightness (see Fig. 19-7 and Fig. 19-8 for thoracic stretches). Instead, it should be an energetic lift that is gentle and not forced. This posture will also promote and enhance proper breathing.

CASE STUDY

CASE STUDY 19-1 ■

A 25-year-old right-dominant woman was holding her 4-month-old baby when she fell on tile flooring. The baby was uninjured, but the mother sustained a left radial head fracture, non-displaced. She was referred to hand therapy 9 days after injury. She initially presented with greater passive range of motion (PROM) than AROM due to pain. She had no pain at rest, but she had 5/10 pain with active elbow flexion and extension in supination and in forearm neutral and with isolated forearm pronation and supination. Initially her PROM at the elbow in forearm neutral and in forearm available supination was 45-90; PROM of supination and pronation was 0-30. Wrist and digital ROM were within functional limit (WFL).

The patient made steady progress over the next 2 weeks and recovered pain-free active elbow flexion, supination, and pronation. Elbow extension lacked 25-degrees actively and passively with a soft-end feel. In addition to traditional hand therapy treatment, Pilates concepts were applied. She was treated lying supine. The therapist gently, manually-assisted scapular correction, humeral external rotation, forearm pronation, and neutral wrist with the hand domed on a raised surface since she lacked full elbow extension and could not touch the treatment table with her hand. The therapist also positioned the uninjured side for connectedness as described earlier. Immediately the patient reported that this posture provided a calming and "open" feeling. With this connectedness, she relaxed her finger-grabbing tendency and experienced elongation of extrinsic flexors and extensors while the therapist performed soft tissue work including myofascial release (MFR) (see Video 4 of spiral soft tissue mobilization for external rotation with pronation on the Evolve website). The patient was taught to practice the position of UE connectedness at home in bed. She continued to make progress, and in the next 2 weeks she had full elbow extension and was independent in all ADLs including holding and dressing her baby.

Do I Have to Be a Pilates Instructor to Use These Concepts in Hand Therapy?

One of the authors (Brenda Nealy) is a Pilates instructor with a physical therapy background. The other author (Cynthia Cooper) is a hand therapist who takes Pilates private lessons once a week with Brenda. We feel that the classical Pilates concepts of connecting through the hand (described earlier) add value to hand therapy and elicit favorable tissue responses that are less easily achieved when the UE being treated is not connected proximally. In the context of a hand therapy session, therapists who are not Pilates instructors are not "doing Pilates," but rather they are using classical Pilates concepts to promote favorable tissue responses.

Conclusion

Applying Pilates concepts to hand therapy contributes to improved posture and promotes better neuromuscular responses to our tissue-specific interventions. This approach adds variety to the repertoire of hand therapy treatment and restores a wholeness to the patient physically and psychologically that is unique and powerful.

References

1. Pilates JH, Miller WJ: *Return to Life*, Boston, 1960, The Christopher Publishing House.
2. Friedman P, Eisen G: *The Pilates Method of Physical and Mental Conditioning*, New York, 2005, Viking Studio.

Yoga Therapeutics: A Biopsychosocial Approach

Matthew J. Taylor, Ranay Yarian and Cynthia Cooper

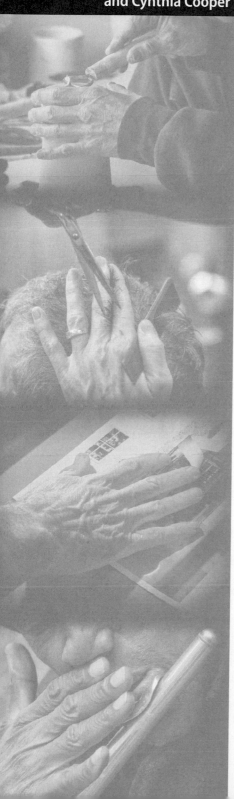

Yoga Therapeutics

"Down-dog for my hand patients?… You don't know my patients!" That's the usual response when professionals first consider the possibility of yoga and rehabilitation mixing. Unfortunately in the West, the caricature our society has about yoga is a fitness class with peculiar poses and acrobatic displays of physicality. The inclusion of the *International Journal of Yoga Therapy* to the US National Library of Medicine, National Institutes of Health (PubMed.gov) in 2011 illustrates how inaccurate that caricature is and why this chapter is included in a fundamentals textbook. With that thought in mind, let's start with defining yoga and yoga therapeutics.

Yoga doesn't equal stretching or poses (asanas). Yoga involves far more and is an evolving, complex 5000-year-old set of principles, precepts, and technologies that originated in India.[1] It continues to grow and adapt as a science of life that is both philosophical and practical in application. It is not a religion, but a spiritual practice in that it invites the practitioner to consider and answer for themselves what they are, who they are, and based on those answers, how they should act or move. In 150 CE yoga was defined by the ancient sage Patanjali in Yoga Sutra[1,2] as, "Yoga is the control of the fluctuations of the mind." The word "yoga" is from the Sanskrit word "yuj," which means "yoked or union," referring both to the act of connection of body-mind-spirit and also the realization that they are already connected and there is nothing to do.

In addition to the familiar asanas, there are behavioral/self-care principles, breathing practices, non-reactivity exercises, concentration drills, hand movements (mudras), imagery lessons, and deep somato-emotional-sensory integration practices. Yoga therapeutics is defined as "… the process of empowering individuals to progress toward improved health and well-being through the application of the philosophy and practice of Yoga."[2] The remainder of this chapter addresses how all of these psychospiritual technologies apply to hand therapy in a busy, modern, conservative rehabilitation practice.

How Is Yoga Therapeutics Different from Conventional Rehabilitation

Conventional rehabilitation is beginning to embrace the complex dynamics of both movement and pain revealed in the emerging neuroscience literature and practices, largely made possible by technological advances in imaging. The blurring of the edges of physical/emotional/mental disciplines in determining comfort and mobility heralds a call to regional interdependence[3] or biopsychosocial approaches. The practical application of yoga therapeutics to hand therapy arises from what were traditionally considered secondary outcomes of having attained control of one's mind and subsequent spiritual development. Yoga is designed to control the *fluctuations* of the mind (think fear avoidance, catastrophization, muscle guarding, and so on) with the physical body serving as just one tool toward that end. As the power of the mind is properly harnessed and focused (stable, without fluctuation) the physical outcomes are enhanced flexibility, posture, balance, strength, and physical health.[4]

While conventional rehabilitation is moving through its arc from a predominantly biomechanical model to a complex biopsychosocial model, yoga first described such a model in the Taittiriya-Upanishad of the Indian Vedanta doctrine of the sheaths, or koshas, over 3000 years ago. This source values the understanding that not only is physical regional interdependence important in optimizing health, but so too are all of the other aspects of the human experience, including social, emotional, psychological, and spiritual influences.[1] The kosha model bears many similarities to both the regional interdependence model and the biopsychosocial model as used in rehabilitation. Historically, it would be more accurate to say these modern day models actually resemble the kosha model. So how does this ancient model developed over the millennia and its technologies fit in with hand rehabilitation?

Presently we have this new understanding of the need for such a robust model, but we are short on techniques and interventions to accommodate the new paradigm. The hand is particularly complex and subject to these influences as made evident by this very book. Dysfunction of the hand impacts quality of life, occupation, self-image, and vulnerability to many pain complications.

> ◎ **Clinical Pearl**
>
> In yoga the hands are described as "doing the heart's work," and when we're denied that ability, the whole of the person is impacted.

Yoga has many practical techniques for addressing this need for an integrative approach, offering a phenomenological framework of care with an emphasis on the person's illness experience in total beyond just upper extremity pathology. Prior to describing those techniques, how this all fits in evidence-based practice (EBP) and the basic science supporting yoga therapeutics will be summarized.

Yoga Therapeutics within an Evidence-Based Practice

Too often EBP is misconstrued to equate to the notion that "if there isn't a randomized controlled trial (RCT) study demonstrating efficacy of the intervention, it shouldn't be used." While research evidence is one leg of the three-legged stool of EBP, within this leg are the various levels of evidence from RCTs, through foundational science to single case studies. Frequently overlooked are the other two legs of the EBP stool, clinical mastery and patient values. Recognizing how yoga therapeutics is situated with each of these legs will facilitate understanding for readers, their patients, and their referral sources. Utilization of just more "techniques" fractures the integrity of the system, generates barriers to incorporation, and restricts the potential for healing. Hand therapists need to appreciate the following context development of the fabric of the whole, or union, before proceeding to actual techniques as parts of the yoga.

Research Evidence and the Science of Yoga

There is very limited evidence to date on upper extremity conditions per se and yoga therapy (for a thorough review and discussion see Taylor et al.[4]). There is only one RCT to date on carpal tunnel syndrome (CTS) and yoga, which was performed by Garfinkel et al.[5] This study compared the effectiveness of Iyengar yoga with the use of orthoses for patients with CTS. The researchers utilized eleven yoga postures that were designed for strengthening, stretching, and balancing each joint in the upper body. After eight weeks, the results revealed that the yoga-based group had greater improvement in hand grip strength as well as symptoms (pain) and signs (Phalen's test) associated with CTS compared to either the wrist orthotic or no intervention control groups.[5] In 2008, O'Connor et al. compared the effects of

a yoga-based therapy program and CTS bracing and found that yoga was significantly more effective in improving reports of pain, nocturnal waking, and grip strength while reducing positive results from CTS special tests as compared to current bracing techniques.[6] These studies had small sample sizes and variability in measurement. More randomized clinical trials are needed that seek to compare yoga to other treatment options for CTS.

Garfinkel et al.[7] also looked at yoga for hand osteoarthritis in a small study and found it may be beneficial for reducing pain and disability. Beyond those studies, we move to scientific discussion of how yoga may influence hand function. Certainly radiculopathy, central nervous system (CNS) lesions, vascular disorders, complex regional pain syndrome (CRPS), and other generalized peripheral neuropathies may all manifest with signs and symptoms of the hand. Further, psychological factors may contribute to increased perception of symptoms, such as pain and stiffness. Yoga has been proposed as a potential intervention, because it is believed that practicing better positioning and joint posture may help to decrease intermittent compression of the median nerve, while the stretching involved during performance of asanas may help to relieve upper extremity entrapment and compression. Such relief of compression may help to improve blood flow thus decreasing any ischemic effects on nerves. Additionally stress and fatigue may cause psychological changes that may influence the manner in which an individual perceives the world around them. An individual who is depressed or extremely stressed may feel pain at a greater intensity than one who is not experiencing such things. The meditation component of yoga practice may help in reducing some of these psychological influences thus serving to regulate pain perception in hand therapy populations.[7-9]

Broadening our lens of scientific relationship even further, the function of the upper extremity and hand is regionally dependent on the function and alignment of the spine and thoracic cage, and there is growing evidence of yoga's efficacy in complementing back pain care.[10] Recent findings have extended our understanding of the complex relationship of postural stability between the thoracic outlet to include the glottis, the diaphragm, and the pelvic floor.[11-17]

> ◎ **Clinical Pearl**
>
> Succinctly, generating stability for the hand doesn't stop at the shoulder or chest wall, but through the pelvic floor, and from there down through the entire lower extremity kinetic chain to the great toe.

The details of this biomechanical relationship are illustrated in the accompanying Video 20-1 (see Evolve website) entitled "The 3 Diaphragms Model." Any alteration in function at one or more of the three levels affects the stability and control of the whole to include the extremities. Try it for yourself now: Sit up straight, both feet on the floor, looking straight ahead. Repeatedly flex your right shoulder fully overhead noting your natural end range. Now adduct and internally rotate your left femur, hold it there as you repeat the right shoulder flexion, noting any change in both quantity and quality of range. Return left femur to neutral, and repeat. Does your pelvic floor affect your upper extremity function? Indeed that proximal control then affects the entire length of the upper extremity to the finger tips. It works in the opposite direction as well. Abduct and externally rotate your left femur to sense natural end range, and then make a fist with your right hand and retest your hip mobility against your baseline. Release the right hand, and retest. These experiential exercises are simple but illustrate an important mechanical relationship or linkage for patients and colleagues.

While the concept of linkage is fascinating, the real "magic" as depicted in Video 20-1 is the elaborate interplay between the structural arrangement, the influence that has on the autonomic nervous system (ANS), and how cognition and emotions are influenced by, feedback to, and drive structural alignment and ANS function. The recursive cycles of these dynamic systems relationships are the bridges to understanding the biopsychosocial connections of hand therapy. Like nested Russian dolls, each layer contains new layers that fit within the other. An example would be the patient with a Colles fracture that is breathing from the upper chest post-fall, complaining of sleep difficulties, generalized anxiety, and abnormal sensitivity to touch. Walking these biopsychosocial bridges, the clinician can discover that the transference of the 700+ breaths per hour signals the ANS to sustain a hypervigilant sympathetic output, which influences limbic system arousal and subsequent patient narrative from the cognitive centers that send feedback down the chain in a positive feedback cycle—creating more ANS hypervigilance, destabilization of affected proximal extremity stability, poor movement performance, that drives a worsening narrative, and so on in a true Rube Goldberg machine fashion. The therapist's ability to articulate this process for themselves, their patients, and colleagues from any point in the process will generate a flexibility of perspective and intervention options worthy of yoga's stereotypical Gumby-renown flexibility. As a point of interest, the 3 diaphragm relationship isn't some new understanding, rather it is what yogis have described as the three bandhas and their relationship to the earlier described kosha model, which is now spelled out in Western medical terminology.

Returning to the example of the patient with a Colles fracture, the ANS responses described earlier, along with the physiological impact of the injury itself, contribute to sluggishness of the lymphatic system. Remember that it takes a high amount of interstitial fluid to occur before edema is actually visible. Do not wait for visible signs. The faster that normalizing interventions are initiated, the fewer the problems associated with lymphatic sluggishness, including fibrotic changes of soft tissues, articular tightness, and poor quality of motion. If not contraindicated, this patient needs lymphatic stimulation with manual edema mobilization (MEM) (see Chapter 3 and the Evolve website), which, like yoga practice, helps interrupt the cycle described earlier. Resting on this evidence to date, we now turn to the other two legs of EBP.

Clinical Mastery

Hand therapists who incorporate yoga therapeutics experience a freedom to explore patients' real-life issues and to intervene with an expanded repertoire leading to more meaningful solutions. For example, a traditional way to learn about self-care limitations is to use an activity of daily living (ADL) checklist or a standardized outcome measure limited to predetermined items that may be irrelevant to your particular patient. The practice of yoga therapeutics facilitates patient awareness leading to connections that extend beyond an isolated self-care task. A patient who cries when telling you she cannot prepare a meal might go on to explain how important it is to her to be able to do this because this is how she shows her love to her family.

Therapists who practice yoga therapeutics experience a personal enrichment in and from their patient interactions. We must be clear of mind and focused on the patient, present with and caring about the patient. This type of engagement is invigorating and calming at the same time, and patients recognize that something special is happening even if they cannot articulate exactly what it is. This quality of interaction typically elicits a compliment from the patient that they feel comfortable with you and that they feel you are helping them. For these and other reasons, therapists who practice this way are much less likely to experience professional burnout. They are also more likely to be open to trying new ways of treating and experience their careers as a lifelong education about their patients and themselves.

The practice of yoga therapeutics exemplifies and integrates concepts from each chapter in Part 2 of this textbook. Quieting the ANS reduces pain (see Chapter 12). Being present with the patient is a prerequisite for developing rapport (see Chapter 13). Creating acceptance dispels stigmas and eliminates obstacles that interfere with resolution of symptoms (see Chapter 17). Choosing our words thoughtfully promotes patient self-awareness and participation (see Chapter 14). Conveying respect to our patients helps them feel safe to address fears that feed autonomic hypervigilance (see Chapter 11). Promoting awareness of and integrating core musculature maximizes upper extremity health and function (see Chapter 19).

How Yoga Therapy (Asana, Breathing, Meditation, Mudra, and so on) Links to Your Current Skill Set

Which Hand Therapy Patients Are Appropriate for Yoga Therapy

A central feature of yoga therapy is that each practice can be modified depending on the participant's abilities and state of health. These characteristics make yoga therapy an ideal form of practice for all age groups, making it accessible and easy to utilize.

Clinical Pearl

The only prerequisite for participating in yoga therapy is that the participant be breathing.

Yoga therapy stresses the importance of the participant's developing awareness of how what they think, believe, perceive, and have been told influences their physical posture and mobility, their quantity and quality of breathing, and the level of CNS vigilance. All of these ultimately affect flexibility, health, and vitality. In addition to breathing, here are some intake questions to ask to clarify which patients could be most in need of the augmentation that yoga therapy can offer:

1. Do you have difficulty falling to sleep or staying asleep?
2. Do you worry about the outcome of your condition?
3. Do you find it difficult to sit still?
4. Have you had any change in mood or felt anxious or depressed?
5. Are headaches or neck pain a challenge?
6. Have you lost your sense of humor since this started?
7. Do you catch yourself taking deep breaths, holding your breath, or yawning more than you used to?

8. Do you work at a desk?
9. Do you have any low back, pelvic, or hip pain issues?
10. Do you have any history of physical, verbal, or sexual abuse?

"Yes" to one or more of these questions supports the potential need for a broader approach than just a biomechanical model.

What to Look at in Your Exam from a Yoga Therapy Perspective

> **◎ Clinical Pearl**
>
> What you have always done shifts slightly more in perspective rather than technique to become yoga therapy.

A video recording of your session might look the same to you and your patient, but your experience and that of the patient would be very different. The softening of your grip because of your diaphragmatic breath rather than your harder grip from a habitual chest breathing pattern would allow the patient to relax their forearm as you mobilize their carpals, both videos might look the same but have very different internal experiences for both of you. Consider these ways of examining and assessing patients with hand challenges. The following principles will suggest entry points for the reader to begin a seamless integration of yoga into the most conservative or traditional hand therapy rehabilitation practices.

Examination Principles

Postural assessment is the first pillar of a yoga therapy examination and begins from the base(s) of support (BOS) in all standard postures (sitting, standing, gait, supine, and prone) and is considered to be foundational rather than complementary. Before the primary complaint is addressed, imbalances in the BOS are identified first by the individual and then, if not recognized or sensed, illuminated by the therapist both through proprioception and visual feedback. A fundamental principle of yoga is that alignment of structure dictates the flow or communication of prana (the basic life force) or what in present day language would be described as ground reaction forces and Newton's third law of motion. To initiate movement or treatment without assessing and intervening to bring awareness and balance to the BOS first would be anathema to the yogic understanding of regional interdependence.

Postural holding habits are a related area of assessment where the individual discovers postural holding patterns with open-ended questions, such as "Where do you feel the most tension in your body in this position?," and "Which leg is tighter and denser feeling than the other?," and so on. The therapist's questions empower the individual to develop an internal awareness rather than merely listing the therapist's observed patterns. The therapist is helping to identify not only postural also but breathing, emotional, and spiritual patterns that reflect a hypervigilance on the part of the individual. These patterns become the touchstone for home care programs.

Postural awareness and accuracy is fundamental to a yoga therapy assessment. The individual learns the ability to accurately describe observed asymmetries in their various postures without first looking or merely repeating what they have been told but by what they can sense in the moment. This includes regional areas, such as which foot is turned in or out, higher shoulder, shorter rib

cage, greater seat pressure right or left, which shoulder is higher off the table, which palm faces more backward, and so on. This active participation by the individual during assessment generates an introspective attitude as they sense, then confirm visually, and then re-sense if they were initially inaccurate to begin their embodied therapy. During this process, the therapist may introduce topics, such as neuroplasticity as their awareness corrects on the spot, homuncular smudging[18] and its importance in motor planning, and the importance of restoring accurate interface between the sensing mind and structural body.

Breath assessment forms the second pillar of a yoga therapy examination. Inclusive of all the Western parameters of rate, volume, and quality, the therapist studies closely the regional movements associated with the act of respiration. The yoga therapist may ask him/herself or the patient, "Is there movement in the abdomen? How much and in which directions?" There are similar questions for the upper quarter, "Is there lateral movement of the rib cage that generates upper extremity movement? The sternum, scapula, head, or clavicles? Tone of the tongue, eyes, facial musculature? A thoracic or diaphragmatic recruitment?" As before, rather than list these observations, the therapist queries the individual to first sense and assess. This continued pattern of recursive observation, sensing, and education weaves throughout the assessments interlacing with the other principles. During this time the therapist can introduce the importance of respiration patterns around both the state of hypervigilance of their CNS and how with over 17,000 repetitions of these movements a day, failure to provide an efficient and stable BOS around breathing will make all other attempts to alter function much more difficult or impossible.

Self-assessment of the organs of sensing is a critical assessment. Yoga Sutra 1:2 defines yoga as the "stabilization of the mind." A preponderance of focus on the thoughts (one of the senses in yogic theory) generates a lack of awareness of the other sensing fields or an "instability" in function of the mind. Therefore, in yoga therapy individuals are made aware of these fields to initiate moving the mind off the fixation to thinking. If the therapist notes areas of tension or constriction around any of the organs of sensing, further questions are asked or expanded. Again the process of assessment moves activation from primarily the prefrontal cortex and limbic systems to sensory centers of interception and visceroception, generating ease and CNS acquiescence during the evaluation to facilitate optimal motor learning in the "intervention" phase.

These highlighted principles of assessment represent only a small percentage of the available tools of assessment for the yoga therapist. Many of those include observation of movement patterns, strength, and flexibility, which are redundant to traditional rehabilitation assessments. Others require extensive training and study beyond the scope of this chapter. These examples illustrate the manner in which adopting an integral approach to rehabilitation quickly blurs the boundaries of evaluation, assessment, and interventions as well as the roles where the individual becomes a partner in assessment. The therapist also takes on the role of learner in addition to the role of expert. The next section suggests how these assessments generate interventions both in the clinic and at home as a treatment plan that develops through a truly collaborative patient-centered process.

Intervention Principles

Manual therapy/neuromuscular re-education in yoga therapy is not considered a unidirectional intervention from the therapist to the individual. Manual contact in yoga therapy is seen as an intimate intermingling of consciousness/mind, or in the language of Siegel, intrapersonal attunement.[19]

> ## Clinical Pearl
>
> The state of the therapist's mind-body is an equal concern in determining the effectiveness of the intervention.

If the therapist is harried, distracted, breathing shallowly, and so on the quality of the procedure will be affected. The yoga therapist self-monitors their own state, their own intention, and also that of the individual throughout hands-on care. A sense of reverence of touch, intention, and gentleness create a state of therapeutic presence allowing for greater sensitivity and decreased overload or unintentional violence (yamas) to either party.

Therapeutic exercises can be adapted using yoga therapy's focus on the precision of movement facilitated through careful concentration and control of specific movement patterns in exercises. Traditional therapeutic exercises become asana when synchronized with the breath and studied for the relationship between the distal and proximal segments of the extremities and the relationship between the extremities and the spine. With each movement, the intention of the action is held, the mind scans for sensations, emotions, and thoughts that arise, and all are performed while maintaining the posture. Thus, yoga therapy asana is a very busy process in comparison to counting repetitions or striving to reach some end point of movement in traditional rehabilitation.

Directed therapeutic activities build upon the awarenesses described earlier. Individuals stay engaged in scanning their entire experience beyond just gross movement to include awareness around the BOS, their thoughts, emotions, and other sensations. If the activity reveals breaches in awareness or new insights, these are explored, and the intervention is adjusted in real time. For instance, difficulties in a dressing situation, like donning a jacket, reveal a lack of side-bend and rotation to the opposite side. In response, an asana that incorporates those components is introduced to enhance weight shifting and side bend. The activity is then revisited holding that regional awareness. If the process fails to transfer, a discussion around any perceived fear or hesitancy may yield additional insight. The limitation is used as the teaching point with successive layers of inquiry going beyond just biomechanics. The simple activity quickly becomes a deep, rich experience of exploration and discovery rather than a repetitive task of frustration as new strategies are unearthed within the tapestry of past movement learning. Tying one's shoes, reaching for the seatbelt, and grooming one's hair take on a playful sense of discovery and seemingly infinite levels of exploration, experimentation, and discovery about one's self. Intention, attention, and action blend together in a myriad of patterns creating fun and invoking ongoing cycles of inquiry for both the patient and therapist.

Home exercise programs are determined collaboratively. The program is composed of the various technologies and chosen to reinforce new learning. They may also be chosen to invite new awarenesses that the therapist believes will foster additional understanding and possibilities. For example, an individual with persistent left temporomandibular disorder has a habit of clenching the right hand at rest. An asana that opens and stretches the right palm and arm may enhance the mind-body connection to a level that the clenching becomes an activity that raises the patient's awareness, thus making conscious the previously unconscious habit and offering the possibility to change that deleterious habit. Whatever is learned in the process informs the next session of interventions as the individual and therapist work together to ease suffering associated with the presenting complaint.

Beyond the formal home program, the individual is encouraged to regularly return to awareness throughout their day, especially in instances of frustration or exacerbation to use the situation for further learning. Referred to as "off the mat" yoga, the individual is expected to return with a full list of experiences to explore and introduce into the session rather than wait for the therapist to create the agenda. Passivity and apathy in yoga therapy have their own set of therapeutic protocols and would be employed if encountered during rehabilitation before pursuing the entry complaint.

Internal "passive" exercises include the technologies of bhavana (to be introduced later) and yoga nidra (yogic rest) that augment the qualities of non-reactivity and equanimity to various stimuli and environments. Whether used in isolation as separate activities or blended with other interventions, the specific techniques and languaging vary widely. They require participation by the individual as well to match their lexicon and life experiences. Bhavana and yoga nidra can also be incorporated during otherwise passive modalities, such as ice, electrical stimulation, or ultrasound. The individual is encouraged to broaden their own vocabulary of description of sensation, movement, and activities along the guidelines within motor imagery studies and the use of precise, detailed visioning. This "movement" of the mind from frontal cortex to memory with its interplay in the limbic center and self-regulation of the breath develops a resiliency or stability of the mind and is anything but passive when fully engaged by the individual. In yoga, it is said that it is in this active exploration that the seeds of fear and suffering are discovered, and within the light of awareness the seeds wither and make way for integration and healing. In modern rehabilitation, an interesting juxtaposition to overcoming and pushing through pain is often utilized when dealing with fear avoidance, depression, and anxiety. Some of the most frequently used technologies available to the rehabilitation professional are described in the following paragraphs.

Asanas (Ah·sah·nas), or physical postures, are the third limb of Patanjali's classical eight-limbed system and have been demonstrated to generate greater cardiovascular fitness, strength, mood modification, and flexibility (see Table 20-1). Each posture teaches increased body awareness and optimal biomechanical positioning of the body in space, both in static and dynamic movement. Each asana has a unique purpose of enhancing awareness of and skill in harnessing the effect of thoughts, emotions, memories, and breathing on comfort and stability. The selection of the asana is far more complex than just a biomechanical assessment to address stability and inflexibility of the musculoskeletal system. Postures for deep relaxation are introduced from the beginning in order to facilitate perception, reflection, and calming of the CNS.[4] Asanas are often slowly repeated with focused attention and then sometimes are held for an extended period of time. Maintenance of selected postures allows for the elongation of muscles safely and naturally with gravity assistance and the further discovery of previously unknown postural patterns of holding and tension.[4] The selection and sequencing of asana includes not only principles that correlate to therapeutic exercise progression, but also those that affect breathing patterns, thoughts, emotions, and spiritual

TABLE 20-1   Eight-Fold Limbs of Raja Yoga

Limb	Description
Yamas	Moral precepts: Non-harming, truthfulness, non-stealing, chastity, greedlessness
Niyamas	Qualities to nourish: Purity, contentment, austerity (exercise), self-study, devotion to a higher power
Asana	Postures/movements: A calm, firm steady stance in relation to life
Pranayama	Breathing exercises: The ability to channel and direct breath and life energy *(prana)*
Pratyahara	Decreased reactivity to sensation: Focusing senses inward; non-reactivity to stimuli
Dharana	Concentration: Unwavering attention, commitment
Dhyana	Meditation: Mindfulness, being attuned to the present moment
Samadhi	Ecstatic union: Flow, "in the zone," spiritual support/connection

insights inherent in the asana. Keep in mind the following list of principles about asana that is vitally important in differentiating yoga therapy from traditional rehabilitation:

- Mindful procedures are followed for entering into, holding, and emerging from each asana.
- Movements are slow and coordinated with breathing for ease and comfort throughout the asana.
- Noting breath sensation and other bodily sensations is prescribed to decrease the agitation and distraction of the thinking mind (prefrontal cortex) in order to become aware of the deeper patterns of fear, attraction, and revulsion (limbic system).
- Every asana has a counter-asana. The deliberate careful movements between the polarities of experience are ancient processes known as "pacing, scaling, graded exposure, and desensitization" and are helpful in addressing fear avoidance, hyperesthesia, and kinesiophobia.
- Asana selection is by an understanding similar to traditional therapeutic progression in terms of load and perturbations, while remembering there are emotional, intellectual, and spiritual responses. The selection of postures is covered in detail by respective lineages of yoga much as the conventional schools of neurological rehabilitation have their Bobath, Brunnstrom, proprioceptive neuromuscular facilitation (PNF), and so on approaches to ordering and sequencing activities.
- Asanas are adapted with props (such as, belts, blocks, and blankets) in order for the individual to approximate a more complex posture in the same way orthotics, assistive devices, and prostheses are employed in traditional rehabilitation.

Pranayama (prah·Nah·yah·ma) is the fourth limb of yoga. There are over one hundred different combinations of yoga breathing patterns that may be employed. Each is designed to enhance awareness and experience of this vital bodily function that is tied to not only respiration but consciousness and action.[4] Breathing techniques in yoga therapy are energy management tools to curb the effects of increased stress, mood imbalance, and pain.[4] These patterns of inhalation and exhalation bridge the connection between breathing, the mind, and emotions.

Germane to rehabilitation is the interplay of respiration and the autonomic state of the patient. In a thoracic, sympathetic chest-breathing pattern utilizing accessory respiratory musculature of the cervical spine and thoracic cage, there is a significant impact on the individual at a rate of over 17,000 breaths per day. The obvious load and postural imbalances on the upper kinetic chain and lumbopelvic basin are readily apparent. In yoga therapy, alternative breathing patterns through pranayama decrease these loads and assist in deeper self-reflection and awareness to discover the source of the threat (real or perceived) to the individual that elicits the sympathetic response. This yoga therapy approach to fear empowers the individual to address the etiology rather than just "tough through" the rehabilitation or overcome the biomechanical limitations of the moment. The development of such introspective reflection yields new understanding for the individual and therapist. The process generates new strategies for action (that is, movement with intention).

Pratyahara (Prut-yah-hah-ruh) (withdrawing of the senses) and dharana (Dhah-ruh-**nah**) (concentration) are important skills that increase attention and awareness, and they are the fifth and sixth limbs of yoga. The practice of these enhances awareness during both rehabilitation and ADLs. Their outcomes are still the CNS from its level of hypervigilance by augmenting the integration of the limbic system with the prefrontal cortex, thus enhancing the interplay with the sensory and motor homunculi. Outcomes include decreased reactivity to stimuli, increased concentration and focus, and creative motor strategies beyond the habituated levels. The individual can sense their own physical limitations with clarity, accuracy of perception, and execution, not clouded by habitual thought patterns or unexamined biasing fear patterns. These concepts are being employed by the US Army and Marine Corp to address post-traumatic stress disorder (PTSD) and other symptoms of CNS hypervigilance. These techniques are more volitional and differ from the practice of dhyana, the seventh limb of yoga, which creates uninterrupted concentration.[4]

Dhyana (dhy·ah·na), or meditation, is described as a conscious mental process that induces a set of integrated physiological changes. This practice of meditation results in uninterrupted concentration aimed at quieting the mind and body. Siegel of the UCLA Mindfulness Research Center defines the mind as "[a] process that regulates the flow of energy and information" (see *The Mindful Brain* by Siegel[19] for an extensive summary and compendium of the research documenting the neurophysiology and integration that generates an intra and interpersonal "attunement"). Such attunement increases awareness of movement, enhancing the perception of any aberrant movement patterns that may exist. Increased awareness promotes muscle relaxation, encouraging the adoption of more beneficial postures and patterns of movement, resulting in the prevention of misalignment, cumulative stress, and pain. The relaxation component of yoga therapy also counteracts the negative effects induced by prolonged stress and chronic pain.

Meditation is an active state of awareness of all the processes of the mind to include sensations, images, feelings and thoughts—not the abolition of all thoughts.

Siegel has extensive commentary on the implications such practice has for both the therapist and patient in a therapeutic relationship. He specifically cites the deleterious effects on the patient's ability to breathe well and attain mindfulness if the therapist is stressed, distracted, and lacking in personal integration. Consequently, the state of the mind of the therapist influences the patient's ability to integrate the intervention. Amazingly, the literature indicates that directing not only meditation, but all of the yoga therapy technologies, the therapists themselves have a tendency to assume similar introspective, self-reflective qualities that mirror the desired outcomes.[19]

Mudras are precise ways of holding the hands, fingers, tongue, and/or body to produce specific effects in the mind and body. The integral yoga therapy perspective understands the fingers and the hand to be far more than just a tool of manipulation and acquisition.

How we greet, touch, communicate, and support one another with our hands provides for an experiential connection between one another that generates meaning and community. The loss of hand function offers a gateway to discovering this subtle reality for the patient, and mudras provide a practical tool of appreciation and a road back to full engagement with their world. The incorporation of mudra generates a natural segue to visual and motor imagery as the perception of these experiences is often most easily described by images and metaphor rather than abstract conceptual language.

Bhavana (imagery) and yoga nidra (deep rest) are technologies that provide for hemispheric integration of the mind and body as well as conscious and subconscious integration of memories, emotions, and conceptual limitations of the individual. Closely related to motor imagery in current rehabilitation, yoga therapists have long used these tools of mental representation of sensation and movement without any body movement and in conjunction with movement. In all of the technologies reviewed, there is purposeful use of image, metaphor, imagination, visualization, and sensation to invite whole brain participation and discovery. The therapist's language facilitates creativity in the experience for the individual while vocalization of experience by the individual deepens their embodied experience and communicates potential clinical information for decision-making by the therapist.

Yoga therapy uses these tools to address fear. The yogic texts contain natural extensions to employ such imagery in assisting motor performance individuals who exhibit fear avoidance and kinesiophobia. In context with current visual and kinesthetic imagery tools, there is the potential for complementing factors in designing protocols and discovering additional applications specific to an individual's clinical presentation, life circumstances, and history. The individual can also be taught how to create their own applications as a part of their home exercise, testing and modifying them based on their lived experience, and bringing this information back to inform the therapist during the next treatment session.

In conclusion, these technologies of yoga therapy may have seemed far removed from traditional rehabilitation, but closer study yields many commonalities between them. To some degree, an integrative, biopsychosocial approach to rehabilitation both revisits the very old and also becomes the new evolution of yoga as it incorporates the insights of modern imagery and research. Its rich traditions offer hand therapists concepts and treatments that strengthen a biopsychosocial approach to hand therapy.

CASE STUDY

CASE STUDY 20-1 ■

SM, a 37-year-old left-dominant woman, sustained a right non-dominant comminuted olecranon fracture with mild-to-moderate displacement of the fracture fragments. The injury occurred at a water park where she had taken her children. She underwent open reduction and internal fixation (ORIF) and was referred to therapy elsewhere about 5 days post-operation. She describes significant diffuse right upper extremity edema with "sausage fingers" and limited active range of motion (AROM)/passive range of motion (PROM) of right shoulder, elbow, forearm, wrist, and digits at her first therapy visit elsewhere. Pain was not significant. She describes the place where she was evaluated as a busy clinic environment, and she was given a tight-fitting elastic glove, told to elevate her arm, and instructed to come back in a week. At her next appointment, she was then instructed to perform pulley exercises and isolated elbow and forearm and wrist active assistive range of motion (AAROM). She reports that she never received any hands-on soft tissue work, manual therapy, or any instruction in breathing. At her next visit, she was fitted with a pre-fabricated hinged elbow orthotic to wear as a static progressive orthosis for elbow flexion during the day at all times except for hourly removal for home exercises. She was provided with a custom-fabricated anterior elbow orthotic for elbow extension to wear throughout the night. Her therapist told her that she should ideally come back in a few days for recheck, but unfortunately the clinic was too busy to see her since they were already double-booked all day; so she was scheduled to return in one week. SM reported that she never felt that the therapist cared about her or her situation and that they were too busy and just struggling to get through the day. She tried the night orthosis, but she only slept 2 hours that night because of discomfort.

SM spoke with colleagues and friends, and she decided to try a different therapist at a different therapy clinic. She presented with an anxious expression, shallow rapid breathing, elevated right shoulder posturing, moderate diffuse edema of upper arm, forearm, wrist, and hand, but she had achieved functional right shoulder, forearm, and digital AROM. Pain was not a problem. Vasomotor instability was noted, but no hyperhidrosis or other autonomic signs were seen. Posterior incision was well-healed but diffusely edematous and indurated with no skin or scar mobility. Right elbow AROM was 35-55 in forearm supination and 35-60 in forearm neutral position. PROM was equal to AROM. Biceps tightness, brachioradialis tightness, triceps tightness, and elbow articular tightness were noted. Wrist flexion was 0-25 primarily due to musculotendinous tightness.

At the first therapy visit after changing clinics, 5 weeks post-operation, SM was evaluated without provoking pain. Breathing exercises were performed, along with manual edema mobilization and gentle scar mobilization. SM immediately reported that the hands-on work was extremely comfortable and made her arm "feel alive again." She described her anguish at losing her right upper extremity function and explained she was not even able to use it to wash her face, groom her hair, or feed herself. She has two young active children, and she has not been able to function in the kitchen at all, putting the burden of this on her husband. SM stated that she had given up hope of recovering the use of her right upper extremity, which she used as a dominant arm to play tennis, which was one of her passions. While practicing breathing and relaxation, and while explaining to SM that she still had good potential to recover right upper extremity function, pain-free AROM and AAROM for shoulder flexion, external rotation, elbow flexion and extension, forearm supination and pronation were practiced. A home exercise program was written and reviewed, to be pain-free, and to focus on calm breathing and active motion in comfortable ranges. She was educated about clinical strategies for remodeling collagen using controlled stress in physiologic planes. Repeated remarks were made to the patient to reinforce the idea that she was going to recover. She was instructed to try to start picturing using her right upper extremity normally in the future and to think of her current situation as temporary. At the end of the first session, she had gained 10 degrees in active and passive right elbow flexion and extension. She cried as she told us that she felt so happy to sense that we cared about her as a human being, and she knew she was going to get better care this way.

Practical Issues: Billing, Documentation, and Peer Interface

Documentation

Because the incorporation of yoga therapeutics is largely a subjective refocusing of attention and awareness, there is little need to alter your documentation. Describe any asana not by a Sanskrit name, but as you would any therapeutic exercise. Again the available 3 Diaphragms Model video offers the bridging language of both interregional dependence and neurological motor learning rationales. Keep in mind the audiences you are writing for: other treating colleagues, third-party payers, and hopefully not, attorneys. Therefore use accepted terminology, offer the evidence-based clinical rationales for treatment where indicated, and use standard coding. For example, "Patient was instructed in breathing techniques supine with AAROM to promote pain relief, decrease guarded UE posturing to generate decreased CNS hypervigilance and facilitate improved ROM, motor learning, and function of the R UE."

Billing

In the previous example, therapeutic exercise could be charged. If the breathing was being performed as a component of manual edema mobilization, it could be charged as manual therapy. For ADL training, either therapeutic activities or neurologic re-education can be used depending on your emphasis regarding verbal instruction, focus of attention, or manual facilitation. The choice of the code billed is determined by the emphasis or purpose of that intervention, just as it is in conventional rehabilitation.

How to Market Yoga Therapeutics

The term "yoga" carries a great deal of preconceived images. In MT's experience, placing marketing emphasis on the benefits to the consumer is more effective than struggling to overcome misperceptions. Some consumers may be less receptive to terminology that is unfamiliar to them, whereas others may be excited and receptive to the holistic implications of yoga therapeutics as part of your treatment approach. If your patients are improving and speaking highly of you to their referrers, that is what matters most to them and the payers. Some referrers may not want all the details of how your practice is different and unique, as long as it works on their patients. Certainly you can direct your marketing differently extolling the yoga to consumers that you know would embrace this and respond especially favorably because of it. For example, some physicians are very involved in yoga and incorporate it into their patients' treatment. These referral sources would most likely want to know explicitly that you are using yoga therapeutics in your rehabilitation. Table 20-2 lists some examples of terminology to consider for the respective consumers of your service.

Justifying Time Spent on Yoga Therapeutics

Actually, if you are currently treating patients without first attending to the autonomic state of both yourself and the

TABLE 20-2 Marketing Terminology for Consumers

Consumer Group	Terminology
Patients	• Gentle • Non-violent • Personal • Immediate changes • Less pain during exercise • Fun • Fascinating • Real world problem-oriented • Utilizes the latest mind–body science • Fresh and useful for a lifetime • Feels good • Life changing (Yes, this is the most frequent feedback Matthew Taylor gets on patient surveys.)
Referrers	• Adjunct for your difficult/fragile patients • Helps to ease medication dependency • Evidence-based • Increases self-care adherence • Offers an alternative when traditional sources fail to provide satisfactory results • Comfortable for even your most conservative patients
Payers	• Increased home exercise adherence • Reduces red and yellow flag issues to prevent more expensive and complex claims • Evidence-based • Requires fewer and less intensive interventions • No additional cost or charges

patient, you are wasting time and resources trying to affect change on sympathetically-biased nervous systems. The brief time and redirected attention that it takes to start from a more parasympathetic state and end with the same via the previously described interventions, as well as enhanced home exercise adherence, are all time savers, not expenders. Patients, payers, and referrers may need to be educated in this regard to better appreciate the value of yoga therapeutics in hand rehabilitation. Patient testimonials will certainly be powerful. Payers will be happy if your combination of interventions leads to fewer treatments and improved outcomes. Referral sources will be happy if their patients recover. Emphasize these aspects as needed so the pertinent details fit the role of the person with whom you are communicating, remembering the cardinal marketing rule: Sell benefits, not features!

Conclusion

If we limit ourselves to traditional hand therapy indoctrination, we restrict our scope of practice, limit the potential for our patients to recover, and stifle our personal growth and well-being. Yoga therapeutics offers therapists a broad array of techniques to elicit individualized authentic experiences for our patients and for ourselves. The old becomes the new, and the new enhances the old practices for the next generation of hand therapy.

References

1. Feuerstein G: *The yoga tradition*. Presscott, 1998, Hohm Press. 178.
2. Taylor MJ: What is yoga therapy? An IAYT definition, *Yoga Therapy in Practice* 3:3, 2007.
3. Wainer RS, Whitman JM, Cleland JA, et al: Regional interdependence: a musculoskeletal examination model whose time has come, *J Orthop Sports Phys Ther* 37(11):658–660, 2007.
4. Taylor MJ, Galantino ML, Walkowich H: The use of yoga therapy in hand and upper quarter rehabilitation. In Skirven, et al, editors: *Rehabilitation of the hand and upper extremity*, ed 6, Philadelphia, 2011, Mosby Elsevier, pp 1548–1562.
5. Garfinkel MS, Singhal A, Katz WA, et al: Yoga-based intervention for carpal tunnel syndrome: a randomized trial, *JAMA* 280(18):1601–1603, 1998.
6. O'Connor D, Marshall S, Massy-Westropp N: Non-surgical treatment (other than steroid injection) for carpal tunnel syndrome, *Cochrane Database Syst Rev*(1):CD003219, 2003.
7. Garfinkel MS, Singhal A, Katz WA, et al: *The effect of yoga and relaxation techniques on outcome variables associated with osteoarthritis of the hands and finger joints*, Philadelphia, 1992, Temple University.
8. Van Baar ME, Dekker J, Lemmens JA: Pain and disability in patients with osteoarthritis of hip or knee: the relationship with articular, kinesiological and psychological characteristics, *J Rheumatol* 25:125–133, 1998.
9. Smith J, Kelly E, Monks J: *Pilates and yoga: a high-energy partnership of physical and spiritual exercise techniques to revitalize the mind and body*, London, 2004, Hermes House.
10. Sherman KJ, Cherkin DC, Erro J, et al: Comparing yoga, exercise, and a self-care book for chronic low back pain: a randomized, controlled trial, *Ann Intern Med* 143(12):849–856, 2005.
11. Knox JJ, Hodges PW: Do you know where your arm is if you think your head has moved? *Exp Brain Res* 173(1):94–101, 2006.
12. Hodges PW, Sapsford R, Pengel LHM: Postural and respiratory functions of the pelvic floor muscles, *Neurourol Urodynam* 26(3):362–371, 2007.
13. Smith MD, Coppieters M, Hodges PW: Postural response of the pelvic floor and abdominal muscles in women with and without incontinence, *Neurourol Urodynam* 26(3):377–385, 2007.
14. Massery M: Multisystem consequences of impaired breathing mechanics and/or postural control. In Frownfelter D, Dean E, editors: *Cardiovascular and pulmonary physical therapy evidence and practice*, ed 4, St Louis, 2006, Elsevier, pp 695–717.
15. Massery M: *Theoretical model: the interaction and inter-dependence of breathing and postural control*. Provo, UT, 2003, Unpublished manuscript for doctoral classwork at Rocky Mountain University of Health Professions. pp. 1–15.
16. Hagins M, Lamberg EM: Natural breath control during lifting tasks: effect of load, *Eur J Appl Physiol* 96:453–458, 2006.
17. Hagins M, Pietrek M, Sheikhzadeh A, et al. The effects of breath control on intra-abdominal pressure during lifting tasks, *Spine* 29(4):464–469, 2004.
18. Butler DS: *The sensitive nervous system*, ed 1, Minneapolis, 2006, Orthopedic Physical Therapy Products.
19. Siegel DJ: *The mindful brain: reflection and attunement in the cultivation of well-being*, New York, 2007, W.W. Norton & Company, Inc.

21 Wound Care

Christine M. Wietlisbach

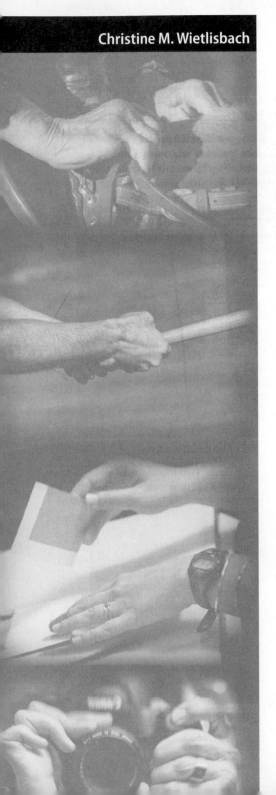

Introduction

Therapists specializing in upper extremity rehabilitation see and treat a wide variety of wounds, including abrasions, lacerations, skin tears, blisters, punctures or penetrations, human-animal-insect bites, de-gloving, surgical incisions, open surgical wounds, burns, and skin grafts. The significance of this aspect of hand therapy cannot be understated. Understanding how to properly care for a hand wound gives you the ability to reduce pain and swelling, speed wound closure, and minimize superficial scar tissue formation. When these factors are controlled, your client is much more likely to participate in all other aspects of the hand therapy program that lead to successful outcomes.

Both the American Occupational Therapy Association (AOTA) and the American Physical Therapy Association (APTA) definitively state that wound care is within the scope of practice of occupational therapists and physical therapists, respectively.[1-2] Many state practice acts also define wound care as within our scope of practice, but states vary with regard to what specific wound care procedures can be performed by occupational and physical therapists. As such, you should always consult your state licensing board on the legal parameters of providing this service in your state.

This chapter introduces the basics of proper wound care. You will learn how wounds heal, the many factors that can influence wound healing, how to cleanse and debride wounds, and how to choose dressings that maintain the optimal environment for wound healing. Additionally, you will learn how to measure, describe, and document wounds along the healing continuum. This chapter does not cover the specifics of treating burns or skin grafts. These are special-circumstance wounds and while many principles of basic wound care will also apply to burns and skin grafts, the appropriate handling of these wounds is more complicated and beyond the scope of this chapter.

Diagnosis

For the purposes of this text, we will consider a wound as any sort of open traumatic or surgical damage to the skin. The skin consists of two layers: the **epidermis** and the **dermis** (Figure 21-1).

The epidermis is the outermost surface of the skin. It is avascular and made up primarily of **keratinocytes**—cells that produce the protein keratin. Although it is only about 0.5 mm thick, the epidermis is a rather dense and tough covering that helps shield the body from infection, trauma, and rapid dehydration.

The dermis lies directly below the epidermis, is about 3 mm thick, highly vascular, and made up mostly of **fibroblasts.** Fibroblasts are cells that produce collagen and elastin, which give skin strength and flexibility. Other cells found in the dermis include **macrophages** that destroy debris and bacteria within the skin and **mast cells** that secrete substances that initiate inflammation to help fight infection. The dermis helps regulate body temperature, protects the body from infection when foreign substances

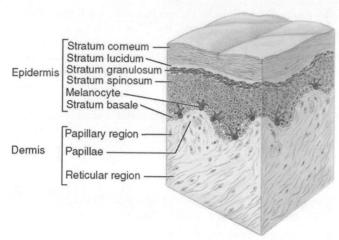

Epidermis
- Stratum corneum
- Stratum lucidum
- Stratum granulosum
- Stratum spinosum
- Melanocyte
- Stratum basale

Dermis
- Papillary region
- Papillae
- Reticular region

FIGURE 21-1 The skin consist of two layers: the epidermis and the dermis. (From Today's Medical Assistant, 2009.)

break through the epidermis, and provides sensory information via receptors located there.

Timelines and Healing

Normal Wound Healing

When the skin is wounded, it normally undergoes a predictable sequence of events consisting of three overlapping phases: inflammation, proliferation, and maturation (also called remodeling). Collectively, these three phases are known as the *wound healing process*. This process is a very complicated vascular and cellular response to tissue injury. What follows here is a very basic description of these events. Understanding the wound healing process can assist you in evaluating and planning a course of treatment for upper extremity wounds.

Inflammation is the initial response to tissue injury. During the **inflammatory phase of wound healing**, the body is working to control blood loss and to clean the wounded area. Blood loss is controlled, in part, when the blood vessels in the injured area immediately constrict. This is known as **vasoconstriction.** At the same time, a protein-based fluid leaks out of the vessels and swelling begins at the injury site. Additionally, the body begins sending specialized clean-up cells to the area that work to break down and destroy damaged tissue, foreign matter, and bacteria. Within about 30 minutes, mast cells release histamine, which causes blood vessels to open, or **vasodilate.** This vasodilation pushes more fluid into the tissue spaces and causes increased pain, swelling, and discoloration (red, blue, or purple) in and around the wound.

The inflammatory phase begins the moment of injury and continues until the injured area is free of debris and bacteria. It is a normal and necessary phase of tissue healing. The acute inflammatory phase usually lasts 2 days to 2 weeks. During this time, physicians and therapists should strive to control only *excessive* inflammation and edema, because these issues result in severe pain and potentially decreased circulation, which can cause further tissue damage. However, it is important to remember that some amount of inflammation and swelling is normal and necessary to prepare the wound for the proliferative phase of healing.

The **proliferative phase of wound healing** begins once the injured area is clean and free from damaged tissue, foreign matter, and bacteria. At this point, the body starts repairing the open space created by the wound. Proliferation consists of granulation, angiogenesis, wound contraction, and epithelialization. Granulation occurs when the body forms a matrix of connective tissue, including collagen, in the wound bed. This tissue is known as **granulation tissue** and builds on itself to fill the "hole" of the wound. **Angiogenesis** is the growth of new blood vessels. Very small capillary networks are formed in the granulation tissue of the wound and give healthy wounds their distinctive pink-red color. **Wound contraction** occurs when specialized cells in the wound bed act to pull the edges of the wound together. Finally, epithelial cells migrate across the top of the granulation tissue and completely cover the wound. This is known as **epithelialization.** The proliferative phase may take up to a few weeks to complete. It is completed more rapidly in a moist and protected environment, which becomes important for you to remember when choosing appropriate wound dressings.

Newly epithelialized wounds are still quite fragile and must go through the **maturation phase of wound healing** (also called the remodeling phase). During this final phase, water and amino acids are squeezed out of the granulation tissue matrix as collagen fibers continue to be produced. This new tissue, dense with collagen, is called *scar tissue.* Scar tissue is not as elastic or as cosmetically appealing as skin, but it serves as an adequate wound cover.

> **◎ Clinical Pearl**
>
> Although scar tissue becomes stronger over time, at full maturity it is only about 80% as strong as skin. The maturation phase can take up to 2 years to complete. Throughout the maturation phase, collagen fibers change and reorient as a result of stress in and around the wounded area. During this time, therapists can influence final scar quality through the tension of exercise and orthoses, as well as scar mobilization techniques.

Factors Affecting Wound Healing

Although most wounds progress through the three phases of healing without incident, there are certain factors that can influence both the rate and quality of healing. These factors include:
- Circulation
- Debris in the wound bed
- Infection
- Chemical stress
- Temperature of the wound bed
- Amount of moisture in and around the wound
- Medications and other medical conditions
- Nutrition
- Age

Neither the therapist nor the client has control over all factors affecting wound healing. However, to the extent that it is possible, all factors that can be modified to improve wound healing should be addressed. Familiarizing yourself with these variables will help you and your clients create an optimal environment for wound healing. Understanding these variables will also help explain why some wounds take longer to heal.

Adequate circulation is essential to wound healing. Wounds will not heal unless an adequate supply of oxygenated blood reaches the wound bed. Many things can reduce blood flow to the hands, such as peripheral vascular disease, diabetes, smoking,[3] excessive edema, and mechanical stress from orthotics or dressings. It is the therapist's responsibility to assure that all wound dressings and orthotics fit correctly. Dressings that are wrapped too tightly or orthotics that cause pressure areas can affect circulation in the hand.

In addition to having adequate circulation, a wound must be clean before it can heal. A wound is considered "clean" when it is free from infection and debris. **Wound debris** is anything embedded in the wound bed that should not be there: sutures, gauze fibers, dog hair, dead tissue, and so on. When a wound is infected or contains debris, the body's natural reaction is to clean it up by initiating an inflammatory response, sending specialized clean-up cells to the area that work to destroy foreign matter and bacteria. The wound will remain stuck in the inflammatory phase of healing until it is clean. As a hand therapist, you play an important role in monitoring wounds for infection and in removing debris from the wound bed to facilitate more rapid healing.

Chemical stress occurs when a toxic substance makes contact with granulation tissue forming in the wound bed. Cells that make up granulation tissue are very fragile and must be treated with care. When chemical stress occurs, the new cells die, and this slows the rate of wound healing. Many products that have traditionally been used to clean wounds, such as hydrogen peroxide and povidone-iodine, are **cytotoxic** and can kill tissue cells.[4] You must use care in choosing wound cleansing products, and educate your clients to do the same.

The temperature of the wound bed also influences healing. Wounds heal best when the wound surface temperature is kept relatively constant and close to the normal core body temperature range of 36° C to 38° C (96.8° F to 100.4° F).[5] The temperature of the wound bed drops, on average, 2 degrees Celsius (3.6° F) when the dressings are removed and the wound is cleansed with room temperature saline. It can take up to 3 hours for the temperature of a wound to return to pre-dressing change temperature once a new dressing is applied.[6] Strategies that reduce the frequency of dressing changes help keep the wound warm and the temperature more constant, and this assists with healing.

Another factor that assists with wound healing is moisture balance. A wound that is either too wet or too dry will not heal as quickly as a properly-balanced moist wound. A moist wound provides the optimal environment for cell growth and migration of epithelial cells over the wound bed. Wounds with a high level of **exudate** (drainage) can become too wet, and this often leads to breakdown of the wound bed and surrounding skin. Wounds with little or no exudate can become too dry, and this slows the action of regenerative cells in the wound.[7]

> ◎ **Clinical Pearl**
>
> Selecting the right dressings to balance wound moisture is the key to promoting efficient wound healing.

Finally, there are a few factors specific to the uniqueness of each client that will interact and affect wound healing. Wounds in younger clients tend to heal more quickly than wounds in older clients. This is generally due to the presence of medical conditions, medications, and inadequate nutritional intake more likely to be found in older clients. However, when these factors are present in younger clients, the effect on wound healing is the same. Chronic diseases, such as peripheral vascular disease and diabetes, will slow wound healing. Clients with cancer or AIDS or those with autoimmune disorders who require immunosuppressive drug therapy will also demonstrate slower wound healing.[8] Additionally, clients with chronically poor nutritional intake will demonstrate less efficient wound healing because malnutrition affects cell production, collagen synthesis, and wound contraction.[9]

Non-Operative Treatment: Basic Wound Management

With so many variables affecting wound healing, what can you do to help heal your clients' wounds? We already know that some factors affecting healing are out of both the therapist's and the client's control. However, there are a few factors that we can manipulate to facilitate better wound healing. It is helpful to think of basic wound management in terms of the three hallmarks of therapy-assisted wound care: 1) wound debridement, 2) proper wound cleansing, and 3) maintenance of proper moisture balance in and around the wound.

Wound Debridement

Debridement is the removal of necrotic tissue from a wound so that healthy tissue is exposed in the wound bed. Remember, a wound will not heal as long as it contains debris. It will be stuck in the inflammatory phase of wound healing until it is clean. Dead tissue is a type of wound debris, and it can take two forms: slough or eschar. **Slough** is a moist composite of fibrin, bacteria, dead cells, and exudate. It is whitish or yellowish in color and usually somewhat adhered to the wound in the form of stringy tissue. **Eschar** is dead tissue that is usually hard and dry but will occasionally be moist in appearance. It is black in color and firmly attached to the wound.

Both slough and eschar are breeding grounds for bacteria and increase the risk of wound infection. Removal of this devitalized tissue will both speed healing and reduce the risk for wound infection, so it is generally one of the first actions that should be considered as part of the wound care plan. However, not all wounds should be debrided. Any wound in an area where blood flow is impaired should be debrided cautiously, if at all. *You should always discuss with the physician any plans to debride a wound in an area with compromised circulation.*

There are four traditional methods of wound debridement: autolytic, enzymatic, sharp, and mechanical. Autolytic debridement is the method of choice in the hand therapy clinic. Occasionally, you may need to resort to enzymatic or sharp debridement. Mechanical debridement is no longer used by most therapists and physicians, and it should be avoided.

Autolytic debridement occurs when the body breaks down necrotic tissue on its own. We can encourage this by choosing wound dressings that keep the wound moist and trap the body's natural enzymes that break down dead tissue. Film and hydrogel dressings are excellent for promoting autolytic debridement. A discussion of these and other dressings will be covered later in this chapter. Autolytic debridement is comfortable and usually effective, but it can take longer to accomplish than the other methods of debridement. Therapists should take care to maintain a proper moisture balance when using this method. A wound that is too wet can result in macerated wound edges, which is a weakening of healthy tissue around the wound caused by too much fluid absorption. **Macerated skin** can easily break down and cause the wound to enlarge.

Enzymatic debridement uses topical enzymes to break down slough and eschar. Therapists should check their state practice act for legal guidance on the application of topical medications. Some states do not allow therapists to do this. The most widely-used enzymatic treatment is collagenase ointment, which is sold under the brand name Santyl and is available with a physician's prescription. Collagenase ointment is applied to necrotic tissue once or twice daily and covered with a dressing. Very dry eschar should be cross-hatched first to help the enzymes penetrate the tissue. Enzymatic debridement is selective, in that it breaks down necrotic tissue without harming healthy granulation tissue in the wound bed. This method is very effective, but may cause some discomfort and irritation in clients who are hypersensitive to the enzyme.

Sharp debridement is the use of any sharp instrument, such as scissors or a scalpel to selectively remove necrotic tissue. Again, therapists should refer to their state practice act for legal guidance on this. Some states allow occupational and/or physical therapists to perform sharp debridement; other states do not. Sharp debridement is the fastest and most effective method of debridement, but it should only be done by a skilled clinician. Once you cut something out, it is permanent. It can sometimes be difficult for an inexperienced therapist to distinguish between adipose tissue, slough, and tendon. If in doubt, never cut! This method of debridement can also be uncomfortable for the client and may require topical or local anesthetic. Because of these factors, many therapists defer sharp debridement to the physician.

Mechanical debridement is the removal of dead tissue using methods, such as whirlpool agitation, high pressure fluid irrigation, or wet-to-dry dressings. Wet-to-dry dressings are made by wetting gauze and inserting it into the wound. The dressing is allowed to dry inside the wound, and the gauze is then ripped out quickly so that tissue within the wound is pulled out along with the gauze. This method will, of course, remove some necrotic tissue every time it is performed. The problem is that any new granulation tissue forming in the wound bed is also pulled out with the gauze. Removing healthy tissue along with dead tissue is called *non-selective debridement*, and it is disruptive to wound healing. Mechanical debridement methods, especially wet-to-dry dressings, slow wound healing and are unnecessarily painful for clients. Therefore, they are not recommended. There are much more comfortable and effective methods to debride wounds in the hand clinic.

Sometimes you will utilize a combination of debridement methods. For example, the surgeon may surgically remove most of the necrotic tissue, and you will remove the rest with autolytic or enzymatic debridement. No matter what form of debridement you employ, the goal is always the same. You want to remove all devitalized tissue so that only a healthy, well-vascularized, pink-red wound bed remains.

There is one more thing to mention about preparing the wound for healing through the removal of unwanted tissue. A healthy wound bed is pink-red. However, there is a certain type of tissue that forms in the wound bed that is red-colored but undesirable. This tissue develops when there is an overgrowth of granulation tissue, possibly due to infection or excessive moisture in the wound.[10] It is called *hypergranulation tissue.*

Hypergranulation tissue normally looks like shiny, deep-red balls of tissue that grow taller than the wound margins. Some therapists think it looks like little red raspberries (Figure 21-5). The tissue is soft and will often bleed easily when touched. This tissue must be treated in order for the wound to heal normally. An effective way to treat this tissue is to apply silver nitrate to the hypergranular areas.[10,11] Use silver nitrate sticks and roll the treatment end of the stick over the abnormal tissue. As you treat the tissue, it will turn gray in color. After treating with silver nitrate, you can bandage the wound as you normally would. Repeat the procedure at each dressing change until the hypergranulation tissue is controlled.

Wound Cleansing

Wounds should be cleansed every time the dressing is changed. The purpose of cleansing the wound is to remove loose debris and surface contaminants from the wound bed. Gauze fibers, loose sutures, liquefied necrotic tissue, and bacteria are all commonly found in wounds and must be washed out. Ideally, this should be done without causing trauma to any new tissue forming in the wound bed. The therapist must decide two things: 1) what solution to use to cleanse the wound, and 2) how to apply the solution.

The best solutions for cleansing wounds in the hand clinic include normal saline, sterile water, and drinkable tap water.[12] Avoid using solutions such as hydrogen peroxide, Dakin's solution, povidone iodine/Betadine, soap, or bleach on clean wounds. These solutions contain chemicals that are toxic to granulation tissue, and use of these solutions will slow wound healing. Using a product like hydrogen peroxide is really only appropriate in the home setting for cleaning cuts and scrapes immediately after an injury. Hydrogen peroxide is fine for cleaning a dirty superficial wound at home once or twice. However, once that wound is free of injury-related debris like dirt, asphalt, and grass, it should be cleansed with saline, sterile water, or drinkable tap water so as not to impede the healing process.

> ◎ **Clinical Pearl**
>
> A good rule of thumb is to never cleanse an open wound with anything that you would not be willing to put into your eye.

The method you use to apply the cleansing solution is also important. You want to use enough pressure to remove surface debris and contaminants without causing trauma to any new tissue forming in the wound bed. To date, research has failed to identify the ideal method of wound cleansing.[13] However, most practitioners have discarded the practice of whirlpool wound cleansing and replaced that method with syringe irrigation. Syringe irrigation is more convenient and carries less risk of cross-contamination between clients than whirlpool cleansing. Much of the available literature indicates that wounds seen by the hand therapist should be irrigated with pressures at or below 8 psi.[13,14] A 35 mL medical syringe with a 25-gauge needle will produce 4 psi, and a 35 mL/19 gauge combination will produce 8 psi.[15] This equipment is readily available in most health care settings. You can cleanse all wounds in the clinic with either of these syringe/needle combinations filled with saline, sterile water, or drinkable tap water.

> **◎ Clinical Pearl**
>
> When your clients will be performing dressing changes at home, a saline squeeze bottle like those used to clean contact lenses works great to cleanse the wound. Squeezing saline out of this type of bottle produces 4.5 psi.[16]

Maintenance of Moisture Balance

Moisture in the wound bed is critical to efficient wound healing. A moist wound will heal much faster than a wound that is either too wet or too dry. Maintaining an appropriate moisture balance depends on one thing: your choice of wound dressing. Every wound is different and will require different dressings or dressing combinations to keep it moist. If a wound has a lot of exudate, you will want to choose a dressing that can absorb the drainage. On the other hand, if a wound is too dry, you will want to choose a dressing that will add moisture to the wound bed.

Choosing the right dressing is somewhat of an art form that requires practice. The more wounds you see, the better you will get at selecting the right dressing. However, understanding the different categories of available dressings, and the characteristics of each, will help guide you.

Dressings are sometimes described as non-occlusive, semi-occlusive, or totally occlusive. This nomenclature has to do with the relative ability of a dressing to block water, water vapor, and bacteria from passing through the dressing. A completely **non-occlusive dressing** will allow the free passage of water, vapor, and bacteria. A completely **occlusive dressing** will not allow any passage of water, vapor, and bacteria. A **semi-occlusive dressing** falls in the middle of this continuum—generally allowing the passage of water vapor, but not water or bacteria. In truth, there is no completely occlusive or completely non-occlusive dressing, but dressings are described with the term that most accurately describes its ability to keep water, vapor, and bacteria from passing through.

When occlusive dressings first arrived on the scene, many physicians feared that their use would cause infection. This myth is still prevalent in some settings. However, research has shown that occlusive dressings do *not* increase the risk for infection.[17] The goal is to find a dressing that will keep bacteria out, retain some moisture, but still absorb any excess fluid if needed.

Standard dressing choices generally fall into the following categories: transparent films, impregnated low-adherence dressings, hydrogels, hydrocolloids, gauze, foams, and alginates. There are other types of specialty dressings available, but the typical hand therapist will make his or her selection from these standard dressing choices. Every medical supply company has these types of dressings available, but they will be identified by different brand names. When looking for a specific type of dressing, ask your supplier for the names of the available dressings in that category. The dressing categories described below are listed in order from least absorptive to most absorptive.[18-21]

Transparent Films

These versatile dressings are exactly what they sound like: thin, see-through films (Figure 21-2). Films come in a variety of shapes and sizes and easily conform to the contours of the hand. They adhere right to the skin and can be used either as a **primary dressing** (making contact with the wound) or as a **secondary dressing** (holding a primary dressing in place). Transparent films

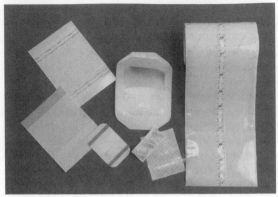

FIGURE 21-2 Transparent film dressings. (From Acute and Chronic Wounds, 2007)

are semi-occlusive in that they are permeable to water vapor, but impervious to liquids and bacteria.[19] Therefore, they are waterproof in the shower and good at keeping bacteria out of the wound. Another advantage of transparent film dressings is our ability to see the wound without removing the film. Films are non-absorptive, and because these dressings hold most moisture in, they are excellent for promoting autolytic debridement of slough or moist eschar. Transparent films must be changed if too much fluid builds up under the film and starts to leak out the edges. However, dry or very low draining wounds can tolerate a film dressing in place for up to 7 days.

Brand names of transparent films include OpSite (Smith & Nephew), Tegaderm Transparent Film (3M), and Suresite (Medline).

Impregnated Low-Adherence Dressings

These non-occlusive to semi-occlusive dressings are designed to make contact with the wound and reduce sticking and tearing of wound tissue during dressing changes. Low-adherence dressings are almost always used at the time of surgery in preparation for the first post-operative dressing change. These dressings are generally made of gauze or mesh impregnated with paraffin or a petroleum-based ointment; and they require a secondary dressing to keep them in place. A few low-adherence dressings contain antibacterial agents, and there is some evidence that application of these particular types of non-stick dressings in the operating room reduces the risk of surgical site infections, including methicillin-resistant *Staphylococcus aureus* (MRSA) infections.[22] Impregnated low-adherence dressings are indicated for use in the hand clinic when the wound is very superficial, not draining much, and expected to heal without incident in a matter of a few days. They are easy to use and conform well to the contours of the hand.

Brand names include Adaptic (Johnson & Johnson) and Xeroform (Kendall).

Hydrogels

Hydrogels are non-occlusive to semi-occlusive dressings made mostly of water and are available in sheet, impregnated gauze, or gel form (Figure 21-3). They are designed to hydrate wounds, but some newer hydrogels have additives that allow them to also absorb a little exudate while keeping wounds moist.[20] Hydrogels are very soothing and can therefore offer some pain relief. They are excellent for promoting autolytic debridement, especially of

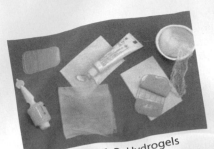

FIGURE 21-3 Hydrogels

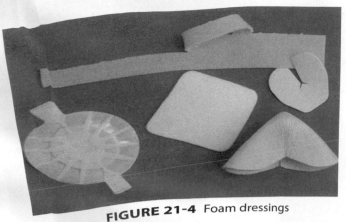

FIGURE 21-4 Foam dressings

small amounts of eschar. Hydrogel sheets do not conform well to the contours of the hand but will conform to the forearm area. Gels and impregnated gauze can easily be kept in place on the hand with a secondary dressing. Hydrogels usually need to be replaced every 24 to 72 hours, but this will depend on how much exudate, if any, is being produced by the wound.

Brand names include Intrasite Gel and 3-d Site Wound Gel (Smith & Nephew), ...gel Hydrogel Wound Filler (3M).

Hydrocolloids

Hydrocolloid dressings are occlusive ... ...semi-occlusive and are made of ingredients like cellulose, gelatin ... ... Hydrocol... ...while holding on to natural growth factors in the wound ... ...er the wound bed as it absorbs ... ...experts claim that this gel is resistant to wound exudate that assist with efficient wound repair.[20] Hydrocolloids absorb moderate amounts of exudate while hydrating the wound bed, so they can assist in autolytic debridement if needed. These dressings come in a variety of shapes, sizes, and thicknesses. Depending on the specific hydrocolloid, it may or may not conform well to the contours of the hand. However, hydrocolloid adhesive is stronger than in most dressings, so it can usually stand alone without a secondary dressing. The strong adhesive around the edge of the dressing helps keep fluids and bacteria from entering. Additionally, hydrocolloids feel cool and comforting to the client, so they are well-received. One thing to be aware of is that hydrocolloids take on an unpleasant odor when they absorb exudate. During dressing changes, this odor is very noticeable and is sometimes mistakenly interpreted as a sign of infection.[20] When using hydrocolloids, be sure to cleanse the wound thoroughly before assessing for infection.

Brand names include DuoDERM (ConvaTec), Tegaderm Hydrocolloid (3M), and RepliCare (Smith & Nephew).

Gauze

Woven gauze is the most widely-available and probably the most commonly-used dressing material in the hand clinic. Every hand therapist has worked with gauze. It comes in a variety of sizes and forms, from pads to rolls. It is easy to obtain, moderately absorptive, and easy to work with. Gauze can be used to clean around wounds, to pack wounds, and to cover wounds. It can be inexpensive to use if not many dressing changes are needed. Gauze is an important material in every hand therapist's clinic.

The problem with using gauze as a primary dressing is that it cannot easily create a moist wound environment on its own because it is relatively non-occlusive. Some therapists try to wet gauze with saline to keep wounds moist, but it is difficult to gauge how much moisture is needed to create that optimal healing environment. Often, we add too much water and end up with macerated wound edges. Other times, we add too little water and

the dressing becomes dry and adhered to the wound—causing trauma to the wound bed during the next dressing change. Gauze also tends to shed its fibers. If we do not thoroughly irrigate wounds between dressing changes, fibers left behind can irritate the wound and slow healing.

When it comes to upper extremity wound care, gauze works best for loosely packing larger wound cavities and as a secondary dressing for keeping other types of dressings in place. When packing wounds, you should try to have any gauze in direct contact with the wound bed be the low-adherence impregnated type of gauze. Standard dry gauze is fine for packing the remainder of the wound cavity. When gauze is used to pack a wound, sterile gauze should be used. If gauze is used as a secondary dressing over a wound, clean gauze can be used. Sterile gauze has been processed to kill all living germs and microorganisms, and it is usually packaged in units of one dressing per package. Clean gauze is not sterile, but it is free from environmental contaminants, such as dirt and other foreign material. Multiple rolls of clean gauze are usually contained within one package.

Brand names include Kerlix (Kendall) and Kling (Johnson & Johnson).

Foams

Foam dressings are made of mostly polyurethane and are used to absorb moderate amounts of exudate[21] (Figure 21-4). Some foams can adhere directly to the wound area, while other foams require a secondary dressing to hold them in place. The thicker foams can even provide a little protective cushioning over the wound. Additionally, most are semi-occlusive in that the outer cover of foam dressings are usually waterproof and will act as a bacterial barrier.[20] However, one of the difficulties with using foam dressings is that, despite the wide variety of shapes and sizes available, they never seem to conform well to the contours of the hand.

Brand names include Allevyn (Smith & Nephew), PolyMem (Ferris), and Mepilex (Molnlycke).

Alginates

Alginate dressings are non-occlusive to semi-occlusive, highly absorbent, and made to manage moderate to large amounts of exudate (Figure 21-5). These dressings are made primarily of seaweed derivatives, and the fibers are spun into ropes or sheets. As the alginate absorbs fluid, it is converted to a gel that provides moisture to the wound bed. Alginates always require a secondary dressing to keep them in place. Alginates conform well to the

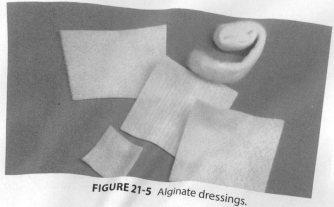

FIGURE 21-5 Alginate dressings.

contours of the hand. In rope-form, they are also great for filling small, draining wound cavities.

During dressing changes, you must be sure to irrigate the wound thoroughly to remove all of the alginate before applying a new dressing. If you find that not all the alginate has gelled, you are either changing the dressing too soon, or the wound is not draining enough to warrant an alginate dressing. It is important to reserve alginates only for moderate to severely draining wounds. Using an alginate on a wound with minimal exudate will dry out the wound bed.

Brand names include AlgiSite M (Smith & Nephew), Sorbsan (Bertek), and SeaSorb (Coloplast).

Operative Treatment

Almost every wound that we see in the hand clinic has first been addressed by a physician. When a client presents to a physician with a wound, the physician must decide how to best clean and prepare the wound so that it can heal. In the case of trauma-related hand wounds, the wound is often part of an environment that includes tendon and nerve injuries. Traumatic and infected wounds often need to be addressed in surgery before the client is followed by the therapist in the hand clinic. Some clients will require more than one surgical procedure to address wound issues throughout the course of hand therapy.

A common procedure performed by hand surgeons is surgical irrigation and debridement. During this procedure, the client is placed in a sterile environment within the surgical suite and administered an anesthetic. Intravenous antibiotics are usually administered during the procedure to help treat or reduce the risk of infection. The surgeon will then use a scalpel and forceps to remove any wound debris, including non-viable tissue, and the wound is thoroughly irrigated with saline. Assuming no other structures need repair, the surgeon must then decide whether to close up the wound or to leave it open.

When a wound is closed with sutures or staples, it is said to heal by **primary intention.** Since the wound edges are approximated (brought together), these wounds heal by fibrous adhesion with little to no granulation tissue formation. Healing is quick and usually without incident.

When a surgeon leaves the wound open and allows it to heal through the granulation process, this is called healing by **secondary intention.** These wounds require close monitoring and skilled wound care to assure they heal without complications. Deep open wounds are traditionally loosely packed to assure they

heal from the inside out. The common understanding is that if a wound is allowed to close over too early, the inside cavity is susceptible to infection and abscess. There is some recent evidence that wound packing may be unnecessary,[23] but more research is required to validate this assertion.

Some clinicians rely on the use of negative pressure therapy, like the vacuum assisted closure device (V.A.C.), to assist with healing large open wounds. Wounds do tend to granulate better with the use of negative pressure therapy,[24] but the disadvantage for hand wounds is that the cumbersome tubing and machine must stay attached to the hand at all times. Because this interferes so drastically with hand function, many hand therapists tend to use the wound V.A.C. for only the most difficult wounds or for wounds on people who are substantially immobilized in the hospital—as in the case of severe trauma victims.

Occasionally, a surgeon will leave a wound open after the irrigation and debridement procedure with the plan to return the client to surgery for wound closure in a few days. This is known as delayed primary wound closure, although the wound is said to heal through **tertiary intention.** This is most commonly done for very dirty or infected wounds. The surgeon will want to wait a few days before closing the wound to make sure all infection is under control and healing is underway.

? Questions to Discuss with the Physician

Close collaboration between the referring physician and the hand therapist is strongly encouraged during hand rehabilitation, and this is especially true when wound care is part of the treatment plan. With regard to your client's wound, you will want to have the following types of discussions:

- If you start to notice any signs of infection, you will want to ask the physician to evaluate. If an infection is present, it is important to start medical treatment as soon as possible. Common wound infections include those caused by MRSA, *Streptococcus pyogenes* (strep), and *Pseudomonas aeruginosa.* Wound infections generally require systemic antibiotics.

- Also, know that sometimes a wound just will not heal and no one suspects infection because the wound is not red, inflamed, odorous, or draining pus. Although typical signs of infection are usually present, occasionally the only sign of an infection is the non-healing wound. If wound healing stops progressing for a couple of weeks, contact the physician and discuss the possibility of infection. The physician may want to culture the wound to see if it is, indeed, infected.

- If there is an infection, ask if it is ok to move the joints surrounding the infected area. Some physicians will want to limit movement until an infection is controlled, for fear of spreading the infection. It depends on the physician, the type of the infection, and the severity of the infection.

- If debridement is necessary, discuss the type of debridement you plan to perform.

- Autolytic debridement should be your first choice, but the physician will need to know that this type of debridement may take some time to complete. If the physician wants faster debridement, then you will need to discuss either enzymatic or sharp debridement. Enzymatic debridement requires a prescription enzyme. Sharp debridement may require a topical anesthetic. If you are at all uncomfortable or

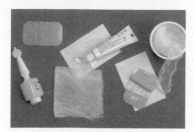

FIGURE 21-3 Hydrogels

small amounts of eschar. Hydrogel sheets do not conform well to the contours of the hand but will conform to the forearm area. Gels and impregnated gauze can easily be kept in place on the hand with a secondary dressing. Hydrogels usually need to be replaced every 24 to 72 hours, but this will depend on how much exudate, if any, is being produced by the wound.

Brand names include Intrasite Gel and SoloSite Wound Gel (Smith & Nephew), and Tegagel Hydrogel Wound Filler (3M).

Hydrocolloids

Hydrocolloid dressings are occlusive to semi-occlusive and are made of ingredients like cellulose, gelatin, and pectin. Hydrocolloids create a gel-like substance over the wound bed as it absorbs exudate.[21] Some wound experts claim that this gel is resistant to bacterial growth while holding on to natural growth factors in the wound exudate that assist with efficient wound repair.[20] Hydrocolloids absorb moderate amounts of exudate while hydrating the wound bed, so they can assist in autolytic debridement if needed. These dressings come in a variety of shapes, sizes, and thicknesses. Depending on the specific hydrocolloid, it may or may not conform well to the contours of the hand. However, hydrocolloid adhesive is stronger than in most dressings, so it can usually stand alone without a secondary dressing. The strong adhesive around the edge of the dressing helps keep fluids and bacteria from entering. Additionally, hydrocolloids feel cool and comforting to the client, so they are well-received. One thing to be aware of is that hydrocolloids take on an unpleasant odor when they absorb exudate. During dressing changes, this odor is very noticeable and is sometimes mistakenly interpreted as a sign of infection.[20] When using hydrocolloids, be sure to cleanse the wound thoroughly before assessing for infection.

Brand names include DuoDERM (ConvaTec), Tegaderm Hydrocolloid (3M), and RepliCare (Smith & Nephew).

Gauze

Woven gauze is the most widely-available and probably the most commonly-used dressing material in the hand clinic. Every hand therapist has worked with gauze. It comes in a variety of sizes and forms, from pads to rolls. It is easy to obtain, moderately absorptive, and easy to work with. Gauze can be used to clean around wounds, to pack wounds, and to cover wounds. It can be inexpensive to use if not many dressing changes are needed. Gauze is an important material in every hand therapist's clinic.

The problem with using gauze as a primary dressing is that it cannot easily create a moist wound environment on its own because it is relatively non-occlusive. Some therapists try to wet gauze with saline to keep wounds moist, but it is difficult to gauge how much moisture is needed to create that optimal healing environment. Often, we add too much water and end up with macerated wound edges. Other times, we add too little water and

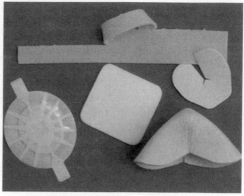

FIGURE 21-4 Foam dressings

the dressing becomes dry and adhered to the wound—causing trauma to the wound bed during the next dressing change. Gauze also tends to shed its fibers. If we do not thoroughly irrigate wounds between dressing changes, fibers left behind can irritate the wound and slow healing.

When it comes to upper extremity wound care, gauze works best for loosely packing larger wound cavities and as a secondary dressing for keeping other types of dressings in place. When packing wounds, you should try to have any gauze in direct contact with the wound bed be the low-adherence impregnated type of gauze. Standard dry gauze is fine for packing the remainder of the wound cavity. When gauze is used to pack a wound, sterile gauze should be used. If gauze is used as a secondary dressing over a wound, clean gauze can be used. Sterile gauze has been processed to kill all living germs and microorganisms, and it is usually packaged in units of one dressing per package. Clean gauze is not sterile, but it is free from environmental contaminants, such as dirt and other foreign material. Multiple rolls of clean gauze are usually contained within one package.

Brand names include Kerlix (Kendall) and Kling (Johnson & Johnson).

Foams

Foam dressings are made of mostly polyurethane and are used to absorb moderate amounts of exudate[21] (Figure 21-4). Some foams can adhere directly to the wound area, while other foams require a secondary dressing to hold them in place. The thicker foams can even provide a little protective cushioning over the wound. Additionally, most are semi-occlusive in that the outer cover of foam dressings are usually waterproof and will act as a bacterial barrier.[20] However, one of the difficulties with using foam dressings is that, despite the wide variety of shapes and sizes available, they never seem to conform well to the contours of the hand.

Brand names include Allevyn (Smith & Nephew), PolyMem (Ferris), and Mepilex (Molnlycke).

Alginates

Alginate dressings are non-occlusive to semi-occlusive, highly absorbent, and made to manage moderate to large amounts of exudate (Figure 21-5). These dressings are made primarily of seaweed derivatives, and the fibers are spun into ropes or sheets. As the alginate absorbs fluid, it is converted to a gel that provides moisture to the wound bed. Alginates always require a secondary dressing to keep them in place. Alginates conform well to the

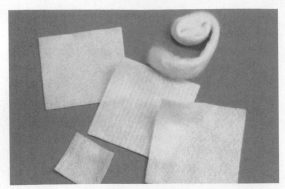

FIGURE 21-5 Alginate dressings.

contours of the hand. In rope-form, they are also great for filling small, draining wound cavities.

During dressing changes, you must be sure to irrigate the wound thoroughly to remove all of the alginate before applying a new dressing. If you find that not all the alginate has gelled, you are either changing the dressing too soon, or the wound is not draining enough to warrant an alginate dressing. It is important to reserve alginates only for moderate to severely draining wounds. Using an alginate on a wound with minimal exudate will dry out the wound bed.

Brand names include AlgiSite M (Smith & Nephew), Sorbsan (Bertek), and SeaSorb (Coloplast).

Operative Treatment

Almost every wound that we see in the hand clinic has first been addressed by a physician. When a client presents to a physician with a wound, the physician must decide how to best clean and prepare the wound so that it can heal. In the case of trauma-related hand wounds, the wound is often part of an environment that includes tendon and nerve injuries. Traumatic and infected wounds often need to be addressed in surgery before the client is followed by the therapist in the hand clinic. Some clients will require more than one surgical procedure to address wound issues throughout the course of hand therapy.

A common procedure performed by hand surgeons is surgical irrigation and debridement. During this procedure, the client is placed in a sterile environment within the surgical suite and administered an anesthetic. Intravenous antibiotics are usually administered during the procedure to help treat or reduce the risk of infection. The surgeon will then use a scalpel and forceps to remove any wound debris, including non-viable tissue, and the wound is thoroughly irrigated with saline. Assuming no other structures need repair, the surgeon must then decide whether to close up the wound or to leave it open.

When a wound is closed with sutures or staples, it is said to heal by **primary intention.** Since the wound edges are approximated (brought together), these wounds heal by fibrous adhesion with little to no granulation tissue formation. Healing is quick and usually without incident.

When a surgeon leaves the wound open and allows it to heal through the granulation process, this is called healing by **secondary intention.** These wounds require close monitoring and skilled wound care to assure they heal without complications. Deep open wounds are traditionally loosely packed to assure they

heal from the inside out. The common understanding is that if a wound is allowed to close over too early, the inside cavity is susceptible to infection and abscess. There is some recent evidence that wound packing may be unnecessary,[23] but more research is required to validate this assertion.

Some clinicians rely on the use of negative pressure therapy, like the vacuum assisted closure device (V.A.C.), to assist with healing large open wounds. Wounds do tend to granulate better with the use of negative pressure therapy,[24] but the disadvantage for hand wounds is that the cumbersome tubing and machine must stay attached to the hand at all times. Because this interferes so drastically with hand function, many hand therapists tend to use the wound V.A.C. for only the most difficult wounds or for wounds on people who are substantially immobilized in the hospital—as in the case of severe trauma victims.

Occasionally, a surgeon will leave a wound open after the irrigation and debridement procedure with the plan to return the client to surgery for wound closure in a few days. This is known as *delayed primary wound closure,* and the wound is said to heal through **tertiary intention.** This is most commonly done for very dirty or infected wounds. The surgeon will want to wait a few days before closing the wound to make sure all infection is under control and healing is underway.

? Questions to Discuss with the Physician

Close collaboration between the referring physician and the hand therapist is strongly encouraged during hand rehabilitation, and this is especially true when wound care is part of the treatment plan. With regard to your client's wound, you will want to have the following types of discussions:

- If you start to notice any signs of infection, you will want to ask the physician to evaluate. If an infection is present, it is important to start medical treatment as soon as possible. Common wound infections include those caused by MRSA, *Streptococcus pyogenes* (strep), and *Pseudomonas aeruginosa.* Wound infections generally require systemic antibiotics.
- Also, know that sometimes a wound just will not heal and no one suspects infection because the wound is not red, inflamed, odorous, or draining pus. Although typical signs of infection are usually present, occasionally the only sign of an infection is the non-healing wound. If wound healing stops progressing for a couple of weeks, contact the physician and discuss the possibility of infection. The physician may want to culture the wound to see if it is, indeed, infected.
- If there is an infection, ask if it is ok to move the joints surrounding the infected area. Some physicians will want to limit movement until an infection is controlled, for fear of spreading the infection. It depends on the physician, the type of the infection, and the severity of the infection.
- If debridement is necessary, discuss the type of debridement you plan to perform.
- Autolytic debridement should be your first choice, but the physician will need to know that this type of debridement may take some time to complete. If the physician wants faster debridement, then you will need to discuss either enzymatic or sharp debridement. Enzymatic debridement requires a prescription enzyme. Sharp debridement may require a topical anesthetic. If you are at all uncomfortable or

feel you do not have the skill to perform sharp debridement, you must speak up. Sharp debridement may need to be performed by the physician.

- If the wound is covered with eschar, but the underlying tissue has decreased circulation, discuss the pros and cons of debridement with the physician. In the case of poor blood flow to the wound area, immediate debridement is not always a good idea. Other medical interventions, like revascularization surgery, may need to be considered first.

- It is also worth noting that debridement of uninfected dry fingertip necrosis caused by vascular insufficiency, such as in patients with Raynaud disease, systemic lupus erythematosus, and scleroderma is rarely performed. In these unfortunate cases, the usual course of treatment is to allow the fingertip to auto-amputate.

- If a physician asks for a less-than-ideal wound treatment, offer a wound care plan that meets the current standard of care.

- Therapists still get orders for wet-to-dry dressings and for whirlpool treatments. In these instances, you have a responsibility as a licensed clinician to discuss better alternatives for wound debridement and cleansing with the physician. Once a physician is aware of more effective and safer options, he or she will almost always agree with your plan of care.

- If a wound just isn't healing and infection has been ruled-out, discuss the client's lab work with the physician.

The following lab values are indicators of malnutrition or poorly-controlled blood sugar and may indicate that nutritional status is interfering with wound healing:[11]

Serum albumin levels below 3.5 g/dL
Serum prealbumin levels below 16 mg/dL
Serum transferrin levels below 170 mg/dL
Total lymphocyte count (TLC) below 1800/mm³
Blood glucose levels greater than 110 mg/dL

While malnutrition is a rare factor in clients coming to an out-patient hand clinic, you may see malnutrition interfering with wound healing in hospitalized patients or residents of long-term care facilities. When nutrition might be a factor in poor wound healing, a dietitian should be part of the care team.

(•) What to Say to Clients

You will want to give your clients as much information as possible so that they become partners in the wound healing effort. Many clients have misconceptions about wound healing, but once educated, most will do everything possible to help their wounds heal. The following topics should be discussed with every client who has a wound.

Schedule for Dressing Changes

As the therapist, you will decide how frequently to change the dressings. If you see clients in an outpatient setting, you will decide if the dressing changes will be done at home or in the clinic. Many things factor into your decision: how much the wound is draining, what dressing you plan to use, the client's anxiety about the wound, the client's ability to follow directions, support systems available to the client, and reimbursement issues. The more wounds you treat, the better you will get at making this decision.

Once you decide how often the dressing should be changed, you must clearly communicate this to your client. Make it very clear that the dressing should not be changed more frequently, unless it becomes soiled or saturated. In the event that the dressing must be changed early, have a plan, and communicate this to your client. If your client is an outpatient, decide if the client should come into the clinic for a dressing change or if he/she should go ahead and change the dressing at home. You can say, "I am going to see you back here in the clinic in a couple of days. I want you to keep this dressing clean and dry. If the drainage from your wound starts to seep through the dressing, or if you accidentally get your dressing wet or very dirty, I want you to call me as soon as possible so that we can have you come in for a dressing change."

Cleansing

One of the biggest misconceptions therapists encounter has to do with wound cleansing. If your client will be doing dressing changes at home, make it very clear that only saline, sterile water, or drinkable tap water should be used to cleanse the wound. Many clients are surprised to learn that hydrogen peroxide or soap should not be used to cleanse open wounds. Educate your clients that using these substances will slow the healing process by killing healthy cells that build the granulation tissue. Because we do not give out needles and syringes for home wound cleansing, clients performing home dressing changes usually cleanse their wounds with drinkable tap water running slowly from the faucet, or a squeeze-bottle contact lens saline solution. Tell your clients, "I want you to rinse your wound well every time you change your dressing. Put your hand under warm (not hot) slowly-running tap water, or rinse the wound by squeezing contact lens saline solution from a bottle. Rinse the wound for 30 seconds. Do not use anything else to clean your wound. Some things, like hydrogen peroxide and soap, actually slow down healing by killing 'good' cells that are helping to close the wound."

Moist Wound Healing

The second biggest misconception that therapists encounter concerns moist wound healing. Most of us were taught as children to expose our wounds to the air and sun in order to dry them. Our parents and grandparents told us that this would help our wounds heal faster. We now know that this could not be further from the truth. You must educate your clients on the efficacy of moist wound healing. All you usually need to say is that, "Research has shown that moist wounds heal faster than dry wounds, and moist wound healing occurs when wounds stay covered. Keep your dressing on, and try not to change it any more often than we have discussed."

(•) Clinical Pearl

If you need a boost in convincing your client to keep his or her wound covered, let him/her know that a moist wound heals with less scarring and therefore will look better when fully healed.[25]

Hygiene

Clients need to know that it is important for their dressings to stay clean and dry between dressing changes (unless you are using a waterproof dressing like a transparent film). Most dressings are not waterproof and must be covered in plastic for bathing. A wet dressing is a breeding ground for bacteria and can cause maceration of the skin around the wound. Clients who are sports enthusiasts should also be cautioned about exercising. Body sweat can saturate a dressing from the inside out. *Whatever the cause, a dressing that is wet to the touch must be changed.* Tell your client, "You must keep your dressing dry to help avoid infection and skin breakdown. Cover it with plastic in the shower, and try to avoid house-cleaning tasks that involve water. Also, avoid activities that will cause you to sweat a lot. Sweating can make your dressing wet from the inside out. Just remember—if your dressing is wet to the touch, it must be changed."

Additionally, although dressings are designed to keep debris and bacteria out of the wound, clients must use common sense in their daily activities. Not many upper extremity dressings can withstand the stress of activities like cleaning the garage, working in the yard, or changing the oil in the car. If a dressing gets too dirty or too worn from activity, there is an increased risk for wound infection. *A dirty or damaged dressing must be changed.* Say, "You must protect your dressing from damage to reduce the risk for infection. Avoid heavy hand use for things like cleaning, working in the yard, or working with heavy equipment. If your dressing gets dirty or worn, it must be changed."

◎ *Clinical Pearl*

Teach your clients this trick for keeping dressings dry in the shower: Wrap the hand/dressing in a small towel before covering everything with a plastic bag. Seal the plastic bag around the arm with hypoallergenic tape. If any water leaks inside the bag, it will be absorbed by the towel, not the dressing!

Cigarette Smoke

If your client smokes cigarettes, you should educate him/her that nicotine decreases the delivery of oxygen to tissues and can increase the risk for wound-healing complications.[26] Smoking just one cigarette can reduce blood flow to the hand.[3] You should encourage your clients to temporarily stop smoking until their wound is healed. However, for many clients, this is not a realistic expectation. If you get the sense that your client will not stop smoking during the wound healing process, you should tell your client that if he or she cannot stop smoking entirely, that there may be some benefit in cutting back on the number of cigarettes smoked per day. Most clients are willing to at least cut back on smoking until their wound is healed. You can say, "I am not going to give you a lecture about smoking, but you should know that your wound will heal better if you stop—or at least cut back—on your smoking until your wound is healed. Smoking just one cigarette decreases oxygen to the hand, and your wound needs all the oxygen it can get to heal."

Diet

Although we are not dieticians, we can encourage our clients with wounds to eat well and drink plenty of fluids. Tell your clients, "Try to eat a balanced diet and drink plenty of water right now. Nutrition plays an important role in wound healing. Your wound especially needs protein to heal."

Signs and Symptoms of Infection

All clients should be educated about the signs and symptoms of infection. If a client does have any indication that an infection may be present, encourage him or her to call the physician immediately. You should use plain and simple language with your clients. Say, "These are the signs and symptoms of infection that I want you to watch for: feeling generally unwell, running a fever, increased pain in the wound area, redness around the wound, red streaks leading away from the wound, warmth in the wound area, a bad odor coming from the wound, or any discharge that is white, thick, and yellow, or greenish/blue." *Tell your clients not to be shy about reporting a possible infection because it is important to catch infections early.* Say, "If you suspect you have an infection, call your doctor or me right away—even if you are not sure. I would rather you be safe than sorry. Wound infections can be serious, and we must catch and treat them early."

Evaluation Tips

Wound evaluation is important for treatment planning, for documenting the progression of wound healing, and for communicating with other caregivers. You must know what you are looking at and how to record it. Additionally, your assessment methods and terminology must remain consistent in order to accurately track progress. Never rely on your memory to gauge the progress of a wound. Wound evaluation is the basis for every intervention you choose, so the wound must be evaluated at every dressing change.

A good evaluation of an upper extremity wound will include the following:

- The location and size of the wound
- The condition of the periwound skin and wound margins
- Wound characteristics that might include granulation tissue, hypergranulation tissue, debris, or dead tissue
- The amount of wound exudate
- Any signs or symptoms of infection

Location and Size of Wound

When describing the location of a wound, do so in terms of anatomical position. For example, "The wound is on the anterior medial aspect of the distal forearm, 2 cm proximal to the pisiform." The more precise you can be, the better.

The size of the wound is usually recorded in millimeters or centimeters. Size is described in terms of length, width, and depth. There are a couple of ways to measure length and width. Some therapists will sit across from their client and view the wound in terms of a clock face. The length of the wound would be the measurement from 12 o'clock to 6 o'clock. The width of the wound would be the measurement from 9 o'clock to 3 o'clock. Another way to measure length and width is to measure the longest proximal to distal points of the wound, and then the widest medial to lateral points of the wound. Whichever way you choose to measure wound length and width, always do it the same way. This will assure consistency of comparative wound size over time.

Wound depth is measured by inserting a moistened sterile cotton-tipped applicator (that is, a sterile cotton swab) into the deepest part of the wound. Next, slide your gloved fingers down the length of the applicator until your fingers are at the level of the surrounding intact skin. Keep holding the applicator in this spot while lifting the applicator out of the wound. Measure the distance between the tips of your fingers to the tip of the cotton applicator. This is your wound depth.

Occasionally, in the forearm or upper arm, you will notice that a wound is very deep in a particular direction. If you gently try to push a moistened sterile cotton-tipped applicator into this area, you will note a narrow and deep hole—like a small tunnel that runs away from the main part of the wound. This is a condition called "**tunneling.**" Tunnels create open areas called "dead space" and increase the risk of abscess formation, so you want to keep the tunnel very clean. Record the depth of the tunnel as the distance that the sterile applicator can be gently inserted into the hole. Record the location of the tunnel using the clock face method. For example, "There is a 3 cm tunnel at 7 o'clock."

Condition of Periwound Skin and Wound Margins

When you look at the edges of the wound, you want to note its color and condition. Healthy **wound margins** look pink and flat. This tells you that epithelial tissue is being generated at the wound margins and that the wound is healing normally. If the wound margins appear grey or slightly turned under, that is a sign that the wound is not healing in a timely or efficient manner.

Wound margins should be firmly attached to the tissue underneath. If you notice that there is space under the wound edge, this is known as **undermining.** Undermining is another sign that the wound is not healing efficiently. There is a breakdown of tissue under the wound margins and the result is a relatively smaller wound opening with a larger wound underneath. It is difficult to see undermining, so if you do not clearly see that the wound edges are attached to the wound, try to gently slip a moistened sterile cotton-tipped applicator horizontally under the wound edge. If you have undermining, record the depth of the undermining as the distance that the sterile applicator can be pushed under the wound edge. Record the location of the undermining using the clock face method. For example, "There is 1 cm of undermining between 4 and 7 o'clock."

The skin around the wound, or **periwound skin,** should be skin-colored or maybe a little pink. Redness, inflammation, or hardening of the periwound skin could indicate infection. Small lesions of the periwound skin could indicate damage from adhesive dressings. If the periwound skin is soft and white, this indicates that the skin has absorbed too much fluid. We call this macerated skin, and it is the result of wound exudate not being adequately absorbed by the wound dressing. Macerated skin is fragile and easily damaged. If the epidermis around the wound starts to break down, we call this **denuded skin.**

Wound Characteristics

One of the simplest ways to describe the wound itself is to use the "red-yellow-black" system. To use this method, simply estimate what percentage of the wound is covered by each color. For example, "The wound is 50% red, 25% yellow, and 25% black." In this system, red represents a healthy wound bed, yellow represents slough, and black represents eschar. This is a common method of describing wounds, and many health care professionals who treat wounds understand this terminology.

Digital photos are extremely helpful in documenting what the wound and periwound skin looks like. When using a digital camera to record wound healing progression, be as consistent as possible with your picture-taking technique. For example, always taking the picture after cleansing and/or debriding the wound. Use the same camera and camera settings for all photos, and try to take the picture from the same distance and angle every time. Always include a patient identifier, date, and scale reference (like a centimeter tape measure) in every picture. Finally, try to approximate the same lighting conditions for each picture if possible.

> ◎ **Clinical Pearl**
>
> Do not use a flash when using a digital camera to record the image of a wound. You will be able to see more detail when the flash is turned off.

Wound Exudate

Wound exudate should be described in terms of type and amount. Terms used to describe the type of exudate are based on the color and consistency of the discharge. Color can range from clear to red to tan to green. Consistency can range from thin and watery to very thick and creamy. The following terms to describe exudate are commonly used and well-understood by healthcare professionals:

- **Serous**—clear and watery. This is normal.
- **Serosanguinous**—thin and pink. This is normal.
- **Sanguinous**—thin and bright red. This may or may not be normal, depending on the amount and type of tissue in the wound bed.
- **Purulent**—thick or thin, tan to yellow. This is a sign of possible infection.
- **Foul purulent**—thick, yellow to green, bad odor. This is a sign of infection.

Remember if you are using a hydrocolloid dressing, you will notice a thick, foul-smelling gel during dressing changes. This is normal and needs to be cleansed away before you can assess for foul purulent discharge.

The amount of wound exudate can range from nothing to large amounts. Describing the amount of drainage is subjective, but the following terms are typical:

- None—dry wound
- Scant amount—wound is moist but not draining
- Minimal amount or moderate amount—easily managed with your standard dressing choices
- Large amount—requires alginate dressing to control drainage
- Copious amount—so much drainage that it is difficult to manage with any dressing; this is rare

Infection

The cardinal signs and symptoms of infection include increased pain, foul odor, purulent drainage (pus), **erythema** (redness), **calor** (warmth), **induration** (hardening) around the wound, **lymphangitic streaking** (red streaks), **malaise** (feeling unwell), and **febricity** (fever). When documenting signs and symptoms of infection, it is acceptable and common to use lay terms so that what you are seeing is very clear to all members of the team. Only the physician can formally diagnose an infection. However, you are the care provider who sees the wound most often. It is your responsibility to assess for signs and symptoms of infection every time you see your client. If you have any indication that a wound is infected during your assessment, this should be immediately reported to the referring physician.

◎ Clinical Pearl

Not all infections smell bad. A wound that smells sweet and that has a distinctive neon-green discharge is very likely infected with *Pseudomonas aeruginosa*.

Diagnosis-Specific Information That Affects Clinical Reasoning

In summary of what we have already learned in this chapter, clinical reasoning in wound care is guided by the following principles:

1. Moist wound healing is the standard of care. Choose the right dressing to create a moist wound environment.
2. A wound will not heal until it is free of anything that should not be there: dead tissue, dressing debris, hypergranulation tissue, and so on. Strive to create a wound bed that is a healthy pink-red in color.
3. The regenerating wound bed is fragile. Do not stress a healing wound with cytotoxic chemicals, high pressure irrigation, or dressings that stick to the wound bed.
4. Infection must be identified and addressed early. Assess for infection at every dressing change and report any signs to the physician immediately.
5. Above all, do no harm. Never cut anything from an open wound that has not been positively identified.

♡ Tips from the Field

If you are able to assimilate everything presented in this chapter, you will have the basic skills necessary to care for your clients' upper extremity wounds. However, here are a few more pieces of advice:

1. Keep in mind that even if wound care is legally within your scope of practice, you still must be competent to provide the service. Most state licensing laws include language stating that therapists must be *competent* to perform any service within his or her scope of practice. No one wants to find themselves in front of a licensing board or jury box supporting a claim of competence to provide wound care services, but this does happen. Most of us get very little information about wound care in school. Therefore, you will want to gain additional knowledge and skill in this area through post-professional continuing education courses and/or mentorship. Keep all documentation of your training in wound care in a safe place.
2. Keep the lines of communication open with your referring physicians. Ask for help if you need it, and educate when you must. Never allow yourself to be pressured into providing a wound care procedure that you know is not the standard of care.
3. It is absolutely critical to keep exposed tendons moist. Hydrogel in gel form works great for this. If a tendon is allowed to dry, it will be damaged beyond repair. Monitor these clients closely.

⊳ Precautions and Concerns

When you perform wound care procedures, you will want to keep yourself and your clients safe from cross contamination by using **standard precautions.** Standard precautions are basic infection prevention guidelines and include the following: 1) hand hygiene, 2) use of personal protective equipment, 3) proper cleaning and use of medical equipment, 4) and proper environmental cleaning.[27]

You should perform proper hand hygiene before and after donning gloves for a wound care procedure. Using alcohol-based hand rub is the preferred method of hand decontamination except when your hands are visibly soiled, in which case soap and water should be used. During the wound care procedure, you should wear whatever personal protective equipment is needed to protect you from contact with your clients' body fluids. This will always include clean or sterile gloves, and may include disposable gowns, face masks/shields, and goggles. Any medical equipment that will come in contact with the wound itself (for example, scalpels, forceps) should be single-use or properly sterilized between clients. Equipment that will not come in contact with the wound (such as bandage scissors) should be disinfected between patients. Finally, all tabletops and client chair armrests should be disinfected between clients.

There has been a long-standing debate in the literature regarding the use of sterile gloves versus non-sterile (clean) gloves for clinical wound care outside of the surgical suite. A majority of the evidence suggests that there is no difference in infection rates or wound healing based on the use of either sterile or clean gloves.[28] However, proponents of using sterile gloves will point out that the evidence is not clearly convincing, and recommend erring on the side of caution by using sterile gloves for all dressing changes.[29] More research is needed in this area. Many hand therapists use clean gloves for all but their most high-risk patients. Sterile gloves should always be used if a patient is immune-compromised, has a resistant infection, or has a history of multiple infections.

One thing that you can do to reduce the chance of contaminating a wound is to apply dressings using a "no-touch" technique. It works like this:

- *Don a pair of clean gloves, and remove your client's "dirty" dressing.*
- *Remove your gloves, decontaminate your hands with an alcohol-based hand rub, and then apply a fresh pair of gloves.*
- *Do not touch anything except the new dressing materials and a decontaminated pair of bandage scissors.*

This technique works best with an assistant present to open the dressing packaging. After your assistant opens the packaging, you can reach in and grab the sterile dressing that will make contact with your client's wound. *Only a sterile dressing should make contact with the wound bed.* You don't want to open the package yourself, because the outside of the package may be contaminated, but the inside of the package will be sterile. After the wound bed is covered with the sterile dressing, any secondary dressing that is required can be clean/non-sterile. However, continue with the no-touch technique until all the dressings have been applied.

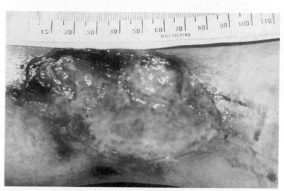

FIGURE 21-6 Upper extremity wound resulting from trauma.

CASE STUDY

CASE STUDY 21-1 ■

Wound Assessment

Figure 21-6 represents a typical upper extremity wound resulting from trauma. Wounds like this can be seen on the forearms of patients who have been in high speed motorcycle accidents. Upon presentation, you note the wound to be tri-colored. It contains approximately 80% slough (yellow), 15% eschar (black), and 5% granulation tissue (pink-red). The wound appears to be very superficial – although you will not know for sure that there is no tunneling or cavities under the eschar until the black tissue has been removed. When documenting the size of this wound, measure the longest proximal to distal point of the wound and call that the wound "length." Then, measure the widest medial to lateral point of the wound and call that the wound "width." The periwound skin looks healthy – a pinkish tan color. There is little discharge and the wound does not have a foul odor. Based on these observations, you would not suspect a wound infection at this point.

Treatment planning

In order for this wound to heal, you must remove the eschar and slough from the wound bed. Your goal is to remove all dead tissue until only healthy pink-red granulation tissue is present. The safest and easiest way to try to remove the eschar and slough is through autolytic debridement. You can encourage the body to break down its own dead tissue by choosing a dressing that keeps the wound moist. At first, there will be some trial and error as you look for the most effective dressing. Because this wound is superficial and has little discharge, you might first try applying a transparent film over the wound. Irrigate the wound well with sterile saline, pat it dry with a sterile piece of gauze, and then use a "no-touch" technique to apply the transparent film. Your client should keep this dressing in place until he returns in 3 to 5 days. Transparent films are waterproof in the shower, so your client may shower with the dressing in place. When your client returns to the clinic, remove the transparent film and note how much of the dead tissue has liquefied under the dressing. Irrigate the wound with saline and decide on the most appropriate dressing to try next. If there has been little change in the amount of eschar and slough, you need to add moisture and might consider a little hydrogel under the transparent film. If there was a lot of liquification of dead tissue under the film and the periwound skin is turning white, the wound is now too wet. You may need to change the film dressing more frequently. At each dressing change, continue to choose dressings based on the amount of moisture in the wound. Once the eschar and slough are gone, continue to use dressings that keep the wound moist until it is completely healed. Monitor for any sign of infection or non-healing at each dressing change, and report these situations to the referring doctor.

References

1. American Occupational Therapy Association: The role of occupational therapy in wound management: a position paper, *AOTA* (white paper online): http://www.aota.org/-/media/Corporate/Files/AboutAOTA/OfficialDocs/Position/Wound%2020Management.ashx. Accessed May 6, 2013.
2. News Now Staff, American Physical Therapy Association: New APTA resource on active wound care management available online, *PT in Motion for members of the American Physical Therapy Association* (website): http://www.apta.org/PTinMotion/NewsNow/2011/7/14/WoundManagementFAQs/. Accessed July 2, 2012.
3. Mosely LH, Finseth F: Cigarette smoking: impairment of digital blood flow and wound healing in the hand, *Hand* 9(2):97–101, 1977.
4. Wilson JR, Mills JG, Prather ID, et al: A toxicity index of skin and wound cleansers used in vitro fibroblasts and keratinocytes, *Adv Skin Wound Care* 18:373–378, 2005.
5. Alvarez OM, Rogers RS, Booker JG, et al: Effect of noncontact normothermic wound therapy on the healing of neuropathic (diabetic) foot ulcers: an interim analysis of 20 patients, *J Foot Ankle Surg* 42:30–35, 2003.
6. McGuiness W, Vella E, Harrison D: Influence of dressing changes on wound temperature, *J Wound Care* 13:383–385, 2004.
7. Okan D, Woo K, Ayello EA, et al: The role of moisture balance in wound healing, *Adv Skin Wound Care* 20:39–53, 2007.
8. Hess CT: Checklist for factors affecting wound healing, *Adv Skin Wound Care* 24:192, 2011.
9. Langemo D, Anderson J, Hanson D, et al: Nutritional considerations in wound care, *Adv Skin Wound Care* 19:297–303, 2006.
10. Hampton S: Understanding overgranulation in tissue viability practice, *Br J Community Nurse* 12:S24–S30, 2007.
11. Myers BA: *Wound management: principles and practice*, New Jersey, 2004, Prentice Hall.
12. Fernandez R, Griffiths R: Water for wound cleansing, *Cochrane Database Syst Rev* 15:CD003861, 2012.
13. Chatterjee JS: A critical review of irrigation techniques in acute wounds, *Int Wound J* 2:258–265, 2005.
14. Hess CT: *Wound care*, ed 5, Philadelphia, 2005, Lippincott, Williams & Wilkins.

15. Stevenson TR, Thacker JG, Rodeheaver GT, et al: Cleansing the traumatic wound by high pressure syringe irrigation, *JACEP* 5(1):17–21, 1976.

16. US Department of Health and Human Services: Quick reference guide for clinicians: pressure ulcer treatment clinical practice guideline, *HHS.Gov Archive* (online archive from 1994 December 21): http://archive.hhs.gov/news/press/1994pres/941221a.txt. Accessed May 6, 2013.

17. Panuncialman J, Falanga V: The science of wound bed preparation, *Surg Clin N Am* 89:611–626, 2009.

18. Fulton JA, Blasiole KN, Cottingham T, et al: Wound dressing absorption: a comparative study, *Adv Skin Wound Care* 25:315–320, 2012.

19. Worley CA: So, what do I put on this wound? Making sense of the wound dressing puzzle: part III, *Medsurg Nursing* 15:251–252, 2006.

20. Worley CA: So, what do I put on this wound? Making sense of the wound dressing puzzle: part II, *Medsurg Nursing* 15:182–183, 2006.

21. Worley CA: So, what do I put on this wound? Making sense of the wound dressing puzzle: part I, *Medsurg Nursing* 15:106–107, 2006.

22. Mueller SW, Krebsbach LE: Impact of an anti-microbial-impregnated gauze dressing on surgical site infections including methicillin-resistant *Staphylococcus aureus* infections, *Am J Infect Control* 36:651–655, 2008.

23. Kessler DO, Krantz BS, Mojica M: Randomized trial comparing wound packing to no wound packing following incision and drainage of superficial skin abscesses in the pediatric emergency department, *Pediatr Emerg Care* 28:514–517, 2012.

24. Taylor CJ, Chester DL, Jeffery SL: Functional splinting of upper limb injuries with gauze-based topical negative pressure wound therapy, *J Hand Surgery* 36:1848–1851, 2011.

25. Wigger-Alberti W, Kuhlmann M, Ekanayake S, et al: Using a novel wound model to investigate the healing properties of products for superficial wounds, *J Wound Care* 18(3):123–128, 131, 2009.

26. Bartsch RH, Weiss G, Kastenbauer T, et al: Crucial aspects of smoking in wound healing after breast reduction surgery, *J Plast Reconstr Aesthet Surg* 60:1045–1049, 2007.

27. Centers for Disease Control and Prevention: Guide to infection prevention for outpatient settings: minimum expectations for safe care, *CDC.gov Healthcare-associated Infections* (website article written May 2011): http://www.cdc.gov/HAI/settings/outpatient/outpatient-care-guidelines.html. Accessed August 13, 2012.

28. Flores A: Sterile versus non-sterile glove use and aseptic technique, *Nurs Stand* 23(6):35–39, 2008.

29. St Clair K, Larrabee JH: Clean versus sterile gloves: which to use for postoperative dressing changes? *Outcomes Manag* 6(1):17–21, 2002.

22 Common Shoulder Diagnoses

Mark W. Butler

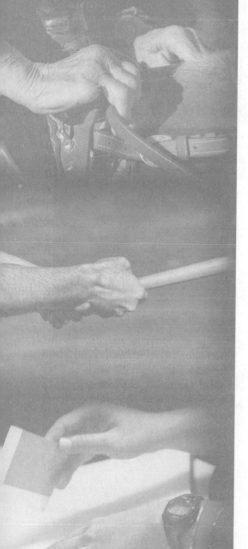

Introduction

Positioning the hand in space to allow for interaction with the environment is the primary function of the shoulder. Accordingly, dysfunction of the shoulder complex often results in profound impairment of the entire upper extremity (UE).[1] The shoulder will compensate for decreased mobility of the wrist and elbow, which can lead to shoulder dysfunction as the individual tries to perform normal activities of daily living (ADLs). *Consequently, when treating a client with elbow or wrist dysfunction, the therapist needs to monitor the health of the shoulder.* Therefore a thorough understanding of the shoulder is imperative for therapists treating clients with UE dysfunction.

Clinical Pearl

The shoulder has the greatest range of motion (ROM) of any joint in the body. This ROM is the result of the aggregate movement of a series of articulations that comprise the shoulder complex. These articulations work in concert to provide a unique balance between mobility and stability with the emphasis on mobility. A shift in this balance often results in (or can be caused by) the pathological processes we will review in this chapter.

Anatomy

The shoulder complex consists of:
- Three bones: The humerus, the clavicle, and the scapula
- Three joints: The glenohumeral (GH), acromioclavicular (AC), and sternoclavicular (SC)
- One "pseudo joint": The scapulothoracic (ST) articulation

Glenohumeral Joint

The GH joint is a multi-axial, synovial, ball-and-socket joint that moves around three axes of motion: internal/external rotation around a vertical axis, abduction/adduction around a sagittal axis, and flexion/extension around a frontal axis (Fig. 22-1). The humeral head forms roughly half a sphere with the glenoid fossa forming the socket component of the joint. The glenoid fossa covers only one third to one fourth of the humeral head (Fig. 22-2). The glenoid labrum, a ring of fibrocartilage, surrounds and deepens the glenoid socket by about 50% and increases joint stability by increasing humeral head contact 75% vertically and 56 % transversely.[2]

The **open-packed position** (joint position in which the capsule and ligaments are most lax and separation of joint surfaces are greatest) of the GH joint is 55° of abduction and 30° of horizontal adduction. The **close-packed position** (joint position in which the capsule and ligaments are under the most tension with maximal contact between joint surfaces) of the joint is full abduction and lateral rotation. At rest, the humerus sits centered in the glenoid cavity; with contraction of the rotator cuff (RC) muscles, the humeral head translates anteriorly, posteriorly, superiorly, inferiorly, or any combination of these movements. These translations are very small, but full motion of the GH joint is impossible without them because the combined actions of the RC muscles contribute to the overall stability of the GH joint during ROM.[3] It is the motion of the GH joint that contributes the most to shoulder movement.

Acromioclavicular Joint

The AC joint is a **plane synovial joint** (joint with a synovium-lined capsule and relatively flat surfaces) that augments the ROM of the GH joint; this is the joint around which

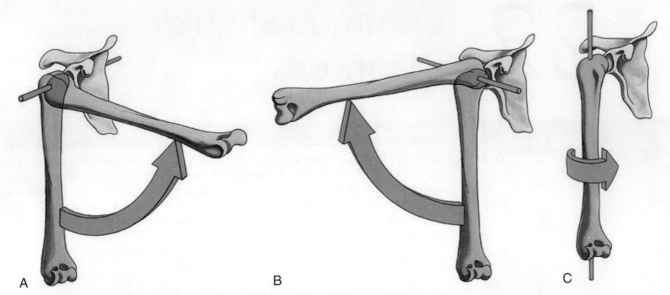

A   B   C

FIGURE 22-1 **The three degrees of freedom of the glenohumeral (GH) joint. A,** Flexion/extension; **B,** abduction/adduction; **C,** internal/external rotation. (From Standring S: *Gray's anatomy e-book,* ed 40, St Louis, 2012, Churchill Livingstone.)

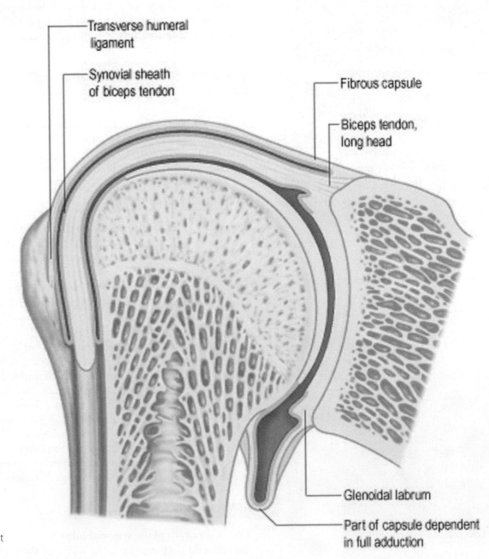

Transverse humeral ligament

Synovial sheath of biceps tendon

Fibrous capsule

Biceps tendon, long head

Glenoidal labrum

Part of capsule dependent in full adduction

FIGURE 22-2 Coronal section of the left shoulder joint through the long head of the biceps tendon. (From Putz R, Pabst R: *Sobotta—atlas of human anatomy single volume edition: head, neck, upper limb, thorax, abdomen, pelvis, lower limb,* ed 14, St Louis, 2008, Elsevier.)

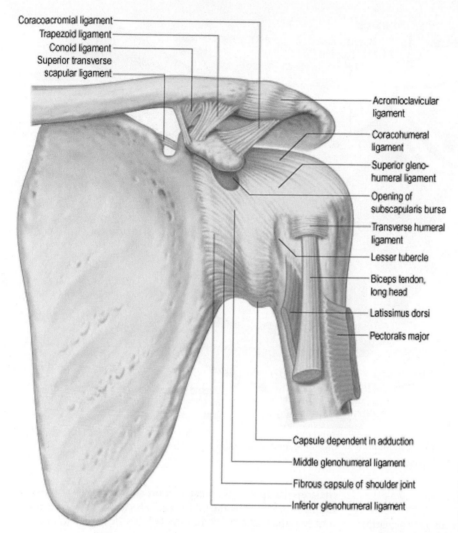

Coracoacromial ligament
Trapezoid ligament
Conoid ligament
Superior transverse
scapular ligament

Acromioclavicular
ligament

Coracohumeral
ligament

Superior gleno-
humeral ligament

Opening of
subscapularis bursa

Transverse humeral
ligament

Lesser tubercle

Biceps tendon,
long head

Latissimus dorsi

Pectoralis major

Capsule dependent in adduction

Middle glenohumeral ligament

Fibrous capsule of shoulder joint

Inferior glenohumeral ligament

FIGURE 22-3 Anterior aspect of the left shoulder showing the joint capsule and acromioclavicular (AC) ligaments. (From Standring S: *Gray's anatomy e-book*, ed 40, St Louis, 2012, Churchill Livingstone, p. 802.)

the scapula moves. The bones that comprise the AC joint are the acromion process of the scapula and the distal end of the clavicle. The AC joint moves around three axes resulting in three **degrees of freedom** (direction or type of motion at a joint): pure spin around a longitudinal axis for abduction/adduction of the shoulder, a vertical axis for protraction/retraction of the shoulder, and a horizontal axis for shoulder elevation/depression.

The AC and coracoclavicular (CC) ligaments support the AC joint (Fig. 22-3). The AC ligaments contribute the least to joint stability; they function mainly to support the joint capsule and check anterior/posterior translation of the clavicle on the acromion. The AC ligaments are damaged in grade I shoulder separations. The CC ligaments have no attachment to the acromion and consist of the conoid and trapezoid ligaments. They transmit scapular motion to the clavicle and check superior clavicular displacement.[4] As all fibers of the upper trapezius insert on the clavicle,[5] the CC ligaments play an integral role in the transmission of force from the upper trapezius to the scapula.[6] Complete rupture of these ligaments represents a grade III separation resulting in a step deformity at the AC joint (Fig. 22-4).

The open-packed position for the AC joint is with the arm by the side. The close-packed position is at 90° of shoulder abduction.

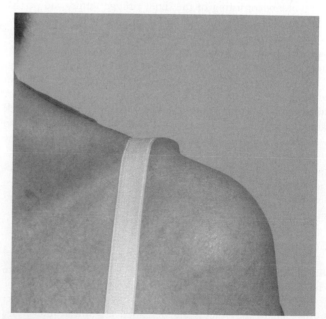

FIGURE 22-4 Chronic grade III acromioclavicular (AC) separation showing step deformity indicating disruption of the coracoclavicular (CC) ligaments.

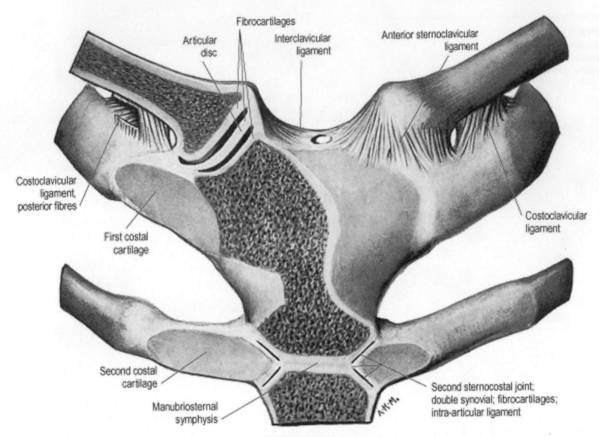

FIGURE 22-5 Sternoclavicular (SC) joints: Right joint in coronal section. (From Standring S: *Gray's anatomy e-book*, ed 40, St Louis, 2012, Churchill Livingstone, p. 802.)

Sternoclavicular Joint

The sellar (saddle) shaped SC joint is the only direct articulation between the shoulder complex and the **axial skeleton** (skeletal components consisting of the skull, ribcage, spine, and pelvis). The articulations of the SC joint are between the medial end of the clavicle, the clavicular notch of the sternum, and the cartilage of the first rib. Interposed between the clavicle and the sternum is an articular disc that enhances stability of the joint (Fig. 22-5). Movement between the disc and clavicle is greater than movement between the disc and sternum. The joint is further stabilized by the joint capsule and ligaments that primarily check superior and anterior translation.[7] The SC joint is stabilized so well by the disc and ligaments that trauma to the clavicle usually results in fracture instead of dislocation.[8] The motion of the SC joint mirrors that of the AC joint: elevation/depression, protraction/retraction, and rotation (spin). The open-packed position for the SC joint is with the arm by the side. The close-packed position is full UE elevation.

Scapulothoracic Articulation

As the scapula has no direct bony or ligamentous connections to the thorax, the ST articulation cannot be considered an anatomic joint. Scapular movement results in movement of the shoulder girdle. These movements are described as: upward/downward rotation around an axis perpendicular to the scapular body, internal/external rotation around a vertical axis along the medial border, and anterior/posterior tilt around a horizontal axis along the scapular spine.[9] Scapular motion allows for elevation above the 120° provided by the GH joint.[2] The scapula's bony articulation is with the AC joint, but the stability of the ST joint comes from muscular attachments to the scapula.

Much like a street performer balancing a ball on the end of a stick, the scapula must change position during shoulder elevation to keep the humeral head balanced in the glenoid fossa, thus allowing for the most efficient length-tension relationship of the RC. With shoulder elevation, the majority of motion occurs at the GH joint during the initial (0° to 60°) and final (140° to 180°) phases of motion. It is during these phases that the ST articulation plays a subtler balancing or stabilizing role. Throughout the middle or critical (60° to 140°) phase of shoulder elevation, the ratio of GH to ST motion shifts, with more emphasis on ST movement[10] (see Video 22-1 on the Evolve website).

This movement of the scapula is the result of force couples between groups of muscles that run from the thorax to the scapula (Table 22-1). A **force couple** is defined as two resultant forces of equal magnitude in opposite directions that produce rotation of a structure. The upward rotation of the scapula that occurs during shoulder elevation is primarily the result of the **concentric** (muscle contraction resulting in approximation of the origin and insertion) actions of the upper and lower trapezius and the lower portion of the serratus anterior muscles with the levator scapulae, rhomboids, and pectoralis minor acting **eccentrically** (muscle contraction to stabilize movement resulting in increased distance between the origin and insertion) to produce smooth motion.

In the normal resting position, the scapula sits angled 20° to 30° forward relative to the frontal plane, 20° forward in the

TABLE 22-1   Scapular Force Couples

Movement	Concentric Force Couple	Eccentric Stabilizers
Upward rotation (GH elevation)	Upper trapezius Lower trapezius Serratus anterior	Levator scapulae Rhomboids Pectoralis minor
Retraction	Trapezius Rhomboids	Serratus anterior Pectoralis major Pectoralis minor
Protraction	Serratus anterior Pectoralis major Pectoralis minor	Trapezius Rhomboids
Elevation	Upper trapezius Levator scapulae	Serratus anterior Lower trapezius
Depression	Serratus anterior Lower trapezius	Upper trapezius Levator scapulae
Downward rotation	Levator scapulae Rhomboids Latissimus dorsi Pectoralis minor	Upper trapezius Lower trapezius Serratus anterior

GH, Glenohumeral.

sagittal plane with the medial border angled at 3° top to bottom from the spinous processes. This position, combined with the orientation of the glenoid fossa, results in elevation of the arm in a plane that is 30° to 45° anterior to the frontal plane. This motion is termed *scapular plane abduction* or **scaption.**[11] The scapula extends from the level of the T2 spinous process to the T7 or T9 spinous process based on size. Since the ST articulation is not an anatomic joint, there is no close- or open-packed position.

Proximal (Cervical) Screening

Because of the proximity of the cervical spine to the shoulder, the cervical spine must be screened for contribution to the client's symptoms. It is essential to the screening process to have a basic understanding of cervical anatomy and of the structures that refer symptoms to the shoulder and UE.

Anatomy

The cervical structures that refer symptoms to the shoulder and entire UE that are cleared via cervical screening are the following:
- Cervical nerve roots
- Cervical discs
- Cervical facets
- Cervical intrinsic soft tissue (muscles, ligaments, joint capsules)
- Cervical extrinsic musculature

Cervical Nerve Roots

The C4 to C7 nerve roots supply structures that overlie or comprise the shoulder complex (Fig. 22-6). The C5 and C6 nerve roots innervate most of the GH joint structures with the C4 nerve root innervating the AC joint.

Because of their location and path of travel, the cervical nerve roots are susceptible to injury. A **disc herniation** (damage

to the annular wall of the disc resulting in disc deformity as the nucleus displaces into the lesion) can entrap the nerve root against the vertebral lamina and encroach upon the dorsal root ganglion. Hypertrophy of the facet joints, spurring of the vertebral end plates, and spurring of the **uncinate processes** (winglike projections from the superior portion of the cervical vertebrae that articulate with the inferior portion of the vertebrae above) will narrow the **intervertebral foramen (IVF)** (bony canal that contains the spinal nerve) resulting in compression of the cervical nerve roots. Degenerative loss of cervical disc height further enhances this process.

Cervical Discs

The cervical spine contains five discs with the most superior disc located between C2 and C3, and the most inferior disc located between C7 and T1. The disc consists of three parts: the **annulus fibrosis** (multi-layered ligamentous exterior of the disc), the **vertebral end plate** (cartilaginous interface between the vertebral disc and the vertebral body), and the **nucleus pulposus** (pulpy semi-liquid center of the disc). The cervical discs are morphologically quite different from lumbar discs, because they essentially lack a posterior annular wall.[12] The posterior longitudinal ligament mainly supplies that role. Also, the cervical disc develops horizontal annular clefts or tears in the lateral portion by age 15 that progressively extend across the back of the disc.[12] It is likely due to these differences that the cervical discs degenerate more quickly than the lumbar discs.[13]

The onset of neck and arm pain with cervical disc herniation is usually insidious and often starts in the neck and medial scapular border before radiating to the shoulder and arm. Symptoms can spread as far as the hand depending on the involved nerve root.

Cervical Facets

The **facet joints** of the cervical spine are paired synovial joints with fibrous capsules. The capsules are heavily innervated by **mechanoreceptors** (specialized nerve endings that transmit information regarding position and motion) and **nociceptors** (specialized nerve endings that transmit pain signals), which likely modulate protective muscle reflexes that are important in preventing joint instability and degeneration.[14]

Studies on normal individuals and clients with neck pain demonstrated pain referral patterns from the cervical facets to the cervical and shoulder regions.[15,16] These studies demonstrated a consistent pain referral pattern to the top and lateral parts of the shoulder, extending to the inferior border of the scapula from the C6 to C7 facet joints.

Cervical Intrinsic Soft Tissue

The intrinsic soft tissue structures of the cervical/thoracic region include the muscles that do not originate or insert on the clavicle or scapula. Of these muscles, the scalenes demonstrate **trigger point** (palpable taut muscle bands that refer pain when compressed) pain referral patterns to the shoulder (Fig. 22-7). There are substantial anatomical variations in the attachments of the scalene muscles. In general, the proximal portions attach to the transverse processes of the cervical vertebrae. The distal attachments of the anterior and medial scalene are the first rib; the distal attachment of the posterior scalene is the second rib. The trigger points refer pain to the anterior lateral aspect of the shoulder and medial scapular border.[17]

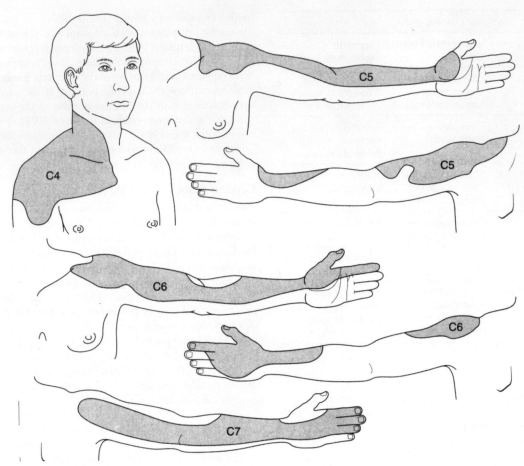

FIGURE 22-6 Cervical dermatomes affecting the shoulder. (From Magee DJ: *Orthopedic physical asssessment,* ed 5, Philadelphia, 2008, Saunders, p.183.)

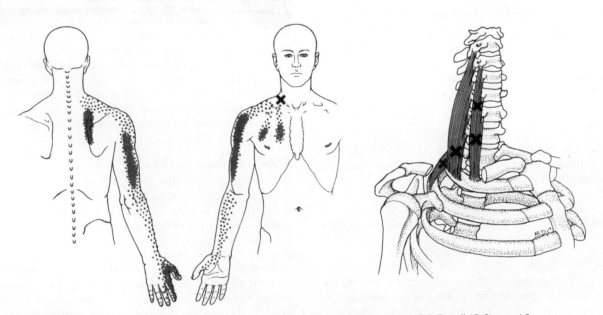

FIGURE 22-7 Scalene trigger point location and referral pattern. (From Simons DG, Travell JG, Simons LS: *Travell & Simons' myofascial pain and dysfunction: the trigger point manual,* vol. 1, ed 2, Baltimore, 1998, Lippincott Williams & Wilkins, p. 506.)

Cervical Extrinsic Muscle

The extrinsic muscles are those that have attachments to the shoulder structures (scapula and clavicle) and cervical spine. Of these, the trapezius and levator scapulae demonstrate trigger point pain referral patterns to the shoulder.

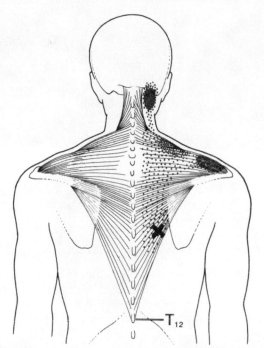

FIGURE 22-8 Lower trapezius trigger point location and referral pattern. (From Simons DG, Travell JG, Simons LS: *Travell & Simons' myofascial pain and dysfunction: the trigger point manual,* vol. 1, ed 2, Baltimore, 1998, Lippincott Williams & Wilkins.)

The trapezius extends down the midline from the occiput to T12, anteriorly to the clavicle, laterally to the acromion and superior medial scapular angle, and superiorly to the scapular spine. Six trigger points with distinctive pain patterns are located in the upper, middle, and lower fibers. The trigger point located in the lower trapezius refers pain to the mastoid area and the posterior acromion (Fig. 22-8).[17]

The levator scapulae attaches proximally to the transverse processes of the first four cervical vertebrae and distally to the superior medial scapular angle. The trigger point refers pain to the angle of the neck and often projects to the posterior aspect of the shoulder (Fig. 22-9).[17]

Diagnosis and Pathology

The primary goal of the cervical screening examination is to efficiently screen for cervical pathology that may be contributing to or causing shoulder symptoms. If screening indicates cervical pathology, the examiner must perform further testing of the cervical spine. There are numerous examination procedures described in the literature that are beyond the scope of this chapter. *The following screening procedures are not a substitute for a complete examination of the cervical spine.*

Cervical Screening Examination

Range of Motion Testing—Intrinsic versus Extrinsic Restrictions

Having your client perform active movements of the cervical spine is an excellent beginning point for the screening examination. By changing the relative position of the shoulder and cervical spine during testing, you can begin to differentiate between intrinsic and extrinsic restrictions to cervical motion.

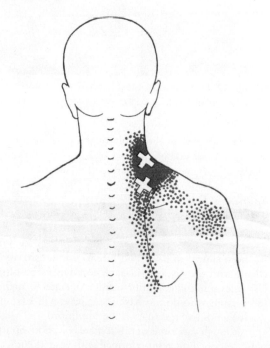

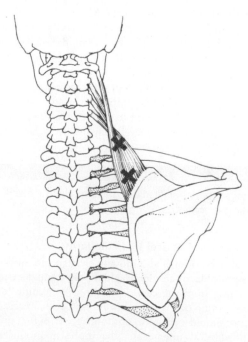

FIGURE 22-9 Levator scapulae trigger point location and referral pattern. (From Simons DG, Travell JG, Simons LS: *Travell & Simons' myofascial pain and dysfunction: the trigger point manual,* vol. 1, ed 2, Baltimore, 1998, Lippincott Williams & Wilkins.)

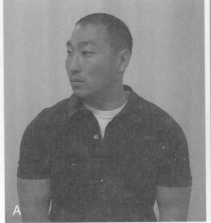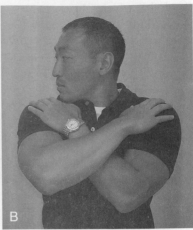

FIGURE 22-10 Cervical rotation testing. **A,** Arms at rest; **B,** cross-arm position.

Your client performs the basic motions of the cervical spine (flexion/extension, rotation, lateral flexion) from a corrected neutral seated posture with the arms unsupported. Next, he/she performs the same motions in a crossed arm position (Fig 22-10; see Video 22-2 on the Evolve website). Your client grasps as close to their AC joints as possible and then relaxes their arms and shoulders, letting their arms rest against their chest wall.

This position effectively elevates the scapulae; and by having your client grasp their shoulders, the scapular elevators are allowed to relax. An improvement in ROM in this position implicates the extrinsic cervical structures as contributing to motion loss. No change in motion implicates the intrinsic structures. However, the extrinsic structures may still be limiting motion. The test is designed to rule out intrinsic restrictions if a difference exists between the two test positions.

Repeated Motion Testing—the Search for a Directional Preference

Repeated motion testing is the basis of the McKenzie model of examination. By having your client perform the cervical motions of protrusion, retraction, retraction plus extension, flexion, lateral flexion, and rotation in groups of 5 to 10 repetitions, the therapist looks for a **directional preference.**

A directional preference exists if any of these movements centralize and/or decrease your client's symptoms, and/or improve any ROM restrictions. It is important to note that with centralization, your client's proximal pain levels may intensify.

Ⓒ **Clinical Pearl**

Worsening and/or peripheralization of your client's distal symptoms indicate cervical pathology.[18]

Test Clusters to Detect Cervical Radiculopathy

Since the cervical nerve root is the most likely structure of the cervical spine responsible for **cervicobrachial pain** (shoulder and arm pain originating from the cervical region),[19] screening for cervical nerve root pathology is critical in ruling out the cervical spine as a source of shoulder pain. An optimum group of four test items was identified by Wainner, et al.[20] that if present, produced a **post-test probability** (the probability of the condition being present compared to pretesting) of 90%. These items were the Spurling's test, cervical distraction test, cervical rotation ROM

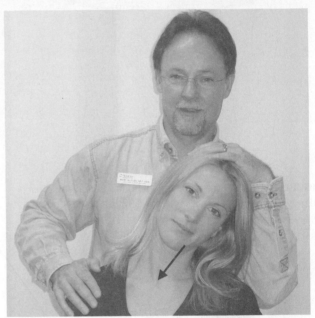

FIGURE 22-11 Spurling's A test. Consists of lateral cervical flexion to end range followed by axial compression of approximately 7 kg.

less than 60° toward the involved side, and the upper limb neurodynamic test (ULNT) (described in the following "Thoracic Outlet Syndrome/Brachial Plexopathy" section).

Spurling's Test

Spurling's test has been described as a screening test to detect cervical radiculopathy (CR) (disease of the cervical nerve roots) in numerous studies considered to be good.[20-23] The Spurling's test has been shown to have moderate to low **sensitivity** (few if any clients with the disease will have negative test results; a negative test rules out the condition) and moderate to high **specificity** (all persons who do not have the disease will have negative test results; a positive test rules in the condition).

Although variations of this test are common, Spurling[24] originally described the test performed with your client seated and the examiner passively side-bending his/her client's neck toward the symptomatic side to end range, next adding axial compression of approximately 7 kg directed toward the base of the cervical spine (Fig. 22-11; see Video 22-3 on the Evolve website). The examiner executes these steps sequentially, stopping with reproduction or worsening of his/her client's symptoms. Variations of the test include the additional movements of extension and rotation toward the painful side prior to adding compression of cervical spine (Fig. 22-12; see Video 22-3 on the Evolve website).[23] With the cervical spine in this position, the IVF diameter closes down by approximately 70%,[25] decreasing the available space for an inflamed nerve root; the presence of a space-occupying lesion (such as, a disc herniation or osteophytic spur) will intensify the test result. Axial loading at the end range of extension, lateral flexion, and rotation also stresses the facet joints, provoking symptoms if pathology is present.

Cervical Distraction Test

The examiner performs this test seated at the head of the plinth with his/her client supine. The examiner grasps his/her client's chin and occiput, flexes their neck to a position of comfort, and applies an axial distraction force of approximately 14 kg (Fig. 22-13; see Video 22-4 on the Evolve website). A positive test results in reduction or elimination of his/her client's symptoms. With distraction of the cervical spine in this manner, the IVF diameter increases by approximately 120% effectively relieving pressure on the inflamed nerve root, resulting in symptom reduction.[25]

Cervical Rotation Range of Motion

The examiner performs this test utilizing a standard goniometer standing behind his/her client seated in a chair with back support to stabilize the thoracic spine. The examiner positions the axis of the goniometer over the vertex of the client's head, the stationary arm of the goniometer perpendicular to his/her shoulders, and the movable arm in line with the client's nose (Fig. 22-14). Rotation ROM of 60° or less toward the involved side results in a positive test.

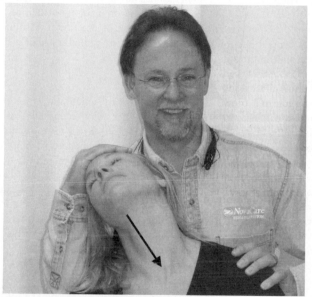

FIGURE 22-12 Spurling's B test. Consists of lateral cervical flexion to end range—cervical extension to end range with the addition of axial compression here of approximately 7 kg, or adding ipsilateral rotation followed by axial compression.

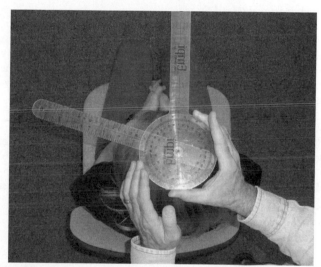

FIGURE 22-14 Cervical rotation range of motion (ROM) measurement technique.

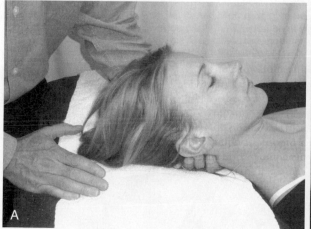
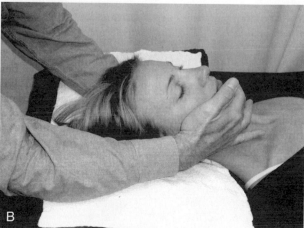

FIGURE 22-13 Cervical distraction test. A, Therapist hand position on client's occiput. **B,** Final hand position with the addition of 14 kg axial traction pull.

Thoracic Outlet Syndrome/Brachial Plexopathy

The term *thoracic outlet syndrome (TOS)* encompasses an assortment of clinical entities involving the shoulder region. *The thoracic outlet provides the pathway for the neural and vascular structures to and from the upper limb, therefore pathology of this area has profound and often disabling results.* As vascular presentations of TOS are relatively uncommon (3% to 5%), the great majority of TOS clients, in fact, have brachial plexopathies.[26]

Anatomy

The Thoracic Outlet

The thoracic outlet (TO) can be divided into four regions: the sternocostovertebral space, the scalene triangle, the costoclavicular space, and the pectoralis minor (coracopectoral) space. Each region has distinct boundaries, contents, and potential pathologies that result in neurovascular compression and/or entrapment (Fig. 22-15).

Sternocostovertebral Space

The sternocostovertebral space is bordered anteriorly by the sternum, posteriorly by the spinal column, and laterally by the first rib. The contents are the roots of the plexus; the subclavian artery and vein, jugular vein, and neck lymphatics. Compression of the contents is usually caused by tumors of the lung (Pancoast), thymus, parathyroids, and lymph nodes.

Scalene Triangle

The scalene triangle is bordered anteriorly by the anterior scalene, posteriorly by the middle scalene, and inferiorly by the first rib. The contents are the roots and trunks of the plexus and subclavian artery. Compression and entrapment of these structures are caused by variations in scalene anatomy and the presence of congenital fibrous bands that may interdigitate with the plexus.[27]

Costoclavicular Space

The costoclavicular space is bordered superiorly by the clavicle and inferiorly by the first rib. The contents are the divisions of the plexus and the subclavian artery and vein. Compression of these structures between the clavicle and first rib occur as a result of postural deficits, resulting in shoulder girdle depression, clavicular and first rib fractures, and the presence of a cervical rib.

Pectoralis Minor (Coracopectoral) Space

The coracopectoral space is bordered superiorly by the coracoid process, anteriorly by the pectoralis minor, and posteriorly by the chest wall. The contents are the cords of the plexus and the subclavian artery and vein. Compression of these structures is caused by hypertrophy and contracture of the pectoralis minor and hyperabduction of the arm as they are pulled up against the pectoralis minor tendon.

The Brachial Plexus

The brachial plexus is net-like in design, which allows for the individual neurons from the spinal nerves to eventually reach their respective peripheral nerve. It also serves as a force distributor to dissipate traction forces from the peripheral nerve, helping to prevent traction injuries of the lower cervical nerve roots.

Although anatomical variations exist, the brachial plexus is fairly consistent in its organization. Moving proximal to distal, the plexus is organized into roots (C5 to T1); trunks (upper, middle, lower); divisions (anterior, posterior); and cords (medial, lateral, posterior). Trunks are supraclavicular; cords are infraclavicular with the divisions occurring under the clavicle.

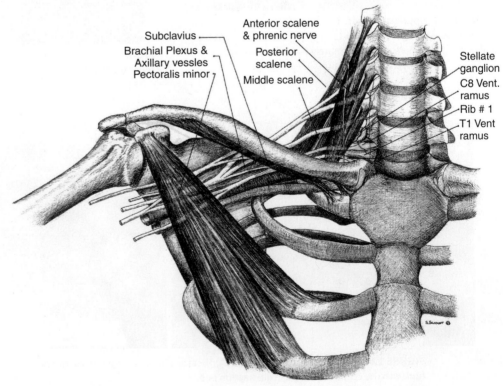

FIGURE 22-15 The thoracic outlet (TO). (From Edgelow PI: Neurovascular consequences of cumulative trauma disorders affecting the thoracic outlet: a patient-centered treatment approach. In Donatelli RA, editor: *Physical therapy of the shoulder,* ed 4, St Louis, 2004, Churchill Livingstone. Courtesy of Peter Edgelow.)

- Of the five nerve roots that supply the plexus, the top two make up the upper trunk, the bottom two make up the lower trunk, and the middle root makes up the middle trunk.
- The upper trunk supplies the scapular musculature and scapular stabilizers.
- The lower trunk supplies the hand intrinsics.
- Anterior division of the lower trunk supplies the medial cord.
- Anterior divisions of the upper and middle trunk supply the lateral cord.
- Anterior divisions supply the elbow and wrist flexors with the exception of the brachioradialis, which is supplied by the posterior cord.
- Posterior divisions of all trunks supply the posterior cord.
- Posterior cord supplies the elbow and wrist extensors.

Diagnosis and Pathology

There are nearly a dozen surgical and medical specialties that see TOS clients. Unfortunately these various specialties have disparate views regarding diagnosis and treatment of the condition. The most up-to-date thoughts on TOS are that it is comprised of five discrete subgroups. These groups consist of: 1) arterial vascular, 2) venous vascular, 3) true neurologic, 4) traumatic neurovascular, and 5) disputed.[26] Groups 1 to 4 are rare and beyond the scope of this chapter. The disputed subgroup is considered to be fairly common and primarily involving the brachial plexus. As a result, wide ranges of clinical presentations are common and confusing to clinicians.[26,28]

Vascular Component

The diagnosis of TOS vs. brachial plexopathy is somewhat controversial. TOS, being a syndrome, by definition is a collection of symptoms related to pathology of an anatomical space (the TO). Brachial plexopathy by definition is pathology of a specific anatomical structure (the brachial plexus). The vascular component of TOS ought to be diagnosed via vascular studies, because there is often a sympathetic nervous system component to the brachial plexopathy that presents clinically with vascular symptoms.

Unfortunately the clinical tests for vascular compromise that are advocated in the literature (such as the Adson's and Wright's tests, which rely on obliteration of the radial pulse while in the test position) have a high incidence (as high as 87%) of positive results in normals.[28-33] Therefore drawing conclusions based on the results of these tests in the clinic should be questioned.

Neural Component—Brachial Plexopathy

Due to the paucity of diagnostic tests that detect mild to moderate brachial plexopathies, the best way to identify a brachial plexopathy is through careful and thorough evaluation. This should include a detailed history that covers the onset of symptoms and mechanism of injury. Onset of symptoms is often traumatic in nature with trauma involving forced lateral cervical flexion with the shoulder held in a fixed position (as in a seat belt injury), forced depression of the shoulder combined with forced lateral cervical flexion (as in a sports injury, such as "burner" or "stinger" syndrome), or even dislocation of the shoulder. Symptoms may be delayed for months as adhesions form between the neural tissue and surrounding nerve bed. This leads to restricted **neural mobility** (the ability of the neural structures to adjust to changes in the nerve bed length through a combination of gliding and elongation), ultimately resulting in loss of UE motion and function.

Onset can be insidious in nature with genetic and morphologic predisposition combined with poor postural and movement habits leading to the development of the condition. During the growth phase into adolescence, the scapulae gradually descend down the posterior thorax with the descent being greater in women. A strain with resulting weakness of the scapular suspensory muscles that lengthen during this process is associated with the development of brachial plexopathy. This helps to explain the rarity of insidious onset brachial plexopathy before puberty and the increased incidence of the disease in women.[34]

Clients with brachial plexopathy will often complain of unilateral headaches in the occipital region with facial pain from the angle of the jaw to the zygomatic region to the ear. They may complain of shoulder and chest wall pain from the trapezius ridge down the medial border of the scapula, in the supra/infraclavicular fossa, and from the sternum to the axilla to the epigastric region. These clients are often seen in the emergency room for a suspected cardiac event but misdiagnosed with costal chondritis or gastritis.[35]

> **Clinical Pearl**
>
> Arm and hand involvement often includes complaints of pain, paresthesias, and weakness. A strong clue that the plexus is involved is that these symptoms do not follow dermatomal or peripheral nerve distributions. Other strong indications that the plexus is involved are intolerance to overhead activities, reports of dropping objects, cramping of the hand intrinsics while writing, waking with a "dead arm," and intolerance of straps across the top of the shoulder.

Timelines and Healing

Full recovery from a brachial plexus injury is rare. However, clients can often achieve enough of a reduction in symptoms to allow for a return to restricted activity. The level of restriction is related to the severity of the original injury, **neural sensitization** (activation of the small diameter pain fibers within the nerve itself)[36] and the amount of **intraneural** (contained within the nerve) and/or **perineural** (between the nerve and the nerve bed) scarring. This is a lifelong injury, and your client must be instructed in management of the condition. Unfortunately, the condition is characterized by periods of high and low neural irritability based on your client's activity level and the degree of pathology. As these clients have experienced an injury to the nervous system, most progress to a condition known as **central sensitization** (loss of brain-orchestrated pain inhibitory mechanisms and hyperactivation of ascending pain pathways).[37] Specifically, the problem is not just due to a peripheral nerve injury, but symptoms are driven from changes within the brain—not a bottom-up, but a top-down issue. This fairly recent way of looking at clients with chronic nerve pain has led to treatments that take advantage of the brain's **neuroplasticity** (the ability of the brain to adapt and

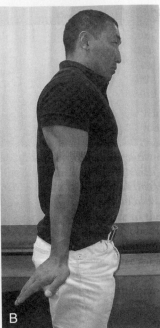

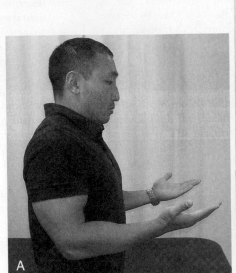

FIGURE 22-16 Nerve glide biasing the medial and lateral cords via the median nerve. **A,** Starting and ending position. **B,** Midpoint of the glide.

change neuronal connections based on a variety of stimuli) and are beyond the scope of this chapter.

Non-Operative Treatment

The theme that provides the underpinning of treatment for brachial plexus injured clients is that the nerves need three conditions to optimize healing: 1) space, 2) motion, and 3) minimally-sustained tension or strain. The most important step to begin healing is to teach your client how not to irritate the injured plexus. Through neural mobility assessment, clients can be taught where the safe boundaries of motion are. If your client is able to follow these movement guidelines and plexus irritation drops to a stable level, they can attempt to regain plexus mobility through gliding and stretching exercises. As plexus mobility improves, the safe boundaries of motion increase, resulting in improved ADL function.

Clients must be taught how to breathe using the diaphragm, minimizing the use of the scalenes; and they must be instructed in safe sleeping positions to avoid stretching or compressing the plexus. *Most importantly, your client must be taught to maintain a posture that minimizes stress on the brachial plexus while maximizing the apertures of the TO.*

These clients will rarely tolerate conventional weight training at the gym, but guided exercises to strengthen the scapular stabilizers and elevators are essential. With direct supervision, clients can use resistance bands and/or weights to strengthen the upper, middle, and lower trapezius; as well as the levator scapulae, rhomboids, and serratus anterior. Doing the exercises in sets of three repetitions allows the therapist and client to assess for increased plexus irritation signs between sets, thereby avoiding overstressing the TO contents.

Clients can regain scapular proprioception through visual feedback exercises. Your client stands facing the mirror while performing scapular motions, targeting points of the clock. With 12:00 being superior, 9:00 anterior, and 3:00 posterior; your client symmetrically elevates the shoulders to the 12:00, 1:00, and 2:00 positions (see Video 22-5 on the Evolve website). These are

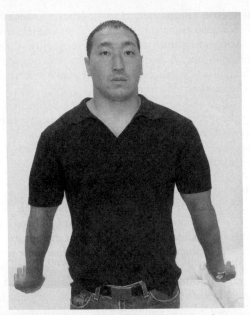

FIGURE 22-17 Midpoint of the nerve glide biasing the posterior cord via the radial nerve.

performed in straight lines of motion as smoothly as possible. After each cycle your client assesses their level of irritation and adjusts the exercise accordingly.

Your client performs gliding and stretching exercises in front of the mirror as well. He/she begins the glide exercise with the arms against the side and elbows flexed to 90° with the palms facing up. Next your client elevates the shoulders while slowly extending the elbows. To bias the medial and lateral cords of the plexus via the median nerve, he/she maintains supination while extending their wrists (Fig. 22-16; see Video 22-6 on the Evolve website). To bias the posterior cord of the plexus via the radial nerve, your client pronates their forearms and flexes their wrists (Fig. 22-17; see Video 22-6 on the Evolve website).

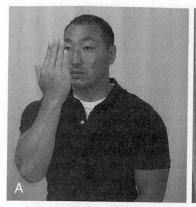
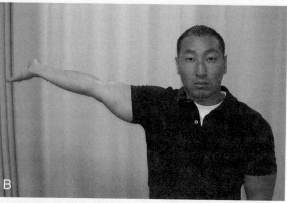

FIGURE 22-18 The oscillating brachial plexus nerve stretch. A, Starting position and ending position. **B,** Maximal stretch position.

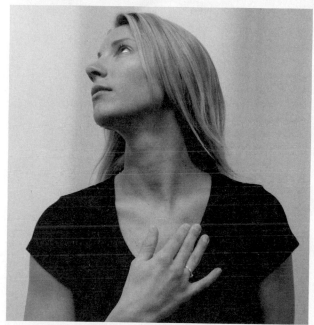

FIGURE 22-19 Scalene stretch of the left scalenes. Note stabilization of the first rib to enhance the stretch and protect the brachial plexus.

Your client begins the stretch exercise with the palm of the hand brought to eye level in front of the face and the elbow held close to the body. While maintaining the hand at eye level, your client moves their shoulder into abduction and external rotation (ER) with the forearm held in supination. Again keeping the hand at eye level, your client slowly extends their elbow just until a stretch is felt or a slight increase in symptoms occurs. At this point he/she backs off slightly on his/her elbow extension and alternately flexes and extends the wrist three times (Fig. 22-18; see Video 22-7 on the Evolve website). Your client attempts to straighten their elbow further with each cycle of the exercise. The nerve gliding variation of this exercise consists of cervical lateral flexion toward the ipsilateral arm with wrist extension (see Video 22-6 on the Evolve website). The glide and stretch exercises are performed in sets of three as well.

Your client performs all exercises from a neutral posture position. They achieve this by lifting their sternum through increasing their lumbar lordosis and elevating their rib cage. This effectively corrects the forward head rounded shoulder posture relieving stress from the TO contents.

Clients who demonstrate tight scalenes and pectoralis minor muscles must be taught stretching exercises. *Since these muscles lie against the brachial plexus, the therapist must watch for an increase in their client's symptoms during stretching.* The rule of threes works here as well—sets of three stretches held for three seconds. As your client demonstrates good tolerance to the stretch, the stretch can be held for longer periods and/or the number of sets can be increased.

Many of the scalene stretches described in the literature and in exercise kits often bias stretch the brachial plexus and should therefore be avoided. They usually instruct the client to depress their shoulder while stretching, frequently causing further irritation to the injured plexus. The scalenes, which have no attachment to the shoulder and are intrinsic to the cervical and thoracic regions, should be stretched with the shoulder held elevated—thereby relieving tension from the brachial plexus during stretching. Anchoring the first rib at its sternal attachment further enhances the scalene stretch (Fig. 22-19; see Video 22-8 on the Evolve website).

The doorway stretch is ideal for stretching the pectoralis minor (Fig. 22-20). An important component of this stretch is the addition of the shoulder shrug before stepping into the doorway. This initiating maneuver serves two purposes: first, lifting the shoulders increases the origin-to-insertion length of the pectoralis minor, enhancing the stretch; second, lifting the shoulders increases the aperture of the costoclavicular space by elevating the clavicle away from the first rib, minimizing the potential for neurovascular compression once the stretch is commenced. *Having your client perform nerve glides as previously described between each stretch helps to minimize neural irritation that may occur as a result of tissue stretching.*

Operative Treatment

The primary goal of TOS surgery is decompression of neurovascular contents or **neurolysis** (the removal of scar tissue from the nerve) of the entrapped brachial plexus. Clients who fared the best were those with confirmed vascular or neurological compromise in the TO via diagnostic testing.[38] Unfortunately, surgical outcomes have been disappointing; therefore surgery is reserved as a last resort.[28,39] The most common procedures are transaxillary first rib resection and **supraclavicular scalenectomy** (surgical removal of the anterior scalene) with neurolysis.

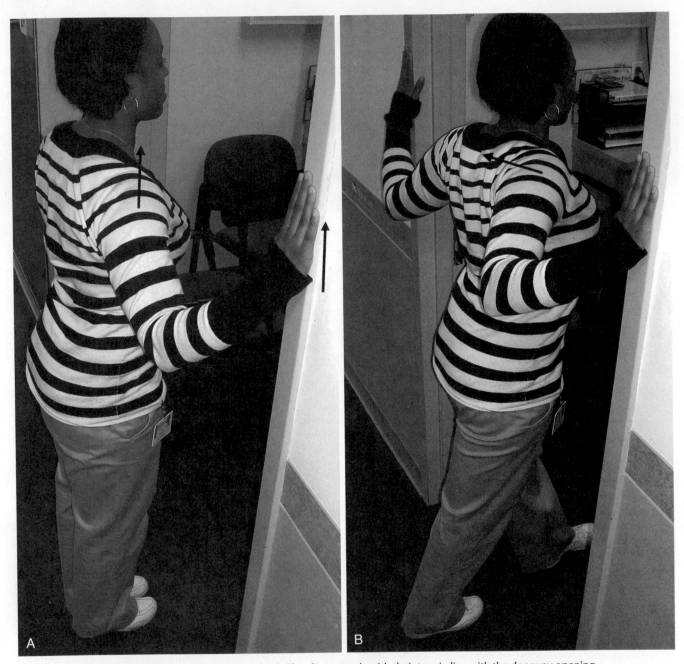

FIGURE 22-20 The doorway stretch. A, The client stands with their toes in line with the doorway opening. They shrug their shoulders and raise their hands along the doorframe to shoulder height, or just below the point of symptom provocation, whichever happens first. **B,** While holding this posture, the client takes a half step into the doorway.

? Questions to Discuss with the Physician

Postoperative Client
- How soon can ROM exercises begin?
- Are there any restrictions to movement of the neck or shoulder?

( ) What to Say to Clients

About the Condition

"Here is a drawing of your thoracic outlet. You can see the nerves and blood vessels that supply the arm travel through here. The areas of possible damage are here in your neck (the scalenes), between the collar bone and first rib, or under the muscles of your chest wall (pectoralis minor)."

About the Home Exercise Program

"In order for you to move your arm comfortably, your nerves must be able to slide through the thoracic outlet smoothly. You may have developed restrictions that prevent this from happening. Maintaining good posture is critical as you place excessive strain on the nerves with poor posture habits. Your exercises are designed to reinforce proper posture and help the nerves slide through the thoracic outlet, much like sliding a string through a straw."

Evaluation Tips

- Assess your client's ability to achieve the corrected posture position described earlier.
- Check for asymmetry of scapular/shoulder position.
- Look for swelling over the supraclavicular fossa.
- Monitor your client's UE for evidence of **autonomic instability** (sympathetic nervous system irritation) during testing, such as reticular mottling, color changes, temperature changes, and so on.
- Palpate along the course of the brachial plexus and peripheral nerves for tenderness and evidence of a **Tinel's sign** (production of tingling or paresthesia with percussion over the nerve).
- Neural mobility testing of the brachial plexus can be graded as follows (Fig. 22-21; see Video 22-9 on the Evolve website):
  - 0/5: Shoulder in internal rotation (IR), elbow flexed to 90° with arm across stomach, wrist and fingers in neutral (see Fig. 22-21, *A*)
  - 1/5: Shoulder in neutral, elbow flexed to 90°, wrist and fingers in neutral (see Fig. 22-21, *B*)
  - 2/5: Shoulder in approximately 100° of abduction, neutral rotation, elbow flexed to 90°, wrist and fingers in neutral (see Fig. 22-21, *C*)
  - 3/5: As earlier with the shoulder in approximately 90° of ER, forearm in supination, and fingers in neutral (see Fig. 22-21, *D*)
  - 4/5: As earlier with the elbow extended to 0° (see Fig. 22-21, *E*)
  - 5/5: As earlier with the wrist and fingers extended to end range (see Fig. 22-21, *F*)

- Use +/– for positions between each grade. If movement into the test position is less than halfway to the next grade position, the (+) is added the level achieved. If the position achieved is more than halfway but falls short of the next level, the (–) is added to the next level to aide in documentation.
- Block shoulder elevation during testing at 45° of shoulder abduction moving from the 1/5 test position to the 2/5 test position; *do not depress the shoulder* (Fig. 22-22).
- Use **elevated arm stress test (EAST)** (Roos Test) and record the time to provocation of symptoms. Described as a 3-minute test;[40] in my experience, clients with plexopathy will not tolerate more than 1 minute (Fig. 22-23). Having your client open/close their hands during the test is optional, because it tests for fatigue of the forearm and hand muscles.
- During myotomal screen, focus on scapular elevators for upper trunk lesions and hand intrinsics for lower trunk lesions.
- Using a safety pin flagged with tape to check for acuity to sharp sensation keeps the level of pressure applied during testing constant (Fig. 22-24). Clients with brachial plexopathy will show differential sensation of the middle finger vs. ring finger for clients with carpal or cubital tunnel syndrome. Decreased acuity along the medial half of the ring finger indicates medial cord involvement; decreased acuity along the lateral half of the ring finger indicates lateral cord involvement.[35] Differences found with testing of the ring finger concurrent to positive findings of the long finger could indicate the presence of a **double** or **multiple crush syndrome** (areas of more than one compressive lesion along the injured nerve).

"Your postural exercises are to be performed hourly to help reinforce good postural habits. Set your cell phone to 'beep' on the hour to remind you to exercise. Your gliding and stretching exercises are to be performed a minimum of three times a day. Tie these exercises to meal times so that you will remember to do them."

Diagnosis-Specific Information that Affects Clinical Reasoning

◎ Clinical Pearl

Clients who cannot tolerate the corrected posture position, have a positive EAST result in less than 30 seconds, and/or neural mobility of the plexus lower than 3/5 have a poorer prognosis, because they will easily irritate their condition during ADLs.

Achieving these basic parameters should be the initial goals of treatment. Base the speed and intensity of the rehabilitation program on your client's level of symptom irritability/stability. Inform your clients with chronic restrictions that they may experience increased symptoms for up to 48 hours after treatment. *If their level of post treatment irritation persists for greater than this, the intensity of the treatment needs to be decreased.*

♡ Tips from the Field

Constantly stress proper posture when your clients are in the clinic. Instruct them to notice the poor posture of people they encounter during their day and to use these observations as a reminder to correct their own posture. *The inability of your client to achieve stable symptoms at correct posture is one of the best predictors of treatment failure.*

Clients will often complain that their home exercises are increasing their symptoms. Have them demonstrate their home program on a regular basis and correct any modifications they have made. Adjust the amount of movement during the home exercises to keep symptoms stable.

The application of heat prior to exercise helps to calm symptoms. Riding the stationary bike for 10 to 15 minutes while using proper posture with the involved arm supported is an excellent warm-up exercise.

➤ Precautions and Concerns

- *Avoid over-stretching the brachial plexus during treatment.*
- *Be careful with overhead exercise, such as wall pulleys.*
- *Use of an upper body ergometer (UBE) is not recommended for these clients.*
- *Progress strengthening exercises cautiously.*
- *Watch exercise positions to avoid overstressing the brachial plexus.*

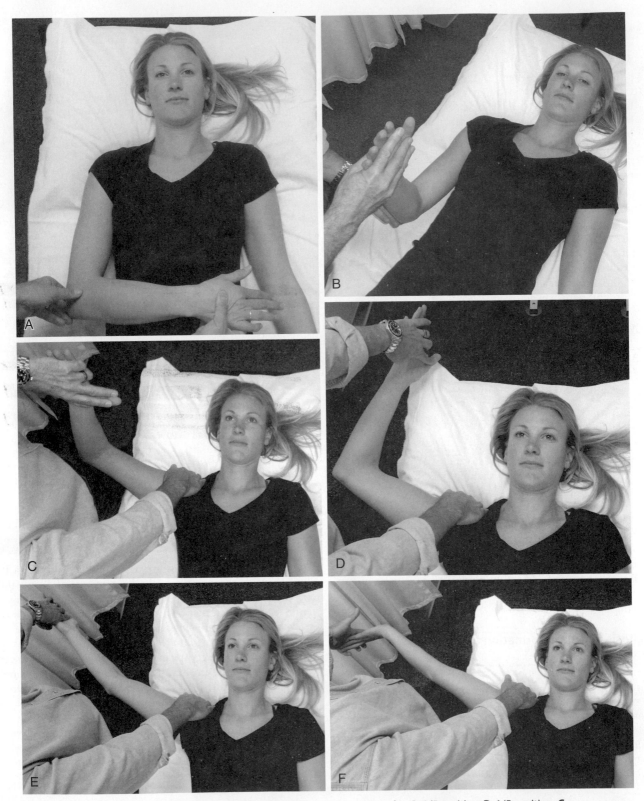

FIGURE 22-21 Brachial plexus mobility graded on a 0/5 to 5/5 scale. **A,** 0/5 position; **B,** 1/5 position; **C,** 2/5 position; **D,** 3/5 position; **E,** 4/5 position; **F,** 5/5 position.

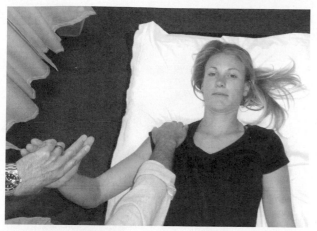

FIGURE 22-22 Blocking shoulder elevation at 45° of abduction prevents shoulder hiking, which will reduce neural tension and affect the testing outcome, reducing test-retest reliability.

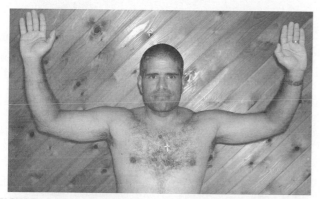

FIGURE 22-23 Test position for the elevated arm stress test (EAST), or Roos test.

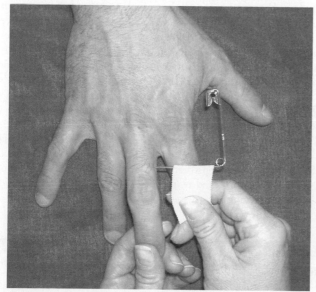

FIGURE 22-24 Example of a tape-flagged safety pin used to maintain constant pressure to check for sensation difference between the medial and lateral aspect of the long finger.

Anatomy

Proximal humerus fractures are the most common fracture of the humerus and may involve the articular surface, greater tuberosity, lesser tuberosity, or the surgical neck. These four regions are described as the four major fracture fragments that occur and are the basis of the classification systems for proximal humerus fracture.[41,42]

Diagnosis and Pathology

The majority of proximal humerus fractures occur as a direct result of a fall on the involved shoulder in the elderly population or a direct blow to the humeral region and are stable one-part fractures involving the surgical neck of the humerus.[41,43]

One-part fractures as classified by the Neer system are described as no fracture fragments being displaced more than 1 cm and no more than 45° of angulation. Two-part fractures exceed these position limits and can involve the humeral head and surgical neck or the humeral head and greater tuberosity. Three- and four-part fractures involve the humeral head, greater tuberosity, and lesser tuberosity.[41,42]

Timelines and Healing

One-part fractures are treated by sling immobilization initially for 1 to 3 weeks. Clients can start passive movements when the humeral shaft and head move as a unit, which can be as early as a couple of days.[41] Two- to four-part fractures, being more complex, usually require 4 to 6 weeks of immobilization, except in clients with hemiarthroplasties, who begin passive range of motion (PROM) exercises on postoperative day one.

Non-Operative Treatment

Your client begins treatment while still in the immobilizer by performing gripping exercises and active range of motion (AROM) of the elbow and wrist to prevent edema and joint stiffness. Once clinically stable, your client starts PROM exercises in the clinic and pendulum and tabletop PROM exercises at home. He/she should continue to wear the sling immobilizer in public and while sleeping for support and protection the first 6 weeks postinjury or surgical repair.

The therapist can start more aggressive stretching and the client begins AROM exercises around 4 to 6 weeks. The focus here should be on proper GH and ST movement to prevent the substitution patterns of early scapular elevation and trunk leaning to achieve UE elevation. Substitution patterns discourage proper recruitment of the RC muscles, so they need to be avoided at all costs.

The therapist plays a significant role here by having the client perform hand-to-hand active assisted range of motion (AAROM) progressing to AROM mirroring exercises in a seated position while the therapist prevents early scapular elevation (Fig. 22-25; see Video 22-10 on the Evolve website). Once your client understands the movement concept, they can perform the same exercise through self-scapular stabilization and wall walking (Fig. 22-26; see Video 22-11 on the Evolve website). These motions are performed in the scapular plane initially to provide the RC muscles the best length-tension relationship to encourage coordinated activity.

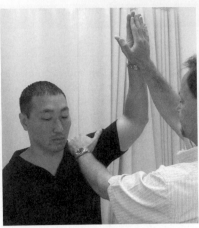

FIGURE 22-25 Range of motion (ROM) exercise with the client mirroring the therapist while the therapist stabilizes the shoulder to prevent early scapular elevation.

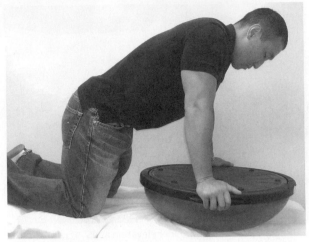

FIGURE 22-27 Example of closed chain exercise for the shoulder in quadruped on a rocker surface.

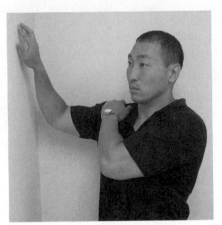

FIGURE 22-26 Wall walking exercise with the client self-stabilizing to prevent early scapular elevation.

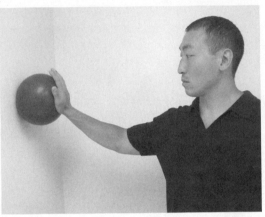

FIGURE 22-28 Example of closed chain exercise for the shoulder rolling a weighted ball against the wall.

At 8 to 12 weeks post-injury/repair your client can begin resisted strength training. The focus is on the RC muscles and scapular stabilizer/force couple muscles. Therapist-provided manual resistance in diagonal planes of motion is essential at this stage of the program to encourage functional movements and to discourage substitution movements.

A mixture of open and closed chain exercises must be included at this stage, because the shoulder functions in both situations. **Open chain exercises** are defined as working against resistance where the extremity is free to move in space resulting in movement of the distal segment. **Closed chain exercises** are defined as working against resistance with the extremity working against a stationary or mobile but motion-constrained object or surface. Closed chain exercises impart a degree of stability during the exercise motion.

Closed chain exercises include wall pushups, seated press-ups, weight shifting in quadruped, prone press-ups resting on elbows, and advanced exercises including box walk overs in a press-up position (see Videos 22-12 through 22-15 on the Evolve website). Variations include ball rolling against the wall or tabletop and use of a tilt board for weight bearing in quadruped (Fig. 22-27 and Fig. 22-28; see Videos 22-16 through 22-18 on the Evolve website).

If at 12 weeks post-injury/repair your client has achieved functional ROM and normal movement patterns, they can begin

plyometric (exercises that link strength and speed of movement to produce an explosive-reactive type of muscle response) (see Video 22-19 on the Evolve website) and sport-specific activities to prepare them for return to full function. It is therefore important to understand your client's goals of rehabilitation and their **premorbid** (prior to injury) activity level.

Operative Treatment

Proximal humerus fractures graded as two- to three-part will usually require surgical intervention of open reduction and internal fixation (ORIF) to reduce the displaced fracture fragments. **Hemiarthroplasty** (prosthetic replacement of one joint surface) is usually indicated to replace the avascular, compromised humeral head in four-part fractures.

? Questions to Discuss with the Physician

Regarding Operative Clients
• What structures were repaired? Ask for a copy of the operative report.
• How soon can active motion start?
• When can I begin lifting weights?

Regarding Non-Operative Clients
• When can I begin to take off the sling?
• How much longer do I need to wear the sling to sleep?
• How soon can I begin moving my shoulder?
• When can I begin lifting weights?

( ) *What to Say to Clients*

About the injury

If the fracture is classified as one-part: "Your fracture is considered stable, so you are allowed to begin moving your arm while the healing process continues. In fact the motion will help the healing process. All motions must be passive—meaning motion provided by the therapist, by gravity, or on a supported surface, such as a tabletop. You are not to attempt to raise your arm by itself for the next couple of weeks, because this could affect the healing fracture."

If the fracture has been surgically repaired or if it is a two-part fracture and is now considered stable: "Your doctor has determined that the fracture is healed enough to begin motion exercises. Movement will make a big difference in how quickly you recover, and it is critical to your recovery."

About Exercise

"You need to move your arm as often and much as possible. The motion helps to lubricate the joint and keeps it healthy."

If your client is doing tabletop exercises: "By using your fingers to pull your arm forward, you will avoid stressing your shoulder during this exercise. Keep your shoulder relaxed while moving; at the end of tolerable motion, rest your hand flat on the table surface while you sit back upright, dragging your arm back to the starting position."

If your client is doing pendulum exercises: "Do your exercises next to a table or counter. Using the table for support with your uninjured arm, bend at the waist as far as you can and let your injured arm swing forward as if it were a piece of rope. Now rock your body side-to-side and in circles. Do get your arm swinging just as you would do with your hand to swing a rope side-to-side or in a circle."

For all ROM exercises: "It is not how hard you push your stretches, but how often you stretch and how much cumulative time you spend at the end of motion that counts. Try for a minimum of 15 minutes of total end range time by doing 50 stretches a day, each held for 20 seconds."

Evaluation Tips

Take PROM measurements with your client seated. Make sure motions are slow and gentle, because your client will be very apprehensive about moving their arm. Often, when you attempt to return your client's arm to neutral after full elevation, he/she will experience sharp pain as the deltoid and humeral head elevators reflexively contract causing sharp pain. By having your client actively lower their arm against your resistance, this reflex is inhibited and the motion will be considerably more comfortable.

Measure functional IR by seeing which bony landmark on the pelvis or spinous process your client can touch with their thumb (for example, anterior superior iliac spine (ASIS), iliac crest, posterior superior iliac spine (PSIS), L5, and so on).

Diagnosis-Specific Information that Affects Clinical Reasoning

Obtaining information on the type of fracture from the doctor is crucial. This information is also available from radiology and operative reports.

◎ *Clinical Pearl*

The type of fracture directly affects how aggressively you may rehabilitate your client.

Alignment of the humeral head to the shaft will affect how much ROM your client will ultimately recover. For example, if the shaft is in 45° extension relative to the humeral head, your client's expected flexion ROM will be 135° (180° – 45° = 135°). The same holds true for rotational deformities.[42]

♡ *Tips from the Field*

Clients beginning therapy a few weeks after a one-part proximal humerus fracture will usually be apprehensive to move their arm due to fears about fracture instability. There are two ways to calm their fears. First tell them that as you rotate their arm, the humeral head will not move if the fracture is unstable. Have them place their hand over their injured humeral head while you gently rotate the arm from IR to ER; they should feel the humeral head move. The second and rather novel technique involves using a stethoscope. Explain to your client that sound will not travel across an open fracture. Next have your client listen through the stethoscope placed on the humeral head of their healthy shoulder while you tap on their lateral epicondyle. Do the same to their injured shoulder, where the intensity of sound should be the same. This will often decrease their apprehension about moving their shoulder and speed recovery.

Scapular position and posture have a direct effect on shoulder ROM. These clients must be given postural exercises as previously described for brachial plexus clients.

➤ *Precautions and Concerns*

• *RC injuries are often overlooked at the time of injury. Watch for evidence of rotator cuff tear (RCT) during rehabilitation.*
• *These clients are at a high risk of developing adhesive capsulitis (frozen shoulder). Movement must be the basis of any therapy program.*
• *Many of these clients will have a concurrent axillary nerve or brachial plexus injury. Screen for this during the initial examination by checking sensation over the deltoid (axillary distribution) and by asking if the client is experiencing paresthesias in the hand or arm (possible brachial plexus involvement).*

Frozen Shoulder/Adhesive Capsulitis

Anatomy

The fibrous capsule that envelopes the GH joint is lined with synovial tissue. It is attached medially to the glenoid margin and

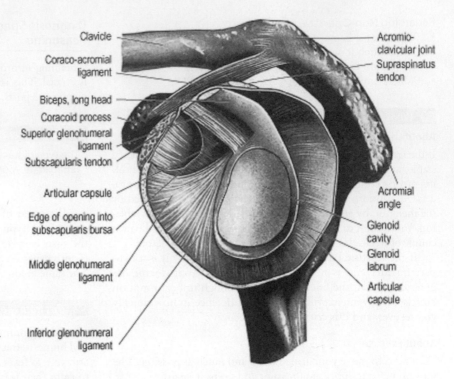

FIGURE 22-29 Interior view of the left shoulder joint, looking into the glenoid fossa and joint capsule. (From Putz R, Pabst R: *Sobotta—atlas of human anatomy single volume edition: head, neck, upper limb, thorax, abdomen, pelvis, lower limb,* ed 14, St Louis, 2008, Elsevier.)

encompasses the glenoid labrum and long head of the biceps. Laterally it attaches to the anatomical neck of the humeral head near the articular surface. The inferior portion attaches laterally about 1 cm distal to the articular surface on the humeral shaft. The capsule is slack enough that the GH joint surfaces can be distracted up to 3 cm.[2]

The capsule has three distinct thickened areas known as the GH ligaments (superior, middle and inferior) that help stabilize the GH joint. These ligaments become taut at various portions of GH motion as their fibers run in both radial and circular directions. During abduction and rotation, the capsule becomes shortened, producing both a compressive and centering force of the humerus on the glenoid.[44] During abduction and rotation, the inferior GH ligament forms a sling providing anterior, posterior, and inferior stability to the joint. With the arm at rest, this portion of the capsule forms the dependent axillary pouch, which is often obliterated with frozen shoulder (FS) (Fig. 22-29; see Fig. 22-2).

The coracohumeral ligament extends from the base of the coracoid process as two bands that blend with the capsule running to the greater and lesser tuberosities. Parts of the ligament form the tunnel for the biceps tendon and reinforce the **rotator interval** (the region between the superior edge of the subscapularis and anterior edge of the supraspinatus tendons).

The tendons of the subscapularis, supraspinatus, infraspinatus, and teres minor fuse with the lateral part of the joint capsule forming the RC. With contraction of the RC muscles, the lax capsule is pulled away from the movement path of the humeral head preventing capsular impingement.[2]

Diagnosis and Pathology

The terms *adhesive capsulitis* and *FS* are used interchangeably in the literature. The condition is characterized by a progressive loss of GH ROM usually in the capsular pattern of ER being most limited followed by abduction and IR. Magnetic resonance

imaging (MRI) studies demonstrate capsular thickening with loss of the axillary recess.[45,46] The disease appears to be periarticular with most authors finding little to no capsular adhesions during arthroscopic examination.

The condition is found in 2% to 5% of the US population[47] most commonly in the fourth through sixth decades of life.[48] However, one author[49] who has studied this disease extensively feels it is over diagnosed. Bunker provides a compelling argument that the prevalence of FS is about 0.75%. It is more common among women, with one study reporting women comprising 70% of the FS client.[48] FS is usually classified as primary or secondary adhesive capsulitis with the course of the disease following three phases: the freezing phase, the frozen phase, and the thawing phase.[47,48,50-52]

> ⊙ **Clinical Pearl**
>
> The condition is characterized by a progressive loss of GH ROM usually in the capsular pattern of ER being most limited followed by abduction and IR.

Primary Adhesive Capsulitis

Primary FS is idiopathic in nature. There is considerable debate over the pathogenesis of FS with possible causes being inflammatory, immunologic, endocrine alterations, or biochemical. This form of the disease is over-represented in clients with diabetes with rates three to six times that of the normal population.[51,52]

Histological findings in a group of primary FS clients revealed active fibroblastic proliferation of the coracohumeral ligament and rotator interval with the absence of inflammation or synovial involvement, much like that of **Dupuytren's disease** (disease process resulting in thickening and contracture of the palmar fascia).[46] In examining the hands of 58 clients with FS, Smith, et al.[53] found that 30 patients had a pit, nodule, or band of Dupuytren contracture. Bunker noted the same finding in 58% of clients with FS.[49]

Secondary Adhesive Capsulitis

Secondary FS is characterized by a precipitating event (such as, surgery or trauma to the shoulder) or specific shoulder pathology (such as, bursitis, impingement syndrome, or tendonitis). Although the same pattern of motion loss occurs, these clients may not go through all the stages of freezing, frozen, and thawing.[51]

The Freezing Phase

This phase is characterized by shoulder pain interrupting sleep, pain with ADLs (such as, brushing one's hair or tucking in one's shirt), and often pain at rest. It is difficult to distinguish FS pathology from that of RC tendonitis, shoulder bursitis, or impingement syndrome.

Examination of your client during this phase reveals ROM to be close to full with pain occurring often before the end of motion. Palpation reveals non-specific tenderness at the anterior, lateral, and posterior aspects of the shoulder. Strength is often normal or slightly decreased with pain on resisted testing.

Clients tend to limit the use of the affected extremity because all movements are painful, leading to further loss of motion. Over the next 2 to 9 months, the pain subsides, and the client is left with the typical FS with pain occurring at the end of motion.

The Frozen Phase

This phase may last up to 1 year. It is characterized by distinct pathological movement patterns as your client attempts to substitute ST motion to compensate for the lack of GH mobility. In this phase, pain occurs with stretching of the joint capsule at the end of motion.

The Thawing Phase

This phase is characterized by a gradual return of motion and lasts on average up to 26 months. The idea that clients will obtain full motion once they have completed the thawing phase is unclear in the literature. In an earlier study, Shaffer, et al.[54] reported that 30% of primary FS clients exhibited some degree of motion loss compared to the uninvolved shoulder at an average follow-up of 7 years. A relatively recent study was more optimistic, reporting 94% of clients with primary FS achieved motion and function equal to their uninvolved side without treatment.[55]

Timelines and Healing

As noted earlier, there are average time lines for each phase of the disease. The majority of clients complete the thawing phase within 18 months to 3 years from onset.[55]

Non-Operative Treatment

There is no evidence to suggest that therapeutic modalities (such as, ultrasound or interferential electric stimulation) affect the outcome of the disease; in fact the use of passive modalities may prolong recovery.[48] Treatment should be directed at the process occurring during each phase of the disease. *Over stretching the capsule during the freezing phase may enhance the inflammatory process stimulating further capsular fibrosis.* When the joint has achieved the frozen and thawing phases the stretching exercises can be more aggressive. *However, pushing to the point that reinitiates the inflammatory process should be avoided.*[51]

The role of the occupational therapist (OT) in assisting clients with bilateral FS in ADL modifications or adaptive equipment for grooming, bathing, and dressing cannot be overestimated.

Clients with unilateral FS may benefit from workstation modification to help them remain productive during the protracted course of the disease.

The use of intra-articular corticosteroid in the freezing phase of the disease may be helpful in stabilizing the synovial tissue, allowing for better tolerance to stretching exercises.[56]

Operative Treatment

For FS cases that fail to progress after protracted conservative treatment, manipulation under anesthesia and arthroscopic release of the GH capsule ligaments are two of the most common surgical interventions. Of the two, arthroscopic release of the anterior GH ligament and coracohumeral ligament currently has the most promising outcome.[57]

? Questions to Discuss with the Physician

Operative Clients
- What was the intra-operative ROM?

( ) What to Say to Clients

About the Injury

"Here is a diagram of your shoulder, and this is the joint capsule. Normally the capsule is loose and develops a redundant pouch at the bottom when your arm is at your side. Having this extra capsule space allows you to raise your arm above your head. Think of your shoulder capsule as an accordion with its folds glued together. That accordion would be unusable because it could not expand; your shoulder is restricted in motion and function as well."

About Exercises/Activities of Daily Living

"Moving your shoulder regularly to the end of comfortable motion helps to prevent motion loss. Avoid positions and activities that cause your shoulder to hurt for more than a few minutes afterward. Sleeping on your back is the best position. If you must sleep on your side, keep your arms to your sides if possible to prevent shoulder irritation. Using a body pillow may help you find a comfortable sleeping position."

"You have to watch your posture. Having your shoulders rounded will place more stress on the supportive tissue and will slow the healing process."

Evaluation Tips

- Take careful baseline and follow-up ROM measurements with your client supine to stabilize the trunk and scapula. This will allow for careful tracking of the progress of the condition.
- Loss of rotation ROM must be present for a diagnosis of FS. Specifically loss of ER must be observed. The loss of IR without the loss of ER ROM constitutes glenohumeral internal rotation deficit (GIRD), which is not the same clinically as FS.[58]
- If all passive and resisted motions are painful throughout the ROM, your client is still in the freezing stage.
- If resisted motion is pain free and pain occurs only at end ROM, your client is in the frozen or thawing phase.

Diagnosis-Specific Information that Affects Clinical Reasoning

The intensity of the therapy program is directly proportional to the phase of the condition. The primary treatment goal of the freezing phase is to prevent motion loss. The primary treatment goal of the frozen and thawing phase is to restore functional ROM.

♡ *Tips from the Field*

Proper posture and normal **scapular kinematics** (scapular movement in sequence and proportion to humeral movement) must be stressed during exercise at all times. Clients with FS quickly develop the pathological motion of early scapular elevation to raise their arm. This movement pattern can lead to secondary cervical problems further complicating the recovery process.

◎ *Clinical Pearl*

Proper posture and normal **scapular kinematics** (scapular movement in sequence and proportion to humeral movement) must be stressed during exercise at all times.

▷ *Precautions and Concerns*

- *Do not push ROM during the freezing phase to the point of pain that lasts more than a few minutes. This will only enhance the inflammatory and fibrosing process.*
- *These clients must avoid self-imposed immobilization.*

Glenohumeral Instability

Anatomy

GH instability could be considered the antithesis of adhesive capsulitis. However, laxity of the GH joint is a quality that allows full ROM; *laxity is not synonymous with instability*. When laxity leads to pain with loss of power and shoulder function, then GH instability exists.

The concepts and structures that contribute to GH stability can be categorized as static and dynamic. The static stabilizers have a larger role when the shoulder is at rest, while the dynamic stabilizers playing a larger role when the shoulder is in motion.

The static restraints include **negative intracapsular pressure** (air pressure inside the joint capsule being lower than pressure outside the capsule), the suction effect of the glenoid labrum acting on the humeral head like a "plunger," and cohesion-adhesion between the wet smooth surfaces of the humeral head and glenoid fossa. The orientation of the humeral head and glenoid fossa contribute to the static stability of the GH joint as well. With proper postural positioning of the scapula, the dynamic stabilizers need minimal effort to maintain GH congruency.[2]

The dynamic restraints include the RC, which provides a compressive and positioning force, and to a certain degree the long head of the biceps tendon. Although the GH ligaments are passive structures, they are under relatively little tension with the shoulder at rest. These ligaments serve as a restrictive leash to check force and limit ROM at various positions of the GH joint during movement. Of these ligaments, the inferior GH ligament is the most crucial to dynamic GH stability. As mentioned in the section covering adhesive capsulitis, during abduction and rotation, the inferior GH ligament forms a sling providing anterior, posterior, and inferior stability to the joint; affording stability when the GH joint is potentially at its most vulnerable position for dislocation.

Diagnosis and Pathology

Two major categories are useful in understanding shoulder instability. They are known by the mnemonics of AMBRII and TUBS.[58] The meaning of the mnemonics are summarized in Table 22-2. The pathology and treatment of AMBRII and TUBS shoulders are quite different.

AMBRII shoulders have no history of dislocation or subluxation. The client's major complaint is pain with activity, usually in overhand throwing motions. This pain is often a result of **impingement** (compression of soft tissue between bony structures), which is related to your client's inability to adequately stabilize the ST and/or GH joint due to RC pathology, capsular laxity, and altered **proprioception** (awareness of joint position).[59] Budoff, et al.[60] described this condition as primary instability leading to secondary impingement.

Primary instability is often a combination of global capsular laxity and pathological imbalances of the RC and shoulder muscles. Weak and/or proprioceptively compromised RC muscles cannot effectively oppose the upward pull of the deltoid muscle during UE elevation. The result is superior migration of the humeral head and impingement of the greater tuberosity and RC against the underside of the acromion and coracoacromial (CA) ligament (Fig. 22-30).

TUBS shoulders have a history of dislocation, usually in the anterior direction. The mechanism of injury is a fall or blow to the arm while in the position of abduction and ER. Recurrent subluxation or dislocation results when your client places their arm in the position of injury, leading to apprehension and dysfunction. These clients often have a resulting **Bankart lesion,** which consists of damage to the anterior GH capsule glenoid labrum and possibly the glenoid; and a **Hill-Sachs lesion,** which consists of an osseous defect of the posterolateral portion of the humeral head, caused during traumatic anterior dislocation. Both conditions usually require surgery to restore stability to the GH joint.

TABLE 22-2 TUBS vs. AMBRII	
TUBS or "Torn Loose"	**AMBRII or "Born Loose"**
Traumatic etiology **U**nidirectional instability **B**ankart lesion is the pathology **S**urgery is required	**A**traumatic or microtrauma with no specific episode **M**ultidirectional instability (MDI) may be present **B**ilateral: asymptomatic shoulder is also loose **R**ehabilitation is the treatment of choice **I**nferior capsular shift, and **I**nterval between the supraspinatus and subscapularis closed surgically if conservative measures fail

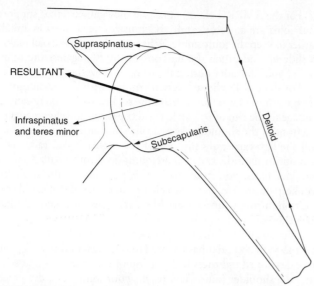

FIGURE 22-30 Force couple between the rotator cuff (RC) and deltoid resulting in inferior glide of the humeral head during elevation of the arm. (From Donatelli RA, editor: *Physical therapy of the shoulder*, ed 4, St Louis, 2004, Churchill Livingstone. Courtesy of Peter Edgelow.)

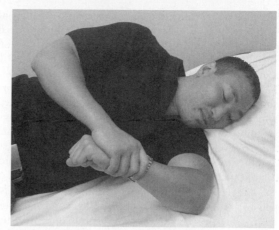

FIGURE 22-31 **Example of the sleeper stretch.** Gentle pressure applied in the direction of internal rotation (IR) while the body weight stabilizes the scapula.

Between these categories of shoulder instability are a group of shoulder pathologies related to asymmetrical capsular tightness.[61] This occurs from the excessive distraction force on the GH joint during the deceleration phase of throwing leading to thickening and contracture of the posterior-inferior portion of the capsule.[62] The sequelae of this asymmetrical capsular tightening is a loss of GH IR resulting in a cascade of events that may lead to impingement syndrome as well as pathology of the biceps tendon, labrum, and RC.[58,63]

The long head of the biceps tendon helps stabilize the GH joint during the overhand throwing motion.[2] The unstable and asymmetrically tight shoulder places extra stress on the biceps tendon leading to bicipital tendon irritation and **superior labrum anterior to posterior (SLAP) lesions.**[63] The SLAP lesion is hypothesized to be a result of increased torsional force from the biceps tendon that "peels back" the biceps and posterior labrum from the glenoid rim.[64] The SLAP lesion then enhances the dynamic and static instability of the already unstable shoulder. All the conditions described above can contribute to the development of impingement syndrome and RC disease described in the next section.

Timelines and Healing

For your client with a non-surgical unstable shoulder, 4 to 8 weeks of rehabilitation is common. The length of rehabilitation depends on their ability to gain control of the instability. Once stable, they are released to a sustained home exercise program that they will continue indefinitely. Surgically-corrected unstable shoulders require more time for rehabilitation. After a period of immobilization lasting 2 to 4 weeks, 3 to 6 months of rehabilitation is common. These clients will also require a sustained home exercise program. Most postoperative clients report that it takes 6 months to 1 year before their shoulder feels "normal."

Non-Operative Treatment

Treatment focuses on strengthening the RC and scapular stabilizers. Strengthening starts with shoulder isometrics in the safe position of the arm at the side. The motions resisted include shoulder flexion/extension, internal/external rotation, and abduction/adduction, and also elbow flexion and extension. While performing isometrics, it is important that clients "set" their scapula against their rib cage in a corrected posture position to engage the scapular stabilizers.

Once your client demonstrates fair to good control of the instability, the next step in the rehabilitation program is progression to isotonic exercises in a sub-impingement range using light resistance and high repetitions. For clients with anterior instability, the focus is on strengthening the internal rotators, adductors, and biceps. For clients with global instability, the focus is on the RC, scapular stabilizers, deltoid, biceps, and triceps.

It is essential at this stage to incorporate open and closed chain exercises as previously described for proximal humeral fractures. The intensity of the closed chain exercises can be increased by using weighted medicine balls against the wall, by moving the body into a more horizontal position, or even working off the exercise ball while in prone UE weight-bearing position.

Therapist-applied manual resistance can be used throughout each phase of the rehabilitation process. Starting with isometrics and AAROM and then progressing to concentrics and eccentrics, the therapist controls the speed of movement and amount of force. The major benefit of manual resistance is the immediate feedback that the therapist receives from his/her client during rehabilitation.

For clients with posteroinferior capsule restrictions, stretching exercises to restore IR are critical. Use of towel behind back stretches and the sleeper stretch work well (Fig. 22-31).

Operative Treatment

Surgical correction of the multidirectionally unstable shoulder should be considered only after a minimum of 3 months of conservative therapy has failed.[65] The two surgical procedures that are most often recommended in the literature are the **open inferior capsular shift** (surgical detachment and superior advancement of the inferior GH ligament)[66] and **arthroscopic capsular plication** (suturing folds into the GH capsule).[67] A third procedure, **thermal capsulorrhaphy** (selective heating of portions of the joint capsule, resulting in capsular shrinkage) also exists.[68] Each of these procedures has advantages and disadvantages.

There is greater surgical morbidity with the open inferior capsular shift, but the repair has good and predictable outcomes and allows for repair of the glenoid fossa if needed. Surgeons usually recommend the open inferior capsular shift procedure for moderate-to-severe multidirectional instability (MDI) with concurrent injury to the glenoid fossa. They recommend arthroscopic capsular plication for mild-to-moderate MDI without involvement of the glenoid fossa. In cases of mild-to-moderate MDI, the open and arthroscopic techniques yielded comparable results with less morbidity occurring with the arthroscopic procedure.[67]

Thermal capsulorrhaphy can trace its origins to Hippocrates' time. He describes inserting a hot iron into the axilla to cauterize the unstable joint. Treatment has improved a lot since then; this is now an arthroscopic procedure. However, there is a paucity of long-term studies about surgical outcomes. Complications include return of the instability, axillary nerve damage, and adhesive capsulitis.[69] Hawkins, et al.[70] found a high failure rate (up to 60%) on 2-year follow-up for clients having this as a stand-alone treatment for MDI. They recommended against this surgery as a stand-alone procedure but state it may be used in combination with arthroscopic capsular plication. *Great care must be taken in the rehabilitation of these clients to avoid* **attenuating** *(weakening, stretching) the healing capsule.* Your client can initiate AROM exercises earlier because the RC structures are left intact, but return of motion needs to be supervised carefully by the therapist.

For clients with traumatic anterior dislocation, the need for surgical repair of the Bankart lesion varies based on your client's age range and the physical demands on the shoulder. Rates of recurrent dislocation were highest in clients younger than 30 with rates ranging from 79% to 100%. Conservative therapy had little effect on reducing rates of recurrence. Therefore, clients younger than 30 and those over 30 who perform UE labor-intensive jobs should consider surgical repair.[71]

? Questions to Discuss with the Physician

Non-Operative Clients
- What is the nature and direction of the instability?
- Are there any secondary pathologies that need to be addressed (that is, RCT, SLAP lesion, and so on)?
- Is this client a surgical candidate?

Operative Clients
- What type of repair was performed? Ask to see an operative report.
- What are the ROM restrictions?
- How soon can the patient begin strengthening exercises?
- Do you have a specific postoperative protocol for rehabilitation?

( ) What to Say to Clients

About the Injury
"Your shoulder is a ball and socket joint with the ball much larger than the socket. This design allows for a lot of motion, but your shoulder must rely on the muscles and ligaments to keep the joint stable."

For the AMBRII client: "Because the ligaments that support your joint are so loose, your RC muscles need to work much harder to keep the joint stable. When they fatigue, the ball is able to slide up and pinch the tendons of the RC against the bony roof of your shoulder during throwing and overhead activities."

For the TUBS client: "When you fell with your arm out to the side, the ball was forced from the socket, which likely caused damage to the rim of the socket and the supportive ligaments in the front of the shoulder. As a result, your shoulder is unstable, and the ball can easily slip out of the socket if you raise your arm out to the side as if you are going to throw a ball. As your shoulder heals, you must avoid this position, or the problem will keep occurring. There is a chance that even if you avoid this position during your recovery, the damage is great enough that your shoulder will remain unstable."

For the client with the tight posterior capsule: "Because of the way your shoulder has adapted to the stress of throwing, you have developed tightness in a portion of the ligaments that support the shoulder joint. As a result, your joint has a decreased ability to internally rotate. This restriction causes abnormal motion of the ball in the socket when your shoulder is under the stress of throwing, resulting in your pain and loss of function."

About Exercises
For the AMBRII client: "Your exercises are designed to compensate for your unstable shoulder by increasing the strength, coordination, and endurance of your RC and scapular stabilizing muscles. This exercise program is a life-long commitment, because if the weakness returns, your shoulder problems will return as well."

For the TUBS client: "Your exercises strengthen the muscles around your shoulder to support the damaged part of the joint. You must follow the motion restrictions carefully during exercise to avoid disrupting the repair process."

For the client with the tight posterior capsule: "You need to regain the internal rotation motion of your shoulder to restore the normal function. The stretches work best if performed frequently. Three sets a day is not enough. You should try for a minimum total of 15 minutes of total stretch time each day. Remember, it is not how hard you push the stretch, but how much time you spend at the end of motion that counts."

Diagnosis-Specific Information that Affects Clinical Reasoning

The direction of the instability dictates the course of treatment as described earlier. Consequently, you must have a clear understanding of your client's instability pattern. *Applying an incorrect exercise and stretching program may enhance your client's pathology.*

Many of these clients have impingement and/or SLAP lesions as well. If a SLAP lesion is present, your client may need to avoid rotary exercises with the arm above shoulder height. In these cases, overhead throwing exercises are contraindicated.

♡ Tips from the Field

- **Proprioception exercises** (activities to enhance position and movement sense/control of the scapula and shoulder complex) need to be stressed with these clients.
- Manually resisted exercises in diagonal patterns at various speeds using concentric and eccentric force are a valuable component of the rehabilitation program.

Evaluation Tips

- Screening for general connective tissue laxity utilizing the Beighton scale (Table 22-3) assists in identifying the degree of hypermobility that your client exhibits. Clients scoring greater than 4/9 are considered hypermobile[72,73] (Fig. 22-32).
- For the unstable shoulder, the goals are to find the direction(s) of instability and to reproduce the client's symptoms. Their feedback during examination is critical.
- The client must be as relaxed as possible during examination, because muscle guarding will hide the degree of instability.
- Various tests are described in the literature to test for shoulder instability. Basic tests to check for the direction of instability are as follows:
  - Anterior and posterior drawer tests: Your client is supine for both tests. For the anterior test, the therapist stands facing his/her client and fixes the client's hand in his/her opposite axilla (Fig. 22-33; see Video 22-20 on the Evolve website); by holding the client's arm to be tested in this manner, the client is able to relax his/her arm. The therapist grasps the humeral head with the hand opposite the client (the same side holding the client's hand in the axilla) while stabilizing the scapula and clavicle with the other. Next, the therapist applies an anterior subluxing force to the humeral head while assessing the amount of humeral head movement.
  - For the posterior test, the therapist stands level with the affected shoulder and grasps his/her client's proximal forearm while flexing the patient's elbow to 120°. He/she next positions the client's shoulder in 80° to 120°

of abduction and 20° to 30° of forward flexion (Fig. 22-34, *A*). The therapist stabilizes the client's scapula with the opposite hand while resting their thumb over the humeral head (Fig. 22-34, *B;* see Video 22-21 on the Evolve website). To perform the test motion, the therapist horizontally adducts his/her client's arm while simultaneously applying a posterior oblique pressure to the humeral head tangential to the glenoid fossa. If instability exists, the therapist will be able to sense the humeral head's movement as it subluxes posteriorly. The therapist then compares the amount and quality of movement to the opposite side for both tests.[74]
  - Sulcus sign test: With the client seated and their arm supported in 20° to 50° of abduction, the therapist pulls inferiorly on his/her client's arm. A depression of more than a finger width resulting between the acromion and humeral head indicates a positive test. This test indicates MDI[75] (Fig. 22-35; see Video 22-22 on the Evolve website).
  - Apprehension test: With the client supine, the therapist moves their shoulder into 90° abduction and end range ER. If with the application of over pressure his/her client experiences apprehension but not pain, the test is considered positive for anterior instability.[76]
  - Relocation test: With the client positioned as at the end of the apprehension test, the therapist applies posteriorly directed pressure from the anterior aspect of the humeral head. The test is positive if the client's apprehension disappears. This test helps to confirm anterior instability.[76]

- Have your client perform UE exercises to strengthen the RC while concurrently working on balance while in quadruped, sitting, kneeling, and standing positions.
- Stress proper posture as described earlier.

Precautions and Concerns

- *Do not perform end range or grade IV joint mobilization or stretches on your client with MDI.*
- *Clients with anterior instability need their posterior capsule mobilized. Avoid stretching the anterior capsule.*
- *Pay close attention to ROM restrictions for postoperative clients.*

Rotator Cuff Disease

Anatomy

After neck and back pain, shoulder pain is the third most common musculoskeletal disorder. Up to 70% of shoulder disorders are related to RC disease.[77] The structures of the shoulder that are involved in RC disease include the muscles of the RC, the long head of the biceps tendon, the subdeltoid-subacromial bursa, and CA arch.

The supraspinatus, infraspinatus, and teres minor make up the greater tuberosity attachments of the RC. The subscapularis attaches to the lesser tuberosity. All the RC muscles work together to stabilize the head of the humerus in the glenoid fossa during

✗ emphasize

shoulder motion while their tendons form a cuff that surrounds the humeral head.

Along with their primary role of stabilizing the GH joint, each muscle of the RC imparts specific motion to the humeral head. The supraspinatus is an abductor, the infraspinatus is an external rotator, the teres minor is an external rotator and weak adductor of the humerus, and the subscapularis is an internal

TABLE 22-3	**Beighton Score for Assessing Hypermobility**	
Beighton Scale Item	**Highest Possible Score***	**Criteria for a Positive Sign**
Passive hyperextension of fifth finger	2	> 90°
Passive thumb opposition to forearm	2	Thumb touches forearm
Elbow hyperextension	2	> 10°
Knee hyperextension	2	> 10°
Standing trunk flexion with knees fully extended	1	Both palms flat on floor

*Each item is scored bilaterally, except for standing trunk flexion. A score greater than 4/9 is considered positive for hypermobility

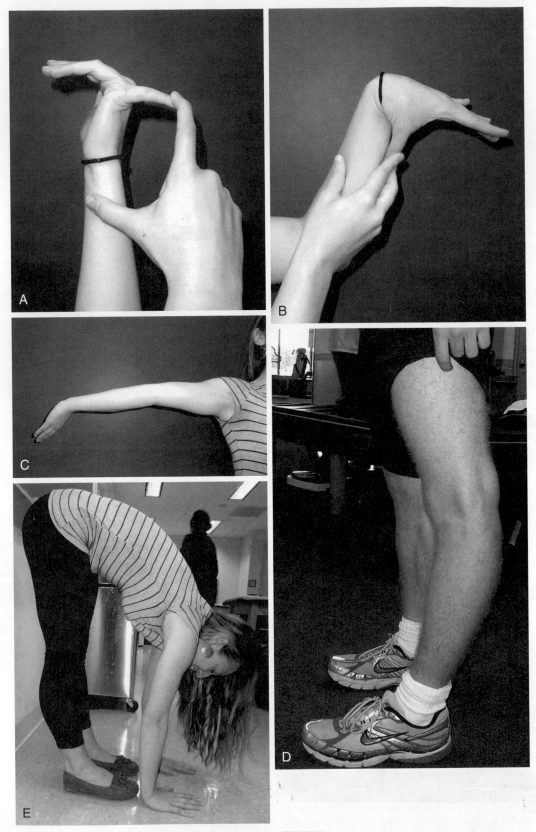

FIGURE 22-32 A, Passive hyperextension of the fifth finger; **B,** passive thumb opposition to the forearm; **C,** elbow hyperextension; **D,** knee hyperextension; **E,** standing trunk flexion with the knees extended.

subscapularis is strong

rotator and the strongest of the RC muscles (Fig. 22-36 and Fig. 22-37).

The stabilizing role of the long head of the biceps tendon is reviewed previously in the section on GH instability. As the arm elevates overhead, the head of the humerus glides along the biceps tendon as it sits in the bicipital groove between the greater and lesser tuberosities. The long head of the biceps plays a role in shoulder flexion, as well as forearm flexion and supination.

The subdeltoid-subacromial bursa is a smooth serosal (a smooth membrane that secretes lubricating fluid that reduces friction) sac that sits between RC tendons and the CA arch. Above, it is adherent to the underside of the deltoid, CA ligament, and the acromion. Beneath, it is adherent to the RC and greater tuberosity. This structure provides a cushioning and low friction interface between the convex humeral head and RC as they rotate below the concave CA arch during arm elevation.

The CA arch consists of the anteroinferior aspect of the acromion process, the inferior surface of the AC joint, and the CA ligament. This structure forms a roof over the RC and humeral head.[11] It not only serves as an attachment site for the deltoid and subdeltoid-subacromial bursa, but it also provides superior stability and protection to the GH joint.

Diagnosis and Pathology

There are two major hypotheses about the etiology of RC disease. One is based on extrinsic causes, and the other is based on intrinsic causes. Current evidence demonstrates that both contribute to the disease process and are affected by age, postural habits, movement quality, and activity level.

Extrinsically caused lesions result from the repeated impingement of the RC tendon against different structures of the GH joint. Neer[78] describes impingement between the long head of the biceps and supraspinatus tendons and the CA arch during UE elevation, resulting in lesions on the bursal side of the RC. His three-stage classification of impingement syndrome is still used today (Table 22-4). Bigliani, et al.[79] described three types of acromion morphology (Fig. 22-38) with cadaver studies demonstrating a 70% incidence of RC tears in subjects with a Type III acromial shape and a 3% incidence in subjects with a Type I

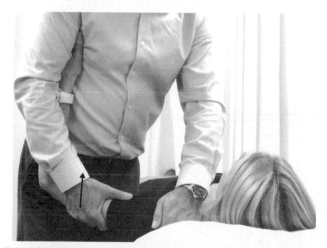

FIGURE 22-33 Starting position for the anterior drawer test. The *arrow* indicates the direction of force applied by the therapist while performing the test.

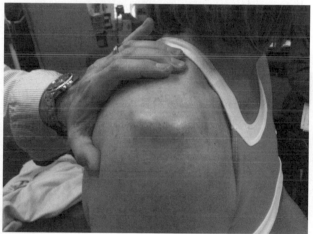

FIGURE 22-35 Example of a positive Sulcus sign test.

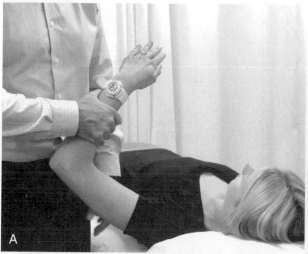

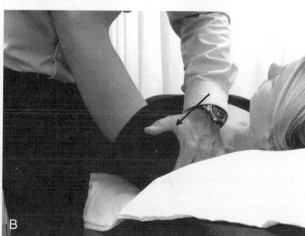

FIGURE 22-34 A, Starting position for the posterior drawer test. **B,** Hand position for performing the test. The *arrow* indicates the direction of force applied by the therapist while performing the test.

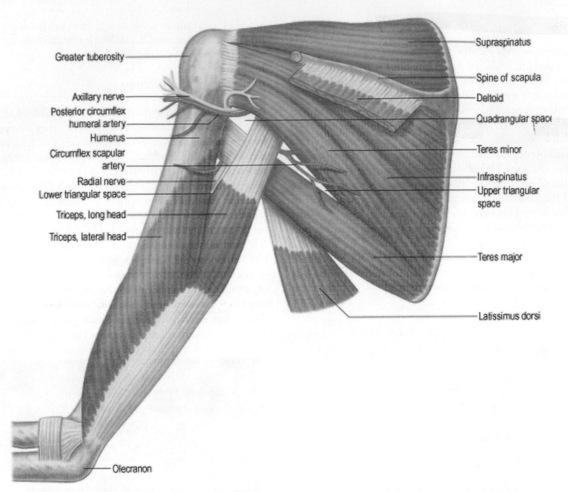

Greater tuberosity

Axillary nerve
Posterior circumflex
humeral artery
Humerus
Circumflex scapular
artery
Radial nerve
Lower triangular space
Triceps, long head
Triceps, lateral head

Olecranon

Supraspinatus
Spine of scapula
Deltoid
Quadrangular space
Teres minor
Infraspinatus
Upper triangular
space
Teres major
Latissimus dorsi

FIGURE 22-36 Dorsal muscles of the shoulder, including the supraspinatus, infraspinatus, and teres minor of the rotator cuff (RC). (From Standring S: *Gray's anatomy e-book*, ed 40, St Louis, 2012, Churchill Livingstone, p. 839.)

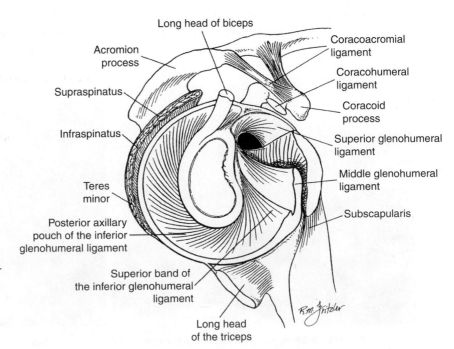

Long head of biceps
Acromion
process
Supraspinatus
Infraspinatus
Teres
minor
Posterior axillary
pouch of the inferior
glenohumeral ligament
Superior band of
the inferior glenohumeral
ligament
Long head
of the triceps

Coracoacromial
ligament
Coracohumeral
ligament
Coracoid
process
Superior glenohumeral
ligament
Middle glenohumeral
ligament
Subscapularis

FIGURE 22-37 Internal view of the right shoulder joint. The tendons of the rotator cuff (RC) and long head of the biceps are indicated. (From Dutton M: *Dutton's orthopaedic examination, evaluation, and intervention*, ed 3, Philadelphia, 2012, McGraw Hill Medical, p. 409.)

acromial shape. Walsh, et al.[80] described a type of impingement between the supraspinatus and infraspinatus tendons in the late cocking phase of throwing on the glenoid rim, resulting in lesions on the articular side of the RC.

Intrinsically caused lesions result from age-related degeneration of the RC tendon. These lesions are related to the vascularization of the RC cuff and are on the articular side of the tendon.[11,59,60] Lindblom was the first to describe an area of hypovascularity of the supraspinatus tendon where it attaches to the greater tuberosity.[81] Codman referred to the same area as the "critical zone" as it appeared to be at greater risk of developing a tear.[82]

As most RC tears are partial-thickness tears,[83] the condition is often progressive in nature and can lead to a full-thickness lesion. As tendon fibers fail, they retract because the RC is under constant tension. This process leads to at least four adverse effects:[84]

- Increased load on intact neighboring fibers—leading to their potential failure
- Loss of muscle fibers attached to bone—leading to decreased strength and function of the RC
- Intact tendon's blood supply placed at risk by distorted anatomy from fiber failure—leading to progressive ischemia and tendon degeneration
- Loss of tendon repair potential as the tendon is exposed to joint fluid containing lytic enzymes, which inhibit hematoma formation that would facilitate healing

Usually beginning in the supraspinatus tendon, the tear may progress to involve the infraspinatus tendon. Once this occurs, the RC's ability to stabilize the humeral head in the glenoid fossa is severely compromised leading to superior migration under the unopposed pull of the deltoid. Humeral head superior migration loads the long head of the biceps tendon leading to tendinopathy and potential failure. Traction spurs develop at the CA ligament attachment on the acromion through repeated loading from the upward displacement of the humeral head, leading to further RC damage. This damage allows the RC tendon to slide down below the axis of joint rotation. Much like a boutonnière deformity of the finger, the buttonholed RC becomes a humeral head elevator instead of a depressor. The RC is then ineffective as a humeral head stabilizer, and the client is unable to elevate the arm above a horizontal position.

Timelines and Healing

Recovery from RC pathology is extremely variable due to multiple presentations of the disease. If the case is uncomplicated, such as a tendonitis, the condition can stabilize in 2 to 6 weeks. If secondary pathologies are present (such as, FS, impingement, instability, and RC tear), recovery time lengthens considerably. Complex cases may take up to 1 year to resolve with or without surgical intervention.

Non-Operative Treatment

Initial treatment focuses on rest and anti-inflammatory modalities to stabilize the disease process. Early ROM exercises (such as, pendulum and wand-assisted elevation in the scapular plane to avoid impingement) help to moderate pain through the analgesic effect of mechanoreceptor stimulation.

> **Clinical Pearl**
>
> Maintaining full pain-free IR and ER are critical to preventing FS.

Strengthening of the healthy portion of the RC and scapular stabilizer muscles, usually in the motions of shoulder IR, adduction, and extension, is safe and encourages the stabilizing function of the RC. The use of isometrics and resistance band exercises are effective during this portion of the program. As pain levels decrease and RC function improves, the next step is to strengthen the UE elevators and external rotators. Throughout this process, you must stress muscle balance and proper scapular kinematics. Incorporating open/closed chain and manual exercises, like those

TABLE 22-4	Neer's Three-Stage Classification of Impingement Syndrome	
Stage	**Age Range**	**Pathology**
I	< 25 years	Reversible edema and hemorrhage from excessive overhead use
II	25 to 40 years	Irreversible fibrotic changes to the RC following repeated episodes of mechanical inflammation
III	> 40 years	Bone spurs and tears (complete and incomplete) of the RC and long head of the biceps tendon

RC, Rotator cuff.

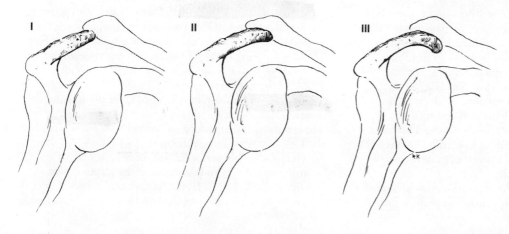

FIGURE 22-38 Acromion morphology types I, II, and III. (From Jobe CM: Gross anatomy of the shoulder. In Rockwood CA, Matsen FA III, editors: *The shoulder*, Philadelphia, 1990, WB Saunders.)

described for proximal humerus fracture and for GH instability, complete the exercise program.

You should focus on strengthening the scapular force couples once your client demonstrates good control of the RC muscles. The addition of sport- and activity-specific exercise is usually the final phase of your client's rehabilitation program.

Operative Treatment

Indications for RC surgery are the presence of a full or partial tear that has not responded to a course of conservative care and that interferes with your client's ADLs. RC surgery is rapidly evolving as more and more physicians perform complex repairs through the arthroscope.

Arthroscopic debridement for freshening of the frayed, partially torn RC tendon stimulates healing. For full thickness tears, the surgeon debrides the tear edges and then closes the defect to provide a foundation to regain RC strength and shoulder function. Acromioplasty is often performed at the time of RC repair to decompress the subacromial space and to prevent impingement of the repaired structures.

Most postoperative therapy programs include a 2- to 4-week period of immobilization while the tissue stabilizes. Your client then starts therapy to regain ROM. For the next 2 to 3 weeks, ROM progresses from passive to active motion exercise. At approximately 8 to 10 weeks postoperative, your client begins strengthening exercises and follows the program for the non-operative client listed earlier.

? Questions to Discuss with the Physician

Non-Operative Clients
- Are there any concurrent pathologies (instability, impingement, and so on)?
- Is surgery a possibility?

Operative Clients
- What structures were repaired? Try to obtain an operative report.
- Do you have a specific rehabilitation protocol?
- Are there any ROM restrictions or precautions?
- How soon can strengthening begin?

( ) What to Say to Clients

About the Injury
"Your shoulder relies on the rotator cuff muscles to stabilize the head of the humerus in the socket and to prevent the humeral head from being pinched against the roof of your shoulder when you raise your arm. Your rotator cuff is damaged, so this protective function has been interrupted, placing your shoulder at risk. If the problem progresses, you may lose the ability to raise your arm."

About Exercise
"By strengthening the healthy portions of your injured rotator cuff, there is a good chance you can regain the ability to use your arm for your daily needs. The exercises are specific and need to be performed on a regular basis."

"When you perform the range of motion exercises, you should not experience sharp sudden pain when raising your arm up. To prevent this from occurring, you must lead the motion with the thumb side of your hand while keeping the point of your elbow facing the ground throughout the motion. Before raising your arm, you must correct your posture.* By following these movement precautions, you will minimize the chance of pinching the rotator cuff under the bony roof of your shoulder."

*As described in the "Thoracic Outlet Syndrome/Brachial Plexopathy" section.

Evaluation Tips

There are a multitude of tests to detect RC disease. The following tests are included because they are easy to perform and because research indicates they have reasonable sensitivity and specificity:

- A quick screening test to detect a large RC tear involving the supraspinatus and infraspinatus is to resist ER with your client's shoulders in neutral and the elbows flexed to 90°. In the presence of a large RC tear, the unopposed deltoid will abduct the arm while the hand dips into IR[85] (Fig. 22-39).
- Client positioning to palpate the RC insertions are as follows:[86]
  - Supraspinatus: With your client's dorsum of their hand resting on their posterior iliac crest, palpate just inferior to the anterior aspect of the acromion (Fig. 22-40).
  - Infraspinatus: With your client's shoulder in ER and their elbow brought to their navel, palpate just inferior to the posterior aspect of the acromion (Fig. 22-41).
  - The long head of the biceps tendon: With your client's arm held in IR and the forearm resting on a pillow in the patient's lap, the tendon should lie in the deltopectoral interval (the sulcus formed by the medial border of the deltoid and the lateral edge of the pectoral muscle belly) (Fig. 22-42).
  - Subscapularis: With your client positioned as described earlier, bring the shoulder to neutral rotation. Palpate

the lesser tuberosity and tendon in the deltopectoral interval (Fig. 22-43).
- Shoulder impingement is a sign of RC disease. The Hawkins-Kennedy and Neer impingement tests are useful in detecting this pathology:[85]
  - Hawkins-Kennedy test:[85,87] With your client's shoulder flexed to 90°, bring the shoulder into full IR. This drives the greater tuberosity under the CA arch and will elicit pain if impingement is present (Fig. 22-44; see Video 22-23 on the Evolve website).
  - Neer impingement test:[85,88] Passively flex your client's shoulder to end ROM. Positioning the shoulder in IR at the start of the test enhances the impingement of the RC on the underside of the anterior third of the acromion and CA ligament (Fig. 22-45; see Video 22-24 on the Evolve website).
- Isometric testing of the specific muscles of the RC and the long head of the biceps aids in detecting tendinopathy. These tests include the Jobe or "empty or full can" tests, the Patte test, the Gerber lift-off test, and the Speed's test:
  - The Jobe or "empty or full can tests:" Your client's arms are brought to horizontal in the scapular plane with the shoulder in IR for "empty can" (see Video 22-25 on the Evolve website) or 45° externally rotated

Evaluation Tips—cont'd

with the thumb point up for the "full can" test (see Video 22-26 on the Evolve website). Next, apply downward pressure while your client provides isometric resistance. Weakness or the inability to hold this position implicates the supraspinatus[89] (Fig. 22-46).

- The Patte test: Your client's arm is positioned in 90° of abduction with neutral rotation in the scapular plane. Apply pressure at your client's wrist to resist shoulder ER while stabilizing the arm at the patient's elbow. Weakness and/or pain implicates the infraspinatus[89] (Fig. 22-47; see Video 22-27 on the Evolve website).
- The Gerber lift-off test: Position your client's arm so that the dorsum of their hand rests against their posterior iliac crest. Have your client actively raise their hand 2 to 5 inches from their back while you apply resistance (Fig. 22-48; see Video 22-28 on the Evolve website). Your client's inability to apply pressure or hold their hand in this position implicates the subscapularis.[89-90]
- The Speed's test: Position your client's shoulder in 70° to 90° of flexion with the elbow in extension and the forearm in supination. Resist shoulder flexion while palpating the long head of the biceps tendon in the bicipital groove. A painful response implicates the long head of the biceps[85] (Fig. 22-49). The test can also be performed without tendon palpation (see Video 22-29 on the Evolve website).
- There is no resistance test specific to isolating the teres minor.
- While performing these tests, watch for patterns that support specific locations of RC lesions.

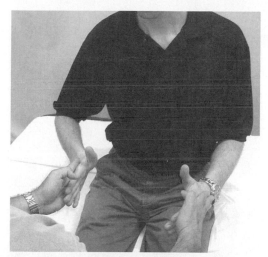

FIGURE 22-39 Quick screening position test for full thickness rotator cuff (RC) tears involving the supraspinatus and infraspinatus. A positive test is pictured. The right shoulder moves into abduction and internal rotation (IR) on resisted external rotation (ER) as the deficient RC cannot stabilize against the action of the deltoid.

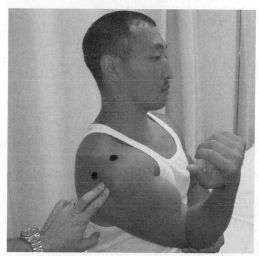

FIGURE 22-41 Palpation position for the infraspinatus insertion. The *black markers* indicate the posterior and anterior aspects of the acromion process.

Diagnosis Specific Information that Affects Clinical Reasoning

The existence of a RCT does not always lead to a surgical repair. Clinical experience shows that many clients function well with RC deficits confirmed via MRI. Clients who are unable to regain pain-free shoulder function are the best candidates for surgical repair.[91]

♡ *Tips from the Field*

Good palpation skills aide substantially in differentiating subacromial-subdeltoid bursitis from RC tendonitis. The bursa lies beneath the therapist's finger as well when palpating the supraspinatus and infraspinatus insertions as described earlier. Since the bursa is a relatively fixed structure, its position changes little during arm movement. Conversely, the palpation locations for the RC tendons change with arm movement. A pain response with palpation implicates both structures. *When your client returns their arm to the resting position, the pain will remain constant if the bursa is the source and will decrease if the RC tendons are the source.*

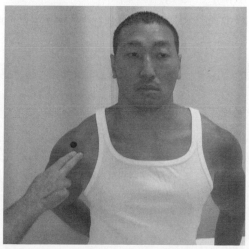

FIGURE 22-40 Palpation position for the supraspinatus insertion. The *black marker* indicates the anterior aspect of the acromion process.

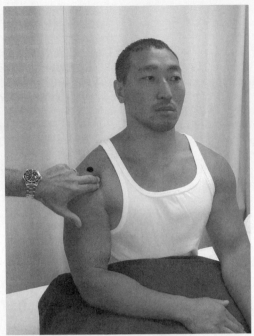

FIGURE 22-42 Palpation position for the biceps tendon in the deltopectoral interval. The *black marker* indicates the anterior aspect of the acromion process.

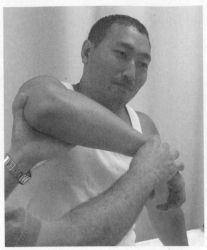

FIGURE 22-44 End test position of the Hawkins-Kennedy impingement test.

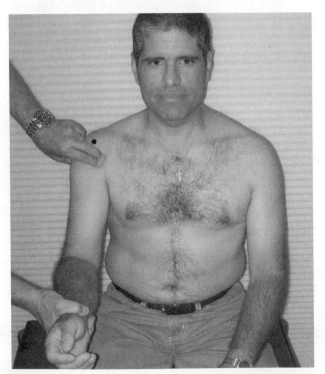

FIGURE 22-43 Palpation position for the subscapularis insertion in the deltopectoral interval. The *black marker* indicates the anterior aspect of the acromion process.

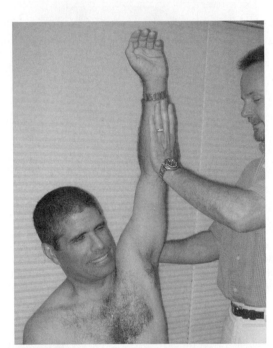

FIGURE 22-45 End test position of the Neer impingement test.

> **Precautions and Concerns**

- *Watch for a tight posterior capsule with these clients and treat accordingly.*
- *In clients showing impingement signs, care must be taken to avoid impinging the shoulder during overhead exercise.*
- *Monitor for excessive scapular elevation during UE elevation. Abnormal movement patterns must be avoided.*
- *Discourage clients from sleeping on their involved side, as this often increases the chance for impingement.*

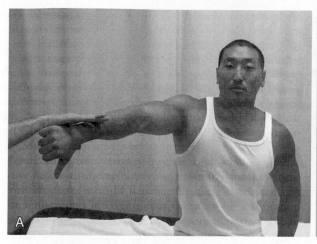
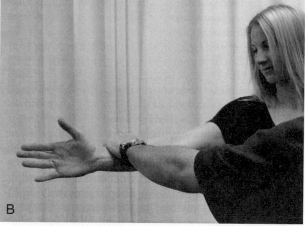

FIGURE 22-46 A, Test position for isometric testing of the supraspinatus or the "empty can" test. **B,** "Full can" test position.

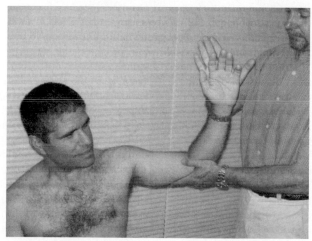
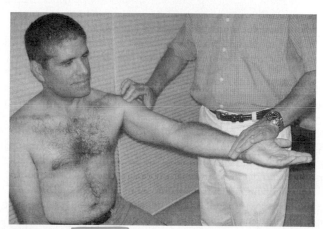

FIGURE 22-47 Test position for the Patte test for isometric strength of the infraspinatus and teres minor.

FIGURE 22-49 Speeds test for pathology of the long head of the biceps tendon and superior glenoid labrum.

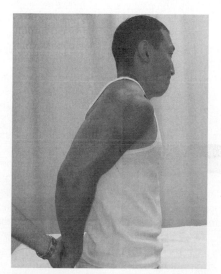

FIGURE 22-48 Test position for the Gerber lift-off test for isometric strength of the subscapularis.

CASE STUDIES

CASE STUDY 22-1 ■

JS is a 48-year-old right dominant stockbroker, non-smoker, who started therapy with a diagnosis of mild brachial plexus stretch injury. He reported symptoms of headache in the C2 distribution, anterior chest wall pain on the left, and pain in the left anteriolateral neck extending to the angle of his jaw and to the anterior aspect of his shoulder. He noted occasional swelling with flushing of the left side of his face, extending to his ear. This symptom became more prevalent when his left upper quarter pain was high. He was experiencing slight numbness of digits 1 to 3 and arm pain on the inside of the proximal humerus of the left UE while sitting at his desk and with overhead activities. He reported difficulty combing his hair because of arm pain.

Symptoms began 2 months ago when he decided to return to surfing after a 15-year hiatus. He stopped surfing about 1 month ago because his face, chest wall, and arm symptoms would increase dramatically during and for days after time spent on his board.

He had a thorough cardiac work-up and was cleared. X-rays and MRI of the cervical spine were unremarkable. He is in excellent physical shape with an unremarkable past medical history (PMH).

During the exam, he demonstrated a drooped left shoulder with a forward-head-rounded-shoulders posture. Cervical ROM was limited 25% only for rotation and lateral flexion to the right. A crossed-arm cervical ROM test showed no improvement in motion. Shoulder ROM was limited in flexion to horizontal by arm pain with IR and ER being full. RC strength was at 5/5 bilaterally and pain-free upon testing. There was muscle spasm in the suboccipital region, across the trapezius ridge, and along the medial scapular boarder.

Palpation at the left supraclavicular fossa was tender with spread of pain into the side of the face to the ear. Palpation at the left infraclavicular fossa and neurovascular bundle was painful with an increase of left UE symptoms. Tinel sign was positive in the same areas.

There was decreased sensitivity to pin prick of the thumb, index, and radial side of the long finger on the left. Roos (EAST) test was positive immediately. Neural mobility of the brachial plexus was at 2–/5 on the left with increase of left upper quarter symptoms and 5/5 on the right.

Impressions

Based on clinical presentation, JS demonstrated evidence of an upper trunk–lateral cord brachial plexopathy with decreased plexus mobility restricting UE elevation. Cervical motion loss implicated scalene tightness.

Facial symptoms with headache combined with shoulder droop implicate the upper trunk. Decreased acuity to pin prick on the radial side of the long finger continuing to the index finger and thumb implicate the lateral cord as well. No change in cervical motion with the cross-arm position combined with the pattern of cervical motion loss implicates the scalenes.

Because JS has full shoulder IR and ER, his limited UE elevation was not likely due to a capsular restriction. RC pathology is unlikely as well since RC strength was 5/5, and he was pain-free upon testing.

Treatment

Treatment on the first visit consisted of instruction in posture correction exercises, modification of computer placement to encourage proper posture while working, and instruction to limit all overhead activities. JS was instructed in nerve gliding exercises to be performed three times a day in sets of three with his posture correction exercises to be performed hourly in sets of ten.

JS's work schedule only allowed for weekly visits, so his treatment program was designed accordingly. On his second visit, JS demonstrated excellent technique with his home program. He had avoided all overhead activity and modified his workstation to encourage proper posture. He reported a 50% improvement in symptoms with no headache for the past week.

Brief exam revealed neural mobility at 3+/5, good postural awareness and less left shoulder drooping.

Treatment consisted of pectoral minor and scalene stretching with nerve glides. Neural mobility improved to 4+/5 by the end of treatment. JS's home program was modified to include scalene stretching and pectoralis minor doorway stretches. He was allowed to perform nerve glide and stretching exercises as long as his symptoms remained stable in sets of three completed three times a day. Scapular clock exercises were added to work on proprioception on an hourly basis.

On JS's visit 1 week later, he again demonstrated excellent compliance with his home program. He had full neural mobility, and his cervical ROM was full. Shoulder position was equal bilaterally. Roos (EAST) test was positive at 45 seconds of testing.

Treatment consisted of home program modification with the addition of scapular strengthening with focus on the upper, middle, lower trapezius, and serratus anterior using resistance bands. All exercises were performed daily in sets of three once through each exercise before starting the next set. JS was instructed to stop exercising if symptoms returned.

On the fourth visit 2 weeks later, JS had been symptom free for 1 week. Exam was normal except for a positive Roos test at 1 minute of testing leading to paresthesia into the thumb and index finger. Since his condition was stable and he had excellent understanding of his home program, JS was discharged from therapy with instructions to call as needed for program progression or if his status changed. He was instructed to avoid surfing.

Because JS was in excellent shape prior to his injury from surfing and was compliant and motivated, he quickly stabilized and returned to a functional baseline. Many clients have difficulty modifying their lifestyle to avoid further injury to their brachial plexus resulting in a protracted recovery period.

CASE STUDY 22-2 ■

FB is a 75-year-old right dominant female who tripped over her cat and sustained a Neer one-part fracture of the proximal humerus. She is 3 weeks post-injury when she comes to therapy in a simple sling for immobilization. Therapy orders are for ROM exercises with no strengthening for the next 3 weeks. FB is very apprehensive about moving her arm, because she feels that the break is still unstable since not enough time has passed from her injury date.

Prior to moving FB's right shoulder, I explained that sound will not travel across an open fracture and use a stethoscope at the humeral head while tapping on the lateral epicondyle to demonstrate to her there is no difference in the sound level. Next I showed her that the head of her humerus was moving as I rolled her arm from IR to ER, again indicating that she is ready to begin ROM exercise.

Exam revealed severe ecchymosis in the axilla and around the elbow. I explained that when she fractured her arm, there was a lot of bleeding from the bone and that blood has run down her arm along the interior tissue planes to collect around her elbow and distal axilla.

Shoulder elevation was 50°, abduction was 40°, and IR was arm across the abdomen and thumb to the iliac crest while attempting arm behind back position. ER was neutral. ROM of the elbow was 20° to 110° with wrist and hand ROM normal. Strength testing was deferred at that time.

I instructed FB in pendulum and tabletop ROM exercises that she was to perform hourly in sets of three to ten with up to three sets each exercise session. She started ROM exercises for her elbow that she was to perform whenever sitting.

FB's treatment over the next 2 weeks focused on ST stabilization via manual resistance applied to the scapula along with scapular mobilization and proprioception scapular clock exercises. PROM of the shoulder was also stressed focusing on avoidance of substitution patterns of excessive scapular elevation and protraction.

Re-evaluation 2 weeks later revealed ROM of elevation at 110°, abduction at 90°, and ER to 30° at 75° of abduction and 40° at neutral shoulder abduction. IR is at thumb to L5 reaching behind the back.

Treatment continued to focus on ROM, stressing active motion in normal movement patterns as FB mirrored my UE elevation while I stabilized her shoulder to prevent early scapular elevation. FB then added wall walking to her program incorporating self-stabilization of the scapula with her left hand.

At 6 weeks post-injury, FB's shoulder elevation is 150°, abduction is 135°, ER at 90° abduction is 50°, ER at shoulder neutral is 60°, and IR behind the back has progressed little at thumb to L3. Elbow, hand, and wrist ROM are full.

As FB was then allowed to begin strengthening, isometrics for all planes of shoulder movement and resistance band exercises of the elbow flexors and extensors were added. Behind the back stretches with good scapular position and upright posture were stressed as well. At this point, the therapy program included joint mobilization and more aggressive stretching to focus on gaining end ROM.

FB attended therapy for a total of 6 weeks. She had 160° of elevation, 150° of abduction, and 70° of ER at 90° of abduction and with the shoulder at neutral. IR behind the back remained restricted with the thumb reaching the L2 spinous process. FB was fully independent in self-care with her right arm, and she was pain-free. Shoulder strength was 4/5 except for abduction and ER which were 4–/5. She never regained full IR, because there may have been a rotary component to her fracture as she healed limiting the potential for normal IR ROM.

CASE STUDY 22-3 ■

TB is an 18-year-old high school football player who sustained a traumatic anterior dislocation of his right (dominant) shoulder. The MRI

results demonstrated a Bankart lesion with anterior glenoid labrum and capsule tear. As TB was a heavily recruited athlete, he opted to have arthroscopic shoulder surgery 4 weeks post-injury.

TB started therapy 2 weeks after surgery with his arm in a sling immobilizer.

Active motion is contraindicated to avoid disrupting the surgical repair. PROM of the right shoulder was 90° of flexion, 40° of abduction, and 10° of ER. IR was arm across stomach. Strength testing was deferred.

Treatment initially focused on protecting the surgical repair by following ER ROM restrictions to 40°. Scapular proprioception exercises were issued for a home program to get a head start on preventing poor scapular kinematics. These consisted of half shoulder rolls in the posterior direction only and clock shoulder elevation to 12:00, 1:00, and 2:00 positions performed in front of a mirror for feedback.

Over the next 4 weeks, treatment consisted of sub-maximal isometrics of the internal and external rotators with ER limited to 40° to avoid disrupting the repaired anterior structures. Scapular stabilization exercises continued during this period. PROM manual therapy was the primary component of treatment.

At 8 weeks, TB had 145° of flexion with active flexion at 135° and ER at 40°. The ER safe zone was now to 60°. The protocol allowed for resistance band exercises of the external and internal rotators. Active shoulder elevation by TB while mirroring the therapist with the therapist preventing early scapular elevation was started. *– keep the scapula "set"*

During the next 4 weeks, the resistance band exercises were progressed to include shoulder elevation and abduction as long as scapular substitution patterns were avoided. Strengthening of the triceps and scapular depressors/stabilizers by doing seated press-ups were added. *→ lat dorsi* Manual resistance exercises in diagonal planes both supine and seated with focus on normal kinematics were started as well. Throughout all phases, ROM exercises were stressed.

By 12 weeks, flexion was 170°, abduction was 165°, and ER was 60° with IR at 70°. Strength of the shoulder is 5/5 for extension with flexion and IR at 4+/5; ER and abduction was at 4/5. By then, all motion restrictions were removed. The focus of the next 4 to 6 weeks was to gain full ROM, full strength, and start sport-specific training. Plyometric drills with two-hand throw/catch activities using weighted balls were started.

By 18 weeks TB has full ROM, and scapular kinematics/shoulder mechanics are normal. He has returned to work out at the gym using a custom program designed to strengthen the anterior shoulder structures and globally strengthen the RC, deltoid, serratus anterior, pectoral, and back muscles. Because of his successful rehabilitation, TB went on to play collegiate football.

→ most common

References

1. Ludewig PM, Phadke V, Braman JP, et al: Motion of the shoulder complex during multiplanar humeral elevation, *J Bone Joint Surg Am* 91:378–389, 2009.
2. Lugo R, Kung P, Ma CB: Shoulder biomechanics, *Eur J Radiol* 68:16–24, 2008.
3. Nam D, Maak TG, Raphael BS, et al: Rotator cuff tear arthropathy: evaluation, diagnosis, and treatment: AAOS exhibit selection, *J Bone Joint Surg Am* 94(6):e34, 2012.
4. Matsumura N, Nakamichi N, Ikegami, et al: The function of the clavicle on scapular motion: a cadaveric study, *J Shoulder Elbow Surg* 22(3):333–339, 2013.
5. Mercer SR, Bogduk N: Clinical anatomy of the Ligamentum nuchae, *Clin Anat* 16:484–493, 2003.
6. Johnson D, Ellis H: Pectoral girdle, shoulder region and axilla. In Standring S, editor: *Gray's anatomy*, ed 39, New York, 2005, Elsevier, pp 817–850.

7. Bontempo NA, Mazzocca AD: Biomechanics and treatment of acromio-clavicular and sternocoavicular joint injuries, *Br J Sports Med* 44:361–369, 2010.

8. Groh GL, Wirth MA: Management of traumatic sternoclavicular joint injuries, *J Am Acad Orthop Surg* 19:1–7, 2011.

9. Kibler WB, Sciascia A, Wilkes T: Scapular dyskinesis and its relation to shoulder injury, *J Am Acad Orthop Surg* 20:364–372, 2012.

10. Donatelli RA: Functional anatomy and mechanics. In Donatelli RA, editor: *Physical therapy of the shoulder*, ed 4, St Louis, 2004, Churchill Livingstone, pp 11–28.

11. Ludewig PM, Braman JP: Shoulder impingement: biomechanical considerations in rehabilitation, *Man Ther* 16:33–39, 2011.

12. Mercer SB, Bogduk N: The ligaments and anulus fibrosus of human adult cervical intervertebral discs, *Spine* 24(7):619–626, 1999.

13. Boden SD, McCowin PR, Davis DO, et al: Abnormal magnetic-resonance scans of the cervical spine in asymptomatic subjects: a prospective investigation, *J Bone Joint Surg Am* 72(8):1178–1184, 1990.

14. McLain RF: Mechanoreceptor endings in human cervical facet joints, *Spine* 19:495–501, 1994.

15. Dwyer A, Aprill C, Bogduk N: Cervical zygapophyseal joint pain patterns. I: A study in normal volunteers, *Spine* 15(6):453–457, 1990.

16. Fukui S, Ohseto K, Shiotani M, et al: Referred pain distribution of the cervical zygapophyseal joints and cervical dorsal rami, *Pain* 68(1):79–83, 1996.

17. Travell JG, Simmons DG: *Myofascial pain and dysfunction the trigger point manual*, vol 1, Baltimore, MD, 1983, Lippincott Williams & Wilkins.

18. Werneke MW, Hart DL, Deutscher D, et al: Clinician's ability to identify neck and low back interventions: an inter-rater chance-corrected agreement study, *J Man Manip Ther* 19(3):172–181, 2011.

19. Salt E, Wright C, Kelly S, et al: A systemic review of the literature on the effectiveness of manual therapy for cervicobrachial pain, *Man Ther* 16(1):53–56, 2011.

20. Wainner RS, Fritz JM, Irrgang JJ, et al: Reliability and diagnostic accuracy of the clinical examination and patient self-report measures for cervical radiculopathy, *Spine* 28(1):52–62, 2003.

21. Shah KC, Rajshekhar V: Reliability of diagnosis of soft cervical disc prolapse using Spurling's test, *Br J Neurosurg* 18(5):480–483, 2004.

22. Tong HC, Haig AJ, Yamakawa K: The Spurling test and cervical radiculopathy, *Spine* 27(2):156–159, 2002.

23. Anekstein Y, Blecher R, Smorgik Y, et al: What is the best way to apply the Spurling test for cervical radiculopathy? *Clin Orthop Rel Resear* 470:2566–2572, 2012.

24. Spurling RG, Scoville WB: Lateral rupture of the cervical intervertebral discs: a common cause of shoulder and arm pain, *Surg Gynecol Obstet* 78:350–358, 1944.

25. Takasaki H, Hall T, Jull G, et al: The influence of cervical traction, compression, and Spurling test on cervical intervertebral foramen size, *Spine* 34(16):1658–1662, 2009.

26. Wilbourn AJ: 10 most commonly asked questions about thoracic outlet syndrome, *Neurologist* 7(5):309–312, 2001.

27. Roos DB: Congenital anomalies associated with thoracic outlet syndrome: anatomy, symptoms, diagnosis, and treatment, *Am J Surg* 132(6):771–778, 1976.

28. Hooper TL, Denton J, McGalliard MK, et al: Thoracic outlet syndrome: a controversial clinical condition: part 1. anatomy, and clinical examination/diagnosis, *J Man Manip Ther* 18(2):74–83, 2010.

29. Gergoudis R, Barnes R: Thoracic outlet arterial compression: prevalence in normals, *Angiology* 31:538, 1980.

30. Costigan DA, Wilbourn AJ: The elevated arm stress test: specificity in the diagnosis of thoracic outlet syndrome, *Neurology* 35(Suppl 1):74, 1985.

31. Warrens AN, Heaton JM: Thoracic outlet compression syndrome: the lack of reliability of its clinical assessment, *Ann R Coll Surg Engl* 69(5):203–204, 1987.

32. Rayan GM, Jensen C: Thoracic outlet syndrome: provocative examination maneuvers in a typical population, *J Shoulder Elbow Surg* 4(2):113–117, 1995.

33. Nord KM, Kapoor P, Fisher J, et al: False positive rate of thoracic outlet syndrome diagnostic maneuvers, *Electromyogr Clin Neurophysiol* 48(2):67–74, 2008.

34. Leffert RD: Thoracic outlet syndrome, *J Am Acad Orthop Surg* 2(6):317–325, 1994.

35. Schwartzman RJ: Brachial plexus traction injuries, *Hand Clinics* 7(3):547–556, 1991.

36. Dilley A, Lynn B, Pang SJ: Pressure and stretch mechanosensitivity of peripheral nerve fibers following local inflammation of the nerve trunk, *Pain* 117:462–472, 2005.

37. Nijs J, van Wilgen CP, van Oosterwijck J, et al: How to explain central sensitization to patients with "unexplained" chronic musculoskeletal pain: practice guidelines, *Man Ther* 16(5):413–418, 2011.

38. Degeorges R, Reynaud C, Becquemin JP: Thoracic outlet syndrome surgery: long-term functional results, *Ann Vasc Surg* 18(5):558–565, 2004.

39. Cherington M, Happer I, Machanic B, et al: Surgery for thoracic outlet syndrome may be hazardous to your health, *Muscle Nerve* 9(7):632–634, 1986.

40. Roos DB, Owens JC: Thoracic outlet syndrome, *Arch Surg* 93(1):71–74, 1966.

41. Handoll HHG, Ollivere BJ: Interventions for treating proximal humeral fractures in adults (review), *The Cochrane Library* 12:1–76, 2010.

42. Neer CS 2nd: Displaced proximal humeral fractures: part I. Classification and evaluation, 1970, *Clin Orthop Relat Res* 442:77–82, 2006.

43. Palvanen M, Kannus P, Parkkari J, et al: The injury mechanisms of osteoporotic upper extremity fractures among older adults: a controlled study of 287 consecutive patients and their 108 controls, *Osteoporos Int* 11(10):822–831, 2000.

44. Gohlke F, Essigkrug B, Schnitz F: The pattern of the collagen fiber bundles of the capsule of the glenohumeral joint, *J Shoulder Elbow Surg* 3(3):111–128, 1994.

45. Emig EW, Schweitzer ME, Karasick D, et al: Adhesive capsulitis of the shoulder: MR diagnosis, *Am J Roentgenol* 164(6):1457–1459, 1995.

46. Tasto JP, Elias DW: Adhesive capsulitis, *Sports Med Arthros Rev* 15:216–221, 2007.

47. Favejee MM, Huisstede BM, Koes BW: Frozen shoulder: the effectiveness of conservative and surgical interventions—systemic review, *B J Sports Med* 45(1):49–56, 2011.

48. Jewell DV, Riddle DL, Thacker LR: Interventions associated with and increased or decreased likelihood of pain reduction and improved function in patients with adhesive capsulitis: a retrospective cohort study, *Phys Ther* 89:419–429, 2009.

49. Bunker T: Frozen shoulder, *Orthopedics and Trauma* 25(1):11–18, 2011.

50. Zuckerman JD: Definition and classification of frozen shoulder, *J Shoulder Elbow Surg* 3:S72, 1994.

51. Kelly MJ, McClure PW, Leggin BG: Frozen shoulder: evidence and a proposed model guiding rehabilitation, *J Orthop Phys Ther* 39(2):135–148, 2009.

52. Milgrom C, Novack V, Weil Y, et al: Risk factors for frozen shoulder, *Isr Med Assoc J* 10(5):361–364, 2008.

53. Smith SP, Devaraj VS, Bunker TD: The association between frozen shoulder and Dupuytren's disease, *J Shoulder Elbow Surg* 10(2):149–151, 2001.

54. Shaffer B, Tibone JE, Kerlan RK: Frozen shoulder. A long-term follow-up, *J Bone Joint Surg Am* 74(5):738–746, 1992.

55. Vastamaki H, Kettunen J, Vastamaki M: The natural history of idiopathic frozen shoulder: a 2- to 27-year followup study, *Clin Orthop Relat Res* 470(4):1133–1143, 2012.

56. Hannafin JA, Chiaia TA: Adhesive capsulitis. A treatment approach, *Clin Orthop Relat Res*(372)95–109, 2000.

57. Ogilvie-Harris DJ, Biggs DJ, Fitsialos DP, et al: The resistant frozen shoulder. Manipulation versus arthroscopic release, *Clin Orthop Relat Res*(319)238–248, 1995.

58. Wilk KE, Macrina LC, Fleisig GS, et al: Correlation of glenohumeral internal rotation deficit and total rotational motion to shoulder injuries in professional baseball pitchers, *Am J Sports Med* 39:329–335, 2011.

59. Guerrero P, Busconi B, Deangelus N, et al: Congenital instability of the shoulder joint: assessment and treatment options, *J Orthop Sports Phys Ther* 39(2):124–134, 2009.

60. Budoff JE, Nirschl RP, Guidi EJ: Débridement of partial thickness tears of the rotator cuff without acromioplasty. Long-term follow-up and review of literature, *J Bone Joint Surg Am* 80(5):733–748, 1998.

61. Tyler TF, Nicholas SJ, Lee SJ, et al: Correction of posterior shoulder tightness is associated with symptom resolution in patients with internal impingement, *Am J Sports Med* 38:114–118, 2010.

62. Nakamizo H, Nakamura Y, Nobuhara K, et al: Loss of internal rotation in little league pitchers: a biomechanical study, *J Shoulder and Elbow Surg* 17:795–801, 2008.

63. Shanley E, Rauh MJ, Michener LA, et al: Shoulder range of motion measures as risk factors for shoulder and elbow injuries in high school softball and baseball players, *Am J Sports Med* 39(9):1997–2006, 2011.

64. Burkhart SS, Morgan CD: The peel-back mechanism: its role in producing and extending posterior type II SLAP lesions and its effect on SLAP repair rehabilitation, *Arthroscopy* 14(6):637–640, 1998.

65. Zazzali MS, Vad VB, et al: Shoulder instability. In Donatelli RA, editor: *Physical therapy of the shoulder*, ed 4, St Louis, 2004, Churchill Livingstone, pp 483–504.

66. Neer CS 2nd, Foster CR: Inferior capsular shift for involuntary inferior and multidirectional instability of the shoulder: A preliminary report, *J Bone Joint Surg Am* 62(6):897–908, 1980.

67. Jacobson ME, Riggenbach M, Woodbridge AN, et al: Open and arthroscopic treatment of multidirectional instability of the shoulder, *Arthroscopy* 28(7):1010–1017, 2012.

68. Hayashi K, Markel MD: Thermal capsulorrhaphy treatment of shoulder instability: basic science, *Clin Orthop Relat Res:* (390) 59–72, 2001.

69. Ritzman T, Parker R: Thermal capsulorrhaphy of the shoulder, *Current Opinion in Orthopaedics* 13:288–291, 2002.

70. Hawkins RJ, Krishnan SG, Karas SG, et al: Electrotheramal arthroscopic shoulder capsulorrhaphy. A minimum 2-year follow-up, *Am J Sports Med* 35(9):1484–1488, 2007.

71. Godin J, Sekiya JK: Systemic review of rehabilitation versus operative stabilization for the treatment of first time anterior shoulder dislocations, *Sports Health* 2(2):156–165, 2010.

72. Cameron KL, Dufffey ML, DeBerardino TM, et al: Association of generalized joint hypermobility with a history of glenohumeral joint instability, *J Athl Train* 45(3):253–258, 2010.

73. Johnson SM, Robinson CM: Shoulder instability in patients with joint hyperlaxity, *J Bone Joint Surg Am* 92(6):1545–1557, 2010.

74. Gerber C, Ganz R: Clinical assessment of instability of the shoulder with special preference to anterior and posterior drawer tests, *J Bone Joint Surg Br* 66(4):551–556, 1984.

75. Tzannes A, Paxinos A, Callahan M, et al: An assessment of the interexaminer reliability of tests for shoulder instability, *J Shoulder Elbow Surg* 13(1):18–23, 2004.

76. Farber AJ, Castillo R, Clough M, et al: Clinical assessment of three common tests for traumatic anterior shoulder instability, *J Bone Joint Surg Am* 88:1467–1474, 2006.

77. Longo UG, Berton A, Papapietro N, et al: Epidemiology, genetics and biological factors of rotator cuff tears, *Med Sport Sci* 57:1–9, 2012.

78. Neer CS 2nd: Anterior acromioplasty for the chronic impingement syndrome in the shoulder: a preliminary report, *J Bone Joint Surg Am* 54(1):41–50, 1972.

79. Bigliani LU, Morrison D, et al: The morphology of the acromion and its relationship to rotator cuff tears, *Orthop Trans* 10:228, 1986.

80. Walch G, Boileau P, et al: Impingement of the deep surface of the supraspinatus tendon on the glenoid rim, *J Shoulder Elbow Surg* 1:239–245, 1992.

81. Lindblom K: On pathogenesis of ruptures of the tendon aponeurosis of the shoulder joint, *Acta Radiologica* 20:563–567, 1939.

82. Codman EA: *The shoulder*, ed 2, Boston, 1934, Thomas Todd.

83. Finnan RP, Crosby LA: Partial-thickness rotator cuff tears, *J Shoulder Elbow Surg* 19:609–616, 2010.

84. Matsen FA III, Arntz CT: Rotator cuff tendon failure. In Rockwood CA Jr, Matsen FA III, editors: *The shoulder*, vol II, Philadelphia, 1990, WB Saunders Co, pp 647–677.

85. Park HB, Yokota A, Gill HS, et al: Diagnostic accuracy of clinical tests for the different degrees of subacromial impingement syndrome, *J Bone Joint Surg Am* 87:1446–1455, 2005.

86. Mattingly GE, Mackarey PJ: Optimal methods for shoulder tendon palpation: a cadaver study, *Physical Therapy* 76:166–174, 1996.

87. Kelly SM, Brittle N, Allen GM: The value of physical tests for subacromial impingement syndrome: a study of diagnostic accuracy, *Clin Rehabil* 24(2):149–158, 2010.

88. Alqunaee M, Galvin R, Fahey T: Diagnostic accuracy of clinical tests for subacromial impingement syndrome: a systematic review and meta-analysis, *Arch Phys Med Rehabil* 93(2):229–236, 2012.

89. Longo UG, Berton A, Aherns PM: Clinical diagnosis of rotator cuff disease, *Sports Med Arthrosc Rev* 19:266–278, 2011.

90. Gerber C, Krushell RJ: Isolated rupture of the tendon of the subscapularis muscle. Clinical features in 16 cases, *J Bone Joint Surg Br* 73(3):389–394, 1991.

91. Kijima H, Minagawa H, Nishi T, et al: Long-term follow-up of cases of rotator cuff tear treated conservatively, *J Shoulder Elbow Surg* 21(4):491–494, 2012.

23

Elbow Diagnoses

Carol Page

Function of the Elbow

The elbow serves as the essential functional link between the hand and the shoulder, allowing the hand to be brought inward toward the body and outward into the surrounding environment. It also transfers force through the upper extremity (UE) during weight bearing on the hand. The functional range of motion (ROM) required at the elbow is reported to be 30° of extension, 130° of flexion, and 50° each of pronation and supination.[1] However, because functional demands vary, the range required will differ somewhat among individuals. In general, it is easier to compensate for limited extension by moving closer to objects during reach than it is to compensate for limited flexion. Because the most common complication of elbow trauma is stiffness, it is essential that therapists treating individuals with elbow injuries be well versed in effective treatment approaches. To "push harder" or "be more aggressive" is not an effective solution and may instead cause more damage and stiffness. In addition to being mobile, the elbow must also be stable so that it can withstand the forces of daily activities. Maintaining the most effective balance between minimizing stiffness through early motion, preserving stability, and protecting healing structures is a challenge even for experienced therapists.

◎ Clinical Pearl

Elbow stiffness is the most common complication of elbow trauma.

Elbow Anatomy

Three bones contribute to the **elbow joint,** the distal humerus, proximal ulna, and proximal radius (Fig. 23-1). They form the three articulations of the elbow: the ulnohumeral, radiohumeral, and proximal radioulnar joints. The distal humerus has two articular surfaces: the spool-shaped **trochlea** medially and the convex **capitellum** (also known as the *capitulum*) laterally. The **ulnohumeral joint** is the close articulation of the trochlea with the rounded **trochlear notch** formed by the **coronoid** and **olecranon** of the proximal ulna. In full elbow flexion the **coronoid fossa** on the anterior distal humerus receives the coronoid process of the anterior trochlear notch. In full extension, the **olecranon fossa** on the posterior distal humerus receives the olecranon process of the posterior trochlear notch. The **radiohumeral joint** is the articulation of the capitellum of the distal humerus with the shallow concavity on the proximal aspect of the **radial head.** The radial head and the **radial notch** of the ulna form the **proximal radioulnar joint.**

Due to the oblique orientation of the trochlea of the humerus, in full extension the elbow has a **valgus** angle, known as the **carrying angle.** It has been widely reported that men have a carrying angle of approximately 5° to 10°, while women have a slightly greater carrying angle of approximately 10° to 15°. However, measured radiographically, the normal carrying angle in adults is reported to be 17.8° on average with no significant difference between men and women.[2]

◎ Clinical Pearl

The most reliable way to determine if the carrying angle of an injured elbow is normal is to compare it to the individual's uninjured elbow.

Ligaments

The three elbow articulations share a common joint capsule. The medial and lateral collateral ligament complexes of the elbow are essentially thickenings of the joint

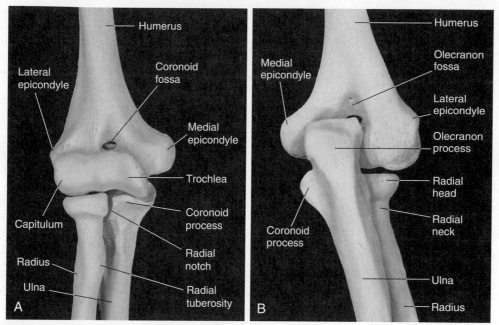

FIGURE 23-1 A, Anterior view of the elbow joint. **B,** Posterior view of the elbow joint. (From Thibodeau G, Patton K, editors: *Anatomy & physiology,* ed 8, St Louis, 2013, Mosby.)

capsule. Portions of the collateral ligament complexes remain taut throughout elbow flexion and extension, making an essential contribution to static elbow stability. The **medial collateral ligament complex** (Fig. 23-2) has three components, the anterior bundle, posterior bundle, and the transverse ligament. This ligament complex, particularly the anterior bundle, stabilizes the elbow against valgus (abduction) forces. The **lateral collateral ligament complex** (Fig. 23-3) has four components, the **lateral ulnar collateral ligament (LUCL),** the radial collateral ligament, the annular ligament, and the accessory lateral collateral ligament. The lateral collateral ligament complex is considered to be one of the primary stabilizers of the elbow. It provides restraint from **varus** (adduction) forces. The LUCL, one of the four components of this ligament complex, also provides posterolateral stability to the ulnohumeral joint.

> ### ◎ *Clinical Pearl*
>
> Edema often affects all three joints of the elbow because they share a common joint capsule.

The **interosseous ligament,** fibrous tissue lying obliquely between the radius and ulna, transfers forces from the radius to the ulna during weight bearing on the hand. Although not part of the elbow complex, injury to the interosseous ligament can alter the mechanics of the elbow. If the radial head is fractured or excised, the interosseous ligament is critical to load sharing. If it is disrupted, the entire force is shifted to the ulna rather than being shared between the ulna and radius.

Muscles

The muscles that cross the elbow provide it with active power and dynamic stability. Biceps brachii, brachialis, and brachioradialis are the primary elbow flexors. Biceps brachii is the primary

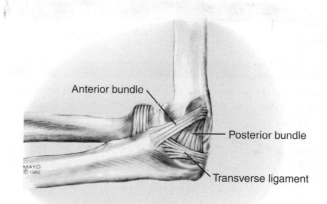

FIGURE 23-2 The medial collateral ligament complex of the elbow. (From Morrey BF, Sanchez-Sotelo J, editors: *The elbow and its disorders,* ed 4, Philadelphia, 2009, Saunders.)

supinator of forearm with supinator acting as an additional, weaker supinator. Triceps is the primary elbow extensor. Pronator teres is the primary forearm pronator with pronator quadratus in the distal forearm acting as another, weaker pronator. The other muscles crossing the elbow joint serve as secondary movers and contribute to dynamic joint stability.

Nerves and Blood Vessels

The muscles that move the elbow are innervated by the musculocutaneous, radial, and median nerves. The musculocutaneous nerve innervates biceps brachii and brachialis. The radial nerve innervates brachioradialis, triceps, and supinator. The median

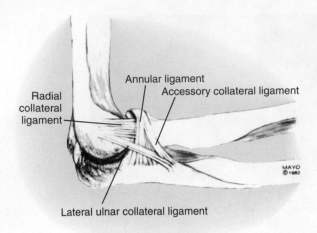

FIGURE 23-3 The lateral collateral ligament complex of the elbow. (From Morrey BF, Sanchez-Sotelo J, editors: *The elbow and its disorders,* ed 4, Philadelphia, 2009, Saunders.)

nerve innervates pronator teres. The median, ulnar, and radial nerves and the brachial artery all lie close to the elbow joint and as a result are susceptible to injury in elbow fractures and dislocations. The ulnar nerve is particularly susceptible to injury as it passes posterior to the medial epicondyle through the **cubital tunnel.**

Clinical Pearl

Abnormal stress on the ulnar nerve can result from an elbow injury, a direct blow, or prolonged direct pressure (such as, when leaning on the elbow or prolonged or repetitive elbow flexion) that stretches the nerve. Numbness and tingling in the small finger and ulnar aspect of the ring finger and grip weakness can be signs and symptoms of ulnar **neuritis** or compression of the ulnar nerve in the cubital tunnel.

Elbow Biomechanics

Motion at the elbow occurs in two axes: flexion-extension and pronation-supination. The elbow acts as a hinge during flexion-extension. However, rather than occurring in a single plane, flexion-extension is accompanied by slight rotation and medial-lateral motion, which results in the carrying angle of the elbow. Normal elbow ROM is approximately 0° extension to 140° flexion. Because flexion is limited by soft tissue approximation, end range is variable. Hyperextension of up to 10° is observed more commonly in women. During pronation-supination, the radius rotates around the ulna. Normal forearm ROM is approximately 85° pronation and 90° supination. ROM varies among individuals, and a variety of normal values are reported in the literature.

Clinical Pearl

Determination of normal elbow and forearm ROM for an individual is best made by comparison to the uninvolved UE rather than to published norms.

Stability at the elbow is provided by both static and dynamic constraints. The osseous structures provide static stability. The highly congruent ulnohumeral joint is the primary stabilizer of the elbow. The radial head also acts as a stabilizing structure. The joint capsule, medial collateral ligament complex, and lateral collateral ligament complex provide additional static stability. The muscles that cross the elbow, when contracted, contribute dynamic stability to the elbow.

Elbow Fractures

The elbow is a complex joint, vulnerable to fracture from falls on an outstretched hand as well as from direct trauma. Elbow fractures are frequently challenging to treat, often requiring operative intervention. The most common complication of elbow fracture is stiffness. Failure to regain elbow ROM can result in significant functional impairment. To minimize this risk, it is important that mobilization begin early. The necessary stability to safely allow early mobilization of displaced and unstable elbow fractures requires operative management.

Radial Head Fractures

Radial head fractures are the most common elbow fracture in adults. The most common mechanism of injury is falling onto an outstretched hand with the forearm pronated. These fractures can also result from falling directly onto the elbow. The most common complication of both stable, non-operatively managed radial head fractures and those requiring operative stabilization is **elbow flexion contracture,** the loss of full elbow extension.

Clinical Pearl

In the presence of radial head fracture, the forearm and wrist should also be carefully evaluated, because there may be associated injuries to the interosseous ligament and the distal radioulnar joint, known as an **Essex-Lopresti lesion.**

Olecranon Fractures

Olecranon fractures are another relatively common elbow fracture in adults. These fractures usually result from a fall onto a bent elbow or a direct blow. The olecranon is particularly vulnerable to direct trauma due to its location just below the skin where it has minimal protective soft tissue coverage. The majority of olecranon fractures are displaced with a tendency to be widely separated because of the pull of the triceps insertion. Most olecranon fractures require operative management. Severe, unstable olecranon fractures are usually associated with trauma to other structures and can be very complex and challenging to treat.

Clinical Pearl

The ulnar nerve is susceptible to injury in olecranon fractures due to its adjacent location.

Distal Humeral Fractures

Fractures of the distal humerus are relatively uncommon, accounting for only 2% of all fractures. They occur most frequently in young males and in females over 80 years of age. In younger individuals, distal humeral fractures are usually associated with higher velocity injuries, such as motor vehicle and sports-related accidents. In the elderly with poor bone stock, they can occur from a simple fall onto an outstretched hand.[3]

Timelines and Healing

To minimize the risk of elbow stiffness following an isolated elbow fracture, gentle active motion in the stable range is usually initiated within the first week following injury or surgery. While early motion is highly desirable, fracture stability is the prerequisite. Isolated elbow fractures that are stable and non-displaced are usually referred to therapy several days after injury. Displaced or unstable fractures are treated operatively to restore bony alignment and stability; this is to ideally allow controlled motion within the first week following surgery. Open fractures must be treated operatively to clean the wounds and minimize the risk of deep infection, to restore alignment and stability, and to allow early mobilization.

During the healing process, fractures must be protected from excessive or uncontrolled forces that could disrupt alignment and lead to malunion or nonunion. *Strengthening exercises are not initiated until there is evidence of fracture consolidation,* usually 8 to 12 weeks following the injury or surgery. Return to all previous activities is allowed when the fracture has fully consolidated and normal or near normal strength has been regained, 3 to 6 months following injury.

Non-Operative Treatment

Elbow fractures that are stable and well aligned are usually referred to therapy within the first few days following injury. Unstable and poorly-aligned fractures are treated operatively and then referred to therapy. The initial goal of therapy is to restore motion while protecting the elbow from harmful stresses that could compromise fracture alignment and healing. A removable thermoplastic orthosis is the most common means of protective immobilization. The orthosis is removed, usually within the first week, for initiation of gentle active and active-assisted elbow and forearm motion in the arc that does not compromise stability. Educate your patient in precautions, such as any initial restrictions to the arc of motion necessary to protect fracture stability and the avoidance of weight bearing and lifting with the involved UE. Active motion of the digits, wrist, shoulder, and shoulder girdle should be performed to preserve the motion of these uninvolved joints. Elevation, cold packs, light compression wraps, and light massage are useful for the control of pain and edema. In addition to preventing digit stiffness, active digit motion helps to minimize edema in the hand and entire UE.

The rate of treatment progression is dependent on fracture healing. *Discuss the degree of fracture stability with the referring physician before proceeding.* Once the physician determines that there is evidence of fracture union and sufficient stability, introduce gentle passive motion, joint mobilization, and soft tissue mobilization with the goal of restoring full motion. Scar management for operatively-managed fractures should begin once the surgical incision is fully healed. As healing progresses, encourage gradual return to use of the involved UE for light functional activities. The protective orthosis is discontinued except for sleep, travel, and other circumstances that might put the elbow at risk.

Following fracture consolidation, instruct your patient in resistive exercises to strengthen the involved UE. The ultimate goal of therapy and best outcome is restoration of the previous level of function with a mobile, stable, and pain-free elbow. If your patient reaches a plateau before achieving end range motion, a static progressive orthosis or serial static orthosis may be required to address joint stiffness (see "The Stiff Elbow" section later in this chapter).

Operative Treatment

The goal of surgery is to restore alignment and stability to the displaced or unstable elbow fracture. When achieved, elbow motion can be initiated within a few days, minimizing the risk of joint stiffness. *However, stability must never be sacrificed for the sake of mobility.* Motion is initiated once the referring physician has determined that sufficient stability has been restored through surgery or fracture healing.

Complications of elbow fractures are more common when there is articular involvement. In addition to stiffness, the most common postoperative complications of elbow fractures are infection, malunion, nonunion, ulnar **neuropathy,** and **arthrosis.**

Displaced radial head fractures with comminution or mechanical block to forearm rotation require operative treatment. The presence of one or more associated injuries at the elbow including capitellum fracture, olecranon fracture, ligamentous injuries, and elbow dislocation, is also an indication for operative treatment. Approximately one in three radial head fractures is associated with another injury.[4] Options for the operative treatment of radial head fractures include internal fixation with plate and screws, radial head excision, and radial head replacement. Comminuted fractures are treated with radial head excision or replacement. Displaced fractures with mechanical block to forearm rotation are treated with internal fixation or radial head excision. Note that due to important stabilizing function of the radial head, it must be replaced rather than excised in radial head fractures with associated injuries that compromise elbow stability.

Most olecranon fractures require open reduction and internal fixation. A posterior approach is typically used. The type of internal fixation is chosen depending on the individual characteristics of the fracture. Options include Kirschner wires, tension band wiring, compression screws, and plate fixation. With appropriate management, outcomes of olecranon fractures are typically good to excellent.[5] In addition to the complications common to all elbow fractures, hardware on the posterior aspect of the elbow is not always well tolerated. Chronic irritation can result in olecranon bursitis and may require excision of the hardware.[6]

Distal humeral fractures that are comminuted, displaced, involve the trochlea or capitellum, or have neurovascular involvement require operative treatment. There is a higher risk of complications in high-energy mechanisms of injury, open fractures, and non-operatively managed fractures. In addition to the complications common to all elbow fractures, **heterotopic ossification,** bone in nonosseous tissues, may develop following fractures of the distal humerus. Although these fractures are frequently challenging to manage, the majority heal within 12 weeks without significant complications.[3] Most are stabilized surgically with open reduction and internal fixation with plates and screws. A posterior surgical approach is most commonly used for visualization of the fracture. The triceps is split or elevated and reflected, or an olecranon **osteotomy** is performed. Following an olecranon osteotomy, the olecranon is reattached with Kirschner wires and screws or plating.[7] An **anterior ulnar nerve transposition** is sometimes performed during surgery for fracture repair to lessen the likelihood of postoperative ulnar neuropathy. Elderly individuals with complex distal humerus fractures and osteoporotic bone present a particular challenge to the surgeon. **Total elbow arthoplasty** may be necessary in these individuals if screws cannot obtain adequate bony purchase for fracture fixation.[8]

? Questions to Discuss with the Physician

- Which bone was fractured, and what was the nature of the fracture? Ask for the radiology report.
- Were there any associated injuries?
- Was the fracture treated surgically, and if so, how? Ask for the operative note.
- Is the fracture stable enough to begin active motion?
- Are there any movement limitations or other precautions?
- What are the preferred type, position, and wearing schedule for the protective orthosis?

As the Patient Progresses

- When can the protective orthosis be discontinued?
- When can passive motion be initiated?
- When can the use of static progressive orthoses be initiated (if necessary to increase motion)?
- When can resistive exercises be initiated?

( ) What to Say to Clients

About Stable Elbow Fractures

"You may be surprised to start motion exercises so soon after breaking a bone, but elbow stiffness is the most common problem after an injury like yours. Your fracture is stable enough now to safely do the gentle exercises that I'm going to teach you. They will help you maintain and improve your elbow motion."

About the Home Exercise Program

"You'll get more benefit from doing your motion exercises slowly and fully than from doing lots of them quickly. It's best to do the exercises throughout the day. For example, do a set when you first get up in the morning, another at lunch, another after work, and a last set before bed. It's normal to feel tighter in the morning and looser later in the day. When your elbow feels stiff, breathe deeply and relax as you slowly move your elbow as far as it will go. Forceful or quick motions will tend to make all your muscles contract and fight the movement you're trying to do."

◎ Clinical Pearl

When the elbow is viewed from behind in 90° of flexion, the medial and lateral epicondyles of the distal humerus and the tip of the olecranon of the ulna should form an inverted equilateral triangle. With the elbow in full extension, these landmarks should form a straight line.

Evaluation Tips

- When assessing motion, strength, sensibility, and edema, compare the measurements to those of the patient's uninvolved UE to determine what is normal for that individual.
- Do not measure passive range of motion (PROM) or strength until cleared by the referring physician.
- Ask your patient to complete a self-report questionnaire at initial evaluation, re-evaluation, and discharge. These measures are useful for tracking and reporting progress as well as for highlighting functional problems that may require attention in therapy. The Disabilities of Arm, Shoulder, and Hand (DASH) questionnaire and the Patient-Rated Elbow Evaluation (PREE) are self-report measures commonly used for elbow injuries. The DASH documents UE function, whereas the PREE documents pain and function and is specific to the elbow. Although both are scored from 1 to 100, 100 on the DASH represents maximum functional disability, whereas 100 on the PREE represents least pain and best function.

Diagnosis-Specific Information That Affects Clinical Reasoning

Radial head fractures that are non-displaced or minimally displaced are treated non-operatively, unless there is a mechanical block to forearm rotation. These fractures have a favorable prognosis as long as motion is begun early. Active motion is usually initiated within the first several days following injury. *Be sure to emphasize elbow extension, because this motion is most frequently lost after radial head fracture.* Immediate mobilization has been shown to result in less pain and better elbow function at 1-week follow-up as compared to motion initiated 5 days following radial head fracture; although results were similar with respect to pain, ROM, and function at 4-week follow-up.[9] Non-displaced and minimally displaced radial head fractures treated non-operatively do not require as long of a period of protective immobilization as other elbow fractures and radial head fractures treated operatively. The use of a sling or orthosis for comfort during the first week is usually sufficient. Not all individuals with non-operatively managed radial head fractures require repeated therapy visits to achieve good results. However, to minimize the risk of elbow flexion contracture, it is important to provide a structured therapy program to individuals who are reluctant to move or who are stiff after several weeks of performing a home exercise program.

Some olecranon fractures with minimal or no displacement can be treated non-operatively. The elbow is immobilized full-time in a cast or orthosis at 60° to 90° of flexion and neutral forearm rotation for 1 to 2 weeks. Therapy should then be initiated to minimize the risk of elbow stiffness.

Most distal humeral fractures require operative treatment. However, some non-comminuted, stable fractures with minimal or no displacement can be treated with closed reduction followed by immobilization in a cast or orthosis. To minimize the risk of stiffness, gentle motion must be started after no more than

2 weeks of full-time mobilization. If the distal humerus is not stable enough to tolerate motion after this period of initial immobilization, it is best treated surgically to achieve the necessarily stability to allow early motion.[6] When treating a patient referred to you following surgery for a distal humerus fracture, initiate elbow motion exercises with passive or gravity-assisted extension and active flexion. Depending on the type of surgical exposure that was used, either the triceps mechanism or the olecranon osteotomy may require protection for the first 6 weeks or so. *Therefore, check with the surgeon before beginning active elbow extension and passive elbow flexion.*

♡ Tips from the Field

Orthoses

- You will usually fabricate a thermoplastic posterior elbow orthosis to provide protection and support to the recently fractured elbow. Braces, casts, and slings are sometimes used as alternatives to orthoses.
- Most isolated elbow fractures are immobilized with the elbow in 90° of flexion with the forearm in neutral rotation. Olecranon fractures that are managed non-operatively or have tenuous fracture fixation may require immobilization in more extension to minimize the pull of the triceps at its insertion on the olecranon.
- Instruct your patient to remove the orthosis several times daily for active motion exercises unless contraindicated due to instability. Daily removal of the orthosis for hygiene is usually permissible, although initially wearing it covered with a plastic bag or cast cover while showering or bathing offers greater protection.
- Even with optimal treatment, regaining full or at least functional motion following elbow fracture can be challenging. If your patient's elbow motion plateaus, fabricate or provide a static progressive or serial static orthosis once the fracture has healed sufficiently (see "The Stiff Elbow" section).

Motion Exercises

- Unless contraindicated, it is often most comfortable for your patient to begin elbow flexion and extension in supine with the upper arm supported on a pillow or folded towel alongside their torso. Progress to other gravity-assisted positions, such as elbow extension while seated and elbow flexion in supine with the shoulder flexed at 90°.
- Instruct your patient to gently support the involved UE with their uninvolved hand while performing gentle motion exercises to increase comfort and control.
- It is common to compensate for limited forearm ROM by leaning to the side or substituting shoulder motion. Minimize this by having your patient support the upper arm against their torso while they pronate and supinate the forearm. Maintaining erect posture may be easier initially if forearm rotation is performed bilaterally.
- Longer holds at end range are more effective for increasing motion than performing a greater number of fast repetitions.
- An early means of increasing motion is through active-assisted "place and hold" exercises in which the joint is placed at its end range position followed by an active holding of the position.
- Precondition soft tissues with moist heat to make active and passive motion exercises more comfortable and effective.

Strengthening Exercises

- When the physician determines that there has been sufficient fracture healing, begin strengthening with isometric exercises and progress to isotonic exercises. In addition to addressing strength deficits of triceps and the elbow flexors, also address any strength deficits of the shoulder girdle, shoulder, wrist, and hand.
- Be sure not to overlook triceps, which tend to be weak following elbow injury. An effective exercise for initiating activation and strengthening of the triceps is elbow extension in supine with the shoulder flexed at 90°.

◎ Clinical Pearl

Most individuals will be more comfortable if you include their wrist when you fabricate the protective orthosis. Make sure that they perform active wrist motion each time they remove the orthosis to prevent loss of wrist motion.

➢ Precautions and Concerns

- *Adhere to precautions related to your patient's fracture, surgery, and phase of healing, and be sure that your patient understands them. Don't sacrifice stability for the sake of mobility.*
- *Progress treatment based on the healing of your patient's fracture as determined by their referring physician and on their individual response to therapy.*
- *Passive motion and stretching should be performed slowly and gently. Forceful passive motion may damage rather than lengthen soft tissues.*
- *Be alert for symptoms of ulnar neuritis, such as numbness or tingling in the small finger and ulnar aspect of the ring finger, and if present, report them to the referring physician.*

Elbow Dislocation

Despite its inherent stability, the elbow is the second most commonly dislocated joint, following the shoulder. Mechanisms of injury include falling onto an outstretched hand, motor vehicle accidents, and direct trauma to the elbow. The direction of dislocation is almost always posterior. Severity ranges from **simple elbow dislocation,** joint displacement without associated fractures, to **complex elbow dislocation,** joint displacement with accompanying fracture or fractures. The most common complication of elbow dislocation (as of elbow fracture) is stiffness. While early motion is important for the optimal outcome, mobilization cannot begin without adequate elbow stability.

The approach used in managing an elbow dislocation depends on the structures damaged and the resulting degree of elbow stability. O'Driscoll's description of the sequential progression of soft tissue disruption occurring in simple elbow dislocation is widely cited.[10] Following a fall onto an outstretched hand in shoulder abduction, tissue disruption at the elbow occurs laterally to medially in three stages. The first stage is disruption of the lateral collateral ligament complex. This results in **posterolateral rotatory subluxation** in which the ulna externally rotates on the trochlea of the humerus, causing partial displacement of the ulnohumeral and radiohumeral joints. The subluxation is transient and resolves spontaneously when the elbow is flexed.

In the second stage, the anterior and posterior joint capsule is also disrupted resulting in incomplete posterolateral elbow dislocation. The third, most severe, stage of soft tissue disruption includes disruption of the medial collateral ligament complex in addition to soft tissues injured in the initial two stages. This results in complete posterior elbow dislocation. There are different considerations for managing elbow dislocations with associated fractures. Management of these complex elbow dislocations is discussed in the "Elbow Instability" section.

Timelines and Healing

Simple elbow dislocations of all stages, despite disruption to the joint capsule and ligaments, can usually be treated non-operatively. Most individuals can return to their previous activities within 8 to 12 weeks following injury. Outcomes for most simple dislocations are good with achievement of full or near-full motion, normal strength, and stability reported at 6 to 18 months. However, if immobilized for more than 3 weeks, contracture is a likely complication.[10]

Screening of the UE for associated injuries is essential following elbow dislocation. Fractures of the radial head, coronoid, and/or olecranon commonly accompany elbow dislocation. These complex elbow dislocations, in which both the bony and soft tissue stabilizers of the elbow are disrupted, are inherently unstable and require operative treatment.

Both simple and complex elbow dislocations carry the risk of neurovascular injuries. The ulnar nerve is most commonly affected. In addition, associated hand, wrist, and shoulder injuries may be present. Late complications of elbow dislocation include flexion contracture, heterotopic bone formation, arthrosis, and recurrent instability.

◎ Clinical Pearl

The ulnar nerve is susceptible to traction injury during elbow dislocation.

Non-Operative Treatment

Simple elbow dislocations can almost always be managed non-operatively with closed reduction followed initially with protective immobilization in flexion in an orthosis or sling. Despite disruption to the ligaments and capsule, if there are no associated fractures, active motion in the stable arc can usually be initiated within the first week of injury without compromising stability and healing. If there is residual instability, elbow extension is initially limited to the stable range and gradually increased as stability is regained through soft tissue healing.

Operative Treatment

Operative management of elbow dislocation is required when stability is inadequate to safely allow early active motion in a protected arc. Unstable dislocations usually have associated elbow fractures. Although uncommon, some simple elbow dislocations, although they do not have associated fractures, may also require surgery for restoration of stability. The operative and postoperative management of unstable elbow dislocations is discussed in the "Elbow Instability" section.

◎ Clinical Pearl

Fracture of the ulna associated with radial head dislocation is known as a **Monteggia fracture.** This injury requires operative management and careful progression in therapy due to its inherent instability.

? Questions to Discuss with the Physician

- Which structures were injured? Were there associated fractures or nerve injuries?
- What is the preferred type and position of immobilization?
- How stable is the elbow?
- What is the initial safe arc of elbow motion?
- Are there any other precautions?

As the Patient Progresses

- When can protective immobilization be discontinued?
- When can unrestricted motion and resistive exercises be initiated?

( ) What to Say to Clients

After a Simple Elbow Dislocation

"When you dislocated your elbow, you injured the ligaments and other soft tissues that support the joint. Your elbow needs to be protected from stresses that could prevent it from healing properly. This usually requires wearing a sling or orthosis for support for up to 3 weeks. Injured elbows have a tendency to quickly become stiff. So while your elbow is healing, it is also important to move it in a controlled way. I'm going to teach you specific motion exercises to prevent stiffness without putting stress on the structures you injured. After an injury like yours, most people have a good recovery and can go back to their usual activities within 2 or 3 months."

Evaluation Tips

- The evaluation tips listed for elbow fractures also apply for elbow dislocations.
- If there is residual elbow instability, do not measure ROM in a way that would compromise stability. For example, if the elbow is unstable in end range extension, delay assessment of extension beyond the prescribed range until the precaution is discontinued by the referring physician.

Diagnosis-Specific Information That Affects Clinical Reasoning

Simple elbow dislocations are usually stable following reduction. There may, however, be some residual instability in elbow extension. Complex elbow dislocations are inherently unstable due to disruption of both the bony and soft tissue stabilizers, requiring a different management approach than the one described in this section.

Orthoses

- For support and comfort following a simple elbow dislocation with minimal or no residual instability, the patient initially uses either a sling or a protective orthosis in 90° of flexion.
- The orthosis or sling is removed for controlled motion exercises beginning within the first week following a simple elbow dislocation. It is discontinued within 3 weeks after the injury.

Therapeutic Exercise

- With the exceptions that follow, the exercises for management of stable, simple elbow dislocation are similar to those for isolated elbow fractures.
- Active motion of the elbow and forearm is initially performed in supine with the upper arm supported next to the trunk on a pillow or folded towel. However if stability is a concern, initiate motion in the supine overhead position as described in the "Elbow Instability" section.
- Instruct your patient to avoid shoulder abduction with internal rotation for the first 3 weeks after injury or longer as this position places varus stress on the lateral collateral ligament complex.
- It may also be necessary to limit elbow extension to 30° for the first 2 or 3 weeks after injury in simple elbow dislocations with residual instability.
- Stretching and strengthening exercises can usually be safely initiated by 6 weeks following simple elbow dislocations.

- *Avoid combining end range elbow extension and supination for the first 6 weeks.*
- *If there is residual elbow instability, some individuals may be required to initially limit end range extension or to perform the supine overhead exercises described later.*
- *Once permitted, passive motion and stretching should be performed slowly and gently. Excessive force may contribute to the formation of heterotopic ossification, which is a common complication of elbow dislocation.*
- *Unstable, complex elbow dislocations have additional precautions and require different management strategies than simple elbow dislocations (see the "Elbow Instability" section).*

Elbow Instability

To function effectively the elbow must be stable as well as mobile. It is subject to varus (adduction) loads during many of our routine daily activities. Gravity imparts this varus load to the elbow as the UE is moved away from the body with the shoulder abducted and internally rotated. Varus forces stress the collateral lateral ligament complex, which are damaged in complex elbow dislocations and essential for elbow stability. **Varus instability,** or lateral collateral ligament insufficiency, usually results from elbow dislocation. It can range from gross instability following acute, complex dislocation to subtle, chronic **posterolateral rotatory instability** due to lateral ligamentous laxity. Posterolateral rotatory instability is recurrent posterolateral rotatory subluxation in which the ulna and radius rotate externally and displace relative to the humerus.

Valgus (abduction) loads on the elbow are far less common in routine daily life than varus loads. Valgus loads occur in activities that stress the medial elbow, such as overhead throwing. **Valgus instability,** or medial collateral ligament insufficiency, tends to be chronic in nature. Repetitive valgus stresses, such as those experienced by throwing athletes, can result in chronic instability.

Timelines and Healing

Before motion can begin following an acute, unstable elbow dislocation, stability must be surgically restored. This allows protected active motion in the stable arc to begin within the first week following surgery. When protected from damaging stresses, ligamentous injuries and fractures of the elbow heal sufficiently for strengthening to begin in approximately 6 to 8 weeks. Return to all previous activities is usually allowed after 4 to 6 months when normal strength has been recovered. Full recovery may take a year or more after severe injuries. Timelines for healing and progression of treatment following reconstruction for recurrent instability are similar to those following surgery for acute instability, but the outcomes are less predictable.

Even with the early initiation of motion, elbow stiffness is a common complication after complex elbow dislocation. *Stability must never be sacrificed in the attempt to gain motion.* If necessary, contracture release and/or excision of heterotopic bone can be performed to address motion deficits once the injured structures have fully healed (see "The Stiff Elbow" section).

Elbow dislocation with associated fractures of the radial head and coronoid is known as the **terrible triad of the elbow** because it is so challenging to treat. Although with optimal operative and postoperative management, most have good to excellent outcomes, stiffness, recurrent instability, and the need for secondary intervention are common complications.[11]

Isolated coronoid fractures are uncommon. They are usually associated with elbow dislocation.[12]

Non-Operative Treatment

Provision of safe and effective therapy for the unstable elbow requires an understanding of how to protect the injured structures while initiating early, protected motion to avoid stiffness. Treatment progression is dependent on the timing of both soft tissue and fracture healing, and it requires close communication with the referring physician. Standard edema and scar management techniques should be used as needed.

Therapy for the acute, unstable elbow typically begins postoperatively with fabrication of a thermoplastic orthosis in elbow flexion and pronation. As soon as stability permits, ideally within the first week following surgery, active motion is initiated in the limited arc of motion in which the elbow remains stable. The supine, overhead motion protocol, described in detail by Wolff and Hotchkiss,[13] allows early, protected motion while preserving elbow stability. Elbow and forearm motion are initially performed supine with the shoulder flexed at 90°. This position allows gravity

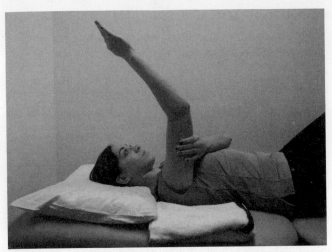

FIGURE 23-4 Supine, overhead elbow extension with the forearm pronated, initially limited to 30°.

to stabilize the elbow and also positions triceps so that it can act as a joint stabilizer. To protect elbow stability, supination and elbow extension should not be combined until the injured structures have healed for at least 8 weeks following surgery. Elbow extension, performed in pronation, should initially be limited to 30° or the stable end range (Fig. 23-4). Initiate active ROM of the shoulder girdle, shoulder, wrist, and digits immediately to preserve their motion, but note that *shoulder abduction with internal rotation must be strictly avoided because it places a significant varus stress on the damaged lateral collateral ligaments.*

Joint stability begins improving during the fibroplastic phase of soft tissue healing, 2 to 6 weeks following surgery. When stability permits, active elbow and forearm motion are progressed to positioning the upper arm next to the torso while sitting or standing. Combined elbow extension and supination must still be avoided. While gentle passive motion can be initiated, avoid both end range elbow extension and forearm supination. Add gentle strengthening exercises for the wrist and grip.

Motion precautions can be discontinued and progressive strengthening initiated during the scar maturation phase, 8 to 12 weeks following surgery, once stability has been regained.

Operative Treatment

Acute elbow dislocation with fractures of the radial head, coronoid, and/or olecranon is the most common origin of lateral elbow instability. To restore elbow stability following these complex dislocations, the fractures are repaired with open reduction and internal fixation. When associated with dislocation, radial head fractures that are too severe to be repaired are replaced rather than excised to prevent chronic instability. In addition to addressing the fractures, the lateral collateral ligament complex must be repaired due to its critical role in elbow stability and the ubiquity of varus loads in daily activities. The medial collateral ligament complex does not routinely require repair unless the elbow remains unstable following fracture fixation and repair of the lateral collateral ligaments. If the elbow remains unstable despite these procedures, a **hinged external fixator** can be placed in the distal humerus and proximal ulna for approximately 6 to 8 weeks to maintain joint reduction while allowing early elbow motion.

Chronic lateral elbow instability, although uncommon, may be a late complication of elbow trauma. More rarely, it is a complication of overuse or of iatrogenic injury following surgical treatment of lateral epicondylitis, other surgeries to the lateral elbow, or multiple steroid injections. Individuals with this condition report lateral elbow pain and clicking, catching or locking most frequently in elbow extension and supination against resistance. On examination, it may present as a subtle posterolateral rotatory elbow instability in which the ulna and radius rotate externally relative to the humerus causing a transient posterior subluxation. The operative treatment is reconstruction of lateral ligamentous support with a free tendon graft, most commonly palmaris longus. Hinged external fixation may also be necessary when the treatment of a complex elbow dislocation has been delayed or has failed to restore stability. The hinged external fixator, inserted in the proximal ulna and distal humerus, provides varus and valgus stability while allowing elbow flexion and extension.

For chronic medial instability that does not sufficiently resolve with non-operative management, a free tendon graft, most commonly palmaris longus, is used for reconstruction of medial ligamentous support.

? Questions to Discuss with the Physician

- Which structures were injured? Were there associated fractures or nerve injuries?
- Was surgery performed, and if so, what was done? Ask for the operative notes.
- What is the preferred position of immobilization?
- How stable is the elbow?
- What is the initial safe arc of elbow motion? Should motion be initially performed in the supine overhead motion position or can it be safely performed with the upper arm next to the trunk?
- Are there any other precautions?

As the Patient Progresses

- When can protective immobilization be discontinued?
- When can unrestricted motion and resistive exercises be initiated?

( ) What to Say to Clients

About the Condition

"To function properly, your elbow needs to be both flexible and stable. Stability is provided by the bones that make up the elbow joint and the ligaments and other soft tissues that surround it. Because you injured these structures, your elbow has lost stability. It is important to protect these healing structures so that your elbow regains stability."

About the Supine, Overhead Motion Exercises

"I'm going to teach you motion exercises to prevent your elbow from becoming too stiff. As long as you do them correctly, the healing structures in your elbow will be protected. Perform the exercises lying on your back with your upper arm and elbow pointing directly up to the ceiling. Use your other hand to support your injured arm. The specific exercises are forearm rotation with your elbow bent, and elbow bending and straightening with your forearm rotated so that your palm faces toward the ceiling. I'll show you how to do them correctly and how far you can safely straighten your elbow at this time."

- The evaluation tips listed for elbow fractures also apply for unstable elbows.
- If there is residual elbow instability, do not measure ROM in a way that would compromise stability. For example, if elbow and forearm motion must initially be performed in the overhead supine position, perform the motion measurements with the UE in this position, noting it in your documentation.

Diagnosis-Specific Information That Affects Clinical Reasoning

The safest forearm position for immobilization and motion depends on which ligaments were injured and require protection. Pronation with elbow flexion has been demonstrated to stabilize elbows with insufficient lateral collateral ligament support and resultant instability.[14] Therefore, the pronated position is recommended for orthoses and motion activities for unstable elbows with lateral collateral ligament disruption. In contrast, elbows with medial collateral ligament damage are more stable in supination. When both the medial and lateral collateral ligaments require protection, neutral forearm rotation with flexion is preferable.

Elbow instability almost always requires operative treatment. The exception is chronic medial instability as seen in overhead throwing athletes. If treated early, this condition can be managed non-operatively with a period of rest from provoking activities and anti-inflammatory medication and modalities. This should be followed with a strengthening program for the UE muscles including the flexor-pronator muscles to improve their dynamic support of the medial aspect of the elbow.[15,16]

Tips from the Field

Orthoses
- The protective thermoplastic orthosis is fabricated in the position of greatest stability. Because joint reduction and stability is greatest in elbow flexion, the elbow is immobilized in at least 90° of flexion. In many cases, 120° or more of elbow flexion is preferred. Positioning in full pronation protects the lateral collateral ligaments. However, if a medial collateral ligament repair was performed in addition to lateral collateral ligament repair, neutral forearm rotation is indicated. As alternative to an orthosis, a hinged brace with an extension stop may be ordered.
- When the injured structures have healed and the elbow is stable, approximately 8 weeks after surgery, static progressive orthoses may be necessary to address remaining motion limitations. For individuals making poor progress with elbow extension, use of a serial static night extension orthosis may be initiated 4 to 6 weeks postoperatively if stability permits (see "The Stiff Elbow" section). Discuss the timing for safely introducing these orthoses with the referring physician.

Supine, Overhead Motion Exercises
- During the supine, overhead exercises for unstable elbows, the shoulder should be maintained at 90° of flexion and not be allowed to abduct.

- Elbow flexion and extension are performed in full pronation. Full flexion is allowed. In most cases extension should initially be limited to 30° (see Fig. 23-4) and then gradually progressed when stability has improved.
- Forearm rotation is performed with the elbow flexed at 90°. Full pronation and supination, within tolerance, are allowed.

Hinged External Fixation
- If a hinged external fixator has been used to stabilize the elbow, it is unlocked for active elbow and forearm motion exercises. Because of the stability provided by the device, exercising in the supine position is not required. In the locked position the fixator is used for passive elbow flexion and extension. Rather than performing multiple repetitions, the elbow is gradually positioned and held for several hours at comfortable end range flexion and extension.
- Following the removal of the fixator 3 to 6 weeks postoperatively, loss of motion is common. Prompt use of static progressive or serial static orthoses is essential to maintain/gain end range elbow motion.

Clinical Pearl

Some individuals require several therapy sessions to learn to perform the supine, overhead elbow exercises correctly. The exercises should not be performed as a home program until they can be performed as instructed.

Precautions and Concerns

- *Do not combine elbow extension with supination for at least 8 weeks.*
- *Protect lateral collateral ligaments repairs from varus stresses by instructing your patient to avoid shoulder abduction with internal rotation for at least 12 weeks. The shoulder should not be allowed to abduct and internally rotate during removal of the protective orthosis and performance of supine, overhead motion exercises.*
- *Be alert for ulnar nerve symptoms and report them to the referring physician.*

The Stiff Elbow

Elbow stiffness is so common that therapists treating individuals with UE disorders will inevitably face this challenge. Elbow stiffness is a frequent complication of elbow dislocation, elbow fracture, head injury, and burns. The more severe the trauma and the longer the period of immobilization, the more likely is the loss of elbow motion. Elbow flexion contracture is particularly common.

Multiple factors contribute to the propensity of the elbow to become stiff following injury. Because the elbow is a highly congruent joint, it is not tolerant of disruption of the articular surfaces. There is a tendency for formation of heterotopic ossification in the surrounding soft tissues, such as the medial and lateral collateral ligaments and joint capsule. The thin anterior joint capsule of the elbow is particularly susceptible to injury and **hypertrophy**. The muscle belly of brachialis lies directly over the anterior capsule. Bleeding in brachialis associated with elbow injury can cause it to scar and adhere to the capsule and can contribute to formation of bone in the muscle. Muscle guarding, adaptive soft tissue shortening, and scarring can also contribute to loss of elbow motion, particularly extension.

> ### ◎ Clinical Pearl
>
> Following injury, the elbow tends to posture at 70° to 80° of elbow flexion, which is the open packed position in which the joint capsule is most lax. Prolonged immobilization in this position of comfort can contribute to the development of an elbow flexion contracture, which is a common complication of elbow trauma.

There are a number of structures lying within and outside of the elbow joint that can limit motion. Elbow stiffness of relatively short duration with extra-articular causes, such as soft tissue shortening and muscle **cocontraction,** can usually be managed non-operatively. However, if motion is not regained after optimal non-operative management, surgical contracture release may be necessary. Heterotopic ossification and intra-articular sources of elbow stiffness, such as joint incongruity, deformity, and impinging hardware from previous surgery, are indications for operative management.

Timelines and Healing

Recovery of a functional ROM following elbow trauma is often challenging even with good management. If a significant contracture persists beyond 6 months in an individual who has received appropriate therapy including orthoses to increase motion, a contracture release may be required. Without surgical intervention, significant improvement is unlikely after 6 months of non-operative management, and heterotopic ossification, if present, will have matured sufficiently by this time to be safely removed.[17]

Following elbow contracture release, the importance of therapy cannot be overemphasized. Positive outcomes depend on the coordinated and concerted efforts of the injured individual, therapist and surgeon. Individuals unwilling or unable to actively participate in an extensive postoperative therapy program are not good candidates for this procedure. It is not unusual for therapy to be required for 3 months following this surgery.

While most individuals make significant gains in motion following elbow contracture release, complications including recurrent stiffness are not rare. In a study of 52 individuals treated for post-traumatic elbow stiffness with open contracture release and therapy including static progressive orthoses, the average arc of elbow motion was found to increase by 59° at 18.7 months average follow up. However, 27% of the individuals required follow up with closed manipulation to address acute recurrence of stiffness with 5 of them ultimately requiring a second contracture release.[18] In addition to recurrent stiffness, other complications of open contracture release include instability, infection, and ulnar neuropathy.

Non-Operative Treatment

The same techniques for increasing elbow motion are useful for the prevention and treatment of elbow stiffness in non-operatively and operatively managed elbow injuries. Treatment progression following elbow injury must always reflect the phase of soft tissue healing and degree of joint stability. If stiffness is due to elbow fracture, progression may need to be slower since the phase of bony healing must also be considered.

In the initial, inflammatory phase of healing, effectively controlling edema and pain is crucial for preventing or minimizing stiffness. Edema management techniques include elevation, cold modalities, light compression, active digital motion, and manual edema mobilization techniques. Active motion of the uninvolved joints should be initiated early, and gentle active elbow and forearm motion initiated as soon as healing and stability permits. Passive motion should always be performed slowly and gently to avoid provoking involuntary muscle guarding and damaging healing tissues.

A variety of techniques for increasing motion are useful during the fibroplastic and scar maturation phases of soft tissue healing. *Avoid aggressive approaches, such as forceful stretching, that may provoke inflammation, damage healing tissues, and increase* **fibrosis** *and stiffness.* Superficial heat prepares soft tissues for motion and is most effective for increasing motion when applied with the elbow positioned at end range. Ultrasound, used for deeper heating, should be combined or followed with end range motion. There are a variety of useful manual techniques for increasing motion including gentle stretching, soft tissue mobilization, joint mobilization, and proprioceptive neurofacilitation techniques, such as contract-relax and hold-relax. Follow the techniques and exercises used to increase passive motion with active motion and functional activities that focus on use of the full available range. Strengthening exercises, which are initiated during the scar maturation phase, should emphasize the end ranges of motion. Triceps tend to be weaker than the elbow flexors and require greater attention in functional activities and strengthening exercises.

Serial static elbow orthoses, which are molded with the joint at end range and remolded as motion improves, are generally well tolerated early in the soft tissue healing process. Use of static progressive orthoses is ideally initiated during the fibroplastic phase and is also effective during the scar maturation phase. Static progressive orthoses have been demonstrated to be effective for increasing motion in elbows that are stiff following trauma.[19]

Operative Treatment

Elbow contracture release is usually performed as an open procedure through a medial and/or lateral approach. The structures limiting motion are identified and excised. These may include the anterior and posterior joint capsule, **osteophytes,** scarring within the coronoid and olecranon fossas, scarring around the radial head and capitellum, the tip of the olecranon, heterotopic ossification, and hardware from previous surgery. While some parts of the medial collateral ligament complex can be excised without compromising joint stability, the lateral collateral ligaments are preserved whenever possible. The ulnar nerve is often released from scar tissue and heterotopic ossification and transposed to an anterior position to minimize the risk of postoperative irritation.

If there is substantial articular damage, an **interposition arthroplasty,** which is the insertion of soft tissue between the joint surfaces, may be performed. In cases in which the elbow is unstable following contracture release or when distraction is required to protect soft tissue placed between the joint surfaces, a hinged external fixator is applied for approximately 6 to 8 weeks. This device allows maximum gains in motion to be made while stability is regained through soft tissue healing.

Therapy is essential following elbow contracture release and is typically initiated the day following surgery. The primary goal of therapy is postoperative motion equal to that obtained in the operating room.

? Questions to Discuss with the Physician

- What structures were addressed surgically? Ask for the operative notes.
- How much motion was obtained intra-operatively?
- Is the elbow stable postoperatively?
- Was an ulnar nerve transposition performed?

( ) What to Say to Clients

After Contracture Release

"Your surgeon released the structures that were keeping your elbow from moving freely. Right after your surgery your elbow was able to move this far (demonstrate patient's intra-operative ROM). Swelling and the gradual formation of scar tissue tend to make your elbow become stiff again. To keep that from happening, it is very important that you come to your therapy sessions and follow your home program. Some swelling is normal but to keep it to a minimum, elevate your arm and apply ice or cold packs as we have discussed. To get the most motion, your elbow will need a lot of your attention for the next several months. Think of doing your exercises and wearing your orthosis (or orthoses) as a full-time job."

About Static Progressive Orthoses

"The purpose of your orthosis is to gradually improve your elbow motion. When you put the orthosis on, adjust it to hold your elbow as straight (or bent) as possible but only to the point that it does not cause pain. After you've had the orthosis on for a while, try to readjust it for more of a stretch. The orthosis works by applying gentle force over long period of time. Using it for a brief, intense stretch will not be as effective. After you take the orthosis off, do your exercises to straighten and bend your elbow as far you can."

Evaluation Tips

- Unless the elbow is unstable following contracture release, it is generally permissible to begin measuring passive and active motion at the first visit.
- While early assessment of strength is not prohibited unless there is postoperative instability, initially pain will be more limiting than weakness. Delay manual muscle testing until after the inflammatory phase when it will be better tolerated.

Diagnosis-Specific Information That Affects Clinical Reasoning

- Biceps brachii and the other elbow flexors have a tendency to co-contract when the injured elbow is extended or positioned

in extension.[20] This involuntary muscle guarding is a common source of limited elbow motion that when not addressed early can contribute to persistent stiffness. Placing a weight on the wrist or in the hand to stretch the elbow into extension is counterproductive if it causes the flexors to contract. While performing passive motion, stretching, and other techniques to increase elbow extension, manually monitor the elbow flexors to make sure they stay relaxed. Avoid rapid and forceful movements. If flexor co-contraction is persistent, biofeedback is a useful tool for increasing awareness and reestablishing normal firing patterns.

- Elbow stiffness that worsens or fails to improve 2 or 3 weeks following contracture release has variable causes and should be reported to the referring physician. Hotchkiss[17] has described a common source of the recurrence of elbow stiffness, usually limited flexion, during this period as "gelling." The usual cause of the loss of flexion gains made in the operating room appears to be pain in the distal triceps against the surface of the posterior humerus. Gentle manipulation under anesthesia is used to restore motion and must be followed immediately with therapy, including orthoses to maintain gains in end range motion.

◎ Clinical Pearl

Motion loss beginning 2 or 3 weeks following elbow contracture release can be an indication of a recurrence of heterotopic ossification. Localized tenderness, swelling, erythema, and warmth are early signs and symptoms of this condition. While postoperative inflammation has a similar appearance, it has usually diminished by this time.[21]

♡ Tips from the Field

End Range Positioning with Thermal Modalities

While using moist heat to precondition soft tissues prior to other treatments, position the elbow at or near its end range of flexion or extension. When using a cold pack at the end of a therapy session, end range positioning can help maintain gains made during the session.

Orthoses

- Orthoses that position the elbow at end range are essential in the treatment of stiffness. Use a custom-made or prefabricated static progressive flexion orthosis to address limited flexion (Fig. 23-5). For a mild limitation of extension, a static orthosis molded at end range and serially remolded as extension improves, can be used (Fig. 23-6). For extension limited by more than 30°, static progressive extension orthoses (Fig. 23-7) are more effective.[22] Wearing schedules vary and depend on individual progress and tolerance to orthotic wear. In general, the more severe the stiffness and limitation into a particular end range, the more time that the elbow will need to be positioned at that end range. It has been demonstrated in stiff joints that the greater the total end range time, the greater the improvement in motion.[23-25] However, always consider individual response to therapy and tissue tolerance to orthotic wear. Extension orthoses are generally better tolerated than flexion orthoses and are therefore commonly worn while sleeping at night. If an ulnar nerve transposition was not performed, carefully monitor for signs and symptoms of ulnar neuritis.

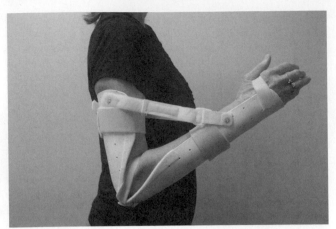

FIGURE 23-5 Static progressive elbow flexion orthosis.

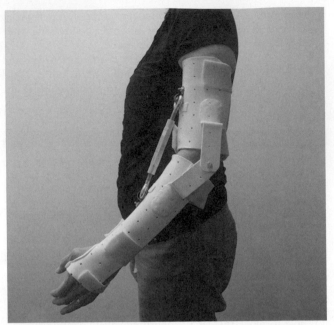

FIGURE 23-7 Static progressive elbow extension orthosis.

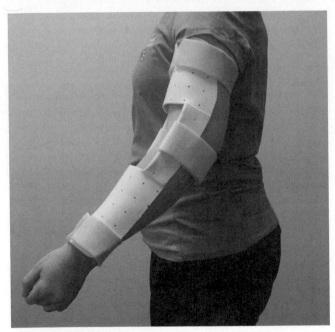

FIGURE 23-6 Serial static elbow extension orthosis.

If they occur, inform the referring physician and limit wearing time for flexion orthoses.
- It may be necessary to use a serial static or static progressive forearm supination orthosis or, less commonly, a pronation orthosis to assist in restoration of limited forearm motion that is not improving with other therapeutic interventions, such as active and passive mobilization techniques.

Therapeutic Exercise

Instruct your patient to follow each session of serial static or static progressive orthotic use with active motion exercises and light functional exercises that focus on end ranges. Doing so will help maintain passive gains made through orthotic wear and will encourage active use of the elbow through the full available range.

Therapy Considerations Following Elbow Contracture Release

Continuous Passive Motion

The effectiveness of continuous passive motion (CPM) machines in the postoperative treatment of elbow contracture release is questionable with research demonstrating mixed results.[26,27] Hotchkiss[17] has described the use of the CPM machine during the first few weeks following contracture release as a slow, intermittent passive positioning device. He advocates its use to position the elbow in end range flexion and extension alternating 20 to 30 minutes in each direction.

Orthoses: A static extension orthosis should be fabricated within the first day or two following surgery. It should be worn at night and intermittently during the day. Use of static progressive orthoses for extension and flexion, if necessary, can be initiated as early as the first week following surgery.

Hinged External Fixation

Therapy follows a different course if a hinged external fixator is applied during surgery. Instruct your patient in using the device to gradually passively position the elbow at end-range flexion and extension. Initially, flexion and extension may be alternated daily. Within a few days they can be alternated several times each day. Within the first week following surgery, instruct your patient to unlock the hinge for active ROM exercises and light functional activities with a focus on end ranges of motion.

> ◎ **Clinical Pearl**
>
> To capitalize on motion gains made during a therapy session, ask your patient to apply their orthosis positioned at the new end range when the session concludes.

> ◎ **Clinical Pearl**
>
> Following the removal of a hinged external fixator that was used to treat an elbow contracture, the immediate use of static progressive orthoses is critical to minimize loss of motion gained while using the fixator.

- *Avoid prolonged positioning of the elbow at comfortable mid-ranges.*
- *Do not use an orthosis to apply a strong or painful force to the elbow in an attempt to gain motion. Instead, use the orthosis to position the joint at end range. Gradually progress the end range by applying a load low provided over a prolonged period. Improvements are typically gradual and with continued orthotic use may continue over a period of 6 to 12 months.[28]*
- *The forces applied by the spring or elastic components of dynamic orthoses are not as controlled as those applied by serial static and static progressive orthoses. Therefore, although dynamic orthoses may be as effective for improving elbow motion, they are not always well tolerated.[28]*
- *Do not use excessive or uncontrolled force when performing passive motion, stretching, and other mobilization techniques. Forceful attempts to increase elbow motion can inflame or damage healing tissues. Gentle passive motion and orthoses used for end range prolonged positioning are effective tools for coaxing more motion from a stiff elbow. Despite the historical belief that passive motion and orthoses can cause or exacerbate heterotopic ossification around the elbow, there is no evidence that this is the case when applied in a controlled manner.[21]*
- *Be alert for signs and symptoms of ulnar neuritis. Potential causes include irritation related to injury or surgery, repetitive or prolonged stretch of the nerve during flexion activities, and flexion orthotic wear if an anterior ulnar nerve transposition was not performed. Later onset of ulnar neuritis can be caused by compression of the nerve by heterotopic ossification.*
- *Monitor the skin over the tip of the olecranon, where the thin soft tissue that covers it is placed under tension during flexion. The potential for delayed wound healing or necrosis is more of a concern following release of long-standing contractures.*

CASE STUDIES

CASE STUDY 23-1 ■

R.M. is a 45-year-old, right-dominant male who works as an information technologist. His only prior medical history is hypertension controlled with medication. He sustained a right posterior elbow dislocation in a fall from a 3-foot high wall onto his outstretched hand. His elbow was relocated and subsequently immobilized in the local emergency room. Two days later R.M. was seen by an orthopedic surgeon who referred him to therapy for non-operative management with a protective orthosis and protected supine overhead motion with extension initially limited to 30°. The surgeon reported that there were no associated fractures or neurovascular injuries, but due to disruption of the collateral ligaments, the elbow was unstable in full extension.

R.M. came to therapy following his visit to the surgeon. He reported 7 out of 10 elbow pain at rest. There was moderate localized edema in his elbow. His sensation was intact. I fabricated R.M. a posterior elbow orthosis in 120° of flexion and full pronation for maximum elbow stability for him to wear. R.M. was unwilling to begin moving his elbow at this time. I reassured him that I would teach him only exercises that were safe for his elbow. I encouraged him to perform active motion of his digits and to intermittently apply ice or cold packs. I explained the precaution of avoiding shoulder abduction with internal rotation. He agreed to return the following day to begin protected elbow and forearm motion exercises.

The following day R.M. appeared less fearful, had less pain, and was willing to fully participate in therapy. I reviewed his precautions and emphasized that he should perform only the exercises instructed, avoiding full elbow extension and combined elbow extension and pronation. The orthosis was to be worn continuously except during his home exercise program, which was to be done four times a day. I taught him protected supine, overhead motion exercises, which were active-assisted elbow flexion and extension to maximum of 30° in full pronation and supination and pronation in elbow flexion. I also instructed him in active motion of his digits and wrist. At this time R.M. had 70° of active pronation, 60° of active supination, 95° of active elbow flexion, 40° of active-assisted elbow extension, and normal active motion of his wrist, digits, and shoulder into flexion. His DASH score was 80.

After 3 weeks of attending therapy and performing the supine overhead exercise program, R.M.'s active motion had improved to full pronation, 70° of supination, 120° of flexion, and 30° of extension. His pain and edema were well controlled with superficial heat and cold modalities. He followed up with the referring surgeon who cleared him for motion exercises, including unlimited extension with his upper arm next to his trunk. The orthosis was now required only for protection while sleeping or going outside. R.M. returned to work and continued attending therapy twice weekly. I instructed him in forearm and elbow motion exercises standing upright next to a wall with a towel roll behind his upper arm to prevent substituting with shoulder motion. I explained that he should continue to avoid shoulder abduction with internal rotation and end range elbow extension in supination. I instructed him in gentle isometric elbow flexion and extension with his elbow flexed at 90°. At 4 weeks he began using the UE ergometer with minimal resistance. After 6 weeks of therapy, his active motion had improved to 15° of elbow extension and full pronation, supination, and elbow flexion. At this time he returned to the referring surgeon who cleared him for progressive resistance exercises and discontinued the orthosis. After an additional 3 weeks of therapy of motion and progressive resistance exercises, R.M. had near normal strength throughout his UE and normal UE motion with the exception of 10° of elbow extension. He returned to his prior functional activities and had a final DASH score of 20. I discharged R.M. from therapy with an independent home exercise program focused on UE strengthening.

CASE STUDY 23-2 ■

A.L. is a 28-year-old, right-dominant, healthy female childcare worker. She came to the surgeon with a chief complaint of a stiff right elbow. Eight months earlier, she had sustained a right olecranon fracture resulting from a fall directly onto the elbow. The fracture was treated 3 days after the injury with open reduction and internal fixation (ORIF). She had attended therapy twice a week for 10 weeks, performed her home exercises regularly, and continued to wear a static progressive extension orthosis at night. Despite appropriate treatment, she had a persistent elbow flexion contracture of 40°. Her flexion had gradually worsened and was now limited to 120°. Her active forearm motion was within normal limits, her forearm and elbow strength good to normal within the available range, and her sensation intact. She reported that limited elbow motion made it difficult to perform her job duties and that she was strongly motivated to participate in whatever intervention was required to improve her elbow motion.

An open contracture release was performed on A.L.'s right elbow. The procedures included anterior and posterior capsulectomies, excision of soft tissue from the olecranon and coronoid fossas, excision of the tip of the olecranon, removal of hardware from the previous surgery, and decompression and anterior transposition of the ulnar nerve. Following surgery while still under anesthesia, her elbow was stable and had a passive range of 10° to 135°.

A.L. received inpatient therapy for 2 days following surgery prior to discharge home. Her pain was well controlled by the postoperative pain management team. Edema was managed with elevation, light compression wraps and intermittent use of ice. On postoperative day 1, a therapist instructed A.L. in active motion exercises for her digits, wrist, and shoulder, and both active and gentle passive motion exercises for her elbow and forearm. The therapist fabricated a custom-molded static elbow extension orthosis at 15°, which was A.L.'s maximum passive elbow extension at that time. A.L. began using a CPM machine for 6 hours a day, alternating 20 minute holds in end range flexion and extension and letting the machine cycle for brief periods in between. While hospitalized, she wore the extension orthosis when sleeping and whenever she wasn't performing motion exercises or using the CPM machine. At discharge, she was instructed to continue ice application, elevation, motion exercises, CPM machine use, and the extension orthosis at night.

At her first outpatient session, which was 5 days following the contracture release, A.L. reported that her elbow was still stiff and that she had constant, localized pain, ranging from 4 to 7 on a scale of 10. She reported that she was using the CPM machine at home for 2 hours, three times a day, alternating 20 minute holds at end range flexion and extension; she was wearing the extension orthosis at night; and she was performing motion exercises as instructed while in the hospital. She had not been consistent with elevation. On examination, A.G. had an intact surgical incision with no drainage, moderate edema at the elbow, minimal edema in her hand, and normal findings on neurological screening. Her DASH score was 75. Her elbow motion was 30° to 115° actively and 20° to 120° passively. Active pronation was normal, and supination was 10° less than on the left side. ROM of the uninvolved joints was within normal limits. Strength tested was deferred due to pain and recent surgery.

A.L. attended therapy two times a week. During the first week, we focused on edema and pain control with elevation, light compression wraps, intermittent use of ice and cold packs, and active digit motion. I also educated A.L. in the correct performance of active and active-assisted "place and hold" elbow and forearm exercises, emphasizing that she take the time necessary to reach maximum end ranges rather than simply going through the exercises to get them done. Initially, to minimize biceps brachii co-contraction, I instructed A.L. to perform her exercises slowly while lying in supine with the upper arm supported next to her trunk on a towel roll.

Two weeks following surgery, A.L.'s pain had decreased, her forearm motion was within normal limits, and her elbow extension had improved to 25° actively and 15° passively. Her elbow flexion had not improved, so I fabricated a static progressive flexion orthosis and instructed A.L. to wear it for a minimum of 2 hours a day with her elbow flexed to the point of a mild stretch but no increase in pain. By the next session her elbow motion was 120° actively and 125° passively, which was an increase of 5°. Home use of the CPM machine was discontinued, and the importance of continuing use of the flexion and extension orthoses was emphasized. At the start of each therapy session, I applied moist heat with her elbow positioned in either extension or flexion, and I used soft tissue and joint mobilization and other manual techniques, such as hold-relax and a contract-relax, to decrease muscle guarding and increase passive motion. I encouraged A.L. to use her right UE for light functional activities and incorporated reaching activities into her therapy sessions. Active elbow extension in supine with the shoulder flexed to 90° and reaching activities were used to target triceps and improve active extension. Overhead pulleys, which later progressed to an upper body ergometer (UBE) with minimal resistance, were used for repetitive elbow motion through the gradually increasing available range. When I applied cold packs to her elbow following treatment, I positioned it in comfortable extension. When A.L.'s surgical incision was fully healed, I instructed her in scar mobilization and the use of a silicone product to minimize scarring.

From 6 to 12 weeks following the contracture release, during the scar maturation phase, the A.L.'s elbow motion and function continued to gradually improve, and her pain became mild and less frequent. At 8 weeks, I remolded the extension orthosis to 10°, which was her current passive end range. In addition to the treatment techniques initiated in the fibroplastic phase, I added resistance exercises with a focus on performing them through the full range of motion and on isolating triceps. Twelve weeks after surgery, A.L. had active elbow motion from 10° to 135°, which was equal to her intra-operative motion; she was functionally independent and had good to normal strength throughout her right-dominant UE. She had successfully returned to work the previous week. Her DASH score had improved to 15. After discussing the plan with A.L. and her referring physician, I discharged her from therapy with instructions to continue wearing her orthoses and performing her home exercise program for another 2 to 3 months.

References

1. Morrey BF, Askew LJ, Chao EY: A biomechanical study of normal functional elbow motion, *J Bone Joint Surg Am* 63(6):872–877, 1981.

2. Beals RK: The normal carrying angle of the elbow: a radiographic study of 422 patients, *Clin Orthop Relat Res* 119:194–196, 1976.

3. Robinson CM, Hill RM, Jacobs N, et al: Adult distal humeral metaphyseal fractures: epidemiology and results of treatment, *J Orthop Trauma* 17(1):38–47, 2003.

4. van Reit RP, Morrey BF, O'Driscoll SW, et al: Associated injuries complicating radial head fractures: a demographic study, *Clin Orthop Relat Res* 441:351–355, 2005.

5. Karlsson MK, Hasserius R, Karlsson C, et al: Fractures of the olecranon: a 15- to 25-year followup of 73 patients, *Clin Orthop Relat Res* 403:205–212, 2002.

6. Beredjiklian PK: Management of fractures and dislocations of the elbow. In Fedorczyk JM, Amadio PC, editors: *Rehabilitation of the hand and upper extremity*, ed 6, Philadelphia, 2011, Elsevier Mosby.

7. Coles CP, Barei DP, Nork SE, et al: The olecranon osteotomy: a six-year experience in the treatment of intraarticular fractures of the distal humerus, *J Orthop Trauma* 20(3):164–171, 2006.

8. Ring D, Jupiter JB: Fractures of the distal humerus, *Orthop Clin North Am* 31(1):103–113, 2000.

9. Liow RY, Cregan A, Nanda R, et al: Early mobilization for minimally displaced radial head fractures is desirable: a prospective randomized study of two protocols, *Injury* 33(9):801–806, 2002.

10. O'Driscoll SW: Elbow dislocations. In Morrey BF, Sanchez-Sotelo J, editors: *The elbow and its disorders*, ed 4, Philadelphia, 2009, Saunders Elsevier.

11. Pugh DM, Wild LM, Schemitsch EH, et al: Standard surgical protocol to treat elbow dislocations with radial head and coronoid fractures, *J Bone Joint Surg Am* 86(6):1122–1130, 2004.

12. Regan WD, Morrey BF: Coronoid process and Monteggia fractures. In Morrey BF, Sanchez-Sotelo J, editors: *The elbow and its disorders*, ed 4, Philadelphia, 2009, Saunders Elsevier.

13. Wolff AL, Hotchkiss RN: Lateral elbow instability: nonoperative, operative, and postoperative management, *J Hand Ther* 19(2):238–243, 2006.

14. Dunning CE, Zarzour ZD, Patterson SD, et al: Muscle force and pronation stabilize the lateral ligament deficient elbow, *Clin Orthop Relat Res* 388: 118–124, 2001.

15. Cohen MS: Elbow instability: surgeon's management. In Fedorczyk JM, Amadio PC, editors: *Rehabilitation of the hand and upper extremity*, ed 6, Philadelphia, 2011, Elsevier Mosby.

16. Park MC, Ahmad CS: Dynamic contributions of the flexor-pronator mass to elbow valgus stability, *J Bone Joint Surg Am* 86(10):2268–2274, 2004.

17. Hotchkiss RN: Treatment of the stiff elbow. In Wolfe SW, Hotchkiss RN, Pederson WC, Kozin SH, editors: *Operative hand surgery*, ed 6, Philadelphia, 2011, Elsevier Churchill Livingstone.

18. Tan V, Daluiski A, Simic P, et al: Outcome of open release for post-traumatic stiffness, *J Trauma* 61(3):673–678, 2006.

19. Doornberg JN, Ring D, Jupiter JB: Static progressive splinting for post-traumatic stiffness, *J Orthop Trauma* 20(6):400–404, 2006.

20. Page C, Backus SI, Lenhoff MW: Electromyographic activity in stiff and normal elbows during elbow flexion and extension, *J Hand Ther* 16(1):5–11, 2003.

21. Casavant AM, Hastings H 2nd: Heterotopic ossification about the elbow: a therapist's guide to evaluation and management, *J Hand Ther* 19(2):255–266, 2006.

22. Chinchalkar SJ, Pearce J, Athwal GS: Static progressive versus three-point elbow extension splinting: a mathematical analysis, *J Hand Ther* 22(1):37–41, 2009.

23. Flowers KR, LaStayo P: Effect of total end range time on improving passive range of motion, *J Hand Ther* 7(3):150–157, 1994.

24. Glasgow C, Wilton J, Tooth L: Optimal daily total end range time for contracture: resolution in hand splinting, *J Hand Ther* 16(3):207–218, 2003.

25. Glasgow C, Fleming J, Tooth LR, et al: The long-term relationship between duration of treatment and contracture resolution using dynamic orthotic devices for the stiff proximal interphalangeal joint: a prospective cohort study, *J Hand Ther* 25(1):38–46, 2012.

26. Lindenhovius AL, van de Liujtgaarden K, Ring D, et al: Open elbow contracture release: postoperative management with and without continuous passive motion, *J Hand Surg Am* 34(5):858–865, 2009.

27. Higgs ZC, Danks BA, Sibinski M, et al: Outcomes of open arthrolysis of the elbow without post-operative passive stretching, *J Bone Joint Surg Br* 94(3):348–352, 2012.

28. Lindenhovius AL, Doornberg JN, Brouwer KM, et al: A prospective randomized controlled trial of dynamic versus static progressive elbow splinting for posttraumatic elbow stiffness, *J Bone Joint Surg Am* 94(8):694–700, 2012.

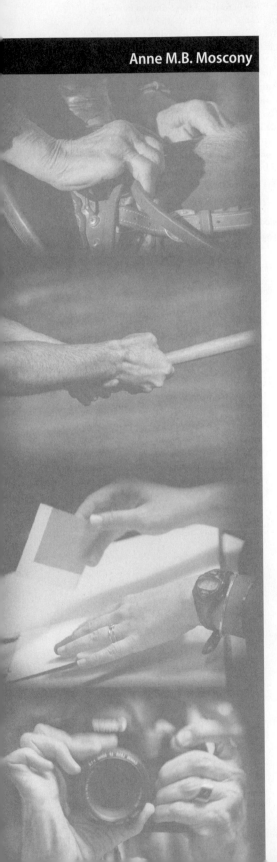

24

Peripheral Nerve Problems

Anne M.B. Moscony

Introduction

Functional recovery from a peripheral nerve injury requires the cooperative efforts of the physician, therapist, and client. The potentially grave consequences of these injuries are well known to surgeons and therapists but may not be obvious to our patients. For example, loss of sensation in the hand can result in difficulties performing such simple tasks as safely reaching into one's pocket to retrieve an item or manipulating an object like a safety pin—especially if vision is occluded. Muscle weakness or paralysis can result in decreased strength and endurance for household and work tasks with monetary consequences that include lost work time and/or lost job skills. Pain is usually a sequela of nerve injury, and nerve pain is itself a costly and difficult condition to treat. Inadvertently, clients may further damage their nervous system if they are not properly educated about their injury and relevant precautions. Full participation in their rehabilitation is essential to optimal recovery.

Appreciating the normal static and dynamic aspects of the nervous system is vital to understanding our client's peripheral nerve pathology. We must understand how changes in one part of the nervous system can cause changes throughout the entire system and how these changes can result in functional problems for our clients. The art of hand therapy is anticipating and assisting our clients in remediation of these functional deficits.

Many of us learned about the nervous system as consisting of the peripheral nervous system (PNS) and the central nervous system (CNS); that is, two segregated systems with similar functions but very different presentations following injury to one or the other.

> #### ◎ Clinical Pearl
>
> The nervous system is actually one system that crosses multiple joints and moves through various muscular and fibrossesous tunnels. It consists of various tissue types interconnected electrically and chemically. All nerve tissue has the same elementary function of continuous electrochemical communication. This system is complex and highly organized. When one part of the system changes, there are repercussions throughout the system—even at parts that are metrically distant.

There is an ongoing plasticity within our nervous system. This means the nervous system can change, learn, and adapt or maladapt throughout the individual's life span. Sensory receptors of peripheral nerves will become less sensitive to stimuli that is not harmful to the body if the stimuli is present for a long enough period of time. For example, if you walk into a room where there is a strong odor, say a baby's diaper, your olfactory sensory receptors will eventually habituate, or decrease their responsiveness to this smell. Your PNS has *temporarily* changed its sensitivity to this odor. Still, if you leave the room and come back later, the strength of the stimulus (the bad smell) returns. The intensity of that stimulus is the same as when you entered the room the first time; your habituation to the stimulus was short lived. On the other hand, if your nervous system is exposed to that stimulus for a long enough time, your nervous system could alter, modulate, or *permanently* change. A gradual and long-lasting change in both the CNS and PNS is called **modulation.** Your sensitivity to a strong odor might permanently decrease (or increase) depending upon your nervous system's attempt to maintain **homeostasis.** The capacity of our nervous system to modulate or change permanently is called **neuroplasticity.** This is the cornerstone of neurorehabilitation.[1]

Neuroplasticity is predicated upon interactions with the environment. Our nervous system is dynamic and is continually changing throughout our lifespan. An injury or change in one part of this system will affect other parts of the system, even if those tissues are not physically close to the site of injury. Efficient motor coordination (for prehension, for example) is based upon a continual stream of sensory input used to guide coordinated motor actions or output. Consider how an injury to the brain (CNS) can affect both strength and sensation in the contralateral arm and leg resulting in gross limb paresis (or weakness) and loss of efficient motor control or coordination. Information in the sensory receptors of the joints of the involved extremity would not be able to supply accurate or reliable proprioceptive information. This person would find it challenging to accurately open and close his fingers just the right amount to grasp a coffee mug and would have difficulty recruiting motor units and using the right amount of force to pick up the mug and bring it smoothly to his mouth to drink.

Likewise, if there is an injury to a peripheral nerve (PNS) (for example, let's say the median nerve), there would be muscle paralysis and loss of sensory feedback to the CNS. In this case, the patient would not be able to actively position his thumb in opposition to grab the cup handle due to paralysis of the opponens pollicus, nor would he be able to feel if the cup was too hot to handle safely. Such deficits in sensorimotor control lead the brain to rapidly attempt to reorganize to the reduction in sensory input and motor output.[2] The CNS will quickly reorganize its cortical representations of the hand following an alteration of skin sensory inputs induced by a peripheral nerve injury.[2] Neglect of a body part (for example, following a nerve injury with consequent motor paralysis) will also lead to changes in cortical organization. In fact, how the cortex reorganizes following a peripheral nerve injury has been proposed as a major factor in final functional outcomes, including whether or not our patient will develop chronic pain.[2-5]

> ### ◎ Clinical Pearl
>
> The therapist must consider how the entire nervous system has been impacted following a PNS or CNS injury during both evaluation and treatment planning.

This chapter reviews normal nerve anatomy and looks at factors that can pervert the nerve and hence the nervous system itself. The chapter explains how the nerve responds to injury and how we as clinicians can assist our clients in modifying the potentially deleterious effects of commonly seen peripheral nerve injuries of the upper extremity (UE). The chapter concludes with case studies using critical reasoning to determine how to treat these clients.

Overview of Neuroanatomy

The **neuron** is the basic unit of the nervous system; it consists of a cell body (the **soma**), some **dendrites,** and usually one **axon.** A chain of communicating neurons is called a **pathway.** Within the CNS, a bundle of pathway axons is called a **tract** or a **fasciculus.** Outside the CNS, a bundle of pathway axons is called a **nerve.**

The CNS is well-organized with an intricate system of motor and sensory pathways arranged to reflect and respond to the continual input of information from our interaction in the environment. Cortical information is processed somatotopically with a homunculus or mapping in both the frontal lobe (for the motor pathways) and the parietal lobe (for sensory pathways) to specifically handle compartmental information and assure very quick feedback for movement and sensory integration. This

cortical representation or homunculus mapping in the brain is arranged to reflect the amount of neuronal input and output demand; thus, the hand is represented as a much bigger part of the homunculus than is the elbow.[5]

All upper motor neurons originate in the frontal lobe and terminate on the anterior horn cells (or lower motor neurons) in the gray matter of the spinal cord. All peripheral motor nerves originate from these lower motor neurons. All peripheral sensory nerves have their cell bodies in the dorsal root ganglia, located adjacent to the intervertebral foramen of the vertebral column. Sensory information arrives here and is initially processed at the spinal cord level. This information must pass upward through the thalamus into the contralateral parietal cortex for further processing or perception. If sensory information does not reach the cortex for processing, the brain will not consciously perceive or recognize the sensory experience (including the sensation of pain). This has implications for pain management.

The sensory and motor roots join together to form a **spinal nerve** (Fig. 24-1). Sympathetic nerve axons from autonomic ganglia also join the spinal nerve by way of the rami communicans. Therefore, spinal and somatic peripheral nerves are usually mixed with sensory, autonomic, and motor axons. Shortly after merging, the spinal nerve splits into dorsal and ventral rami. The ventral rami of all spinal nerves, except for T2 to T12, form networks of nerves called **plexuses.** There are four main plexuses; the largest are the brachial plexus and lumbar plexus.

The brachial plexus (Fig. 24-2) is formed by the anterior rami of cervical roots C5 to T1. This plexus emerges from the anterior and middle scalene muscles and passes deep to the clavicle before entering the axilla. In the distal axilla, the axons from the plexus

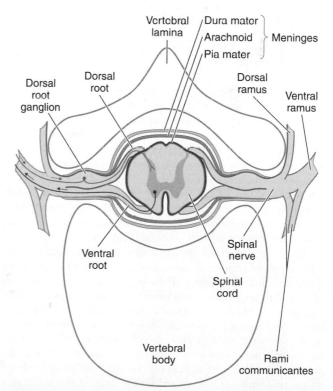

FIGURE 24-1 Schematic of a typical spinal nerve formed from the dorsal and ventral roots of the spinal cord. (From Lundy-Ekman L: *Neuroscience: fundamentals for rehabilitation*, Philadelphia, 1998, WB Saunders.)

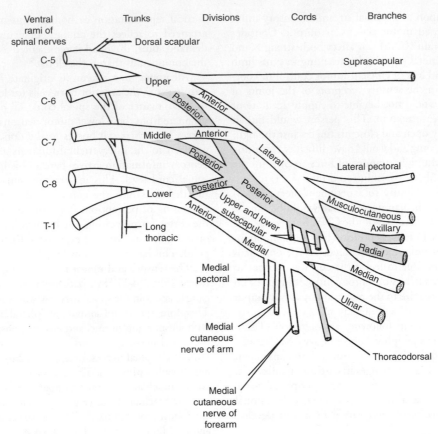

FIGURE 24-2 Diagram of the brachial plexus. (From Jenkins DB: *Hollinshead's functional anatomy of the limb and back,* ed 8, Philadelphia, 2002, Saunders.)

become the radial, median, ulnar, axillary, and musculocutaneous nerves. The entire upper limb is innervated by branches from this brachial plexus.

The peripheral nerve is composed of many very long cells that originate in the spinal region and progress distally in bundles, surrounded by multiple tissue coverings. These nerve cells are designed to be conduits for transmitting impulses—no matter how or in what position the body moves. We know that joints move in a matter of degrees, that muscles contract, and that tendons slide. Nerves also move; they move relative to the tissues that surround them.[4] The nerve cell itself must stretch and slide within its protective tissue coverings, and the nerve trunk must glide relative to the surrounding external tissues while continuing to perform its essential duty, impulse conduction.

The normal nervous system is designed to protect its neurons and their peripheral axons during movement. It has been speculated that the gliding of the peripheral nerves across our joints and through anatomical tunnels promotes axoplasmic flow and enhances blood circulation to neural tissue.[4] However, certain movements or postures can increase the amount of pressure within the nerve trunk, and if enough pressure is placed on the nerve trunk, temporary anoxia from diminished blood flow to the nerve will result. We've all experienced our foot "going to sleep" after sitting with our legs crossed for too long. In this scenario, a local compression of the peroneal nerve that runs behind the knee results in a temporary loss of blood flow to that nerve. This results in transitory sensory loss and brief muscle paresis. As blood flow is restored to this nerve, we experience pins and needles, burning,

and a gradual return in ability to weight bear on our involved leg. However, given the right circumstances, this type of innocuous insult can turn into significant nerve pathology.

Axoplasmic flow within the nerve's axon allows for a constant and controlled flow of substances that serves to maintain neural health and allow the nerve to function normally through electrochemical messaging.[1,6,7] There is a constant flow of materials in each nerve fiber from the nerve cell body to its end organs (anterograde flow) and from the end organs in the muscles or sensory receptors to the nerve cell body (retrograde flow). Various substances and organelles are synthesized in the nerve cell body and are transported within the axon to and from its terminal. This requires a continuous energy supply of oxygenated blood flow. Compromised blood flow to a nerve will result in diminished axoplasmic flow. Impaired axoplasmic flow will lead to compromised neural function, including slowed and/or decreased synaptic activity, and trophic changes in the tissues served by that nerve.[4,8,9]

Peripheral nerves are ensheathed, protected, and at times constrained by multiple layers of connective tissue coverings: the endoneurium, perineurium, epineurium, and **mesoneurium.** These coverings create a nerve "bed." Within this nerve bed, individual nerve fibers sit gently coiled in a wavy pattern. These fibers change position within the nerve bed, frequently entwining and separating into different fascicles as they course in an undulating fashion to their final destination. This meshing serves as a protective mechanism, allowing some play in the overall length of the nerve[9] (Fig. 24-3). Thus, peripheral nerve fibers

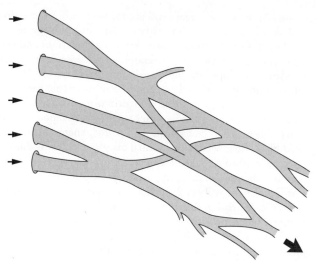

FIGURE 24-3 The peripheral nervous system (PNS) forms many plexuses and subdivisions, allowing sensory, motor and autonomic fibers to combine, separate, and recombine. These subdivisions and plexuses are good force distributors. (From Butler DS: *Mobilisation of the nervous system*, Melbourne, 1991, Churchill Livingstone.)

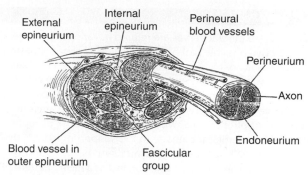

FIGURE 24-4 External protective tissue coverings surrounding a segment of a peripheral nerve. (From Trumble TE, McCallister WV: Physiology and repair of peripheral nerves. In Trumble TE, editor: *Principles of hand surgery and therapy*, Philadelphia, 2000, Saunders.)

are capable of some degree of elastic stretch, or compression, allowing the longitudinal length difference needed when a joint moves into an end range posture. The **ulnar nerve,** for example, must stretch around the medial epicondyle of the humerus during full elbow flexion, and adapt to the slack or shortening that occurs during full elbow extension. This elongation and slack uptake is distributed evenly throughout a healthy peripheral nerve.[9]

Generally, peripheral nerves are protected from injury by their external protective connective tissue coverings (Fig. 24-4). The outermost covering, the **epineurium,** functions to surround and cushion nerve fascicles, especially in locations where the peripheral nerve is vulnerable to compression.[9,10] There is a greater percentage of epineural tissue present where the nerve is more superficial and/or located near a joint. For example, the ulnar nerve (because it traverses under the medial epicondyle of the humerus) is typically protected from contusions and compression by the large percentage of epineurial tissue present in that part of the nerve. The deeper layers of epineurium function like packing material to protect the fascicular groups of nerve fibers. Each fascicle is surrounded by a mechanically strong sheath called the **perineurium.** This connective tissue layer serves as a diffusion barrier, helping to preserve the specialized microenvironment inside the fascicles.

The fibers inside the fascicles are embedded in a loose connective tissue called the **endoneurium,** or basement membrane. Around each nerve fiber (or axon), however, the endoneurium becomes closely packed, forming a supporting wall. The endoneurium serves to electrically insulate individual nerve fibers from each other. Some of these nerve fibers are myelinated. A **myelinated nerve fiber** is one that has a longitudinal chain of concentrically wrapped **Schwann cells** surrounding it, creating an insulating tube that promotes fast impulse conduction. The Schwann cell tissue together with the closely packed endoneurial tissue constitutes the **endoneurial tube.**[1] Along a myelinated nerve fiber, there are discrete areas not covered by the column of Schwann cells. These nodes or bared sections are called **nodes of Ranvier.** Portals, called **ion channels,** are located at these nodes. Conduction of an impulse along a myelinated nerve fiber can occur very rapidly as these channels open, allowing an infusion of charged ions that depolarize whole sections of the nerve fiber, from node to node, like a fuse that is continually being relit at each node.

Within the outermost covering, the epineurium, is a well-developed, longitudinally oriented vascular system that feeds the nerve fibers. Peripheral nerves are vulnerable to vascular changes as a result of altered circulation or blood flow within the epineurium of the nerve. Butler aptly describes nerves as "blood thirsty"[9] with the nervous system consuming 20% of the available oxygen in circulating blood, even though this system consists of only 2% to 5% of the body mass. Lundborg and Rydevik demonstrated that when a nerve is stretched to about 8% (in a range of 5% to 10%) of its original length, venous stasis develops. The vulnerability of axons in the PNS to vascular changes is well-documented.[8,11,12] The effects vary depending on the duration as well as the magnitude of the trauma. Prolonged stretch or compression with consequent compromised circulation will result in edema within the nerve's connective tissue coverings once circulation is restored. This swelling will lead to nerve pathology.

Mechanism of Nerve Injuries: Incomplete versus Complete Injuries

Knowing the mechanism of the nerve injury is helpful for estimating prognosis, need for, and type of medical and/or therapeutic intervention. Etiology of the injury can include compression or entrapment from internal sources, such as a tumor or scar tissue or compression from an external source (such as, crutches or a cast). Nerve injury may occur via traction or stretching to the nerve, by avulsion or laceration, by chemical or electrical burns, or by radiation. Nerve injuries are classified by whether the nerve fibers are severed or whether the nerve fibers and/or their endoneurial tube remain in continuity despite various degrees of damage to the nerve's connective tissue coverings and to the nerve fiber itself. Nerve injuries where the nerve is completely severed or where the nerve shows serious internal disorganization are considered to have the poorest prognosis for functional recovery.[10,14] Typically, these cases require surgical intervention to allow for some amount of functional recovery.

> ### Clinical Pearl
>
> Although peripheral nerves are injured in various ways, there are only two possible pathological responses: **demyelination** and/or axonal loss.[4, 7,8, 20] Segmental demyelination (or neurapraxia) results in a transient state of disrupted nerve conduction along the injured segment. More severe degrees of injury to a nerve in continuity will always involve some amount of axonal disruption. Those with significant axonal disruption and with concomitant damage to the supporting connective tissue will usually require surgical intervention.[14,17, 20, 21] Often, an injured peripheral nerve will manifest as a mixed pattern of demyelination and axonal loss. This is because each peripheral nerve is composed of thousands of axons, some of which are more vulnerable at the particular lesion site than others.

Incomplete Injuries (Injuries Where the Nerve is Still in Continuity)

Neuropathy is the term used to describe pathologic conditions of the peripheral nerve. Incomplete injuries to a nerve are defined as those where the external connective tissue coverings remain to some degree intact. An incomplete injury has important therapeutic implications. **Mononeuropathy** involves damage to a single nerve.[15] An example would be compression of the median nerve at the carpal tunnel, or **carpal tunnel syndrome (CTS)**. **Multiple mononeuropathy** is a multi-focal asymmetrical involvement of multiple nerves.[15] Compression of the right median and ulnar nerves as a complication of occupational stresses that require repetitive elbow and wrist flexion is an example of multiple mononeuropathy.

Altered axoplasmic flow in a peripheral nerve that results from diminished blood flow can cause the entire nerve to become sick and thus to become vulnerable to more than one site of irritation along its axon. Increased susceptibility for a secondary impingement may develop in areas where the nerve must traverse through spaces of increased friction (for example, fibroosseous tunnels). When the nerve has serial impingements or dual sites of pathologic manifestations that developed without a history of acute trauma, it is called **double** or **multiple crush syndrome**.[15]

Metabolic changes can result in neuropathies as well. Typically, one sees **polyneuropathy,** or bilateral extremity damage to two or more peripheral nerves. Peripheral polyneuropathy may involve the feet as well as the hands, and it occurs most frequently in people who smoke, who have nutritional deficiencies secondary to alcoholism, and who have autoimmune disease and/or difficulty controlling their blood sugar levels.[10,15] Often such nerve damage is in a stocking and/or glove distribution. Neuropathies secondary to pregnancy will often resolve gradually as the woman's body returns to its prenatal metabolic state.[16] Other polyneuropathies may be stable with medications or may be progressive as the disease advances.

The effects of compression on peripheral nerves may be attributed to alterations of blood circulation to and from the nerve compromising the energy needed for normal axoplasmic flow, or to direct injury to the nerve's axonal transport system. Nerve fibers have a well-developed micro-vascular system that ensures circulation throughout the nerve trunk. The middle connective tissue layer, the perineurium, provides a diffusion barrier to keep toxins away from nerve fibers while allowing blood supply to flow to and from the nerve fibers. When there is sustained compression or trauma to the nerve, edema will accumulate within the endoneurial sheath or basement membrane that surrounds the nerve fibers. The diffusion barrier created by the perineurium and the lack of lymphatic vessels in the endoneurial space means that once edema develops, the increased pressure cannot be dissipated, resulting in impaired endoneurial microcirculation. The accumulation of edema in the endoneurium results in increased intraneural pressure and a reduction or cessation of blood flow to the nerve fiber. When circulation is impaired, energy from oxygenated blood flow needed for normal axoplasmic flow is diminished. This is called a *metabolic conduction block.*

If this metabolic conduction block is of long enough duration and/or intensity, it will result in functional deficit, pain, and/or anesthesia in the region that that nerve supplies.[7,11,12,13,17]

Venous blood flow from the peripheral nerves is shown to be reduced at 20 to 30 mm Hg. A classically sited study by Gelberman, et al.[13] demonstrated that with 90° of wrist flexion or extension, carpal tunnel pressure in those persons *without* CTS rose to 30 mm Hg on average. Thus, compressive forces on a peripheral nerve can be exacerbated by certain provocative postures, such as holding the wrist in end range flexion or extension. If these forces are augmented by concomitant pathology, such as swelling in the carpal tunnel area following a wrist fracture, a metabolic block or compression neuropathy may develop. If compression is of long enough duration (that is, if the compression is long standing but of a comparatively low level), one will see diminished microvascular flow in the nerve's fascicles, resulting in a chronic reduction of the nerve's axoplasmic flow and slowing of the nerve's conduction of impulses (slowed conduction velocity). Function will fail sequentially in the following order: motor, proprioception, touch, temperature, pain, and then sympathetic function. Recovery occurs sequentially in the reverse order following timely conservative or surgical intervention.

Timelines and Healing (Incomplete Nerve Injuries)

> ### Clinical Pearl
>
> Compressive neuropathies, of either acute or chronic nature, often can be treated successfully via nonsurgical methods, which include rest, activity modification, nonsteroidal anti-inflammatory drugs, corticosteroid injections, and orthotics.[19]

Following compression and temporary loss of blood flow to a nerve, one will experience sensory loss, and thankfully, only short-lived motor paralysis. If the pressure on the nerve is of high enough magnitude, a local conduction block could ensue. There may be some damage to the myelin sheaths, which would result in an extended local conduction block. This is called a **neuropraxia,** and this type of nerve compression problem usually resolves within weeks or months. A classic example of this neuropractic lesion (also classified as a Sunderland type 1 nerve injury) is a **Saturday night palsy,** which is a radial nerve injury at the humeral level that results from compression from some hard external source.

If the compression was of a severe enough nature, the axons distal to the lesion would degenerate, but the endoneurial tubes of the axons could remain. In this type of nerve injury, called an **axonotmesis,** or Sunderland type 2 nerve injury, axonal regeneration would occur with good recovery of function because the endoneurial tubes would serve as guidelines to the appropriate end organ of the axon.

Nerve compression initially results in a loss of proprioception and discriminative touch, followed by a loss of pain and temperature sensation. This loss of proprioception occurs first because compression of a nerve affects the large myelinated fibers (that carry information about proprioception and discriminative touch) prior to affecting the smaller, unmyelinated fibers. If the compression persists or is severe enough, the smaller fibers that carry information about pain and temperature also are lost.[8]

When the compression resolves, abnormal sensations called **paresthesias** occur as the blood supply to the nerve resumes. The client may complain of burning, tingling, or pricking sensations. Sensation gradually returns in the reverse order in which it was lost: dull, diffuse aching pain; perception of heat; sharp, stinging sensations; cold perception; conscious proprioception; and finally, discriminative touch.[18]

> **Precautions and Concerns**

General Comments Following Nerve Injury

- *If the patient has diminished or lost protective sensation, you will need to teach them to protect the insensate part from temperature extremes (including hot bath water) as well as from situations where the insensate part might accidentally be injured because they are not visually attending to the injured part.*
- *Any patient with diminished or loss of protective sensation in the hand or in a part of the UE should be strictly cautioned against exposing this body part to moving machinery, because they could reinjure that body part without immediately realizing it.*

? Questions to Discuss with the Physician

- What nerve was injured?
- What was the mechanism of injury? Was it a clean injury or a crush injury?
- Were an electromyelogram and nerve conduction study done? What were the results?
- Is surgical decompression indicated at this time?

Complete Nerve Injuries (Injuries Where the Axon Is Transected and/or There Is Significant Loss or Disorganization of the External Connective Tissue Layers)

Grave consequences in terms of motor and/or sensory loss will occur following an injury where the peripheral nerve is severed, or where a segment of the nerve is severely traumatized with serious internal disorganization. Following such an injury, the nerve is divided into two parts: a proximal part attached to the nerve cell body, and a distal part, which undergoes degeneration. Functional recovery depends upon replacement of the lost distal portion by the outgrowth of new axonal processes growing to reach their corresponding original peripheral targets.[17]

In cases where a nerve suffers severe compression, one sees increasing involvement of the external connective tissue layers of the nerve. A Sunderland type 3 injury, for example, involves destruction of the endoneurial tubes, and a type 4 injury involves destruction of the perineurium. In the latter case, significant internal scarring occurs within the nerve trunk that impairs functional recovery. Resection of the fibrotic segment of the nerve trunk followed by nerve repair with a graft would probably be required.

A complete nerve injury (Seddon's neurotomesis or Sunderland's type IV and V injury categories) is defined as a physiologic disruption of the entire nerve or a section of a nerve. It may or may not include actual nerve transection (or laceration), but it does require surgical intervention because there is too much damage to the axon and its external connective tissue layers. It cannot repair itself. Surgical intervention might involve surgical **decompression,** or a neurolysis or a surgical repair.

When a nerve is severed, an immediate consequence is loss of its vital axoplasmic fluid.[21] The axon itself contains 90% of the axoplasmic fluid present in that nerve cell. The axoplasmic transport system (with its retrograde and anterograde flows) allows the neuron to maintain its structure and health at its synapses. This system also allows the soma (or nerve cell body) to get feedback about the axon's overall health including the health of the nerve's distally located synaptic clefts. When this communication and transport system fails, the muscle and sensory receptors associated with that nerve change. There is a loss of or decrease in these receptors' ability to receive or generate impulses. One will also see **trophic changes** in the target tissues: that is changes in the tissues served by that nerve that include abnormal hair growth, nail bed changes, cold intolerance, and soft tissue atrophy.

◎ Clinical Pearl

A completely severed peripheral nerve presents as loss of sensation, loss of muscle control, and a loss of reflexes in those structures distal to the nerve injury that are innervated by that specific peripheral nerve.

Another consequence of axonal transection is that the soma, or cell body, swells, and the cell's nucleus is displaced peripherally. This reflects a change in the metabolic priority from production of neurotransmitters to production of structural materials needed for axon repair and growth. The more proximal the site of injury, the more intense the cell body's reaction, which peaks about 2 to 3 weeks post injury.[17] The proximal axon undergoes traumatic degeneration within the zone of injury (that is, to the next node or nodes of Ranvier). The endoneurial tubes of the proximal axon lie empty. Distal to site of injury, **Wallerian degeneration,** or the breakdown of the axon distal to the site of injury, occurs. This process begins about 48 to 96 hours after transection and concludes about 3 weeks post injury. During this time, there is progressive deterioration of the myelin, and the distal axon becomes increasingly disorganized. This one of the reasons that best prognosis for surgical repair is when the surgery can be performed within that 48 to 96 hours.[14,17]

> **Precautions and Concerns**

General Comments Following Nerve Laceration

- *The development of disuse osteoporosis in adjacent bone is a common occurrence following nerve laceration. Be cautious with initial loading of nearby bone and joints once strengthening is permitted, especially if your patient has a history of osteopenia or osteoporosis.*
- *The development of stiff and fibrotic joints and soft tissue in the adjacent areas may also be expected following a period of immobilization to protect the nerve repair site. Check with the surgeon to insure you are immobilizing the fewest joints and soft tissues possible without compromising the repair.*

- *Muscle tissue atrophy and interstitial fibrosis in the tissue innervated by the involved nerve will occur with an initial weight loss of 30% in the first month and 50% to 60% by 2 months. Muscle atrophy reaches a relatively stable state at 60% to 80% weight loss by approximately 4 months.[17]*

◎ Clinical Pearl

An orthotic fabricated in the initial month post-surgery will need to be regularly checked and refitted to accommodate this dramatic decrease in muscle fiber volume.

Overview of Postoperative Management—Decompression versus Nerve Repair

Surgical intervention is always necessary if the nerve is severed and may be necessary if the nerve has enough internal disorganization and scarring. Intervention might include surgical repair, a decompression, and/or a neurolysis. A **primary nerve repair** refers to operative nerve repair performed within the first week after injury. Primary repairs are associated with better results.[20] A **delayed** or **secondary nerve repair** is one performed a week or more after injury. **Nerve grafting** is a type of nerve repair performed when a primary repair cannot be completed without undue tension on the nerve's cut ends.[21] The nerve graft acts to provide a source of empty endoneurial tubes through which the regenerating axon can be directed. A nerve graft can be performed using a commercially available **conduit**, or by using an autograft or allograft. An **autograft** is graft material harvested from typically dispensable sensory nerves and used to repair large mixed nerves. An **allograft** is graft material harvested from human cadavers, for example. Both allografts and autographs are used to address large nerve gaps.

A **neurolysis** is the surgical dissection and exploration of a damaged nerve with the goal of freeing the nerve from local tissue restrictions or adhesions.[20] Peripheral **nerve decompression** surgery is performed when the nerve has become trapped or impinged in some way. This surgical procedure decreases the compressive forces or pressure on a nerve. It may involve cutting tissue that is constricting the nerve, or physically moving the nerve to a different site.

Timelines and Healing Following Complete Nerve Injuries

In general, nerve cells have limited powers of regeneration (the ability to replicate or repair themselves). Around 6 months after injury, virtually all developing neurons lose their ability to undergo mitosis.[1] This means that when a neuron is damaged or destroyed, it cannot be replicated by daughter cells from other neurons. A destroyed neuron is permanently lost, and only some types of damage to a peripheral nerve may be repaired.

Complete peripheral nerve lesions can achieve full or partial recovery following injury if certain conditions exist. First, the soma, or nerve cell body, must be viable. Certain severe injuries, such as nerve root avulsions, can kill the motor neurons in the spinal cord and the dorsal root ganglion cells located adjacent to the spinal cord. Damage to the soma results in the death of the entire nerve cell.

Second, the physiologic environment in and around the nerve lesion must support axonal sprouting and peripheral growth. Ideally, there is an intact endoneurial tube with undamaged Schwann cells distal to the level of the injury. Schwann cells produce nerve growth factor, which is key to allowing peripheral nerve damage

to resolve.[15] Peripheral growth ceases if the sprouting axons meet scar tissue or bone that blocks access to the empty Schwann sheaths and endoneurial tubes or to the end organ of the axon.

A third condition for recovery is that the regenerated axon must connect to the appropriate end organ, and that end organ still must be viable. The motor nerve fiber must grow to its original motor end plate, and the sensory nerve fiber must connect with its appropriate receptor organ. If a sensory axon is misdirected into a motor distal tubule, the axonal growth will be wasted. Therefore, nerve injuries in which the nerve remains in continuity with intact endoneurial tubes have a better prognosis than **neurotmesis,** which is when the whole nerve is disrupted. In the latter case, there are many chances for misguided axons to enter the wrong endoneurial tube. Even if the proper nerve fibers get to the correct sensory end organ and motor end plate, the receptors and muscle tissue must be viable. Sensory end organs have no end plate, and therefore they retain the potential for reinnervation for 1 to 3 or more years.[17,21] However, denervated muscle tissue loses the ability to support axonal regeneration as the motor end plate degenerates. The muscle becomes hypersensitive and fasciculates clinically. The chances of functional reinnervation diminish if the nerve does not reach the motor end plates within approximately 12 months of denervation.[20]

◎ Clinical Pearl

For practical purposes, the maximum length that a nerve can grow to restore motor function is approximately 35 cm or 13 to 14 inches.[21]

A final condition for peripheral nerve recovery is that the CNS must perceive and interpret the injured PNS signals appropriately. The CNS will need to reorganize its cortical representations of the hand, for example, following alteration of skin inputs induced by a peripheral nerve injury. This is an exciting topic in itself and one that is explored briefly in a later "Tips from the Field" box with the heading of "Sensory Reeducation." The classification systems that are used following nerve injury are summarized in Tables 24-1 and 24-2.

♥ Tips from the Field

Nerve Injury

If surgery can be avoided, it should. Typically, there is pain after surgery. In addition, postoperative swelling can exacerbate a compression injury. Thus, try conservative management first if possible. For example, compression of the median nerve at the wrist (CTS) often may be ameliorated with splinting at night, ergonomic interventions, and client education about provocative positions to avoid.[22]

If surgery is necessary, allow the injured nerve time to recover from the trauma of surgery. The amount of time that is necessary for healing depends on a number of factors, including the severity of the nerve injury before surgery and the type of surgery. An endoscopic **carpal tunnel release (CTR)** is typically less traumatic than the traditional open CTR, for example, but there are certain risks. Other factors may include the presence of systemic diseases, such as rheumatoid arthritis or diabetes, which can slow or permanently compromise healing, or the presence of concomitant injuries that may exaggerate the early phases of tissue healing. Gentle active range of motion (AROM) in the area of the nerve injury usually can begin when the client has moved beyond the inflammatory stage of healing. The typical timeline for this ranges from 2 to 3 days postoperatively to 2 to 3 weeks postoperatively. Avoid strengthening exercises until the remodeling phase of healing, which is typically 2 to 5 weeks postoperatively. Knowledge about the phases of wound healing enables the therapist to devise an appropriate postoperative program for each client. Again, the reader is cautioned to address each client as an individual, observing that person's tissue response to exercise and adjusting each program accordingly.

? Questions to Discuss with the Physician

- What was the date of the repair?
- Was the nerve repair under tension? Was there need for a nerve graft?
- Was there a delay from the time of injury to the time of the nerve repair?
- Are there other structures that were injured and repaired?
- Do you have a particular postoperative therapy protocol you would like to be followed? How long do you want the nerve repair to be protected by immobilization?
- Can we begin range of motion (ROM) of the parts distal and proximal to the repair site to maintain joint suppleness and tissue length and gliding?

Diagnosis-Specific Information that Affects Clinical Reasoning

- Repaired peripheral nerves heal at a rate of about a 1 to 3 mm/day after an initial 3- to 4-week latency period.[14,21] Additional delays may occur as the regenerating axon attempts to cross the injury site and reinnervate the end organ.
- Sensory end organs remain viable because there is no end plate like there is in muscles. Thus, these organs retain the potential for reinnervation. Nerve grafting a digital sensory nerve defect (in the finger) may provide protective sensation even many years after the initial injury.[21]
- Proximal nerve lesions have a worse prognosis for full sensory and motor recovery than distal nerve lesions.
- The presence of scar tissue in and around the healing peripheral nerve can significantly impair the surgical and therapeutic goal of accurate nerve regeneration.
- Nerve regeneration and functional outcomes are age-related. Better functional outcomes in the young may be due to greater cortical plasticity.[2,5,17]
- Still, cells that fire together will wire together. According to Merzenich and Jenkins[5] and others,[2,23-25] practice strengthens and expands the somatosensory cortical representation of the area that is used. Sensory reeducation and cortical retraining may be helpful, even in cases in which the outcome of surgical intervention is poor.

Evaluation Tips

Distinguishing among Central Nervous System, Spinal Segment, and Peripheral Nerve Lesions

- CNS lesions show motor spasticity/flaccidity and whole limb sensory changes, which are frequently on the side of the body contralateral to the injury site.
- Spinal segment lesions show myotomal and dermatomal changes in the corresponding area. Typically, several adjacent spinal levels must be affected before a dermatomal and myotomal pattern can be appreciated.
- Peripheral nerve lesions show sensory or motor loss specific to the involved nerve with symptoms and signs at and distal to the site of injury.

TABLE 24-1   Seddon's Classification

Classification	Description
Neuropraxia	A conduction block; no anatomical disruption—all components intact.
Axonotmesis	Disruption of axons and myelin sheaths, but endoneurial tubes are intact.
Neurotmesis	Complete severance or serious disorganization; no spontaneous recovery.

TABLE 24-2   Sunderland's Classification

Degree	Description	Mechanism of Injury	Prognosis
1°	All structures remain intact; local conduction block and demyelination	Acute compression (Seddon's neuropraxia)	Complete recovery (days/months)
2°	Axonal disruption with distal (Wallerian) degeneration; however, endoneurial tubes are intact	Mild traction or moderate compression (Seddon's axonotmesis)	Typically, complete recovery (months), limiting factor is distance of regeneration required (viable end organ)
3°	Disruption of axons and endoneurial tubes; mild to moderate functional loss; fascicles remain intact	Moderate-severe traction or crush (Seddon's neurotmesis)	Axons may regenerate but in "wrong" endoneurial tube; many result in nerve-target organ mismatch; poor prognosis for proximal injuries
4°	Loss of fascicular integrity within the nerve; only epineurium is intact	Severe traction or crush (Seddon's neurotmesis)	Moderate to severe functional loss; may be improved by fascicular repair; neuroma in continuity is common; regenerating axons lost in scar
5°	Complete nerve transection	Severe traction or crush; laceration (Seddon's neurotmesis)	Severe functional loss; requires surgery

General Considerations

Begin with the client interview. Gather information about the client's history and mechanism of injury, medical history, current functional status, current living situation, and the client's goals.

Observation and Palpation

Observe the posture of the involved extremity. Observe how the client uses (or avoids use of) this extremity, for example, while the client is taking off his or her coat or filling out forms. Observe for obvious muscle atrophy, skin lesions, edema, color changes (for example, areas of erythema, mottled skin, or skin that has a blanched appearance) and trophic changes. **Precaution.** *Make note of and caution the client about vulnerability to blisters and other signs of hand injury that may occur with use of a vulnerable insensate hand. Document areas of edema,* **hypersensitivity,** *adhesions, and atrophy. Use of a pictorial format in addition to written format may be helpful.*

Precaution. *Always use universal wound precautions around any lesions and rashes.*

Refer to Chapter 5 for specific evaluation protocols. The following sections are meant to serve as a review of the pertinent tests and the procedures used in evaluating clients with nerve injury.

Assessment of Sensory Function

- Semmes-Weinstein monofilament testing: This is a graded light-touch testing instrument consisting of a kit of twenty nylon monofilament probes. The monofilaments are used by the therapist to map light-touch sensibility in the hand. An abbreviated kit is also available.
- Two-point discrimination testing: According to Moberg, a good indicator of eventual fine motor function following a peripheral nerve injury is the return of two-point discrimination.[18] He asserts that 6 mm of two-point discrimination is needed to wind a watch, 6-8 mm for sewing and 12 mm for handling precision tools. Static two-point discrimination and moving two-point discrimination tests assess the client's ability to discriminate between one point and two points of pressure applied randomly to the fingertip. Moving two-point discrimination returns before static two-point discrimination.
- Localization of touch: Neither of the aforementioned tests requires the client to identify the location of the stimulus. Localization requires a more integrated level of perception than simple recognition of a stimulus. Localization is appropriate for testing after a nerve repair because difficulty with localization of a stimulus is a common phenomenon following nerve injury. Poor localization can impair function significantly.
- The therapist can record the client's accuracy in localizing light-touch stimuli by using the lowest Semmes-Weinstein monofilament that can be perceived in the area of dysfunction. Ask the client to close the eyes and to indicate verbally if he or she feels the stimulus. Each time the client answers in the affirmative, ask the client to open the eyes and to point to the exact spot touched. The therapist should record the client's results

on a grid-like map of the hand, indicating the actual location of stimulation and the sites of referred touch perception. The therapist can draw arrows on the grid to indicate referred perception sites. This test has no formal interpretation or scoring; rather, evidence of poor localization is useful when determining the need for and when planning a sensory reeducation program.
- Moberg pickup test: This is a useful test for assessing median nerve function. The test may be helpful for testing children or adults who have cognitive involvement or who may have secondary agendas that prevent them from full participation in other sensory tests.
- Hoffmann-Tinel sign: Following trauma, gentle percussion along the course of the injured, regenerating nerve produces a temporary tingling sensation in the distribution of the injured nerve up to the site of regeneration. The tingling persists several seconds. Test from distal to proximal for best accuracy. If this sign is absent or is not progressing distally as is expected with a healing nerve, there is a poor prognosis for continued nerve recovery. Likewise, a progressing **Tinel's sign** is encouraging but does not necessarily predict complete recovery. Table 24-3 gives a summary of light-touch sensibility testing, standardized tests, and techniques for administration, scoring, and interpretation of scores.

Assessment of Motor Function

- Goniometric assessment: Evaluation of articular motion and musculotendinous function is performed with a goniometer. Passive range of motion (PROM) is defined as a measurement of the ability of the joint to be moved by an external source through its normal arc of motion. Limitations indicate problems within the joint or capsular structures surrounding the joint. AROM is defined as a measurement of the individual's own capability for moving a joint through its normal arc of motion. A limitation in AROM when PROM is full may indicate diminished or lost muscle power resulting from a nerve lesion. Therefore, assess AROM first, and if limitations exist, then assess PROM.
- Manual muscle testing: Muscle paresis or paralysis can result from a peripheral nerve lesion. Careful documentation of muscle strength, using a manual muscle test (MMT), is an important component of the initial evaluation following a nerve injury.[39] If possible, compare strength with the uninvolved side to determine what the normal strength is for that client.
- Test the muscle or muscle group in the middle position using a "brake" test. Tell the client to "hold this position," and say, "Don't let me move you," while exerting a counter-directional force, attempting to move the client's body part out of the test position. Use a grading system that minimizes the amount of pluses and minuses, because that makes it easier for other health professionals to review the documentation and appreciate what was observed. Table 24-4 gives the recommended grading system for manual muscle testing.
- Strength testing—grip and pinch: Gross grip and pinch strength can be assessed using standardized tools, the Jamar dynamometer, and the pinch gauge.[39]

Assessment of Autonomic Function

- Sympathetic function: If sweating (sudomotor function) is still present following a nerve lesion, this suggests that the nerve damage is incomplete, because peripheral autonomic nerve fibers

TABLE 24-3 Light Touch Sensibility Testing–Standardized Tests and Techniques

Test/Purpose	Equipment/Instructions to Client	Testing Procedure	Scoring	Interpretation of Scores*
Semmes-Weinstein monofilament: Threshold test for light touch sensibility	Equipment: Quiet test area, colored pencils and map or grid of the hand for recording results, kit of 20 nylon monofilament probes ranging from 1.65 to 6.65. Alternatively: The minikit containing probes: 2.83, 3.61, 4.31, 4.56, and 6.65. Instructions: Introduce test and familiarize patient with test expectations by demonstrating in proximal area believed to have normal sensibility. Ask subject to say "yes" if the stimulus is felt. Alternatively, obscure subject's vision with blindfold. The test hand should be securely stabilized on the table.	Begin distally, and progress proximally along the peripheral nerve's receptive field. Start with the probe marked 2.83, apply to skin with enough pressure to bow the filament. Apply in 1.5 seconds, hold 1.5 seconds, and remove in 1.5 seconds. Repeat three times at each site; progress to next thicker filament if prior one is not perceived. Filaments marked ≥4.31 should be applied only once at each site.	One response out of three is considered affirmative. 2.83 = Normal light touch 3.22 to 3.61 = Normal light touch 3.84 to 4.31 = Diminished light touch 4.56 to 6.65 = Diminished protective sensation > 6.65 = Absence of all sensation	2.83 = Normal light touch 3.22 to 3.61 = Stereognosis and pain perception intact, close to normal use of hand 3.84 to 4.31 = Mild to moderate impaired stereognosis and pain perception, difficulty manipulating objects 4.56 to 6.65 = Moderate to significant impaired pain and temperature perception, unable to manipulate objects with vision occluded, marked decrease in spontaneous hand use; will need instructions regarding protective care of impaired area > 6.65 = Unable to identify objects or temperature; with visual guidance, capable of gross coordination only
Static two-point discrimination/functional test: For determining two-point discrimination and ability to use hand for fine motor tasks	Equipment: Hand-held disk-criminator or Boley gauge. Instructions: Introduce test and familiarize client with test expectations by demonstrating in the proximal area believed to have normal sensibility. Ask subject to say "one" or "two" in response to perception of one point of pressure or two points of pressure. Ask the subject to close eyes their during testing. Alternatively, obscure the client's vision with a blindfold. The test hand should be securely stabilized on the table.	Typically, only volar fingertips are tested. Begin testing at 5 mm of distance between two points. Apply one or two points randomly with the probes held in a longitudinal orientation to avoid crossover from overlapping digital nerves. Force is applied lightly, just until the skin blanches. If responses are inaccurate, the distance between the ends is increased by increments of 1 to 5 mm. Testing is stopped at 15 mm or sooner if digit length is not adequate.	Score is the smallest distance at which client is able to accurately discriminate between two points of pressure and one point of pressure. Seven out of 10 correct responses are required. Normal ranges: 3 to 5 mm = Normal, ages 18-70 6 to 10 mm = Fair 11 to 15 mm = Poor One point only perceived = Protective sensation only No points perceived = Anesthetic	6 mm = Normal, needed for winding a watch 6 to 8 mm = Fair, needed for sewing 12 mm = Poor, needed for handling precision tools > 15 mm = Loss of protective sensation to anesthetic; above this gross tool handling may be possible but only with decreased speed and skill

*Interpretation of scores is based on information in Bell-Krotoski J: Correlating sensory morphology and tests of sensibility with function. In Mackin EJ, et al, editors: *Tendon and nerve surgery in the hand: a third decade*, St Louis, 1997, Mosby, and in Callahan A: Sensibility assessment for nerve lesions in continuity and nerve lacerations. In Mackin EJ, Callahan AD, Skirven TM, editors: *Rehabilitation of the hand and upper extremity*, ed 5, St Louis, 2002, Mosby.

within the nerve are responsible for sweating. Vasomotor homeostasis is likewise a function of the sympathetic nervous system; therefore, abnormal changes in skin temperature and skin color may indicate involvement of these peripheral nerve fibers.

- Trophic changes: The combination of sympathetic and sensory dysfunction results in characteristic trophic changes in all tissues of the involved area. Specifically, one would expect to see nail changes (blemishes, talon-like appearance), abnormal hair growth (may fall out or become longer and finer), cold intolerance, soft tissue atrophy (most notably in the fingertip pulps), and a slowed rate of tissue healing.

- The O'Riain wrinkle test (1973): This is an objective test that identifies areas of denervation; denervated skin does not wrinkle when soaked in warm water. The denervated hand is placed in warm water (40° C [104° F]) for 30 minutes, and the presence or absence of finger wrinkling is documented. This test is most useful for children or others who may be unable or unwilling to cooperate with sensibility testing.

Assessment of Pain

Pain is almost always a consequence of a nerve injury; therefore acknowledging this fact and aiming to quantify and qualify this multidimensional experience is important to the therapist and the client.[39,53] Many pain assessment tools are one-dimensional, attempting to quantify the pain experience numerically. The benefit of such tools is that they are easy and quick to administer and to score, and they produce repeatable, objective results that can be used to assess treatment outcomes. Performing a pain interview at the time of the initial evaluation, in addition to these other pain assessments, is the best way to provide the therapist with a more complete picture of the client's pain experience. This unstructured interview should include questions about topics, such as current medication regimen, location and frequency of pain, verbal description of pain, and what factors exacerbate or decrease pain.

Table 24-5 summarizes typical pain assessment tools with a brief synopsis of administration and scoring instructions. This is not an exhaustive list of pain assessments but rather a list of those that can be used efficiently during an initial evaluation of a client with a peripheral nerve injury.

Other Assessments to Consider

- Canadian Occupational Performance Measure (COPM): The COPM is a client-centered assessment tool for use by occupational therapists. The COPM is designed to assess a client's self-perceived change in occupational performance problems

TABLE 24-4   Manual Muscle Test Grades and Interpretation

Grade	Interpretation
5, Normal	Able to move body part full range against gravity, holding position with normal strength
4, Good	Able to move body part full range against gravity, holding position with good strength
3+, Fair +	Able to move body part full range against gravity, holding position for short time and/or against some resistance
3, Fair	Able to move body part full range against gravity, unable to hold position against any resistance and/or for any functional length of time
2, Poor	Able to move body part full range in gravity minimized position
2–, Poor minus	Able to move body part through partial range in gravity minimized position
1, Trace	Palpable flicker in muscle, no observable movement at joint
0, Zero	No palpable flicker in muscle, no observable movement at joint in gravity minimized position

TABLE 24-5   Typical Pain Assessment Tools

Name	Description/Administration	Scoring/Interpretation*
Numeric pain scale	Description: Subjective rating of pain intensity using a 10-point numeric scale Administration: Client is asked to rate his current pain on a 0 to 10+ scale, with 0 = no pain and 10 = worst possible pain imaginable. Client may be asked to rate his best and worst pain experienced over the past 30 days or since the onset of pain.	Scoring: Record the number identified by the client. Interpretation: 0 to 2 = Low level of pain 3 to 5 = Moderate level of pain 6 to 10+ = High level of pain
Visual analogue scale	Description: Subjective quantitative measure of pain intensity using a 10-cm line with descriptors (no pain at all; pain as bad as it could be) at each end Administration: Clients are asked to make a mark through the line to indicate the pain they are presently experiencing.	Scoring: The distance is measured on the line from the bottom anchor to the client's mark and recorded in centimeters as the client's pain score. Interpretation: 0 to 2.9 cm = Low level of pain 3 to 5.9 cm = Moderate pain level 6 to 10.5 cm = High pain level
Pain drawing	Description: Subjective drawing of pain diffusion and localization Administration: Clients are given an outline of the body or body part and asked to use symbols (that denote different qualities of pain) to reflect his current distribution of symptoms.	Scoring: No standardized or widely accepted method for scoring exists. Interpretation: Look for patterns of pain diffusion that may indicate radicular symptoms occurring along a specific dermatone. Widespread or non-anatomical pain drawings may indicate chronic pain or poor psychodynamics.

*Interpretations of these scales are based on information in Galper J, Verno V: Pain. In Palmer ML, Epler ME: *Fundamentals of musculoskeletal assessment techniques*, ed 2, Philadelphia, 1996, Lippincott-Raven Publishers.

over time. The COPM is intended for use as an outcome measure. The test is designed to assist the client and the therapist in identifying problem areas of occupational performance and in setting treatment goals. Instructions for administration are indicated clearly in the manual.[51] In a semi-structured interview, the problem areas are identified and then rated in terms of importance to the client. The five most important problems are then the focus of intervention. These problems are rated by the client to determine the client's perception of ability to perform the identified task/activity and the client's satisfaction with that performance. After a period of time, the COPM form is re-administered, and possible changes in the client's perceptions are recorded. The difference between the initial and subsequent scores gives the measure of outcome, with a two-point difference in either direction indicating significant change.

- Reflexes: Complete severance of the efferent or afferent nerve in a reflex arc abolishes that reflex. However, a reflex can be lost even in partial nerve injuries, and so hyporeflexia is not a good guide of injury severity.
- Cold sensitivity: Cold sensitivity or intolerance is a common consequence of peripheral nerve injuries. Cold intolerance is related to functional impairment, and it may adversely affect returning to work and leisure activities in locations where the injured extremity may be exposed to cold. Consider using self-report to document cold intolerance, because many of the available test protocols for assessing temperature tolerance lack standardization.[39]
- Edema measurements: The presence of edema compromises the available space for the nerve as it traverses through fibroosseous tunnels and other tightly confined areas, such as the carpal tunnel. Take edema measurements initially, or once sutures are removed, using a volumeter if there are no wound issues or a tape measure to assess circumference. Establish a baseline before starting therapy.

> ## Precautions and Concerns

An increase in edema following treatment along with degradation in sensory status indicates that your treatment program was too aggressive.

- Provocative testing: Testing to provoke symptoms is used to clarify the site of injury and to exclude the possibility that other non-neural tissues may be sources of pain. Provocative nerve testing is predicated on the fact that irritated nerve tissue is sensitized or hyper-responsive to any manual stimulus applied along its length.[4,50] A manual stimulus is defined as mechanical stimuli acting as percussion along a nerve, or a compressive force to a nerve trunk or a graded force that causes longitudinally directed nerve gliding. In the normal nerve, these forces would not result in an irritated neural response. For example, tapping over a nerve normally would not cause a Tinel sign unless the nerve was injured. Therefore, Tinel testing, or percussion along a nerve that results in an irritated tingling sensation, is considered a positive provocative stress test. Likewise, upper limb tension testing is considered a provocative stress test, because the nerves of the brachial plexus are moved passively and longitudinally. A positive upper limb tension test would present as a pathologic response or symptomatic pain reproduction.[4,6,25]

> ## Precautions and Concerns

Provocative Testing

- *Neural provocative testing, especially upper limb tension testing, must be done carefully and by a skilled therapist who understands the testing technique and the interpretations and who can manage symptoms once provoked. UE provocative tests are not standardized in terms of precise positioning, how long each position is held, or how much force is applied.*
- *Whenever possible, compare the involved to the uninvolved side to appreciate the client's individual normal response.*

Clinical Reasoning: Determining Which Tests to Use

Table 24-6 contains a list of recommendations for determining which assessment tools to use when evaluating a nerve injury in continuity versus a nerve injury not in continuity.

> ## Radial Nerve

Anatomy and Common Sites of Compression

Table 24-7 provides a summary of radial nerve anatomy, common lesion sites, and typical deficits/deformities associated with radial nerve lesions.

TABLE 24-6 Recommendations for Therapist's Evaluation Battery	
Nerve Lesions In Continuity—Non-Operative	**Nerve Lacerations—Postoperative**
• Client history • Observation/palpation of involved tissues • Tinel test at suspected compression site • Semmes-Weinstein monofilament test • Pain assessments (including pain interview) • Provocative stress testing if client reports intermittent symptoms aggravated by certain positions/activities • Moberg pick-up test (for functional assessment with a median nerve injury) • AROM followed by PROM if limitations present with active movement • Strength test: MMT to isolate muscle involvement, grip and pinch testing to assess functional grasp and pinch strength • Modified COPM for goal setting	• Client history • Observation/palpation of involved tissues with special attention to trophic, sudomotor, and vasomotor changes (possible sympathetic dysfunction) • Tinel test to determine distal progression of regenerating axons • Semmes-Weinstein monofilament testing followed by localization (determine light touch sensibility, need for sensory protection techniques and/or sensory reeducation) • Two-point discrimination testing if client is able to perceive ≤ 4.31 monofilament (predicts functional status, need for sensory reeducation) • Pain assessments (Is there a need for desensitization program?) • AROM followed by PROM (if needed) of involved extremity as permitted by postoperative protocol • Modified COPM for goal setting

AROM, Active range of motion; *COPM,* Canadian Occupational Performance Measure; *MMT,* manual muscle test; *PROM,* passive range of motion.

TABLE 24-7	Summary of Radial Nerve
Sensation	*Brachial cutaneous branches* supply the posterior region of the arm and lower lateral arm. An *antebrachial branch* supplies the posterior skin of the forearm. The *superficial sensory branch* of the forearm supplies the lateral two-thirds of the dorsum of the hand, the dorsal thumb and the proximal portion of the dorsal index, and long digits and radial half of the proximal ring.
Motor	*Innervations, proximal to distal:* Triceps (lateral head), triceps (long head), triceps (medial head), anconeous, BR, ECRL, ECRB, supinator, EDC, extensor digiti minimi, ECU, abductor pollicis longus, extensor pollicis longus, extensor pollicis brevis, and extensor indicis proprius
Function	An intact radial nerve allows for elbow extension and is *essential to the tenodesis action that is fundamental to the grasp-release pattern of normal hand function.* The radial nerve powers all wrist extension, all MP joint extension, and thumb extension and radial abduction.
Common sites of entrapment/injury	*Crutch palsy* (axilla level, motor and sensory involvement) *Saturday night palsy/high radial nerve palsy* (mid-humeral compression or shaft fractures—triceps spared, motor and sensory involvement) *PIN palsy* (fracture/dislocations of elbow joint, tendinous edge of ECRB, between two heads of supinator—radial wrist extensors spared, primarily motor involvement) *RTS* (compression between radial head and supinator muscle; primarily a pain syndrome) *Superficial radial sensory nerve palsy* (compression between ECRL and BR tendons or at wrist from tight cast/splint—sensory involvement only)
Results of lesion	*Motor palsy* has significant functional consequences. A lesion to this nerve as it passes medially to laterally across the posterior shaft of the humerus will result in *"wrist drop"* with a loss of all active wrist, digit, and thumb extension. Supination of the forearm will remain functional because the intact biceps brachii is a powerful supinator of the forearm. Likewise, the triceps is spared because it receives its innervation more proximally. Only high lesions to the radial nerve (as in the axilla) result in loss of all active elbow extension as well as the aforementioned problems. Lesions to the *PIN branch* in the forearm spares the BR and radial wrist extensors, but thumb, digit, and ulnar wrist extension are lost. A *lesion to the superficial radial sensory nerve* results in some loss of sensation on the dorsal lateral hand. This is not typically a debilitating problem for clients. Following radial nerve palsy, clients report an inability to use the hand for grasp or release. The loss of stability at the wrist results in an inability to use the long flexors to make a fist. Clients cannot move their thumb away from their hand to grab hold of a cup or utensil, for example, or skillfully to let go of an object once placed in their hand.

BR, Brachioradialis; *ECRB,* extensor carpi radialis brevis; *ECRL,* extensor carpi radialis longus; *ECU,* extensor carpi ulnaris; *EDC,* extensor digitorum communis; *PIN,* posterior interosseous nerve; *RTS,* radial tunnel syndrome.

The radial nerve is the most commonly injured of the three major peripheral nerves in the UE[28] (Fig. 24-5). It is particularly vulnerable about mid-humeral level, because it traverses around the spiral groove of the humerus moving medially to laterally. Injury at this level is called a **high radial nerve palsy.** The triceps muscle is spared, because nerve fibers innervating this three-headed muscle branch off the main trunk at the level of the axilla (or just distal to this). Thus, elbow extension is intact. The supinator and brachioradialis (BR) muscles are paralyzed; however, elbow flexion and forearm supination remain because the musculocutaneous-innervated biceps brachii muscle is a primary elbow flexor and forearm supinator. There is paralysis of all wrist extensors, loss of finger extension at the metacarpophalangeal (MP) joints, and an inability to extend and radially abduct the thumb. This injury is called **wrist drop deformity** (Fig. 24-6), named for its classic dropped or flexed wrist posture.

The most common cause of radial nerve palsy is direct trauma to the nerve, often secondary to fractures of the humerus, elbow dislocations, and Monteggia fracture-dislocations.[29] According to Barton, about one in ten humeral shaft fractures are complicated by a high radial nerve palsy.[28] External compression, such as from a crutch in the axilla or along the mid-humeral level where the nerve runs somewhat superficially between the triceps muscle and the humeral shaft, can also result in neuropathy of the radial nerve. The latter case is frequently referred to as *Saturday night palsy* or *drunkard's palsy.*[7] Depending on the level of injury, triceps paresis

may exist, as well as some posterior arm sensory loss. A therapist will see paralysis of all the wrist and finger extensors and sensory loss along the dorsal lateral aspect of the forearm and hand.

Conservative Management of High Radial Nerve Injuries

Presentations

- Crutch palsy (**axilla level,** motor and sensory involvement) presents with loss of triceps function at the elbow (that is, loss of elbow extension), weakness with supination, loss of digit MP extension, thumb extension, and radial abduction. Gravity can assist with elbow extension for functional tasks; but the therapist should monitor for the development of elbow flexion contractures secondary to the unopposed elbow flexors contracting and adaptively shortening.
- Saturday night palsy/high radial nerve palsy (mid-humeral compression or shaft fractures-triceps function is spared, otherwise motor and sensory involvement is as previously described)

Timelines and Healing

Typically, a radial nerve palsy that results from closed injuries represents a neuropraxia, which resolves spontaneously over a period of a few days to 3 to 4 months.[20] Patients who fail to show clinical improvement after 3 months of conservative management may be considered for surgery.

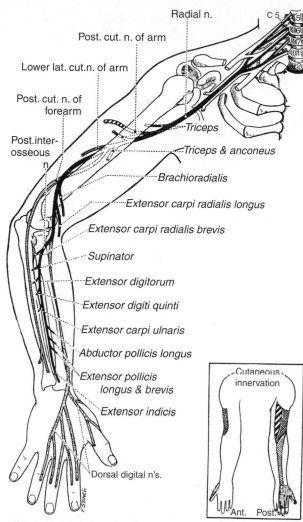

Radial n.

Post. cut. n. of arm

Lower lat. cut.n. of arm

Post. cut. n. of forearm

Post.inter-osseous n.

C 5

Triceps

Triceps & anconeus

Brachioradialis

Extensor carpi radialis longus

Extensor carpi radialis brevis

Supinator

Extensor digitorum

Extensor digiti quinti

Extensor carpi ulnaris

Abductor pollicis longus

Extensor pollicis longus & brevis

Extensor indicis

Dorsal digital n's.

Cutaneous innervation

Ant. Post.

FIGURE 24-5 Schematic of the radial nerve. (From Stanly BG, Tribuzi SM, editors: *Concepts in hand rehabilitation*, Philadelphia, 1992, FA Davis.)

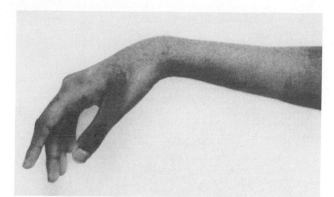

FIGURE 24-6 Wrist drop deformity resulting from radial nerve palsy. (From Stanly BG, Tribuzi SM, editors: *Concepts in hand rehabilitation*, Philadelphia, 1992, FA Davis.)

➤ Precautions and Concerns

If using a wrist cock up orthosis to improve function and stabilize the wrist, you will need to monitor for digit MP and thumb flexion contractures. Extensor muscles that are not innervated may become overstretched by unopposed flexors, resulting in biomechanical issues as the nerve heals and muscles are reinnervated. An alternative is to fabricate a forearm-based wrist orthosis with index through small finger MP extension, thumb in extension, and abduction crossing the IP.

➤ Precautions and Concerns

Care should be taken when gauging the appropriate force needed to provide adequate digit extension while allowing full flexion of digits. When designing this orthosis, use less dynamic extension force on the fourth and fifth digits, because their digit flexors are exceptionally powerful and needed for gross grip. Also, make certain that the normal distal palmar arch is maintained.

❪❫ What to Say to Clients

About Radial Nerve Palsy

"You have an injury to the nerve that powers all the wrist and finger extensor muscles; in other words, those muscles that allow you to straighten your wrist and fingers at the same time. This loss of wrist stability means that you will have a lot of difficulty using this hand for functional grasp. Your physician feels that you have an (excellent/good) prognosis for full recovery, but it will take time—perhaps as long as 3 to 4 months. During this time, it will be necessary to protect your weak muscles from being overpowered and overstretched by those muscles that are working normally. Therefore, you will need to use a brace to stabilize your wrist. There are a few options available."

These options should be reviewed with the client using pictures or prototypes. You will need to help guide your patient in choosing the best option given their lifestyle, hand dominance and side of injury, financial situation, and ability to return to therapy for occasional orthotic adjustments.

Conservative Management of Low Radial Nerve Injuries (Posterior Interosseous Nerve Syndrome)

In the forearm, about the level of the radial head, the radial nerve divides into a superficial sensory branch and a motor branch, the

♡ Tips from the Field

Orthotic Options for High Radial Nerve Palsy

- A wrist immobilization orthosis with the wrist in a functional position of 30°- extension is an option. The client can usually extend the fingers to release an object using hand intrinsic muscles and wrist flexion. Some of the advantages of using this type of orthotic include cosmetic reasons. A wrist cock up orthosis is less conspicuous than a dynamic orthosis, and it is more comfortable without problems of an outrigger bulk when used during sleep. Furthermore, this orthosis is less costly and easy to take on and off. It is a reasonable choice for some patients when the injury is on the non-dominant side.[27]

- A low profile mobilization orthosis that dynamically holds the MP joints in extension but allows for full digit flexion can be used to substitute for absent muscle power and promote functional use of the injured hand, leaving the palmar surface of the injured hand free for sensory input (Fig. 24-7).

- An advantage of a Colditz tenodesis mobilization splint is that the wrist is not immobilized, but rather it moves with the natural tenodesis effect. The potential disadvantages include the expense and time to fabricate[28] (Fig. 24-8).

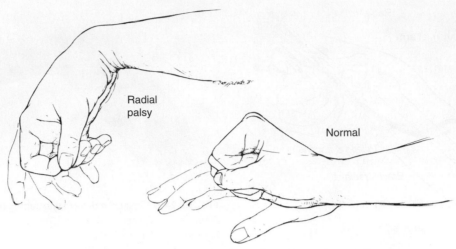

FIGURE 24-7 Radial nerve palsy results in a loss of normal tenodysis action.

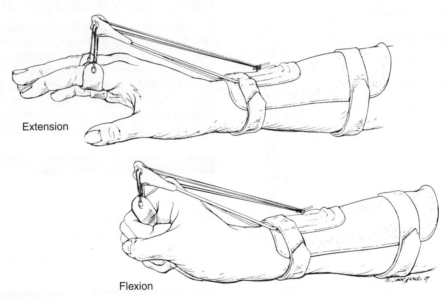

FIGURE 24-8 A, Low profile radial nerve palsy orthotic. **B,** Colditz radial nerve palsy splint. (Both from Colditz
J: Splinting for radial nerve palsy. *J Hand Ther* 1:19, 1987.)

posterior interosseous nerve (PIN). This motor nerve branch of the radial nerve courses deep beneath the supinator muscle, traveling through the radial tunnel of the forearm. This tunnel is about 3 to 4 fingers' breadth in length, lying along the anterior aspect of the proximal radius. An injury to this motor branch will spare the radial wrist extensors, which receive their innervation above the level of the elbow joint. Injuries to the nerve at this level can occur secondary to compression of the nerve between the humeral and ulnar heads of the supinator muscle (called the *arcade of Frohse*), from radial head fracture-dislocations, tumors, or from a history of repetitive and strenuous pronation and supination. In the latter cases, men are affected twice as often as women, and the dominant arm is involved twice as often as the non-dominant arm.[29]

The clinical presentation of PIN syndrome is as follows: paralysis or paresis (weakness) of ulnar wrist extension, digit extension and thumb extension and radial abduction. Since the terminal, branch of the PIN supplies pain and proprioception fibers to the dorsum of the wrist, clients may also present with vague dorsal wrist pain. Patients with PIN syndrome typically present with dropped fingers and thumb, secondary to weakness or paralysis of

the supinator, extensor carpi ulnaris (ECU), and extrinsic digital extensors. Since the function of the extensor carpi radialis longus (ECRL) is preserved, the wrist is able to extend and radially deviate even in cases of severe neuropathy. There may be vague dorsal wrist pain, and the electromyogram (EMG) is usually positive for nerve compression at the radial tunnel.

♡ *Tips from the Field*

Orthotic Options for Pin, Low Radial Nerve Palsy

Combined positions of elbow flexion, supination, and wrist extension place the least stress and strain on the radial tunnel.[30] However, this position is not well-tolerated by patients, because it seriously limits activities of daily living (ADLs) and instrumental activities of daily living (IADL) tasks. Patients may be more comfortable using a wrist brace that positions the wrist in extension and avoiding prolonged positions of pronation with elbow extension and wrist flexion during daily and work tasks to reduce strain on the radial nerve. Patient education is the key to compliance with this approach.

Conservative Management of Low Radial Nerve Injuries (Radial Tunnel Syndrome)

Radial tunnel syndrome (RTS) is a condition caused by compression of the radial nerve in the proximal forearm.[19] The clinical picture is one of dull aching or burning pain along the lateral forearm musculature rather than one of frank muscle weakness and/or sensory loss. Etiology is most often compression of the nerve at the fibrous edge of the supinator muscle from an external source (such as, counterforce bracing used to treat lateral epicondilitis) or from repetitive forceful supination with concurrent wrist extension.

Symptoms may be confused with but can coexist with lateral epicondylosis. Lateral epicondylosis is a degenerative process that primarily involves the tendinous origin of the extensor carpi radialis brevis (ECRB). With lateral epicondylosis, there is pain localized over, or just distal to, the lateral epicondyle. This pain is provoked by palpation over the lateral epicondyle area and/or by resisting wrist extension. With RTS, placing the wrist in flexion and resisting long finger extension will provoke symptoms of dull pain or aching and burning in the lateral forearm. Symptoms may also be reproduced when forearm supination is resisted while the elbow is extended. Pain associated with RTS is located 3 to 4 cm distal to the lateral epicondyle in the area of the mobile wad and radial tunnel. Compression and symptoms are aggravated by placing traction on the nerve—extending the elbow, pronating the forearm, and flexing the wrist.

◎ Clinical Pearl

RTS and PIN are both compressions of the radial nerve at the radial tunnel; however, clinical presentations are very different. Patients with RTS present with mobile wad and lateral forearm pain without motor involvement. Dang, et al.[19] suggests that the difference may be attributed to a difference in the degree of compression of the nerve. There is a negative EMG result with RTS.

♡ Tips from the Field

Orthotic Options for Radial Tunnel Syndrome

As with PIN syndrome, treatment involves rest, splinting, activity modification, gentle stretching/nerve sliding, and anti-inflammatory medications. If splinting the elbow and forearm/wrist, fabricate a long arm orthosis with the wrist in extension, elbow in flexion, and forearm in supination to neutral rotation; this is the classic position recommended in our literature. However, most people will not wear a long arm orthosis that limits elbow and forearm use during the day; therefore, consider recommending a wrist immobilizing orthosis for waking hours.

➣ Precautions and Concerns

If patient has RTS, do *not* use elbow clasp splints or straps, and be cautious with compression sleeves for the elbow. Elbow clasp splints can further compress the radial nerve at the radial tunnel.

Conservative Management of Low Radial Nerve Injuries (Superficial Sensory Branch of Radial Nerve [Dorsal Radial Sensory Nerve] or Wartenburg's Syndrome)

The dorsal radial sensory nerve (DRSN) courses distally into the forearm deep to the BR muscle. At approximately 9 cm proximal to the radial styloid, the DSRN becomes subcutaneous, traveling between the BR and ECRL tendons. The DRSN compression can occur at two potential sites. The greatest risk for compression is at the posterior border of the BR, because the nerve transitions from a deep to a subcutaneous structure. When the DRSN emerges between the tendons of the BR and ECRL, pronation of the forearm causes these two tendons to come together, thus, compressing the nerve. Repetitive pronation-supination results in scissoring of the tendons over the DRSN. The other site of compression is where the DRSN runs in the subcutaneous tissue in the distal forearm. Compression occurs at this site secondary to the lack of excursion of the nerve during repetitive wrist flexion and ulnar deviation. This low radial nerve lesion presents with pain and dysesthesia on the dorsal radial forearm emanating to the dorsal thumb and index finger.[19]

♡ Tips from the Field

Orthotic Options for Dorsal Radial Sensory Nerve Compression

Although spontaneous resolution is common, an orthosis may be helpful. A volar forearm-based thumb orthosis maintaining the wrist in extension and thumb in retroposition, may minimize tension on the DRSN.

◎ Clinical Pearl

Monitor the position of the distal forearm strap and consider cutting out the radial styloid area (Figure 24-9).

Postoperative Management Following Radial Nerve Laceration and Repair above the Elbow, Below the Axilla

Consider the following guidelines:[31,32]

- Fit your patient with a static elbow orthosis, positioning the elbow in 90° to 100° of flexion and the forearm in neutral, wrist in extension, and MP joints in 10° to 20° of flexion. (The collateral ligaments of the MP joints are slack when these joints are held in 0° extension; therefore, it is necessary to place the joints in some degree of flexion to mitigate joint capsule tightness.)
- At 4 weeks, extend the elbow to 60° of extension.
- At 5 weeks, extend the elbow to 30° of extension.
- At 6 weeks, discontinue use of the orthosis altogether to allow full elbow extension. Initiate AROM and PROM exercises to the elbow, forearm, wrist, and hand. At this time, fabricate a radial nerve palsy orthosis to facilitate functional grasp and release and to prevent adverse tissue changes, including wrist joint contractures and soft tissue adaptive shortening.
- Have the patient continue using the radial nerve palsy orthosis until adequate motor return occurs or tendon transfers are done.

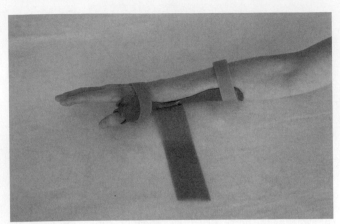

FIGURE 24-9 Orthotic thumb spica design that leaves radial styloid and distal radial sensory nerve free from external compression. (Used with permission of Anne Moscony)

Postoperative Management Following Radial Nerve Laceration and Repair at the Elbow or Forearm

Consider the following guidelines:[31,32]

- Within the first or second postoperative week, fabricate a static wrist extension orthosis positioning the wrist in 30° of extension to protect the nerve repair juncture. Dynamic extension outriggers can be fabricated for the digit MP joints and for thumb extension. Initiate AROM exercises for the digits.
- At 4 weeks postoperatively, adjust the wrist immobilization orthosis to 10° to 20° of extension.
- In the fifth week postoperatively, have the client begin active and active assistive range of motion (AAROM) exercises. The wrist should continue to be splinted between exercise sessions until there is adequate wrist extensor muscle strength to maintain the wrist in extension against gravity.

Postoperative Management Following Decompression for Radial Nerve Injuries

Compression resulting in motor weakness that does not improve with several months of splinting, anti-inflammatory medications, and activity modification is usually treated with surgical decompression. Results after radial nerve decompression are not as favorable as those following CTR or cubital tunnel release.[19,33]

The optimal duration and efficacy of conservative regimens versus surgical interventions has not been determined.[19] The general consensus at this time is that if there is no improvement in motor dysfunction by approximately 3 months, spontaneous recovery is not likely and surgery is recommended.

Decompression of the posterior interosseous branch of the radial nerve (PIN) at the level of the ligament of Frohse, or deep to the superficial head of the supinator, has been reported to have good results[19] with up to 75% to 94% of patients showing good to excellent results with full motor recovery. The recovery period is approximately 9 months if the diagnosis is correct with motor return occurring within 6 months on average, and with wrist pain taking up to 9 months to abate.

A dynamic wrist and MP joint extension orthotic, as described earlier, can facilitate function while the patient awaits motor return.

Educating your patient to avoid repetitive gripping and forearm rotation tasks is necessary to prevent increased nerve tension and compression following surgical release of the PIN.

Following decompression of the radial tunnel, the use of an orthosis to support the wrist varies among surgeons. Given the amount of dissection, an over-the-counter wrist cock up splint or a long arm orthosis may be helpful for pain management when used intermittently within the first 10 to 14 days postoperative. Dang and Rodner reviewed current relevant literature in 2009 and reported that, surgical decompression had good results in 86% of patients with a single diagnosis of RTS, but it was only 40% successful in patients with concomitant tennis elbow.[19] Full AROM is encouraged within the first postoperative week; however, maximum recovery may take 3 to 4 months.

Instruct the patient to avoid full forearm pronation, elbow extension, and wrist flexion as this position places excessive tension on the radial nerve and surrounding soft tissue.

Decompression of the DRSN is performed to free the nerve from any sites of compression if conservative management is not successful. If an orthosis is ordered, the wrist should be splinted in neutral and the thumb in radial abduction. Cut out the radial border at the distal wrist level to prevent irritation from the rigid material at the scar site. Use soft strap material at the distal wrist. Patients should be encouraged to begin AROM of the fingers, wrist, and elbow and desensitization may be necessary to address hypersensitivity at the decompression site.

Median Nerve

Anatomy and Common Sites of Compression

Table 24-8 provides a summary of median nerve anatomy, common lesion sites, and typical deficits/deformities associated with median nerve lesions.[35-37]

The median nerve arises from the lateral and medial cords of the brachial plexus (Fig. 24-10). It runs distally in the anteromedial compartment of the arm. In the cubital fossa of the anterior elbow and in the forearm, the median nerve lies medial to the brachial artery. Just distal to the elbow joint, the median nerve passes below the bicipital aponeurosis and between the two heads of the pronator teres. The median nerve gives off a purely motor branch, the anterior interosseous nerve (AIN), to the flexor pollicis longus (FPL), to the flexor digitorum profundus (FDP) tendon, to the index finger, and to the pronator quadratus.

The main trunk of the median nerve traverses under the fibrous origin of the flexor digitorum superficialis (FDS) and then emerges to become a more superficial structure in the distal forearm. Just proximal to the wrist, the palmar cutaneous (or sensory) branch arises and runs superficial to the flexor retinaculum to innervate the midpalm. The terminal portion of this nerve, along with the nine extrinsic digit flexor tendons, runs under the flexor retinaculum, and then through the carpal tunnel and under its roof, the volar carpal ligament.

TABLE 24-8	Summary of Median Nerve
Sensation, includes the palmar cutaneous branch	Volar hand: Thumb, index, long, radial aspect of ring, volar radial palm, dorsal 20% to 35% of terminal dorsal thumb, index, long, and radial ring rays
Motor	*Innervations proximal to distal in this order:* Pronator teres, flexor carpi radialis, palmaris longus, FDS, radial two FDP, FPL, pronator quadratus, abductor pollicis brevis, FPB (superficial head), opponens pollicus, index lumbrical, and middle digit lumbrical
Function	The median nerve allows for forearm pronation; thumb, index, and long digit flexion; and thenar palmar abduction and opposition. These movements combine to position the hand for grasping (as a piece of candy off the table, for example) and allow for precision pinch. The sensory contribution of the median nerve is huge; without intact sensation along the radial volar aspect of the hand, fine motor coordination is not possible.
Common sites of entrapment/injury	*Pronator syndrome:* Compression at ligament of Struthers, lacertus fibrosis, hypertrophy of pronator teres muscle or at arch of FDS; pain syndrome, sometimes sensory involvement *Anterior interosseous syndrome:* Compression of deep motor branch, paralysis of FPL and FDP to index, sensory symptoms absent, forearm pain present *CTS:* Compression at carpal tunnel resulting from provocative positioning, anatomic anomalies, metabolic conditions, trauma to wrist, space occupying lesions; nocturnal pain and dysesthesia and thenar weakness
Results of lesion	Loss of median nerve integrity at the elbow *(high-level lesion)* results in *ape hand deformity* with loss of precision pinch, loss of thenar opposition, paralysis of FDS and radial two FDP muscles. Forearm pronation is significantly compromised secondary to paralysis of both pronator muscles. Pronation can occur only by abduction of the shoulder and the assistance of gravity. A *lesion to the AIN* results in paralysis of the FPL and index and (sometimes) long digit FDP, making it difficult to make an "O" when attempting to pinch *(Ballentine's sign)*. A more distal *(low-level) lesion* of the nerve, as at the *carpal tunnel*, results in loss of thenar opposition with frequently observable thenar muscle wasting. The thumb lies to the side of the radial palm, and a web space contracture may develop secondary to the unopposed pull of the thumb adductor. The *loss or diminution of sensation* in the tips of the thumb, index, and long digits results in significant functional deficits with regard to all fine motor tasks (such as, writing, winding a watch, tying a shoe, or picking up a small object) particularly if vision is occluded. Clients will complain about nocturnal dysesthesia, dropping objects, diminished fine motor coordination, and debilitating numbness

AIN, Anterior interosseous nerve; *CTS,* carpal tunnel syndrome; *FDP,* flexor digitorum profundus; *FDS,* flexor digitorum superficialis; *FPB,* flexor pollicis brevis; *FPL,* flexor pollicis longus.

> ### Precautions and Concerns

In the shallow carpal tunnel, the nerve sits superficially in relation to these tendons, making it particularly vulnerable to compression in this area because it is sandwiched between these tendons and the volar carpal ligament.

The distal thenar motor branch of the median nerve innervates the thenar intrinsic muscles; the common digital branches innervate the first two lumbrical muscles to the index and long digits. The nerve continues through the palm as sensory branches that primarily provide sensation to the volar thumb, index, long, and medial half of the ring digits.

Conservative Management of High (Proximal) Median Nerve Palsy (Anterior Interosseous Nerve Palsy and Pronator Syndrome)

Compressive neuropathies of the median nerve in the proximal forearm are unusual lesions.[37] The two major compression neuropathies of the proximal median nerve occur with similar symptoms. Both syndromes involve entrapment of the nerve in the proximal forearm, and both are associated with pain in the proximal (volar) forearm that typically increases with activity.

The more proximal entrapment is called **pronator syndrome.** Compression of the median nerve occurs as it passes between the two heads of the pronator teres muscle or under the proximal edge of the FDS arch. Diffuse pain in the medial forearm or distal volar arm along with dysesthesia in the radial three and one-half digits of the hand (similar to sensory alterations commonly seen with CTS) are hallmarks of this syndrome. Symptoms may be provoked by resisting elbow flexion, and may be exacerbated with concurrent resisted forearm pronation. Provocation of symptoms with isolated resistance to the long finger FDS indicates pronator syndrome with the site of compression likely to be at the arch of the FDS. Symptoms have an insidious onset and often are not diagnosed for months to years.[37]

Four possible sites of nerve entrapment are associated with pronator syndrome. The first is at the distal third of the humerus, which is between the ligament of Struthers and the humeral supracondyloid process. The second site is at the elbow joint, because the nerve courses under the lacertus fibrosis. A third potential site of compression is within the pronator teres, especially if that muscle is hypertrophied. The final site occurs at the arch of the FDS, because the median nerve passes deep to it.[37]

Anterior interosseous syndrome is an entrapment neuropathy of the motor branch of the median nerve. This syndrome presents as nonspecific, deep aching pain in the proximal forearm that increases with activity. Usually there are no sensory symptoms. Paralysis of the FPL to the thumb and the FDP to the index and long finger results in collapsed distal interphalangeal (IP) joints when attempting to pinch or make the "okay" sign (called **Ballentine's sign**; Fig. 24-11, *A*). Although paresis of the pronator quadratus may be present, it is difficult to appreciate, given the overlapping action of the stronger pronator teres. Potential sites and sources of compression are the same as with pronator syndrome and include local edema, hypertrophy of the pronator teres, or prolonged and excessive elbow flexion (120° or greater).[40]

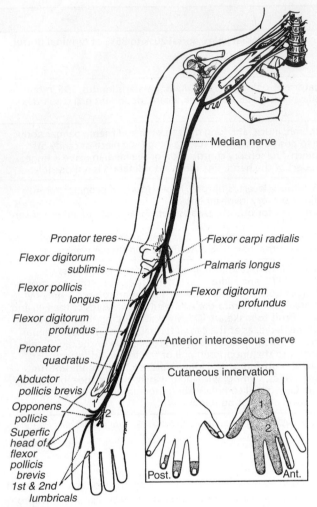

FIGURE 24-10 Schematic of median nerve. (From Stanly BG, Tribuzi SM, editors: *Concepts in hand rehabilitation*, Philadelphia, 1992, FA Davis.)

Evaluation Tips

- Both of these syndromes present with a negative Tinel's sign at the carpal tunnel and symptoms are not provoked with wrist flexion. Nocturnal symptoms, as seen with CTS, do not occur.
- Pronator syndrome typically occurs with diffuse forearm pain aggravated by resisted elbow flexion and forearm pronation and sensory changes along the volar radial three and one-half digits of the hand.
- Anterior interosseous syndrome typically presents with diffuse forearm pain, a positive Ballentine's sign with tip pinch, and no sensory changes.

Timelines and Healing

Many clients have vague symptoms for months or even years before a definitive diagnosis is made. This is frustrating for the client and may require serial clinical examinations and repeat electrodiagnostic studies to confirm anterior interosseous syndrome or pronator syndrome. Furthermore, prolonged compression of the median nerve indicates a poor prognosis for full recovery, even following surgical decompression.[35,37,40]

Ideally, clients with proximal median nerve entrapment neuropathies are evaluated and are given a home exercise program and a short course of in-clinic pain management, followed by interim therapy visits every 2 to 4 weeks until resolution of symptoms occurs. Insurance and financial constraints may necessitate altering this timeline.

♡ Tips from the Field

Orthotic Options for High (Proximal) Median Nerve Injuries

Most patients with anterior interosseous syndrome or pronator syndrome improve with conservative management of rest, splinting, and anti-inflammatory medications.[37,40]

- Orthotics for anterior interosseous syndrome involve stabilizing the IP joint of the thumb, and often the index finger, using custom tip orthoses or commercially available figure-eight splints to enhance function/tip pinch with activities, such as holding a pen for writing (see Fig 24-11, *B*).

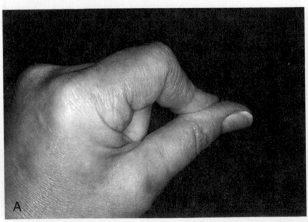
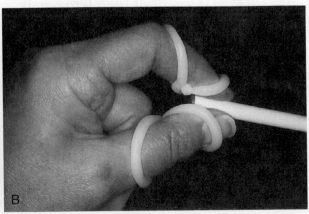

FIGURE 24-11   A, Anterior interosseous palsy. **B,** Tip splinting for anterior interosseous palsy. (From Mackin EJ, Callahan AD, Skirven TM, editors: *Rehabilitation of the hand and upper extremity*, ed 5, St Louis, 2002, Mosby.)

- Conservative management for pronator syndrome includes fabricating an orthosis to rest the irritated tissues with instructions to use it as much as possible over the initial 2 to 3 weeks, removing it for hygiene and gentle AROM only.
- If compression is at the fibrous arch of the heads of the FDS (resistance to FDS of the long finger aggravates symptoms), fabricate a resting hand orthosis with the forearm included.
- If compression is at the pronator teres, pain/parasthesias will be aggravated by resistance to forearm pronation and will be enhanced as the elbow is extended. In this case, fabricate an orthosis with the forearm in neutral, the wrist in neutral, and the elbow in flexion. This long arm orthosis will rest the elbow at 90° to 100° of flexion.
- If symptoms are aggravated by resisted flexion of elbow with forearm in full supination, compression is likely at the lacertus fibrosus, and the orthosis should limit elbow flexion and forearm supination. Consider an anterior long arm orthosis with the forearm neutral rotation, using the lightest thermoplastic material option possible.

Conservative Management of Low (Distal) Median Nerve Palsy (Carpal Tunnel Syndrome)

CTS is the most common nerve entrapment in the UE with a 1% to 3% incidence rate in the general population.[38,49] Etiology is typically idiopathic; however, pathology is clearly related to increased pressure in the carpal tunnel. Symptoms of CTS are well known—paresthesias in the thumb index and middle fingers, loss of dexterity, exacerbation of symptoms at night, worsened by repetitive forceful hand motion, and an improvement in symptoms after shaking or straightening the affected hand.

Evaluation Tips

Discriminating between CTS and pronator syndrome can be difficult, because both of these syndromes present with pain in the volar wrist and forearm, and numbness or parathesias in the median nerve-innervated radial 3½ digits. The palmar cutaneous branch of the median nerve arises 4 to 5 cm proximal to the transverse carpal ligament. This branch of the median nerve provides the sensory input from the mid-volar and radial palm. Therefore, a patient presenting with CTS-like symptoms in addition to decreased sensation over the mid-volar palm and the thenar eminence should be evaluated for a more proximal lesion, such as pronator syndrome. Likewise, individuals with pronator syndrome should not have a Tinel sign over the wrist, nor should their symptoms be provoked with wrist flexion.[37]

Pregnancy-induced CTS is relatively rare and is usually diagnosed in the third trimester. Symptoms typically respond to conservative treatment of orthotics (with or without steroid injection) and/or resolve postpartum.[38]

♥ Tips from the Field

Orthotic Options for Low (Distal) Median Nerve Palsy

Conservative management for mild CTS has been well-documented, including orthotics to decrease carpal tunnel pressure by positioning the wrist in neutral. Evans describes the position of 2° of wrist flexion and 3° of ulnar deviation as the position where carpal tunnel pressure is optimally minimized. Splinting is most effective if utilized within 3 months of symptom onset.[16] A custom-made orthosis or an over-the-counter splint should be used at night. Bracing the wrist during the day is only necessary to control work postures that worsen carpal tunnel pressure.

Recent studies have suggested a role for the lumbrical muscles in CTS, because these muscles are intermittent space-occupying structures within the carpal tunnel. The lumbrical muscles are a unique group of intrinsic muscles of the hand that originate on the tendons of the FDP. When our fingers are in extension, these lumbrical muscles sit distal to the transverse carpal tunnel ligament. When the fingers flex, the FDP tendons glide through the carpal tunnel, taking their associated lumbrical muscles with them. Lumbrical muscles glide approximately 3 cm during full fisting and will lie within the carpal canal during fisting, thus increasing the carpal tunnel contents and possibly contributing to median nerve compression. This is further exacerbated with the wrist positioned in flexion. **Berger's test** can be used to identify possible lumbrical contribution to CTS. Have the patient hold a full fist position with the wrist in neutral for 30 to 40 seconds. This creates lumbrical incursion into the carpal canal. The test is positive if pain and paresthesias occur within 30 to 40 seconds. If Berger's test is positive, Evans suggests that an MP flexion block be added to the traditional wrist orthosis. This orthosis would position the wrist in neutral and block the MP joints at 20° to 40° of flexion to prevent lumbrical migration into the carpal tunnel during grasp or fisting.[16]

Baker, et al.[22] evaluated the effectiveness of a custom-made lumbrical block carpal tunnel orthosis with traditional wrist bracing and a home program of stretches. They concluded that traditional wrist splinting combined with stretches targeting the lumbrical muscles was a more effective long-term treatment for functional gains than splinting or stretches alone in patients with mild to moderate CTS[22] (Fig. 24-12).

( ) *What to Say to Clients*

About Carpal Tunnel Syndrome

"You have an injury to the median nerve, which is one of the nerves of your wrist and hand. As this nerve travels down your arm and enters into your hand, it has to travel through a tight space called the *carpal tunnel*. There are other structures that also run through this space. If for some reason, the space becomes congested (as by swelling) or if the space becomes smaller (as can happen following bony changes from arthritis), the carpal tunnel nerve may get pinched or squished in this tight area. If you bend or straighten your wrist frequently, or if you hold your wrist in a stretched extended or bent position, you may be further aggravating this nerve."

- Try to keep your wrist in a neutral position with daily activities.
- Avoid sustained pinch or gripping, particularly prolonged pinching when your wrist is in a flexed or bent posture.
- Avoid repetitive overuse of the wrist in activity
- Avoid positioning your wrist in a bent or flexed posture (the fetal position) when sleeping. Use your orthosis at night to help keep your wrist in the safe, neutral position.
- Whenever possible, use tools in the kitchen, the workplace, the garden, and so on, that have larger grips contoured to the

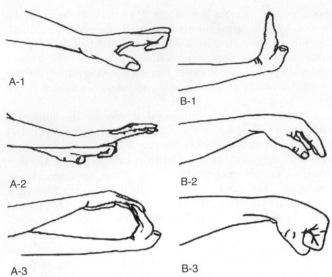

A-1
B-1
A-2
B-2
A-3
B-3

FIGURE 24-12 Lumbrical stretches (A-1) Rest the hand, palm down on the thigh with the PIP and DIP joints fully flexed. (A-2) The opposite hand then presses downward over the MCP joints. (A-3) The wrist, MCP, PIP and DIP joints are then pulled into maximal extension with the opposite hand. (B-1) Hold a position of composite wrist and finger extension (B-2) followed by a 5 second rest period, (B-3) then place hand into composite wrist and digit flexion, followed by another 5 second rest period. (From Baker et al: The comparative effectiveness of combined lumbrical muscle splints and stretches on symptoms and function in carpal tunnel syndrome. *Arch Phys Med Rehabil 93:1-10, 2012.*)

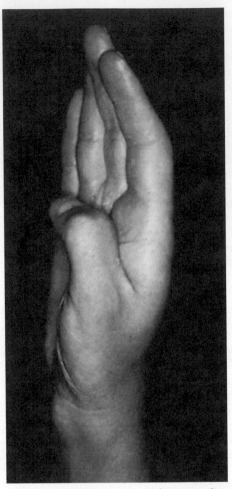

FIGURE 24-13 Ape hand deformity secondary to median nerve palsy. (From Mackin EJ, Callahan AD, Skirven TM, editors: *Rehabilitation of the hand and upper extremity,* ed 5, St Louis, 2002, Mosby.)

arches of your hand. Your hand should easily close around the handle. You don't want one that is too big or too small for your hand. The grip handle can be adjusted with dense foam to increase the diameter (if necessary) and to pad the surface somewhat so that it is easier on the structures, like your nerve, that lie underneath the skin of your hand.

- Look at a workstation design handout to figure out how to set up your home office or your work office. These ergonomic workstation designs are available and free on the Internet.

Postoperative Management Following High (Proximal) Median Nerve Lacerations and Repairs—Elbow to Wrist Level

Severance of the median nerve in the forearm typically occurs from knife or glass lacerations. The clinical presentation is one of sensory and motor involvement with specific deficits depending on the site of injury. Loss of median nerve integrity at the elbow or proximal forearm (high-level lesion) results in an **ape hand deformit**y (Fig. 24-13 with loss of precision pinch, loss of thenar opposition, and paralysis of the FDS and radial two FDP muscles and their corresponding two lumbrical muscles. The thenar eminence is atrophied with the thumb lying to the side of the palm. Loss of ability to oppose and palmarly abduct the thumb occurs. Index finger metacarpal and proximal interphalangeal (PIP) joint flexion is lost, as is thumb IP joint flexion. Forearm pronation is significantly compromised because of paralysis of the pronator teres and the pronator quadratus. Some forearm pronation can occur however, with the assistance of gravity when the shoulder is

abducted slightly. Sensory loss typically includes the radial three and one-half digits and the radial volar palm.

Timelines and Healing Following Surgical Repair

Consider the following guidelines:[32]

- Remove the bulky compressive dressing, and apply a light compressive dressing for edema control.
- Fabricate a custom-made dorsal wrist blocking orthosis with the wrist in approximately 30° of palmar flexion but not more than 45° of palmar flexion. The amount of wrist flexion is predicated upon the amount of tension at the nerve repair site. Replicate the wrist position of the postoperative cast if the surgeon is not immediately available to give you guidelines.
- Have the client wear the orthosis continuously for 4 to 6 weeks except for protective skin care. Hygiene should occur with the orthosis on.
- Begin AROM and PROM of the digits and thumb; do ten repetitions every waking hour within the brace. Instruct the client in active tendon glide exercises so that the extrinsic flexor tendons glide separately and do not become adherent at the area of surgical repair.[57] (Fig. 24-14 depicts tendon glide exercises.)
- Scar massage and scar mobilization techniques may begin 24 to 48 hours after sutures are removed but should be gentle initially.

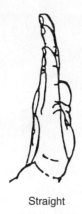
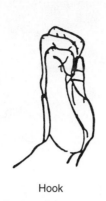
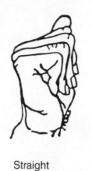
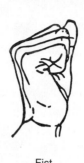

| Straight | Hook | Straight | Fist |

FIGURE 24-14 Tendon glide exercises. (From Mackin EJ, Callahan AD, editors: *Hand clinics: frontiers in hand rehab*, Philadelphia, 1991, WB Saunders.)

- At 4 weeks postoperatively, adjust the dorsal wrist blocking orthosis to 20° of palmar flexion.
- At 5 weeks postoperatively, adjust the dorsal wrist blocking orthosis to 0° to 10° of palmar flexion.
- By 6 weeks postoperatively, discontinue use of the dorsal wrist blocking orthosis and initiate progressive strengthening for the hand and wrist. Begin by having the client incorporate the postoperative hand into daily activity use. Strengthening can be as simple as setting a table, tying a shoe, or writing a grocery list.
- By 8 weeks postoperatively, the client can begin a work rehabilitation program designed to address residual strength and coordination deficits that adversely affect return to work.

> ◎ **Clinical Pearl**
>
> In the adult client with a high median or ulnar nerve injury, return of normal motor and sensory function is rare.[34] Therefore, splinting to maintain PROM may be necessary in preparation for tendon transfers.

Postoperative Management Following Laceration of the Median Nerve at the Wrist

Typically, an isolated laceration and repair of the median nerve at the wrist will require a dorsal-block wrist splint protection to be worn for a period of 3 to 6 weeks. An isolated median nerve laceration at the forearm or wrist is rare. More commonly, concurrent flexor tendon injuries occur. In this situation, you will need to address postoperative protocols for flexor tendon repairs as well as for the nerve repair.[32,39]

An isolated laceration of the median nerve at the wrist presents with paralysis of the intrinsic thenar muscles that allow for opposition and palmar abduction of the thumb. Wasting of the thenar eminence may develop, and the thumb will lie to the side of the radial palm because of the unopposed pull of the thenar adductor pollicus. Loss of sensation to the volar thumb, index, and long tips (and radial half of the ring finger) results in loss of fine motor coordination and an increased risk for soft tissue injuries in this area, such as burns or lacerations, especially during prehension tasks where vision is occluded.

Client education is critical regarding sensory impairment. Teach the client protective sensation techniques, including visually monitoring all activities performed with the insensate hand until there is adequate protective sensory return.

> ▷ **Precautions and Concerns**

With a high or low median nerve injury, thenar web space or adduction contractures of the thumb are the most common and preventable deformity that should be addressed by proactive orthotic use.

A rigid hand-based or short opponens orthotic that positions the thumb in palmar abduction and opposition should be fabricated and provided (Fig. 24-15). An orthosis made of neoprene or leather can be used to hold the thumb in a stable and opposed, if not fully abducted, position during the day if function is retarded with a rigid orthosis. This semi-rigid orthosis can be fabricated or purchased from one of the commercial splint catalogs. The advantage to this type of orthosis is that it does not block the index finger MP joint from flexion, thereby diminishing the possibility of an extension contracture developing at that joint.

Postoperative Management for Decompression of High Median Nerve Injuries (Anterior Interosseous Nerve or Posterior Interosseous Nerve Syndrome)

Surgical decompression of the median nerve to address pronator syndrome is uncommon and occurs only after 2 to 3 months of conservative measures have failed to provide relief.[33,37] When surgery is necessary, the success rate in the treatment of pronator syndrome approaches 90%.[37] Early active motion is recommended after this surgery.

> ▷ **Precautions and Concerns**

If the pronator teres muscle is released and reattached, avoid active pronation and end range supination for 4 to 6 weeks.

Surgical decompression for AIN syndrome is also rarely performed. There is a paucity of literature supporting the appropriate duration of conservative treatment for this condition. Spontaneous full recovery has been reported even as long as 12 to 18 months after onset of symptoms. Etiology and pathophysiology for AIN palsy is not clearly understood. Compression is a theory based upon analogy with carpal and cubital tunnel syndrome. Resolution of weakness is atypical for idiopathic compressive neuropathies.[37] If surgery is performed, the patient is encouraged to begin AROM immediately.

Orthoses are used to improve fine motor function, such as the Oval-8 orthosis to stabilize the thumb and index for tip pinch.

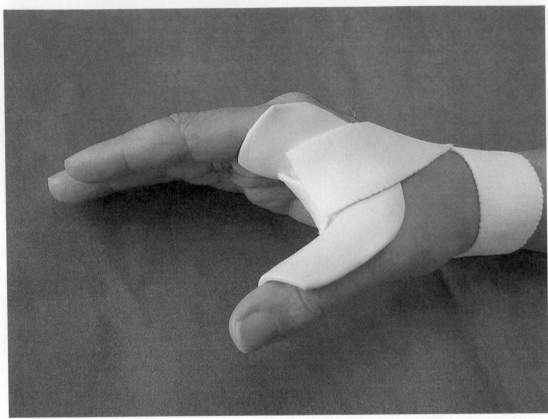

FIGURE 24-15 Static thenar web spacer splint to prevent adduction contracture following median nerve palsy. (From Mackin EJ, Callahan AD, Skirven TM, editors: *Rehabilitation of the hand and upper extremity,* ed 5, St Louis, 2002, Mosby.)

Exercises should focus on gradually restoring full elbow extension and supination during the first 2 weeks after surgery.

Postoperative Management for Decompression of Low Median Nerve Injuries (Carpal Tunnel Release)

If CTS is moderate to severe with muscle atrophy or significant sensory impairment, conservative management has not been proven to be successful, and surgical decompression has been shown to be more cost effective than orthotic positioning.[38,39] The procedure involves transection of the transverse carpal ligament (called a *carpal tunnel release [CTR]*). CTR is estimated to be among the ten most commonly performed operations in the United States.[38] Traditional open CTR surgery or a less invasive endoscopic release may be performed. The latter technique has the advantage of less postoperative pain, a quicker recovery of strength, and faster return-to-work time. However, endoscopic release also is associated with increased complications including accidental severance of or injury to the ulnar nerve, the palmar cutaneous branch of the median nerve, the ulnar artery, and the flexor tendons. Incomplete release of the transverse carpal ligament with consequent reoccurrence of CTS following surgery is another complication of this surgical method.

The traditional open CTR is always performed if the surgeon suspects that a flexor tenosynovectomy or a neurolysis may be needed. The goal of the tenosynovectomy is to remove the diseased synovial tissue so that there will be better gliding between the tendons and the nerve and to decompress the nerve further within the hand. A neurolysis is performed to resect constricting scar tissue

that is affecting the circulation within the nerve adversely. In either of these cases, the therapist will see a larger scar postoperatively.

♡ Tips from the Field

Postoperative Management of Carpal Tunnel Release

When surgery is uncomplicated after a short incision CTR, many patients do not need therapy. When therapy is needed, it is often a minimal program with emphasis on the home program. Skilled therapeutic intervention should be considered for the following:

- Wrist control positioning to decrease incisional tension and to prevent overuse and inflammation for 2 to 3 weeks postoperative. The wrist should be positioned in about 25° of extension, because this prevents wound site tension.[16]
- Patients with diabetes or other systemic illnesses may need skilled therapy intervention to address wound care to promote uneventful healing. These clients are at a higher risk for infections or wound dehiscing.
- Modalities are helpful in addressing scar tenderness. Scar tenderness is the most common problem seen postoperatively following an open CTR.[16]
- **Pillar pain,** or pain on either side of the CTR incision, is a normal postoperative occurrence. This pain can be debilitating, making it difficult to grip or perform palmar weight-bearing activities. Return to work is often delayed because of pillar pain.[16] The exact cause of pillar pain is unknown; the various theories suggest that it is ligamentous or muscular in

TABLE 24-9 Summary of Ulnar Nerve

Sensation:Dorsal cutaneous branch and superficial sensory branch	Ulnar/medial side of palm (both volar and dorsal); entire fifth digit and ulnar aspect of fourth digit (both volar and dorsal)
Motor	*Innervations, proximal to distal:* FCU, FDP to digits 4 and 5, abductor digiti minimi, opponens digiti minimi, FDM, fourth and third lumbrical muscles, three palmar interossei muscles and four dorsal interossei muscles, deep head of the FPB, and adductor pollicis
Function	The ulnar nerve allows for simultaneous strong wrist flexion and ulnar deviation, as well as power grip via full flexion of the ulnar two digits. This is necessary for tasks, such as swinging a golf club or a hammer. Ulnar nerve integrity is necessary to allow for powerful tip and lateral or key pinch, because the adductor pollicis and first dorsal interossei assist in stabilizing the thumb and index during pinching. The hypothenar muscles and the interossei muscles allow the hand to powerfully cup an object, such as a doorknob or a basketball.
Common sites of entrapment/injury	*Cubital tunnel syndrome:* Causes include direct compressive trauma, repetitive or sustained elbow flexion, cubitus valgus deformities, second-degree supracondylar fractures, disease processes; symptoms include pain, dysesthesia, and motor weakness *Guyon's canal compression:* Causes include pisiform or hook of hamate fractures, arthritis, thrombus, and mass/ganglion; symptoms include pain, intrinsic muscle weakness, and dyesthesia
Results of lesion	Motor ulnar palsy has significant functional consequences. The balance between extrinsic and intrinsic muscles is lost, secondary to paresis of most of the intrinsic muscles of the hand. This results in a flattening of the normal arches of the hand. Low-level lesions, as at the wrist, produce the *classic claw deformity* of the digits with hyperextension of the MP joints and flexion of the IP joints. (This posture is less noticeable in the index and long digits because the lateral two lumbrical muscles, which serve to flex the MP joints, remain innervated by the median nerve.) There is wasting of the interosseous muscles, of the thenar adductor, and of the hypothenar eminence. Paralysis of the thenar adductor causes *significant loss of pinch strength.* If the client attempts to pinch, the distal phalanx typically assumes a position of flexion *(Froment's sign),* and the proximal phalanx may hyperextend *(Jeanne's sign)* as the unimpaired FPL and the extensor pollicis brevis attempt to stabilize the thumb. High-level lesions, for example lesions to the nerve proximal to the innervation of the FCU, result in all of the aforementioned deficits and loss of simultaneous wrist flexion and ulnar deviation. Typically a client complains about significant loss of grip strength (that is, for swinging a golf club or a hammer), difficulty with gross grasp (that is, unable to effectively grasp a doorknob), and loss of ability to perform such in-hand manipulation tasks, such as shaking dice or moving coins into position to place into a slot. The client may report difficulty with lateral pinch (that is, unable to turn a key in the ignition) and difficulty donning gloves and typing (resulting from paresis of the interossei). Sensory loss, although problematic, is not as severely disabling as with the median nerve. Clients tend to complain of difficulty gauging the force needed to hold an object (such as a glass).

FCU, Flexor carpi ulnaris; *FDM,* flexor digiti minimi; *FDP,* flexor digitorum profundus; *FPB,* flexor pollicis brevis; *FPL,* flexor pollicis longus; *IP,* interphalangeal, *MP,* metacarpophalangeal.

origin or a result of an alteration of the carpal arch. Typically, this pain decreases over the first year after surgery. Intervention strategies may include gel pads that are positioned across the irritated site, education about the etiology and prognosis for pain resolution, and manual therapy/scar massage.

Ulnar Nerve

Anatomy and Common Sites of Compression

Table 24-9 gives a summary of ulnar nerve anatomy, common lesion sites, and typical deficits/deformities associated with ulnar nerve lesions.

The ulnar nerve (Fig. 24-16) arises from medial cord of the brachial plexus (C7 to T1 roots). The nerve runs medial to the humeral artery, travels through the medial intermuscular septum, and passes superficially between the medial epicondyle of the humerus and the olecranon at the elbow joint. The ulnar nerve enters the forearm between the two heads of the flexor carpi ulnaris (FCU) and descends within the anteriomedial forearm under the cover of the FCU. In the lower third of the forearm, the ulnar nerve gives off a dorsal cutaneous branch, which supplies the skin

of the ulnar half of the dorsum of the hand. At the wrist, the ulnar nerve sits medially to the ulnar artery and runs with this artery in the osseofibrous carpal canal called **Guyon's canal,** which is a superficial passageway between the pisiform and hamate bones of the carpus. Just distal to the pisiform, the ulnar nerve divides into two terminal branches: the superficial (palmar) cutaneous branch and the deep motor branch. The motor branch winds around the hook of the hamate and innervates the three intrinsic hypothenar muscles (opponens digiti minimi, abductor digiti minimi and flexor digiti minimi), the ulnar two lumbrical muscles, and the three palmar adductors and four dorsal abductors. The ulnar nerve terminates at the adductor pollicis and the deep head of the flexor pollicis brevis (FPB). The sensory branch supplies the skin of the ulnar half of the volar hand and the fifth digit and the medial half of the fourth digits.

Conservative Management of High (Proximal) Ulnar Nerve Compression (Cubital Tunnel Syndrome)

The cubital tunnel is a fibrosseous space bound by the medial epicondyle anteriorly, the ulnohumeral ligament laterally, and the fibrous arcade of the two heads of the FCU posteromedially. A fibrous band extending from the olecranon to the medial

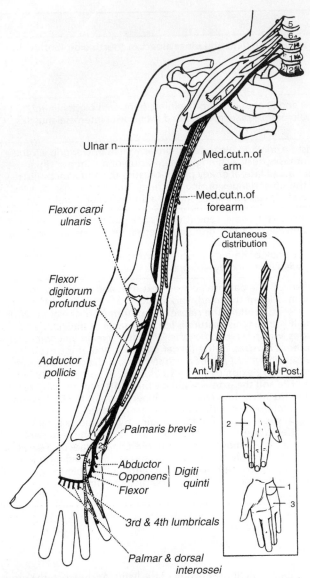

FIGURE 24-16 Schematic of the ulnar nerve. (From Stanly BG, Tribuzi SM, editors: *Concepts in hand rehabilitation*, Philadelphia, 1992, FA Davis.)

epicondyle of the humerus forms the roof of this tunnel. The ulnar nerve can be palpated easily within this superficial tunnel. Compression of the ulnar nerve within this tunnel is called **cubital tunnel syndrome.** It is the second most common peripheral compression neuropathy in the UE.[41]

The elbow has five potential sites for ulnar nerve entrapment. They are under the arcade of Struthers, at the medial intramuscular septum, at the medial epicondyle, within the cubital tunnel itself, and beneath the deep aponeurosis of the FCU.

There are a variety of causes for the development of ulnar nerve compression at the elbow.[41,42,43] Systemic disease (such as, diabetes or chronic alcoholism) may predispose one to compression neuropathies. External sources of compression can include tourniquets or pressure from a hard surface on which the elbow was leaning. Occupational activities (such as, in assembly line work) that requires repetitive or sustained elbow flexion can induce compression. Fractures and dislocations of the medial epicondyle and supracondylar area of the humerus may lead to acute or chronic nerve compression. Elbow deformities, either

congenital or because of a posttraumatic cubitus valgus deformity (essentially, too much lateral angulation of the forearm), can result in nerve compression. Gelberman reported that the most significant ulnar nerve pressure increases occur with flexion of the elbow greater than 100° to 110° degrees. Studies also show that increasing pressure and traction develop in the ulnar nerve with concomitant shoulder abduction.[43-45] Wrist extension, pronation, and radial deviation also increase tension on the ulnar nerve.

The clinical picture depends on the severity and duration of the compression. Cubital tunnel syndrome may present with sensory symptoms and/or motor dysfunction. Pain quality can be sharp or aching in nature. Pain may be located primarily on the medial side of the proximal forearm, or it can be diffuse and radiate proximally and distally in the arm. Paresthesias, decreased sensation in the ulnar digits, a feeling of coldness, muscle weakness, and atrophy may be present along the ulnar nerve distribution. Motor weakness and wasting of the ulnar-innervated intrinsic muscles are present in more severe cases. This muscle involvement results in decreased power grip and decreased pinch strength. In advanced cases, one sees clawing of the ring and small fingers, the resulting paralysis of the ulnar-innervated interossei and lumbrical muscles. When the balance between extrinsic and intrinsic muscles is lost, you can expect to see a flattening of the normal arches of the hand. The ability to cup the hand around an object is lost. The unopposed extensor digitorum communis (EDC) pulls the MP joints into hyperextension, and the IP joints assume a position of flexion. This is called a **claw hand deformity** (Fig.24-17, *A*). (This posture is less noticeable in the index and long digits because the lateral two lumbrical muscles, which serve to flex the MP joints, remain innervated by the median nerve.) If the MP joints are passively held in flexion, the EDC force will be shunted distally, allowing IP joint extension (see Fig. 24-17, *B*).

Wasting of the interosseous muscles, thenar adductor, and hypothenar eminence occurs. The client will lose the ability to abduct and adduct the digits, which are needed for typing or playing the piano. Paralysis of the thenar adductor causes significant loss of pinch strength, especially lateral or key pinch. If the client attempts to perform this type of pinch, the distal phalanx typically assumes a position of flexion (**Froment's sign**) and the proximal phalanx may hyperextend (Jeanne's sign) as the unimpaired FPL and the extensor pollicis brevis attempt to stabilize the thumb.

Evaluation Tips

- Froment's sign: When the client attempts powerful lateral pinch, one sees flexion of the IP joint of the thumb as the FPL attempts to compensate for the paralyzed or weak adductor pollicis and FPB.
- **Wartenberg's sign:** This sign is present if the fifth finger is postured or held in an abducted position from the fourth finger. This indicates interosseous muscle weakness (specifically paresis of the palmar adductor interossei).
- **Elbow flexion test:** This provocative maneuver is designed to reproduce the symptoms of ulnar nerve compression. The elbow is flexed fully, and the wrist is held in neutral for up to 5 minutes. A positive test is a reproduction of symptoms.

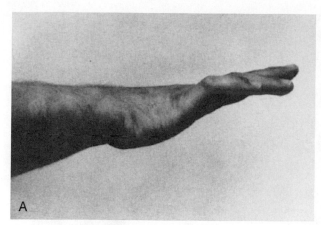

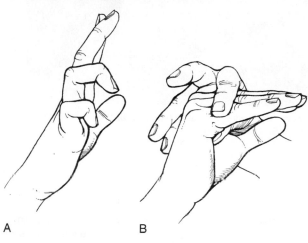

FIGURE 24-17 A, Claw hand deformity secondary to ulnar nerve palsy. **B,** Drawing of the clawing posture of the fourth and fifth digits following ulnar nerve palsy, that results from paralysis of the lumbrical muscles and the unopposed pull of the antagonist muscle, the extensor digitorum communis (EDC). If the metacarpophalangeal joints are passively blocked in flexion, the force of the EDC will translate distally, allowing interphalangeal joint extension. (**A,** From Stanly BG, Tribuzi SM, editors: *Concepts in hand rehabilitation,* Philadelphia, 1992, FA Davis.)

◎ *Clinical Pearl*

The muscle strength of the ring and small finger FDP can be an important diagnostic tool to help determine the level of compression along the ulnar nerve. Normal strength of these muscles indicates a distal or low-level entrapment, most likely at Guyon's canal.

♡ **Tips from the Field**

Orthotic Interventions for Cubital Tunnel Syndrome

- Nocturnal elbow splinting to restrict the elbow from acute elbow flexion is a common intervention.[44] A literature review indicates recommendations for a long arm orthosis, with the elbow positioned at 30° to 70° flexion, forearm and wrist in neutral, and digits free. However, patients have a difficult time complying with use of a rigid elbow orthosis during the day and even sometimes at night while sleeping. If necessary, make a long arm orthosis with the lightest material possible (for example, perforated ³⁄₃₂ inch thermoplastic) on the volar or anterior aspect of the arm/forearm. If the cubital tunnel is particularly sensitive to external compression, such as pressure from the mattress of the bed, consider fabricating this night orthosis over a padded elbow pad or Heelbo.

- There are various commercially available prefabricated splints that patients can purchase to limit elbow flexion when sleeping if a custom-made orthosis is not an option.

- Another economic solution to immobilize the elbow is to use a large bath towel fastened circumferentially around the elbow and secured with duct tape. In a 2006 study, this customized towel splint was shown to decrease symptoms of cubital tunnel as effectively as some of the commercially-available splints.[44]

- During the day, consider use of a prefabricated padded elbow sleeve to prevent external sources from increasing pressure at the cubital tunnel (as when one leans the elbow on the table). Demonstrate elbow pads to clients. If the clinic does not have elbow pads, small pillows lightly ace-wrapped to the volar elbow may substitute.

- Corrective orthotics for intrinsic weakness/claw deformity may be necessary. Also consider an orthotic to stabilize the thumb during lateral pinch tasks, especially if the compression is on the patient's dominant side.

When making an anticlaw orthosis for a hand with ulnar nerve palsy, take care to fabricate the splint so that the MP joints do not buckle or pop out of the splint inadvertently when the client attempts digit extension. Make sure that the palmar bar is form-fitting and wide enough to cover the entire MP joint. Also, make sure the carefully molded dorsal hood of the orthosis extends all the way to the PIP joints, ending at the axis for PIP joint movement. At the same time, the splint should allow full finger flexion of all digits.

◎ *Clinical Pearl*

Those who prefer to sleep on their stomach with their hand above their head may be exacerbating their cubital tunnel issues. Since we cannot comfortably (or easily) control the position of the shoulder when sleeping, look to modifying the position of the elbow, forearm, and wrist. Try to avoid elbow flexion while sleeping.

◎ *Clinical Pearl*

To prevent a fixed claw deformity of the ring and small fingers, a dorsal MP joint blocking orthotic with the MP joints in flexion should be fabricated. This helps to redistribute force *from the EDC to the IP joints* to allow full IP joint extension (see Fig. 24-18).

◖◗ **What to Say to Clients**

About Cubital Tunnel Syndrome

"You have an injury to your nerve at your elbow. You know when you hit your funny bone? It doesn't feel funny. Does it? That's

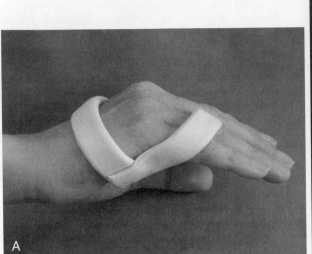

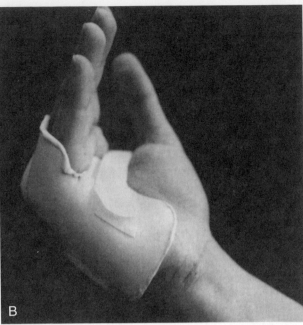

FIGURE 24-18 A, Hand-based splint designed to prevent clawing secondary to ulnar nerve palsy. **B,** Hand-based ulnar nerve anticlaw splint with good volar support. (**A,** From Mackin EJ, Callahan AD, Skirven TM, editors: *Rehabilitation of the hand and upper extremity*, ed 5, St Louis, 2002, Mosby; **B,** From Stanly BG, Tribuzi SM, editors: *Concepts in hand rehabilitation*, Philadelphia, 1992, FA Davis.)

because you're actually hitting your nerve, which is like a live wire close to the surface. You need to be careful and protective of that nerve, especially right now, when it's so sensitive. One way to protect the nerve is to avoid what I call the 'telephone position.' That is the elbow position you assume when you're holding the phone receiver up to your ear. This is a provocative position for your nerve; it doesn't like this posture. If you have to use the phone a lot, you should consider getting a headset so that you can avoid that position. Also, you'll need to avoid that bent elbow position when you sleep. We can talk about some brace options that will help you in avoiding this posture when sleeping."

Conservative Management of Low (Distal) Ulnar Nerve Injuries (Ulnar Tunnel Syndrome or Entrapment at Guyon's Canal)

The ulnar tunnel at the wrist, called *Guyon's canal,* contains the ulnar nerve and artery and fatty tissue. The canal is bounded by the pisiform and tendinous insertion of the FCU ulnarly and the hook of the hamate radially. The roof of the canal is the flexor retinaculum. After giving off the dorsal cutaneous branch about 5 to 6 cm proximal to the wrist, the ulnar nerve enters Guyon's canal medial to the artery. Within the canal, the ulnar nerve divides into two branches: the superficial sensory branch and the deep motor branch.

The most common cause of ulnar nerve compression at the wrist is a space-occupying lesion (such as, a tumor, lipoma, or ganglion) followed by occupational neuritis. Other causes include a pisiform or hook of hamate fracture, pisotriquetral arthritis, thrombus, or vessel anomalies. Smoking or the use of a pneumatic drill can predispose the client to ulnar artery thrombosis.

Hamate fractures and prolonged compression of the hypothenar eminence from activities (such as, holding onto a handlebar of a bike) can contribute to symptoms.[42]

The clinical picture is one of sensory loss and motor paresis affecting the intrinsic ulnar-innervated muscle, including the interossei and the adductor pollicis. Occasionally, the hypothenar opponens, abductor, and flexor digiti minimi (FDM) muscles are spared. The sensory deficit involves the palmar ulnar aspect of the hand, both sides of the little finger, and the ulnar border of the ring finger. The dorsal, ulnar aspect of the hand is spared, because it is supplied by the more proximal dorsal cutaneous branch. Sensory symptoms of pain and paresthesias are usually worse at night and exacerbated by prolonged wrist flexion or extension.

Motor ulnar palsy has significant functional consequences. The balance between extrinsic and intrinsic muscles is lost, a consequence of paralysis of most of the intrinsic muscles of the hand. This produces a flattening of the normal arches of the hand, with loss of the ability to cup the hand around an object, such as a door knob. The unopposed extensor digitorum produces the classic claw hand deformity (described earlier) with hyperextension of the MP joints and flexion of the IP joints. As with high ulnar nerve lesions, there will be wasting of the interosseous muscles, thenar adductor, and hypothenar eminence.

Evaluation Tips

A detailed sensory exam (such as, Semmes-Weinstein monofilament testing) of the volar and dorsal hand assists the clinician in detecting the site of compression.

Sensory loss on the dorsal and volar hand would indicate a lesion proximal to Guyon's canal, whereas intact dorsal hand sensation with diminished sensation of the volar hand and small digit and ulnar half of the ring digit would indicate compression within or just distal to Guyon's canal.

♡ *Tips from the Field*

Orthotic Options for Low (Distal) Ulnar Nerve Palsy (Ulnar Tunnel Syndrome)

Design an ulnar nerve palsy orthosis, also called an *anticlaw orthosis,* to prevent overstretching of the denervated lumbrical muscles and interossei of the ring and small fingers (Fig. 24-18). Instruct the client to remove the orthosis for hygiene only. Continue use of the brace until the muscle imbalance resolves or until tendon transfers are performed. If PIP flexion contractures of the involved digits have developed, a dynamic PIP extension orthosis is needed to address joint contractures before using the static anticlaw orthosis. I have found commercially available spring coil splints effective for mild contractures (about 30° or less).

A padded antivibration glove, a bicycle glove that has a gel pad that crosses the wrist crease, or a custom-made padded glove can be used to protect Guyon's canal from further external irritation during activities, such as riding a mountain bike, using a lawn mower, or grasping hand bike brakes.

Ergonomic tools that are designed to minimize or eliminate stress on the ulnar wrist are good choices for clients with **ulnar tunnel syndrome.** An ergonomic hammer, for example, has a shaft that is designed to conform to the arches of the hand and has the tool head angled so that hammering can occur with the wrist in neutral. Remember that you can use splinting material to create an ergonomic handle for many of the tools that our clients use, if the acquisition of a commercially available option is not available or economically feasible. Educate the client about provocative postures and activities. Tell the client to avoid prolonged positions of simultaneous ulnar deviation and wrist flexion, for example. For the biking enthusiast, suggest foot brakes or having the hand brakes repositioned to avoid this posture. Have the client avoid vibratory input as much as possible, or at least to use dampening splints, such as gel pads or padding on the handles of the equipment (lawn mower, vacuum, motorcycle).

◎ *Clinical Pearl*

If a joint contracture occurs, (for example, because a client did not seek medical intervention immediately), then splinting should focus on restoring maximum joint PROM before addressing orthotic interventions for muscle imbalance.

Postoperative Management Following Ulnar Nerve Laceration and Surgical Repair—Elbow to Wrist Level

Lacerations to the ulnar nerve can occur following injuries from a knife or glass. Typically, these injuries occur with concurrent flexor tendon injuries or ulnar artery injuries. Postoperative protocols need to consider all injured structures.

Consider the following guidelines:
- Fabricate a dorsal blocking orthosis with the wrist in 20° to 30° of flexion, depending on the amount of tension at the nerve repair junction. If in doubt, position the wrist in the same amount of flexion as in the postoperative cast. Incorporate into the splint an MP dorsal block that limits MP joint extension to 45°. This further minimizes tension on the nerve repair by limiting nerve excursion during digit extension and simultaneously blocks clawing or hyperextension at the MP joints of the ring and little digits.
- Wound care should reflect wound healing timelines and can commence as soon as the client is referred and evaluated. Begin by assessing the incision site and documenting your findings. Immediately report the presence of clinical signs of infection (such as, foul-smelling exudate or pus present at the incision site) to the physician. Once the sutures are removed, gentle scar massage may begin. The goal of scar management is to facilitate optimal scar formation that can withstand external friction stresses (that is, not hypersensitive to non-noxious cutaneous stimuli) and that does not impede the normal gliding of underlying structures, such as tendons or the neurovascular bundle.
- If there is no concurrent tendon injury and repair, AROM and PROM can begin immediately within the orthosis.
- Desensitization for hypersensitive scar tissue may begin after sutures are removed and wounds are healed.
- Between weeks 3 and 5 to 6 postoperatively, gradually adjust the dorsal blocking splint at the wrist, bringing it closer to neutral or 0° extension. Progression is dictated by the surgeon, surgical procedure, and the client's relevant medical history.
- By week 6 the dorsal blocking splint is discharged. A hand-based anticlaw splint may be needed until intrinsic muscle function returns.
- AROM of the wrist and hand outside the orthosis can begin by week 6. Progressive strengthening exercises and resumption of self-care activities can occur over the next 2 weeks.
- By week 8, address residual strength issues that limit return to work in a work-conditioning program.

Postoperative Management Following Decompression for High Ulnar Nerve Lesions (Cubital Tunnel Syndrome)

Cubital Tunnel Release In Situ

An in situ cubital tunnel decompression consists of releasing the fascial roof of the cubital tunnel to decompress the nerve, thus opening up the cubital tunnel space at the elbow. All restricting fibrous bands are excised. This eliminates the restriction and pressure that has occurred along the ulnar nerve at the elbow. This procedure is done if the symptoms do not respond to conservative management and if the ulnar nerve does not dislocate around the medial epicondyle groove of the humerus.[43,45] Therapy postoperatively will focus on addressing pain or hypersensitivity. There are typically no ROM restrictions.

An **endoscopic release** may be utilized for in situ decompression of the ulnar nerve. This is an option for patients with mild to moderate preoperative symptoms. Postoperative splinting is usually not ordered, and the patient is encouraged to begin AROM and nerve gliding within the symptom-free range.[45]

Anterior Transposition of the Ulnar Nerve: Subcutaneous versus Submuscular

A number of surgical options are available to address persistent cubital tunnel syndrome that may be aggravated further by painful subluxation of the ulnar nerve. Typically, the nerve is exposed, elevated from its bed, and transferred anterior to the medial epicondyle. With a **subcutaneous ulnar nerve transposition,** the nerve is transferred anteriorly and positioned below the subcutaneous fascia of the anterior forearm, medial to the median nerve. In a **submuscular ulnar nerve transposition,** the nerve is placed in a well-vascularized muscular bed. Traditionally, the flexor-pronator muscle origin was separated and then reattached to its origin on the medial epicondyle. In 2004, Lee Dellon and J. Henk Coert described the results of a musculofascial lengthening technique for submuscular transposition of the ulnar nerve at the elbow.[46] This technique allows submuscular nerve transposition *without* cutting the flexor-pronator muscle origin.

> **Precautions and Concerns**

- *If the flexor-pronator muscle origin was reflected and reattached in surgery, the initiation of gentle AROM of the elbow, forearm, and wrist typically is delayed for about 3 to 4 weeks to allow the reattachment to heal enough to withstand active motion.*
- *If the flexor-pronator muscle origin was reattached, passive forearm supination with elbow, wrist, and finger extension is contraindicated, because this will stress the repair site.*
- *Premature stretching and strengthening activities can result in avulsion of the flexor/pronator origin. Regarding initiation of strengthening, it is always best to err on the cautious side with clients who have had a submuscular transposition.*
- *Following any of these procedures, strong gripping and lifting are contraindicated for 3 to 8 weeks, depending on the procedure and the client's individual response to the trauma of surgery.*
  Precaution. *Know which surgical technique for ulnar nerve transposition was employed, because this will help you predict the postoperative protocol. The need for orthotics, activity restrictions, and the postoperative therapy program are based on the type of surgery performed. Ultimately, the surgeon will dictate the need for and course of rehabilitation.*

> **Tips from the Field**

Subcutaneous and Submuscular Transposition

- Subcutaneous transposition: Use of a long arm orthotic appears to be surgeon specific. If the surgeon requests a long arm orthotic, fabricate one on the posterior aspect of the arm/forearm with the elbow in 90° of flexion. If unable to avoid including the area of the incision site in the brace, carefully pad this area to prevent chaffing or irritation from the rigid material. Inclusion of the wrist in this orthotic depends on patient comfort. Typically, patients may remove their orthotics to begin exercise immediately. Full active elbow extension is expected by 4 weeks.
- Submuscular transposition: A long arm orthotic is used for 4 to 6 weeks post surgery to protect the flexor-pronator

mass. Place the elbow in 90° of flexion, forearm in neutral to slight pronation and wrist in neutral to slight flexion. Passive ROM may be initiated for the elbow, forearm and wrist, but aggressive end range stretching should be avoided. Initiation of AROM is up to the surgeon; typically, it is allowed at 4 to 6 weeks post surgery.
- Submuscular transposition utilizing a musculofascial lengthening: This z-lengthening technique of the flexor-pronator fascia allows for full AROM immediately postoperatively. Proponents of this technique report that only intermittent use of a sling for comfort (as during the nighttime and/or when the patient is walking or standing for extended periods of time) is necessary. For the rest of the time, the arm may be placed on a pillow in a comfortable position.[46] Nonetheless, it is my experience that some surgeons have continued to prescribe intermittent use of a long arm orthosis for 4 to 6 weeks post this procedure to provide support and protection of the soft tissue structures (nerve, fascia) effected by the surgery.

Postoperative Management Following Decompression of Low (Distal) Ulnar Nerve Palsy (Ulnar Tunnel Syndrome)

Surgical exploration and decompression is recommended with ulnar tunnel syndrome because of the high incidence of space-occupying lesions.[42] Surgery involves decompressing the ulnar nerve within the tunnel. Postoperative therapy involves use of orthotics as described before, wound/scar management as appropriate, and activity modification as described before. A post-surgical wrist immobilization orthosis typically is not needed following decompression; rather a bulky dressing serves the purpose of resting the tissues for the first 3 to 10 days postoperatively. Full ROM is usually allowed immediately postoperative.

> **Tips from the Field**

Severe Ulnar Nerve Compression with Intrinsic Muscle Paralysis

Intrinsic function does not commonly return in adults following severe ulnar nerve compression with intrinsic muscle paralysis. Tendon transfers are typically necessary to correct the muscle balance that results from an ulnar nerve palsy. In this scenario, the use of an orthosis to prevent joint contractures will be necessary until tendon transfers have been performed.

Postoperative Management Following Tendon Transfers for Nerve Palsies

When it is clear that the muscles are not going to be reinnervated, tendon transfers may be performed to restore some balance of the wrist and/or hand. [32] The tendonous insertion of an innervated muscle is rerouted or transferred to a different site to compensate for the paralyzed muscle. For example, the insertion of the pronator teres, which is a frequent donor choice to provide wrist extension, is surgically cut, repositioned, and anchored to allow for active radial wrist extension. The goal of this procedure is to redistribute the available motor power in an attempt to improve function (see Chapter 32). Consider the following guidelines for intervention following tendon transfers for nerve palsies:[32]

- Clients undergoing tendon transfers are usually immobilized for 3 to 6 weeks in a protected cast or orthosis that minimizes tension on the repair.
- Begin brief sessions of active muscle contractions and place-and-hold exercises by week 5 or 6. Clients will need muscle reeducation to help them learn how contracting the donor muscle results in a new movement. Biofeedback and electric stimulation of the donor muscle can be used to help increase the client's awareness and isolated control. Splinting is continued between exercise sessions so as not to overload the healing tendon.
- Resistive exercises can begin by week 7 or 8, and the daytime protective orthosis can be discontinued at this time. Typically, by week 12, the client may resume all prior activities without restrictions.

Postoperative Management Following Digital Nerve Repairs

Digital nerves are the most frequently injured upper limb nerve. Ideally, surgical repair of acute digital nerve lacerations is performed with a primary tension-free repair. Rehabilitation following such a repair has been less clearly defined. Cast immobilization for 3 weeks has been the standard of care for almost a century.[47]

Following peripheral digital nerve surgery, common functional impairments include poor two-point discrimination, cold intolerance, and hyperesthesias.[39] Evidence indicates that immobilization of a limb or joint will lead to joint stiffness, impaired tendon gliding, and muscle-tendon shortening secondary to loss of muscle sarcomeres.

Use of a hand-based dorsal block orthosis for 3 weeks versus free AROM following primary tensionless repair of a digital nerve injury has been studied.[47,48] Results indicated that immobilization did not improve the integrity of the repair from a sensibility standpoint or in self-reported function/limitation. Certainly, not requiring immobilization with a cast or orthosis would be an advantage for patients and their wallets.

> ### Precautions and Concerns

Follow the conservative protocol of 3 weeks of immobilization following digital nerve surgery unless the surgeon requests otherwise.

All patients undergoing a digital nerve repair, whether treated with a traditional orthosis or allowed early AROM, should be advised to avoid full passive wrist and digit extension during the initial 3 weeks after surgery.

The traditional protocol involves using a dorsal block custom-made orthosis with MP joints at 70° to 90° of flexion and IPs in extension; if the thumb is involved, CMC at 15° flexion, MP at 30° flexion, and IP in extension. AROM is allowed within the orthosis. The orthosis is continued for the initial 3 weeks after surgery.[47]

> ### Precautions and Concerns

Scar massage and ultrasound should not be performed over a nerve conduit.[55]

Therapy should include edema control, massage, and desensitization once sutures are removed. Light strengthening can be initiated at 3 weeks after surgery for tension-free digital nerve repairs.

> © **Clinical Pearl**
>
> There is a correlation between patients' reports of hyperesthesia (or hypersensitivity) and their own estimation of recovery/functional status.[47] Therefore, hypersensitivity should be addressed early on in therapy.

Conservative Management of Double Crush Syndrome

Dellon[52] suggests that the injured nerve could have more than two sites of compression, each being insufficient in itself to cause clinical symptoms, but with the effects of each summating to create symptomatology. These clients would present with diffuse UE complaints and multiple sites of minor peripheral nerve irritation or entrapment. Mononeuorpathy may predispose the rest of the nerve trunk to irritation and thus secondary neuropathies. Minor, serial impingements along a nerve have been proposed to have an additive effect that can cause a nerve entrapment lesion distal to the initial lesion site. Since the peripheral nerve is one long continuous cell, injury in one part of the cell will likely have consequences in other areas of the cell, especially at those more vulnerable sites, such as where the nerve must traverse through spaces of increased friction (for example, fibrosseous tunnels).[3,9] Increased vulnerability of the nerve cell is likely due to impairment in axoplasmic flow and disruption of the axon's neurofilament architecture.[3,9] This is called *double crush syndrome*. Likewise, patients with "multiple crush" syndrome would present with diffuse UE complaints and multiple sites of minor peripheral nerve irritation or entrapment.

If the flow of a nerve's axoplasm is slowed, adverse consequences include an alteration in the quality and quantity of synaptic transmissions, and damage to the nerve cell body and to the axon itself. The important point here is that the nerve does not need to receive a specific injury, such as a crush or a stretch injury. Rather, over time, altered axoplasmic flow in a nerve that results from diminished blood flow to the nerve can cause the entire nerve to become sick and to become vulnerable to multiple sites of irritation along its axon.[3,4,9]

Typically, electrodiagnostic testing (such as, an electromyography) will objectively demonstrate and quantify abnormal peripheral nerve function. However, minor changes in the nerve fibers may not register as abnormal on electrodiagnostic tests, or these tests may not be specific enough to identify the presence of multiple sites of (mild) nerve irritation.[9] Therefore, the clinician may need to utilize the non-standardized exams, such as nerve tension testing, to assess the presence of and the exact locations of multiple-site nerve irritation. Typically, patients with double crush syndrome will complain of an intermittent and varying intensity diffuse UE pain with a spread of symptoms from one area to another (for example, from the wrist to the elbow).[3] Pain and paresthesias may be induced with specific postures of the arm that place the involved neural structures on tension.[3,9] As the nerve irritation progresses, the patient may assume a protective posture of the involved extremity that minimizes tension on the irritated nerve or nerves and/or may develop a disuse atrophy as a means of coping with a chronic pain that seems to "have a mind all of its own."[4,6,9]

The most commonly studied double crush syndrome is the CTS-cervical spine injury,[3,9,49] followed by cubital tunnel syndrome and thoracic outlet syndrome.[3] Metabolic conditions (such as, alcoholism, diabetes, and thyroid dysfunction) may predispose the PNS to double or multiple crush syndromes.[3]

Conservative and Postoperative Management of Double Crush Syndrome

There isn't much written about the non-operative and postoperative treatment of double crush syndrome. As with any peripheral nerve irritation, the therapist must follow protocols for tissue tolerances and wound care. Dellon notes that release of one compression site may relieve the patient's symptoms without the need to release all sites.[3] If surgical decompression is performed, the postoperative protocols should follow those specific for that surgery. For example, if a CTR is done, follow the postoperative protocols for this surgery, and augment with interventions aimed at addressing the other, more proximal "crush" site(s).[49] If multiple sites of entrapment are decompressed, then the timeline for healing is lengthened. Below are some additional tips that may assist the clinician in designing an appropriate and successful intervention program. Please refer to Chapter 22 for further information and suggestions.

- Early compression stage: Patients in this stage will have intermittent and position-dependent symptoms with on slight provocation of symptoms upon physical examination. There may be a hypersensitive response to vibratory stimuli. Surgery is not recommended unless the symptoms fail to improve after at least 3 months of conservative management. Appropriate splinting and instructions to decrease those activities that cause repetitive compression of the nerve are most helpful.

- Moderate compression stage: Patients in this stage will have intermittent symptoms, though these are more pronounced than in the earlier stage. For example, motor weakness is evident and measurable. Sensory threshold testing will indicate changes from normal sensibility perception. Symptoms may interfere with daily activity performance and occupational roles. Surgery is still not indicated until a 3-month conservative management program has been tried and deemed unsuccessful. Dellon suggests steroid injections at the site of compression may be temporarily helpful.[3]

- Severe compression stage: Patients in this stage have persistent symptoms with muscle wasting, finger numbness, abnormal two-point discrimination, and significant limitations in role performance secondary to pain. Surgery is recommended, because these patients will not improve without surgical intervention.[3] Following surgery, it is important that the decompressed nerve not be immobilized for more than 1 week. ROM exercise at the joint crossed by the released nerve and nerve gliding exercises should be introduced early. The postoperative patient may not be able to return certain previous repetitive activities nor to using vibratory or pneumatic impact tools.[3]

♡ *Tips from the Field*

Double Crush Syndrome

- *Patient education and cooperation are keys to successful management.* Educate the client about the underlying pathology

and about conditions that can further pervert the already irritable nervous system. Encourage the client to find a safe and comfortable imaginary "zone" in which she can move her arms without pain/increased symptoms. Have her practice "staying within the box" when performing self-care and work tasks. Reinforce concepts by reviewing the patient's responses to "staying within the box." Later, as the nerve irritation diminishes, the boundaries of the "box" can be increased.

- *Ergonomics can help lessen the external stresses on the irritable nerve.* Avoid repetitive UE movements in the ranges and postures that aggravate the nerve. For example, instead of reaching overhead to put dishes away, use a sturdy step stool and keep the shoulder close to the body. Instead of bending the elbow to hold the receiver to the ear, use a headset. Avoid using vibratory or pneumatic impact tools; if they are necessary, use an anti-vibration glove with a palmar gel pad to absorb some of the vibratory shock. Educate clients about their syndrome and about modifications needed for sleep and work habits. An ergonomic assessment of the work place may be helpful in identifying those tasks that contribute to perpetuation of symptoms. Good posture and frequent stretch breaks from repetitive or sustained provocative positions are key components to managing symptoms.

- *Nerve gliding should never be painful; find a way to encourage movement without irritating the nerve further.* Even a little bit of movement at a joint where the nerve crosses is better than none. If, for example, the patient is unable to perform the entire brachial plexus glide without pain, adapt the glide so that the proximal joints remain still, minimizing some of the tension on the nerve, while the distal joints move, creating nerve glide in the distal extremity. Then hold the distal joints still, in a position that minimizes tension on that nerve, as the proximal joints move to create proximal nerve gliding.

- *Sometimes incomplete symptom resolution is the best that it gets.* Not all patients will recovery completely from double or multiple crush syndrome. In fact, many will not. Help the patient make the psychological adjustment necessary to living with a chronic and painful condition by teaching the patient pain management strategies and by allowing the patient to verbalize his grief about this. Listen, acknowledge his grief, and when necessary, refer the patient to a psychologist and/or psychiatrist.

❓ *Questions to Discuss with the Physician*

- Does nerve testing (EMG/NCS) support the diagnosis of double crush syndrome?
- Where are the proximal and distal sites of entrapment?
- Is the patient a candidate for CTR (or some other decompression surgery)? What is the likely outcome of surgical intervention (incomplete symptom resolution)?

Treating Nerve Injuries—Conservative and Postoperative

Therapeutic intervention for any nerve injury will likely incorporate techniques to address pain, hypersensitivity, nerve gliding, patient education, and possibly sensory reeducation. The following interventions may be useful.

Nerve Gliding[4,6,25,34,56,57]

Nerve health is predicated upon motion. Motion is lotion to the nerves! All movement produces nerve gliding to some degree, because the nerve accommodates to changes in the length of its bed produced by joint motion. Wilgis and Murphy (1986)[58] reported that the average median nerve glide was 7.3 mm and the average ulnar nerve glide was 9.8 mm during full flexion and extension of the elbow. Wright et al. (1996)[59] reported a total longitudinal excursion of the median nerve (proximal to the carpal tunnel) of 19.6 mm when the wrist was moved from 60° of wrist extension to 65° of wrist flexion. However, if nerve movement was restricted at one location, then one would expect increased neural tension or stretch at and distal to the site of compression during normal joint motion. Therefore, care must be taken when designing a nerve gliding program to ensure that the prescribed exercise fosters gentle nerve longitudinal sliding, not nerve tensioning or stretching.

If a nerve is constrained or compressed, surgery may be necessary. Once the nerve is decompressed, therapeutic exercises should be introduced as soon as possible to restore and maintain the normal longitudinal excursion of the nerve. Thus, one goal of a **nerve gliding** program is to alter the formation of motion limiting adhesions between the nerve and its surrounding tissue (Totten & Hunter 1991[60].

Another goal of nerve gliding is to enhance blood flow to the nerve and to facilitate axoplasmic flow, hence encouraging nerve homeostasis.[9] A nerve gliding program attempts to maximize the excursion of the nerve while minimizing the strain on the nerve. Stretching a nerve more than 8% of its resting length will result in venous congestion and inhibit blood flow. The patient will feel a burning sensation.

The concept of **nerve sliding** was initially introduced by Butler, Shacklock and Slater[4] in 1994). Essentially, nerve sliding involves encouraging gliding of the nerve within its tissue bed while decreasing the tension at the proximal or distal ends of the range. Presumably, a slider will allow better movement and present less challenge and less generation of tension; thus, it is more likely to reduce neural symptoms and protective muscle guarding while facilitating nerve health. The concept of nerve slides as a treatment technique may be visualized as sliding a piece of floss through teeth. When one end (of the floss) is pulled, the other end is relaxed or free from tension. Likewise, as the peripheral nerve is pulled across a joint or through a tunnel, tension must be eased at one end or the other so as not to create or increase adverse nerve tension.

Echigo, et al.[55] noted that the position of the elbow, forearm, wrist, and digits should be considered when designing the optimum nerve sliding exercise. For example, forearm supination produces the most distally oriented median nerve gliding, while active full finger flexion produces the most proximally oriented median nerve gliding at the carpal canal.[56]

Nerve sliding should be done slowly, moving the extremity as if one was a dancer. Advise the patient to pay attention to how these exercises feel and to stop at any point in the sequence if numbness, discomfort, or pain increases.

Precaution. *It is important to instruct the patient that nerve gliding can increase symptoms and nerve irritability if it is not done carefully and correctly. Creating nerve tension by pulling on both ends of a nerve to complete an exercise or activity will surely increase symptoms.*

> **Clinical Pearl**
>
> Incorporating the movements of the nerve slide into a functional activity makes the nerve slide easier to remember. Remember that the goal of these exercises is to gently slide the nerve through its available range to promote axoplasmic flow and general nerve health. These exercises should *never* be painful.

Sensory Reeducation[2,5,6,10,24]

An important part of rehab for patients with sensory loss associated with peripheral nerve damage is sensory reeducation. Peripheral nerve lesions can result in a shuffling of skin "addresses" or end organ sites with respect to CNS addresses. In other words, individual regenerating axons may not end up reinnervating the exact same end organs as prior to the injury. This will result in an altered, and likely diminished, pattern of input coming from this area of the periphery to the somatosensory cortex. The cortex will reorganize in response to this altered pattern or picture.

The goal of sensory reeducation is to improve the patient's perception of sensory information arising from receptors in the hand so that the patient can correctly interpret the (altered) pattern of incoming sensory signals. Assuming that the higher cortical somatosensory pathways for object recognition are intact, once a patient has achieved sufficient return of protective sensation, sensory reeducation can begin.

A sensory reeducation program includes incorporation of localization tasks, graded stimulus tasks and recognition tasks. Sensory reeducation may be divided into two stages—a protective and a discriminative stage. The goal of protective sensory reeducation is to educate the patient in techniques of compensation for loss of sensory protection. These patients are unable to discriminate protective sensation; they are unable to evaluate the potential harmfulness of hot/cold or of sharp objects. They are at significant risk for unknowingly injuring their insensate hand, especially when vision is occluded. Education about the injury, the potential risks for re-injury, and about compensation strategies can typically be performed in one to two sessions. Tell the patient to avoid working around machinery, or anything with moving parts, and to avoid situations where the environmental temperature is below 60° F. The patient should be advised to use vision to compensate for sensory loss. Reaching into a pocket becomes a potentially harmful situation for a patient without protective sensation.

> **Clinical Pearl**
>
> Keep the body part warm, because cold exposure damages muscle and leads to fibrosis. Compression dressings must not cause venous congestion and edema.

The goal of discriminative sensory reeducation is the recovery of discriminative sensibility. Following nerve injury there is a predictable pattern of sensory recovery, beginning with pain perception and progressing to vibration of 30 cps, moving touch, and constant touch. The return proceeds from proximal to distal. This phase of sensory reeducation will incorporate graded training tasks involving localization and discrimination of textures, shapes and objects. A visual-tactile matching process can be used; the patient attempts to correctly identify the stimulus location or modality type, first with eyes closed. If the patient is wrong, then the stimulation is repeated with eyes open, and the patient concentrates on matching what he feels with what he sees.[18,52]

For successful carryover of newly developed discriminative sensory skills, the patient must have the motor skills for object manipulation. The patient must ultimately be able to hold onto and manipulate an object for a short time without the object slipping through the fingers, even with vision occluded.

Cortical plasticity, or the brain's ability to change representations of the body surface, is dependent upon tactile experiences with the environment. Specific cortical and subcortical reorganization can occur within minutes of a peripheral nerve injury and can be long standing if not permanent. Rosen and Lundborg[24] recommend a two-phase sensory reeducation program with initiation of "phase one" within 3 weeks of nerve repair, focusing on maintaining the cortical hand representation by using the brain's capacity for sensory imagery as well as cortical visual-tactile interaction. "Phase one" lasts until some protective sensation is present (6.65 in Semmes-Weinstein monofilament testing).

In "phase one", visual and auditory cues are used to minimize synaptic reorganization of the somatosensory mapping of the insensate aspect of the hand. Functional MRIs [24] have confirmed that there is a continous cortical interplay within the brain, with polymodal association areas 'lighting up' during a single modal sensory or motor task. For example, when a blind person reads Braille, the primary visual cortex is activated along with the somatosensory cortex. Imagining a movement will activate the premotor cortex. When imaging music, the auditory cortical areas are recruited. While there is need for further evidenced based research, current work in this area suggests that we can minimize adverse cortical mapping by asking patients to visualize movement of the wrist and hand; and to imagine how it feels to touch and massage the involved area. Observing movement and/or touch of the uninvolved hand in a mirror while thinking about both hands performing the same movment, or feeling the massage may 'fool' the brain and mimimize early synaptic reorganization.[24]

In "phase two," desensitization may need to be addressed. Sensory relearning and desensitization can influence sensory recovery as well as the pain that is typically seen after a nerve injury. During "phase two," training for sensory localization is critical to the outcome, with localization improving with time, use, and sensory reeducation.

Using the injured hand/limb in functional tasks as opposed to exercises only facilitates faster return of function and discourages disuse atrophy. Appropriately challenging and motivating activities with familiar objects and environments aid return of motor control.[2] Sensory relearning and desensitization can influence both sensory recovery and pain after injury. Cortical changes are facilitated or modulated by the strength of the behavioral reinforcement. In other words, sensory reeducation is more successful if the exercise or reeducation program is functionally oriented and appropriately challenging to the patient.[5]

To be successful, both protective and discriminative sensory reeducation should begin as soon as possible after a nerve injury in order to encourage the patient to use the affected extremity before abnormal use patterns can develop. This minimizes compensatory use of the uninvolved arm with resultant neglect of the involved extremity. It is more difficult to do this if the deficit is on the non-dominant side.

The treatment for sensory deficits and retraining for fine motor skills requires functional use of the involved hand and a high degree of motivation and commitment from the patient. Repetition and motivation are key concepts; therefore, task completion must be meaningful to the patient and must have just enough degree of difficulty, yet possibility of success, for the therapy to be successful. Research indicates that without a sensory reeducation program, the prognosis for recovery of discriminative sensibility following a proximal (or high level) peripheral nerve injury is poor for adults, though better for children.[5,10,52]

Desensitization

Immediately after injury to tissue, the local neural tissue will lower its sensory stimulus threshold in response to the sensitizing effects of inflammation.[6] In other words, it is easier for the sensory nerve to achieve an action potential. Sensory input that is non-noxious, such as palpation or percussion along the nerve, may be perceived as irritating or painful. Prolonged irritation to the neural tissue can result in a state of **hyperalgesia,** or hypersensitivity, with local sensitivity changes that will be reflected in the way the central somatosensory system processes sensory inputs. Patients with hyperalgesia may complain of extreme discomfort or irritability with tactile stimulation to their involved body part. For example, hypersensitivity of the skin around the radial styloid and proximal thumb is a fairly common phenomenon occurring with radial sensory nerve irritation. Interestingly, even when the source of irritation (such as, a tight cast or splint) is removed, the hypersensitivity may remain. This can result in significant functional problems for patients, because wearing a watch or allowing the sleeve of a shirt or coat to touch the area may be unbearable.

Desensitization is the systematic process of applying nonnoxious stimuli to peripheral tissues to reeducate and retrain the nervous system. As with sensory reeducation, the ideal patient must be motivated to participate in a home program. For desensitization to be successful, frequent sessions with various tactile stimulations must occur throughout the day. The more treatment the patient does, the quicker the results are. Initially, patients may need to apply the stimulus around the irritated tissues rather than directly on these tissues. The patient applies the stimulus herself, so the amount of pressure that is tolerable is under the patient's control.

❲❳ *What to Say to Clients*

About Hypersensitivity and Desensitization

"Your nerve is irritable at this time, and that's why things that shouldn't be painful feel painful. To improve your sensation, you will need to reeducate your sensory process.. To help it recover, you will need to touch the irritated skin regularly. Try short sessions at first, say 5 to 10 minutes. Try to touch the irritated skin every waking hour or every other hour. Make sure you are relaxed when you do this. You can put on nice music, watch a favorite TV show, or go into a quiet room—whatever works for you. Try touching or tapping your skin with a towel or a piece or cotton or massaging the area with cream. Any type of cream is fine. Or, you could use a soft brush, such as a toothbrush or baby's hair brush, and gently brush over the irritated area—always moving in the same direction (that is, fingertip to elbow or elbow to fingertip). The key to getting better is to do this treatment often and every day. If you wait, your brain will learn that this pain is normal and the pain message may become permanently fixed, like a memory."

Pain Management

According to Paul Brand,[53] pain can be diminished if the patient understands the cause of pain and loses fear associated with such unknown variables as healing expectations and timelines. This is an opportunity for us as therapists to be powerful pain relievers. The following may also be helpful in mitigating the patient's pain experience.

Modalities

The subsequent list is not meant to be an exhaustive accounting of available modalities, nor of the parameters for using these modalities. Therapists should seek out and follow guidelines for modality use as listed by the appropriate state regulating agency for his/her profession occupational therapist (OT) versus physical therapist [PT] versus occupational therapy assistant [OTA] versus physical therapy assistant [PTA]). Ongoing courses in modality use will keep the practitioner up to date on current research and practice issues.[54]

- Continuous wave ultrasound, a deep heat modality, has been shown to increase tissue extensibility, to improve blood flow and tissue permeability, and to increase the pain thresholds. Ultrasound can reach tissue depths of 5 cm or more; therefore this is a good modality choice for addressing pain emanating from structures deep to the skin.
- Pulsed ultrasound can facilitate the resolution of the inflammatory phase of healing; therefore, this is a good choice in the acute phase of tissue healing. Michelovitz[55] notes that ultrasound in the area of a peripheral nerve repair to facilitate nerve regeneration has been studied using a rat sciatic nerve model. Using low intensity ultrasound, there was statistically significant acceleration of functional recovery. The effects of ultrasound in enhancing nerve regeneration in humans has not been defined at the time of this publication.
- Iontophoresis, the use of direct current to introduce topically applied ions to underlying tissue, may alter pain perception and reduce edema.
- Transcutaneous electrical nerve stimulation (TENS) can be an effective modality for addressing both acute and chronic pain. I think of TENS as providing "white noise" or a safe distraction that can dampen those unhelpful pain messages that interfere with function. There are various theories about how TENS is effective in controlling pain. The **Gate theory,** proposed by Melzack and Wall in the mid-1960s,[54] is perhaps the most widely recited. Recent research has led to modifications of this theory. Gating off pain by using TENS is predicated upon the fact that a message of pain is brought to the spinal cord by small- diameter, slow conduction nociceptive nerve fibers with little or no myelin (type A-delta or C fibers). Large diameter, myelinated, A-beta sensory fibers can inhibit the activity of these nociceptive nerve fibers in the spinal cord by activating local interneurons in the substantia geltinosa of the dorsal horn of the spinal column. These interneurons depress the transmission of nociceptive signals to the brain by releasing a neurotransmitter that dampens the nociceptor nerve cell activity.[1] Activation of the cutaneous mechanoreceptors by light touch/massage, percussion, vibration and/or stretch will stimulate A-beta nerve fibers. TENS that provides a low level, cutaneous stimulation may therefore provide temporary pain relief at least until the patient acclimates to that TENS setting. Eventually, humans will acclimate to any non-noxious cutaneous stimulation. Use of large electrode pads may help recruit a more optimum number of A-beta nerve fibers than use of small pads.

> ### ◎ *Clinical Pearl*
>
> TENS can create a kind of "white noise" or static at the spinal cord level that blocks the pain message from getting to the brain for perception. When setting up your patient on a TENS unit, keep this in mind. The static or "white noise" input should be comfortable, but of high enough intensity to block at least some of the pain. Like a white noise machine designed to block out external environmental noises so you can sleep, the treatment level should be high enough to distract your client from pain, but still comfortable. After a while, your client may report that she cannot feel the intensity of the output as much. There is *no* need to turn up the TENS output at this point. Rather, explain to your client that as she becomes accustomed to the TENS, both the intensity of this stimuli and the pain intensity will decrease. For example, once you have started to fall asleep, you wouldn't get up to turn up your "white noise" machine. In the same vein, you do not need to turn up the intensity of the TENS unit during this pain management session.

The application of **superficial heat,** as with a hot pack, prior to ROM exercises or stretching can diminish stiffness and muscle spasms. Do not use superficial heat if the patient has sensory loss as there is a greater risk of burning the tissue when sensation is compromised.

- Fluidotherapy, a type of superficial convection heat, is a dry whirlpool that has the added advantage of desensitizing irritable scar tissue while simultaneously heating this tissue prior to stretch and exercise.
- A paraffin bath, another type of superficial heat modality, is advantageous because the patient can be taught how to use this pain relief modality at home. Paraffin baths are relatively inexpensive and readily available at many department stores and pharmacies.
- Cryotherapy, or cold therapy, is a modality frequently used to address pain that results from muscle spasms. Post exercise pain and some types of edema can be managed effectively by cold packs or ice massage.

Manual therapy techniques, designed to increase blood flow and reduce pain, are also helpful. Therapeutic touch can be augmented by discussions about stress management, relaxation, visualization, and activity pacing. Incorporating these cognitive-behavioral techniques with manual therapies, in my experience, facilitates pain reduction by acknowledging the presence of pain and by gently and supportively instructing the patient in pain-management strategies. Discussion of soft tissue mobilization and myofascial release techniques are beyond the scope of this chapter. The reader is encouraged to seek out courses in these areas to develop appropriate knowledge and skills before applying these techniques.

- Brushing: When TENS is not accessible to a patient, it may be possible to get a similar (temporary) analgesic response by using anything that stimulates the A-beta sensory fibers. Vibration, massage, or brushing may do this. The patient should use a soft baby's hairbrush and brush the irritated limb, moving along the entire peripheral nerve. Initially, have the patient move from proximal to distal, using large, firm but gentle sweeping motions to recruit as many large A-fibers as possible. Later, a more random pattern of brushing, using circular motions for example, may be used so that it is more difficult for the patient to acclimate to the brushing sensation.

- Patient education: Patients are often fearful about their injury, about life changes that have occurred or may still occur secondary to their injury, about re-injury, and/or about expectations for recovery. These fears will frequently present as pain and pain behaviors, both in and outside the clinic.[53] Therapists are in the best position to address many of these concerns simply because we spend more time with the patient than the physician can. Therefore, patient education is an integral part of any treatment program. Therapists should anticipate some of these concerns and fears and be prepared to address them.

- Occupation-based interventions: Research supports the concept that pain management is most effective when it is client centered and when the therapy program allows the patient to be actively engaged in both goal setting and intervention planning.[53] Interventions should be meaningful and motivating for each individual client. Using the COPM to elucidate areas of performance difficulty and/or dissatisfaction will assist the therapist in developing an appropriate collaborative intervention program.

▷ Precautions and Concerns

Our job as health care providers is first: do no harm. Our patients may often think they are supposed to work through pain or tolerate painful situations/stretches because they have been indoctrinated to think this way. It is our responsibility to instruct them that pain is an indication of tissue injury and pain is to be avoided. Make certain that you are clearly and regularly stating to your patients that the mantra, "no Pain, no gain," is not true.

◊ What to Say to Clients

Typical Concerns
- Why is my hand/wrist/forearm/elbow still swollen?
- *Typical Answer:* "Swelling is a normal part of healing. Your body is producing the cells that are needed for healing. Following an injury or surgery to a nerve, you can see swelling initially, but we will reduce it with hand therapy treatment as quickly as possible."
- Will my scar open up if I massage over it?
- *Typical Answer (once sutures are out and the wound is showing adequate tensile strength):* "No, your wound won't break open if you apply cream and massage your scar. You can begin gently, using any kind of lotion. I prefer something with an oily feel, because while the nerve is healing, it can't maintain the skin's normal healthy elasticity."
- Why do I have pain? *Or* why do I still have pain? Should I keep exercising if I have pain?
- *Typical Answer:* "Pain is your body's normal mechanism for telling you that something is wrong. It's actually one of our

senses, like smell or taste. Usually that's a good thing, letting you know that you're doing too much or that something is amiss. Sometimes this warning mechanism continues to alert you, even when you've taken care of the initial problem. Your brain comes to expect pain, even when what you're doing should not be painful. When that happens, you need to learn how to self-manage your symptoms. Knowing the difference between pain that is a 'good' warning pain and pain that needs to be self-managed is difficult. I can help you with this. You should always tell me if you have pain with anything I give you in therapy (or with anything you are trying to do at home). Do not work through pain. You can actually injure yourself further if you push through pain. Early on in the healing process, discomfort is quite common during exercise or activity; however, working through pain is not okay. The mantra, "no Pain, no gain," is erroneous. Part of my job is to identify appropriate activities and exercises for you that will be introduced at the right time to assist with tissue healing and functional gains."

♡ Tips from the Field

Orthoses
The rationales for choosing and providing an orthosis for our patients are well known. Deciding which type to use (an over-the-counter splint, a prefabricated custom orthosis, or a low temperature orthosis) requires an understanding of the pathology, appreciation of the economic and time constraints of the therapist and patient, and attention to the psychosocial issues unique to each of our patients. The first two rationales (protection and prevention) address the biological issues. The last rationale is where clinical reasoning comes into play: Why choose one design over another?

- For protection: To diminish neural tension to create a healing environment. It is used to abate acute symptoms or symptoms that are observed at rest and increased with activity.

- For prevention: To prevent motions that result in additional compression to the nerve, reducing potential inflammation that could lead to worsening of symptoms. To prevent contractures secondary to muscle imbalance. **Myoplasticity** is the principle that muscle tissue will adapt structurally and functionally to changes in activity level and/or to prolonged positioning. Overstretched muscles result in an increase in sarcomeres (the functional unit of the muscle). An increase or decrease in sarcomeres means that the muscle adapts to its new resting length. Muscles can only generate optimal force at their resting length. Furthermore, muscles will contract about 50% of their resting length to generate this optimal force.[1] Thus, overstretched reinnervated muscles to the wrist/hand will demonstrate a decreased ability to generate optimum strength during functional activities/use.

- For functional enhancement: To substitute for, or enhance impaired function. When we stabilize an arthritic joint, as with the CMC joint of the thumb, we expect improved stability and strength at that joint and a decrease in joint pain during activity. When we develop a static progressive orthotic that provides a slow and steady stretch to the tissues, we expect to see improved tissue extensibility and thus improved motion and function at that joint. When we provide our client with a dynamic radial nerve palsy brace that provides passive MP joint extension, but allows digit flexion, we intend to improve the client's functional grasp following a radial nerve palsy. Orthotics can be custom fabricated or ordered. They may contain rigid parts, or not, and may come in different colors, thicknesses, and shapes. How does one decide which to use? Choosing the right orthotic requires a collaborative effort between the therapist and client. Begin by assessing the patient's needs and wants. Educate that client about how this orthosis will improve his function within his unique environment. If possible, give your client options and/or allow him to have input into the process. If appropriate, encourage the client to add to the cosmesis of the orthosis, using glued on 'bling' or duct tape to give the brace a different appearance.

> ### ◎ Clinical Pearl
>
> A review of our literature indicates that it is usually up to the surgeon to dictate the length of time the patient is immobilized postoperatively, the splint position specifications, the point at which ROM exercises are initiated, what the limits of motion are, and, in some cases, how quickly a patient progresses.[43]

> ### ◎ Clinical Pearl
>
> If a joint contracture occurs (for example, because the client did not seek medical intervention immediately), then orthotics should be fitted to focus on restoring maximum joint PROM before addressing muscle imbalance.

> ### ◎ Clinical Pearl
>
> Successful application of an orthotic must address biological factors, psychological factors, and social factors using a biopsychosocial approach to orthotic intervention.

♡ Tips from the Field

Range of Motion Exercises—Management of Nerve Injury with Grade Fair Plus to Normal Muscle Strength

- AROM exercises are introduced as soon as safely possible to prevent tendon adherence or joint stiffness and to facilitate blood and lymphatic flow. Instruct the client in PROM and active/active assistive range of motion (A/AAROM) exercises in the clinic, and have the client continue these daily at home. (I recommend six to eight sets per day with ten repetitions of each set to start, and then adjust according to the client's response.) The goal is to prevent joint contractures and to promote general joint health by encouraging frequent movement through the normal available arc of motion.

♡ Tips from the Field

Range of Motion Exercises—Postoperative Management of Nerve Injury with Muscle Paresis or Muscle Strength of Grade Fair or Less

- Begin with active assistive motion (place and hold, bottle roll for digit extension) with gravity minimized when possible,

and progress to motions against gravity to facilitate muscle activation and movement.
- Place and hold, and active motion foster muscle activation. The focus is on motor relearning and adaptive strategies.
- Consider pool therapy to decrease the role of gravity.
- As muscle strength returns and the client is able to demonstrate full movement in the gravity minimized plane (MMTs are 2/5 strength), begin place-and-hold exercises (or isometric contractions) in the against-gravity plane. Initially, these exercise sessions will be brief because the muscle fibers will fatigue quickly.
- Begin isotonic strengthening exercises to correct proximal weakness and muscle imbalance once there is adequate muscle strength to hold the body part against gravity for a functional period (MMT is 3+/5). As noted before, these initial isotonic strengthening sessions should be short but frequent.
- Begin muscle retraining as soon as possible. Encourage the client to use the involved extremity as normally as possible during the day whether the client needs an orthotic to assist or not. Use of the involved extremity can become part of the client's daily home exercise regimen. It is important for the client not to develop a habit of performing daily activities with the uninvolved arm only because the brain will forget how to incorporate the impaired extremity even when motor power returns.

CASE STUDIES

CASE STUDY 24-1 ■

PR is a 32-year-old, right hand dominant female executive who sustained puncture injuries to her right third and fourth digits, volar surface, from her cat's claws. She was seen by her family physician, who prescribed antibiotic medication to prevent infection. She continued to complain of pain, numbness, stiffness, and swelling at her follow-up appointment. Her physician referred her for a course of hand therapy to address her complaints.

At her initial visit, which was approximately 1 month post injury, PR had significantly swollen and stiff long, ring, and small digits per circumference measures. The volar puncture wounds had healed with minimal observable scar tissue, although PR reported some hypersensitivity with gentle palpation to these areas. AROM measurements were taken; isolated joint motion indicated that all extrinsic flexor tendons were intact. Active flexion-to-the-distal palmar crease ranged from 2.2 cm (small digit) to 4.5 cm (long digit). Semmes-Weinstein monofilament testing indicated normal light touch (2.83) at the tip of the fifth digit, tip of the index, and along the ulnar aspect of the fourth digit. The radial aspect of the ring finger responded with diminished light touch (3.61) at the base of the digit to diminished protective sensation (3.84) at the tip. The ulnar aspect of the long finger responded with diminished protective sensation (3.84 to 4.31). The radial aspect of the long finger responded with diminished light touch (3.22 to 3.61). PR reported tingling radiating to the tips of both her ring and long fingers with percussion to the digital nerves about 1 cm distal to the puncture sites. PR reported that her finger "numbness" had not improved since the date of injury. She reported concerns about the integrity of her nerves and voiced concern that she might need surgery to "fix them." The sensory findings were explained to PR as consistent with the physician's diagnosis of a nerve injury in continuity. Persistent sensory symptoms were likely aggravated by venous stasis.

A modified COPM was performed to establish patient goals. It became clear that PR was avoiding normal use of her right hand during work and at home because "it hurts." She was typing one-handed and utilizing her left hand to cook and clean whenever possible. She was observed being hesitant to grip her briefcase with a hook fist, preferring to use a modified grasp (between the index and thumb) to secure the handle.

PR was instructed in tendon glide exercises and blocking exercises for the digits to encourage better pull through and gliding of the extrinsic flexor tendons. She was also instructed in edema control measures, including use of 1-inch Coban, retrograde massage and in active fisting to assist the overwhelmed venous system. She was instructed in the likely repercussions of continuing to avoid using her right hand, and she was encouraged to begin to incorporate her hand in such activities as holding onto the toothbrush while brushing her teeth. Cylindrical foam was provided, and PR was instructed in application of the foam to her toothbrush, her eating utensils, and even her briefcase handle so that she could comfortably and securely grip these items during use. Finally, PR was educated about how nerves respond to trauma and was given an expected timeline and guideline for what she could expect as the nerves continued to heal. Protective sensory education strategies were discussed and appropriate cautions (such as not reaching into a suds-filled basin for a knife) were reviewed.

PR returned to therapy 1 week later. Although she did not have a complete fist, she was now able to touch her palm with each fingertip after a few warm up exercises. Her swelling was less noticeable, and she demonstrated correct application of Coban. She requested another roll, indicating consistent use of it. She continued to complain of some scar hypersensitivity and of intermittent "zinging" up to the tips of her involved fingers. She was assured that this was a normal response as the nerves healed, and she was told to continue with scar massage and normal hand usage. She also reported some cold intolerance with marked change in the fingers' ability to tolerate the air conditioner blowing on them. This would appear to indicate a concomitant digital vascular injury. She was instructed to continue her tendon glide exercises even after full digit motion was achieved to encourage nerve gliding within the digits.

PR was seen once a week for short sessions over the next 3 weeks. She was now approximately 9 weeks from her injury. Digit motion was full. She reported that she had resumed all pre-injury work and home activities using her right hand. Sensory testing showed moderate improvements in light touch sensibility with both the ring and long neurologically-impaired areas responding with diminished light touch (3.61). Since it was likely that the digital nerves would continue to heal at a rate of about 1 mm/day, and since she had successfully returned to all pre-injury activities and had achieved the goals she had set for herself (via the COPM), a final but optional visit was offered (1 month later) to document continued nerve healing. PR reported that she would call if she had further issues; she was satisfied that her hand would continue to heal as she had been instructed.

CASE STUDY 24-2 ■

LE was an 11-year-old, right hand dominant boy at the time of his injury. He was playing with his brother when he fell into a plate glass door. He suffered numerous lacerations and punctures, including a

severe puncture to his right axilla. Almost immediately, he was covered in blood. His mother's cousin, an ER nurse, happened to be visiting that day, and she was able to pinch off the impaired artery until the trauma team arrived. LE was transported by helicopter to the nearest trauma center, where he underwent several hours of surgery. Because of the severe blood loss, his parents were told that he might not survive.

LE arrived at the outpatient clinic with his parents and a health maintenance organization (HMO) referral 6 weeks after surgery. The HMO referral stated, "Evaluate and treat, splint fabrication." LE was wearing a long arm half cast that had been removed to date "only by the surgery team." The prescription from the hand surgeon requesting a long arm splint and bearing a diagnosis of right axillary artery laceration and repair was eventually produced. A telephone call to the surgeon to further qualify orders and surgical procedures was not successful; the surgeon was in surgery. The half cast was, therefore, carefully removed with attention paid to minimizing movement at the shoulder. LE's arm and forearm showed significant atrophy of the triceps (posterior compartment of the arm), and of the lateral-posterior compartment of the forearm. His unsupported wrist and digits fell into the classic wrist drop posture. Muscle strength of the triceps was 0/5. Sensory loss included the posterior lateral aspect of the distal arm and the dorsal radial hand. His skin appeared dry and inelastic. Surgical incisions, although closed and suture-free, presented as raised and red-purple with evidence of early hypertrophy.

A long arm orthotic replicating the position of the half cast was fabricated and provided with wear and care instructions. The family was instructed to begin a regime of scar massage and mobilization. A follow-up appointment was made for several days later. Aggressive telephone calling was necessary to reach the busy surgeon prior to LE's next visit. Concerns about a high-radial nerve palsy were addressed. The surgeon reported that he was one of a team of surgeons who worked on LE, and that the brachial plexus had been visualized and appeared to be intact at the time of this surgery. It was possible that the posterior cord of the plexus was now acutely compressed from edema and/or from scar tissue. The surgeon instructed the therapist to monitor the radial nerve palsy with appropriate testing and proceed with appropriate splinting and therapy.

At LE's next therapy visit, a dynamic extension assist splint was fabricated. LE was allowed to come out of his long arm splint for initially short exercise sessions, and the dynamic splint was to be worn during this time to prevent overstretching of the paralyzed muscles and to encourage LE to use the right dominant arm with light activities. Already LE had (competently) switched to his left hand to complete many tasks; he was at risk for a disuse atrophy. Therapy sessions focused on age-appropriate play activities, such as playing a board game where the right hand had to move the pieces.

LE was weaned from the long arm splint over the first 3 weeks of therapy. A nighttime static volar splint was fabricated to hold his wrist, thumb, and digit MP joints in extension, and the dynamic splint was to be used during the day. LE preferred the static short arm splint, because the outrigger of the dynamic splint got in his way with dressing. Therapy continued to focus on incorporating the right arm into ADLs; however, the loss of stability at the elbow and wrist secondary to muscle paresis was a strong hindrance MMTs continued to show no palpable muscle fiber contractions in the triceps or in any of the radial wrist extensors. LE's scar, although mobile, was hypertrophic, despite use of scar-compression gel pads.

Because of the extraordinary nature of the injury, LE's parents were able to get an HMO extension beyond the typical 2 months of therapy. At 3 months post injury, electrodiagnostic testing was conducted. No activity was seen in the radial nerve. Surgery options were discussed; however, the family and the vascular surgeon felt the risks of an exploratory neurolysis of the radial nerve outweighed the benefits. Therefore, approximately 5 months from the initial injury, LE underwent tendon transfers to correct his wrist drop. At this point, it was clear that switching dominance made sense, since the left unimpaired arm had better strength overall and good elbow stability in particular. Postoperative rehabilitation, therefore, included change of dominance training and was uneventful. Again, therapy focused on age-appropriate activities, including playing with a yoyo, a paddleball, and eventually bouncing a basketball to facilitate strength and motor reeducation of the transferred muscles.

Post-script: Two years after the injury, LE did undergo an exploratory neurolysis. The radial nerve was found to be bound down in scar tissue and adhered to the brachial artery. Repair was attempted in hopes that LE would get some triceps return. He went through another course of therapy, but no functional strength return of the triceps muscle was seen.

CASE STUDY 24-3 ■

TB is a 52-year-old, left hand dominant machine shop worker with bilateral CTS. He underwent a CTR for his right hand; then 6 weeks later had his left carpal tunnel released. Past medical history includes insulin-dependent diabetes, cardiac issues, sleep apnea, and obesity. TB lives with his sickly wife, on whom he clearly dotes, and with his mother in-law, whom he describes as demanding and lazy. Because of his wife's illness and his mother-in-law's presence, he is solely responsible for cooking, cleaning, shopping, and household maintenance. His grown son lives in the area, has been in some recent legal trouble, and has had his driver's license temporarily revoked. TB is on call to drive him to and from work. He is helping his son fix the motor on his car so that once the driving restrictions are lifted, the son can drive himself. TB is also the self-appointed guardian of his neighborhood. Because of his size (and he is indeed a large, imposing man), neighbors call him to deal with errant teenage children. He has been known to take a disrespectful teenager on a tour of the local prison. Leisure interests include hunting with a bow and arrow. He wants to return to work and to return to hunting as soon as possible.

TB arrived late at the clinic for his initial evaluation; he got lost. He became agitated and was quite vocal with the receptionist. He was quickly taken back to the evaluation room, where he immediately complained of serious left hand pain, swelling, and weakness. He insisted that he had no trouble when recovering from surgery with his right (non-dominant) hand. A couple of discrete questions allowed the therapist to glean the earlier personal, social, and community demands upon TB, while also allowing him some time to calm down.

TB was 12 days postoperative of a left CTR. The sutures were still in place, and he was wearing a beaten-up, prefabricated wrist splint that did not quite close around his swollen hand and wrist. Both hands were quite large and clean but had calluses. There was some yellow exudate oozing from the incision site on the left hand, indicating possible infection. The old splint was thrown out. The incision area was cleaned and dressed with a sterile, non-adherent dressing. The physician was called and notified that the incision appeared infected. The physician instructed the therapist to fabricate a new wrist

orthotic that the patient was to wear full time until his next doctor's appointment. A prescription antibiotic was called in to the patient's pharmacy.

The new splint was fabricated, and it was provided with wear and care instructions reviewed both verbally and in written format. Activity restrictions were clearly outlined with repercussions emphasized in case TB should not follow through. He was told that his right hand likely healed better because he wasn't using it as much. (Remember, he is left hand dominant.) He was told that he would need to give his left hand similar "time off" if he wants it to heal. The real issue for TB, though, was when he was told that he would not be able to engage in hunting in the next 2 or 3 months, given his response to surgery and postoperative recovery. TB had a hunting trip scheduled for early Fall, and he desperately wanted to go. Rigid adherence to the activity restrictions provided by the surgeon and therapist would be a necessary prerequisite; although, no promises were made.

TB was seen 3 days later. The wounds were clean, and the orthotic showed signs that TB had been using it regularly. The evaluation was completed. TB had limited finger flexion to the distal palmar crease and was unable to oppose his thumb past his long finger. A sensory evaluation indicated diminished light touch to diminished protective sensation in all fingertips. This is not an uncommon finding for someone with diabetes. There appeared to be significant edema in the hand, but the sutures precluded volumetric measurements. Wrist ROM was not assessed per the physician's orders. TB was instructed in tendon glide exercises and thumb opposition exercises. Activity restrictions were reviewed again. Time was spent instructing TB about tissue tolerances, wound healing time tables, and the need to balance rest with the stimulation of AROM exercises.

TB was seen three times a week for the next 3 months. He continued to periodically overdo his home program and/or to overdo his activities at home. He developed significant scar hypersensitivity and pillar pain in the left hand, which was probably exacerbated by his postoperative infection. Modalities for pain relief were tried, including iontophoresis. However, the iontophoresis played havoc with his blood sugar, and he reported a bad headache after the first trial session; therefore, this modality was not used again.

TB's job was considered a medium physical demand level, meaning he must be able to perform a maximum lift of 50 lbs. Strength issues and general body mechanics were addressed in preparation for return to work. TB reported that he might be required to hammer between 8 to 288 nails into a board that is approximately 2 inches thick, although he believed he would be allowed to pace himself. Ergonomic leather gloves with the palmar surface padded and the fingertips free were procured for use at work. TB demonstrated good tolerance for hammering with the gloves on.

As the date of the hunting trip loomed closer, TB anxiously explored his options. Apparently, shooting a bow and arrow requires considerable bilateral hand strength and endurance, which TB did not have at that time. There was a particular bow design, called a *cross bow*, that would allow him to participate in hunting with less stress to his hands. He would need special medical approval to get a permit to use this design. His physician was contacted, the prescription written, and TB successfully attended his hunting trip with his new cross bow. (Unfortunately, because of the weather that year, there were no deer to be had.)

TB did successfully return to work. For the next year and a half, he popped up at the clinic about every 4 to 6 months requesting new work gloves, because his gloves regularly wore out with the tough work tasks in which he was engaged.

References

1. Lundy-Ekman L: *Neuroscience: fundamentals for rehabilitation*, ed 4, St Louis, 2013, Elsevier Saunders.
2. Duff S: Impact of peripheral nerve injury on sensorimotor control, *J Hand Ther* 18:277–291, 2005.
3. Dellon AL: Client evaluation and management considerations in nerve compression. In Rayan GM, editor: *Hand clinics: nerve compression syndromes*, Philadelphia, 1992, WB Saunders.
4. Butler DS: *Noigroup Publications, The sensitive nervous system*, Adelaide, 2000, Australia.
5. Merzenich MM, Jenkins WM: Reorganization of cortical representations of the hand following alterations of skin inputs induced by nerve injury, skin island transfers, and experience, *J Hand Ther* 6(2):89–104, 1993.
6. Elvey RL: Physical evaluation of the peripheral nervous system in disorders of pain and dysfunction, *J Hand Ther* 10:122–129, 1997.
7. Jacoby SM, Eichenbaum MD, Osterman AL: Basic science of nerve compression. In Skirven T, Osterman L, Fedorcyzyk J, et al: *Rehabilitation of the hand and upper extremity*, ed 6, St Louis, 2011, Elsevier, pp 649–656.
8. Smith KL: Nerve response to injury and repair. In Skirven T, Osterman L, Fedorcyzyk J, et al: *Rehabilitation of the hand and upper extremity*, ed 6, St Louis, 2011, Elsevier, pp 601–610.
9. Butler DS: *Mobilisation of the nervous system*, Melbourne, 1991, Churchill Livingstone.
10. Lundborg G: Peripheral nerve injuries: pathophysiology and strategies for treatment, *J Hand Ther* 6(3):179–188, 1993.
11. Rydevik B, Lundborg G, Bagge U: Effects of graded compression on intraneural blood flow, *J Hand Surgery Am* 6(1):3–12, 1981.
12. Gelberman RH, Szabo RM, Williamson RV, et al: Tissue pressure threshold for peripheral nerve viability, *Clin Orthop Relat Res*(178)285–291, 1983.
13. Gelberman RH, Hergenroeder PT, Hargens AR, et al: The carpal tunnel syndrome: a study of carpal canal pressures, *J Bone Joint Surg Am* 63(3):380–383, 1981.
14. Slutsky DJ: New Advances in Nerve Repair. In Skirven T, Osterman L, Fedorcyzyk J, et al: *Rehabilitation of the hand and upper extremity*, ed 6, St Louis, 2011, Elsevier, pp 611–618.
15. Gutman S: *Quick reference neuroscience for rehabilitation professionals*, Thorofare, NJ, 2001, SLACK.
16. Evans RB: Therapist's management of carpal tunnel syndrome: a practical approach. In Skirven T, Osterman L, Fedorcyzyk J, et al: *Rehabilitation of the hand and upper extremity*, ed 6, St Louis, 2011, Elsevier, pp 666–677.
17. Lee SK, Wolfe SW: Peripheral nerve injury and repair, *J Am Acad Orthop Surg* (8)243–252, 2000.
18. Callahan AD: Sensibility assessment for nerve lesions in continuity and nerve lacerations. In Skirven T, Osterman L, Fedorcyzyk J, et al: *Rehabilitation of the hand and upper extremity*, ed 5, St Louis, 2002, Mosby, pp 214–239.
19. Dang AC, Rodner CM: Unusual compression neuropathies of the forearm, part I: radial nerve, *J Hand Surg Am* 34(10):1906–1914, 2009.
20. Isaacs J: Treatment of acute peripheral nerve injuries: current concepts, *J Hand Sur Am* 35(3):491–497, 2010.
21. Slutsky DJ: A practical approach to nerve grafting in the upper extremity, *Hand Clin* 10:73–92, 2005.
22. Baker NA, Moehling KK, Rubinstein EN, et al: The comparative effectiveness of combined lumbrical muscle splints and stretches on symptoms and function in carpal tunnel syndrome, *Arch Phys Med Rehabil* 93:1–10, 2012.
23. Duff SV, Estilow T: Therapist's management of peripheral nerve injury. In Skirven T, Osterman L, Fedorcyzyk J, et al: *Rehabilitation of the hand and upper extremity*, ed 6, St Louis, 2011, Elsevier, pp 619–633.
24. Rosen B, Lundborg G: Sensory reeducation. In Skirven T, Osterman L, Fedorcyzyk J, et al: *Rehabilitation of the hand and upper extremity*, ed 6, St Louis, 2011, Elsevier, pp 634–648.
25. Porretto-Loerke A, Soika E: Therapist's management of other nerve compressions about the elbow and wrist. In Skirven T, Osterman L, Fedorcyzyk J, et al: *Rehabilitation of the hand and upper extremity*, ed 6, St Louis, 2011, Elsevier, pp 695–712.
26. Galper J, Verno V: Pain. In Palmer ML, Epler ME, editors: *Fundamentals of musculoskeletal assessment techniques*, ed 2, Philadelphia, 1998, Lippincott-Raven.
27. Hannah S, Hudak P: Splinting and radial nerve palsy: a single-subject experiment, *J Hand Ther* 14:195–201, 2001.
28. Colditz JC: Splinting for radial nerve palsy, *J Hand Ther* 1:18–23, 1987.
29. Eaton CJ, Lister GD: Radial nerve compression. In Rayan GM, editor: *Hand clinics: nerve compression syndromes*, Philadelphia, 1992, WB Saunders.
30. Cleary C: Management of radial tunnel syndrome: a therapist's clinical perspective, *J Hand Ther* 19:186–191, 2006.
31. Colditz JC: Splinting the hand with a peripheral nerve injury. In Mackin EJ, Callahan AD, Skirven TM, editors: *Rehabilitation of the hand and upper extremity*, ed 5, St Louis, 2002, Mosby, pp 622–634.
32. Cannon N, editor: *Diagnosis and treatment manual for physicians and therapists*, ed 4, Indianapolis, 2001, Hand Rehabilitation Center of Indiana.
33. Abzug J, Martyak GG, Culp RW: Other nerve compression syndromes of the wrist and elbow. In Skirven T, Osterman L, Fedorcyzyk J, et al: *Rehabilitation of the hand and upper extremity*, ed 6, St Louis, 2011, Elsevier, pp 686–694.
34. Keir PJ, Rempel DM: Pathomechanics of peripheral nerve loading: evidence in carpal tunnel syndrome, *J Hand Ther* 18:259–269, 2005.
35. Eversmann E: Proximal median nerve compression. In Rayan GM, editor: *Hand clinics: nerve compression syndromes*, Philadelphia, 1992, WB Saunders.
36. Omer GE: Median nerve compression at the wrist. In Rayan GM, editor: *Hand clinics: nerve compression syndromes*, Philadelphia, 1992, WB Saunders.
37. Dang AC, Rodner CM: Unusual compression neuropathies of the forearm, part ii: median nerve, *J Hand Surg Am* 34:1915–1920, 2009.
38. Amadio P: Carpal tunnel syndrome: a surgeon's management. In Skirven T, Osterman L, Fedorcyzyk J, et al: *Rehabilitation of the hand and upper extremity*, ed 6, St Louis, 2011, Elsevier, pp 657–665.
39. MacDermid JC: Measurement of health outcomes following tendon and nerve repair, *J Hand Ther* 18:297–312, 2005.
40. Chi Y, Harness N: Anterior interosseous nerve syndrome, *J Hand Surg Am* 35(12):2078–2080, 2010.
41. Rayan GM: Proximal ulnar nerve compression: cubital tunnel syndrome. In Rayan GM, editor: *Hand clinics: nerve compression syndromes*, Philadelphia, 1992, WB Saunders.
42. Moneim MS: Ulnar nerve compression at the wrist: ulnar tunnel syndrome. In Rayan GM, editor: *Hand clinics: nerve compression syndromes*, Philadelphia, 1992, WB Saunders.
43. Lund AT, Amadio PC: Treatment of cubital tunnel syndrome: perspectives for the therapist, *J Hand Ther* 19:170–179, 2006.
44. Apfel E, Sigafoos GT: Comparison of range of motion constraints provided by splints used in the treatment of cubital tunnel syndrome—a pilot study, *J Hand Ther* 19:384–392, 2006.
45. Rekant MS: Diagnosis and surgical management of cubital tunnel syndrome. In Skirven T, Osterman L, Fedorcyzyk J, et al: *Rehabilitation of the hand and upper extremity*, ed 6, St Louis, 2011, Elsevier, pp 678–685.
46. Dellon AL, Coert JH: Results of the musculofascial lengthening technique for submuscular transposition of the ulnar nerve at the elbow, *J Bone Joint Surg Am* 86:169–179, 2004.
47. Vipond N, Taylor W, Rider MR: postoperative splinting for isolated digital nerve injuries in the hand, *J Hand Ther* 20:222–231, 2007.
48. Yu RS, Catalono LW 3rd, Barron OA, et al: Limited protected post-surgical motion does not affect the results of digital nerve repair, *J Hand Sur Am* 29(2):302–306, 2004.
49. Vaught MS, Brismée JM, Dedrick GS, et al: Association of disturbances in the thoracic outlet in subjects with carpal tunnel syndrome: a case-control study, *J Hand Ther* 24(1):44–52, 2011.
50. Topp KS, Boyd BS: Peripheral nerve: from the microscopic functional unit of the axon to the biomechanically loaded macroscopic structure, *J Hand Ther* 25:142–152, 2012.

51. Law M, et al: *Canadian occupational performance measure manual,* Toronto, 1991, CAOT Publications ACE.
52. Dellon AL: *Somatosensory testing and rehabilitation,* Bethesda, MD, 1997, American Occupational Therapy Association.
53. Brand P: Pain—It's all in your head: a philosophical essay, *J Hand Ther* 10(2):59–63, 1997.
54. Bracciano A: *Physical agent modalities: theory and application for the occupational therapist,* Thorofare, NJ, 2000, SLACK.
55. Michlovitz SL: Is there a role for ultrasound and electrical stimulation following injury to tendon and nerve? *J Hand Ther* 18:292–296, 2005.
56. Echigo A, Aoki M, Ishiai S, et al: The excursion of the median nerve during nerve gliding exercise: an observation with high-resolution ultrasonography, *J Hand Ther* 21(3):221–228, 2008.
57. Rozmaryn LM, Dovelle S, Rothman ER, et al: Nerve and tendon gliding exercises and the conservative management of carpal tunnel syndrome, *J Hand Ther* 11(3):171–178, 1998.
58 Wilgis S, Murphy R: The significance of longitudinal excursions in the peripheral nerves, *Hand Clinics* 2:761–768, 1986.
59. Wright TW, Glowczewskie F Jr, Wheeler D, Miller G, Cowin D: Excursion and strain of the median nerve, *J Bone Joint Surg Am.* 78:1897–1903, 1996.
60. Totten PA, Hunter JM: Therapeutic techniques to enhance nerve gliding in thoracic outlet syndrome and carpal tunnel syndrome, *Hand Clin* 7:505, 1991.

25

Wrist Fractures

Anne M.B. Moscony and Tracy Shank

"Thank goodness it's only a fracture. I thought it might be broken."

Client quote, with thanks, from Paul LaStayo, Kerri Winters, and Maureen Hardy[1]

Introduction

Bone fractures are common injuries; in fact, in 2002, the American Academy of Orthopedic Surgeons estimated that on average, each of us will experience two bone fractures over our lifetime. A **fracture** results in impairment of the skeleton's mechanical integrity, which typically leads to functional deficits and pain, especially when the hand is involved. Bone stability is one of the prerequisites for initiation of hand therapy following a fracture. Therefore, an understanding of the biological process of bone healing and the various methods for surgically enhancing bone stability (and thus healing) is important.

General Timelines and Healing

"The goal of fracture healing is to regenerate mineralized tissue in the fracture area and restore mechanical strength to the bone. Ultimately, all fractures must heal with new bone, not scar tissue."[1]

Bones are covered by a dense fibrous connective tissue membrane called the **periosteum.** This strong membrane is united firmly to the shaft of the bone and merges with **articular cartilage** that covers the ends of the bone. The periosteum has two layers: a relatively vascular outer layer and a more cellular and delicate inner layer. The cells (osteoblasts) of this inner layer are capable of producing new bone. Other bone forming cells line the medullary cavity of mature bone, forming the **endosteum.** When a fracture occurs, these osteoblasts begin to lay down bone across the break, forming an enlargement or callus where the fracture occurred.

Following a non-displaced fracture (that is, a fracture where the periosteum remains intact), the body initiates a three-phased organized and predictable process of bone healing. The initial **inflammatory phase** lasts 1 to 7 days. At this time, immediate cellular and vascular responses to the injury promote the formation of a hematoma, which in turn provides some early fracture stabilization. This stage is followed by a **repair phase** where the damaged cells (including the hematoma) are removed and replaced with callus bone (Fig. 25-1, *A* and *B*). This soft callus is characterized by fibrous or cartilaginous tissue within the fracture gap and a significant increase in vascularity. At this point, the fractured ends are no longer freely moveable. The soft callus is gradually converted to hard callus, or woven bone tissue by a process of mineralization called **enchondral ossification** (see Fig. 25-1, *C* and *D*). The repair phase can last up to 4 months, although it is usually complete by 6 weeks after the injury. Finally, there is a **remodeling phase** where the repaired tissue is replaced and reorganized over months to years to provide the bone with its pre-injury strength and structure. This ordered process of bone tissue repair and reorganization is called **secondary healing** (also called *callus healing, indirect healing,* or *enchondral ossification*).

Secondary fracture healing spans an average of 7 or more weeks depending on the location and type of fracture.[3] The initiation of active range of motion (AROM) with these fractures depends on a number of factors, including associated soft tissue injuries and the client's overall health and lifestyle. Often, controlled AROM can begin sometime between the third to sixth week after immobilization (that is, before there is radiographic evidence of bone healing).[1,3] These fractures will continue to need intermittent protection, which is usually accomplished by an interim removable orthosis.[1] By 8 to 10 weeks after the injury, most clients can begin progressive resistive exercises (or more forceful work) and leisure or homemaking tasks using the involved extremity.

Healing of a bone fracture requires stability at the injury site. Without stability, healing may be delayed, or nonunion of the fracture fragments may result. Non-displaced fractures (that is, those where the bone fragment(s) remain correctly aligned and the periosteum is intact) do not require medical intervention to restore normal bony configuration. Other fractures require some type of manipulation by the physician in order to get the bone fragments normally, or near normally, aligned. This is called **reduction.** Physicians use various techniques to realign the fracture ends.

Once a displaced fracture is appropriately realigned, it must be rendered stable either by external or internal support to ensure healing. **Unstable fractures** are those that displace spontaneously or with motion; these will require some type of fixation method to ensure that healing occurs without malunion, angulation, or rotation of the bone. The medical goal of maintaining anatomical reduction of the fracture ends is achieved by various internal and/or external means, including plates, screws, pins, casts, or orthoses.

If the physician can secure the bone fragments using stiff metal (plates and/or screws) with enough integrity that there is essentially no movement and good vascularity at the fracture site, fracture healing will bypass the typical three phases described earlier. This is called **primary healing.** Primary healing permits direct regrowth of bone because there is adequate compression across the fracture line (that is, all interfragmentary gaps are eliminated) and adequate stability (no motion between the fracture fragments). The internal rigid stability offered by a plate and/or screws serves as a substitute external callus, ensuring the absence of motion that is required for bone healing.

The advantages of rigid fixation of a fracture and consequent primary healing include avoidance of callus formation (and possible local tissue adherence), immediate access by the therapist to the fracture site for wound care and edema control, and early initiation of motion. Fracture healing timelines, soft tissue tolerances, and the client's personal interests, lifestyle, health, and functional goals will dictate progression in therapy and the choice of therapeutic activity or exercise.

> ## ◎ *Clinical Pearl*
>
> If the physician uses a rigid internal fixation to secure the fracture, AROM can and should begin within the first week post-surgery.

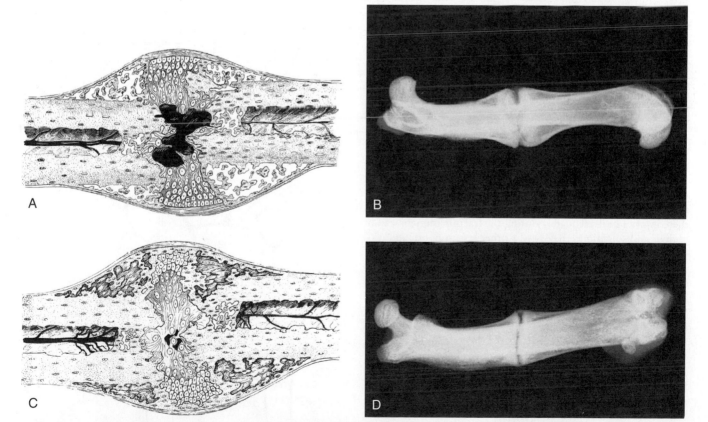

FIGURE 25-1 **A** and **B,** During the early part of the repair phase of bone fracture healing, soft callus forms in the region adjacent to the fracture ends. Dense fibrous tissue covers the central region, forming a new periosteum, which is not radiographically evident. **C** and **D,** Abundant osteoblast activity occurs during the latter part of the repair phase of bone fracture healing. Mature bone develops when the callus converts from fibrocartilaginous tissue. This early bone formation may be very thin and appears less opaque than mature bone. The central region is still the bulk of the bridging tissue. (From Browner BD, Jupiter JB, Levine AM, et al: *Skeletal trauma: basic science, management, and reconstruction,* ed 3, Philadelphia, 2003, Saunders.)

Resistive exercises require the healing bone to be structurally capable of tolerating high muscle forces across it.[1,3] Gripping forces in particular are amplified as they cross the distal radius. Lifting heavy objects or using moderate to maximal grip strength may be enough force to disrupt bony alignment or cause plate failure. Therefore, during the first 6 weeks after surgery, clients should be restricted from gripping more than 31 psi (pounds per square inch) if using an external fixator, or 36 psi if they have a volar or dorsal plate.[4,5] The therapist can teach what this amount of gripping feels like by demonstrating on the uninjured hand with the dynamometer. The introduction of resistance into the therapy plan must always be approved by the physician.

> ### Precautions and Concerns

Early resumption of resistive or repetitive work, homemaking or vocational tasks, and/or premature introduction of progressive resistive exercises will likely result in pain and increased swelling and may compromise the integrity of the healing bone.

Instead, encourage clients to use their involved hand early on for pain-free, light activities of daily living (ADLs), work, and/or leisure interests. Clients may need help in identifying and grading these tasks appropriately so that they do not overuse the injured extremity.

> ### Clinical Pearl

Most daily activities (such as, buttoning, zippering, or using utensils) require about 20 lbs of grip strength and 5 lbs to 7 lbs of pinch strength.[30,31]

Associated Soft Tissue Injuries Following Bone Fracture

A wise orthopedic surgeon observed that "…a fracture is a soft tissue injury that happens to involve the bone."[4] Fractures to the forearm are diagnosed in the emergency room by x-ray with little difficulty; however, associated soft tissue trauma may not be as easily recognized. Given the forces required to break a bone, concomitant soft tissue injuries can be expected. Sometimes these injuries heal adequately during the fracture immobilization period, and sometimes they need further rest, support, and protection requiring up to 12 weeks or more to fully heal.

Soft tissue injuries commonly associated with wrist fractures may include injury of the **triangular fibrocartilage complex (TFCC),** peripheral nerve injury/injuries, ligament sprain or tear, and/or an aggravation of pre-existing osteoarthritis.[7] Early detection of these conditions allows the therapist to explain associated symptoms to their clients, aids the therapist in determining appropriate modifications in the plan of care, and leads to more successful treatment outcomes. It is important to communicate these findings to the client's referring physician through telephone calls and/or written reports.

If surgery is required to reduce the fracture, the surgery itself produces a soft tissue disruption or "injury." Like bone healing, soft tissue healing follows a predictable three stage process. The inflammatory phase lasts between 1 and 5 days and is characterized by a cascade of healing cells (cytokines, histamines, prostaglandins, and fibrinogen) entering the injured area. Resultant edema is usually resolved within 10 days. The second phase of soft

tissue healing lasts from 2 to 6 weeks and is called the **fibroblastic phase.** During this phase, cells called *fibroblasts* polymerize, forming a diffuse collagen network of interstitial scar. Gains in range of motion (ROM) are most easily attained at this time. During the last phase, termed **maturation**, the scar tissue becomes more organized and acts to provide stability to the traumatized area. The maturation phase continues from 6 weeks up to 2 years. As interstitial scar becomes more organized, ROM limitations due to adhesions will become increasingly resistive to change.[4]

Distal Forearm Fractures

Anatomy

The **wrist** is the common term used to describe the multiple articulations that exist between the distal radius, ulna, and eight carpal bones (Fig. 25-2). The distal radius articulates with the scaphoid and lunate; and this is called the **radiocarpal joint.** It is a biaxial ellipsoid joint, meaning it has two axes of motion: (wrist) flexion/extension and radial/ulnar deviation. The normal radiocarpal joint has a slight palmar tilt or angulation (of about 10° to 15°) when viewed laterally by x-ray. Maintaining this palmar tilt following fracture of the radius has been linked to functional outcomes, including return of pain free normal ROM.[8]

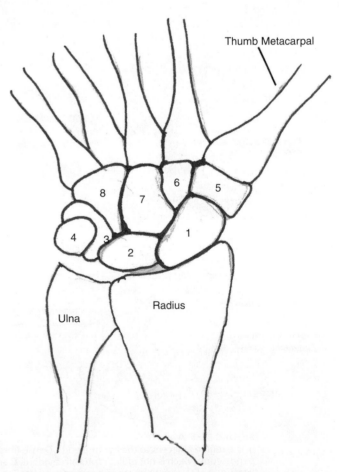

FIGURE 25-2 Schematic of the bones and multiple articulations of the wrist. *1,* Scaphoid; *2,* lunate; *3,* triquetrum; *4,* pisiform; *5,* trapezium; *6,* trapezoid; *7,* capitate; *8,* hamate.

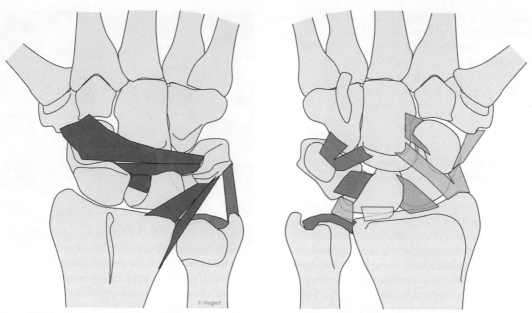

FIGURE 25-3 Triangular fibrocartilage complex (TFCC). Dorsal and Volar view. From Slutsky DJ: *Principles and practice of wrist surgery,* Philadelphia, 2010, Saunders.)

The ulna does not directly articulate with the proximal carpal row. Instead, the TFCC, a hammock-like structure composed of cartilage and ligaments, suspends the ulnar carpus and acts as both a force distributor between the ulna head and triquetrum, and a primary stabilizer for the **distal radioulnar joint (DRUJ)** (Fig. 25-3). The central portion is an articular disc that provides a smooth gliding surface for the ulnar carpus. It has no blood supply; therefore, it will not heal if torn. The peripheral portions are ligamentous and capable of bearing tensile loads generated during gripping or weight bearing on the wrist. These portions have fair-to-excellent blood supply and accordingly have a fair-to-good capacity to heal following injury. When bearing weight on the wrist, or gripping, about 80% of the load traveling through the carpal bones is transferred to the radius and 20% is transferred to the ulna by way of the TFCC.[9] Therefore, injury to the TFCC may have significant functional repercussions for our clients, including loss of grip strength and pain with loading of the wrist and/or distal forearm.

The distal radius articulates with the distal ulna to form the DRUJ (Fig. 25-4). This is an important joint because it is a major site of persistent symptoms and residual disability after fracture of the distal radius.[10] The DRUJ is a **uniaxial pivot joint** that allows rotatory motion called *supination and pronation of the forearm.* The action of forearm rotation involves the radius pivoting around a relatively stable ulna. However, the ulna is not completely stationary. There is a "proximal-distal" translation of the ulna with regard to the radius during pronation. In fact, the ulna slides distally up to 2 mm in relation to the radius during pronation.[9] This subtle movement is relevant in that a fracture (of the radius or ulna) can result in changes in the relationship between the length of the radius and ulna and/or in how much the ulna translates or moves during pronation.

◎ Clinical Pearl

A change in the proportion of force distributed to the radius or ulna during gripping or loading of the wrist often results in pathology and pain.

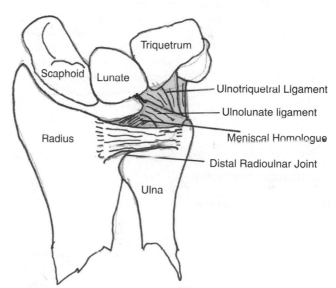

FIGURE 25-4 Anatomy of the distal radioulnar joint (DRUJ). The head of the ulna covers 80% of the surface and articulates with the sigmoid notch of the distal radius (radially) and with the inferior surface of the triangular fibrocartilage complex (TFCC). *L,* Lunate; *S,* scaphoid; *T,* triquetrum. (Copyright the Mayo Foundation. From Cooney WP, Linscheid RL, Dobyns JH, editors: *The wrist: diagnosis and operative treatment,* St Louis, 1998, Mosby, p. 775.)

It is more common to see distal radius/ulna fractures as opposed to shaft fractures because of the difference in the density of the bone. The **shaft** of a long bone (such as, the radius) has more cortical bone, which is denser and thus more difficult to break. It also has less blood flow and on average takes longer to heal. The enlarged distal end of the radius has more cancellous bone, which is less dense (that is, more susceptible to fracture). On the other hand, cancellous bone has a greater blood supply, which contributes to faster healing as compared to fractures of the shaft of a bone.[14]

In general, distal forearm fractures fall into three categories based on the degree of bone displacement and damage. The fracture requiring the least amount of intervention is typically the **extra-articular fracture** that is non-displaced. This means that the fractured bone is still in place and that the fracture did not cross into joint space, interrupting the cartilage at the end of the bone. These typically stable fractures heal with immobilization from a cast or orthosis brace with relatively few complications. Ulnar styloid fractures frequently fall into this category and, thus, require minimal treatment. If the ulnar styloid is displaced and interrupts the TFCC, medical intervention will be needed. Minimally displaced **intra-articular fractures** occur when the fractured bone segment shifts and crosses into the joint space. The result is greater soft tissue damage with a possible change in angulation of the bone's articular or joint surface. This type of fracture will require some type of reduction, such as a closed reduction followed by tight casting, or by pinning, external fixation or internal fixation. Chauffeur's fracture (fracture of the radial styloid) falls into this category. Following reduction, these fractures are usually secured with percutaneous pins unless there is an associated disruption of the scapholunate space. In this case, additional fixation may be needed.

A **comminuted** extra-articular fracture is usually a high-energy injury, resulting in the bone breaking into multiple segments. Once reduced, these fractures are secured with pins, wires, plates, and/or screws. This type of injury is less stable than those described earlier and the length and angulation of the bone's articular surface may be altered with adverse functional ramifications. Similarly, a comminuted intra-articular fracture is a high-energy injury characterized by multiple bone fragments, some of which shift or protrude into the joint space. These are highly unstable fractures that require surgical reduction and stabilization techniques (Fig. 25-5).[13]

Diagnosis and Pathology

Distal Forearm Fractures

Distal forearm or wrist fractures usually (47%) result from impact to the outstretched hand and wrist during falls (Fig. 25-6). This mode of injury is sometimes referred to as a **fall on out-stretched hand (FOOSH).** Distal forearm fractures account for approximately 44% of upper extremity fractures[11] and 15% of all fractures in adults in the United States.[10] The likelihood of falls resulting in a distal radius fracture is greatest in two groups. The first group consists of those between the ages of 5 and 14 years who sustain a high-energy, sports-related fall. Increased participation in sports (such as, soccer, rugby, and snowboarding) seems to be correlated with this relatively high incidence of wrist fractures. The second group consists of seniors who sustain a low-energy fall and have resultant fracture(s) due to osteoporotic bone. The incidence of distal forearm/wrist fractures is expected to increase by 50% over the next 20 years due to the growth of the elderly population.[12]

There are several types of distal forearm fractures. A **Colles' fracture** is the most common type; and is also one of the most common fractures seen in the human body.[10,11] It is defined as a complete fracture of the distal radius with dorsal displacement of the distal fragment and radius shortening (Fig. 25-7 *A*). It is usually extra-articular, minimally displaced, and stable—meaning the fracture will stay reduced when placed in a cast or a fracture brace. The majority of these fractures occur in postmenopausal

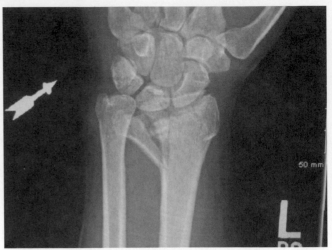

FIGURE 25-5 Intra-articular distal radius fracture. (Courtesy of Kevin Lutsky, MD.)

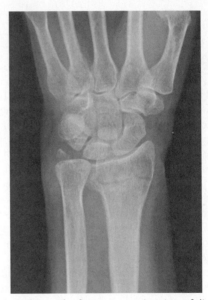

FIGURE 25-6 Radiograph of anteroposterior view of distal radius fracture. (From Skirven T, Osterman AL, Fedorczyk J, et al: *Rehabilitation of the hand and upper extremity*, Philadelphia, 2011, Elsevier.)

women with osteoporotic bone.[12] See Table 25-1 for a list of common forearm fractures and their clinical features.

> ◎ **Clinical Pearl**
>
> Therapists should be aware that the label "Colles fracture" is frequently applied to more complex types of dorsally-displaced forearm fractures that may require more than reduction with casting to restore anatomic alignment.

Smith's fracture is a complete fracture of the distal radius with volar displacement of the distal fragment (see Fig. 25-7 *B*). This is the second most common distal radius fracture. A Smith fracture is frequently unstable and requires some type of internal fixation to hold the displaced distal fragment in correct alignment for healing.

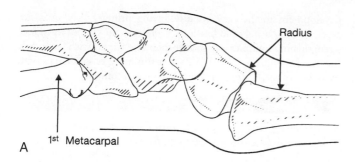

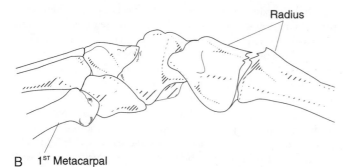

FIGURE 25-7 **Schematic of two types of distal radius fractures.**
A, Colles' fracture with dorsal displacement of distal fragment.
B, Smith's fracture with volar displacement of distal fragment. (From
Stanly BG, Tribuzi SM, editors: *Concepts in hand rehabilitation*, Philadel-
phia, 1992, FA Davis.)

Non-Operative Treatment for Distal Radius Fractures

The goal of therapy for any distal forearm fracture is restoration
of pre-injury function. This is achieved by facilitating the return
of strength and of maximum pain-free ROM of the joints of the
involved extremity, including the shoulder.

> ◎ **Clinical Pearl**
>
> Monitor the motion, strength, and function of the shoulder after
> a distal forearm fracture. Protective posturing of the involved
> extremity can lead to adaptive shortening of the shoulder's
> internal rotators, as well as elbow stiffness, making it difficult for
> the client to reach up and back to put on a coat, for example.

Extra-articular, stable fractures are usually treated with closed
reduction and casting for a period of 2 to 8 weeks.[13,15] The position of immobilization is one of moderate wrist flexion and ulnar
deviation, because this position uses the surrounding intact soft
tissue to help maintain the fracture reduction.

> ➢ **Precautions and Concerns**
>
> *This position can cause or aggravate carpal tunnel symptoms, be-
> cause prolonged moderate wrist flexion will increase carpal tunnel
> pressures to potentially dangerous levels.[15] It is therefore important
> to monitor the client's sensory complaints during the period of cast
> immobilization and promptly report concerns to the physician.*

TABLE 25-1	Common Forearm/Wrist Fractures
Type of Fracture	**Clinical Feature**
Colles' fracture (see Fig. 25-6, *A*)	A fracture of the distal radius with dorsal displacement (from hyperextension of the wrist). Managed surgically with closed reduction and casting or ORIF with volar plate and sometimes simultaneous carpal tunnel release as indicated. Will typically need temporary orthosis for support and protection and some therapy to regain full ROM.
Smith's fracture (see Fig. 25-6, *B*)	A fracture of the distal radius with volar displacement (from hyperflexion of wrist). Surgical and therapeutic management is same as Colles' fracture.
Barton's fracture	Fracture-dislocation of rim of radius along the carpus caused by shearing forces from the proximal carpus translating across the radius. Surgical management with plate or screw. Therapy indicated to regain ROM and for protective orthosis.
Chauffeur's fracture	Fracture of the radial styloid. Typically surgically managed with pinning. Minimal therapy needs. Check for irritation of DRSN.
Salter-Harris fracture	Fracture of the growth (epiphyseal) plate of children and teens. At least nine variations/types have been described. These injuries are potentially serious and necessitate a visit to a hand surgeon versus general practitioner and may require some follow-up by a hand therapist.
Galeazzi's fracture	Unstable fracture of radial shaft and DRUJ disruption. Usually the result of a FOOSH and seen most often in males. Need to check for AIN palsy and trauma to the radial nerve. Higher risk of malunion than other forearm fractures. Usually treated with closed reduction in children and always with ORIF in adults due to the otherwise chronic dislocations of the ulna. Requires skilled therapy post-surgery.
Monteggia's fracture	Unstable fracture of ulnar shaft and radial head dislocation. Usually the result of a FOOSH or blunt trauma (nightstick injury). In children these usually heal readily with closed reduction and casting. In adults, ORIF is typically preferred and skilled therapy is required due to high risk of complications.
Greenstick fracture	Incomplete fracture common in children. Concave side of bone may be intact or buckled. Convex side has fracture. Typically casted for 3 to 5 weeks and does not require therapy.
Torus (buckle) fracture	Incomplete fracture common in children. Concave side of bone compresses (buckles). Convex side is intact. Pain and/or swelling occurs at the fracture site. Movement may be painful. Typically casted for 3 to 5 weeks. Therapy is frequently not needed.

AIN, Anterior interosseous nerve; *DRSN,* dorsal radial sensory nerve; *DRUJ,* distal radioulnar joint; *FOOSH,* fall on out-stretched hand; *ORIF,* open reduction and internal
fixation; *ROM,* range of motion.

Operative Treatment for Distal Forearm Fractures

Unstable distal radius fractures may be treated with percutaneous pinning alone or in conjunction with casting, external fixation, or arthroscopic reduction. More commonly, these fractures are treated with a volar or dorsally fixed metal plate secured to the bone fragments with screws. The biomechanics of reduction with plating are complicated by the goals of maintaining radial length through traction and manipulation, addressing ligament continuity, and allowing for periosteal injury reduction.

Complex distal radius fractures, such as a volarly displaced fracture-dislocation of the distal radius (a Barton's fracture), or those fractures who have a concomitant open wound with soft tissue damage will usually require an open reduction and internal fixation (ORIF) of the fracture with a plate (Fig. 25-8). In this case, stability should be adequate to allow early active motion of the wrist, starting within the first week or so postoperatively. Control of edema, wound care and scar management, pain management, and restoration of digit motion are priorities along with return of wrist and forearm motion during the first 2 months of therapy. Close communication between the therapist and the physician is necessary for at least 8 to 10 weeks postoperatively.[4]

The internal rigid stability offered by a plate and/or screws serves as a substitute external callus, providing the motionless environment required for bone healing. The many advantages to rigid fixation of a fracture include avoidance of callus formation with potential local tissue adherence and early initiation of motion (within 1 week of surgery). A significant disadvantage is that plates or screws, particularly dorsally-placed ones, can cause long-term client discomfort and problems with tendon gliding, inability to extend the IP joint of thumb due to trapping of the EPL beneath the plate, and rubbing of the tendon against the plate may result in tendon rupture. In these cases, a secondary surgery may be necessary to remove the hardware. Other disadvantages include greater scarring and potential for infection. Finally, tensile strength development in the new bone following primary healing is not accelerated by using rigid fixation;[1] therefore, one cannot introduce strengthening exercises any sooner than one would with secondary fracture healing. See Table 25-2 for a summary of guidelines with each type of medical/surgical management technique.[16]

> ### ⮞ Precautions and Concerns

Strengthening exercises cannot be introduced any sooner with primary healing versus secondary healing.

Over the past 5 or more years, there has been a transition from surgeons' preference for an external fixator to use of a rigid internal fixation device, or plate, to treat unstable distal radius fractures. There are a plethora of plate and screw options that are commercially available. Plates are largely selected based upon matching fragment configuration to available options, surgeon preference, cost, and maybe even what a hospital happens to have in stock. The aims of reduction are to maintain radial length through traction and manipulation, to maintain ligament continuity, and to minimize periosteal injury.

The original plates came out in the early 1970s and were T-shaped and held in place by screws. Concerns developed with regard to dorsal plating, including issues with tendon adherence, tendon rupture, and tenosynovitis. This has led to the development of lower profile designs. Bone fragments, while stabilized via screws and/or a plate, require time for the fragments to unite firmly by new bone. New bone remodels over time with increased fracture site stiffness that will gradually mature such that the bone is able to withstand increased loads during gripping and lifting. Mature bone requires exposure to regular mechanical stress to maintain optimal health and strength. However, plates do not get stronger when exposed to mechanical stress; rather they will weaken and eventually bend or break once the metal fatigues. Therefore bone beneath a plate must have adequate strength to absorb external loading forces before much resistance is introduced to the injured

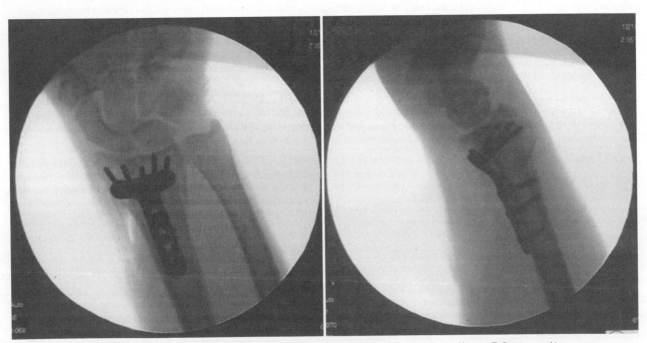

FIGURE 25-8 Two views of fixation of a distal radius extra-articular fracture. (From Skirven T, Osterman AL, Fedorczyk J, et al: *Rehabilitation of the hand and upper extremity*, ed 6, Philadelphia, 2011, Elsevier.)

area. Slutsky and Herman[4] discuss fracture site forces that can disrupt a plate, noting that grip forces during therapy should remain less than 159 N (less than 36 lbs) during the initial four weeks post fracture plating of the distal radius. Given how difficult it would be to explain to our clients just how to limit their grip forces—both at home and in the clinic—it is best to introduce strengthening exercises only after the physician has seen radiographic evidence of bone healing under the plate.

"Despite a lack of compelling clinical data proving its superiority, open reduction and volar locked plate fixation of distal radius fractures has increased in popularity in recent years. External fixation remains, however, a viable treatment option for patients with distal radius fractures. In particular, external fixation can be useful as an adjunct to pin fixation in fractures with significant comminution in which direct fixation or buttressing of the fracture fragments cannot be obtained, or as temporary or definitive fixation in fractures associated with severe soft tissue contamination or vascular injury."[2]

If traction across the fracture site cannot be achieved with a plate and screws, an **external fixator** may be used. Various types of external fixators are commercially available. These devices consist of pins, wires, or screws that attach the appropriately aligned and stabilized injured bone to an external low profile scaffold. Tension can be adjusted relatively easily by the physician. Reduction by means of an external fixator allows the therapist access to the hand and wrist for hygiene and edema control. Without a bulky cast, the client may have an easier time performing AROM of uninvolved

adjacent joints. These devices are removed after a period of 4 to 6 weeks, once the risk of loss of reduction is resolved or minimized. At this point, wrist ROM can begin. There is a high complication rate associated with these devices. Complications include median neuropathies, irritation of the dorsal sensory branch of the radial nerve, damage to finger and/or wrist tendons, finger stiffness, musculotendinous tightness, and most commonly, pin tract infections.[15] If the client has an external fixator, a removable forearm based ulnar wrist orthosis to support the ulnar wrist and the mobile transverse arch of the hand (Fig. 25-9), will improve client comfort.

> ## Clinical Pearl
>
> If a bridging external fixator was used, the client is more prone to extensor and intrinsic tightness. Exercises should aggressively address both MP flexion and PIP/ distal interphalangeal (DIP) flexion (with MP extended) especially of the index finger,[4] once the fixator is removed.

Clients who have percutaneous pins and/or external fixator devices need careful monitoring for proper pin care. This is because the pin provides direct access for bacteria to enter the subcutaneous tissues and the healing bone. Doctors have different preferences for pin sites and wound care; so, ask the referring physician for his/her protocol and be sure to reinforce this with the client.

TABLE 25-2 Types of Fixation Following Distal Radius Fracture and Associated Rehabilitation Guidelines

Type of Fixation or Immobilization	General Rehabilitation Guidelines
Cast	• Early pain and edema control using positioning (elevation of extremity), retrograde massage, and AROM of uninvolved joints • Cast on for 4 to 6 weeks; then orthosis for comfort and support for the next 2 to 4 weeks • Static progressive splinting to address joint contracture/muscle-tendon tightness after 6 weeks
External fixation	• Early pain and edema control • Pin site care • Immediate AROM of uninvolved joints; forearm rotation difficult/expect limitations, AROM of wrist not possible • Desensitization program for irritated RSN when indicated • Once hardware is removed, A/PROM to wrist and forearm can begin; focus on digital flexion, wrist extension, ulnar deviation, and supination • Static progressive orthoses can be introduced as needed to regain ROM • Advance activity and ADLs as tolerated
Dorsal plating	• Early edema control and scar management • Resting static wrist orthosis; use between exercise sessions for 4 to 6 weeks • Immediate AROM of all joints • Guarded early active wrist motion (place and hold for wrist extension) for 4 to 6 weeks may be necessary if EDC integrity is compromised by type of plate or by surgical placement of plate • Once fracture is adequately healed (as identified by physician), may begin static progressive orthosis to regain wrist motion, if needed • Advance activities and ADLs after 6 weeks
Volar fixed angle plating	• Early edema control and scar management • Immediate AROM of wrist and uninvolved joints allowed • Light ADLs to tolerance, out of orthosis • Wrist extension immobilization orthosis in slight extension for 4 to 6 weeks for comfort and for protection if in uncontrolled environment with risk of fall • Once fracture is adequately healed (as identified by physician) begin static progressive orthosis to regain wrist and forearm motion, if needed • Advance activities and ADLs after 6 weeks

ADLs, Activities of daily living; *A/PROM,* active/passive range of motion; *AROM,* active range of motion; *EDC,* extensor digitorum communis; *ROM,* range of motion, *RSN,* radial sensory nerve.
Modified from Smith D, Brou K, Henry M: Early active rehabilitation for operatively stabilized distal radius fractures, *J Hand Ther* 17(1):43-49, 2004.

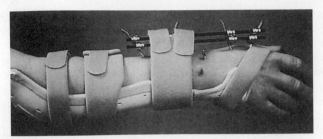

FIGURE 25-9 Ulnar gutter support orthosis, elbow included, for use with an external fixator. The orthosis supports the transverse arch of the hand and allows full motion of the thumb and fingers but limits forearm rotation. The length of the orthosis can vary, from short arm to above the elbow, depending on the need to limit forearm rotation. (From Laseter G, Carter P: Management of distal radius fractures *J Hand Ther* 9:122, 1996.)

> ◎ **Clinical Pearl**
>
> When using sterile cotton swabs, make sure the client is using one swab per pin per application. The client should never use the same swab on more than one pin. This carefulness minimizes the chances of developing infection.

Be sure to educate the client on the signs and symptoms of infection: fever, a foul smell, increased pain, heat or temperature and redness at the pin site, and the presence of **purulence** or viscous, yellowish-white colored pus that oozes from the pin site. Have the client contact his physician if he feels his pin site(s) has (have) become infected.

Maximum functional improvement may take months following a distal radius fracture: up to 6 months for uncomplicated fractures and up to 1 to 2 years for complicated fractures. Given our current atmosphere of managed care and capitation for treatment, therapists and clients may be confronted with completing rehabilitation within a timeframe that is not compatible with anatomical healing and functional recovery.

Diagnosis-Specific Information That Affects Clinical Reasoning

It is helpful to know if the fracture is extra-articular or intra-articular, because an intra-articular fracture would indicate at least some disruption of the articular cartilage, putting the joint at risk for traumatic arthritis. If it is an intra-articular fracture, it is also helpful to know which joint(s) is/are involved: the DRUJ and/or the radiocarpal joint.

Over 50% of the time, fractures of the ulnar styloid occur in conjunction with distal radius fractures; however, these ulnar styloid fractures do not typically require formal medical intervention. They do not tend to impede function or cause lasting discomfort for the client, even though many of these go on to a non-union.[9] While a fracture of the distal tip of the ulnar styloid typically poses no long term problems, it is helpful to be aware of its presence or absence in explaining early-on versus later-developing ulnar sided wrist pain. If the client is aware of the presence of an ulnar styloid fracture, it may be helpful to reassure him that these fractures are usually treated with benign neglect and that early ulnar-sided wrist pain may be indicative of nothing more than the body's attempt to assimilate to this fracture.

A wrist immobilization orthosis that stabilizes the ulnar side of the wrist may help manage the pain associated with these fractures.

A fracture to the proximal or middle one-third of the ulnar styloid may involve the TFCC, and possibly the insertion of the ECU tendon. If the fracture is non-displaced, a long arm cast or brace is worn for 3 to 4 weeks to prevent wrist and forearm motion until the fracture is healed. If the fracture is displaced, ORIF is necessary, followed by immobilization in a long arm cast for about 3 to 4 weeks.[9,16]

Distal ulnar shaft fractures can also disrupt the DRUJ; these may require either open or closed reduction and some type of fixation (for 4 to 6 weeks) to achieve stability.[9]

> ◎ **Clinical Pearl**
>
> Prolonged pain at the distal ulnar wrist area, aggravated by appropriately introduced AROM and strengthening exercises may be indicative of injury to soft tissue structures rather than to the bone itself. Client education about the necessity for slowing down the introduction of strengthening exercises, respecting pain, and using compression sleeves or neoprene wrist wrap splints to provide some external support of the irritated soft tissues is helpful.

> **? Questions to Discuss with the Physician**
>
> - Is there any disruption in radial length, inclination, or tilt?
> - Is the TFCC injured?
> - Are there any restrictions in AROM parameters?
> - What is the preferred protocol for pin care?
> - When does the physician plan to remove hardware, if at all?
> - Are there any other soft tissue considerations?
> - Does the client have pre-existing thumb or wrist arthritis that would affect rehabilitation?

Complications Following Distal Forearm Fractures

A number of factors affect the outcome of a distal forearm fracture including demographic issues, psychosocial complications, and anatomical problems. Demographic factors include hand dominance and age. For example, a middle-age manual laborer with a dominant distal radius fracture will have different standards for satisfaction than a more sedentary middle-age man with a non-dominant hand injury, or than an elderly, retired man with the same injury. Several psychosocial factors relating to patient satisfaction have been identified in the literature including aesthetics, persistent pain, ability to resume ADLs, and the ability to resume previous work roles.[17,23] A satisfactory outcome may be hindered by an individual's inability to manage pain/stress, or by loss of ability to actively participate in life roles. Maintaining a "patient," or sick, role has also been identified as a factor when assessing outcomes following a distal radius fracture.[24] Likewise, anatomical complications with persistent pain experienced during the recovery stage of distal radius fracture can be extremely frustrating to the patient and contribute to unsatisfactory results. Hand therapists must be vigilant for the development or presence of several physical complications, including chronic pain syndromes, post traumatic arthritis, and soft tissue issues, including tendinopathies and/or ligament sprains.

Complex regional pain syndrome (CRPS) is a complication sometimes seen following a distal radius fracture. Observe for signs of increased sympathetic activity and vasomotor instability. Look for discoloration of the skin, especially over the dorsal joints. Observations, such as the development of a shiny, wax-like characteristic of the skin, temperature differences in the involved hand as compared with the uninjured hand, the presence of brawny edema, increased sweating (hyperhidrosis), and persistent, unrelenting stiffness, should all be documented and reported to the treating physician, because these may be harbingers of CRPS. Often this condition presents with pain that is out of proportion to the injury. Early treatment of these symptoms increases the chance of resolving this syndrome and preventing the well-known dysfunctional consequences of CRPS.[25]

Normally there is a variance between the relative lengths of the distal articular surfaces of the radius and ulna. During forearm rotation, the ulna translates or slides, subtly changing the relationship between the distal radius, ulna, and carpus. Maximum forearm pronation results in a shift or translation of the ulna distally; this is described as an increase in positive ulnar variance. Maximum forearm supination results in a subtle decrease in ulnar variance. Following a distal radius fracture, the lengths of the radius and ulna may be altered through injury/surgical reduction. If the ulna is shortened, it can result in a pathological **negative ulnar variance,** which can cause the radius to impinge on the proximal carpal row during forearm rotation. Dorsal and radial wrist pain may develop, and there is an increased chance of developing DRUJ arthrosis and/or Kienbock disease. If the radius heals shorter than its pre-injury length and is shorter than the ulna, a pathological **positive ulnar variance** will develop (Fig. 25-10). In this scenario, the ulna can impinge on the TFCC, particularly during forearm pronation. This kinematic alteration can cause a "wear and tear" injury to the TFCC. TFCC degeneration due to positive ulnar variance is known as **ulnocarpal abutment syndrome** (also called **ulnar impaction syndrome**). This syndrome is characterized by the development of pain and traumatic arthritis of the ulnar wrist, restricted ulnar deviation of the wrist and diminished grip strength.[9] Furthermore, radial shortening of greater than 10 mm can result in 47% pronation loss and 27% supination loss.[4] Imaging techniques as well as quantitative measures, such as the gripping rotatory impaction test (GRIT), may be helpful in describing ulnar impaction. The GRIT test, as described by LeStayo and Weiss, uses a dynamometer to test strength in neutral, supinated, and pronated positions. The strength ratio of supination to pronation is calculated and compared to the contralateral side. A ratio of greater than one is indicative of ulnar impaction.[26] Restoration of the length relationship between the radius and ulna is therefore an important goal of the physician in order to preserve normal pain-free motion at the wrist joint.[4]

<table>
<tr><td>◉   Clinical Pearl</td></tr>
</table>

If ulnar abutment is present or suspected, start exercises in a supinated position to unload the ulnocarpal forces.

Fractures of the distal radius that heal with an incongruity (incompatibility) of the articular surfaces between the distal radius and the proximal carpus and/or between the distal radius and the distal ulna at the DRUJ will often develop painful degeneration

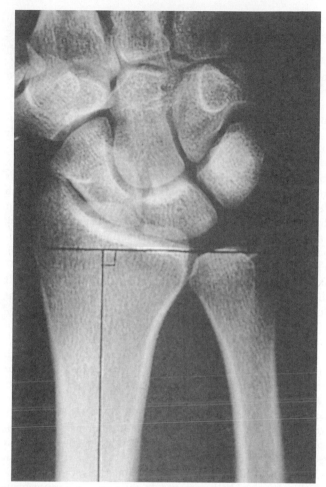

FIGURE 25-10 Standard posteroanterior x-ray view showing 1 mm positive ulnar variance. (From Jaffe R, Chidgey L, LaStayo P: The distal radio-ulnar joint: problems and solutions. *J Am Acad Orthop Surg* 3:95-109, 1995.)

or post-traumatic arthritis. Radiocarpal arthrosis presents as pain exacerbated by wrist flexion and extension. DRUJ arthrosis presents as pain that increases with forearm rotation.[9]

A **malunion** of the distal radius following a fracture infers that the fracture healed with greater than 10° of dorsal angulation of the distal radius, rather than its normal volar angulation. When this happens, one can expect to see painful gripping and difficulty with ADLs because of loss of AROM.

Non-union of a distal radius fracture means that the fracture did not heal despite adequate time and immobilization. This can occur because of metabolic issues or unsuccessful reduction. It is often associated with persistent pain and swelling. In this scenario, the patient should avoid resistive activities and seek physician's advice regarding further testing (blood, x-ray, bone scan) and the use of a bone growth stimulator.

Soft tissue complications include TFCC injury, DRUJ strain, and carpal instability. These all have functional ramifications. They can sometimes be seen on magnetic resonance imaging (MRI), although this costly testing may be limited in use due to insurance and co-pay issues. These soft tissue issues can sometimes be diagnosed by the skilled physician using provocative testing in the office. Soft tissue problems, such as a ligament strain or sprain, necessitate delaying the onset of progressive stretching and resistive activities. Protective orthoses may be needed for an extended period of time depending on the level of trauma and the patient's activity level. This is very frustrating to most patients, and they must be cautioned not to overwork the injured wrist. In some cases, diagnostic arthroscopy and surgical intervention may be required.

Tendinopathy may also occur following a distal radius fracture. Two common sites of irritation to be aware of are the extensor pollicis longus (EPL) because it winds around Lister's tubercle (a prominent bony projection on the distal radius) and the extensor carpi ulnaris (ECU) as it crosses the distal ulna. Occasionally, the EPL will rupture due to its anatomical proximity to Lister's tubercle and the resulting friction forces that occur with thumb flexion and extension. Monitor the patient's complaints about difficulty or pain with thumb motion, and adjust the therapy program accordingly. The ECU muscle is unique because it demonstrates some level of contraction in all planes of wrist motion. The ECU has its own fibro-osseous sheath tying into the TFCC and stabilizing the ECU as it course across the ulnar styloid. If this sheath is damaged, the ECU may have increased movement and friction along the distal ulna, resulting in attenuation/tendinosis. Other extensor tendinoses sometimes occur because of adhesions related to dorsal plating of the radius.

Nerve compression and/or irritation are also associated with distal radius fracture. This can occur at the median nerve, ulnar nerve, or dorsal radial sensory nerve (DRSN). If casted, the patient should be monitored for changes in sensation. The position of the cast along with post injury swelling may cause DRSN irritation and/or carpal tunnel syndrome symptoms. These symptoms can be managed with improved positioning, desensitization techniques, and nerve gliding exercises. Occasionally, the surgeon will anticipate median nerve irritation and release the carpal tunnel during volar ORIF surgeries. In this case, scar management and desensitization techniques should be added to the patient's home exercise program (HEP). Less frequently, patients complain of tingling in their fourth and fifth digits following distal radius fracture. Depending on the nature of the fracture, this could be due to positioning that is provocative to the ulnar nerve at Guyon's canal or may be due to swelling and/or adhesions.

Carpal Fractures

The eight small carpal bones are highly mobile and largely covered by articular cartilage. They can be divided into two rows: a proximal row consisting of the scaphoid, lunate, triquetrum, and pisiform; and a distal row consisting of the trapezium, trapezoid, capitate, and hamate (Fig. 25-11).[13]

➢ *Precautions and Concerns*

Blood supply is tenuous to the carpal bones, and after injury, avascular necrosis (AVN) can develop even in the best of circumstances.[27]

Most carpal fractures occur from a force applied with the wrist in extension.[27,28] Carpal fractures occur one-tenth as often as distal radius fractures with the scaphoid bone accounting for 70% to 90% of carpal fractures.[28,29] There are few outcome studies that address non-scaphoid carpal fracture treatment, since these fractures are so rare. Nonetheless, the strategy for treating

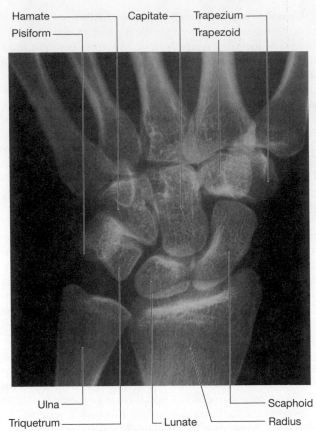

FIGURE 25-11 Posteroanterior x-ray film of a normal wrist with the carpal bones identified. (From Drake RL, Vogl W, Mitchell AWM: *Gray's anatomy for students,* Philadelphia, 2005, Churchill Livingstone.)

these fractures is the same as with any fracture: make an accurate diagnosis, determine the degree of displacement and severity of symptoms, restore stability, and address concomitant injuries.

Scaphoid Fracture

Anatomy

The scaphoid is the second largest carpal bone, shaped somewhat like a kidney bean. It has names for different areas: there is a proximal pole, a distal pole (or tubercle) and a waist, which separates the two poles. Even though it is considered a proximal carpal row bone, it actually spans the midcarpal joint. Proximally, it sits in a shallow facet located at the distal end of the radius, where, along with the lunate bone, it makes up the radiocarpal joint. The blood supply enters at the dorsal, distal pole; therefore, a fracture that disrupts the blood supply to the proximal pole can cause a delay in bone union, an **avascular necrosis (AVN)** of the bone fragment or a nonunion.[28]

Diagnosis and Pathology

The mechanism of injury for a scaphoid fracture is usually a FOOSH with the wrist extended and radially deviated. The proximal portion of the scaphoid is well-stabilized by radiocarpal ligaments as compared to the distal segment of the scaphoid. Thus, if a high force is directed to the radial carpus, the stress will most often center at the middle of this bone, culminating in a fracture of the waist of the scaphoid.[28] The typical client is a young adult, most often male. It is not unusual for this type of injury to go unreported for a period of time, because the client may feel it was "just a sprain." The client with a scaphoid fracture has symptoms of tenderness and pain over the scaphoid, aggravated by palpation of the **anatomic snuffbox** (the dorsal wrist distal to the radial styloid process). ROM, particularly wrist extension, is restricted and grip strength is reduced by more than 50% following this type of fracture.[28]

Diagnosis-Specific Information That Affects Clinical Reasoning

Radial wrist pain can be aggravated or caused by a number of things, including dorsal radial sensory neuritis, acute scaphoid fracture, thumb basal joint arthritis, a scaphoid non-union, or de Quervain's tenosynovitis. A client whose injury entailed a high-energy impact with no evidence of a scaphoid fracture or a distal radius fracture despite repeat x-rays may have injured the scapholunate ligament. The doctor makes this diagnosis, based in part on a positive **Watson's test,** (also known as the *scaphoid shift test*).[27]

> **Precautions and Concerns**

Acute scaphoid fractures may not be evident upon initial x-rays. Therefore, if there is a history of a FOOSH and pain with axial compression of the thumb, treat this injury as a fracture (with immobilization) until symptoms have resolved and there is repeat radiographic or MRI evidence to the contrary.[27]

Non-Operative Treatment for Scaphoid Fractures

Conservative management of a non-displaced scaphoid fracture consists of 6 weeks or more of immobilization with a cast or orthosis. Herbert recommends a short arm cast, leaving the thumb completely free, since incorporation of the carpometacarpal (CMC) and metacarpophalangeal (MP) joints of the thumb do not seem to adversely affect the results,[28] although others recommend a thumb spica cast leaving only the interphalangeal (IP) joint of the thumb free to move.[27]

Typically, a distal pole fracture will heal in 8 to 10 weeks, waist fractures will heal in 12 weeks, and proximal pole fractures (where vascularity is poor) will heal in 12 to 24 weeks.[27] Non-operative management of scaphoid waist or proximal pole fractures require 6 weeks in a long arm thumb spica cast (one that includes the elbow, thus preventing forearm rotation) followed by 6 weeks or more of a short arm thumb spica.[27] As you might imagine, significant stiffness and intra-articular adhesions result from this prolonged immobilization.

Hand therapy may begin while the client is still casted. During these sessions, the therapist should address edema control of the digits and AROM of the uninvolved joints, including the ipsilateral shoulder.

Once the cast is removed, the client is typically fitted with a forearm-based thumb spica orthosis with the IP joint free. The purpose of this brace is to provide intermittent protection and support of the scaphoid and local soft tissue between exercise sessions and when the client is engaged in strenuous activities with the involved hand for the following 2 weeks. The client is instructed in a HEP of AROM of the wrist and thumb. Because stiffness is often a problem following the long period of immobilization needed for the scaphoid healing, frequent exercise sessions of hourly or every other hour are recommended. The client is encouraged to use his hand to perform familiar functional tasks, resuming self-care and household maintenance over the first month after immobilization. Strengthening exercises can be gradually introduced once he is medically cleared by the physician.

Operative Treatment for Scaphoid Fractures

Displaced fractures, comminuted fractures, or those with associated soft tissue injuries are frequently treated with surgical fixation. Immobilization following surgery is dependent on the location of the fracture, whether or not a bone graft was utilized, the method of internal fixation, and the stability of the fracture following surgery. The immobilization time can range from 2 to 16 weeks after surgery.[11,14]

A client who has been treated for weeks or months in a cast before it is decided that the fracture is unstable, or a client whose fracture has developed into a non-union requiring an ORIF or a vascularized bone graft followed by another lengthy period of immobilization begins therapy with significant joint stiffness and (often) pain. These persons usually need dynamic or static progressive splinting, beginning 6 weeks postoperatively[15] to regain mobility; and they may require a work rehabilitation or conditioning program if they are returning to a job that requires heavy lifting and/or manual labor.

> **? Questions To Discuss with The Physician**

- In what area of the scaphoid is the fracture site?
- Do you want the thumb included in the post-cast orthosis? If so, should the IP joint be free?
- When was the date of injury? Was there any prior treatment for this injury?

For Operative Clients
- What type of fixation was used? Was there a vascular bone graft?
- What is your splinting protocol following cast removal for postoperative clients?
- What exercise precautions are there?

Carpal Fractures Other than the Scaphoid

Fractures of the other carpal bones are less common and are typically treated the same way as scaphoid fractures.[15,29] Up to 90% occur as a result of a force applied when the wrist is in extension.[9] Care should be taken to appropriately diagnosis and treat these injuries.

Diagnosis and Pathology

The trapezium is located in the distal carpal row. It articulates proximally with the scaphoid and distally with the metacarpal of the thumb, where it forms a highly movable tapeziometacarpal or thumb CMC joint. Trapezium fractures account for 3% to 5% of all carpal fractures.[29] Fractures of this bone occur most commonly with a fall on a hyperextended and radially deviated wrist with the thumb in abduction. Clinically, there is point tenderness at the base of the thumb. Resisted wrist flexion will typically aggravate the pain, and there may be associated carpal tunnel syndrome.

The trapezoid is one of the smallest carpal bones; it is interposed between the trapezium and the capitate. The incidence of trapezoid fractures is exceedingly rare, occurring in less than 1% of carpal fractures. The injury is usually the result of high-velocity force pushing the index metacarpal into the trapezoid, causing either a fracture or a fracture-dislocation of the trapezoid. Likewise, capitate fractures are rare, occurring at a rate of 1% to 2% of carpal fractures. The capitate is the largest carpal bone; it is considered the keystone of the carpus. Like the scaphoid, there is a tenuous blood supply to the proximal portion of the capitate, and so post-traumatic AVN can develop following a fracture. Typically capitate fractures are seen in combination with other wrist injuries,[28] particularly scaphoid fractures.[29] The hamate is one of the larger carpal bones. It forms the ulnar border of the distal carpal row. It has a volar protrusion, called the *hook of the hamate.* Fractures of the hamate account for 2% to 4% of carpal fractures with fractures of the hook occurring more commonly than fractures of the body. Hook fractures may occur from a fall on an extended wrist or in association with a forceful swing of a (golf) club or bat.[27] These fractures present clinically with pain when holding a racket or club, acute tenderness over the hook of the hamate, and discomfort with resisted abduction or adduction of the little finger.[28] Pain is exacerbated with ulnar deviation of the wrist because of fracture movement.[29] Paresthesias may occur in the fifth and ulnar aspect of the ring fingers, because the hamate hook serves as the radial attachment for the roof of Guyon's canal. (The ulnar nerve and artery pass through this ulnarly located tunnel as they enter the hand.) The pisiform is a sesamoid bone that resembles a pea; it is situated in the proximal ulnar carpal row. It serves as the attachment for the flexor carpi ulnaris tendon and is the origin site of the abductor digiti minimi muscle. The pisiform forms the ulnar wall of Guyon's tunnel. Pisiform fractures account for 1% to 3% of carpal injuries. The mechanism of injury is typically direct trauma to the volar ulnar aspect of the wrist, or a chip avulsion caused by the pull of the flexor carpi ulnaris against strong hyperextension of the wrist. These fractures present with acute tenderness over the pisiform. Associated ulnar nerve palsy may develop.

The triquetrum is a small irregularly-shaped bone located in the proximal ulnar carpal row, adjacent to the lunate, and just distal to the ulnar styloid. This is the second most common carpal bone fracture. The triquetrum can be palpated when the wrist is radially deviated, allowing the triquetrum to move from the beneath ulnar styloid. Fractures can occur following a direct blow to the dorsum of the hand or from a fall resulting in extreme extension of the wrist. Typically this results in a peripheral chip fracture with dorsal avulsion or (less commonly) in a break through the body of the triquetrum.

The lunate is named for its lunar, or moon-like, shape. It is wedged between the scaphoid and triquetrium in the proximal carpal row. Seventy percent of the lunate sits in a shallow fossa on the distal radius, whereas 30% articulates with the TFCC.[29] Like the scaphoid bone, the lunate has a tenuous blood supply with vascular viability dependent on its ligamentous attachment.[27] Isolated lunate fractures are rare; rather, 50% of lunate fractures are associated with injuries to the distal radius, the carpus, or the metacarpals. Fractures of the lunate are more likely to result from repeated compression or stress than from a single force.[27] There is a strong association between lunate fractures and the development of AVN, or **Keinböck's disease.**

Non-Operative Management of Carpal Fractures Other than the Scaphoid

Most carpal fractures are treated with cast immobilization and heal within 6 to 8 weeks if they are non-displaced and have a good blood supply. During the acute phase of fracture healing, instruct the client in AROM exercises of all the uninvolved joints of the injured arm to minimize stiffness and reduce swelling. Once the fracture is stable enough to permit controlled active motion and the cast has been removed, a removable thermoplastic orthosis should be fabricated to offer continued intermittent protection between exercise sessions. Light self-care/ADL activities can be introduced during this time to encourage motion and resumption of normal hand use.

When the fracture is fully healed, passive range of motion (PROM) and dynamic or static progressive splinting can be introduced if needed, to regain wrist and/or thumb motion. Grip strengthening can also be introduced at this time.

Non-displaced trapezium and trapezoid fractures can be treated with a short arm thumb spica cast for 4 to 6 weeks. Treatment for a non-displaced isolated capitate fracture involves immobilization with a short arm thumb spica cast for 6 to 8 weeks. Small non-displaced isolated lunate fractures are usually managed with immobilization in a short arm cast for 6 weeks.[29] Inclusion of the thumb IP joint in the cast for these fractures is based on physician preferences.

Non-displaced or minimally displaced fractures of the hamate are treated with rigid immobilization for 6 weeks. Most patients with a pisiform fracture can be treated with cast immobilization for 4 to 6 weeks. Conservative management for non-displaced triquetrum body fractures or dorsal chip fractures involves a short arm cast for 4 to 6 weeks.

Operative Management of Carpal Fractures

If the carpal fracture is unstable with displaced fragment(s), a closed reduction with percutaneous pins or an open reduction with internal fixation will likely be necessary to restore articular anatomy. Chronic cases of carpal nonunion, AVN, and arthritis may require a salvage procedure to address pain and accompanying dysfunction.

Displaced trapezium fractures, while rare, can lead to permanent impairment in pinch and grip strength if not adequately treated. These injuries often occur in association with other injuries, such as fracture-dislocations of the first metacarpal, scaphoid fractures, and distal radius fractures. Displaced fractures require an ORIF to restore articular anatomy.

Excision of the pisiform is the treatment for cases of chronic, symptomatic non-union of the fractured pisiform, pisotriquetral arthritis, or in the case of ulnar nerve palsy that has not spontaneously recovered after 8 weeks.[29] "No significant adverse effects have been shown by total pisiform excision."[29] A displaced hamate hook fracture requires surgery; this usually involves excision of the fractured segment. However, a cadaver study published in 2003 revealed a 15% reduction in grip strength with hook fragment excision.[29]

If carpal instability is present following a triquetrum fracture secondary to a concomitant ligament avulsion, surgical reduction with internal fixation will be required. In cases of chronic lunate injury or severe comminution, a salvage procedure may be necessary to relieve symptoms, including partial fusion or a proximal row carpectomy.

Be aware that pain is frequently an ongoing problem and the possibility of refracture always exists with the carpal bones.[28] Therefore, restoration of ROM and strength should be within the client's pain tolerance, and aggressive therapy should always be avoided.

♡ **Tips from the Field**

Remember that the **carpus** is composed of eight small, mobile bones. Following a wrist fracture, the ligaments that restrain and support these bones may be compromised (see Chapter 26). The job of a ligament is to provide stability at a joint. Aggressive stretching, exercising, or splinting of the forearm and wrist that does not protect the vulnerable ulnar carpal ligaments can result in ligamentous laxity that will give the appearance of greater supination. Encouraging supination at the carpus (rather than at the DRUJ) is detrimental to the client in the long run, because he loses stability and strength at the wrist in exchange for more motion.

⊳ **Precautions and Concerns**

Be careful to support the ulnar carpus with an orthosis when trying to stretch the forearm with joint mobilizations or with resistive exercises.

Complications Associated with Carpal Fractures

Misdiagnosed or untreated carpal fractures may lead to nonunion, malunion, AVN, articular incongruity that progresses to osteoarthrosis, carpal instability, nerve compression, or late tendon ruptures, among other conditions. While rare in occurrence, these fractures require timely and accurate diagnosis and treatment to minimize risk of complications.

Sometimes these clients are sent to hand therapy with a diagnosis of "wrist sprain/strain." In these circumstances, a careful evaluation needs to be performed with documentation of the history of the injury, as well as a good biomechanical evaluation of the tissue. Note active motion, pain, volumetrics, and grip strength. An important role of the hand therapist is to use clinical reasoning to help monitor progress or lack thereof. Volumetrics taken pre- and post-exercise can provide information about tissue tolerances for exercise. Remember to take volumetric measures of both the involved and uninvolved hand so that you can compare the client's individual response to activity. One would not expect to see a large increase in both swelling and pain reports following light activities if the involved hand was healed enough to tolerate such loads.

⊳ **Precautions and Concerns**

If light exercise and/or activity consistently aggravate the involved extremity, stop loading the injured hand/wrist, and notify the referring physician.

DRSN compression is a condition that can develop secondary to the extensive immobilization required for carpal fracture healing and/or secondary to irritation from a tight thumb spica cast or orthosis. The symptoms are pain, numbness, tingling and/or burning over the dorsal radial wrist, which are aggravated

by percussion of this area or by wrist flexion and ulnar deviation and thumb flexion, because these postures stretch the radial sensory nerve. Instruct the client with these symptoms to perform radial nerve gliding gently five times per day. Please refer to Chapter 24 for recommendations on teaching radial nerve gliding.

A "non-union" refers to a fracture that has not shown signs of healing despite adequate time and immobilization. Because many of the carpal bones have tenuous blood supply, one of the complications following a carpal fracture is a non-union that goes on to develop AVN or death of part or all of the bone. AVN is common in the wrist, where the blood supply to many of the carpal bones is tenuous. If AVN develops, the injury is treated with prolonged casting and may require salvage procedures, such as bone grafting or arthroplasty or some type of partial or total wrist fusion.[27,28] The consequence of AVN includes an alteration of the wrist joint biomechanics and the development of arthritis. A scaphoid non-union, for example, results in an abnormal position at the ends of the scaphoid with the joint surfaces no longer making proper contact at their respective articulations. Instead of having a broad contact surface between the distal radius and the proximal scaphoid, there is an edge-on-edge contact that results in a wearing down of the articular cartilage and the development of a predictable pattern of arthritis. This is termed a **scaphoid non-union advanced collapse (SNAC) wrist.** Patients have symptoms of pain, swelling along the radial wrist, and some loss of wrist extension. Treatment varies, depending upon various factors, including the patient's age, comorbidities, and current symptoms. Typically, some type of surgical intervention will be required to restore scaphoid alignment. In advanced cases, a wrist reconstruction or salvage procedure may be necessary to address pain while maintaining a functional wrist.

AVN of the lunate (Keinböck's disease) is typically the result of repetitive microtrauma that compromises the blood flow to this bone. It is also associated with negative ulnar variance (that is, an abnormally shorter ulna as compared to the radius at the carpus).

Fractures of the hook of the hamate are difficult to diagnosis on routine radiographs. A non-union typically presents with pain located directly over the hook and may be associated with ulnar nerve neuropathy. Following excision of the hook, there may be significant tenderness at the surgery site aggravated by gripping a rigid surface, such as a hammer or tennis racquet. Clients may benefit from a gel pad placed directly over the incision site to act as a shock absorber during grip tasks.

Distal Forearm and Carpal Fractures

As with any injury, an evaluation should start with a good medical history. It is essential to know about systemic illnesses, medications, and previous injuries before you lay hands on the patient. Hearing the patient's story of how the injury occurred is also an important part of rapport building. This story will give the therapist information on personality issues, activity level, family support, work demands, and the patient's concerns and goals for therapy. In addition, it is helpful to collect information from the physician or the operative report regarding the bony alignment, soft tissue integrity, type of reduction, and stability.

In this age of same-day outpatient surgeries along with an increase in older patients with more comorbidities, the therapist must make time for an adequate systems review and medical screen as part of the evaluation. This is not only to protect ourselves from doing something that would be unsafe for the patient, but also to identify and properly triage patients to the appropriate health prevention specialist and/or education source. As part of this process, when you are interviewing an older patient with an injury sustained from a FOOSH, consider a balance screen and provide education related to fall precautions.

Client-rated outcome measurement tools are an important component of the evaluation, because they facilitate identification of the client's interests and concerns. This information is collected and evaluated in a standardized format and used to develop goals and to demonstrate positive functional outcomes following therapy. The Disabilities of the Arm, Shoulder, and Hand (DASH) is an easy-to-administer, client-friendly outcome tool with excellent validity and reliability measures. It identifies client-specific disabilities that either proximal or distal arm impairments can engender; and it allows the therapist to easily evaluate the outcome of single or multiple treatment sessions in mitigating these disabilities. The Patient-Rated Wrist Evaluation (PRWE) is a similar popular, client-rated outcome tool; as with the DASH, it is quick to administer and easy to score with low scores indicating little or no perceived upper extremity disability[15] (see Chapter 8). Other evaluation measures are also important.

Evaluation Tips

- Check for shoulder AROM and pain. Identify and address secondary shoulder problems immediately in order to prevent complications, such as a frozen shoulder.
- Observe the client's arm and hand posture. Some clients keep their arm in a sling with the shoulder adducted and internally rotated, the elbow and wrist flexed, and the hand hanging out of the end of the sling. This can cause increased distal swelling and elbow/shoulder stiffness. Document elbow AROM and posture.
- Observe wrist motion in both planes (flexion/extension and ulnar/radial deviation) when the wrist is no longer immobilized. Document AROM and report of pain during movement. Remind the patient that stiffness is to be expected after immobilization and that it is a normal part of the healing process.
- Poor finger motion can occur from limited tendon gliding at the wrist, from adhesions that may form following surgery (such as, after an ORIF), and/or from swelling. Check this, and document it.
- Take composite measurements (such as, digit flexion to the distal palmar crease [DPC] and digit extension) off the table with the wrist held in a steady neutral position. This will give you a hint about whether extrinsic flexor and/or extensor tendon tightness has developed.
- Passively flex the MPs (gently) to assess capsular tightness that may have developed secondary to the cast immobilization, especially when the distal volar portion of the cast extends too far distally or is too bulky to allow full MP flexion.
- The EPL tendon changes direction as it wraps around the dorsal bony tubercle on the distal radius called *Lister's tubercle.* Sometimes, just by virtue of its location, the EPL can become attenuated or can rupture following a distal radius fracture. Assess the function of the EPL tendon by having the client position his involved hand with the palm flat on the table and instructing the client to "raise his thumb to the ceiling" (Fig. 25-12). Report pain and/or problems extending the IP joint of the thumb to the physician.

- When measuring forearm rotation at the DRUJ, have the client sit with his elbow flexed to 90° and with his arm close to the side of the body. Maintaining this arm position is important to avoid substitution movements at the shoulder. Align the goniometer's stability arm parallel to the humerus. For supination, align the mobility arm parallel to the proximal volar wrist crease. The axis is just medial to the ulnar styloid. For pronation, the stability arm remains the same; the mobility arm is placed on the dorsum of the wrist at the level of the styloid processes (Fig. 25-13). Measuring forearm rotation this way allows the therapist to appreciate true forearm rotation, as opposed to rotation at the carpus.
- Observe the ulnar side of wrist for swelling, and palpate the ulnar side of the wrist for pain. Ask the client about pain experienced during forearm rotation. Document your findings. Remember that ulnar-sided wrist pain following a distal radius fracture is a frequently observed complication that typically resolves with time. If this pain and swelling is not improving over the first few months of therapy, report your findings to the physician.
- Perform sensory testing as appropriate. Use the Semmes-Weinstein monofilament test to identify or rule out sensory nerve problems. Communicate findings immediately with the client's physician, and discuss guidelines regarding modifications in treatment.
- If edema is present, document circumferential measurement with precise location (for example, the distal wrist crease) and compare to the uninjured side. Alternatively, measure and record volumetric data if no open wounds/cast/external fixation devices are present.
- Skin integrity should be monitored and documented. Observations of scarring, bruising, incision healing, rashes, skin color and temperature (both hot and cold could be problematic), shininess, dryness, and changes in hair growth are all relevant.
- Inquire about pain (which is part of PRWE and DASH) if not already assessed. You can use a simple visual analog scale (VAS) or a numeric pain scale to gather information about

pain perception, or to augment information obtained via the DASH or other patient-rated disability assessment tool.

- After bone has healed sufficiently and the physician gives approval, grip and pinch strength can be tested using a Jamar dynamometer and pinch meter.
- Good thumb abduction is needed for cylindrical grasp; this movement can be compromised following prolonged splinting. Therefore, when evaluating the thumb, consider the following functional measurements: thumb radial abduction, palmar abduction, and opposition. Compare abduction measurements to the uninvolved side to help determine normal range for that client.
- Once strengthening is allowed, volumetric measures taken pre- and post-exercise sessions can help to estab-

lish safe guidelines for exercise and tissue loading. The effect of exercise on the asymptomatic hand was studied by McGough and Surwasky.[18] This study, although done on a small sample of uninjured hands, provides some idea of what the normal response to exercise is and, hence, what could be considered an abnormal response. Their results indicate that females demonstrate a 3.6% increase in volumetrics post-exercise, and males demonstrate a 5.2% increase in volume. Volume changes that exceed these numbers, especially when combined with complaints, may indicate more resistance and/or repetitions during exercise than the healing tissues can tolerate. Further research on post-exercise edema in patients with injured extremities would be very helpful.

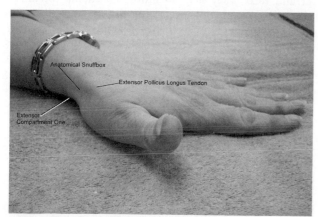

FIGURE 25-12 Test to determine extensor pollicis longus (EPL) patency.

A primary therapy treatment goal for any wrist fracture is restoration of pre-injury function. Facilitating return of strength and maximum pain-free ROM of the joints of the involved extremity (including the shoulder) is the foundation of this goal. Return of pre-injury strength and motion requires resolution of the bone and concomitant soft tissue impairment. A good outcome, as defined by the client, may not be possible if there is shortening of the radius following a distal radius fracture.[4,13] A review of the literature[4,8,10,13,15,17,19] suggests that therapy management of distal radius and carpal fractures is diverse, and that treatment planning is dependent upon the clinical decision-making of the therapist. The following "Tips from the Field" boxes describe some recommendations for intervention strategies.

♡ Tips from the Field

Active Range of Motion

Remember to instruct the client in exercises for all joints of the injured arm, introducing wrist and forearm active exercises as soon as the physician gives clearance. Have the client hold the end range position for a sustained 5-second stretch. Begin with three to four sets per day of ten repetitions of each exercise; the number of repetitions and sets should be adjusted according to the client's response. For example, if

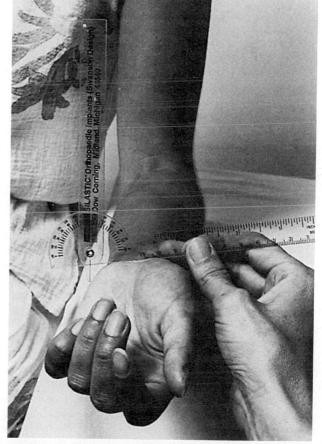

FIGURE 25-13 To assess forearm supination (and pronation) correctly, position the client with the test arm in adduction and elbow flexed to 90°. The axis of the goniometer is just medial to the ulnar styloid. The movable arm is placed across the volar aspect of the wrist for supination, at the level of the ulnar styloid. The stationary arm is aligned with the humerus. (From Cambridge-Keeling CA: Range of motion measurement of the hand. In Mackin EJ, Callahan AD, Skirven TM, et al, editors: *Rehabilitation of the hand and upper extremity*, ed 5, St Louis, 2002, Mosby.)

the client develops shoulder stiffness during the fracture healing phase, the number of sets of shoulder exercises should be increased. As the client resumes functional activities using the injured extremity, the number of sets and/or repetitions of AROM of non-stiff joints can be reduced or stopped altogether.

Weakness of the radial wrist extensors allows the wrist flexors to overpower them during attempted grasp. This flexed wrist position further limits finger flexion and weakens grip. Furthermore, unless cautioned otherwise, clients will often substitute with the digital extensors to initiate wrist extension (Fig. 25-14). Therefore, it is important to isolate the radial wrist extensors during early controlled AROM and to add target strengthening exercises when appropriate. Instruct the client in active wrist extension exercises by having the client make a gentle fist when performing wrist extension. Encourage tenodesis with simultaneous wrist extension and finger flexion, and concomitant wrist flexion and finger extension. Instruct the client in individual tendon gliding exercises for the flexor digitorum superficialis and flexor digitorum profundus tendons. The "hook fist position" isolates the MP extensor, the extensor digitorum communis (EDC), and simultaneously addresses IP flexion while stretching the intrinsic muscles of the digits. Active and passive finger extension with wrist held in about 20° of extension facilitates nice extensor gliding with little tension in zones 5 and 6.[4]

Instruct the client in thumb opposition exercises, as well as abduction and extension exercises. To minimize friction of the EPL sheath, the wrist should be held in neutral with slight ulnar deviation.[4]

Pain

You don't need to be the expert in interpreting what exactly is causing ulnar-sided wrist pain when it develops after a distal radius or proximal carpal fracture. Instead, carefully document your findings, indicating conditions in which the pain is exacerbated, and report this to the physician. Remember that sometimes even the best therapy cannot ameliorate pain and dysfunction that is secondary to bony alignment issues.

Normal versus Functional Range of Motion

Sometimes it is not possible to achieve "normal" pain-free ROM of the wrist following a distal radius or carpal fracture. It may be necessary to assist the client in refocusing his goal to gaining pain-free ROM within a functional range. Typically, if the injured hand is the dominant hand, a greater ROM will be necessary for return of function. To determine how much functional ROM is necessary for your client, assist the client in identifying those specific activities that he wants to do and/or that he needs to do with the involved hand. Therapy sessions should incorporate practicing these specific activities, which can be graded in terms of repetition and/or load.

Edema[19]

Elevate the affected extremity above the heart. Use positioning devices, such as pillows, when the client relaxes at home. Avoid slings whenever possible, because these encourage the protected posture (internal rotation and adduction of the shoulder, and flexion of the elbow) that is often assumed by clients after injuring their upper extremity. This posture promotes shoulder and

elbow stiffness and discourages functional use of the involved extremity. Furthermore, the weight of the arm in a sling is born by the contralateral neck in the vulnerable area where the brachial plexus exits the scalenes. *Upper extremity elevation is not appropriate if there is arterial compromise.*

Compressive dressings and/or wraps can temporarily help reduce edema. Use must be monitored carefully to prevent compromised circulation and to make sure the dressings do not restrict movement unnecessarily. Compression wraps should not be tight because doing this collapses the delicate lymphatic network. Compression is contraindicated when there is arterial compromise or with skin grafts or unhealed burns.

Application of cold packs during the first 48 hours after injury/surgery (the inflammatory stage of healing) is indicated if there is no arterial compromise.

Active muscle pumping is a key part of edema control. The simplest approach would be to elevate the arm and pump the fist twenty-five times per hour. As muscles contract and relax, they help to move the edema proximally through the lymphatic system. Ideally one would exercise the larger proximal muscles first to clear any proximal edema and follow that with gentle exercise of the distal muscles. The goal of these exercises is to create muscle pumping and movement within the lymphatic vessels, not strengthening (see Chapter 3).

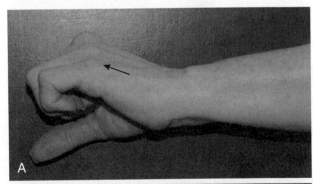
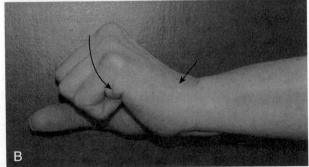

FIGURE 25-14 A, Many distal radius fracture patients have a well-established substitution pattern of using the digital extensors—particularly those in the ring and small fingers—to extend the wrist. **B,** Independent wrist extension is critical to developing the ability to make a fist and in regaining power grip after a distal radius fracture. (From Laseter G: External and internal fixation of unstable distal radius fractures. In Burke S, Higgins J, McClinton M, et al, editors: *Hand and upper extremity rehabilitation: a practical guide,* ed 3, St Louis, 2005, Churchill Livingstone.)

> **Precautions and Concerns**

Caution the patient that this is not exercise to get stronger. Injured tissue is not ready for that level of activity at this stage.

Lymphatic Stimulation

Lymphatic stimulation needs to be performed correctly in order to prevent collapse of superficial lymphatic capillaries. Lymphatic massage is contraindicated if there is a known or suspected deep vein thrombosis, pulmonary embolism, infection, cancer, congestive heart failure, or renal failure. See Chapter 3 for specifics.

♡ **Tips from the Field**

Scar Management/Desensitization

Assess the scars that formed at pin sites and/or at surgical sites (where an ORIF was performed) to determine if the underlying tissues are adherent and restricting normal tendon gliding. Adhesions that form beneath cutaneous scars should be addressed with scar massage and tendon gliding exercises. Topical scar compression dressings designed to improve scar cosmesis can be introduced within 24 to 48 hours of suture removal or when all eschar (scabs) are gone. Scar hypersensitivity can be addressed with a desensitization program that encourages the client to regularly touch and massage the irritable area with various non-noxious stimuli throughout the day.

Client Compliance

Clients may be fearful about re-breaking their wrist when performing exercises or activities at home. If your client is not compliant with the prescribed exercises, consider the possibility that he might be fearful of reinjury. Reassure him that his bone is healed adequately to tolerate these exercises and that these exercises will serve to further strengthen the newly healed bone. If fear and/or pain are not the limiting factors, the therapist must reconsider the prescribed program. If the exercises are not meaningful and/or if it is not clear to the client how these exercises will allow him to resume an activity that is important to him, the client may not be invested in the program and may refuse to "comply." The true art of therapy is to engage the client and incorporate his interests in treatment planning.

Orthoses

Once the cast is taken off, a removable forearm-based wrist orthosis offers intermittent continued protection of the fracture site and of the local soft tissue during the first 2 weeks of controlled active motion. If the physician has not prescribed an orthosis, consider requesting one for the client to use for a period of 1 to 2 weeks to address end-of-the-day pain and fatigue that is typical for clients with newly healed wrist fractures. When orthotic devices are recommended, the patient should be fully informed about the purpose and wearing schedule and should be taught how to care for both the brace and the skin. It is optimal to include the patient in decision making regarding the usefulness and cosmesis of the orthosis because this will improve compliance.[18] Extended use of the orthosis beyond the therapeutic interval will delay the recovery of motion and functional hand use. These clients may need gentle encouragement to wean from their orthosis.

Identify signs of extrinsic flexor tightness and use a night extension resting pan orthosis that can be serially adjusted with the fingers and wrist positioned in extension. The client should feel only a light stretch to the finger flexors when the orthosis is adjusted in the clinic. Clients will not be able to tolerate aggressive stretching from an orthosis while trying to fall asleep, and what feels like a mild stretch when awake can feel intolerable in the quiet of the night. Also, remember that a slow, sustained stretch will allow the tissues to remodel without causing pain, tearing, or other tissue deformation.

Stretching

Stretching must be avoided until cleared by the physician. Even then, therapists must remember that gentle, prolonged, comfortable stretch promotes tissue remodeling, whereas aggressive stretching causes microtears and results in further stiffness. Gentle stretching to regain wrist and/or forearm motion may be introduced 1 week after the cast is removed, or 3 to 4 weeks after plating of the distal radius. Typically, the index MP joint is stiffer than other digits following immobilization by an external fixator for a distal radius fracture. Early on, PROM should target digit MP joint flexion, IP joint extension, and the thumb web space.

The prayer stretch (Fig. 25-15) can be helpful in regaining functional wrist extension. Instruct the patient to perform this stretch gently, making sure the palms of the hand stay together throughout the stretch. The towel stretch (Fig. 25-16) is an easy way to self-stretch the forearm to regain functional forearm rotation. Instruct the patient to keep the elbow close to the side when performing this stretch.

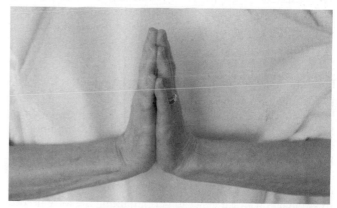

FIGURE 25-15 Prayer stretch.

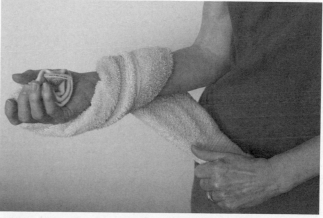

FIGURE 25-16 Towel stretch for supination. Reverse the direction of pull to provide a stretch into pronation.

> **Precautions and Concerns**

Stretching should never increase pain. Teach the patient that the mantra, "no pain, no gain," is not applicable to rehabilitation of the forearm and wrist after a fracture. In fact, painful stretching can result in further injury to the soft tissue and more swelling.

> **Precautions and Concerns**

Resistive exercises should not be introduced without the specific consent of the treating physician, who must determine if the healing fracture is capable of withstanding high muscle forces across it.

♡ **Tips from the Field**

Strengthening

Many therapists use a hammer as a weight to stretch the DRUJ joint and/or to strengthen the forearm muscles (Fig. 25-17, *A*). This exercise can be graded by having the client grasp the shaft of the hammer either closer or further away from the head, thus increasing or decreasing the lever arm and the force generated during forearm rotation. If the client experiences ulnar-sided wrist pain during this exercise, have him perform it while wearing a wrist brace (see Fig. 25-17, *B*) and encourage him to rotate the hammer in the mid-range (between 10:00 and 2:00) only. The brace will protect the vulnerable ulnar carpus, and strengthening in the mid-range is effective and less stressful to the ulnar wrist. As an alternative to the orthosis, the client can support the DRUJ with the other hand while performing forearm pronation/supination AROM.

Resumption of Functional Activities/Activities of Daily Living

Light functional activities that are familiar to the client should be re-introduced as soon as possible to discourage the client from "disuse atrophy." Clients may need help in appropriately adapting and/or grading (and upgrading) activities and tasks. For example, provide the client with some cylindrical tubing and instructions on how to put it on a toothbrush. Enlarging the handle of a toothbrush, pen, hair brush, hand razor or spoon makes it much easier to grasp, limiting the force needed to complete a task, such as brushing one's teeth or signing a check. Most clients relish the return to independence with self-care tasks; encourage and cheer their successes!

Home Exercise Program

HEPs should be encouraged starting at the first visit when possible. The program can address positioning, edema control strategies, pain management strategies, re-engagement in appropriate ADLs, leisure, or work tasks, as well as ROM exercises, use of orthotic devices, and strengthening when appropriate. The HEP should be meaningful and simple and should be upgraded over time to reflect the patient's needs. Allowing the patient to use their cell phone camera to video orthotic donning/doffing procedures, as well as specific exercises, may be useful in addition to written handouts. Be sure to consider the patient's learning style and needs when designing the HEP to maximize compliance. Research has shown that participation in a HEP with good compliance results in fewer total visits needed (that is, lower health care costs) and quicker return to function.[21,22]

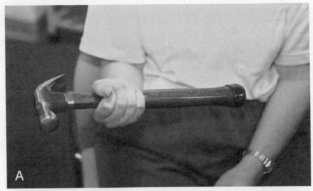

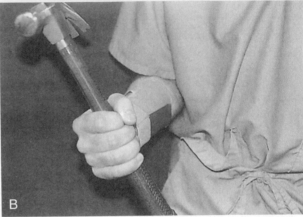

FIGURE 25-17 A, A hammer can be used to passively stretch the forearm and/or to strengthen the muscles of forearm rotation. The torque force can be adjusted by changing the point where the client grasps the handle (thereby increasing or decreasing the lever arm). **B,** Exercising the forearm with a hammer may require the use of a wrist orthosis to protect the vulnerable ulnar carpus. (**A,** From LaStayo PC: Ulnar wrist pain and impairment: a therapist's approach to the triangular fibrocartilage complex. In Mackin EJ, Callahan AD, Skirven TM, et al, editors: *Rehabilitation of the hand and upper extremity,* ed 5, St Louis, 2002, Mosby. **B,** From Jaffe R, Chidgey L, LaStayo P: Distal Radioulnar Joint: anatomy and management of disorders *J Hand Ther* 9:136, 1996.)

Passive Range of Motion/Dynamic/Static Progressive Orthoses

If ROM of the wrist and/or distal forearm plateaus before the client has achieved functional range(s), dynamic and/or static progressive orthoses should be considered.[4,20] Static progressive orthoses apply low-load, prolonged stretch to tight, adaptively-shortened tissues and/or to adhesions to encourage this tissue to grow longer. Typically supination is more impaired than pronation, and loss of functional wrist extension is more a concern than loss of wrist flexion. There are a number of commercially-available dynamic orthoses to address wrist tightness and/or decreased forearm rotation (Fig. 25-18, *A* through *C*). It is also possible to design and fabricate a static progressive orthosis to address decreased motion using thermoplastic orthosis materials and strapping (see Fig. 25-18, *D*). When deciding which orthotic design to use, consider the costs to the patient, because commercially-available -static progressive orthoses or dynamic orthoses may or may not be covered by the patient's insurance, and these are frequently expensive. You will also need to consider fabrication time, and the patient's tolerance for donning/doffing and wearing a particular orthosis.

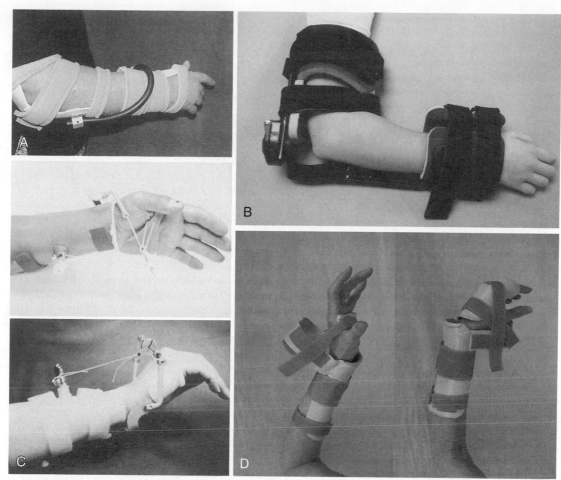

FIGURE 25-18 Dynamic orthoses used to address forearm and wrist ROM limitations after a distal radius fracture. **A,** A dynamic forearm rotation orthosis using components made by Rolyan. **B,** A dynamic forearm supination orthosis. **C,** A static progressive wrist flexion and extension orthosis using the Phoenix wrist hinge and the maximum end range time component. **D,** A static progressive custom-made orthosis for wrist extension. A dorsal hand piece may be fabricated and the volar forearm trough rotated onto the dorsal surface to allow for a static progressive wrist flexion stretch. (**A,** From Jaffe R, Chidgey L, LaStayo P: Distal Radioulnar Joint: anatomy and management of disorders *J Hand Ther* 9:136, 1996. **B,** From Fess EE, Gettle KS, Philips CA, et al: *Hand and upper extremity splinting: principles and methods,* ed 3, St Louis, 2005, Mosby. **C,** From King JW: Practice Forum *J Hand Ther* 5:36-37, 1992. **D,** Courtesy of Anne Moscony.)

◎ *Clinical Pearl*

The concept of **total end range time (TERT)** means that to gain motion, you must hold a joint and it associated muscle/tendons at its available end range for a prolonged period of time. It is not the strength of the force, but rather the amount of time (in a 24-hour period) that results in adaptive lengthening of soft tissue structures.

◖◗ *What to Say to Clients*

About a Fracture

"You fractured the _____ bone. That means it is broken. *(Have a diagram or illustration ready to share with the client/caregiver.)* Here, let me show you where the fractured bone is, using this picture."

"Imagine the amount of force necessary to break a bone. It is likely that some of the adjacent soft tissue (for example, tendons, nerves, muscles, ligaments) were also hurt at the time

of your injury. Therefore, it is important that your wrist be protected and immobilized for the time it takes for your body to heal. Your physician will closely assess the fracture at regular intervals and let us know when we can safely start to move the joints at, or near, the fracture site. During this initial immobilization time, it is important that you move your shoulder normally and maintain the range of motion in the fingers and elbow to speed up your recovery and to avoid further complications when the cast is removed. Once we can begin gentle exercises outside of the cast, you will need to avoid overuse of your hand and wrist so that the soft tissue can adequately heal. We will work together to identify when discomfort with a prescribed exercise is to be expected and when you should limit yourself, so as not to cause further injury to your healing soft tissue."

About Static Progressive Splinting

"This orthosis, or splint, is designed to help you regain motion. You will need to wear it for a total of 3 hours per day, initially.

You can divide up the 3 hours any way you want, just as long as you've clocked-in the total prescribed time. This splint should not increase your pain. It is designed to hold your tight wrist (or forearm) at the end of its available motion. Research has shown that if a joint is stretched to its end available range for a long enough period of time, the tissue will adapt to this and grow longer, translating into more motion. I expect that you will gain 3° to 5° of motion a week, or more, by using this splint for 3 hours a day. If you don't gain motion, we will need to increase the amount of time you are in the splint, not the force or pull of the splint."

About Exercises

"Reducing swelling and improving movement are important goals during the initial phase of hand therapy. We will focus on motion for the thumb, fingers, wrist, forearm, and elbow. I would like you to start by doing your exercises for three to five sets per day. I will adjust the number of repetitions and sets based upon how you respond to these exercises. It is very important to exercise the fingers often during the day to minimize swelling in the hand and promote normal hand motion. It is also very important to learn how to isolate your wrist muscles from your finger muscles. We will practice the exercises together now, and I will give you a handout with pictures of the exercises so that you remember how to do them correctly. Please remember that you should not experience pain with these exercises, although you may have some discomfort related to moving joints that haven't moved in a while. Always do your exercises slowly and hold the end position so that you get a little stretch."

About Swelling

"Swelling is initially a normal bodily response to injury and/or surgery. It means your body is doing what it needs to do to bring the cells necessary for healing, assisting the injured tissue in the repair process, and providing a way to remove the debris and waste products that accumulate as the body heals. If you had no swelling, you couldn't heal. So, thank goodness for swelling! If not treated early and effectively, swelling can last for a long time after an injury, especially if there is a lot of soft tissue trauma associated with the injury. However, we want to resolve swelling as soon as possible, because it contributes to pain and stiffness. Still, morning stiffness is normal and can take a long time to resolve."

"Even though swelling is a healthy and normal initial response to injury to your body, we still want to address it and appropriately reduce the swelling response. Otherwise, you'll find it hard to move your fingers, and you could develop contractures or limitations in movement. Exercises, like I've shown you, will help. Try to limit the amount of time you allow your injured arm to hang by your side; instead, keep your hand above your elbow when possible, using a pillow, for example, to position it comfortably. This allows gravity to assist with recirculating the fluid that accumulates in your hand. If the swelling becomes problematic and exercise, positioning, and proper massage don't seem to control it, we may use some elastic gloves or sleeves or a compressive bandage that will assist your body in resolving it. These elastic sleeves or bandages work like light-support pantyhose that people sometimes wear to assist their leg circulation. They must not be too tight, or the swelling will persist."

CASE STUDIES

CASE STUDY 25-1 ■

K.P. is a 70-year-old male who sustained a right-sided distal radius fracture after a FOOSH. He came to the ER several hours later where x-rays were taken. An extra-articular, non-displaced distal radius fracture diagnosis was confirmed, and he was casted. At the first follow-up visit with the hand surgeon, a new cast was formed due to increased swelling. The patient was referred to hand therapy for digital ROM.

At his first therapy visit, K.P. completed the DASH with a score of 79 points (where the best score is 0 and the worst is 100). On a VAS, he rated his pain a 2 out of 10 (where 10 is the worst). His medical history was positive for high blood pressure, depression, and gastroesophageal reflux disease (GERD). His physical appearance was disheveled. He reported living in a house by himself with no family support. (His wife was recently deceased, and his adult children live in other parts of the country.) He is retired with no current leisure interests but strongly desires to maintain independent living. The patient reported wearing a sling to help him protect the arm. He reported that he was eating out and doing no housework at this time, because the cast made it too difficult. He reported taking prescription pain killers when needed. Physical findings included moderate swelling of the hand and fingers on the right side, and a mildly tight elbow and shoulder that were painful with movement. At this first visit, the therapist recommended discontinuing the sling to allow more natural movement of the elbow and shoulder, to prevent neck strain, and to encourage light use of the hand during the day. Elevation and ice were recommended for the swelling, as well as gentle digital flexion and tendon glides four to six times a day. Because he was at risk for noncompliance, therapy was scheduled two to three times per week.

K.P. was very cooperative during every therapy session but admitted he didn't always follow through at home. He missed several therapy visits during these first few weeks, saying that he overslept. As the therapist got better acquainted with him during this first month, it became clear that he was an alcoholic and was struggling to do everyday tasks, such as laundry and light meal preparation. Community supports, such as a home health aide and meals on wheels, were recommended. The therapist reiterated the importance of good nutrition and sleep during this time of healing. The patient was advised to reduce alcohol consumption to promote better healing and reduce the risk of falls. Basic coping skills/stress management techniques were discussed, which K.P. was open to hearing but continued to lack follow through. Concerns were shared with the physician.

After 6 weeks, the cast was removed. A full evaluation was performed with the following findings:
- Shoulder AROM full, not painful
- Elbow AROM full, not painful
- Forearm AROM supination 15°, pronation 50
- Wrist AROM flexion 10, extension 5, ulnar deviation 15, radial deviation 10
- Able to oppose thumb to ring finger
- Composite flexion (distance to DPC) was:
  - Digit 2 = 5 cm
  - Digit 3 = 4 cm
  - Digit 4 = 4 cm
  - Digit 5 = 3.5 cm
- Persistent distal swelling, observed
- Pain over the dorsal wrist and thumb, reported
- Pain at the wrist, rated 5/10 with movement

The therapist fabricated a custom, removable wrist orthosis for support and protection as needed for the patient. Wear and care instruction were provided. The patient practiced donning and doffing in the presence of the therapist. A new HEP was established: The patient was encouraged to use a compression glove to reduce swelling, to continue light ADLs, a full program of AROM exercises were provided for each joint in a non-painful range, and desensitization techniques were taught for irritation of the DRSN. This program was demonstrated, practiced, and written instructions with pictures were also provided. The patient did attempt to be compliant at that time.

K.P. showed up for twice-weekly therapy over the next 6 weeks with improvements at each visit. He said he had started to go to Alcoholics Anonymous (AA) again, and he appeared less disheveled. His pain was down to a 2/10 with movement, and the DRSN irritation was intermittent and improved. He had discontinued taking pain killers. He gradually weaned from the orthosis with encouragement, and by 6 weeks he was fully weaned. At 6 weeks, however, he had persistent stiffness and ADL dysfunction. His DASH score at this time was 50 points. His grip strength, as measured by Jamar dynamometer, was 15 lbs on the right and 60 lbs on the left. He had discontinued use of the compression glove with new DPC measurements as follows:

- Digit 2 = 2 cm
- Digit 3 = 1.5 cm
- Digit 4 = 0.5 cm
- Digit 5 = 0.5 cm

Wrist AROM was flexion 35°, extension 35°, radial deviation 15°, and ulnar deviation 20°. Active supination was 55°, and pronation was 70°. ADL dysfunction included pain when pushing up from a chair, opening a jar or turning a door knob, and difficulty using a knife to cut meat. These findings were provided to the physician at the patient's 6-week follow-up visit. New x-rays were taken, which showed adequate healing, and the physician wrote a prescription for gentle strengthening and a static progressive wrist splint.

K.P. willingly participated in new strengthening exercises, which included heavier ADL/ instrumental activities of daily living (IADL), and he participated in recommended leisure activities with a social component to a lesser extent. A sample static progressive splint was shown to him, and the estimated wearing schedule was discussed. K.P. decided that this would not be appropriate for him. Self-stretching exercises were chosen instead. K.P. continued therapy once per week at this time for 6 more weeks. He showed gains in both functional strength and ROM when re-evaluated at his last visit, and he felt confident in his ability to continue to maintain his house independently. He was discharged at this visit, which was 12 weeks post injury.

CASE STUDY 25-2 ∎

S.J. is a 68-year-old, right hand dominant, female school psychologist who fell at work on November 3rd. She completed her work day after reporting her fall. Her pain increased over the next few days, and she had an x-ray at the local ER, which was negative for a fracture. The state in which she was injured has a managed workers compensation injury program. Given her persistent complaints, she was eventually sent to a general orthopedic physician, who splinted her with an over-the-counter wrist brace and sent her to physical therapy for 3 weeks. She had persistent complaints of snuffbox pain and was eventually sent to a physician who had

some hand surgery experience. This physician sent S.J. for an MRI, which showed a fracture at the waist of the scaphoid. The physician put S.J. in a long arm cast, immobilizing the elbow, forearm, wrist, and thumb.

S.J. was referred to a certified hand therapist (CHT) for follow up 2 weeks after surgery. She was unable to work because of her injury and needed considerable assistance from her husband to perform many of her routine ADL tasks, including driving, food preparation, and dressing. She came to therapy with a long arm cast, immobilizing her elbow, forearm, wrist, and all thumb joints. The cast was fabricated distal to the DPC, effectively limiting the MP flexion of her digits. Evaluation at this time reported significant general joint effusion of all of her digits, with a red, shiny appearance that she referred to as "looking like sausages." AROM measurements indicated a total digit extension loss as follows:

- Index: −45°
- Long: −46°
- Ring: −41°
- Small: −25°

Numeric pain rating was reported as 3/10 at the time of the evaluation, and 5/10 at its worst (over the past few days). Past medical history was positive for a prior right rotator cuff injury, which had been treated with conservative therapy. She was given a HEP of shoulder AROM, digit AROM within the confines of the cast, and retrograde massage for her digits. At this time, the therapist also discussed positioning between exercise sessions and encouraged S.J. to only use of her sling when she needed to stand for long periods of time.

About 4 weeks from her initial evaluation, S.J. had her cast replaced, freeing her elbow for AROM. She was seen one to two times per week at this time to address persistent pain, finger edema, stiffness and pain, and elbow AROM. There was a concern about the development of CRPS, given the persistent redness, swelling, and shiny appearance of her digits. Shortly after the initial evaluation, she returned to work part time with modified duties. She reported persistent pain, and increased swelling and redness dependent upon the position in which she kept her right upper extremity. She reported that she needed significantly more sleep/naps during the day. The therapist assured her that this was normal and that she needed to allow her body to heal and to take naps when she felt she needed to allow her to function with fewer symptoms. S.J. was seen two to three times per week to address her significant digit swelling, stiffness, and pain symptoms. Messages to the doctor about the level of and persistence of both pain and swelling were left via fax and phone; however, the surgeon did not respond to the therapist's concerns. During this time, the therapist added visualization exercises to S.J.'s program, which consisted of mental visualization of S.J. performing normal forearm, wrist, digit, and thumb motion. This was designed to facilitate cortical firing of the pre-motor cortex and to lessen the development of disuse atrophy as S.J. switched to using her non-dominant hand for many of her ADLs. She was encouraged to use her right upper extremity as much as possible within the confines of her cast. She was given adaptive foam handles for her silverware, for example, to allow her to use her right hand for eating with utensils.

On April 20th, (after 12 weeks of immobilization) the cast was removed, and this patient was given an over-the-counter thumb spica brace by her physician and sent to therapy for three times per week to address ROM and functional limitations. (S.J. was so excited to be out of her cast that she celebrated by bringing the entire therapy office coffee and donuts!) An evaluation at this time showed the following objective measures:

- QuickDASH score = 45 (best = 0)
- Total digit extension loss:
  - Index = −45°
  - Long = −51°
  - Ring = −54°
  - Small = −49°

This was a significant improvement from her active digit extension as measured on February 14th.

Her digit flexion to the DPC was within 1 cm, all digits. Her forearm pronation was 75°, and supination was 50°. Her active wrist motion was 43°, and wrist flexion was 5°. Pain, at its worst in the past few days was rated as 4/10 on the numeric pain scale. The assessment of her presentation in therapy was as follows: "This patient has symptoms of stiff fingers and wrist/forearm, s/p prolonged immobilization in a cast. She responded well to paraffin, and a home paraffin unit was recommended to address her stiff joints. She should continue to make functional gains with both wrist and finger motion and strength needed to perform tasks, such as buttoning, turning a key in the care ignition, pushing open doors at work, and being able to bear weight on an extended wrist to push herself up off of low surfaces." The benefits of adding a static progressive orthosis to address wrist extension tightness and extrinsic flexor muscle tightness were noted. Therapy focused on resumption of all of her self-care tasks, from driving independently to washing her own hair and cutting her food. It also focused on AROM, gentle stretching, and edema management.

S.J. returned to work full time, at the beginning of May. Incorporating suggestions made in therapy, she was able to self-modify some of the more difficult job requirements. Measurements on May 11th indicated no change in active wrist extension. Her DASH score was 41, which improved 4 points—not a significant statistical level of change. Orders were received for a static progressive splint, which was fabricated to address the need for increased wrist extension. She demonstrated ability to don/doff this orthosis independently with some practice in the clinic. (She took pictures of her brace with her

cell phone so that she could accurately don/doff this brace.) She was told to use the orthosis for a total of 180 minutes/day, splitting this time up however she wanted. She was also given a serial static splint to use at night to encourage both wrist and digit extension. On May 18th, her wrist extension was measured at 57°, which was 14° better than after removal of her cast.

On June 13th, a re-evaluation indicated no significant change in her DASH score; however, her total digit extension loss was much improved as follows:

- Index = −31°
- Long = −39°
- Ring = −22°
- Small = −25°

Wrist extension plateaued around 58° to 60°. Grip strength continued to be an issue for her; she reported difficulty opening tight jars, lifting her briefcase for work, and carrying heavy file folders to and from meetings. Grip strength on the Jamar dynamometer, position 2, was (R/L) 25/55 lbs at this time. S.J. expressed concerns about her ability to quickly and efficiently set up, demonstrate, and score the standardized IQ testing that she routinely used with clients at work prior to this injury. Therefore, she was encouraged to bring in the standardized test and to practice in the clinic. Therapy was also adjusted to focus more on functional grip strength and endurance for bearing weight on her extended wrist. Since her interests outside of work included tennis, part of her therapy involved performing ball exercises with her tennis racquet, followed by hitting the tennis ball against her garage door. With time, she was encouraged to lobby the tennis ball back and forth over the net in a friendly game with her husband.

S.J. was discharged to a HEP on July 1st. At this time, she demonstrated full digit flexion to the DPC and small consistent gains in digit total extension. She had weaned from her static progressive splint and was able to maintain both her wrist and digit extension gains. Her DASH score was 30, and her grip strength measured 33 lbs on her affected side. Most importantly, she felt confident that she would continue to see small gains over the year from her surgery, and she felt comfortable with her HEP.

References

1. LaStayo P, Winters K, Hardy M: Fracture healing: bone healing, fracture management and current concepts related to the hand, *J Hand Ther* 16(2):81–93, 2003.
2. Lutsky K, MD: *Personal communication*, July 24, 2012.
3. Hardy M, Freeland A: Hand fracture fixation and healing: skeletal stability and digital mobility. In Skirven T, Osterman AL, Fedorczyk J, et al: *Rehabilitation of the hand and upper extremity*, ed 6, Philadelphia, 2011, Elsevier, pp 361–376.
4. Slutsky D, Herman M: Rehabilitation of distal radius fractures: a biomechanical guide, *Hand Clin* 21:455–468, 2005.
5. Putnam MD, Meyer NJ, Nelson EW, et al: Distal radial metaphyseal forces in an extrinsic grip model: implications for postfracture rehabilitation, *J Hand Surgery Am* 25(3):469–475, 2000.
6. Zelle B, Weiss KR, Fu FH: Pathogenesis of soft tissue and bone repair. In Maxey L, Magnusson J, editors: *Rehabilitation of the postsurgical orthopedic patient*, ed 2, Philadelphia, 2007, Mosby/Elsevier, pp 13–16.
7. Lutsky K, Boyer MI, Steffen JA, et al: Arthroscopic assessment of intra-articular distal radius fractures after open reduction and internal fixation from a volar approach, *J Hand Surg* 33(4):476–484, 2008.
8. Smith D, Brou K, Henry M: Early active rehabilitation for operatively stabilized distal radius fractures, *J Hand Ther* 17(1):43–49, 2004.
9. Bednar J: The distal radioulnar joint: acute injuries and chronic injuries. In Skirven T, Osterman AL, Fedorczyk J, et al: *Rehabilitation of the hand and upper extremity*, ed 6, Philadelphia, 2011, Elsevier, pp 963–973.
10. Davis DI, Baratz M: Soft tissue complications of distal radius fractures, *Hand Clin* 26(2):229–235, 2010.
11. Chung K, Spilson S: The frequency and epidemiology of hand and forearm fractures in the United States, *J Hand Surg* 26(5):908–915, 2001.
12. Figl M, Weninger P, Jurkowitsch J, et al: Unstable distal radius fractures in the elderly patient—volar fixed-angle plate osteosynthesis prevents secondary loss of reduction, *J Trauma* 68(4):992–998, 2010.
13. Medoff R: Distal radius fractures: classification and management. In Skirven T, Osterman AL, Fedorczyk J, et al: *Rehabilitation of the hand and upper extremity*, ed 6, Philadelphia, 2011, Elsevier, pp 941–948.
14. Thompson J: *Netter's concise orthopaedic anatomy*, Philadelphia, 2010, Saunders/Elsevier. pp142–149.
15. Mischlovitz S, Festa L: Therapist's management of distal radius fractures. In Skirven T, Osterman AL, Fedorczyk J, et al: *Rehabilitation of the hand and upper extremity*, ed 6, Philadelphia, 2011, Elsevier, pp 949–962.
16. Cannon N, editor: *Diagnosis and treatment manual*, ed 4, Indianapolis, 2001, The Hand Rehabilitation Center of Indiana, pp 119–141.

17. Marks M, Herren D, Vlieland T, et al: Determinants of patient satisfaction after orthopedic interventions to the hand: a review of the literature, *J Hand Ther* 24(4):303–312, 2011.

18. McKee PR, Rivard A: Biopsychosocial approach to orthotic intervention, *J Hand Ther* 24(2):155–163, 2011.

19. Villeco J: Edema: therapist's management. In Skirven T, Osterman AL, Fedorczyk J, et al: *Rehabilitation of the hand and upper extremity*, ed 6, Philadelphia, 2011, Elsevier, pp 845–857.

20. Lucado AM, Li Z, Russell GB, et al: Changes in impairment and function after static progressive splinting for stiffness after distal radius fracture, *J Hand Ther* 21(4):319–325, 2008.

21. Lyngcoln A, Taylor N, Pizzari T, et al: Relationship between adherence to hand therapy and short term outcomes, *J Hand Ther* 18:2–8, 2005.

22. Valdes K: A retrospective pilot study comparing number of therapy visits required to gain functional wrist and forearm range of motion following volar plating of distal radius fracture, *J Hand Ther* 22(4):312–318, 2009.

23. Schier JS, Chan J: Changes in life roles after hand injury, *J Hand Ther* 20(1):57–69, 2007.

24. Rozental T, Branas C, Bozentka D, et al: Survival among elderly patients after fractures of the distal radius, *J Hand Surg* 27(6):948–952, 2002.

25. Koman L, Zhongyu L, Smith BP, et al: Complex regional pain syndrome: types I and II. In Skirven T, Osterman AL, Fedorczyk J, et al: *Rehabilitation of the hand and upper extremity*, Philadelphia, 2011, Elsevier, pp 1470–1478.

26. LaStayo P, Weiss S, The GRIT: a quantitative measure of ulnar impaction syndrome, *J Hand Ther* 14(3):173–179, 2001.

27. Dell P, Dell R, Griggs R: Management of carpal fractures and dislocations. In Skirven T, Osterman AL, Fedorczyk J, et al: *Rehabilitation of the hand and upper extremity*, ed 6, Philadelphia, 2011, Elsevier.

28. Prosser R, Herbert T: The management of carpal fractures and dislocations, *J Hand Ther* 9:130–147, 1996.

29. Vigler M, Aviles A, Lee SK: Carpal fractures excluding the scaphoid, *Hand Clin* 22:501–516, 2006.

30. Terrano AL, Nalebuff EA, Philips CA: The rheumatoid thumb. In Mackin E, Callahan A, Skirven T, et al: *Rehabilitation of the hand and upper extremity*, ed 5, Philadephia, 2002, Mosby, p 1559.

31. Smaby N, Johanson ME, Baker B, et al: Identification of key pinch forces required to complete functional tasks, *J Rehabil Res Dev* 41(2):215–224, 2004.

26

Wrist Instabilities

Shrikant J. Chinchalkar and
Joey G. Pipicelli

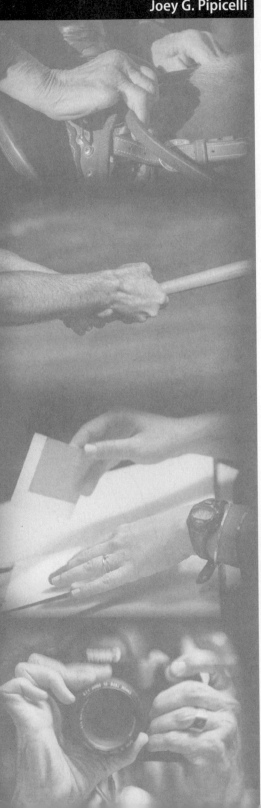

Introduction

The wrist is an intricate joint with complex motion and function and is comprised of several articulations. These articulations are formed by various anatomical structures with varying degrees of curvatures and congruencies supported by the ligamentous elements, controlled by musculotendinous units, and based on precise proprioceptive input from various ligaments. The meticulous normal functioning of the hand is dictated by the stability and mobility of the carpus, allowing the hand to grasp objects in a variety of wrist positions.

Carpal dislocations and instabilities are common injuries, especially in young adults. Most carpal disruptions are caused by trauma; however, conditions such as congenital laxity, infection, inflammatory processes (rheumatoid arthritis), or congenital defects can also be the culprit. Carpal dislocation and instability injury patterns can be easily misdiagnosed, because an exact diagnosis is often difficult to establish. If such injuries are not correctly diagnosed, this can eventually lead to premature degeneration and arthrosis at radiocarpal and midcarpal joints due to altered carpal kinematics.

Carpal instability is defined as dislocation or loss of contact between bones of the distal carpal row over the proximal carpal row in relation to the radioulnar joint. The loss of contact is either static or dynamic, causing a decreased ability to transfer loads across the wrist during motion or function. Common symptoms reported by patients include pain, sudden loss of motion control, and at times clunking associated with pain and weakness. Untimely identification and inadequate management of carpal instabilities will cause abnormal intercarpal and radiocarpal loads, ultimately leading to degeneration at the articular surfaces. In order to understand carpal instability, an understanding of the anatomy of the wrist joint and the kinematics of the carpal bones is imperative.

Osseous Anatomy

The wrist consists of the distal radius and ulna forming the distal radioulnar joint. The distal radius is typically tilted in anterior/posterior (A/P) plane by an average of 11° (Fig. 26-1, *A*) and radioulnar plane by 23° (see Fig. 26-1, *B*). The distal radius is composed of two fossae—a rectangular and shallow fossa for the articulation of lunate, and a deep triangular fossa for the scaphoid (Fig. 26-2). The distal surface of the ulna is covered by the triangular fibrocartilage complex (TFCC). The proximal carpal row is formed by the scaphoid, lunate, and triquetrum, whereas the distal carpal row is formed by the trapezium, trapezoid, capitate, and hamate. The joint formed by both these rows is the midcarpal joint. The midcarpal joint has three articulations: lateral, central, and medial. The lateral segment of the midcarpal joint is formed by the convexity of the distal pole of the scaphoid articulating with the concavity formed by the trapezium, trapezoid, and lateral aspect of the capitate. The central portion of the joint is formed by the proximal concavity of the scaphoid and lunate and distally by the convexity of the head of the capitate and the proximal pole of the hamate representing a "ball and socket" articulation. Medially the joint is formed by the articulation of the hamate and triquetrum. The midcarpal joint is highly synovial, thus allowing for maximal motion in all the planes. The scaphoid bridges both proximal and distal carpal rows. The pisiform, a sesamoid bone, is in the substance of the flexor carpi ulnaris (FCU) tendon, which articulates with the triquetrum. The proximal carpal row has been termed as an intercalated segment between the distal carpal row and the radius. The bones of the proximal carpal row move directly in response to the muscular force regulated by the ligaments that connect to the forearm and the distal carpal rows.[1-4]

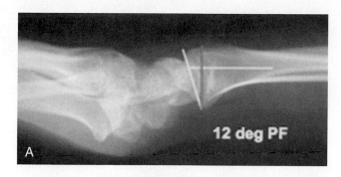

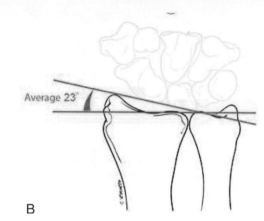

FIGURE 26-1 A, The distal radius is typically tilted an average of 11 degrees in the anterior posterior plane. **B,** The distal radius is tilted an average of 23 degrees in the radial-ulnar plane. This is called radial inclination.

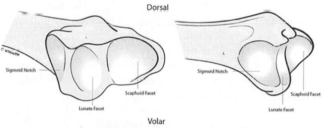

FIGURE 26-2 The fossae of the distal radius.

Ligamentous Anatomy

The ligamentous structures are divided into extrinsic, intrinsic, palmar, and dorsal.[5] The palmar extrinsic ligaments arise from the distal radius and ulna, and they connect to proximal and distal carpal rows. These ligaments are labeled in accordance with their length and insertion.

Palmar Ligaments

> ◎ **Clinical Pearl**
>
> The palmar extrinsic ligaments are stronger than the dorsal extrinsic ligaments and are considered the main stabilizers of the radiocarpal joints.[5]

The radioscaphocapitate (RSC) is the radial most ligament originating from the radial styloid, and it traverses across the distal pole of the scaphoid connecting to the waist of the capitate. This ligament blends into the ulnocapitate (UC) ligament arising from the ulnar side. The RSC ligament is a primary radial stabilizer of the wrist and resists ulnar translation of the carpus over the radius. Lateral to the RSC ligament, the radioscapholunate (RSL) ligament provides neurovascular supply to the carpal bones and has no contribution to carpal stability. Lateral to the RSL ligament, the long radiolunate (LRL) and short radiolunate (SRL) ligaments offer primary resistance to lunate displacement, thereby preventing perilunate dislocation.[6]

On the ulnar side, the palmar ligaments, such as the ulnotriquetral (UT) and ulnolunate ligaments, arise from the TFCC and distal ulna. The medial most ligament, which arises from ulna, is called the *UC ligament.* As previously mentioned, this ligament blends in with the RSC ligament forming an acute structure. These ligaments connect the ulna to the carpus.

Palmar Intrinsic Ligaments

The palmar intrinsic ligaments are named based on their connection between the carpal bones. The proximal carpal bones are stabilized by the scapholunate (SL) ligament on the radial side and the lunotriquetral (LT) ligament on the ulnar side. The SL and LT ligaments have certain characteristics. The SL ligament has three distinct components: palmar, dorsal, and proximal. The dorsal SL ligament is the toughest portion of the ligaments and is responsible for preventing excessive flexion and rotation of the scaphoid, whereas the LT ligament is toughest on the volar side, which prevents ulnar translation of the lunate. Two deltoid or arcuate intrinsic ligaments consist of scaphocapitate and triquetrocapitate ligaments. These ligaments serve as the stabilizer of the midcarpal joint. Trapezio-trapezoid, trapezio-capitate, and capito-hamate ligaments connect the bones of the distal carpal row.

> ◎ **Clinical Pearl**
>
> The space in-between both the proximal and distal carpal rows is termed *the space of Poirier* and is where most common patterns of carpal collapse and instability occur.

Dorsal Ligaments

The dorsal intrinsic wrist ligaments are intracapsular and are not as well-defined and strong as the volar intrinsic ligaments (Fig. 26-3, *A*). The dorsal extrinsic ligaments of the wrist consist of dorsal radiocarpal (DRC) and dorsal intercarpal (DIC) ligaments (see Fig. 26-3, *B*). The DRC originates from the dorsal distal radius at Lister's tubercle crossing, obliquely inserting on the triquetrum. The DRC ligaments prevent ulnar translation of the carpus. The DIC ligament originates from the triquetrum and extends towards the distal pole of the scaphoid and trapezoid where it inserts. This ligament provides stability to the midcarpal joint preventing dorsal dislocation of the capitate from the SL interval.

Similar to the palmar intrinsic ligaments, the intrinsic ligaments on the dorsal side are labeled in accordance with their connection between the carpal bones.

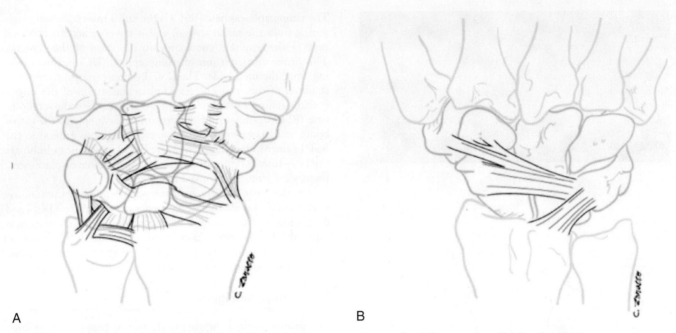

A

B

FIGURE 26-3 A, The dorsal intrinsic wrist ligaments are intracapsular and are not as well defined and strong as the volar intrinsic ligaments. **B,** The dorsal extrinsic ligaments of the wrist consist of dorsal radiocarpal (DRC) and dorsal intercarpal (DIC) ligaments.

Retinacular Ligaments and Tendons Responsible for Wrist Motion

Other attachments to the carpus consist of distinct fascial layers of extensor and flexor retinaculum. The extensor retinaculum consists of two layers: infratendinous and supratendinous. The extensor retinaculum inserts on the palmar margin of the distal radius and ulnarly on the pisiform on the volar aspect. In between two layers of extensor retinaculum, vertical septii divides the extensor tendons into six different compartments. The primary extensors of the wrist include the extensor carpi radialis brevis (ECRB) and extensor carpi radialis longus (ECRL) on the radial side and extensor carpi ulnaris (ECU) on the ulnar side. The digital and thumb extensor tendons also supplement wrist extensor force to some degree.

On the palmar side, the flexor retinaculum attaches to the hook of the hamate and pisiform, and on the radial side, it inserts on the scaphoid tubercle and the tuberosity of trapezium. The flexor retinaculum forms a carpal canal that contains the median nerve and nine flexor tendons shared by the fingers and thumb. The primary wrist flexors consist of the flexor carpi radialis (FCR) and FCU. The FCR inserts on the base of second metacarpal, whereas the FCU inserts on the pisiform with extension in a form of ligaments connecting to the hamate (pisohamate ligament) and the base of the fifth metacarpal (pisometacarpal ligament). Other than the FCU, no other tendinous insertions exist on the carpus, except for the abductor pollicis longus (APL) inserting on the trapezoid, trapezium, and distal pole of the scaphoid as an anatomical variation.

Normal Kinematics of the Wrist Joint

Understanding the complexities of carpal motion is based on various evolutionary studies that identified the instability patterns of the wrist. Navarro[7] originally proposed the column theory. He

suggested that the carpus was made up of three columns: central, radial, and ulnar. This column theory was later modified by Taleisnik.[5] Other studies including work by Lichtman, et al.[2] identified the four-unit concept, whereas Linscheid, et al.[1] introduced a slider crank mechanism of the scaphoid. Linscheid, et al.[1] also identified that regardless of the previously published studies illustrating the normal kinematics, the scaphoid maintains an average of 47° of flexion orientation in relation to the lunate and radius on lateral radiograph. The SL ligament plays an important role in neutralizing the flexion tendency of the scaphoid under physiologic loads. Gillula and Weeks[8] identified that there is a distinct parallelism between the curvatures of the proximal and distal carpal rows on A/P radiograph. The proximal carpal row's behavior during flexion/extension or radio/ulnar motion is based on its central placement between two rigid structures (that is, distal radius proximally and stable distal carpal row distally).

The motion of the carpal bones during flexion/extension and radial/ulnar deviation of the wrist is extremely complex. The motion of the proximal carpal row is dependent on the compressive loads placed by the distal carpal row. The musculotendinous units inserting distal to the distal carpal row produce this physiologic load on the carpus. Having normal anatomic relationship of the proximal carpal row structures along with the radius is critical for normal functioning of the wrist joint to occur.[9]

Flexion/Extension Motion

During extension of the wrist, the lunate extends and translates palmarly, whereas the capitate rotates dorsally.[10] The palmar radiolunate ligament prevents excessive rotation of the lunate, preventing dorsal intercalated segmental instability (DISI). When the wrist is flexed, the lunate translates dorsally and the capitate rotates palmarly. The DRC and DIC ligaments prevent excessive rotation of the lunate, preventing volar intercalated segmental instability (VISI).

Radioulnar Motion

Radioulnar motion of the wrist is more complex than the flexion/extension arc of motion. The radioulnar motion of the wrist influences both of the carpal rows to move in different directions. The distal carpal row rotates in a radial direction, whereas the proximal carpal row slides in an ulnar direction when radial deviation is performed; a reversal mechanism occurs when the wrist is brought into an ulnar deviation posture. These changes occurring in both the carpal rows are influenced by the geometry of the carpus, ligamentous constraints offered by the extrinsic and intrinsic ligaments of the wrist, and the muscles of the wrist acting through the distal carpal row.

Upon radial deviation of the wrist, the distal pole of scaphoid is compressed between the radial styloid proximally and the trapezium-trapezoid distally, forcing the distal pole of scaphoid to flex in almost perpendicular direction to the radius. As the scaphoid flexes, the entire proximal carpal row also assumes a flexed position. The intact SL and LT ligaments cause the entire proximal carpal row to follow the scaphoid's tendency towards flexion. During radial deviation the ulnar ligaments (such as, ulnocarpal, ulnar lunate, and UT) stretch, whereas the ligaments on the radial side become lax. Tensioning of the UT ligament influences the triquetrum, causing it to slide or disengage off the waist of hamate. Besides these changes, the motion of the wrist in a radial direction produces a translatory effect on the proximal carpal row, which then slides in an ulnar direction. A synchronous motion that occurs with radial deviation involves execution of the proximal row in pronation and flexion, whereas the distal carpal row moves in the opposite direction of supination and extension.

As the wrist is moved in ulnar deviation, a compressive force is produced by the hamate over the triquetrum, which forces it into extension, and subsequently the entire proximal carpal row is brought into extension. The entire proximal carpal row slides radially because of tensioning of the RSC, LRL, and SRL ligaments. In addition, as the extension of the proximal carpal row increases with the increment of the deviation, the scaphoid is pulled into extension with lunate and triquetrum. Besides this, the proximal row executes supination and extension, whereas the distal row moves in pronation and flexion.

Motion of the Carpus during Gripping

Studies on load distribution during gripping activities have demonstrated that 80% of the load is transmitted on the radiocarpal joint and 20% on the ulnocarpal region, especially when the radioulnar relationship is in neutral ulnar variance.[11] Out of the 80% radial load, 60% of the load transmission is on the scaphoid, whereas 40% of the load is transmitted on lunate. The load variation changes proportionally, either negative or positive, if ulnar variance is present. In neutral ulnar variance, the forces produced by the flexors and extensors are transmitted from the digits to the distal carpal row upon gripping and then through the proximal pole of capitate to the SL interval. A radiologic investigation using a classic stress test by making a fist is recommended to diagnose partial SL ligament tears, especially in the carpal instability non-dissociative (CIND) category of carpal instability. (This will be discussed later in the chapter.) The carpal motion studies during gripping have shown that the scaphoid demonstrates a tendency to rotate in flexion and pronation; the lunate rotates dorsally, whereas the triquetrum rotates in flexion. The rotatory tendency of the carpus during gripping activities suggest that the proximal carpal row (that is, the intercalary segment) moves together because of the intact SL and LT ligaments. In addition, the dislocation of the carpus is prevented by the palmar intrinsic, as well as the dorsal and palmar extrinsic ligaments.

Dart Throwing Motion

Other physiologic motions of the wrist that are commonly used in activities of daily living (ADLs) involve motion in an oblique plane. The majority of ADLs, such as combing hair or hammering a nail, are performed in a distinct manner. The motion of the wrist involves a combination of wrist extension in radial deviation and flexion with ulnar deviation. This motion has been coined as a *dart throwing motion (DTM)*.[12] The International Federation of Societies of the Hand (IFSSH) Committee[13] recommends the motion taking place at the wrist joint in the so-called DTM be called *radial extension and ulnar flexion*. In vivo investigation of length changes in carpal ligaments during DTM demonstrates that the palmar radiocarpal ligaments' length decreased significantly, whereas the DIC ligaments inserting on the trapezoid lengthened, and the UL and DIC inserting on the scaphoid remained shortest in neutral wrist position. These findings also suggest that DTM does not cause greater loads on the carpal ligaments. In addition, the arcuate ligament (that is, RSC and UC ligaments) resisted excessive motion of the capitate contributing to the midcarpal joint stability.[14] From a carpal motion point of view, the DTM, revealed minimal scaphoid and lunate motion when compared to pure radioulnar or flexion extension arc of motion.[15-17] The muscles that produce DTM are the FCU and the ECU and ECRB and ECRL. DTM will be discussed further later in this chapter.

Muscular Contributions to the Motion of the Wrist and Their Effect on Carpal Stabilization

The motion of the wrist joint in flexion, extension, and radioulnar direction is dependent on various muscular contractions. The palmaris longus, FCR, and FCU produce flexion of the wrist. The digital flexors also contribute secondarily to the flexion of the wrist joint. The ECRB, ECRL, and ECU are the prime extensors of the wrist. Additionally, the digital extensors also contribute secondarily to the extension action at the wrist. Radial deviation is primarily dependent on the action of FCR and ECRL; in addition APL, because of its radial orientation, contributes to radial deviation of the wrist joint. Motion in ulnar deviation is a result of ECU and FCU contraction. The kinematics of the carpus in flexion/extension, as well as the radioulnar arc, were described in the previous section. Based on the kinematics, it is apparent that the deforming forces are produced at the distal pole of the scaphoid, resulting in the intercalary motion of the proximal carpal row. Cadaveric studies by Garcia-Elias[18] and Hagert, Forsegren, & Ljung[19] on the effect on carpal alignment during loading of the muscles have shown that ECU contraction stresses the SL ligament, whereas FCU, FCR, and APL activity reduces the load on the injured SL ligament. In addition, Garcia-Elias[18] identified that FCU and hypothenar muscle contraction produced dorsally directed forces on the triquetrum through the pisiform, which stabilized midcarpal as well as LT joint instability. Based on these cadaveric studies, the authors recommend that the proprioceptive training of these muscles would be beneficial in SL, LT, and midcarpal instabilities. These suggestions are based on cadaveric experimentations, and implementation in clinical situations needs further investigation.

Proprioceptive Input during Motion of the Wrist

As mentioned previously, the motion of the wrist is highly complex.

> © **Clinical Pearl**
>
> In order to move the wrist in various planes, either with or without loading, the wrist joint must maintain entire stability between the radiocarpal and intercarpal joints.

This maintenance of stability during motion is provided by several mechanoreceptors and proprioceptors embedded in the joint capsule and ligaments. These structures are continuously sending feedback to the central nervous system (CNS) about the position of the joint and the speed of motion being performed. In addition, the information regarding pressure, torsion, and sensation of the pain sent to the CNS regulates muscular contraction to maintain the joint stability. A concentration of nerve endings responsible for sending information to the CNS have been found in the dorsal radio carpal ligaments, RSL ligaments, and SL and LT ligaments. The RSL ligament was identified to be responsible for monitoring the SL relationship. The SL and LT ligaments provide continuous sensory feedback during motion of the wrist joint. Upon electrical stimulation of the SL ligament, recruitment of FCR and FCU was recorded with reciprocal activation of ECU and ECRB, suggesting that these muscles guided prevention of instability of the joint. Thus, proprioceptive reeducation may add a benefit in treating ligamentous injuries of the wrist joint.

Carpal Instability Classification

Attempts to simplify our understanding of carpal motion have led to the development of multiple classification systems of carpal instability.[5,20-22] Perhaps the most widely-adopted classification system is the Mayo Classification,[23] which classifies carpal instability into four major categories:
- Carpal instability dissociative (CID)
- Carpal instability non-dissociative (CIND)
- Carpal instability complex (CIC)
- Carpal instability adaptive (CIA)

Carpal Instability Dissociative

CID is caused by fracture or ligament disruption between the same carpal row—usually the proximal row. This form of instability involves pathology to the intrinsic ligaments and includes injuries to the SL or LT ligaments.

Scapholunate Ligament Tears

SL instability occurs most commonly in young- to middle-aged populations and is typically a result of a fall on out-stretched hand (FOOSH). Patients with acute injury often present to the physician's office with a painful and swollen wrist, which may be diffusely tender. With time, pain becomes more localized over the SL ligament dorsally. Clinical examination needs to be exhaustive and systematic. Palpation of maximal areas of tenderness should be noted, and if sharp pain is elicited by pressing on the area just distal to Lister's tubercle, a SL ligament tear is a high probability.[24] Evaluation of the wrist should always include radiographic evaluation. Radiographs will often demonstrate the following in the presence complete SL ligament tears:[5,11,25-27]

- A/P views may demonstrate a SL gap of greater than 2 mm to 3 mm (Fig. 26-4, *A*). This has been termed the *Terry Thomas sign*.
- Scaphoid may be palmarly flexed, giving the appearance of a ring on the AP film (see Fig. 26-4, *B*).
- Lateral views of the wrist may demonstrate the lunate dorsiflexed 15° or greater in relation to the capitate. This deformity is called a *DISI* (see Fig 26-4, *C*).
- Lateral views will also demonstrate an abnormal SL angle of more than 60° to 70° (see Fig 26-4, *D*).
- Long-standing instability may show degenerative changes to the radial styloid and at the capitolunate joint.

Luno-Triquetral Instability

LT instability is far less common than SL instability. This injury typically occurs secondarily to an injury to the ulnar side of the wrist. Patients will often complain of pain over the ulnar aspect of their wrist that is exacerbated by power grip and ulnar deviation. Power grip will increase ulnar variance and thus impingement onto the lunate. Radiographs will often demonstrate the following:
- Lateral radiographs may demonstrate a VISI deformity, which is a capitolunate angle of greater than 30° (Fig 26-5).
- Lateral radiographs will demonstrate that the lunate is more palmarly flexed.
- Lateral radiographs will demonstrate a normal SL angle.

Carpal Instability Non-Dissociative

CIND often results in abnormal motion of the entire proximal carpal row at the radiocarpal and/or midcarpal joint. Thus, it is not specific to a carpal row. CIND involves a large array of disorders, which include midcarpal instability (MCI), ulnar translation of the carpus, capitolunate instability, triquetral hamate instability, and ulnar carpal instability. Patients usually suffer from generalized ligamentous laxity elsewhere (such as, elbows, knees, thumb to forearm, and so on). Patients often visit the physician complaining of wrist pain that is not well-defined or localized. Often pain may be volar or dorsal. Swelling is not usually present. Patients often demonstrate some wrist clicking or clunking as the wrist is moved from radial to ulnar deviation. The capitate can often be subluxated on the lunate when a dorsally-directed force is applied to the hand with the forearm held in neutral position. The reverse maneuver with a palmar-directed force on the hand unit can cause volar subluxation at the midcarpal area. The ligaments are likely to be partially torn or attenuated, keeping the carpal orientation intact. Radiologically, the carpal bones appear in normal orientation, thus making exact diagnosis difficult. Typically, stress views, fluoroscopy, and/or arthroscopy are necessary to establish the diagnosis.

Carpal Instability Complex

With the CIC category both CID and CIND may be present simultaneously. Common findings in this category of instability are perilunate dislocation along with radiocarpal ligament injuries, resulting in SL and LT dissociation with ulnar translation of the lunate.

Carpal Instability Adaptive

This category of instability presents as an adaptive change of the carpus in relation to the radius following malunited distal radius fractures or untreated carpal instabilities.

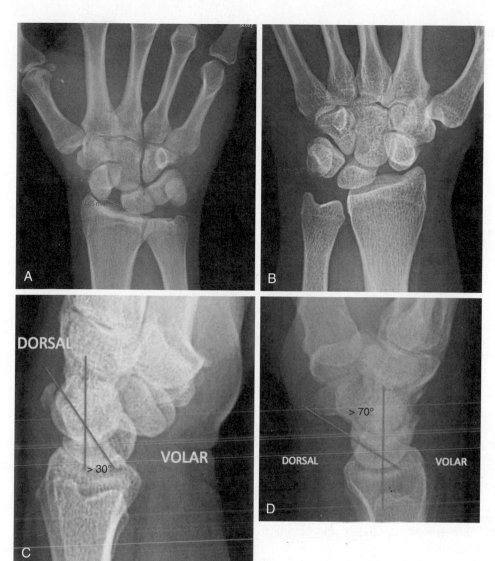

FIGURE 26-4 **A,** Anterior/posterior (A/P) radiograph of the wrist demonstrating a scapholunate gap of greater than 2 to 3 mm. This is called the Terry Thomas Sign. **B,** Scaphoid is palmarly flexed giving the appearance of a ring on A/P radiograph. **C,** Lateral views of the wrist may demonstrate the lunate dorsiflexed 15 degrees or greater in relation to the capitate. This deformity is called dorsal-intercalated segment instability (DISI). **D,** Lateral radiograph of the wrist demonstrating abnormal S-L angle of more than 60 to 70 degrees.

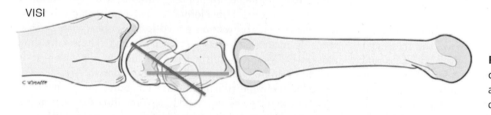

FIGURE 26-5 Lateral radiograph demonstrates (VISI) deformity which is a capitolunate angle of greater than 30 degrees.

Rehabilitation of Carpal Instabilities: Current Practice

The literature describing the rehabilitation of carpal instability is limited. Most rehabilitation programs described are based on author preference and experience.[28-32] These rehabilitation programs are based on sound clinical reasoning; however, they have not been established as best practice, because clinical research studies are lacking. As such, carpal instability rehabilitation should be based on the stages of tissue healing when making clinical decisions regarding the length of time of immobilization, initiation of controlled protected motion, gradual tissue loading, and resumption of unrestricted hand use during functional activity, sport-, and work-related tasks. General rehabilitation following operative or non-operative management of wrist ligament injury should include the following:

- Edema and pain control
  - Through traditional means, including pharmacology, cryotherapy, compression, elevation, and cast/orthotic application
- Maintenance of range of motion (ROM) to the uninvolved joints
- Initiation of controlled, protected mobilization to the involved structures based on stages of tissue healing, observed intraoperative tension to repaired structures, and symptomology of the patient

- Avoidance of exercise or activity that may compromise tissue healing or place undue load to the healing/repaired structures
  - Avoidance of generic wrist ROM and strengthening exercises
  - Avoidance of aggressive ROM and excessive active ROM exercises
- Overall achievement of a stable wrist with functional ROM; functional ROM should be based on the work of Palmer and colleagues,[13] which found that functional wrist ROM is between 5° of wrist flexion to 30° of extension, 10° of radial deviation, and 15° of ulnar deviation

Innovative and Emerging Approaches to Carpal Instability Rehabilitation

New lines of research investigation have elucidated the role of proprioception in stabilization of the wrist. This follows previous investigations of the role of proprioception in the stabilization of other articulations, such as the shoulder, ankle, and knee. However, for therapists to understand these emerging ideas, we must first have a sound foundation of the neuromuscular rehabilitation concepts.

The term *proprioception* has been used since the early twentieth century to describe our body's regulation of posture, balance, joint stability, and audiovisual-motor coordination.[33] Our body maintains appropriate proprioceptive feedback through homeostasis. Homeostasis is defined as a dynamic process by which an organism maintains and controls its internal environment despite disturbances from external forces.[34] The body is composed of many systems that operate automatically and subconsciously to maintain a homeostatic state.[35]

The term *sensorimotor function* was adopted by the participants of the 1997 Foundation of Sports Medicine Education and Research workshop in order to describe the sensory, motor, and central integration and processing components involved with maintaining joint homeostasis during movement.[36] This was an attempt to recognize the portion of proprioceptive research dealing with only joint control.

The process of maintaining joint control and stability is accomplished through the relationship between the static and dynamic joint stabilizers. Ligaments, joint capsule, cartilage, and joint articulation bony geometry comprise the static stabilizers.[37-39] Dynamic contributions to joint stability arise from the skeletal muscles that cross the joint structures. If there is a disruption in the static stabilizers of a joint, the dynamic joint stabilizers must work harder and become smarter and stronger in order to provide enhanced joint stability. However, in order for this to occur we must optimize ligamentomuscular reflexes.

Ligamentous and Muscular Reflexes, Proprioception, and the Wrist

◎ *Clinical Pearl*

Intact wrist ligaments are responsible for wrist stability. However, these ligaments also provide the brain with important sensory input, which enhances the dynamic stability of this complex structure.[20,40-43]

The sensory input provided by the intact wrist ligaments is delivered to the brain through afferent pathways. The sensory end organs that provide this information are the joint mechanoreceptors, because they react to joint pressure, motion, and velocity. The brain then interprets these afferent impulses as joint position sense (JPS), kinesthesia, sense of resistance, motion threshold, and velocity.

The existence of mechanoreceptors in the ligaments of the wrist was first identified by Petrie, et al. in 1997.[44] Since this time, there have been numerous studies on the innervation of the various wrist ligaments.[20,40,41,45-47] These studies found that nerve endings in the various wrist ligaments are predominately located close to the ligament insertion into bone. This ensures firing of the mechanoreceptors only at the extremes of joint motion as the collagen fibers within the ligament have higher stiffness at their insertion into bone.[48] Mechanoreceptors are also found in the DRC and DIC ligaments in the pliant epifascicular regions where they can be readily stimulated and able to provide information throughout the range of wrist motions.[20,42] Interestingly, the ligaments of the radial and volar wrist ligaments have little to no innervation. However, the dorsal and triquetral wrist ligaments (DRC, DIR, dorsal SL, palmar LT, and triquetrocapitate/hamate ligaments) are the most densely innervated.[40,49] What does this mean? The dense mechanically important ligaments that are designed to withstand axial loads are located in the radial column of the wrist. The sensory important ligaments are the dorsal wrist ligaments and ligaments emerging from the triquetrum and should be regarded as key elements in the generation of proprioceptive information required for adequate neuromuscular wrist control (Fig. 26-6).[50]

Dart Throwing Motion

DTM refers to the motion pattern commonly used during ADLs and functional tasks. Palmer and colleagues[13] found that most tasks are performed in a plane from 40° of wrist extension and 20° radial deviation to 0° of flexion and 20° of ulnar deviation. Biomechanical studies of this motion pattern demonstrate that radiocarpal motion is minimized while most of the motion is occurring at the midcarpal joint.[51-53] The relationship this movement pattern has on tension placed to the scapholunate interosseous ligament (SLIL) has also been studied. The results show that the DTM pattern of the wrist produces minimal elongation and thus minimal tension to the volar and dorsal SLIL.[54,55] The clinical implications to hand therapy rehabilitation are that practice-guidelines can be developed implementing early-controlled motion utilizing the DTM pattern following partial SLIL injuries, SL repairs, or potentially other reconstructive procedures. Orthotic application can be utilized to ensure that wrist motion is within the arc of the DTM pattern of movement (Fig. 26-7). Caution must be used in implementing this type of controlled mobilization pattern following partial SLIL injuries and surgical procedures because no studies have determined the optimal time to introduce this pattern of movement following injury or surgery. It is also unknown how long to restrict motion along the DTM path following injury.

Proprioceptive Reeducation to the Wrist

Ligamentous insufficiency within the wrist may distort proprioceptive responses altering the normal reflex mechanism. This has

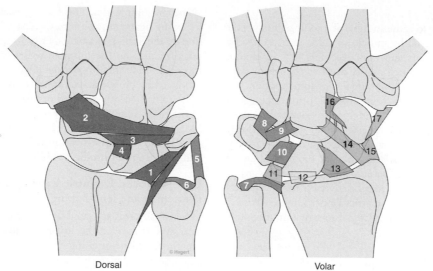

Dorsal   Volar

FIGURE 26-6 Mechanoreceptor and nerve distribution in the wrist ligaments including the Triangular Fibro-cartiliage Complex. Ligaments: dorsal radiocarpal (1), dorsal intercarpal (2), scaphotriquetral (3), scapholunate interosseous (4), ulnar collateral (5), dorsal radioulnar (6), volar radioulnar (7), triquetrohamate (8), triquetrocapitate (9), palmar lunotriquetral (10), ulnolunate (11), short radiolunate (12), long radiolunate (13), radioscaphocapitate (14), radioscaphoid (15), scaphocapitate (16), scaphotrapeziotrapezoid (17). (Courtesy Hagert E, Wrist Ligaments—Innervation Patterns and Ligamento-Muscular Reflexes, Karolinska Institute, 2008.)

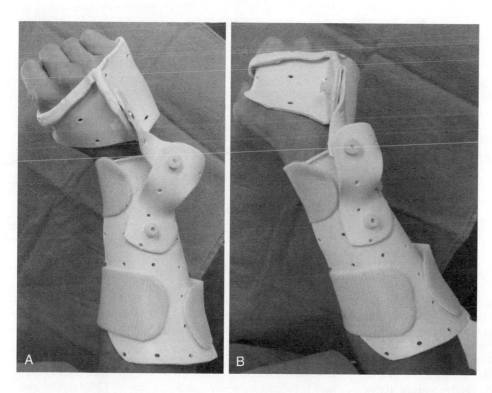

FIGURE 26-7 Custom made dart throw's motion orthosis. **A,** Demonstrating radial deviation with slight extension. **B,** Demonstrating ulnar deviation with slight flexion.

an effect on dynamic joint stability.[56] Although proprioceptive reeducation is a relatively new rehabilitation concept applied to wrist instability, it is a well-established part of the treatment of the unstable shoulder, knee, and ankle joint.[57-62]

Hagert[49] proposed a proprioceptive rehabilitation program for to the unstable wrist joint. The foundation of proprioceptive reeducation is based on identifying muscles that serve a protective function for the specific ligament deficiency and training those muscles to respond more efficiently to prevent injury. Hagert[49] suggests that the three major proprioceptive senses that have therapeutic implications include kinesthesia, JPS, and neuromuscular rehabilitation.

Kinesthesia

Kinesthesia is the ability to sense motion of a joint or limb. This sense is primarily influenced by muscle spindles and secondarily influenced by skin receptors and joint receptors.[63-68] In clinical practice, kinesthesia is measured as the smallest change in joint angle required to elicit conscious awareness of joint motion.[48,69] The common terminology used in proprioception training is "threshold to detection of passive movement."[49] It has been suggested that the joint be placed at a certain angle and then slowly moved passively at a speed of 0.5° to 2° per second until the patient signals that limb motion occurs.[49] The patient should be blinded during initial kinesthesia testing, because limb movement is greatly influenced by visual cues. Also, it may be advisable to use a professional training device (such as, Biometrics Upper Limb Exerciser*) in order to precisely control the speed and degree of joint motion.[49]

Joint Position Sense

JPS is a separate entity from kinesthesia.[70] To describe the differences between JPS and kinesthesia is beyond the scope of this chapter. However, be aware that they differ due to their central processing and interpretation in the brain.[69]

In proprioceptive retraining, JPS is defined as the ability to accurately reproduce a specific joint angle.[49] This form of retraining can be done with visual cues or blinded, as well as with active muscle contraction or through passive motion. Simply, JPS is when the patient is instructed to move the involved wrist to a predetermined joint angle established by using goniometry. This can be performed actively by the patient or passively by the therapist slowly moving the wrist until the patient identifies when the target position is reached. Hagert[49] suggests beginning JPS with visual cues progressing to vision occluded exercises as tolerated by the patient. Patient progress and accuracy can easily be recorded simply by using a goniometer

Neuromuscular Rehabilitation

Hagert[49] suggests that the purpose of neuromuscular wrist rehabilitation is to:

- Regain synchronous and balanced wrist motion following instability
- Use dynamic muscular compression to compensate for ligamentous insufficiency
- Promote ligamentous-friendly muscle contractions to provide joint protection and stability

The design of a neuromuscular rehabilitation program must be custom-tailored for each patient based on which structures are injured or operatively repaired. Furthermore, these techniques should be applied with caution, monitoring the patient's response. As therapists we must ensure that we are not compromising wrist stability; thus, we should monitor for pain, swelling, and signs of instability. The components of a neuromuscular rehabilitation program that may be beneficial include, isometric, concentric, eccentric, isokinetic, co-activation, and **reactive muscle activation (RMA)** exercises.[49]

Isometric Exercises

Isometric strengthening is a static form of exercise in which a muscle contracts and the length of the muscle does not change. The purpose is to increase strength and endurance of the muscles

at specific joint angles. This form of exercise can be applied early following ligamentous injury or repair, because it places no tension on the healing ligaments. Prior to applying this form of resistance training to the unstable wrist, the therapist must have a thorough understanding of the effects of the compressive forces produced by muscle activation, because this may place excessive stress to the recently repaired or healing structures. For example, isometric exercise of the FCR muscle in the presence of a partial SLIL tear may be beneficial. However, in a complete SLIL disruption, isometric FCR activation will further increase the SL angle and enhance this form of instability.

Concentric and Eccentric Exercises: Muscles actively shortening and lengthening

When a muscle is activated to move a joint from flexion to extension and vice versa the involved muscles begin to shorten or lengthen. This shortening and/or lengthening of the muscle is dependent on which direction the joint is moving. Contractions that permit the muscle to shorten are referred to as concentric contractions. Whereas, the muscle that lengthens is called eccentric muscle contraction. This form of muscle activation should be initiated following an initial period of isometric strengthening. The goal of this form of resistance training is to enhance strength, endurance, proprioception and synchronous wrist motion while not placing excessive tension through the healing ligamentous structures.

In concentric contractions, the force generated by the muscle is always lesser than the muscle's maximum. As the load of the muscle is required to lift a joint decreases, contraction velocity increases. This occurs until the muscle finally reaches its maximum contraction velocity. By performing a series of constant velocity shortening and lengthening contractions, a concentric and eccentric relationship is established. Based on the understanding of muscle physiology, it is imperative that we encourage concentric and eccentric strengthening by initiating wrist motion from 15-30 degrees of flexion to 15-30 degrees of extension with increments of 15 degrees on a weekly basis to minimize/prevent excessive articular load and subsequently on the healing ligaments.

Eccentric strengthening is designed to increase strength by applying load while physically lengthening the activated muscle. Eccentric exercises may be beneficial during rehabilitation of carpal instability due to the concurrent shortening on the antagonist muscle(s). For the wrist to produce synchronous motion the muscles must work together in harmony in order to produce joint equilibrium. Following ligamentous injury the muscles which cross the joint are often weak, resulting in a neuromuscular imbalance during dynamic exercise.[49]

Isokinetic Exercise

Isokinetic exercise is when the velocity of limb movement is held consistent by a rate-controlled device. This form of exercise is most frequently used with high level athletes and requires specialized equipment which is often expensive and not typically found in hand therapy clinics. However, isokinetic training has been shown to enhance overall proprioceptive function in athletes with ankle, knee, and shoulder instabilities.[60,71,72] It has been suggested that patients who place extreme demands on the wrist joint (such as professional athletes, gymnasts, or musicians) may benefit from this form of exercise as it may allow for an earlier return to activity specific training.[49]

Biometrics Ltd, Ladysmith, VA.

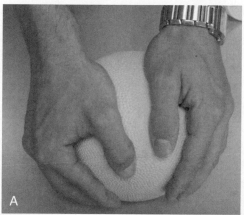

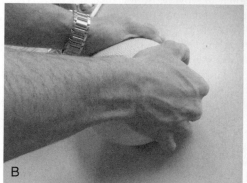

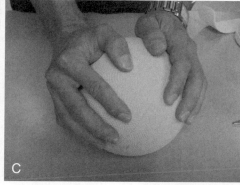

FIGURE 26-8 Demonstration of balance ball exercises. The patient is instructed to perform flexion and ulnar deviation, extension and radial deviation while simultaneously co-activating the musculature involved. **A,** Demonstrates the hand and wrist position at the beginning of the exercise. **B** and **C,** Demonstrates movement pattern on the ball.

Co-Activation Muscle Exercise

Co-activation exercise is the contraction of agonist and antagonist muscles that cross the wrist joint simultaneously. This entails the combination of isometric, concentric, and eccentric exercises in order to improve co-activation efficiency. This form of rehabilitation has been shown to assist with instabilities of the ankle[73,74] and may have a benefit while treating wrist instabilities. A simple method of co-activation training is to perform balance ball exercises in the hand therapy clinic and at home (Fig. 26-8). The patient's hands are placed on a weighted ball. They are instructed to slowly move the ball around the table, which allows for simultaneous activation of the radial extensors and ulnar flexors of the wrist. Co-activation retraining improves wrist stability by increasing proprioceptive awareness during motion. This increased proprioceptive input enables the patient to have greater control of the muscles enhancing stability.

Unconscious Neuromuscular Rehabilitation

The purpose of unconscious neuromuscular rehabilitation is to improve our RMA at the first sense of possible ligamentous strain or instability. The focus of this form of exercise is to:
- Educate the patient on what muscles are ligament-friendly
- Increase the efficiency, endurance, and strength of those muscles
- Increase the ability to sense potentially harmful or unstable motion during ADLs, work, and recreation, which allows a feed-forward response in order to prevent further injury or re-injury

RMA is likely the most beneficial and important wrist proprioceptive function.[49] However, it is also the most difficult treatment approach to apply during proprioceptive reduction.

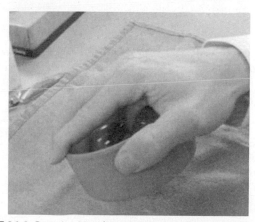

FIGURE 26-9 Reactive Muscle Activation training by placing marbles in a circular container. The patient rotates the container in a clock-wise and anti-clockwise direction.

How to Perform Reactive Muscle Activation Training

RMA training is performed in two stages. In the initial stage, marble exercises are performed progressing to Powerball stimulation, as tolerated. Both of these exercises require varying degrees of muscular control.
- Marble exercises: Marbles are placed in a circular container that is small enough to grasp (Fig. 26-9). The patient is instructed to rotate the marbles by moving the wrist in a circular fashion clockwise and counterclockwise with varying amounts of wrist extension and flexion. This action produces multidirectional forces facilitating RMA.

- Powerball training: Similar to marble RMA exercise, the Powerball exerciser produces variable random multidirectional forces (Fig. 26-10). This exercise is more challenging, because it requires greater muscle control as the central sphere rotates randomly in any direction. This will improve unconscious proprioceptive feed-back and feed-forward through RMA.

A wrist instability proprioceptive guideline has been proposed (Table 26-1).[49] Clinical research on its validity is yet to be confirmed, but it is based on sound clinical reasoning and early research.

Early Controlled Protected Motion Following Surgical Repair

If conservative management of carpal instability is unsuccessful, surgical reconstruction is often indicated to provide stability. SL dissociation is the most frequently diagnosed pattern of carpal

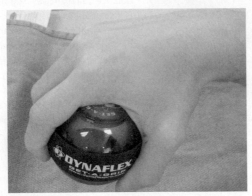

FIGURE 26-10 The Dynaflex Powerball is a gyroscope. The central sphere of this device produces random multidirectional forces stimulating proprioceptive end organs enabling reactive muscle activation for joint stability.

instability.[75] Blatt[75] was the first to describe a dorsal capsulodesis procedure to treat static SL instability. This procedure has also been used to manage dynamic SL instability, and a modified capsulodesis has been used to correct capitolunate instability.[75]

Following such procedures patients are typically immobilized for 6 to 12 weeks in a cast followed by a referral to hand therapy. This long immobilization period often results in significant wrist stiffness, requiring lengthy rehabilitation programs with the emphasis on regaining extension and radial/ulnar deviation. With SL dissociation, the purpose of such capsulodesis procedures is to prevent volar rotation of the scaphoid with a capsular tether from the dorsum of the radius. This tether limits wrist flexion; thus, the treating therapist must not be overzealous with attempts to regain postoperative wrist flexion. It has been proposed that instead of immobilizing the wrist for such lengthy periods, patients be placed in a hinged wrist orthosis within the first few days postoperatively, allowing for controlled wrist flexion and extension.[76] Prior to implementing this early controlled mobilization approach, close communication between the surgeon and therapist is critical. The surgeon must outline to the therapist the details of the surgical procedure, especially the amount of intra-operative tension set to the repair in order to apply controlled mobilization that does not compromise the reconstruction. The intra-operative tension may vary, but it is usually approximately 45° of flexion. With the use of this innovative orthotic design, unrestricted wrist extension can be performed. However, wrist flexion should be limited to 10° the first week postoperatively. The amount of wrist flexion can be increased by 10° per week until the wrist achieves approximately 10° less than the amount of intra-operative tension set. This will ensure that no stress is placed on the repair to prevent attenuation, while preserving wrist extension and reducing lengthy rehabilitation periods. The application of this rehabilitation technique should be reserved for the reliable and motivated patient to ensure compliance. There is limited evidence for the efficiency of this treatment approach. However, it is based on the intra-operative findings and sound

Stages of Proprioception Rehabilitation	Rehabilitation Plan	Purpose	Techniques	Assessment of Outcome
1	Basic rehabilitation	Edema and pain control, promote motion	Basic hand therapy techniques	Visual analog scale (VAS), degree of motion (ROM)
2	Proprioception awareness	Promote conscious joint control	Mirror therapy	VAS and ROM
3	Joint position sense	Ability to replicate a predetermined joint angle	Blinded passive and active reproduction of joint angle	Accuracy of joint motion, measured with goniometer or exercise machine
4	Kinesthesia(threshold to detection of passive movement)	Ability to sense joint motion without audiovisual cues	Motion detection using an exercise machine (preferable)or manual passive motion	Degree of joint angle at which motion was sensed, measured with goniometer ,or exercise machine
5	Conscious neuromuscular rehabilitation	Strengthening of specific muscles to enhance joint stability	Isometric training Eccentric training Isokinetic training Co-activation	Evaluation of specific muscle strength, wrist stability during co-activation, joint stability during isometric exercises
6	Unconscious neuromuscular rehabilitation	Reactive muscle activation	Powerball exercises. Plyometric training	Muscle activation patterns using EMG

TABLE 26-1   Rehabilitation Strategies in Wrist Proprioceptive Reeducation

clinical reasoning. A randomized clinical trial of this controlled mobilization technique is likely to provide evidence that it helps prevent secondary wrist stiffness following capsulodesis procedures.

Rehabilitation Concepts Based on Carpal Instability Patterns

Dissociative instabilities are common and may result from various conditions including SL or LT ligament injuries, inflammatory synovitis, scaphoid non-union or malunion, and Kienböck's disease. These instability patterns are a result of a ligamentous disruption between the bones of the same carpal row.

Scapholunate Instability

> ◎ **Clinical Pearl**
>
> SL dissociation is the most common carpal instability pattern and may appear as an isolated injury or in conjunction with other injuries, such as scaphoid or distal radius fractures.

The precipitating injury pattern is typically a result of a FOOSH that causes wrist hyperextension, ulnar deviation, and midcarpal supination.[77] A spectrum of SL injuries that range from minor SL ligament sprains to complete perilunar dislocations. This spectrum produces alterations to carpal kinematics, which results in varying levels of dysfunction.

SL instability has been categorized into three stages that is defined by arthroscopic, radiographic, and cartilaginous changes as well as reducibility of the scaphoid and the lunate.[78-82]

Pre-Dynamic Instability

The pre-dyamic instability stage is the earliest sign of SLIL pathology.[83] In this stage, the SL membrane is attenuated or partially torn, producing abnormal motion between the scaphoid and the lunate. This kinematic change produces wrist synovitis and pain. If this injury is left untreated in patients with repetitive stress or recurring wrist trauma, there is attenuation of the secondary stabilizers of the wrist and further degeneration of the SLIL leading to

dynamic and static instability.[84] In this stage of injury, plain radiographs are normal. Stress radiographs are typically normal as well.

The kinematic and kinetic consequences of disruption to the SL ligaments have been studied in cadaveric models.[85] It was found that if the palmar SL and proximal membrane are sectioned, only minor kinematic changes are created; this is considered predynamic instability. Complete disruption of the SL membrane and ligaments results in substantial kinematic and force transmission change but does not likely demonstrate carpal malalignment. Static carpal malalignment occurs when there is failure of the SL membrane and ligaments as well as the secondary scaphoid stabilizers, which are the palmar RSC scaphocapitate, and anterolateral STT ligaments. This form of instability may occur acutely as a result of a FOOSH injury or can occur secondarily as a result of progressive attenuation of the secondary stabilizers.[84]

Dynamic Instability

This stage of instability includes ligamentous tears of either the palmar and/or dorsal portions of the SLIL. Static radiographs are most often normal. However, special stress radiographs will often demonstrate instability. Rotatory subluxation of the scaphoid is often not associated with this stage due to the strong scaphotrapezial capsuloligamentous structures.[27,82,86]

Static Instability

In this stage of instability, a SL gap can be seen on a standard A/P radiograph. A SL gap of 3 mm or more has been defined as abnormal.[88-90] Furthermore, lateral radiographs often reveal a SL angle of greater than 60° to 70° (Fig. 26-11, *A*). The lunate has typically rotated dorsally assuming a DISI posture (see Fig. 26-11, *B*). Patients often demonstrate wrist swelling, pain, limited ROM, decreased grip strength, and limited functional use of the hand.

Scapholunate Advanced Collapse Wrist

Long standing DISI deformities result in altered kinetics and radiocarpal load, which causes a sequential deterioration of the carpus leading to degenerative arthritis. This form of arthritis is predictable and begins at the radioscaphoid articulation, particularly at the tip of the styloid. Later advances include capitolunate changes. Further progression results in degeneration throughout the entire carpus.

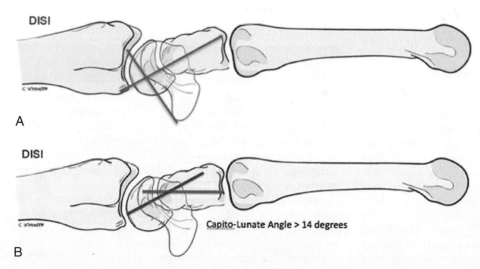

FIGURE 26-11 **A,** Lateral radiographs reveal a scapholunate angle of greater than 60-70 degrees in static scapholunate instability. **B,** The lunate assumes a DISI posture. The capito-lunate angle will measure greater than 14 degrees.

Therapeutic Management of Scapholunate Injury

Management of SL injuries is quite challenging for the surgeon and hand therapist. It is our opinion that the best treatment approach is early surgical intervention performed as soon as the diagnosis of static instability is established. This allows for the restoration of normal carpal alignment while preventing attritional changes to the secondary wrist stabilizers. However, the management of pre-dynamic and dynamic instabilities is controversial.

Pre-Dynamic and Dynamic Instability Therapeutic Management

We feel in all instances where this injury is suspected that patients should be acutely placed in cast immobilization for 7 to 10 days with instruction on edema-control techniques. Following this, the cast is discontinued, and the patient is given a prefabricated orthosis to be used during aggravating activities for an additional 2 to 6 weeks. The purpose of this orthosis is for symptom control and to protect the wrist from inadvertent stresses during ADLs and instrumental activities of daily living (IADLs). During this time the patient is encouraged to perform active range of motion (AROM) exercises to provide recovery from wrist stiffness that may have occurred from the immobilization. However, the patient is instructed to perform ROM exercises in the DTM pattern, because there is minimal tension placed to the SLIL. Once the patient can perform this motion within a pain-free manner, they can be progressed to AROM in all planes. However, the patient must be instructed not to perform rigorous passive range of motion (PROM), because this may disrupt tissue healing by placing too much stress to the carpal ligaments. Once nearly full pain-free wrist ROM can be achieved, the patient can then be progressed to strengthening exercises, beginning with isometric and progressing to isotonic. Furthermore, we should not underestimate the role of proprioception reeducation, because this may allow for the re-establishment of the necessary equilibrium for the dynamic stabilizers to allow for adequate transfer of loads across the wrist (See Table 26-2).

It is our experience that most patients' symptoms resolve within 6 months without surgical intervention. However, in unresolved chronic cases, SL pinning may be performed with or without arthroscopic débridement of any unstable portions of the volar SL ligament and membrane and electrothermal SL ligament shrinkage.[77,90-91]

Proprioceptive Reeducation in the Presence of Pre-Dynamic and Dynamic Scapholunate Instability

The muscles that have been found to play a role in the management of pre-dynamic and dynamic SL instability include the FCR, FCU, ECRB, ECRL, and APL. The FCR tendon uses the scaphoid tuberosity as a hinge toward its insertion into the base of the second metacarpal and may act as a dynamic scaphoid stabilizer.[25] The ECRB may act as a lunate stabilizer by promoting extension of the capitate that increases pressure on the palmar portion of the lunocapitate joint that counteracts the extension tendency of the lunate.[25] Garcias-Elias[25] suggests that in the presence of a pre-dynamic or dynamic instability, the stabilizing capability may be enhanced through proprioceptive training of

these two muscles. However, in the presence of a complete SLIL tear (static instability), the dorsally directed vector produced by the FCR does not control the scaphoid and induces a dorsal translation with further subluxation of its proximal pole. Thus, this form of rehabilitation is not appropriate for static instability management.

Furthermore, the activation of the FCU, FCR, and APL causes scaphoid supination that results in relaxation of the SLIL ligament. However, contraction of the ECU should be avoided, because this has been found to increase the pronation tendency of the distal row of the carpus, which may result in widening of the SL interval and increased tension through the SLIL.[92] Thus, in the presence of pre-dynamic or dynamic SL instability, a sudden ECU contraction may increase the SL gap and tension through the SLIL through excessive torque occurring at the midcarpal level.

> ### ◉ Clinical Pearl
>
> During proprioceptive reeducation and RMA training, we must attempt to enhance the SL protecting muscles while decreasing the tendency to activate the ECU. This can be done through DTM, because the ECU will remain relaxed during this arc of motion. Powerball or marble exercises can also be used.

Why Proprioceptive Reeducation of the Flexor Carpi Radialis?

Instability of the scapholunate (SL) interval is one example of ligament injury where isometric training may be either beneficial or harmful, depending on the degree of ligament injury. If the scapholunate interosseous ligament (SLIL) is intact, the flexor carpi radialis (FCR) is thought to be an important dynamic stabilizer of the scaphoid, most likely through its compressive action on the scaphotrapeziotrapezoid joint.[93] After a complete SLIL disruption with widening of the SL interval, however cadaver studies of FCR kinematics have revealed a significant increase in moment arms, which cause an increase in the load distribution through the radial carpus with further displacement of the scaphoid when contracted.[93] Hence, in a patient with partial SLIL injury or SL laxity, isometric FCR exercises are beneficial through its stabilizing action on the SL interval. In a complete, untreated SLIL injury, however, FCR strengthening exercises are detrimental and only serve to enhance SL instability.

Therapeutic Management of Static Scapholunate Dissociation

Acute static SL instability can present with disruption of the SLIL; however, there is also significant trauma to the secondary stabilizing ligaments. The ideal time frame for acute repair has not yet been defined, but attaining a successful repair is difficult after 2 to 6 weeks post injury, because the intrinsic ligaments tend to undergo rapid degeneration.[77] Thus, early repair (either open or arthroscopically) is preferred.

There are numerous surgical procedures for management of acute static SL instability. Some investigators recommend up to 4 to 6 weeks of casting or splinting of such injuries followed by activity modification for an additional 2 months.[94] It is our experience that acute static dissociations treated by this method is ineffective, because the patient continues to suffer from pain, weakness, and instability upon cast removal. In a study by Tang[95] that compared the outcome of casting alone for the treatment of static SL dissociation in combination with distal radius fractures, he found that at 1 year follow-up all of the patients continued to have signs of instability. Therefore, we recommend that SL dissociation should not be treated by casting alone.

When managing the acute SLIL injury, there are many choices according to the surgeon's preference. Discussion on the pros and cons of the various surgical options is beyond the scope of this chapter. However, some of the options include:

- Arthroscopic repair
- Percutaneous and arthroscopic Kirschner wire fixation
  - Typically, this is completed through a dorsal approach repairing the dorsal SL ligament plus percutaneous Kirschner wire fixation. The Kirschner wires are typically left in situ for 3 to 6 weeks.
- Tendon reconstruction of the scaphoid stabilizers
  - Various surgical techniques using a tendon-graft to reconstruct the scaphoid-stabilizing ligaments. Typically a strip of FCR is used.
- Reduction association of the SL joint (RASL procedure)
  - This method consists of an open reduction, repair of the SL ligaments, and stabilization of the repair by internally fixating the SL joint with one headless screw. The screw fixation is often maintained for 12 months or more.[25]
- Open reduction and internal fixation (ORIF)
- Capsulodesis and secondary ligament repair
  - Dorsal capsulodesis: The most commonly used technique is the Blatt capsulodesis. This procedure consists of tightening the radioscaphoid capsule to prevent excessive scaphoid rotation into flexion and pronation. This is done by creating a capsular checkrein from the dorsal capsule that limits scaphoid rotation. However, there is also a permanent loss of wrist flexion. Typically, patients are limited on average to 20° of flexion.
- Partial carpal fusion
  - Most common partial fusions in clinical practice are the scaphoid-trapezium-trapezoid, scaphoid-lunate, scaphoid-capitate, and radius-scaphoid-lunate fusions with distal scaphoidectomy
  - Four corner fusions with scaphoidectomy is a common procedure for a SL advanced collapse wrist

The overall results of ligament repair are acceptable in the acute phase where no degeneration is present. Patients often report minimal pain with more than 80% grip strength, achievement of 75% of wrist motion to the normal contralateral side, and less than one-third of patients develop slight degenerative changes within the carpus.[96-99]

Postoperative Therapy

Prior to the initiation of rehabilitation, a discussion between the surgeon and therapist should occur outlining the specific details and goals of the surgical procedure to promote the creation of a custom-tailored rehabilitation program.

Primary Scapholunate Repair/Secondary Reconstruction

Following primary SL ligament repair or secondary reconstruction with Kirshner wire fixation, the wrist is typically immobilized in a thumb spica cast for 8 to 12 weeks. During this time,

the patient is instructed in a home exercise program (HEP) consisting of finger, forearm, elbow, and shoulder ROM and edema control techniques. Once the cast is removed, the patient should be placed in a removable custom-made or prefabricated wrist and thumb spica orthosis to be used for an additional 2 to 4 weeks for intermittent protection, support, and pain control.

Upon cast removal, the patient should be instructed in DTM ROM exercises in order to prevent excessive tension to the repaired SLIL. Furthermore, scar desensitization techniques, scar massage, and superficial heating modalities can be utilized. Once the patient can perform nearly pain-free and near-full DTM, they can be progressed to active wrist motion in all planes. The DTM and AROM facilitate proprioceptive training. However, if any alternation in wrist kinematics was performed during the repair, this must be taken in to consideration during the instruction of ROM prescription. Strengthening exercises can be prescribed similarly as outlined for rehabilitation of pre-dynamic and static instability.

Specific Considerations: Ligament Augmentation Procedure—Dorsal Capsulodesis

Following a dorsal capsulodesis, patients are often immobilized in a thumb spica cast for a period of 8 weeks. Upon cast removal, a referral to hand therapy is often made for initiation of AROM of the wrist and forearm. Initially, AROM exercises should be performed in the DTM. A removable thermoplastic custom-made thumb spica or prefabricated orthosis is used for intermittent protection and support during any aggravating activities. Once the patient can perform pain-free near full DTM, they can be progressed to AROM in all planes and passive wrist extension and forearm rotation as needed. Following capsulodesis procedures, the therapist must know what the intra-operative tension to the repair was set to in order to establish appropriate therapy goals. Typically, following such procedures wrist flexion is set intra-operatively to 15° to 20°. Thus, this must be outlined to the patient so that they are aware of the therapy goals and the permanent wrist ROM restrictions. Furthermore, the treating therapist must not be overzealous with attempts to regain postoperative wrist flexion to prevent attenuation to the reconstruction.

Capsulodesis procedures to the wrist often require immobilization for a lengthy period of time that can produce secondary complications, such as wrist stiffness and tendon adhesions in all planes, and these clients often require lengthy rehabilitation programs with the emphasis on regaining wrist extension and radial/ulnar deviation. Limited wrist motion is not the intention of capsulodesis procedures; however, it may be a consequence of relatively lengthy immobilization periods. If the patient is reliable, compliant, and motivated, a protective early mobilization program can be initiated immediately postoperatively to minimize the complications that are often associated with immobilization. Compliance can be enhanced by providing thorough patient education regarding the purpose of the surgical procedure, postoperative precautions, and the consequences of not following the treatment plan.

Close communication between the surgeon and the therapist is critical prior to implementing an early controlled mobilization program. Understanding of the intra-operative finding of the flexion and extension arc of motion forms the basis of the early controlled mobilization program following such procedures. This information minimizes the risk for reconstruction compromise with early ROM exercises within a hinged wrist orthosis during the three phases of healing. With the use of a hinged orthosis the patient can perform full active extension while accurately limiting wrist flexion, ensuring minimal tension is placed on the repair. Thus, a patient who undergoes a capsulodesis could be referred to hand therapy within the first 3 to 7 days postoperatively for fabrication of a custom-made hinged wrist orthosis that allows for unrestricted wrist extension and limits wrist flexion to neutral (Fig. 26-12). Wrist flexion is increased to 10° at 4 weeks postoperatively. At 6 weeks, wrist flexion is increased to 20° within the orthosis. This hinged orthosis is worn at all times, removing it only for skin care with specific instructions not to flex the wrist when not in the orthosis. This hinged orthosis is discontinued at 8 weeks postoperatively, and the patient is provided with a prefabricated wrist and thumb spica splint. DTM is then initiated and continued until this motion can be performed in a nearly pain-free manner. The patient is then progressed to wrist AROM in all planes. At 12 weeks postoperatively, strengthening is initiated, beginning with isometric exercises and progressing to isotonic exercises as tolerated. For all capsulodesis procedures, the patient is restricted to light hand use for approximately 6 months to prevent attenuation of the repair.

Specific Considerations: Intercarpal Fusion—Four Corner Fusion with Scaphoidectomy

Four corner fusion is often performed to manage static SL dissociation with degenerative changes within the carpus. Following such procedures patients are immobilized in a cast for up to 12 to 16 weeks until bony consolidation is observed either through radiography or computed tomography (CT) scan. The purpose of such procedures is to provide pain relief and wrist stability. At final outcome, patients typically achieve approximately 50% of the wrist flexion-extension arc compared to the contralateral wrist.[100,101] Thus, therapists need to be aware of the contralateral wrist ROM measurement in order to achieve approximately 50% on the operative side.

During the initial stages of rehabilitation while the patient is in a cast, they should be instructed in edema control techniques and generalized ROM exercises to the fingers, forearm, elbow, and shoulder to prevent secondary stiffness of these structures. Once bony consolidation is confirmed, the cast is removed, and the patient begins AROM and gentle PROM of the wrist and forearm in all planes. A prefabricated or custom-made wrist orthosis can be provided and worn for an additional 2 to 4 weeks as needed for support and pain control. Typical hand therapy treatments include scar management and superficial thermal

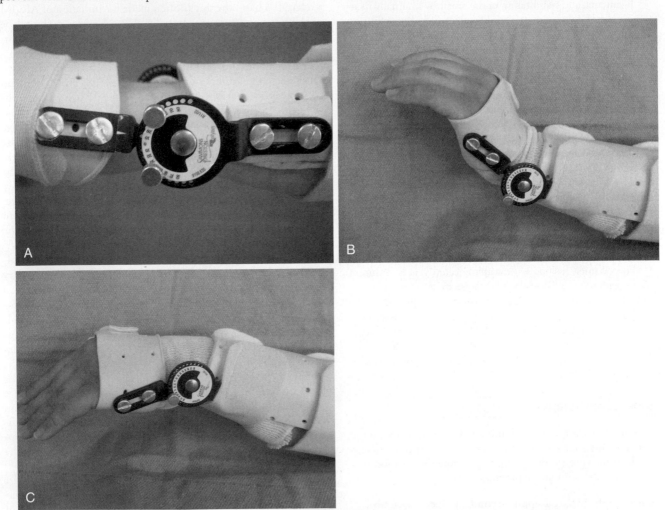

FIGURE 26-12 A, Custom fabricated hinged wrist orthosis which allows the therapist to restrict arc of motion based on intra-operative tension. **B,** Demonstrating unrestricted wrist extension. **C,** Demonstrating restricted short-arc wrist flexion.

modalities. If significant limitations in wrist flexion or extension persist, the patient may benefit from dynamic or static progressive orthotic application that is either prefabricated or custom-made (Fig. 26-13). However, mobilization orthotic intervention should only be applied in consultation with the surgeon to ensure that sufficient boney healing has occurred to tolerate this form of treatment. Proprioceptive rehabilitation techniques would likely play a minimal role in the rehabilitation of these patients, because the surgical procedure has provided sufficient carpal stability.

Lunotriquetral Instability

> ### ◎ *Clinical Pearl*
>
> LT instability is the second most common form of carpal instability and would be classified as a carpal instability dissociative type.[102]

Typically, LT instabilities occur from either a traumatic or a degenerative cause. Radiographically, you may see what is termed a **volar intercalated segment instability (VISI) deformity** (Fig. 26-14). This is when volar rotation of the scaphoid and lunate can be seen on lateral radiograph. Furthermore, on the A/P view the lunate will appear triangular. However, the SL angle remains unchanged.

Most isolated injuries to the LT supporting ligaments occur as a result of a backward FOOSH with the arm being in external rotation, forearm in supination, and the wrist in extension and radially deviated. In this mechanism of injury pattern, most of the impact is concentrated over the hypothenar eminence. However, LT instability can also be a result of a chronic condition, such as ulnocarpal abutment syndrome where increased load and pressure crosses through the LT joint causing strain and attenuation of the ligaments. Either way, these injuries can be managed either operatively or non-operatively.

Acute Lunotriquetral Injuries

If acute LT injuries are diagnosed early, non-operative management may be attempted. Typically patients are immobilized in a short arm cast, a thermoplastic orthosis or an above-elbow cast for a period of 3 to 8 weeks. In the past, treating acute LT injuries conservatively in a carefully molded orthosis or cast with a pad beneath the pisiform and over the dorsum of the distal radius in order to maintain optimal alignment was common.[103] However, failures in this approach were quite common due to insufficient ligament healing and attenuation of the secondary constraints of the LT joint. Garcias-Elias[25] feels that unless pronation and supination is blocked by using an above-elbow cast, the amount of motion that occurs in the LT joint during forearm rotation is substantial owing to the "pistonage" effect of the ulna against the carpus through the TFCC. This micromotion prevents proper healing of the LT ligaments. Thus, Garcias-Elias[25] feels that an above-elbow cast is required in all cases in which conservative management is attempted in the treatment of acute LT injuries.

It has been suggested that acute LT ligament tears are best treated by percutaneous fixation of the LT joint.[25,104] This percutaneous fixation is typically left in situ for a duration of 3 to 6 weeks while the patient is immobilized in a short arm cast or custom-made orthosis. Once the fixation is removed, a referral to hand therapy is initiated for gentle AROM of the wrist in all planes. At approximately 10 weeks postoperatively, PROM can be implemented as needed. The patient is then progressed to a strengthening program beginning with isometric exercises of the ECU and FCU and progressing to isotonic exercises as tolerated.

Proprioceptive reeducation can be implemented with the focus on the FCU and hypothenar muscles to enhance dynamic stability of the LT joint. Isometric concentration of the FCU and hypothenar eminence muscles produces a dorsally-directed force on the triquetrum through the pisiform that helps assist with wrist stability.[25]

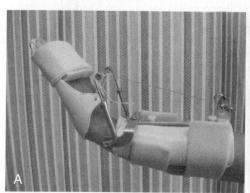

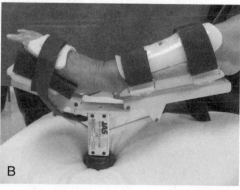

FIGURE 26-13 A, Custom fabricated static-progressive wrist extension mobilization orthosis. **B,** Commercially available static progressive wrist extension/flexion orthosis from Joint Active Systems.

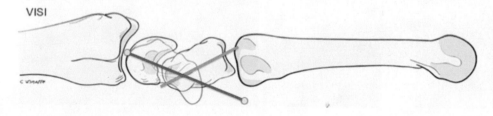

VISI

FIGURE 26-14 Schematic of lateral radiograph measuring the capito-lunate angle demonstrating volar intercalated segment instability occurring following a luno-triquental ligament tear.

Chronic Lunotriquetral Instability

In patients with chronic LT instability who are not surgical candidates, symptom management and joint protection are the focus of hand therapy intervention. Orthoses are used to provide joint protection and symptom control during aggravating activities. The goal of hand therapy is to prevent further discomfort, pain, and to prevent the progression of LT instability and secondary degenerative changes within the carpus. Typically, the chief complaint is ulnar-sided wrist pain with near full wrist ROM and strength. A home program is often sufficient for such patients and should consist of AROM of the wrist in all planes performed in a pain-free manner and isometric exercise of the FCU and hypothenar muscles. A custom-made ulnar boost orthosis may also prove to be useful with symptom control (Fig. 26-15).[105] As symptoms improve, the patient may also attempt ulnar boost taping during work- or sports-related tasks. RMA training exercises by marbles progressing to a Powerball will increase proprioception to the LT joint.

Special Considerations

The therapist should know if a chronic LT instability is part of a degenerative wear pattern, such as in the case of ulnocarpal abutment syndrome. The therapist should educate the patient regarding activities to avoid and what wrist movements and exercises increase abutment, such as gripping with the forearm pronated. This increases ulnar-variance and contributes to the symptoms of ulnar-sided wrist pain.[105]

Surgical Management

When conservative management has failed to provide the patient with symptom control, surgical intervention may be considered. Surgical options include reconstruction of the LT ligaments (either arthroscopically or through open methods), LT partial arthroses, and in advanced cases a proximal row carpectomy. However, proximal row carpectomies are often reserved for patients who have a static VISI pattern of carpal alignment, LT joint degeneration, and a SL dissociation.

Postoperative Hand Therapy

Wrist Arthroscopy

Following wrist arthroscopy and debridement of LT ligament injury, a removable orthosis is typically worn for 1 to 3 weeks postoperatively. This is worn to provide pain control during the inflammatory and fibroplasia phases of healing and to prevent overzealous hand usage. The orthosis can be removed within the first 2 to 5 days postoperatively to initiate gentle active wrist ROM in all planes. The patient is progressed to light loading

and increased hand usage during functional activities, as tolerated, between 2 to 4 weeks postoperatively. The patient is then progressed to isometric exercises of the FCU and hypothenar eminence and instructed in a home proprioception reeducation program. RMA can also be incorporated. The patient is also instructed in co-activation of the FCU and ECU during functional activities to further enhance stability through the ulnar side of the involved wrist.

Lunotriquetral Repair/Reconstruction

Following LT repair/reconstruction, the patient is typically immobilized in a short arm cast for 6 to 8 weeks. The patient should be referred to hand therapy within the first week postoperatively to be instructed in a HEP consisting of finger, forearm, elbow, and shoulder ROM exercises and edema control techniques.

Upon cast removal, which is typically around 6 to 8 weeks postoperatively, the patient is provided with a prefabricated wrist orthosis to be used for protection and is gradually weaned from this, as tolerated, over 2 to 4 weeks. Instruction is given to perform AROM exercise of the wrist in all planes, which begins at cast removal. Light strengthening, beginning with isometric contraction of the FCU and hypothenar eminence, can begin at approximately 10 to 12 weeks post-repair. The patient is instructed to avoid impact loading and forceful forearm rotation for as long as 4 to 6 months. To prevent re-injury, patients should not be overzealous with return to sport or recreational activities.

Lunotriquetral Arthrodesis

Following LT arthrodesis, the patient is immobilized in a short arm cast for 8 weeks or until boney consolidation can be confirmed, either radiographically or by CT scan. These procedures have high-delayed union and non-union rates; thus, patients are immobilized for lengthy periods. Progression of rehabilitation is much the same as for LT repair/reconstruction.

Midcarpal Instability

Midcarpal instability (MCI) is classified as a CIND pattern and refers to instability between the proximal and distal carpal rows.[106] MCI can be a result of extrinsic or intrinsic factors. Intrinsic MCI is characterized by generalized wrist ligament laxity, whereas extrinsic forms are secondary to bone abnormalities outside of the carpus. Examples of extrinsic forms are distal radius fracture malunions and extrinsic ligament injuries found in association with ulnar minus variance. Intrinsic forms can be further classified into dorsal, palmar, or combined dorsal/palmar types.

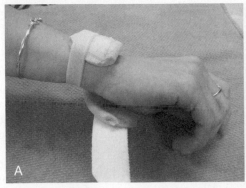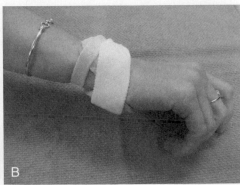

FIGURE 26-15 Custom fabricated ulnar boost orthosis utilizing elastic strapping.

Clinical Examination and Diagnosis

MCI is a common cause of wrist pain and instability. It often results in a sense of wrist instability; significant wrist pain; an abrupt painful click, clunk, or snap during wrist motion; and weakness with gripping. Often the patient history includes a painful clunk that occurs during ADLs, work, and sporting endeavors. This clunk may be a result of trauma to the wrist or could have occurred more gradually with no traumatic history. Many patients who have symptoms of MCI often have generalized ligamentous laxity in other joints, such as the elbows, knees, fingers, and shoulders.

Physical Examination

Observation of a patient's wrist with MCI often reveals a volar sag over the ulnar side that is most noticeable by looking at the affected wrist from the side (Fig. 26-16). Often patients with generalized laxity will have a volar sag bilaterally, however, only suffer from unilateral wrist pain. Physical examination often reveals tenderness over the triquetral-hamate joint (Fig. 26-17). A painful clunk over the midcarpal joint as the wrist is actively moved from radial to ulnar deviation may be felt and observed. Also, passive radial ulnar motion with the forearm positioned in pronation or neutral rotation often reveals a click or clunk within the midcarpal joint. The **midcarpal shift test** is described by Lichtman and colleagues.[107-109] This test is performed by placing the patient's wrist in neutral and the forearm in pronation. A palmar force is applied to the hand at the level of the distal capitate. The wrist is then simultaneously axially loaded and ulnarly deviated. This test is considered positive if a painful clunk occurs that reproduces the patient's symptoms.

Diagnostic Imaging

Imaging the patient with MCI often demonstrates normal plain radiographs including normal radiolunate, capitulonate, and SL angles.[110,111] Lateral radiographs in neutral deviation reveal a VISI resting pattern. Some patients do exhibit a DISI resting pattern, but this is much less common. The MRI often confirms a DISI or VISI resting stance when present; however, it often does not identify any ligamentous disruption.

The most helpful examination is videofluoroscopy combined with a physical examination.[112-116] The lateral fluoroscopic view in palmar MCI often demonstrates a sudden dramatic shift of the position of the proximal carpal row when the wrist moves from radial to ulnar deviation. This is often associated with a clunk. This clunk occurs because the proximal carpal row is not moving synchronously from palmar flexion to dorsal flexion while moving from radial to ulnar deviation. The proximal carpal row gets behind and catches up, which leads to a dramatic clunk back into place. This is termed a **catch-up clunk.** Also, a **reverse catch-up clunk** is often demonstrated under fluoroscopy as the wrist moves from ulnar deviation back to neutral. This clunk pattern represents the wrist returning to its original subluxated position. On the P/A fluoroscopic view, a similar clunk can be seen within the proximal carpal as the wrist moves into ulnar deviation.

Conservative Management

Conservative management of MCI can be challenging for the patient and hand therapist. A sound understanding of carpal kinematics is required by the therapist, and the patient requires motivation to follow the treatment plan. Conservative management should begin with patient education and activity modification. The patient should be advised to avoid activities that require repetitive radial-ulnar motion. The patient should also be educated how to properly contract the FCU, ECU, and hypothothenar eminence muscles during ADLs and aggravating activities in order to provide dynamic stability to the midcarpal joint. Co-contraction of the FCU, ECU, and hypothenar eminence during ulnar deviation may provide sufficient dynamic muscle stabilization during the activities that produce the symptoms of a painful clunk.[107] If the aggravating activities cannot be modified or adapted or the patient reports minimal symptom relief, we recommend the following approach that combines a lengthy period of wrist stabilization within an orthosis followed by a gradual weaning period combined with a structured strengthening program.

Orthotic Application for Midcarpal Instability

If activity modification does not result in symptom reduction or resolution, patients should be placed in a midcarpal stabilization orthosis. This orthosis should provide a dorsally-directed pressure on the pisiform with volar counterpressure over the head of the distal ulna to reduce the volar sag of the carpus and achieve a near neutral carpal alignment.[29,107] Once near carpal alignment is achieved, the goal is to keep the patient in this position for a

TABLE 26-2	Practice Guideline for the Therapeutic Management of PreDynamic and Dynamic Scapho-Lunate Instability	
0-6 Weeks Post Injury **Acute injury/ initial suspicion of injury**	Immobilization in cast for 7 to 10 days Once cast removed patient placed in removable orthosis for additional 2 to 6 weeks.	Treatment Approach Edema Control ROM of unaffected structures (fingers, forearm, elbow, shoulder) Pain free ROM utilizing DTM
8-12 weeks	Orthosis only worn during at risk and aggravating activities	Once DTM can be performed nearly pain free progress to AROM of the wrist In all planes Progress to proprioceptive re-education of the FCR, FCU, APL and ECRL, & ECRB.
10-weeks and beyond	Orthosis discontinued	Progress to isometric and isokinetic strengthening as tolerated Progress to increased hand use as tolerated

TABLE 26-3	Classification of Mid-Carpal Instability (MCI) which is a form of Carpal Instability Non-Dissociative Type

I. Intrinsic:
  -Palmar
  -Dorsal
  -Combined

II. Extrinsic

TABLE 26-4	Practice Guideline for Therapeutic Management of Mid-Carpal Instability		
Weeks	**Orthotic Application**	**Exercise Regime**	**Duration**
0-6	-Rigid forearm based ulnar-boost orthosis (pre-fabricated or custom) -Worn full-time (day and night) removing for skin care and exercise. -Forearm should remain in supination with orthosis removed.	-When pain is minimal can perform isometric exercise of the FCU, ECU, and hypothenar muscles with the forearm in supination	-When pain is minimal 4-5 sets of 5-10 repetitions holding each repetition for 5-10 seconds.
6-12 weeks	-Weaning period during functional activities. Can transition to serpentine orthoses, and ulnar-boost taping. -Night time ulnar boost orthosis continues	-DTM Pattern. -When DTM can be performed pain free with minimal instability the patient can be transitioned to gentle AROM in all planes -Continue with isometric exercise of the ECU, FCU, and hypothenar muscles with variable forearm positions -Can begin Reactive Muscle Activation training -Co-contraction training of FCU an ECU	**-DTM** -begin with short arc of DTM and increase arc as pain and apprehension permit. -this exercise is to be performed 4-8 times per day for 10-120 repetitions **-Isometric Exercise** -4-5 times/day for 5-8 repetitions holding each repetition for 5-8 seconds **-Reactive Muscle Activation** -2-3 times per day beginning for 2 minutes increasing to 10 minutes as tolerated.
12 Weeks and Beyond	-Continue with soft ulnar boost orthosis application or ulnar-boost taping during functional activities.	-Continue with Reactive Muscle Activation and isometric exercises until satisfied with overall hand use and stability of the wrist.	

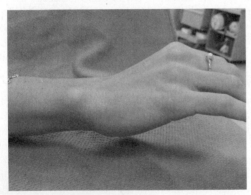

FIGURE 26-16 This wrist demonstrates an ulnar sag of the carpus in relation to the distal radio-ulnar joint.

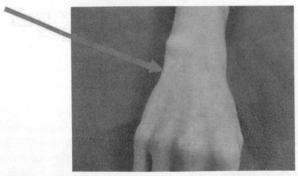

FIGURE 26-17 Physical examination often reveals tenderness over the triquetral-hamate joint.

duration of 6 to 8 weeks full-time to attempt carpal stabilization. The orthosis can be prefabricated (Fig. 26-18) or custom-made (Fig. 26-19). If the MCI is profound upon examination, consideration should be given to above-elbow orthotic application with the forearm positioned in supination, with the wrist in supination, and with an ulnar boost component in a Munster type orthosis.

Otherwise, the orthosis should be forearm-based. If the pain resolves within the first few weeks within the orthosis the patient can be transitioned to a less cumbersome hand-based ulnar boost orthosis that allows for increased motion at the wrist. This orthosis can be custom-made or prefabricated (Fig. 26-20). During the 6 weeks of ulnar boost orthotic use, patients are instructed to use their hand as tolerated for light ADLs. They are not to lift more than 5 lbs to prevent overstress to healing ligaments. The orthosis can be removed for showering; however, they are advised to limit radioulnar motion, as well as to maintain the forearm in supination. Forearm supination places a gravitational load to the carpus proving a subtle ulnar boost, thus maintaining enhanced alignment. Furthermore, forearm supination causes a tightening of the ulnar wrist ligaments due to the ulnar variance change related to the superior glide of the radius in this position.

After 6 weeks of full-time orthotic application, the orthosis will gradually be weaned off for light ADLs over the next 2 to 6 weeks. However, for work and at-risk activities the orthosis should be worn. Alternatively, a "serpentine orthosis" can be fabricated for use with functional activities. This orthosis provides an ulnar boost with limited excessive radioulnar motion while allowing functional wrist flexion and extension (Fig. 26-21). The forearm-based orthosis with ulnar head and pisiform boost is worn to sleep for an additional 6 weeks to promote enhanced carpal alignment.

The patient is instructed in active wrist flexion and extension exercises out of the orthosis four to eight times per day to

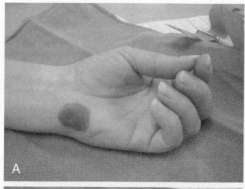

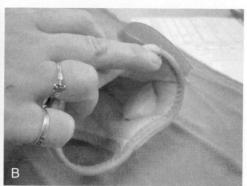

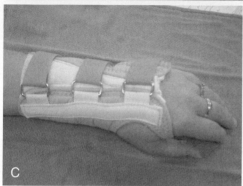

FIGURE 26-18 Pre-fabricated orthosis which is modified by placing a pisiform boost within the orthosis by added a closed cell foam pad. **A,** demonstrates the location of the pisi-form over the ulnar-volar aspect of the wrist. **B,** demonstrates the closed cell foam padding placement. **C,** demonstrates the orthosis application.

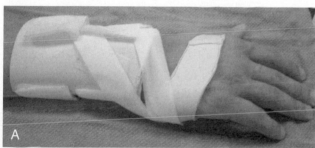

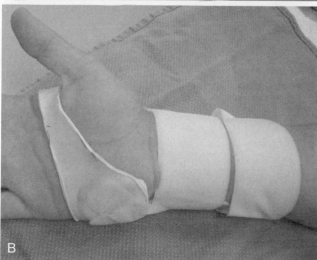

FIGURE 26-19 A, Dorsal view of custom-fabricated forearm-based ulnar-boost orthosis, **B,** Volar view of custom fabricated forearm-based ulnar boost orthosis.

regain any limitations in motion. They are instructed to perform radial-ulnar deviation actively in supination four times a day for ten repetitions within a short-arc. Once the patient can regain nearly full radial-ulnar motion in supination with no symptoms of painful clunking, they are instructed in a specific exercise regime.

Therapeutic Exercises for Midcarpal Instability

The goal of the supervised hand therapy program is to re-establish adequate proprioceptive control of the wrist.[106,109] Salva & Garcia-Elias[117] note that excessive flexion of the proximal carpal row associated with MCI can be dynamically stabilized by the combined contraction of the FCU and ECU muscles.

The exercise program should consist of isometric strengthening of the FCU, ECU, and hypothenar eminence with the wrist in supination. RMA training is performed with marble exercises and progressed to Powerball exercises. Specific consideration must be given to the exercises to avoid that may exacerbate symptomology, such as repetitive radial-ulnar motion ROM exercises, isotonic wrist curls, and repetitive power gripping exercises.

Twelve Weeks and Beyond

If the patient plans to return to aggressive hand use and sports, consideration should be given to either continued ulnar boost orthotic application, soft ulnar boost orthotic application (Fig. 26-22), or ulnar boost taping techniques (Fig. 26-23). This provides added wrist stability and protection during such activities. It is advised, however, to limit return to aggressive hand use for approximately 4 months following this proposed conservative management approach. Further study is needed to identify if this treatment approach is effective at reducing or resolving MCI symptomology. This approach is based on sound clinical reasoning and current practice at our rehabilitation center (See Table 26-4).

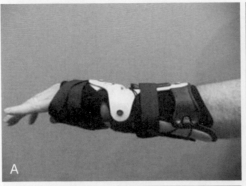

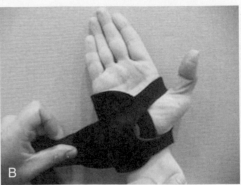

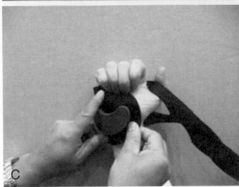

FIGURE 26-20 A, Demonstrates pre-fabricated hinged orthosis which does not allow for radial-ulnar motion, however, allows for wrist flexion and extension. This product is available distributed through Allsport Dynamics Inc, Nacogdoches, Texas (OH2 Wrist Brace). **B** and **C,** Pre-fabricated hinged orthosis provides ulnar boost over the pisiform.

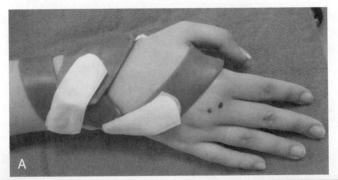

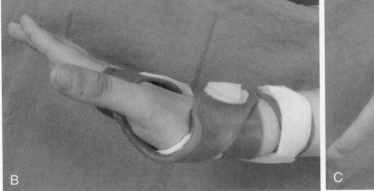

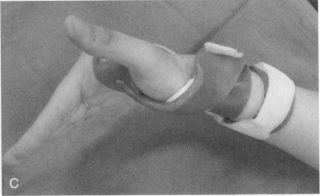

FIGURE 26-21 A, Serpentine orthosis design from the dorsal view. This design limits radio-ulnar motion while allowing functional flexion **(B)** and extension **(C)** of the wrist.

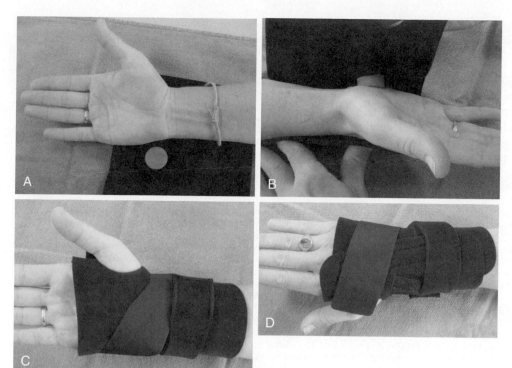

FIGURE 26-22 Soft ulnar boost orthotic application is made of neoprene material with a pisiform component (UlnarBooster™, (www.ulnarbooster.com). **A,** Soft neoprene demonstrating pisiform component. **B,** demonstrating how to don the orthosis. **C** and **D,** demonstrating the volar and dorsal view of this orthoses.

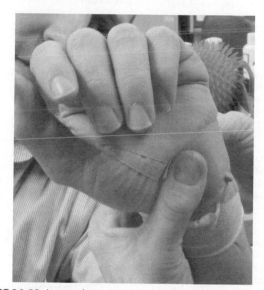

FIGURE 26-23 Image demonstrating ulnar boost taping for midcarpal instability

Surgical Management of Midcarpal Instability

When all conservative measures have failed to control the symptoms of MCI, different surgical options exist. The surgical options can be lumped into two categories consisting of soft tissue procedures or limited midcarpal arthrodesis.

When patients are referred to hand therapy postoperatively, the therapist must communicate with the surgeon to learn the specific procedure performed, goals for the outcome, and stress permitted to the repair site. During the rehabilitation phase, the surgeon and therapist must communicate to ensure that the timing and progression of stress to the carpus will be appropriate and not compromise the surgery.

A common soft tissue procedure is dorsal radiotriquetral ligament reefing. The dorsal radiotriquetral ligament is a major midcarpal joint stabilizer. In the operating room, the surgeon reefs on this ligament and performs the midcarpal shift test. If clunking does not occur with the ligament reefed, the surgeon proceeds to complete this reefing procedure. In the operating room, a dorsal flap is typically made through the DRTL, and this flap is pulled proximally to correct the VISI alignment of the lunate and proximal row. Once this correction is made and confirmed radiographically in the operating room, Kirschner wires are inserted from the triquetrum to the capitate in order to maintain this midcarpal alignment. Following this procedure the patient is casted for 12 weeks. The wires are removed at 8 weeks postoperatively. During the initial period of immobilization, the patient is instructed to perform digital motion and edema control as needed. Upon pin removal, the wrist is typically protected either in a cast or a removable orthosis for an additional 2 to 4 weeks. The orthosis is removed for frequent gentle AROM exercises. Aggressive PROM is avoided to prevent overstress to the healing ligaments. Scar management including desensitization and massage are included in the treatment program as required. Strengthening typically begins at approximately 12 weeks postoperatively and begins with isometric exercises. The physician typically restricts the patient to light hand use and lifting for 4 to 6 months post repair.

Limited midcarpal arthrodesis has also been recommended in the literature for management of MCI.[111,117] Following these procedures the wrist is typically immobilized in a cast until satisfactory bony consolidation occurs. This may take up to 12 to 16 weeks to occur. Emphasis must be placed on maintaining shoulder, elbow, and digital motion. AROM of the wrist is begun only when the surgeon confirms that sufficient healing has occurred at the fusion site. There will be permanent ROM limitations at the wrist, which is dependent on the specific fusion performed.

Typically strengthening can commence once radiographic confirmation of sufficient bony healing has occurred.

Summary

Rehabilitation following carpal ligament injury and reconstruction requires an in-depth understanding of the various instability patterns and their associated pathoanatomy. Close communication between the surgeon and therapist is essential, especially following reconstruction. Rehabilitation must take into consideration the specific injury pattern, phases of healing, muscle contribution, and loading; and its effect on carpal alignment and the demands of the patient. In operative cases, the therapist must be aware of the specific reconstructive procedure performed, intra-operative findings, and the expected outcome. Innovative and emerging concepts are allowing us further enhancement of traditional carpal instability management by increasing our understanding of the role of proprioception, re-education, and neuromuscular rehabilitation.

References

1. Linscheid RL, Dobyns JH, Beabout JW, et al: Traumatic instability of the wrist: diagnosis, classification, and pathomechanics, *J Bone Joint Surg Am* 54:1612–1632, 1972.
2. Lichtman DM, Schneider JR, Swafford AR, et al: Ulnar midcarpal instability—clinical and laboratory analysis, *J Hand Surg Am* 6(5):515–523, 1981.
3. Lichtman DM, Martin RA: Introduction to the carpal instabilities. In Lichtman DM, editor: *The wrist and its disorders*, Philadelphia, 1988, WB Saunders, pp 245–250.
4. Linscheid RL, Dobyns JH: Carpal instability, *Curr Orthop* 3:106–114, 1989.
5. Mayfield JK, Johnson RP, Kilcoyne RK: Carpal dislocations: pathomechanics and progressive perilunar instability, *J Hand Surg* 5:226–241, 1979.
6. Taleisnik J: The ligaments of the wrist, *J Hand Surg* 1:110–118, 1976.
7. Berger RA: The ligaments of the wrist: a current overview of anatomy with considerations of their potential functions, *Hand Clin* 13(1):63–82, 1997.
8. Navarro A: Luxaciones del carpo, *Anales de la Facultad de Medicina* 6:113–141, 1921.
9. Gillula LA, Weeks PM: Post-traumatic ligamentous instabilities of the wrist, *Radiology* 129(3):641–651, 1978.
10. Garcia-Elias M, An KN, Amadio PC, et al: Reliability of carpal angle determinations, *J Hand Surg Am* 14(6):1017–1021, 1989.
11. Kauer JM: The mechanism of the carpal joint, *Clin Orthop Relat Res*(202)16–26, 1986.
12. Patterson R, Moritomo H, Yamaguchi S, et al: Scaphoid anatomy and mechanics: update and review, *Atlas Hand Clin* 9:129–140, 2004.
13. Palmer AK, Werner FW, Murphy D, et al: Functional wrist motion: a biomechanical study, *J Hand Surg Am* 10:39–46, 1985.
14. Moritomo H, Apergis EP, Herzberg G, et al: 2007 IFSSH committee report of wrist biomechanics committee: biomechanics of the so-called dart-throwing motion of the wrist, *J Hand Surg Am* 32(9):1447–1453, 2007.
15. Tang JB, Gu XK, Xu J, et al: In vivo length changes of carpal ligaments of the wrist during dart-throwing motion, *J Hand Surg Am* 36(2):284–290, 2011.
16. Goto A, Moritomo H, Murase T, et al: In vivo-three-dimensional wrist motion analysis using magnetic resonance imaging and volume-based registration, *J Orthop Res* 23(4):750–756, 2005.
17. Crisco JJ, Coburn JJ, Moore DC, et al: In vivo radiocarpal kinematics and the dart thrower's motion, *J Bone Joint Surg Am* 87:2729–2740, 2005.
18. Werner FW, Green JK, Short WH, et al: Scaphoid and lunate motion during a wrist dart throw motion, *J Hand Surg Am* 29:418–422, 2004.
19. Garcia-Elias M: Kinetic analysis of carpal stability during grip, *Hand Clin* 13(1):151–158, 1997.
20. Hagert E, Forsgren S, Ljung BO: Differences in the presence of mechanoreceptors and nerve structures between wrist ligaments may imply differential roles in wrist stabilization, *J Orthop Res* 23(4):757–763, 2005.
21. Hagert E, Persson JK, Werner M, et al: Evidence of wrist proprioceptive reflexes elicited after stimulation of the scapholunate interosseous ligament, *J Hand Surg Am* 34:642–651, 2009.
22. Viegas SF, Patterson RM, Peterson PD, et al: Ulnar-sided perilunate instability: an anatomic and biomechanic study, *J Hand Surg Am* 15(2):268–278, 1990.
23. Taleisnik J, editor: *The wrist*, New York, 1985, Churchill Livingstone.
24. Gilula LA, Mann JH, Dobyns JH, et al: Wrist terminology as defined by the wrist investigators' workshop, *J Bone Joint Surg* 84:1–66, 2002.
25. Dobyns JH, Cooney WP: Classification of carpal instability. In Cooney RL, Linscheid RL, Dobyns JH, editors: *The wrist: diagnosis and operative treatment*, vol 1, St Louis, 1998, Mosby, pp 490–500.
26. Garcia-Elias M: Carpal instability. In Mackin EJ, Callahan AD, Skirven TM, et al: *Rehabilitation of the hand and upper extremity*, ed 6, St Louis, 2011, Mosby.

27. Schimmerl-Metz SM, Metz VM, Totterman SMS, et al: Radiologic measurement of the scapholunate joint: implications of biologic variation in scapholunate joint morphology, *J Hand Surg Am* 24:1237–1244, 1999.
28. Linscheid RL: Scapholunate ligamentous instabilities (dissociations, subdislocations, dislocations), *Ann Chir Main* 3(4):323–330, 1984.
29. Bednar JM, Osterman AL: Carpal instability: evaluation and treatment, *J Am Acad Orthop Surg* 1(1):10–17, 1993.
30. Skirven TM, DeTullio LM: Carpal fractures and instabilities. In Burke SL, Higgins JP, McClinton MA, et al: *Hand and upper extremity rehabilitation: a practical guide*, ed 2, Philadelphia, 2006, Elsevier, pp 461–474.
31. Wright TW, Michlovitz SL: Management of carpal instability. In Mackin EJ, Callahan AD, Skirven TM, et al: *Rehabilitation of the hand and upper extremity*, ed 5, St Louis, 2002, Mosby, pp 1171–1184.
32. Levine WR: Rehabilitation techniques for ligament injuries of the wrist. In Posner MA, editor: *Ligament injuries in the wrist and hand*, Philadelphia, 1992, WB Saunders, pp 669–681.
33. Jeter E, Degnan GG, Lichtman DM: Conservative rehabilitation. In Lichtman DM, Alexander AH, editors: *The wrist and its disorders*, ed 2, Philadelphia, 1997, WB Saunders, pp 699–708.
34. Prosser R: Management of carpal instabilities. In Prosser R, Connolly WB, editors: *Rehabilitation of the hand and upper limb*, Edinburgh, 2003, Butterworth Heinemann, pp 148–159.
35. Sherrington CS: *The integrative action of the nervous system*, New York, 1906, C Scribner's Sons.
36. Clayman CB: *The American Medical Association encyclopedia of medicine*, New York, 1989, Random House.
37. Guyton AC: *Textbook of medical physiology*, ed 8, Philadelphia, 1992, WB Saunders.
38. Lephart SM, Riemann BL, Fu FH: Introduction to the sensorimotor system. In Lephart SM, Fu FH, editors: *Proprioception and neuromuscular control in joint stability*, Champaign, IL, 2000, Human Kinetics, pp 37–51.
39. Lew WD, Lewis JL, Craig EV: Stabilization by capsule, ligaments and labrum: stability at the extremes of motion. In Matsen FA, Fu FH, Hawkins RJ, editors: *The shoulder: a balance of mobility and stability*, Rosemont, IL, 1993, American Academy of Orthopaedic Surgeons, pp 69–89.
40. Tomita K, Berger EJ, Berger RA, et al: Distribution of nerve endings in the human dorsal radiocarpal ligament, *J Hand Surg Am* 32:466–473, 2007.
41. Mataliotakis G, Doukas M, Kostas I, et al: Sensory innervation of the sub regions of the scapholunate interosseous ligament in relation to their structural composition, *J Hand Surg* 34(8):1413–1421, 2009.
42. Johansson H, Sjolander P: The neurophysiology of joints. In Wright V, Radin EL, editors: *Mechanics of joints: physiology, pathophysiology and treatment*, New York, 1993, Marcel Dekker Inc, pp 243–290.
43. Hagert E, Garcia-Elias M, Forsgren S, et al: Immunohistochemical analysis of wrist ligament innervation in relation to their structural composition, *J Hand Surg Am* 32:30–36, 2007.
44. Petrie S, Collins J, Solomonow M, et al: Mechanoreceptors in the palmar wrist ligaments, *J Bone Joint Surg Br* 79(3):494–496, 1997.
45. Lin YT, Berger RA, Berger EJ, et al: Nerve endings of the wrist joint: a preliminary report of the dorsal radiocarpal ligament, *J Orthop Res* 24: 1225–1230, 2006.
46. Hagert E, Ljung BO, Forsgren S: General innervation pattern and sensory corpuscles in the scapholunate interosseous ligament, *Cells Tissues Organs* 177:47–54, 2004.
47. Jew JY, Berger EJ, Berger RA, et al: Fluorescence immunohistochemistry and confocal scanning laser microscopy: a protocol for studies of joint innervation, *Acta Orthop Scand* 74:689–696, 2003.
48. Solomonow M: Sensory-motor control of ligaments and associated neuromuscular disorders, *J Electromyogr Kinesiol* 16:549–567, 2006.

49. Hagert E: Proprioception of the wrist joint: a review of current concepts and possible implications on the rehabilitation of the wrist, *J Hand Ther* 23(1):2–16, 2010.

50. Skirven T: Rehabilitation for carpal ligament injury and instability. In Mackin EJ, Callahan AD, Skirven TM, et al: *Rehabilitation of the hand and upper extremity*, ed 6, St Louis, 2011, Mosby.

51. Calfee RP, Leventhal EL, Wilkerson J, et al: Simulated radioscapholunate fusion alters carpal kinematics while preserving dart-throwers motion, *J Hand Surg Am* 33:503–510, 2008.

52. Werner FW, Green JK, Short WH, et al: Scaphoid and lunate motion during a wrist dart throw motion, *J Hand Surg Am* 29:418–422, 2004.

53. Ishikawa J, Cooney WP III, Niebur G, et al: The effects of wrist distraction on carpal kinematics, *J Hand Surg Am* 24:113–120, 1999.

54. Crisco JJ, Coburn JC, Moore DC, et al: In vivo radiocarpal kinematics and the dart thrower's motion, *J Bone Joint Surg Am* 87:2729–2740, 2005.

55. Upall MA, Crisco JJ, Moore DC, et al: In vivo elongation of the palmar and dorsal scapholunate interosseous ligament, *J Hand Surg Am* 31:1326–1332, 2006.

56. Mataliotakis G, Doukas M, Kostas I, et al: Sensory innervation of the sub regions of the scapholunate interosseous ligament in relation to their structural composition, *J Hand Surg* 34(8):1413–1421, 2009.

57. Riemann BL, Lephart SM: The sensorimotor system. Part II: The role of proprioception in motor control and functional joint stability, *J Athl Train* 37(1):80–84, 2002.

58. Ashton-Miller JA, Wojtys EM, Huston LJ, et al: Can proprioception really be improved by exercises? *Knee Surg Sports Traumatol Arthrosc* 9:128–136, 2001.

59. Holmes A, Delahunt E: Treatment of common deficits associated with chronic ankle instability, *Sports Med* 39(3):207–224, 2009.

60. Wilk KE, Meister K, Andrews JR: Current concepts in the rehabilitation of the overhead throwing athlete, *Am J Sports Med* 30(1):136–151, 2002.

61. Myers JB, Wassinger CA, Lephart SM: Sensorimotor contribution to shoulder stability: effect of injury and rehabilitation, *Man Ther* 11:197–201, 2006.

62. Williams GN, Chmielewski T, Rudolph KS, et al: Dynamic knee stability: current theory and implications for clinicians and scientists, *J Orthop Sports Phys Ther* 31(10):546–566, 2001.

63. Proske U: Kinesthesia: the role of muscle receptors, *Muscle Nerve* 34:545–558, 2006.

64. Gandevia SC, Refshauge KM, Collins DF: Proprioception: peripheral inputs and perceptual interactions, *Adv Exp Med Biol* 508:61–68, 2002.

65. Gandevia SC, Smith JL, Crawford M, et al: Motor commands contribute to human position sense, *J Physiol* 571:703–710, 2006.

66. Proske U, Wise AK, Gregory JE: The role of muscle receptors in the detection of movements, *Prog Neurobiol* 60:85–96, 2000.

67. Sturnieks DL, Wright JR, Fitzpatrick RC: Detection of simultaneous movement at two human arm joints, *J Physiol* 585:833–842, 2007.

68. Edin BB: Quantitative analysis of static strain sensitivity in human mechanoreceptors from hairy skin, *J Neurophysiol* 67:1105–1113, 1992.

69. Riemann BL, Myers JB, Lephart SM: Sensorimotor system measurement techniques, *J Athl Train* 37:85–98, 2002.

70. Proske U, Gandevia SC: The kinaesthetic senses, *J Physiol* 587:4139–4146, 2009.

71. Sekir U, Yildiz Y, Hazneci B, et al: Effect of isokinetic training on strength, functionality and proprioception in athletes with functional ankle instability, *Knee Surg Sports Traumatol Arthrosc* 15:654–664, 2007.

72. Desnica Bakrac N: Dynamics of muscle strength improvement during isokinetic rehabilitation of athletes with ACL rupture and chondromalacia patellae, *J Sports Med Phys Fitness* 43:69–74, 2003.

73. Hoffman M, Payne VG: The effects of proprioceptive ankle disk training on healthy subjects, *J Orthop Sports Phys Ther* 21:90–93, 1995.

74. Richie DH: Jr: Functional instability of the ankle and the role of neuromuscular control: a comprehensive review, *J Foot Ankle Surg* 40:240–251, 2001.

75. Blatt G: Capsulodesis in reconstructive hand surgery. Dorsal capsulodesis for the unstable scaphoid and volar capsulodesis following excision of the distal ulna, *Hand Clin* 3:81–102, 1987.

76. Chinchalkar SJ, Pipicelli JG, Richards R: Controlled active mobilization after dorsal capsulodesis to corret capitolunate dissociation, *J Hand Ther* 23(4):404–410, 2010.

77. Mayfield JK, Johnson RP, Kilcoyne RK: Carpal dislocations: pathomechanics and progressive perilunar instability, *J Hand Surg Am* 5(3):226–241, 1980.

78. Garcias-Elias M: Carpal instability. In Green DP, Pederson WC, Hotchkiss RN, et al: *Green's operative hand surgery*, Philadelphia, 2005, Elsevier Churchill Livingstone, pp 553–565.

79. Nathan R, Blatt G: Rotary subluxation of the scaphoid revisited, *Hand Clin* 166:417–431, 2000.

80. Whipple AJ: The role of arthroscopy in the treatment of scapholunate instability, *Hand Clin* 11:37–40, 1995.

81. Watson HK, Weinzweig J: Zepperi: The natural progression of scaphoid instability, *Hand Clin* 13:39–49, 1997.

82. Wolfe SW: Scapholunate instability, *J Am Soc Surg Hand* 1:45–60, 2001.

83. Watson H, Ottoni L, Pitts EL, et al: Rotary subluxation of the scaphoid: a spectrum of instability, *J Hand Surg Br* 18:62–64, 1993.

84. Moran SL: Acute scapholunate injuries. In Cooney WP, editor: *The wrist: diagnosis and operative treatment*, ed 2, Philadelphia, 2010, Wolters Kluwer Health/Lippincott Williams & Wilkins, pp 617–641.

85. Short WH, Werner FW, Green JK, et al: Biomechanical evaluation of ligamentous stabilizers of the scaphoid and lunate: part III, *J Hand Surg Am* 32:297–309, 2007.

86. Linsheid RL, Dobyns JH: The unified concept of carpal injuries, *Ann Chir Main* 3:35–42, 1984.

87. Dobyns JH, Cooney WP: Classification of carpal instability. In Cooney WP, Linscheid RL, Dobyns JH, editors: *The wrist: diagnosis and operative treatment*, St Louis, 1997, Mosby, pp 490–500.

88. Dobyns JH, Linscheid RL, Chao EY, et al: Traumatic instability of the wrist, *Instr Course Lect* 24:189–199, 1975.

89. Wolfe SW: Scapholunate instability, *J Am Soc Surg Hand* 1:45–60, 2001.

90. Darlis NA, Kaufmann RA, Giannoulis F, et al: Arthroscopic debridement and closed pinning for chronic dynamic scapholunate instability, *J Hand Surg Am* 31:418–424, 2006.

91. Bickert B, Sauerbier M, Germann G: Scapholunate ligament repair using the Mitek bone anchor, *J Hand Surg Br* 25:188–192, 2000.

92. Salva G, Garcia-Elias M: *Role of muscles in carpal stability*, San Francisco, CA, 2009, ASSH/ASHT Combined Meeting.

93. Tang JB, Ryu J, Omokawa S, et al: Wrist kinetics after scapholunate dissociation: the effect of scapholunate interosseous ligament injury and persistent scapholunate gaps, *J Orthop Res* 20:215–221, 2002.

94. Geissler WB, Freeland AE, Savoie FH, et al: Intracarpal soft-tissue lesions associated with an intra-articular fracture of the distal end of the radius, *J Bone Joint Surg Am* 78:357–365, 1996.

95. Tang JB: Carpal instability associated with fracture of the distal radius. Incidence, influencing factors and pathomechanics, *Chin Med J (Engl)* 105:758–765, 1992.

96. Chung KC, Zimmerman NB, Travis MT: Wrist arthroscopy versus arthroscopy: a comparative study of 150 cases, *J Hand Surg Am* 21:591–594, 1996.

97. Cohen MS: Ligamentous repair and capsulodesis for scapholunate ligament injuries, *Atlas Hand Clin* 8:231–241, 2003.

98. Conway WF, Hayer CW: Three-compartment wrist arthrography: use of a low-iodine-concentration contrast agent to decrease study time, *Radiology* 173:56–70, 1989.

99. Conyers DJ: Scapholunate Interosseous recontruction and imbrication of palmar ligaments, *J Hand Surg Am* 15:690–700, 1990.

100. Ashmead D, Watson HK, Damon C, et al: Scapholunate advanced collapse-wrist salvage, *J Hand Surg Am* 19:741–750, 1994.

101. Watson HK, Weinzweig J, Guidera PM, et al: One thousand intercarpal arthrodeses, *J Hand Surg Br* 24:307–315, 1999.

102. Osterman AL, Seidman GD: The role of arthroscopy in the treatment of lunatotriquetral ligament injuries, *Hand Clin* 11:41–50, 1995.

103. Reagan DS, Linscheid RL, Robyns JHL: Lunotriquetral sprains, *J and Surg Am* 9:502–514, 1984.

104. Ambrose L, Posner M: Lunate-triquetral and midcarpal joint instability, *Hand Clin* 8:653–668, 1992.

105. Chinchalkar S, Yong SA: An ulnar boost splint for midcarpal instability, *J Hand Ther* 17:377–379, 2004.

106. Dobyns RL, Linsheid RL, et al: Carpal instability nondissociative, *J Hand Surg Br* 19(6):763–773, 1994.

107. Lichtman DM, Gaenslen ES, Pollock GR: Midcarpal and proximal carpal instabilities. In Lichtman DM, Alexander AH, editors: *The wrist and its disorders*, ed 2, Philadelphia, 1997, WB Saunders, pp 316–328.

108. Feinstein WK, Lichtman DM, Noble PC, et al: Quantitative assessment of the midcarpal shift test, *J Hand Surg Am* 24:977–983, 1999.

109. Lichtman DM, Wroten ES: Understanding midcarpal instability, *J Hand Surg Am* 31:491–498, 2006.

110. Gilula LA, Destouet JM, Weeks PM, et al: Roentgenographic diagnosis of the painful wrist, *Clin Orthop* 187:52–64, 1984.

111. Litchman DM, Bruckner JD, Culp RW, et al: Palmar midcarpal instability: results of surgical reconstruction, *J Hand Surg Am* 18:307–315, 1993.

112. Finsterbush A, Pogrund H: The hypermobility syndrome. Musculoskeletal complaints in 1000 consecutive cases of generalized joint hypermobility, *Clin Orthop* 168:124–127, 1982.
113. Protas JM, Kackson WT: Evaluating carpal instabilities with fluoroscopy, *AJR Am J Roentgenol* 135:137–140, 1980.
114. Sarrafian SK, Melamed JL, Goshgarian GM: Study of wrist motion in flexion and extension, *Clin Orthop* 126:153–159, 1977.
115. Schernberg F: Mediocarpal instability, *Ann Chir Main* 3:344–348, 1984.
116. Schernberg F: Static and dynamic anatomo-radiology of the wrist, *Ann Chir Main* 3:301–312, 1984.
117. Salva G, Garcia-Elias M: *Role of muscles in carpal stability*, San Francisco, CA, 2009, ASSH/ASHT Combined Meeting.
118. Goldfarb CA, Stern PJ, Kiefhaber TR: Palmar midcarpal instability: the results of treatment with 4-corner arthrodesis, *J Hand Surg Am* 29:258–263, 2004.

27

Hand Fractures

Aaron C. Varney

The hand is used in nearly every vocational and avocational human activity. It is often called the *third eye of the body*. As such, it is at times subjected to a wide variety of deforming forces, many of them significant. A **fracture** results when the integrity of a bone is compromised from an external force.[1] Metacarpal and phalangeal fractures are some of the most common fractures that occur in the human body, second only to forearm fractures. Hand fractures account for up to 10% to 20% of all fractures in adults and children.[2,3] Without proper management by a physician and/or therapist, these injuries can become functionally disabling, adversely affecting the patient's work, family, independence, and well-being.

General Timelines and Healing

In order for bone to heal, the body must regenerate mineralized tissue in the fracture area. By healing bone with new bone tissue, mechanical strength to that bone can be restored.

Immediately following a fracture, the body enters a three-phase, bone healing process. The first stage is the **inflammatory phase.** The second stage is the **repair phase.** The third phase is the **remodeling phase.** In the inflammatory phase, the body sets in motion the cellular and vascular activity necessary for hematoma formation and primary stabilization. During the repair phase, the body removes the hematoma and damaged cells and lays down callus bone, further stabilizing the fracture site. In the third phase, the callus is gradually replaced with true bone tissue over the following months and years. Given the right healing environment, the once fractured bone will return to pre-fracture strength. A stable fracture will heal itself via this ordered process of inflammation, repair, and remodeling, which is also known as **secondary healing.**[2]

A fractured bone requires stability at the fracture site in order to heal properly. If there is instability, delayed healing or non-union may result. Some fractures do not require significant medical intervention for normal healing to occur. These fractures are described as non-displaced (that is, the fractured fragments remain properly aligned). Displaced (poorly aligned) fractures require physician manipulation in order to restore proper anatomical alignment, which is also known as **reduction.**[4,1]

After reduction, the physician determines whether or not the fracture is stable. **Unstable fractures** displace spontaneously or with motion and may require some form of internal or external fixation. This allows the bone to heal without any malrotation, angulation, or malunion. External fixation can be achieved via external orthoses or casts. Internal fixation is achieved via internal placement of screws, plates, and or pins across an anatomically aligned fracture. An external cast or custom orthosis may be used to protect the fracture, even after internal fixation. There are instances when a severely comminuted (fragmented) fracture requires traction to realign the bony fragments. An **external fixator** accomplishes this task by attaching a low-profile scaffold system to the proximal and distal portions of the fracture. The physician adjusts the tension to appropriately align the fragments. Advances in internal fixation methods over the past several years have led to less frequent use of external fixators (Fig. 27-1).

Improved internal fixation technology and surgical techniques allow physicians to secure bone fragments through open surgery using metal plates and screws, called **open reduction internal fixation (ORIF).** The healing process, in these cases, bypasses the secondary process of callus conversion to bone. This is called **primary healing.** By securing fracture fragments with plates and screws the physician eliminates interfragmentary gaps and provides the adequate stability required for bone healing, effectively substituting for external callus.[2]

Internal, rigid fixation and the resultant primary healing offer several advantages. First, callus formation (and potential soft tissue adherence) is avoided. Secondly, the therapist can access the injured extremity immediately, thereby allowing for proper wound

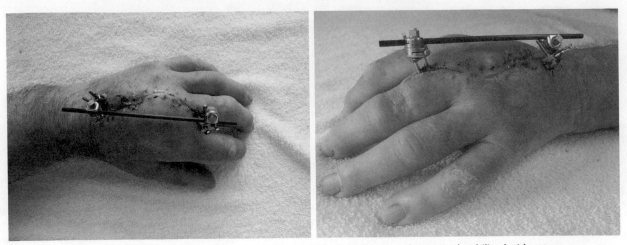

FIGURE 27-1 External fixator. Severe third metacarpal fracture from gunshot wound stabilized with external fixator.

care, accompanied by edema-reduction strategies. Third, rigid fixation allows for protected, active range of motion (AROM) to begin as soon as possible after surgery.

ORIF also has some disadvantages. In order to access the bone, the surgeon must dissect through soft tissue, and as a result scar and potential adhesions will develop. Potential infection is also a disadvantage to internal fixation. Additionally, one cannot underestimate how surgical management affects the intimate nature of the soft tissue in the hand. Plates and screws may interfere with soft tissue mobility, such as tendon gliding. This is especially a problem when the places and screws are placed dorsally.[1-3]

Precaution: *Strengthening initiation following fracture will begin only when solid interval healing has occurred, demonstrated by radiographic evidence. These exercises are not introduced any sooner with primary healing.*

Secondary fracture healing typically requires approximately 7 to 8 weeks. This often depends on location and type of fracture and, therefore, may require a longer duration of healing. Controlled AROM of joints just proximal and distal to the fracture may typically begin around 5 to 6 weeks, and sometimes earlier depending on the patient's health and speed of healing. Light activities of daily living (ADLs) may begin during this time. Approximately 2 weeks after AROM is initiated, and when edema is not a problem, passive range of motion (PROM) may begin, which may include static progressive or dynamic splinting as needed. Resistive exercises may typically begin 8 to 10 weeks after initial reduction and stabilization, but bone healing and absolute stability must be first confirmed by physician prescription.[1]

There has been a recent shift in fracture treatment protocol in the literature with evidence suggesting that early AROM of proximal and distal joints of an extra-articular fracture may assist to prevent stiffness, improve strength and stability of the fracture, and improve alignment of the fracture.[2,5]

Early AROM may sometimes begin before actual radiographic evidence of healing, most often between 3 and 6 weeks. In this situation, the physician must prescribe, the therapist must educate, and the patient must be completely compliant. The therapist may also need to fabricate a fracture brace to provide sufficient stability and protection to the fracture externally in order to avoid displacement during this controlled motion. If the therapist believes that the patient will have poor compliance, then early AROM should not be attempted. In general, fracture

bracing and subsequent early AROM is intended for simple, minimally displaced, extra-articular fractures of long bones.[6] Judy Colditz provides an excellent review of fracture bracing in Chapter 127 of *Rehabilitation of the Hand and Upper Extremity,* edition 6.[6]

The purpose of fracture bracing is to provide sufficient stabilization and alignment to fracture fragments while regional joints are engaging in AROM. The fracture brace provides circumferential support of the long bone and is fabricated to be adjustable in order to accommodate for fluctuations in edema, while allowing for full range of motion (ROM) of the proximal and distal joints[6] (Fig. 27-2). Again, fracture bracing is recommended for extra-articular, stable fractures. More specific details regarding fracture bracing will be discussed in the respective metacarpal and phalangeal sections.

While a philosophical shift has taken place over the past 5 to 10 years, early, controlled AROM is still "generally not recommended during the first 3 weeks of healing."[5] Some clinicians may consider it unsafe, while others may consider it unnecessary, citing that without the intra-articular nature of the fracture, early motion will not provide a functional benefit.[5] Indeed, several authors conclude that clinically, early AROM and fracture bracing makes sense, although the literature still does not support or refute it. They agree that further research needs to be done.[2,5,7] It is the experience of this author that early AROM of both stable and unstable, extra-articular fractures should be on a case-by-case basis. It is of utmost importance that the patient be 100% compliant with the protocol—if compliance is questionable, do not proceed. Furthermore, if there is concern that the patient's joints will increase in stiffness faster than average, then early mobilization should be considered.

As mentioned earlier, the soft tissues in the hand are intimately associated with the bones. The forces required to fracture a bone often and inevitably result in surrounding soft tissue injury.[1,4,5] Soft tissue injuries associated with metacarpal and phalangeal fracture may include peripheral or digital nerve injury, joint capsule and/or ligament injury, and tendon and/or tendon sheath injury, in addition to the sometimes adverse effects of scar formation or reduced tendon gliding. Secondary joint lag, contracture, and decreased muscle strength, endurance, and flexibility may also develop as a result of the soft tissue injury following a fracture in the hand.[1,2] The more complicated the

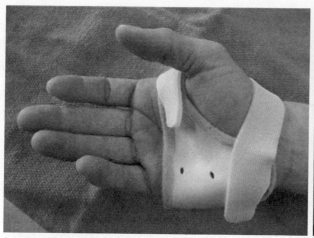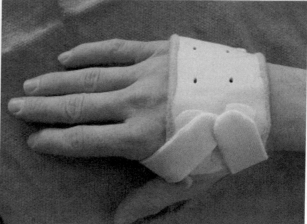

FIGURE 27-2 Volar and dorsal views of completed circumferential metacarpal brace. (From Chinchalkar SJ: Addressing extensor digitorum communis adherence after metacarpal fracture with the use of a circumferential brace, *J Hand Ther* 22:4, 2009.)

injury and/or subsequent surgery, the more important it is to begin therapy early in order to avoid as many complications of immobilization as possible. Indeed, that is typically the purpose of the extensive surgery; to provide significant rigid fixation in order to begin early motion. The therapist needs to recognize complications early and must communicate his or her findings to both the patient and the physician. He or she must also use this information to appropriately modify the plan of care to improve outcomes.

This topic will continue to be discussed and debated over the next several years. For more information see Feehan's work.[2,5]

Early Mobilization

Early mobilization is obviously not appropriate for every hand fracture treated by physicians and therapists. When a patient comes to therapy with a fracture, the therapist needs to be able to identify who is a good candidate to begin early mobilization and who isn't. Typically, early mobilization is considered appropriate for extra-articular hand fractures in one of two situations: 1) a stable, closed, non- or minimally-displaced fracture, and 2) when a fracture has been immobilized with rigid fixation, either externally or internally. Fractures that don't fall into these two categories are generally not recommended for early mobilization due to the increased chance of displacement and subsequent malunion or nonunion.[5] Feehan points out, however, that there may be a place for early mobilization in potentially unstable fractures that are not clear surgical candidates.

Feehan[2] describes several clinical factors that are important to consider before beginning early mobilization:

1. Fracture location: In which bone and where in that bone is the fracture located? The therapist and physician need to know the potential deforming forces that surround the particular fracture (for example, intrinsic and/or extrinsic muscle force vectors).
2. Fracture pattern and amount of displacement: Multiple fracture lines and greater than minimal displacement will require a period of immobilization due to decreased structural stability.
3. Type of fracture reduction and type of hardware used: Was it reduced via open or closed techniques? Is it rigid, coaptive, or stable fixation?

4. Nature of the surrounding soft tissue injury: For example, if a ligament is torn in addition to the fracture, the therapist's treatment plan will need to take this into consideration.
5. Patient's daily functional demands: This information will assist the therapist in predicting the types of daily functional stresses that will be put on the injury. For example, an office worker will have different functional demands than a firefighter.
6. Timing or stage of healing: This will assist the therapist in determining how much additional internal strength has been added by the healing bone.

Early mobilization should be gentle, generally pain-free, supervised, and engaging. The motion of the joint proximal and/or distal to the fracture should be moved through an arc that does not risk reproducing displacement of the fracture.[5] Feehan states that there are many different ways to perform early mobilization. One may delay early mobilization for a few weeks. Fracture bracing may also be used in order to stabilize a fracture while proximal and distal joints are actively ranged. If AROM is not an option, then one may consider gentle PROM with the fracture supported. Feehan states, "The advantage of making this clinical determination (to begin early mobilization or not) early in the fracture healing process is that it is possible to move from categorizing a fracture as either clinically stable or clinically unstable and to think instead in terms of what clinical factors or variables would need to be controlled to maintain fracture structural integrity and still allow for some form of early joint motion."[5]

Evidence-Based Treatment

The landscape of health care is changing. Third-party payers from Medicare, to Labor and Industries, to private insurers are moving toward requiring outcome-based measures to document improvement and necessity for therapy before they issue payment. An objective measurement tool should be used to document need for services. There are several upper extremity based, reliable, and valid outcome measures available for therapist use, including but not limited to the Disabilities of the Arm, Shoulder, and Hand (DASH), QuickDASH, Jebson Taylor Hand Function Test (JTHFT), Minnesota Rate of Manipulation Test, Motor Assessment Scale (MAS), Functional Independence Measure (FIM),

Hand Function Survey (HFS), Michigan Hand Questionnaire (MHQ), Upper Extremity Functional Scale (UEFS), and Arthritis Hand Function Test (AHFT). The most popular assessment seems to be the DASH and the QuickDASH. It is important for each hand therapist and/or clinic to review potential outcomes measures, weigh the pros and cons of each, choose one or two to implement, and then be consistent with its use in the clinic. Future payment may likely depend on it.[8]

Metacarpal Fractures

"Metacarpal fractures are common and account for 18% of all fractures in the hand and forearm."[9] This percentage increases from 30% to 50% when isolated to only the hand.[10,11] Most metacarpal fractures (up to 85%) occur in men, and the most commonly fractured metacarpals are the fourth and fifth, typically from punching-type injuries.[9] The clinician must know and understand the anatomy of the metacarpals and the soft tissues surrounding them, thereby understanding the deforming forces that act on these fractures.

Metacarpal Anatomy

The metacarpal is described as a miniature long bone, composed of a cortical bone **shaft** (or **diaphysis**), and proximal and distal ends composed of cancellous bone. The diaphysis is covered by **periosteum** (the outer lining that envelopes the bone). The proximal and distal ends are called the **epiphyses.** These ends are covered by **articular cartilage** (hyaline cartilage that covers the articular surfaces), which is necessary for smooth, pain-free AROM. Metacarpal bones are concave in nature with the concavity being volar.[11] This concavity allows for space for the long flexors and lumbrical muscles to be "tucked away," as well as to slide over.[10] The rich blood supply to the metacarpals permits fractures of these bones to heal well. Generally, the cancellous bone heals more efficiently than cortical bone.[1,10] The **head** of the metacarpal is located at the distal end, with the **neck**, being just proximal. The most proximal end is called the **base.** The base is connected to the neck and head via the shaft. The five metacarpals vary in length and girth. The longest metacarpal is the index finger, followed by the middle, ring, and small fingers. The thumb metacarpal is the shortest[10] (Fig. 27-3). With the decrease in length, there is also diminution of stability, thereby making the thumb metacarpal the most mobile. The increased mobility on the most radial and ulnar side of the hand allows for a natural curvature of the hand that provides the ability to successfully perform both gross and fine motor hand functions, from grasping a steering wheel to holding and counting change. The arch created by the rigid index and middle metacarpals is the **longitudinal arch.** The rigid nature of these metacarpals is due to the interlocking quality of the metacarpals on their respective carpometacarpal (CMC) joints. There are two **transverse arches** in the hand, a **proximal transverse arch** and a **distal transverse arch** (Fig. 27-4). The proximal transverse arch is created by the interlocking carpal bones. Deep ligaments to the metacarpal heads support the distal transverse arch. Extrinsic and intrinsic muscles also lend support to this functional, skeletal arch system.

When metacarpal fractures occur, disruption of the longitudinal and transverse arches often occurs, because the muscles of the hand are continuing to exert their natural force vectors. The bony support is lost, and deformity occurs. When these arches are disrupted,

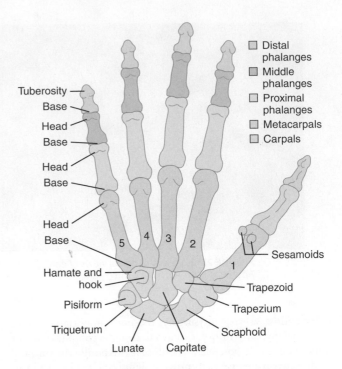

Bones of right wrist and hand (palmar view)

FIGURE 27-3   Hand bones. Volar view of the bones of the hand and wrist. (From Pratt NE: Anatomy and kinesiology of the hand. In Skirven TM, Osterman AL, Fedorczyk JM, et al, editors: *Rehabilitation of the hand and upper extremity,* ed 6, Philadelphia, 2011, Mosby Elsevier.)

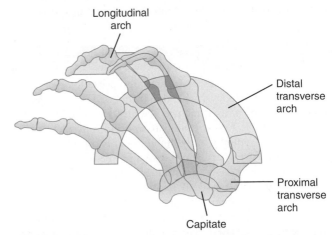

FIGURE 27-4 The longitudinal and transverse arches of the hand. (From Pratt NE: Anatomy and kinesiology of the hand. In Skirven TM, Osterman AL, Fedorczyk JM, et al, editors: *Rehabilitation of the hand and upper extremity,* ed 6, Philadelphia, 2011, Mosby Elsevier.)

there is a loss in hand function. Therefore, medical management of these injuries must work to restore this natural arch system.

Diagnosis and Pathology

Fractures of the metacarpals most often occur in the first and fifth metacarpals. This happens for a couple of reasons. First, they are the border digits and are the most exposed. Second, they are the most mobile.[1,11] Soong, et al. reports that the fourth metacarpal is also frequently fractured because it has the most narrow shaft

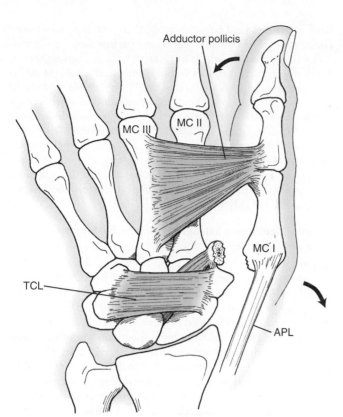

FIGURE 27-5 The deforming forces in Bennett's fracture are the pull of the abductor pollicis longus and the adductor pollicis. (From Lehman T, Hildenbrand J: Fractures and ligament injuries of the thumb and metacarpals. In Trumble TE, Rayan GM, Budoff JE, et al, editors: *Principles of hand surgery and therapy,* ed 2, Philadelphia, 2010, Saunders Elsevier.)

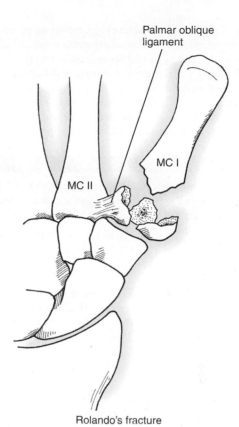

Rolando's fracture

FIGURE 27-6 Rolando's fracture demonstrating the "T" or "Y" fracture pattern that splits the articular surface of the base of the first metacarpal. (From Lehman T, Hildenbrand J: Fractures and ligament injuries of the thumb and metacarpals. In Trumble TE, Rayan GM, Budoff JE, et al, editors: *Principles of hand surgery and therapy,* ed 2, Philadelphia, 2010, Saunders Elsevier.)

diameter. Diagnosis is definitively made with x-ray. The angulation, displacement, and malrotation of the fracture are factors in determining the need for surgery.

Fractures of the metacarpal may occur anywhere along the bone, base, shaft, neck, or head. Each of these areas will be discussed in more detail in the "Timelines and Healing" section. Base fractures are the least common because of their stability. They usually occur as a result of a heavy direct blow or crush injury. Shaft fractures typically occur due to torsion, direct impact, or longitudinal compression. Depending on the number of fragments and/or line of the fracture, it may be classified as transverse, comminuted, or oblique. Malrotation and/or bone shortening often result from an oblique fracture. Dorsal angulation results from a transverse fracture due to the volar vector forces of the interossei and long flexor muscles.[1,2]

There are several specific metacarpal fractures that have identifiable names. The first is a **boxer's fracture** (though a skilled boxer rarely sustains this type of fracture).[9] A boxer's fracture is one in which the metacarpal neck is compromised. Amount of displacement and comminution varies depending on the force that caused the injury. The force tends to be a compressive force that travels proximally from the metacarpal head toward the base, typically occurring when the head of the fifth (and sometimes fourth) metacarpal comes in contact with something solid with the digits in full composite flexion.[1,10]

⊙ **Clinical Pearl**

Structurally, the neck is the weakest point along the metacarpal bone, and when fractured, the metacarpal head will shift volarly.

The second well-known metacarpal fracture occurs at the thumb metacarpal base and is known as a **Bennett's Fracture.** A Bennett's fracture is intra-articular at the first CMC joint (Fig. 27-5). This fracture occurs when there is forced first CMC abduction and an axial blow along the metacarpal shaft when the metacarpal is slightly flexed. A stabilizing ligament, the palmar, oblique ligament, or *beak ligament,* causes an avulsion fracture of the ulnar aspect of the first metacarpal base. Often, these avulsion fractures result in dislocation of the trapeziometacarpal joint. Furthermore, due to the competing forces of the adductor pollicus and abductor pollicus longus tendons, the type of axial blow listed earlier results in dislocation and subluxation of the first CMC joint. **Rolando's fracture** is a fracture of the metacarpal base that presents with a "T" or a "Y" fracture pattern that splits the articular surface of the base of the first metacarpal[1,10,12] (Fig. 27-6).

Timelines and Healing

Metacarpal fractures tend to be quite stable secondary to their multiple muscle and ligament attachments. Metacarpal fractures tend to heal in 3 to 7 weeks with variables of age, nutrition, genetics, stability, and amount of displacement affecting this timeline.[1] If the fracture is not recognized or treated appropriately, the aforementioned normal stabilizing soft tissue forces may cause debilitating deformities. It is important for therapists to recognize this. For example, the volar displacement of the fifth metacarpal head in the boxer's fracture results in a disruption of the normal arch of the hand, which adversely affects hand function and weakens grip strength.

> ### ◎ Clinical Pearl
>
> A malrotated fifth metacarpal head will result in much greater distal deviation of the digit, typically to the radial side, causing a scissoring action. A 5° to 10° shaft rotation results in a 1.5 cm digit overlap in a clenched fist.[10,13]

Base Fractures

As mentioned earlier, base fractures are not common, especially of the second and third metacarpals. If a metacarpal base fracture occurs, it may demonstrate a small amount of rotation. This is significant in that this small rotation will be magnified many times at the distal end of the digit.[10]

Shaft Fractures

Fractures of the metacarpal shafts are typically stable enough that they may tolerate early mobilization well, which is discussed in more detail at the end of this section. The apex dorsal angulation of the fracture can be aesthetically displeasing and may result in impingement or rupture of the extensor digitorum communis (EDC) if left untreated.[10] Any angulation in the index and middle fingers needs to be corrected. As a general rule, angulations greater than 20° in the ring finger and 30° in the small finger need to be corrected. Multiple metacarpal fractures as well as unstable fractures will need to be stabilized by ORIF utilizing plates, lag screws, or Kirschner wires (inserted in either a closed or open manner).[10]

Neck Fractures

A neck fracture is the most common metacarpal fracture seen in the hand clinic. Orthotic fabrication and fitting is required with both conservative and post-surgical treatment. Of course, there is more freedom of movement following ORIF. Surgery is generally required when the dorsal angulation is greater than 15° for the ring and small finger.[10] Decreased metacarpophalangeal (MP) AROM and failure of the small finger to initiate grip result from angulated small and ring finger neck fractures greater than 15°. Some surgeons may avoid surgery with small finger metacarpal neck fractures less than 30° and ring finger neck fractures less than 20°.[13] Displaced, untreated, and/or improperly treated metacarpal neck fractures will often result in a pseudo-claw deformity in addition to decreased ROM at the MP joint. Tenderness in the palm also develops during grip due to the volarly-displaced metacarpal head. These fractures are usually splinted or casted in the intrinsic plus position of MP joint flexion of 70° to 90° with the interphalangeal (IP) joints free to flex and extend. The affected digit will often require buddy taping to the adjacent digit to avoid any malrotation of the metacarpal head.

Head Fractures

Head fractures are uncommon, but serious in nature, because they tend to be intra-articular. If less than 20% of the metacarpal head is involved (and non-displaced), then treatment tends to be conservative. The therapist will fit the patient with an ulnar or radial (depending on which metacarpal head is fractured) wrist, hand, finger, gutter orthosis with the wrist in 0° to 20° of extension, the metacarpal flexed as close to 90° as possible, and the IP joints in 0° of extension. The therapist includes the adjacent digit for increased stability and comfort. ORIF is generally indicated if more than 20% of the articular surface is involved.[10] If ORIF is performed, it is important to begin motion and scar management techniques as soon as possible after surgery. Without immediate motion and scar management, tendon and capsular adhesions may develop from the longitudinal surgical incision, thereby preventing full AROM of the MP joint.[1]

Thumb Metacarpophalangeal Fracture-Dislocation (Bennett Fracture)

In most cases, surgical intervention is required due to the intra-articular nature of these injuries. The stout *beak* ligament mentioned previously is rarely torn; so when forces are strong enough to tear it, the ligament maintains its hold on the first metacarpal base and avulses a piece of bone from the ulnar aspect of the base (see Fig. 27-5). The bony fragments are often greater than 25% of the joint surface or simply irreducible, which are the criteria for internal fixation.[12,13] Stability is compromised significantly with these fractures. Following surgical repair (usually via Kirschner wires), the surgeon immobilizes the fracture for approximately 4 to 6 weeks in a forearm-based thumb spica cast. IP joint AROM may be allowed after 2 to 3 weeks depending on surgeon preference. The surgeon removes the pins after the 4 to 6 week immobilization period. Because the fracture is intra-articular, it should have continued protection in a hand- or forearm-based thumb spica orthosis for another 3 to 6 weeks. If rigid internal fixation has been utilized, IP joint movement may be allowed after 1 week. Resistive exercises are avoided until there is radiographic evidence of stable fracture healing, which is typically after 3 months.[12]

Thumb Metacarpal Shaft Fractures

Due to the high mobility of this particular metacarpal, shaft fractures are rare. Forces strong enough to fracture this bone are often dissipated to the more stable base, where the fracture will occur. Indications for reduction are similar to small finger metacarpal shaft fractures (that is, dorsal angulation greater than 30°). Post fracture treatment (post reduction or ORIF) includes 3 to 4 weeks of immobilization in a thumb spica cast/orthosis with the IP joint included. If the fracture requires more time to heal, IP joint mobilization may be considered after the initial 3 to 4 week time period.[10-13]

Thumb Metacarpal Head Fractures

The most common fracture of the metacarpal head comes from radial directed forces that can tear the ulnar collateral ligament (UCL), which provides lateral stability on the ulnar side of the thumb. Rupture of this ligament often results in an avulsion fracture. This particular fracture is coined *skier's thumb*. Non-displaced injuries are treated with immobilization in a forearm-based thumb spica cast or custom orthosis with the IP joint included. The IP joint portion may be removed to encourage motion after 4 weeks, as long as there is evidence of fracture healing. Displaced fractures need to be stabilized via Kirschner wires or ORIF. This improves joint congruence.[10]

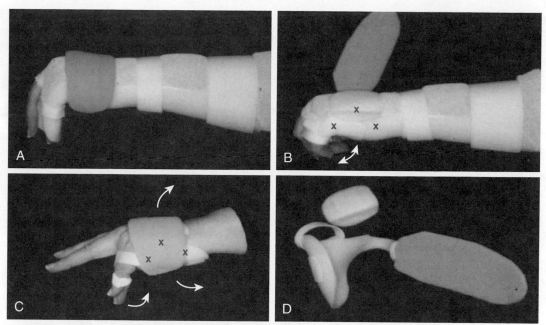

FIGURE 27-7 **Fifth metacarpal fracture: Modified fracture brace. A,** A volar-based orthosis that holds the wrist, hand, and fourth and fifth fingers in a position of function with and adjustable dorsal circumferential strap across the metacarpal region. **B,** The dorsal strap is removed to expose a three-point counter pressure, semi-rigid insert that adds additional fracture support. The orthosis has been serially reduced to allow proximal interphalangeal (PIP) and distal interphalangeal (DIP) motion. **C,** Further serial reduction to free the wrist with a buddy strap distally to control rotation of the finger during motion. **D,** The component parts of the same orthosis shown in **C.** (From Feehan LM: Extra-articular hand fractures part II: therapist's management. In Skirven TM, Osterman AL, Fedorczyk JM, et al, editors: *Rehabilitation of the hand and upper extremity,* ed 6, Philadelphia, 2011, Mosby Elsevier.)

Early Motion for Metacarpal Fractures

The deforming forces, malunion pattern, and common soft tissue complications were discussed previously and need to be considered carefully before deciding to begin early mobilization. The orthotic design for the resting position should hold the MPs in at least 70° of flexion at rest. As the fracture heals, this may be serially reduced to allow for more motion at proximal and distal joints. A fracture brace could also be fabricated in order to provide stabilization to the fracture site, while allowing functional, uninhibited motion of the proximal and distal joints (Fig. 27-7; see also Fig. 27-2). One must be careful with exclusive use of a fracture brace due to skin breakdown from the counterforce pressure points.[13]

Treatment: Non-Operative and Operative

In general, therapeutic management of metacarpal fractures is similar, regardless of the location of the fracture. Initial immobilization is necessary and is achieved by fabricating a radial or ulnar gutter orthosis or cast (depending on which metacarpal was fractured). The orthosis or cast may also be volar-based (see Fig. 27-7). The MP joints are held in a position of 70° to 90° in order to minimize MP joint contractures. The IP joints are held in 0° of extension. The wrist is held in approximately 20° of extension. The surgeon may allow for the IP joints to be free if there is low concern for displacement, such as after rigid fixation or a stable shaft fracture. If IP joints are free, the therapist must take care to allow for unimpeded proximal interphalangeal (PIP) joint flexion by making sure the orthosis sits proximal to the PIP joint. If the thumb metacarpal is fractured, a basic thumb spica orthosis/cast is fabricated with care to maintain the web space. The thumb IP joint is typically included in the orthosis initially and is allowed more controlled motion after sufficient healing has occurred. The therapist must mold the orthoses with care to maintain the longitudinal and transverse arches of the hand.[1,10,12]

Once the patient has been immobilized, he/she needs to be educated on AROM exercises of all uninvolved joints. Edema occurs often following metacarpal injuries and surgeries.

Evaluation Techniques and Tips

1. Clearly educate and explain to the patient what you are doing and why.
2. Compare ROM measurements to the unaffected side.
3. Look for clinical signs of intrinsic or extrinsic vs. joint tightness (see Chapters 1 and 5), and treat accordingly.
4. Look for clinical signs of tendon adhesions.
5. Assess flexor digitorum superficialis (FDS) and flexor digitorum profundus (FDP) bilaterally. Sometimes anatomical anomalies or previous injuries to these tendons affect hand therapy treatment and outcomes.
6. Be aware of skin or tendon adherence at incision or pin sites.
7. Monitor for signs of flexor tenosynovitis, especially as the client regains active, composite digital flexion.

The therapist should educate the patient on proper elevation (for example, elevation above the heart, but without full elbow flexion) and icing techniques. Icing techniques should be utilized in the acute post-injury or post-operative phase. Manual edema mobilization (MEM) is more effective in the sub-acute and chronic phases. AROM of uninvolved joints is also very effective in edema reduction. If percutaneous pinning has been used and the surgeon left the pins exposed, the client must be instructed in pin care (see Chapter 25 for specific pin care instructions).

Closed Reduction

Once the physician has determined sufficient stability at the fracture site, controlled AROM of the wrist and MP joints may begin. This is typically 3 to 5 weeks post injury. As discussed previously, if the fracture is extra-articular and stable, early mobilization should be considered. If the fracture falls into the "gray" area (that is, is not stable) but the patient is not a clear surgical candidate, early mobilization might also begin within 1 to 2 weeks following the fracture. If the therapist, physician, and patient choose this route, 100% compliance must be assured. Typically, between 6 to 7 weeks, gentle PROM may be added to the treatment, both in the clinic and at home. Resistive exercises may be added only after adequate healing has been determined by the physician, typically between 6 and 8 weeks. Resumption of normal activities without restriction is usually around 10 to 12 weeks.[2,10,12,13]

Edema, especially dorsally, may be a complication for patients following metacarpal fractures. If the edema becomes chronic, it is not uncommon for many (if not all) soft tissues to adhere to each other. Compression gloves may be used to treat potentially chronic edema. AROM exercises should be performed hourly and should include EDC exercises, composite flexion, tendon glides, and independent MP joint flexion exercises (often described as "tabletop" or "duck bill" position). If contracture of the thumb web space develops after a first metacarpal fracture, a night web space stretching orthosis may be beneficial in reducing this contracture.

Open Reduction and Internal Fixation

Rigid internal stabilization permits remobilization at 24 to 72 hours after surgery. A very similar orthosis that was discussed earlier is fabricated for protection once the postoperative dressings have been removed. Edema and pain control are primary concerns at this early time. AROM and PROM exercises may begin at this time as well. The exercises discussed in the "Closed Reduction" section will be the same ones in ORIF cases as well. First metacarpal fracture and subsequent rigid fixation AROM exercises should include composite thumb flexion and extension, opposition, IP joint and MP joint flexion and extension, and radial and palmar abduction to maintain web space. A hand-based thumb opponens orthosis should be fabricated for support and protection, but should be removed frequently for AROM (Fig. 27-8).

Scar management techniques may be needed if dorsal scarring results in adhesions that reduce functional use of the hand. These may be started 1 to 2 days following suture removal (typically 10 to 14 days following surgery). Some scar management techniques include silicone gel or elastomer pads within the orthosis, paper tape, ultrasound, and general scar mobilization.[10,12,13]

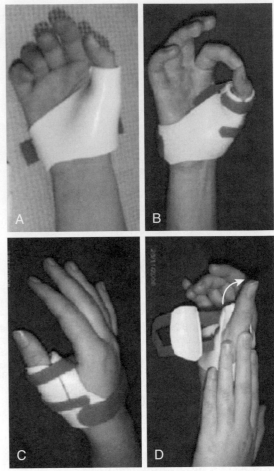

FIGURE 27-8 A, Hand-based thumb spica orthosis with the IP joint free. **B, C,** and **D,** A simple dorsal window cut out over the proximal phalanx that is held in place with straps during functional use and at rest. These straps and dorsal window can be released to allow stabilized MP joint extension exercises for metacarpal fractures in the second through fifth rays. (From Feehan LM: Extra-articular hand fractures part II: therapist's management. In Skirven TM, Osterman AL, Fedorczyk JM, et al, editors: *Rehabilitation of the hand and upper extremity,* ed 6, Philadelphia, 2011, Mosby Elsevier.)

❓ Questions to Discuss with the Physician

Metacarpal Fractures

Asking the physician questions is important if all of the information that you need is not indicated on the referral or if the operative report is not provided. With any of these injuries, it is important for the therapist to have good communication with the physician. Here are some sample questions:

- Where is the fracture located (that is, base, shaft, neck, head)?
- What type of fracture is it (that is, comminuted, displaced or non-displaced, intra-articular or extra-articular, transverse, oblique, and so on)?
- How stable is the fracture fragment(s)?
- Is there a tendon, ligament, or nerve injury (or injuries) that needs to be considered in therapy?
- When can controlled AROM of the wrist and/or MP joints begin?
- Are there any restrictions regarding AROM of the IP joints?
- When can strengthening exercises begin?

About the Injury

"Here is a diagram or model of the metacarpals in your hand. You broke this particular bone. In order to achieve the most functional results (name the treatment method, such as ORIF with plate, screw, pin, or closed reduction with early mobilization, and so on) was performed. Our goal is to maintain stability and alignment of the fracture, thereby improving overall function once it is healed."

About Orthoses

"Dr. _____ has prescribed an orthosis for you to wear (give specifics regarding wearing time, mobilization time, and so on). The orthosis will be custom-molded to you, and you will be in a position that maximizes fracture healing and minimizes stiffness. The position places these (point to patient's MP joints, or refer to your own) joints in as much flexion as we can comfortably get in while keeping these joints (point to PIP and DIP joints) fully extended." (Some physicians, depending on the injury, may allow the IP joints to be free.) If the IP joints are to be included in the orthosis explain to the patient that, "this position keeps the soft tissues (ligaments and tendons) from shortening and causing extreme stiffness at the joint, which is called a *contracture*."

"Wear the orthosis (describe the wearing schedule whether it's supposed to be full time, or whether he/she needs to doff it occasionally for early mobilization)."

If the physician has cleared the patient to doff the orthosis while bathing you may say, "Be extremely careful while you are bathing or showering. The floor of the tub or shower may be slippery with soap. I would recommend getting a shower bench or chair if possible." If percutaneous pins are present, "Be very careful putting on clothes and drying off so that you don't catch the pin on your clothes or towel and accidently pull it out."

About Exercises

If there is direction for AROM, "It is important to begin moving your fingers that aren't involved in the fracture. This range of motion and muscle activation will reduce swelling, prevent joint stiffness, and maintain the motion you currently have. You should avoid pain. Feeling a little discomfort or pulling sensation is all right, but do not push into pain. Painful exercise will tend to increase swelling and result in increased pain, both of which will cause decreased motion and increased stiffness." (If early mobilization has been indicated, more specific exercises should be provided with details for that treatment plan.)

Common Complications and Treatment Tips

Intrinsic Tightness

Orthotic fitting places the hand in the intrinsic plus position (full MP joint flexion and full IP joint extension). This position places the intrinsic muscles in their shortest position. Intrinsic contracture occurs most often following a crushing type injury that has severe and prolonged edema.

This condition is corrected through stretching of the intrinsic muscles, by placing the digits in an intrinsic minus position and

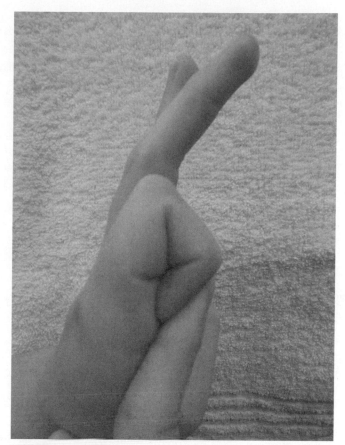

FIGURE 27-9 Passive range of motion (PROM) to stretch the intrinsic muscles of the hand.

applying a passive stretch (Fig. 27-9). One technique is to place the IP joints in a passive stretch position and secure them in that position with 1-inch Coban prior to treating the patient with fluidotherapy or paraffin wax. Be sure that the stretch is not too tight and avoid pain.

Extrinsic Digit Extensor Tightness

A Bunnell-Littler test will assist with determining whether the stiffness is from intrinsic, extrinsic, or joint capsule tightness. The Bunnell-Littler test is performed by flexing the IP joints as far as possible with the MP joints extended and then with the MP joints flexed. If there is IP joint tightness when the MPs are extended but not when they are flexed, then the tightness originates from the intrinsics. If there is IP joint tightness with the MPs flexed, but not when they are extended, the tightness originates from the extrinsic digit extensors. If the tightness in the IP joints is identical when the MPs are flexed and extended, then the tightness originates from the joint capsule (Fig. 27-10). The stretch that helps reduce extrinsic extensor tightness involves making a full composite fist and then gently flexing the wrist. For a more aggressive stretch, fully extend the ipsilateral elbow. Heat may also assist with the extensibility of the tissues. Static progressive or dynamic orthotic fitting and training may be necessary.

Extensor Digitorum Communis Adherence

EDC adherence occurs most often following surgery or if there is a period of immobilization. Complications following this include

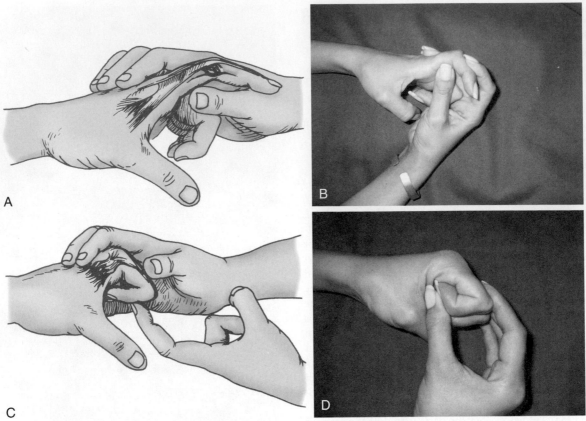

FIGURE 27-10 Intrinsic tightness test. A and **B,** The intrinsic muscles are put on stretch by the examiner, who then passively flexes the proximal interphalangeal (PIP) joint. **C** and **D,** The intrinsic muscles are then relaxed by flexing the metacarpophalangeal (MP) joint. If the PIP joint can be passively flexed more with the MP joint in flexion than when it is in extension, the intrinsic muscles are tight. (From Seftchick JL, Detullio LM, Fedorczyk JM, et al: Extra-articular hand fractures part II: therapist's management. In Skirven TM, Osterman AL, Fedorczyk JM, et al, editors: *Rehabilitation of the hand and upper extremity*, ed 6, Philadelphia, 2011, Mosby Elsevier.)

MP joint extensor lag and/or extensor quadriga (reduction of excursion of uninjured adjacent tendons).

Treatment to correct an extensor lag begins with scar mobilization if this seems to be a contributing factor. Mobilization of the skin with Dycem in the opposite direction of the tendon pull is an effective treatment technique to separate the scar from the skin. This should begin as soon as the therapist suspects that soft tissue adhesions might be preventing tendon excursion.

Fracture bracing is also a documented treatment technique. The fracture brace (see Fig. 27-2) provides circumferential support to the healing fracture and allows for AROM to occur throughout the day allowing for soft tissue excursion while avoiding fracture compromise.[3]

Joint Capsule Tightness

Joint capsule tightness often occurs with prolonged immobilization. Treatment techniques may include AROM, PROM, joint mobilization techniques, and/or static progressive or dynamic orthotic fitting and training.

"Sympathy Pain" or "Sympathy Stiffness"

"Sympathy pain" or "sympathy stiffness," occurs when a digit adjacent to the injured one becomes stiff, swollen, and painful despite not having any injury. This phenomenon occurs due to the interdependence of the three ulnar profundi tendons that share a common muscle belly.[1] This is not an uncommon phenomenon, and patients seem to respond favorably when they understand this. Encourage the patient to perform isolated tendon glides and distal interphalangeal (DIP) blocking exercises for both the injured and non-injured digit when AROM is allowed. Buddy taping may also be beneficial to encourage the digits to move together.

Achievement of full MP flexion is vital to regaining functional grasp for power gripping activities, such as holding onto a steering wheel, broom/mop, or yard tools. MP motion should begin as soon as the physician permits. Communication with the surgeon is vital in order to set up appropriate, individual treatment plans for each patient.

> ### Precautions and Concerns

- *Custom orthoses for metacarpal fractures must keep the hand in the intrinsic plus position with the MP joints held at 70° to 90° of flexion. MP joint contractures occur much more often if this does not occur.*
- *Carefully monitor and manage open wounds, infections, and pin sites.*
- *Patients may experience an increase in inflammation, pain, and edema if they perform finger flexion exercises too aggressively.*

Phalangeal Fractures, Proximal Interphalangeal Fractures, and Fracture Dislocations

In comparison to metacarpals, the hand phalanges have less protection and are therefore more prone to injury. Distal phalangeal fractures are the most common hand fractures (40% to 50% of all hand fractures), followed by proximal phalanx fractures (15% to 20% of all hand fractures). The middle phalanx is the least commonly fractured phalanx (8% to 12% of all hand fractures).[1] Each of the phalanges is similar in anatomy with some varying injury pattern and treatment techniques for each, depending on the injury. This section discusses phalangeal anatomy in general, and then becomes more specific when discussing the pathology and treatment of each phalanx. Because of the difficult nature of PIP joint fractures and fracture dislocations, they will be discussed separately from the general phalangeal fracture discussion.

Anatomy

There are fourteen phalanges in the hand, and like metacarpals, they are considered miniature long bones and have a similar concave shape to them (see Fig. 27-3). The distal epiphysis of the proximal and middle phalanx is called the *head,* and the proximal epiphysis of each phalanx is called the *base.* The neck of the proximal and middle phalanx is located at the junction of the head and the shaft. The distal end of the distal phalanx does not have a head and, therefore, no true neck. The distal pole of the terminal phalanx is called the **tuft.** The FDP inserts onto the volar base of the distal phalanx, whereas the terminal extensor tendon inserts on the dorsal base of the distal phalanx. The rest of the distal phalanx is covered by skin and subcutaneous fat with the nail bed protecting the dorsal surface. This soft tissue has a profusion of sensory nerves that are vital to the dexterity of the hand but also explains why finger injuries can be so exquisitely painful.

The proximal phalanx is surrounded by the extensor mechanism on the dorsal side, and the flexor tendons on the volar side. There are no tendon insertions onto the proximal phalanx. Flexion and extension of the proximal phalanx, therefore, results from an indirect pull of the flexor and extensor tendons, as well as intrinsic muscles acting on the more distal phalanges.[14] Stability of the PIP joint (a hinge joint) is due to both the bony configuration and the ligamentous and tendinous structures that cross and surround the joint. Dorsally, the extensor tendons and lateral bands provide stability. Collateral ligaments provide the lateral stability on both sides of the joint. The conjoined lateral bands also play a role in lateral support to the PIP joint. Volarly, the flexor tendons along with a very strong ligamentous volar plate provide the stability.[1]

The FDS bifurcates at the PIP joint level and inserts on the volar aspect of the base of the middle phalanx. The FDP continues distally to insert on the base of the distal phalanx. The soft tissue anatomy surrounding the proximal and middle phalanges is very complex and intimate. It is beyond the scope of this chapter to discuss the mechanism of these soft tissues and the biomechanics of phalangeal motion. See Chapter 1 in *Rehabilitation of the Hand and Upper Extremity,* edition 6, for more in-depth discussion on this topic. It is extremely important, however, to appreciate and understand this intimate relationship between soft tissue and bone that can cause loss of digital function with soft tissue imbalance following fracture. Maintaining tendon gliding, extensor mechanism mobility, intrinsic balance, and joint mobility following phalangeal fractures is of utmost importance. Disruption of the intrinsic mechanism or other soft tissues, or disruption of the joint stability through fracture or fracture dislocation results in significant functional deficits.

Proximal Phalangeal (P-1) Fractures

Diagnosis and Pathology

"Proximal phalangeal fractures, or P-1 fractures, are most often seen in individuals 10- to 29-years-old, and sports injuries are the leading cause of these fractures."[1] Most often, the fracture occurs at the proximal or midshaft region. Fracture patterns will present with a volar apex pattern because the interossei and lumbricals flex the proximal fragment and the digit extensor mechanism extends the distal fragment (Fig. 27-11).[2,15] This results in a "shortening" of the proximal phalanx, and if the angulation is great enough even with maximal extensor contraction, there is an extensor lag at the PIP joint.

The flexor and extensor tendons basically run flush with the bone. Therefore, any change in bony alignment can adversely affect tendon gliding, particularly where the injured bone forms a callus, or where plates and screws have been placed to reduce the fracture. Oblique fractures at the P-1 level may cause digital rotation or scissoring. In some subtle fractures, this can be more clearly observed during digital flexion.

Timelines and Healing for Non-Operative Treatment

Most closed, non-displaced P-1 shaft fractures are stable enough to effectively be treated with buddy taping and/or splinting of the injured digit to an adjacent uninvolved digit for 4 weeks. A static orthosis (clamshell type or gutter type) that includes the adjacent digit may also be a treatment option if increased stability is needed. If this option is chosen, care should be taken to doff the orthosis every 1 to 2 hours, stabilize the fractured phalanx, and gently perform AROM exercises of the uninvolved joints. Patient education is key.

Minimally displaced fractures are typically splinted in the intrinsic plus position with the MP joint flexed to at least 70° with the IP joints in full extension (intrinsic plus position). Transverse fractures may also be splinted in this position.[14] If more than one digit is involved, then the orthosis should be forearm-based.[1] Splinting usually lasts for 3 to 4 weeks before AROM begins. Callus formation must be visible radiographically as determined by the physician before strengthening exercises are introduced. PROM stretching, dynamic orthotic fitting, and training typically begins around 7 weeks. Strengthening usually begins after 8 weeks, but sufficient healing must be confirmed by the physician.[1]

Other Conservative Management Options
Traction Orthotics

It is estimated that there is a 66% decrease of total AROM after 4 weeks of immobilization of proximal phalanx fractures.[15] The impacts of surgery include additional soft tissue disruption, infection risk, time to heal, edema, and excessive pain. Recent studies support the use of traction splinting to manage proximal phalanx fractures and avoid the adverse effects of immobilization and or surgery. These orthoses can be used to treat fractures around the PIP joint, based on the principle of **ligamentotaxis.** Ligamentotaxis refers to a continuous distraction force distal to a comminuted fracture, which results in an approximation of the fracture

Bone	Region	Regional deforming forces		Pattern of malunion	
Metacarpal (MC)		***Intrinsic muscle:*** distal flexes	Apex dorsal		
Proximal phalanx (P1)		***Intrinsic muscle:*** proximal flexes ***Extensor mechanism:*** distal extends	Apex volar		
Middle phalanx (P2)	Proximal 1/3	***Central tendon:*** proximal extends ***FDS:*** distal flexes	Apex dorsal		
	Distal 1/3	***FDS:*** proximal flexes ***Extensor tendon:*** distal extends	Apex volar		
Distal phalanx (P3)	Shaft	***Extensor tendon:*** N/A (nail bed injury) ***FDP:*** distal flexes	Apex dorsal		
	Tuft	N/A: no tendon insertions	N/A		

Note: All malunions - functional bone shortening +/− digital rotation or lateral angulation distal to fracture

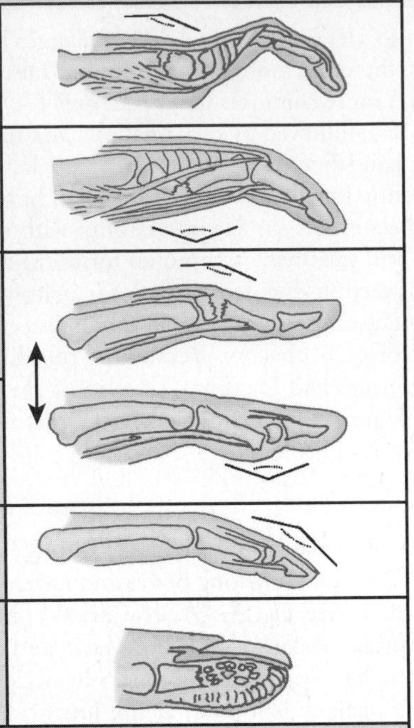

FIGURE 27-11 Regional deforming forces and common patterns of fracture malunion. (From Feehan LM: Extra-articular hand fractures part II: therapist's management. In Skirven TM, Osterman AL, Fedorczyk JM, et al, editors: *Rehabilitation of the hand and upper extremity,* ed 6, Philadelphia, 2011, Mosby Elsevier.)

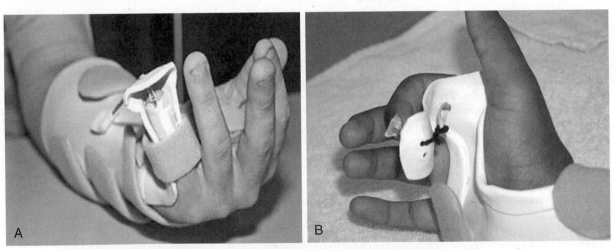

FIGURE 27-12 A, James traction orthosis for proximal phalanx fracture with 300 grams of traction force. **B,** Holes on the volar trough guide the 200 to 300 grams of traction force. (From Goldman SB, Amaker RJ, Espinosa RA: James traction splinting for PIP fractures, *J Hand Ther* 21(2):209-215, 2008.)

fragments.[16] While traction splinting is not a new concept, it is not used frequently in the clinic. Excellent communication is vital between the surgeon and therapist in order to determine the exact MP and PIP joint positions (through radiographic evidence) that optimize fracture reduction alignment. This is often done in the operating room or in the physician's clinic with a portable C-arm system. Koul, et al.[15] report that 23 of the 29 proximal phalanx fractures reviewed attained excellent results, 7 of the 29 attained good results, and 2 of the 29 attained fair to poor results.

The traction orthosis is volar and forearm-based. It includes the affected digit in a volar gutter platform and extends approximately 1 inch beyond the distal end of the distal phalanx. Digital motion is not permitted (Fig. 27-12). The amount of longitudinal force that needs to be applied to the distal end of the affected digit via rubber band attachment to a secured metal hook on the fingernail is 200 to 300 grams. A force gauge must be used in order to ensure that the force is correct. The fracture needs to be assessed under fluoroscopy 24 hours after the orthosis is

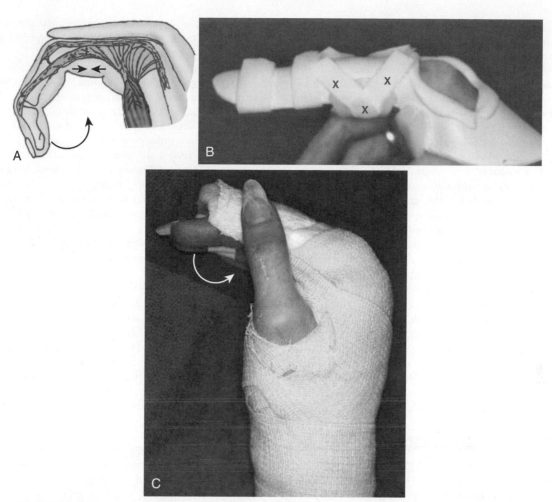

FIGURE 27-13 Proximal phalanx modified fracture orthosis A, Diagram of metacarpophalangeal (MP) joint blocked in flexion with active composite finger flexion, causing distal excursion of the extensor mechanism creating a volar cortical compression that stabilizes P-1 fractures. **B,** A modified proximal phalanx brace design including a distal extension of the dorsal orthosis that holds the interphalangeal (IP) joints in extension at rest with straps that can be released to allow IP flexion. Also shows a three-point (apex volar), semi-rigid thermoplastic volar component and strap that provide additional support to the fracture and a dorsal window over the MP joint that accommodates protruding Kirschner wires *(not shown)*. **C,** Different type of P-1 fracture brace. (From Feehan LM: Extra-articular hand fractures part II: therapist's management. In Skirven TM, Osterman AL, Fedorczyk JM, et al, editors: *Rehabilitation of the hand and upper extremity*, ed 6, Philadelphia, 2011, Mosby Elsevier.)

fabricated to evaluate the reduction and confirm that the fragments are aligning correctly. Weekly radiographs may be used to detect any loss of reduction.[16] See the Goldman, et al.[16] article for step-by-step instructions on orthotic fabrication. The patient wears the orthosis for 2 to 4 weeks depending on the fracture, and AROM begins as soon as indicated by the physician.

Traction orthosis considerations are 1) the patient must be very compliant with orthotic use, and 2) excellent communication between the surgeon and therapist is vital to ensure proper fracture alignment and to modify the orthosis as needed.[16]

Early Mobilization

As mentioned earlier, immobilization can have debilitating effects on the hand. Early mobilization techniques can be utilized in the right situations to avoid stiffness yet protect the proximal phalanx fracture and permit healing.

If early mobilization is a consideration, the patient should be fit with an orthosis that holds the MP joints in at least 70° flexion with the PIP joint held in full extension at rest. A circumferential

portion should surround the proximal phalanx with three-point fracture stabilization. Remember that the apex of a proximal phalanx fracture is typically volar when fabricating the three-point fracture stabilization portion[2] (Fig. 27-13). Freeland, et al.[17] recommends a similar brace, but makes it forearm-based. They recommend that controlled motion may begin 6 to 7 days after immobilization. Remember, if full, early mobilization is not safe, consider partial mobilization with medical clearance to prevent stiffness while allowing for sufficient fracture stabilization.

Edema control is necessary for both non-operative and postoperative treatment to avoid inter-tissue adhesions that result from chronic edema. Edema control may include elevation, compression wraps with Coban or edema gloves, and/or MEM.

Timelines and Healing for Postoperative Treatment

The surgeon may stabilize the fracture with Kirschner wires if it is a minimally-displaced transverse fracture. AROM typically begins 3 to 4 weeks after reduction with emphasis on composite digital flexion and extension, isolated FDS and FDP activation, and gentle passive MP joint flexion with active PIP joint extension. The exercises should be performed six to eight times per day in short sessions, for up to 5 minutes at a time. The hand-based orthosis in the intrinsic plus position mentioned earlier (that is, MP joints flexed to 70° to 90° with IP joints extended) should be fabricated and worn in between exercise sessions, and at night. Early mobilization principles should be considered when the fracture is stabilized with Kirschner wires.[1]

Internal fixation of proximal phalanx fractures usually occurs when the fracture is comminuted or obliquely displaced. Open fractures with subsequent soft tissue damage require irrigation and débridement in addition to ORIF. With rigid fixation AROM and very gentle PROM, exercises may begin 24 to 72 hours following surgery, depending on the surgeon's preference. Hourly exercises should be performed with resting, elevation, and icing performed in between exercise sessions. The same orthotic fitting and training described for non-operative treatment is fabricated and used in between exercise sessions and at night. PROM and strengthening usually begin 8 weeks post-surgery but must be prescribed by the physician.[1]

Scar management and mobilization begins 24 to 48 hours following suture removal. The patient may benefit from an elastomer pad or silicone gel sheeting, which is typically worn throughout the night but may be worn during the day as well if not inconvenient. Thermal agents (such as, fluidotherapy, paraffin wax, and ultrasound) may also be used as to increase the tissue extensibility and assist in improving tendon excursion.[1]

◎ Clinical Pearl

There are two major causes for PIP joint extensor lag after proximal phalanx fracture: 1) soft tissue adhesions between the extensor mechanism and the fracture site, and 2) proximal phalanx shortening secondary to fracture that results in redundancy of the extensor mechanism.[17] When the extensor lag results from option 2, it is not amenable to soft tissue mobilization.

♡ Tips from the Field

When the extensor lag is a result of soft tissue adhesions, the therapist should provide the patient with a home exercise program (HEP) that includes blocked PIP joint extension exercises with the MP flexed. Heating the digit with the modality of his/her choice (for example, hot water, heating pad, microwaved hot packs, and so on), allows for improved soft tissue extensibility. Providing a piece of Dycem to mobilize the skin and scar opposite of the tendon pull is also an effective scar mobilization technique. This method of scar mobilization is much more aggressive and should be used only after sufficient healing has occurred. Monitor the hand and/or affected digit for increased inflammation, and terminate the exercise if this occurs.

Freeland's orthosis is forearm-based and places the wrist in slight flexion to increase tension in the extensor mechanism and simultaneously release the flexor tendon tightness. The forearm-based orthosis may be reduced to a hand-based orthosis after about 3 weeks. The MP joint is placed in flexion, and the dorsal block keeps the extension force focused on the PIP joint to prevent an extensor lag. A volar component may also be added for night use in order to maintain PIP extension and prevent PIP joint flexion contracture.

Dynamic or static-progressive orthoses and serial casting may be used when AROM and PROM exercises prove to be insufficient for joint motion recovery.

A dynamic orthosis utilizes traction devices (such as, rubber bands) to alter the PROM of a joint.[18] Commercially-available dynamic PIP extension splints are readily available (Fig. 27-14). An easy option to regain PIP joint flexion may be fabricated by creating a flexion loop splint out of waistband elastic.[1] The wearing schedule varies by patient and condition. However, the rule of thumb is to make sure that the patient feels only a slight discomfort, thereby allowing a very low-load, long stretch preferably longer than 10 to 15 minutes. This should be performed three to five times per day with increasing duration. PIP extension splints seem to be tolerated better, and they often may be worn through the night. If the contracture begins to worsen during the day, the patient should increase the wearing schedule accordingly. This program should be closely monitored by a skilled hand therapist.[19]

A static progressive orthosis provides a low-load static stretch over a longer duration. The change in soft tissue length is the result of a process called **stress relaxation.** "Stress relaxation occurs when a material is held at a constant deformation. The amount of force required to maintain the deformation decreases with time, as the tissue stretches by plastic deformation until equilibrium is reached."[18] Duration of use will typically be three to four times per day for 30 to 40 minutes at a time. The patient should feel some discomfort but not so much that they need to terminate the orthotic use before end of the wearing time. The patient may adjust the tension as the tissues adapt and lengthen.[20] Shultz-Johnson states that joints with a hard end-feel contracture should wear the orthosis for longer durations, sometimes removing only for hygiene. Gains of 5° to 10° per week indicate success.[21] Static progressive finger flexion slings are also available (Fig. 27-15). Static progressive treatment is usually used after an injury has matured and the end feel of a joint has less give. The same is true for serial static orthoses.

A serial static orthosis immobilizes a joint with the tissue at the end range and is usually used to regain PIP joint extension, but it can be used to regain wrist motion. The joint is stretched to its end range. The cast or orthosis is applied to the extremity in that position. After a period of 1 to 2 days, the tissue has adapted to that length. The therapist will then prepare the tissue again, re-stretch the tissue to its new maximum, and then reapply a new cast or orthosis at that length.[21]

Middle Phalangeal (P-2) Fractures

Diagnosis and Pathology

Non-articular middle phalangeal fractures are rare, and occur most often in high-impact sports or with machinery. The middle phalanx is broader and shorter than the other phalanges making stronger than its neighboring bones.[1] Soft tissue injury is common with middle phalangeal fractures due to the intimate relationship of these tissues to the bone. Often the ligaments surrounding the PIP joint will fail before the bone actually fractures. Middle phalanx fractures deform according to where the fracture occurs along the length of the bone. If the fracture occurs along the proximal third of the joint, the fracture apex is dorsal. The central tendon pulls dorsally on the proximal piece, and the FDS flexes distally (see Fig. 27-11). If the fracture occurs along the

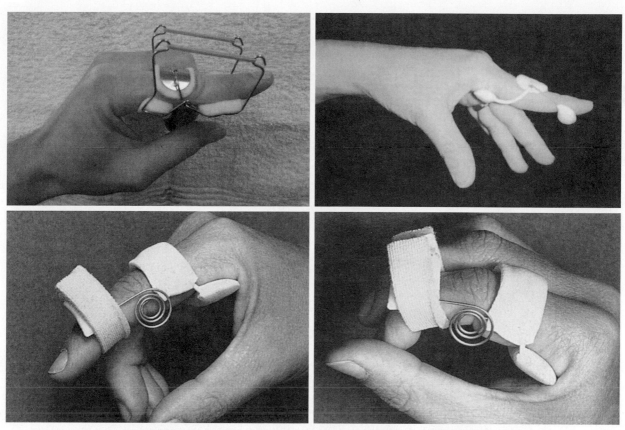

FIGURE 27-14 Examples of commercially-available dynamic extension splints.

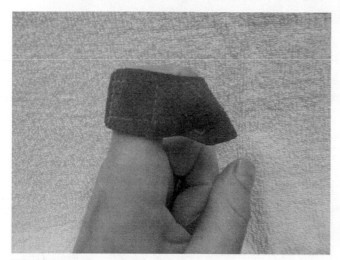

FIGURE 27-15 Finger sling for simple static progressive interphalangeal (IP) stretch.

distal third of the joint, the fracture apex is volar. In this fracture, the FDS flexes the proximal portion of the bone, and the extensor tendon extends the distal portion[2] (see Fig. 27-11).

Timelines and Healing for Non-Operative Treatment

Many of these fractures can be treated effectively with closed reduction. Flexion/extension may be allowed for 10° to 15° in the sagittal plane while only 2° to 3° can be tolerated in the coronal (radial/ulnar) plane.[14] Orthotic or casting treatment is prescribed by the physician. If the fracture is displaced but is reduced,

treatment may consist of a 3-to 4-week immobilization period to allow the fracture to consolidate. The orthosis or cast will typically be a radial or ulnar gutter and immobilize the fracture in the intrinsic plus position with the MP joints in 70° to 90° of flexion, and the IP joints are extended. The ortho may be either hand-based or forearm-based depending on the physician preference.

Early Mobilization

If displacement, malunion, or non-union are of minimal concern or if hypomobility is a concern, then a mobilization orthosis or fracture brace should be considered in order to allow for early motion.[2] This orthosis is a digit-based, dorsal gutter orthosis. The IP joints are held in extension at rest. The orthosis has a padded thermoplastic, volar strap that provides dynamic local stabilization at the fracture site (Fig. 27-16). This orthosis may also be extended proximally to become hand-based if additional fracture support is needed. With this stabilization, the DIP joint and PIP joint can gently be actively moved into flexion without compromising the fracture. Exercises should begin with gentle PROM at the IP joints, followed by gentle AROM (Fig. 27-17).

Timelines and Healing for Postoperative Treatment

Operative treatment usually involves a number of options from Kirschner wire pinning to ORIF. Once the fracture is stabilized with hardware, appropriate AROM and PROM of the PIP and DIP joints should begin.[14] The therapist needs to be aware of what surgical method has been used (for example, if pins cross the DIP joint, AROM and PROM exercises should not be prescribed).

If the physician prescribed early mobilization, then it should be performed as described earlier. If not, AROM of the IP joints

FIGURE 27-16 **A,B Middle phalanx, P2, fracture brace, A,** Dorsal finger-based orthosis with additional volar semirigid thermoplastic orthosis/strap component over P2 providing additional circumferential support to the fracture. **B,** Same dorsal finger-based extension orthosis viewed from the volar side with strap released.

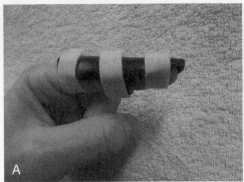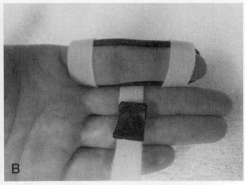

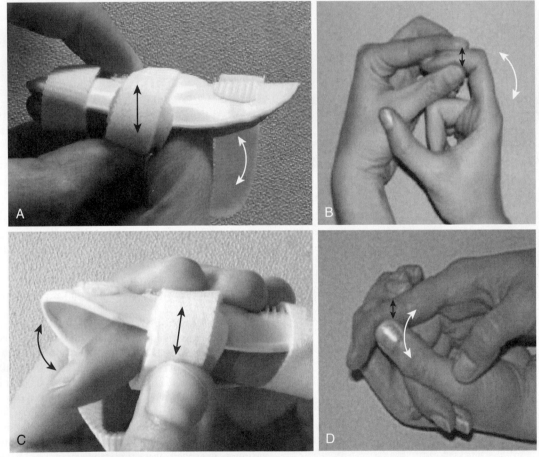

FIGURE 27-17 Middle phalangeal, P2, fracture: stabilized tendon-gliding exercises, **A** and **B,** Stabilized, passive proximal interphalangeal flexion and extension (**A,** in orthosis; **B,** out of orthosis). **C** and **D,** Stabilized active blocked distal interphalangeal flexion and extension. **C,** in orthosis; **D,** out of orthosis (Feehan LM: *Extra-articular hand fractures part II: therapist's management.* In Skirven-Osterman-Fedorczyk-Amadio, editors: *Rehabilitation of the hand and upper extremity,* ed. 6, Philadelphia, 2011, Mosby.)

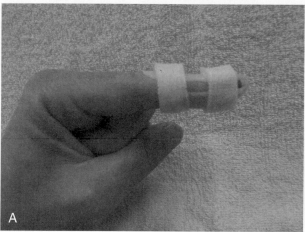 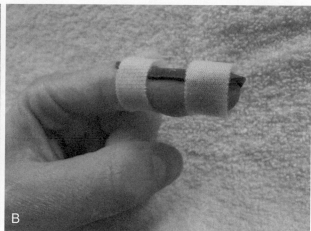

FIGURE 27-18 Mallet finger fracture orthoses, **A,** Clamshell type orthosis, **B,** Dorsal-based orthosis.

will typically begin 3 to 4 weeks after injury. Blocking exercises should be introduced gradually to encourage tendon excursion at the IP joints. A protective, hand-based orthosis may be beneficial in between exercise sessions and at night for an additional 2 weeks. The therapist needs to be vigilant watching for the development of an extensor lag. Nighttime extension orthoses may assist with this. Depending on fracture healing, dynamic or static progressive orthotic fitting (if necessary) may begin.[22]

♡ Tips from the Field

Complications of middle phalanx fractures usually arise due to the intricate nature of the soft tissue and intimate association this soft tissue has to the bone. Complications may include a decreased tendon gliding or extensor mechanism imbalance resulting in a swan neck deformity (PIP joint hyperextension and DIP joint flexion) or a boutonniere deformity (PIP joint flexion with DIP joint hyperextension).

If an extensor lag at the PIP joint and DIP joint develops, a night extension orthosis at the PIP joint and/or DIP joint should be considered. The terminal extensor tendon is thin and extremely weak compared to the stronger FDP tendon. As a result, intermittent splinting may be needed to prevent the FDP from overpowering the terminal extensor tendon, resulting in tendon attenuation and an extensor lag at the DIP joint.

If the DIP joint is limited in flexion, gentle PROM stretching, dynamic or static progressive orthoses, or stretching with Coban may be used. If the joint is supple passively, the therapist should consider FDP excursion motion by blocking the PIP joint in extension, in addition to exercises with theraputty if permitted. A fully functional DIP joint is important to regaining full grip strength.

Distal Phalangeal (P-3) Fractures

Diagnosis and Pathology

Distal phalanges are the most exposed phalanges and are, therefore, fractured more often than other hand fractures. The long finger is the most involved digit, and the thumb is the next most involved.[1] Most distal phalangeal fractures are the result of crush injuries, such as getting the finger shut in a door, sports injuries, or industrial accidents.[14] Associated soft tissue injuries include

nail bed injuries, dorsal skin lacerations, and hematomas. If the fracture is primarily located on the distal phalanx shaft, the apex us usually dorsal due to the volar pull of the FDP tendon.[2]

Avulsion fractures occur both palmarly (flexor tendon) and dorsally (extensor tendon). Avulsion of the FDP occurs when a flexed digit is forcibly extended and is nicknamed **"jersey finger."** This fracture is often seen when a football player holds onto a jersey while trying to make a tackle and his digit is forcibly extended. A **"mallet finger"** occurs when an extended digit is forcibly flexed and the extensor tendon avulses a piece of the dorsal, distal phalanx. This happens, for example, when a basketball or baseball hits the end of his extended digit head on.

Timelines and Healing for Non-Operative Treatment

Bony mallet injuries that are closed, non-displaced, and not comminuted with the articular fragment less than 30% of the joint surface are often amenable to conservative management. Conservative management would include full-time orthotic wear that keeps the DIP joint fully extended or even slightly hyperextended. Tuft fractures or closed non-displaced shaft fractures are typically non-displaced and stable and should be immobilized with an orthosis for at least 2 weeks,[14] after which gentle mobilization may begin. Clamshell type orthoses work well for this. Dorsal based orthoses that keep the DIP joint fully extended with Velcro straps also work well (Fig. 27-18).

Early Mobilization

Early mobilization begins when the physician prescribes it. This may begin approximately 2 weeks following a tuft fracture, as mentioned before. The orthosis is either clamshell-type or dorsally-based, should maintain full DIP extension statically, and should be worn between exercise sessions and at night. The therapist needs to be vigilant for DIP extensor lag formation and should treat accordingly. Mallet injuries are *not* good candidates for early mobilization.[2]

Timelines and Healing for Postoperative Treatment
Mallet Injuries

If the dorsal fragment is greater than 50% of the joint surface, the DIP joint typically becomes unstable. If closed reduction can be obtained, Kirschner wire fixation to secure the fragment is utilized. A 1 mm microfracture screw may be used if closed reduction is unattainable. Full-time orthotic use is recommended for

6 to 8 weeks after any type of surgical fixation. DIP flexion exercises may begin after this time, but the emergence of an extensor lag should be closely monitored. An additional 4 weeks of night orthotic use may be recommended if the patient is involved with heavy lifting or sports activities.[14]

Jersey Finger

FDP avulsions from the distal phalanx frequently involve volar bony fragments. The patient comes to the clinic unable to flex the distal phalanx. Shuler[14] reports that tendon repair with retraction must be done within 10 days from the injury. If the avulsion has not retracted, the tendon can be repaired as late as 6 weeks after the injury. Repair of the tendon is typically done one of two ways 1) through suture anchors, or 2) using drill holes through the nail for a pullout button.

Rehabilitation for a surgically-repaired jersey finger will be similar to a zone 1 flexor tendon repair. Often, however, the repair of the fracture is strong enough that gentle AROM may be performed immediately. This early ROM, of course, pertains to the reliable patient. A dorsal blocking orthosis that holds the wrist in 30° of extension, MPs in 60° to 70° of flexion, and the IP joints in full extension, protects the hand in between exercise sessions and at night. Compressive wraps assist with edema control. Place and hold exercises may begin in the first or second week typically. In these exercises the digit(s) are passively placed in full composite flexion, where they are gently held for 5 seconds, and then released. At around 3 weeks, gentle FDS and FDP gliding exercises may be performed to encourage tendon excursion. Light resistive exercises may begin at 6 weeks, progressing gradually to full resistance and return to sport/work at 12 weeks. Unreliable patients are typically casted in a protected position and allowed PROM for 4 weeks, after which time the cast is removed. A dorsal blocking orthosis similar to the one mentioned earlier is recommended and AROM and tendon gliding exercises are prescribed.[14] Once again, it is vital to communicate with the surgeon to determine the strength of the repair, reliability of the patient, or any other precautions that will affect therapy.

Kirschner Wire Pinning of Shaft Fractures

Skeletal fixation via Kirschner wires typically maintains alignment with the need of rigid orthoses or compressive dressings. The surgeon often requests an orthosis be fabricated for the patient for protection and rest to allow for homeostasis of the tissues. The DIP joint will be held in full extension, and then progressive, gentle ROM may be initiated.[14] Early motion should be in a limited, pain-free arc and gradually progressed to a full arc. The therapist should monitor for development of an extensor lag. Should one develop, treat similar to an mallet injury.[2] Communicate findings with the referring physician.

♡ Tips from the Field

- Edema control is extremely important. Treat edema with MEM, proximal AROM, circumferential, compressive wrapping (such as, with Coban), elevation, and ice if early postoperative.
- If pins were used, educate the patient on proper pin care and signs of infection.
- Successful orthotic fitting and training should include and orthosis that 1) protects the fracture and repair, 2) stays secure at night, and 3) minimizes pressure over the dorsal

DIP joints. Coban or paper tape may assist with securing the orthosis. Use of closed cell foam, perforated orthotic material ($\frac{1}{16}$ inch or $\frac{3}{32}$ inch), or a modification of the orthosis by cutting out a dorsal portion assist to minimize pressure over the DIP joint.

- Progress AROM *gradually*. The FDP is much stronger than the terminal extensor tendon. Aggressive DIP flexion may result in an extensor lag. Stiffness will usually resolve over time due to the strength of the FDP.
- Isometric exercises for DIP extension are sufficient. Instruct the patient to block the MP and PIP joints in flexion and then extend the DIP joint, holding for a count of 5 to 8 seconds. Short sessions every hour are most beneficial.[1]
- The goal is to avoid an extensor lag of greater than 10°. Resume orthotic wear at night and perhaps during the day if an extensor lag begins to develop.

Proximal Interphalangeal Joint Fractures and Dislocations

Diagnosis and Pathology

Injuries to the PIP joint of the hand are not uncommon. The joints in the hand require a balance between mobility and stability in order to allow for functional activities from brushing teeth to operating a chainsaw.[23] Because the hands are virtually always exposed and are used in just about every activity one does, they are frequently subjected to deforming forces that result in injuries ranging from mild strains to joint dislocations to fractured, unstable dislocations. Fracture dislocations are typically caused by axial compression on a semi-flexed or hyperextended digit. This results in a dorsal dislocation of the PIP joint. A dorsal dislocation refers to the direction that the middle phalanx travels in relation to the proximal phalanx. A volar dislocation is much less frequent, in which the middle phalanx moves volarly in relation to the proximal phalanx. Volar dislocations often result in a **boutonniere deformity** due to the disruption of the central slip with PIP joint flexion and DIP joint hyperextension.[1] The following sections are a very basic overview of PIP joint dislocations and fractures. See Chapter 33 in *Rehabilitation of the Hand and Upper Extremity,* edition 6, for a very detailed management program for all intra-articular diagnoses of the IP joints of the hand.[23]

Timelines and Healing for Non-Operative Treatment

In a simple to complex dislocation or fracture dislocation when 25% to 30% or less of the articular surface is involved, conservative management is usually sufficient. A *simple dislocation* is defined as one where the base of the middle phalanx is still in contact with the condyles of the proximal phalanx. Simple dislocations are treated with dorsal-based orthotic immobilization with the PIP joint held in 30° of flexion (preventing PIP joint extension) for 3 weeks. Hourly PIP and DIP joint flexion is permitted and encouraged. After 3 weeks, if stability is confirmed, blocked extension exercises are introduced along with gentle PIP joint extension stretches and static or static-progressive extension splinting as needed and tolerated.[14]

Complex dislocations result when the base of the middle phalanx is no longer in contact with the proximal phalanx condyles. On the x-ray, the affected digit will have a bayonet appearance. If the dislocation is easily reducible, then treatment will be similar

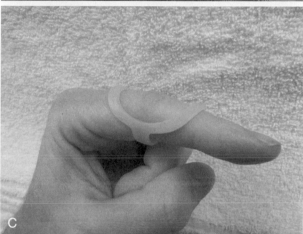

FIGURE 27-19 Figure-eight orthosis, A, Custom figure-eight orthosis, digit extended. **B,** Custom figure-eight orthosis, digit flexed. **C,** Commercially-available figure-eight orthoses.

to that of a simple dislocation (that is, dorsal-based orthotic immobilization with the PIP joint held in 30° of flexion for 3 weeks; gentle PIP AROM flexion is encouraged).

Timelines and Healing for Postoperative Treatment

When greater than 30% of the articular surface is affected, the PIP joint becomes unstable, and surgical intervention is warranted.[14] Multiple surgical techniques may be employed to restore stability to these injuries, but it is beyond the scope of this chapter to discuss them in detail. After surgical reduction and stabilization, the patient will often stay in the bulky dressing for 2 to 3 weeks. Once this is removed, the therapist fabricates a dorsal-blocking orthosis similar to that mentioned in the nonoperative treatment, and encourages active PIP and DIP flexion exercises within the orthosis. The orthosis may be adjusted serially each week to encourage improved extension. Dynamic extension and/or flexion may be initiated at around 6 to 8 weeks with gentle grip strengthening beginning around 8 weeks.

❤ **Tips from the Field**

Goals of Rehabilitation[23]
- Reduce or control edema
- Reduce and control pain
- Prevent infection, and provide proper wound care to achieve full wound closure

- Maintain joint stability
- Obtain complete fracture healing
- Restore joint ROM and muscle tendon-unit length
- Educate patient on correct motor performance in order to avoid compensatory motions
- Improve strength and function
- Maximize independence in the HEP

Remember that articular cartilage is avascular, is not innervated, and therefore relies upon motion for health. Communication with the surgeon is vital since he or she is the one to dictate when AROM may begin, and it is important to begin as soon as possible.

Pain and stiffness are extremely common after PIP joint fracture dislocations. It may take several months to regain full composite flexion. Activity modification and adaptive equipment should be included in the therapy program. Enlarged handles on toothbrushes, yard tools, utensils, and so on will improve a patient's functional independence.

If the reduced joint remains stable and is without fracture, a figure-eight orthosis (Fig. 27-19) may be sufficient for preventing PIP joint extension while allowing full flexion.

Flexion contractures are common complications following PIP joint fracture dislocations. Be sure to not confuse this complication with a boutonniere deformity. In a boutonniere deformity

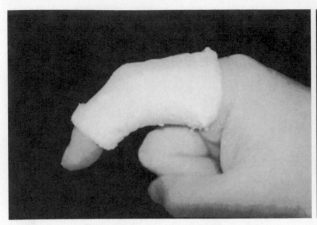 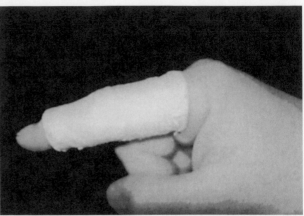

FIGURE 27-20 Serial casting for proximal interphalangeal (PIP) flexion contractures with hard end feel.

the central slip is injured. A flexion contracture following a PIP joint dislocation does not have an extensor tendon injury, and the DIP joint remains flexible. For flexion contractures that have a hard end feel, serial casting of the PIP joint tends to be more effective at correcting the contracture than static progressive or dynamic orthoses[1] (Fig. 27-20).

It is helpful to know where the fracture occurred, and whether or not the joint was involved. Regaining full ROM following articular disruption may be more challenging. Also, AROM and subsequent PROM typically may begin earlier when the fracture is at the base or head/neck region rather than midshaft because cancellous bone tends to heal faster than cortical.[1] The physician always determines when the fracture is clinically healed.

Early edema control is extremely important. Edema produces predictable patterns of deformity with a swollen, moderately flexed PIP joint and an extended DIP joint.[1] If the edema becomes chronic, then adhesions may form between the soft tissues, resulting in a much greater difficulty recovering functional ROM. The therapist needs to educate the patient regarding ice, AROM of uninvolved digits, elevation, and gentle elastic bandaging.

<blockquote>

➤   Precautions and Concerns

- *Do not attempt isotonic strengthening (for example, theraputty) for the terminal extensor tendon. Isometric strengthening is adequate.*
- *The patient should clean exposed pins daily according to the surgeon's preference. Proper cleaning will prevent pin tract infection.*
- *If the pin is exposed, the patient needs to be cautious about inadvertently pulling the pins on towels or clothes.*
- *Do not sacrifice PIP joint extension for full PIP joint flexion. An extensor lag greater than 25° to 30° presents a functional limitation for most patients.[22] An extension assist orthosis (for example, Capener orthosis, see Fig. 27-13) is a good option if an extensor lag or contracture is developing. This allows the patient to actively flex the PIP joint periodically while maintaining PIP extension at rest.*
- *To avoid extensor lag at the DIP joint following a mallet injury, encourage composite flexion and extension of the digit instead of blocked flexion and extension.[1] Permit PROM only when appropriate healing has occurred.*

</blockquote>

?   Questions to Discuss with the Physician

Phalangeal Fractures and/or Dislocations

- What type of fracture is it (for example, comminuted, intra-articular, and so on)? Where is it located? (Obtaining an operative report, if possible, will assist with answering many of these questions.)
- What method of reduction was used?
- Was internal fixation used to maintain fracture reduction? If so, does it cross a joint?
- How stable is the fracture?
- Is early mobilization an option with this patient? (The patient must be very compliant to begin early mobilization if the fracture is not rigidly stable.)

Comminuted Proximal Phalanx Fractures

- Is traction orthotic fitting and training an option?
- What soft tissue structures are involved or compromised?
- When can AROM of the joints immobilized by the orthosis or cast begin?
- When may passive stress at or near the fracture site begin?
- When may strengthening exercises begin?

Evaluation Tips

- Obtain a very detailed history from the patient. This is key in determining all of the tissues involved (soft or bony), the stage of healing, previous treatment, and so on.
- Observe edema. Measure with a circumferential gauge, and document this information along with the location of the swelling. Remember to document the circumference of the contralateral digit.
- Gently palpate and note specific areas of tenderness.
- Note any lateral instability or scissoring of the PIP or DIP joints during active flexion and extension.
- Assess hypermobility and/or lateral laxity of other, non-involved joints. Document findings.
- Assess composite flexion abilities of uninvolved digits and contralateral hand. Document findings.
- Assess intrinsic vs. extrinsic vs. joint capsular tightness via the Bunnell-Littler test.

( ) *What to Say to Clients*

See the earlier "Metacarpal Fractures" section for suggestions.

Conclusion

Hand fractures are commonplace in the hand therapy practice. These fractures can be functionally debilitating if not treated correctly. The therapist must understand the anatomy of the hand, be competent in orthotic fitting and training, be confident in treatment skills and plan, and communicate effectively with the overseeing physician in order to achieve the best outcomes possible.

CASE STUDY 27-1 ■

T.W. is a 60-year-old male who was operating a drill press in his machine shop when the drill bit caught his glove and forcefully rotated his left hand around and slammed it into another portion of the press, resulting in a left index finger non-displaced, intra-articular proximal phalanx base fracture.

T.W. came to hand therapy 8 days after the accident with instructions from the physician to fabricate a custom, radial, hand-based orthosis to stabilize the fracture, yet allow for AROM of noninvolved joints and digits. He came to the clinic in an alumiofoam splint that prevented any left index finger AROM. His hand was extremely stiff. AROM measurement was permitted. Unaffected digit ROM was within functional limits. His left index finger ROM measurements were as follows:

- Left index finger DIP joint: 0° extension, 20° flexion
- Left index finger PIP joint: 0° extension, 35° flexion
- Left index finger MP joint: 0° extension, 25° flexion

T.W. enjoys working in his machine shop and building motorcycles, and he was very eager to begin protective mobilization to regain his hand function.

The physician prescribed a radial gutter, hand-based orthotic to place the left index finger into an intrinsic plus position. Initially, T.W. had extreme difficulty attaining the intrinsic plus position. The therapist warmed T.W's hand in the fluidotherapy machine for 15 minutes to improve tissue extensibility, and then performed gentle PROM stretch to the MP joint of the left index finger. Care was taken to support the fracture manually, and to minimize pain by not aggressively ranging the digit.

Pain-free MP joint flexion of 45° was attained after gentle stretching with emphasis to support the fracture. The therapist then fabricated the orthotic. As stated earlier, it was hand-based in a radial gutter fashion. The MP joint was held in 45° of flexion. The PIP joint was left to move through an AROM from 0° of extension to 50° of flexion. This was pain-free. The PIP joint was blocked from progressing beyond 50° to prevent undue stress on the fracture. The patient was instructed to wear the orthosis at all times except for showering. He was instructed on edema reduction techniques, and gentle AROM of all uninvolved joints.

The patient's insurance required authorization after the completion of the initial evaluation. Three weeks passed before authorization was approved by the insurance company, which was about the same time as the patient followed up with his physician. X-rays were taken at that time, which revealed good interval healing. The patient demonstrated some residual MP, PIP, and DIP joint stiffness and was instructed to follow up with therapy.

At his follow-up appointment the patient demonstrated good improvement in ROM compared to initial evaluation. His measurements were as follows:

- Left index finger DIP joint AROM: 0° extension, 40° flexion
- Left index finger PIP joint AROM: 0° extension, 65° flexion
- Left index finger MP joint AROM: 0° extension, 45° flexion
- Left index finger DIP joint PROM: 0° extension, 55° flexion
- Left index finger PIP joint PROM: 0° extension, 80° flexion
- Left index finger MP joint PROM: 0° extension, 59° flexion

Bunnell-Littler test for intrinsic tightness was negative indicating joint capsule and possibly extrinsic extensor tightness. At this second appointment, the patient was educated on heat modalities to increase the tissue extensibility. He was provided with instructions on IP joint capsular stretching, isolated MP joint PROM, and extrinsic digit extensor stretching for his HEP.

The patient returned 1 week later reporting good compliance with his home program. He demonstrated good progress in that 1 week. MP joint flexion improved 10°. PIP joint flexion improved 10°. DIP joint flexion improved 5° for a total AROM improvement of 25°. The patient reported doing light work in his metal shop without any dysfunction.

Unfortunately, the patient reported during that visit that his wife had just lost her job, and thus he would be losing his insurance. He expressed his confidence with his independence with his HEP. With the good interval healing and independence with his HEP, the therapist provided him with some theraputty and instructed him on gentle grip and pinch strengthening exercises. The patient was appreciative at the time of discharge. It is anticipated that with the client's good motivation, he will continue to progress.

Acknowledgments

Special thanks to David Levy, MS, OTR/L, CHT for his excellent research and article acquisition for this chapter. His assistance is greatly appreciated.

I would also like to thank Anne Moscony, MA, OTR/L, CHT who laid the foundational work for this chapter in the first edition of this book. Writing this chapter was made easier by her excellent efforts.

References

1. Moscony AMB: Common wrist and hand fractures. In Cooper C, editor: *Fundamentals of hand therapy: clinical reasoning and treatment guidelines for common diagnoses of the upper extremity*, ed 1, St Louis, 2007, Mosby Elsevier, pp 251–285.
2. Feehan LM: Extra-articular hand fractures part II: therapist's management. In Skirven TM, Osterman AL, Fedorczyk JM, et al, editors: *Rehabilitation of the hand and upper extremity*, ed 6, Philadelphia, 2011, Elsevier Mosby, pp 386–401.
3. Chinchalkar SJ: Addressing extensor digitorum communis adherence after metacarpal fracture with the use of a circumferential brace, *J Hand Ther* 22(4):377–381, 2009.
4. Hardy M, Wegener EE: Hand fracture management, *J Hand Ther* 16(2):79–80, 2003.
5. Feehan LM: Early controlled mobilization of potentially unstable extra-articular hand fractures, *J Hand Ther* 16(2):161–170, 2003.

6. Colditz JC: Functional fracture bracing. In Skirven TM, Osterman AL, Fedorczyk JM, et al, editors: *Rehabilitation of the hand and upper extremity*, ed 6, Philadelphia, 2011, Elsevier Mosby, pp 1620–1628.

7. Feehan LM, Bassett K: Is there evidence for early motion after an extra-articular hand fracture? *J Hand Ther* 17(1):85–86, 2004.

8. Gabel P: Evidence based medicine for third party (insured) patients using generalized assessment of body and limbs (GABAL) outcome measure protocols, *J Hand Ther* 17(1):85, 2004.

9. Soong M, Got C, Katarincic J: Ring and little finger metacarpal fractures: mechanisms, locations, and radiographic parameters, *J Hand Surg Am* 35(8):1256–1259, 2010.

10. McNemar TB: Management of metacarpal fractures, *J Hand Ther* 16(2):143–151, 2003.

11. Kamath JB, Harshvardhan, Naik DM, et al: Current concepts in managing fractures of metacarpal and phalanges, *Indian J Plast Surg* 44(2):203–211, 2011.

12. Lehman T, Hildenbrand J: Fractures and ligament injuries of the thumb and metacarpals. In Trumble TE, Rayan GM, Budoff JE, et al, editors: *Principles of hand surgery and therapy*, ed 2, Philadelphia, 2010, Saunders Elsevier, pp 35–59.

13. Weinstein LP, Hanel DP: Metacarpal fractures, *J Am Society Surg Hand* 2(4):168–180, 2002.

14. Shuler MS, Slade JF: Fractures of the phalanx. In Trumble TE, Rayan GM, Budoff JE, et al, editors: *Principles of hand surgery and therapy*, ed 2, Philadelphia, 2010, Saunders Elsevier, pp 60–80.

15. Koule AR, Patil RK, Philip V: Traction splints: effective nonsurgical way of managing proximal phalanx fractures, *J Trauma* 66(6):1641–1646, 2008.

16. Goldman SB, Amaker RJ, Espinosa RA: James traction splinting for PIP fractures, *J Hand Ther* 21(2):209–215, 2008.

17. Freeland AE, Hardy MA, Singletary S: Rehabilitation for proximal phalangeal fractures, *J Hand Ther* 16(2):129–142, 2003.

18. Kaplan FTD: The stiff finger, *Hand Clinic* 26(2):191–204, 2010.

19. Colditz JC: Therapist's management of the stiff hand. In Skirven TM, Osterman AL, Fedorczyk JM, et al, editors: *Rehabilitation of the hand and upper extremity*, ed 6, Philadelphia, 2011, Elsevier Mosby, pp 894–921.

20. Doornberg JN, Ring D, Jupiter JB: Static progressive splinting for post-traumatic elbow stiffness, *J Orthop Trauma* 20(6):400–404, 2006.

21. Shultz-Johnson K: Static progressive splinting, *J Hand Ther* 15(2):163–178, 2002.

22. Cannon N, editor: *Diagnosis and treatment manual*, ed 4, Indianapolis, 2001, The Hand Rehabilitation Center of Indiana.

23. Gallagher KG, Blackmore SM: Intra-articular hand fractures and joint injuries: part II—therapist's management. In Skirven TM, Osterman AL, Fedorczyk JM, et al, editors: *Rehabilitation of the hand and upper extremity*, ed 6, Philadelphia, 2011, Elsevier Mosby, pp 417–435.

28

Elbow, Wrist, and Hand Tendinopathies

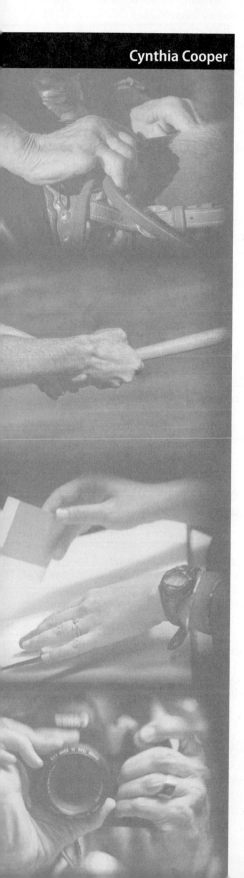

Cynthia Cooper

C lients with tendinitis/tendinosis experience pain that can significantly limit their daily activities. Simply picking up a coffee cup may be a task that is too painful. Stirring food, putting away groceries, or using a computer keyboard may provoke pain, and exercise routines can be interrupted. These clients may put off going to the physician, hoping that the symptoms will pass. Unfortunately, those who wait may develop chronic changes, which can be more difficult to treat.

Symptoms associated with tendinitis/tendinosis include pain with active range of motion (AROM), resistance, or passive stretching of the involved structures. It is very important to identify the activities contributing to the problem and to make as many ergonomic changes as possible. These often can be accomplished with clever improvising and do not necessarily require expensive purchases. For example, simply placing large pillows in the lap to provide forearm and wrist support while reading or knitting can be very helpful. Many clients recover well by improving their posture and upper extremity (UE) biomechanics and by participating in an ongoing exercise program.

General Anatomy

Tendons are viscoelastic structures with unique mechanical properties. They are composed of connective tissues made of collagen, tenocytes, and ground substance, and they are poorly vascularized. Tendons allow muscle to transmit forces that create motion.[1]

The strength of a muscle depends on its cross-sectional area. A larger cross-sectional area provides greater contraction force with transmission of greater tensile loads through the tendon. Tendons with a larger cross-sectional area also are able to bear higher loads.[2]

The factors that most affect tendons' biomechanical properties are aging, pregnancy, mobilization (or immobilization), and use of nonsteroidal anti-inflammatory drugs (NSAIDs). Up to the age of 20, the collagen cross-links in tendons increase in number and improve in quality, which equates with increased tensile strength. With aging, tensile strength decreases.[2]

◎ Clinical Pearl

Tendons remodel in response to the stresses or mechanical demands imposed on them. They become stronger by being exposed to increased stress (e.g., movement). They become weaker when stress is reduced or eliminated (e.g., immobilization, such as orthoses).[2]

General Pathology

Tendinitis is defined as an acute inflammatory response to injury of a tendon that produces the classical signs of heat, swelling, and pain.[3] Physicians and therapists historically have treated tendinitis as a phenomenon of tendon inflammation. However, recent, compelling histologic evidence has resulted in a change of terminology. The term **angio-fibroblastic hyperplasia** or **angiofibroblastic tendinosis** (hereafter referred to as **tendinosis**) describes the pathologic alterations seen in the tissue of clients diagnosed as having tendonitis. A visible change occurs in the gross appearance of the tissue. Microscopically, normal tendon fibers are arranged in an orderly fashion. With tendinosis, the tendon fibers are invaded by fibroblasts and atypical vascular granulation tissue, and the adjacent tissue becomes degenerative, hypercellular, and microfragmented. Typically, only a few, if any, inflammatory cells are seen histologically. Tendinosis now is thought to be a degenerative pathologic condition, not an inflammatory one. Experts currently believe that true tendinitis is rare and that the condition hand therapists see in clients is tendinosis.

This histologic evidence has some intriguing implications for therapists: 1) we should question traditional approaches to the treatment of tendonitis as an inflammatory condition, and 2) we should alter our hand therapy treatments to fit the evidence of a tendinosis pathology.[4]

Individuals most likely to have tendinosis 1) are over age 35; 2) engage in a high-intensity occupational or sports activity three or more times a week for at least 30 minutes per session; 3) use a demanding technique for the activity; and 4) have an inadequate level of physical fitness. Symptoms occur when the tissue is worked beyond its tolerance (i.e., overused).[1]

General Timelines and Healing

The key to promoting healing is to help your clients avoid pain. Timelines and healing vary. Symptoms may persist or recur over years but do not always do so; some clients recover completely. In therapy, some clients may be able to start pain-free isometric or AROM exercises immediately, whereas others may find this too painful initially. Generally speaking, if your client is following therapy guidelines but has not made progress after a few weeks, suggest a return visit to the physician.

General Treatment Suggestions

General treatment suggestions are presented in the following sections. Lateral epicondylitis, medial epicondylitis, de Quervain's tenosynovitis, and digital stenosing tenosynovitis are addressed individually because they are common tendinitis/tendinosis diagnoses. The chapter ends with a table designed to promote structure-specific clinical reasoning and treatment for these and other diagnoses of UE tendinitis/tendinosis.

Posture and Conditioning

Always promote good posture, regardless of which UE structures are diagnosed with the tendinitis/tendinosis. Likewise, proximal UE AROM and tolerable aerobic exercises are valuable for stimulating lymphatic flow and promoting circulation to the distal structures.

Biomechanics and Symptom Management

Instruct clients in biomechanical guidelines promoting physiologic UE motions that are not strenuous. Teach them to keep their elbows at their sides with the forearms and wrists in neutral positions and to use softer force for pinch and grip activities. Encourage the use of padded and enlarged handles on tools. Explain that two-handed activities done frontally put much less strain on distal UE structures than one-handed activities done far away from the body, overhead, or with trunk twisting.

Ergonomic modifications and lifestyle changes, including pacing, can be very beneficial, but convincing clients of this sometimes can be difficult. An even more difficult task is persuading some clients to take better care of their bodies and to delegate more chores or tasks at home if possible. It is essential to learn your client's priorities and goals so that contributory life-style issues can be addressed appropriately and effectively. Adjustments as simple as moving closer to the telephone and using a headset can be quite helpful.

Progression of Treatment

Rest may be necessary initially, depending on the severity of symptoms. Orthoses or soft straps may be helpful for pain, and treatments that relieve pain (e.g., application of superficial heat) should be used. The goal is to bring these clients to the point where they are ready for pain-free isometric and short arc AROM of the involved structures. If exercising the involved structure is too painful, be sure to exercise proximally. Always incorporate aerobic exercise and proximal AROM if possible.

Begin short arc AROM of the involved structures as soon as this can be done without causing pain. If necessary for pain control, eliminate gravity and keep the arc of motion small. Try isometrics with a gentle contraction in a position of comfort and upgrade with varying positions.

Progress to AROM of the involved structures in greater arcs of motion against gravity when this can be done without pain. Gradually add resistance. In most cases, performing more repetitions with a lighter load is better than performing few repetitions with a higher load. Eccentric exercises stimulate the production of collagen and are particularly important for clients who want to return to sporting activities that require eccentric contractions (e.g., tennis). Monitor the client's responses to this upgrade.

As hand therapists, we are taught to believe that we should perform passive stretching of the involved structures. However, this poses a dilemma, because passive stretching can injure tissue. Clients find it difficult to truly relax for passive self-stretching, partly because of an appropriate anticipation of pain. Some experts have found that clients recover full passive stretching capability when pain-free, upgraded exercises are used instead of therapist-assisted passive stretching. This point deserves further research. In the meantime, if you perform passive stretching of involved structures, be very careful to avoid pain and monitor the client's pain after the stretching session. (See Chapter 4 for more information on tissue-specific exercises.)

Precaution. *Always avoid pain with exercise; pain is a sign of injury.*

Lateral Epicondylosis (Tennis Elbow)

Anatomy

The lateral epicondyle of the humerus is the origin of the symptomatic muscle-tendon units in lateral epicondylitis, commonly known as *tennis elbow* (Fig. 28-1). The extensor carpi radialis brevis (ECRB) is most often involved, followed by the extensor digitorum communis (EDC).

Diagnosis and Pathology

Clients usually have point tenderness at the lateral epicondyle, possibly anterior or distal to it. Point tenderness at the supracondylar ridge may indicate involvement of the extensor carpi radialis longus (ECRL). Clients with lateral epicondylitis complain of nighttime aching and morning stiffness of the elbow. Gripping provokes pain, as does resisted wrist extension, supination, digital extension, and wrist radial deviation. Grip strength is reduced when the elbow is extended, and pain may be worse with this position (e.g., when carrying a briefcase). Tightness of the extrinsic extensors is common, and stretching of these muscles causes pain (Fig. 28-2).

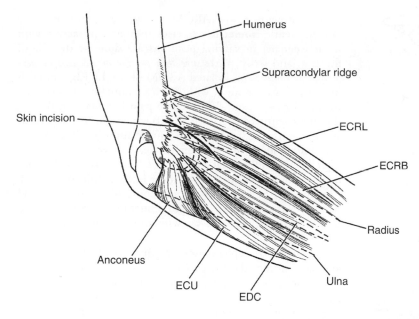

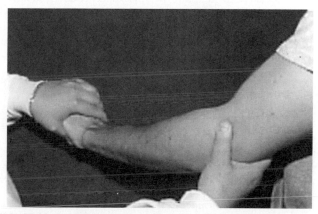

FIGURE 28-1 Muscles that attach at the lateral epicondyle of the distal humerus. (From Trumble TE: Tendinitis and epicondylitis. In Trumble TE, editor: *Principles of hand surgery*, Philadelphia, 2000, WB Saunders.)

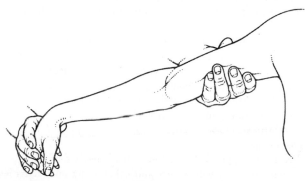

FIGURE 28-2 Stretching of extrinsic extensors. (From Wadsworth TG: Elbow tendinitis. In Mackin EJ, Callahan AD, Skirven TM et al, editors: *Rehabilitation of the hand and upper extremity*, ed 5, St Louis, 2002, Mosby.)

FIGURE 28-3 Cozen's test. (From Fedorczyk JM: Therapist's management of elbow tendinitis. In Mackin EJ, Callahan AD, Skirven TM et al, editors: *Rehabilitation of the hand and upper extremity*, ed 5, St Louis, 2002, Mosby.)

The test for tennis elbow is called **Cozen's test** (Fig. 28-3). The examiner's thumb stabilizes the client's elbow at the lateral epicondyle. With the forearm pronated, the client makes a fist and then actively extends and radially deviates the wrist with the examiner resisting the motion. Severe, sudden pain in the area of the lateral epicondyle is a positive test result.[5]

Mill's tennis elbow test originally was described as a manipulation maneuver, but it can be used as a clinical test. The client's shoulder is in neutral. The examiner palpates the most tender area at or near the lateral epicondyle, then pronates the forearm and fully flexes the wrist while moving the elbow from flexion to extension. Pain at the lateral epicondyle is a positive test result. (For more information on this topic and other provocative tests, see Fedorczyk's work.)[1,5]

Differential diagnoses include cervical radiculopathy, proximal neurovascular entrapment, radiocapitellar joint pain, and radial tunnel syndrome. X-ray films can rule out osseous or articular conditions such as calcification or arthritis. When the triceps is most symptomatic, the condition is called *posterior tennis elbow.*

Radial tunnel syndrome differs from lateral epicondylitis in that the pain is more diffuse and occurs within the muscle mass of the extensor wad rather than at the lateral epicondyle (Fig. 28-4). The middle finger test can be used to detect radial tunnel

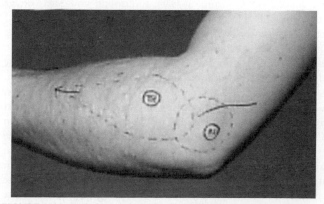

FIGURE 28-4 Radial tunnel syndrome differs from lateral epicondylitis in that the pain is more diffuse and occurs within the muscle mass of the extensor wad rather than at the lateral epicondyle. (From Fedorczyk JM: Therapist's management of elbow tendinitis. In Mackin EJ, Callahan AD, Skirven TM et al, editors: *Rehabilitation of the hand and upper extremity*, ed 5, St Louis, 2002, Mosby.)

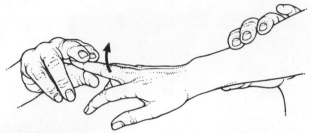

FIGURE 28-5 Middle finger test for radial tunnel syndrome. (From Wadsworth TG: Elbow tendinitis. In Mackin EJ, Callahan AD, Skirven TM et al, editors: *Rehabilitation of the hand and upper extremity*, ed 5, St Louis, 2002, Mosby.)

syndrome (Fig. 28-5). Another test for this syndrome is to tap (percuss) over the superficial radial nerve in a distal to proximal direction. The test result is positive if paresthesias are elicited.[5]

Nonoperative Treatment

Treatment can be divided into two phases, acute and restorative. In the acute phase, the client reports pain at rest that is worsened by daily functional use of the extremity or by range of motion (ROM). The emphasis in this phase is on reducing pain and promoting healing.

> ### ◎ Clinical Pearl
>
> Because lateral epicondylitis is not an inflammatory condition, the traditional use of treatments intended to reduce inflammation (e.g., iontophoresis, phonophoresis, corticosteroid injections, nonsteroidal antiinflammatory drugs) should be questioned.

The application of superficial heat may be beneficial for managing pain and improving tissue extensibility.

Precaution. *Do not use heat if the injury site is inflamed or swollen.*

Ice also may be used for pain relief. The vasoconstrictive effect of ice may help normalize the neovascularization associated with the condition.[6] Continuous-wave ultrasound and high-voltage pulse current (HVPC) have been reported to reduce pain.[1] Although friction massage has been recommended for healing and pain relief, many clients find this technique too painful to tolerate. Fedorczyk[1] notes that more research is needed on the use of soft tissue mobilization to treat tendinosis.

Orthoses are provided in the acute phase to support the wrist extensors. Either a prefabricated or a custom-made volar wrist cock-up orthosis can be used. The wrist should be positioned in 35 degrees of extension. A counterforce brace is worn over the extensor muscle mass, but this should not be used until the client is able to tolerate it comfortably. Most experts suggest removing it at night to avoid nerve compression problems. The counterforce brace is thought to disperse forces and to promote rest of the involved tendon.

Precaution. *Be very careful not to apply a counterforce brace tightly, because this can cause nerve compression. If the client develops sensory symptoms of the superficial radial nerve distribution (dorsal forearm and hand), discontinue use of the counterforce brace.*

In the acute phase, AROM should be within pain-free ranges. Gentle **isometric exercises** (muscle contraction with no movement) in varying positions are done at the elbow, forearm, and wrist. *Make sure that these exercises can be performed without pain.* Isolated AROM of the ECRB can begin in short arcs of motion, with gravity eliminated if necessary, to stimulate and nourish tissue in a pain-free manner. Be sure the client gently contracts the ECRB with a soft fist, to prevent substitution with the EDC. Also make sure the client relaxes the contraction as the motion is released (wrist flexion with digital extension) so that an eccentric ECRB exercise does not occur at this stage, because it most likely would be painful. Proximal ROM and light strengthening of periscapular and hand intrinsic muscles may begin. Functional activities should be included wherever possible with attention given to posture and pacing.

In the restorative phase, the client's pain has improved. AROM and light functional activity are no longer painful. The emphasis in this phase is on helping the extensor mass recover flexibility, strength, and endurance. Periscapular and hand strengthening exercises should be continued, and graded conditioning exercises for the common extensors should be added. Assess ergonomic needs and sports participation with biomechanical modifications as needed.

Isometric exercises are advanced with the use of stronger contractions. As muscle contracts more, the tendon is subjected to greater stress. Progressive resistive exercises with **isotonic contraction** (contraction with muscle shortening) are started with low weight. Gradually, **eccentric contraction** (contraction with muscle lengthening) may be added.

Precaution. *Eccentric exercises should be performed with caution because they are more forceful.*

Eccentric exercise helps restore tissue tolerance of the eccentric loads associated with sports and other functional activities. Eccentric exercise is believed to stimulate collagen production, which is considered the key to recovery from tendinosis. However, favorable responses of eccentric exercise for tennis elbow have not been supported by research to date.[1]

Operative Treatment

Various surgical procedures can be performed for lateral epicondylitis.[7] Orthotic use may be ordered after surgery to support the wrist or elbow or both. ROM guidelines and upgrades for strengthening are determined by the surgeon.

> ### ? Questions to Discuss with the Physician
>
> - Has the client had any corticosteroid injections?
> - Would any x-ray findings affect the progression of therapy?

> ### ◖ What to Say to Clients
>
> #### About Tendinopathy
>
> "Consider this a wake-up call. Your body is telling you that certain structures are overworked and need to recover. Often a few small changes in your body mechanics or improved awareness of posture can make a huge difference in resolving the symptoms. Also, this may be a signal that you should take better care of yourself, get more rest, pamper yourself a little more, exercise more regularly, and delegate more tasks to others if possible.

You know yourself and your body the best, but sometimes clients need to feel permitted to take better care of themselves. So I am instructing you to do so, if possible, because it will help you recover more quickly."

About Orthoses

"The purpose of your orthosis is to rest your muscles so that your pain resolves. Then you will be able to begin gentle, pain-free exercises. However, when tissue is immobilized, it does not get the same blood flow, oxygen, or stimulation; therefore it is important not to use the orthosis more than necessary. As a general guideline, remove the orthosis for any activity you can perform without pain; use the orthosis for any activity that otherwise would be painful."

About Exercises

"You will recover the quickest by avoiding pain. Pain is a sign of re-injury. The best way to heal your tissues is to provide controlled stimulation with exercises that cause no pain. If you cannot tolerate light stimulation, such as a gentle isometric exercise, therapy will focus on resolving the pain so that you become ready to tolerate this stimulation. Thereafter your exercises will be upgraded gradually. If any new exercises cause pain, it is very important to discontinue them."

About Activities of Daily Living

"Your arms and hands work harder when your upper extremity is away from your body. As much as possible, try to keep your elbows at your side when you are using your arms. Use two hands for activities you normally would do with one hand. Do as many of your daily activities as possible in front of you rather than to the side. Avoid reaching whenever possible by moving in closer. Try to use the gentlest force possible when gripping and pinching items such as a pen or the steering wheel. These modifications will promote faster recovery and help reduce your pain."

Evaluation Tips

- Clarify whether the onset of symptoms was due to trauma or was atraumatic.
- Do not cause unnecessary pain with your evaluation.
- Use the Patient-Rated Forearm Evaluation Questionnaire (PRFEQ) (see Chapter 8).
- Find out what activities of daily living (ADL) and recreational activities provoke pain and incorporate this information into your treatment plan.
- Check the client's posture and proximal scapular muscle strength.

Diagnosis-Specific Information That Affects Clinical Reasoning

The smaller, more delicate structures of the upper extremity work harder when the upper arm is unsupported. Biomechanical guidelines for neutral arm position, bilateral frontal UE activity, and softer force with grip and pinch are very helpful.

♥ Tips from the Field

- Built-up and padded handles reduce the forces on joints and tendons. Recommend a sheepskin or padded steering wheel cover, pens with a larger girth, cylindric tubes for toothbrushes, and adapted kitchen implements with larger, padded handles.
- Manual edema mobilization (MEM) techniques promote UE pain relief and can facilitate proximal ROM (see Chapter 3). Light compressive garments may also give comfort. If the lateral epicondyle is quite tender, positioning a chip bag over that area at night may provide relief. The bag usually can be kept in place with a cotton stockinette sleeve.
- The soft, four-finger buddy strap can be helpful for clients with lateral epicondylitis who also have EDC symptoms (see Chapter 1 and the website for more information). This strap helps support the EDC, and clients report that it improves pain-free arcs of motion for digital flexion and extension. The strap can be used in conjunction with a volar wrist orthosis or a counterforce brace. Kinesio Tape has been used successfully for various types of tendinopathy. Courses providing instruction in proper techniques are available.
- Help clients determine which of their daily activities may be provoking pain and suggest changes that promote less strenuous UE biomechanics. Some clients may not realize that they are making progress. Whenever possible, give feedback about objective findings to reassure the client. For example, the arc of pain-free AROM may be greater, the positions of isometric exercises may be upgraded, or the number of exercise repetitions may be increased. A more important point is that clients may now be brushing their teeth with the involved extremity but may not realize that this is a sign of improvement.

≫ Precautions and Concerns

- *Make sure the counterforce brace is not too tight.*
- *Do not encourage any painful exercises.*

Medial Epicondylosis (Golfer's Elbow)

Anatomy

With medial epicondylitis, or golfer's elbow, the medial epicondyle of the humerus is the origin of the symptomatic muscle-tendon units. The pronator teres (PT), flexor carpi radialis (FCR), and palmaris longus (PL) are most often involved, although the flexor carpi ulnaris (FCU) and flexor digitorum superficialis (FDS) also may be implicated.[7]

Medial epicondylitis is less common than lateral epicondylitis. These clients have point tenderness of the medial epicondyle at the common flexor origin. Pain occurs with resisted elbow extension when the forearm is supinated and the wrist is extended. Repetitive or forceful pronation and resisted wrist flexion also cause pain.[8]

Differential diagnoses include cervical radiculopathy, proximal neurovascular compression, and referred pain caused by a shoulder or wrist problem. Ulnar neuropathy or neuritis and ulnar collateral ligament problems are possible associated conditions.[8]

The treatment of medial epicondylitis follows the same guidelines as those for lateral epicondylitis, but the emphasis is on supporting the symptomatic flexor structures rather than the extensors. With medial epicondylitis, the volar wrist orthosis positions the wrist in neutral (Fig. 28-6). Some recommend splinting the wrist in slight flexion, but caution should be used because this position may produce or aggravate symptoms of carpal tunnel syndrome. A counterforce brace is used on the flexor muscle wad. Some clients find the soft, four-finger buddy strap

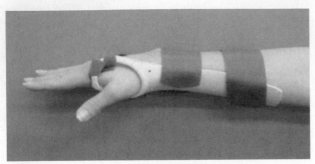

FIGURE 28-6 Volar wrist orthosis with wrist in neutral position.

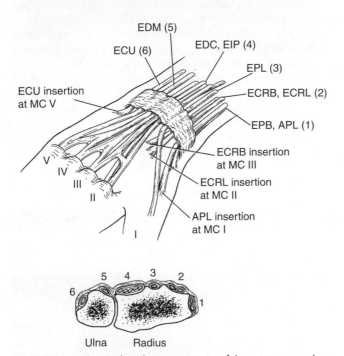

FIGURE 28-7 The six dorsal compartments of the extensor tendons. (From Trumble TE: Tendinitis and epicondylitis. In Trumble TE, editor: *Principles of hand surgery*, Philadelphia, 2000, WB Saunders.)

helpful for pain and gripping function, possibly because it supports the extrinsic flexors.

De Quervain's Disease

Anatomy

The abductor pollicis longus (APL) and the extensor pollicis brevis (EPB) tendons make up the first dorsal compartment of the wrist, where they share a common tendon sheath (Fig. 28-7).

Diagnosis and Pathology

De Quervain's disease is also called *stenosing tenovaginitis* or *stenosing tenosynovitis*. This condition causes pain over the radial styloid process, and the pain can radiate proximally or distally. Pain also occurs with resisted thumb extension or abduction, and Finkelstein's test (Fig. 28-8) frequently has a positive result. Thickening or swelling often is palpable over the symptomatic area. Histologically, clients with de Quervain's disease show fibrotic, thickened tissue with hypervascular changes and tendon degeneration.[3]

The anatomy of the first dorsal compartment varies greatly. The EPB may be absent in 5% to 7% of the population. When present, the EPB may have its own compartment.[9] The APL often has multiple tendinous slips, and these may insert in varying locations.

Forceful, repetitive, or sustained thumb abduction with ulnar deviation of the wrist may contribute to the development of this condition. Activities that may provoke pain include wringing out washrags, opening or closing jars, using scissors, typing on a computer keyboard, playing piano, knitting, racquet sports, or doing needlepoint. Some experts feel that radial deviation of the wrist with pinch is most likely to provoke pain because of the angulation of the involved tendons in this position.[9]

Women are four times more likely than men to have de Quervain's disease. The onset occurs most often between 35 and 55 years of age, but pregnant women in the third trimester and mothers of young children also are at risk.[9] Differential diagnoses include thumb carpometacarpal (CMC) osteoarthritis, scaphoid fracture, wrist arthritis, intersection syndrome, and radial nerve neuritis.

Nonoperative Treatment

A forearm-based, thumb spica orthosis that leaves the interphalangeal (IP) joint free is used to prevent painful motions. Some recommend positioning the wrist in neutral and the thumb in

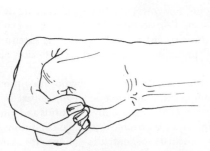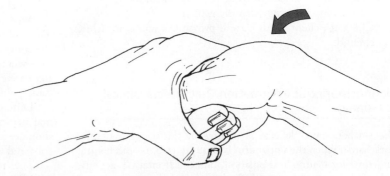

FIGURE 28-8 Finkelstein's test. (From Magee DJ: *Orthopedic physical assessment,* Philadelphia, 2002, WB Saunders.)

radial abduction. Others recommend slight wrist extension of about 20 degrees with the thumb in extension. I suggest finding a pain-free position that allows light thumb function if possible. A radial or volar orthosis may be used. The radial gutter spica orthosis seems to allow more UE function but should not be used unless the client can wear this orthosis without pain. Studies suggest greater clinical success with this condition when an orthosis is combined with corticosteroid injection, compared with splinting alone.[9] As pain resolves, the client may progress to a soft or semirigid orthosis.

Treatments and graded exercises have the same role in de Quervain's disease as in lateral epicondylitis. Isometric exercise of the APL and EPB, short arc AROM of these structures, isolated wrist flexion and extension, and isolated thumb IP flexion and extension should be included.

> ### ◎ Clinical Pearl
>
> Symptom-provoking motions of radial and ulnar deviation and thumb composite flexion and extension should be avoided until the client can perform these movements without pain.

Strengthening exercises for the APL and EPB can be added gradually when pain has resolved. Eccentric exercises have been described, but caution is warranted to avoid causing pain or injury.

Operative Treatment

Surgical release of the first dorsal compartment is an option for clients in whom conservative treatment has failed. High success rates have been reported for this procedure.[4] After surgery, the surgeon indicates the type of orthosis to be used and the precautions to be observed. Generally, the orthosis is weaned over a few weeks with isolated AROM progressing to composite motions of the APL and EPB. Strengthening exercises are begun when they have been approved by the surgeon, usually after a few weeks. Scar management and desensitization are important aspects of therapy.

> ### ⁇ Questions to Discuss with the Physician

(See Lateral Epicondylosis)

> ### 〔〕 What to Say to Clients

About Tendinopathy
(See Lateral Epicondylosis)

About Orthoses
(See Lateral Epicondylosis)

About Exercises
(See Lateral Epicondylosis)

About Activities of Daily Living
"Moving your wrist from side to side [demonstrate radial and ulnar deviation] with your thumb held either straight or bent is likely to cause pain. Try to keep your wrist straight so that the long finger is in line with the middle of your forearm. From this position you may be able to perform light pinch and grip activities without pain."

About Computer Ergonomics
"Try not to deviate your wrist (demonstrate radial and ulnar deviation) when working at the computer keyboard. Instead, keep your elbows at your side and pivot from the elbow, not at the wrist. You may want to investigate computer keyboard designs that make it easier to maintain this neutral position."

> ### Evaluation Tips
>
> - Irritation of the superficial radial nerve may be present (Fig. 28-9). Note this in your evaluation findings.
> - Note whether the client wears a watchband or tight bracelet; if so, suggest that it be worn more loosely on the contralateral side.
> - Clients often test their symptoms by performing a Finkelstein's stretch on themselves to see whether this motion is still painful. I ask them not to do this for at least 1 week. Thereafter, if they must do it, I recommend that they try it once only, as gently as possible. The presence of more pain-free passive stretch than in the previous week is a favorable sign.

Diagnosis-Specific Information That Affects Clinical Reasoning

Most ADL's require combined wrist and thumb motions, which makes de Quervain's disease very challenging to treat. Providing more than one orthotic option often is helpful.

> ### ♡ Tips from the Field
>
> - Pad the dorsal radial wrist area before splinting, because the superficial radial nerve may be irritated or may become irritated. If the client has had surgery, scar sensitivity and hypersensitivity may be noted at this site. Paper tape over the radial wrist can help with hypersensitivity. Splint the client in the position of maximum comfort and function, if both are possible, but be sure the position is pain free.

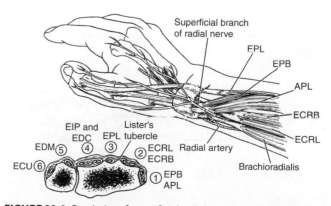

FIGURE 28-9 Proximity of superficial radial nerve and first dorsal compartment. (From Trumble TE: Tendinitis and epicondylitis. In Trumble TE, editor: *Principles of hand surgery*, Philadelphia, 2000, WB Saunders.)

- Provide materials for built-up pens and cylindrical cushions for toothbrushes or kitchen implements. Instruct the client to use the softest force necessary when pinching. The more quickly the client can begin pain-free functional use, the better. Remind the client that pain-free motion most nourishes and stimulates the production and organization of collagen.

Monitor for signs of superficial radial nerve irritation; if these appear, modify the orthosis immediately.

Digital Stenosing Tenosynovitis (Trigger Finger)

Anatomy

With **digital stenosing tenosynovitis,** or trigger finger, a discrepancy exists between the volume of the flexor tendon and the size of the pulley lumen. The site of the problem typically is the first annular pulley (A1), which lies volar to the metacarpophalangeal (MCP) joint in the area of the distal palmar crease (Fig. 28-10). The area between the A1 and A2 pulleys is described as a *hypovascular watershed,* which predisposes the tissue to problems of attrition due to lack of nourishment.[10]

Diagnosis and Pathology

The characteristic symptom of trigger finger is an inability to perform smooth digital flexion or extension. The ring finger and thumb most often are involved, followed by the long, index, and small fingers. Trigger finger can occur in several digits. Most clients describe a painful snapping as they make a fist and an inability to actively extend the affected digit. Palpation in the area of the A1 pulley elicits pain, and crepitus often is heard with active composite digital flexion. When symptoms are more severe, the digit locks in flexion and this can be very painful.[11]

The inflammatory pathology of trigger finger is classified as either nodular or diffuse, based on palpation of the tendon sheath. With nodular inflammation, the swelling is contained and a distinct nodule can be palpated as the digit triggers. With diffuse inflammation, the swelling is less defined. Nodular trigger fingers respond more successfully to conservative treatment. Symptoms that last longer than 6 months are less likely to respond to nonoperative treatment.[11]

Women develop trigger finger more often than men. Differential diagnoses include flexor tendon masses, such as tumors, ganglia, or lipomas. Associated diagnoses include diabetes,

rheumatoid arthritis, gout, carpal tunnel syndrome, and Dupuytren's contracture.[11] Children also can have trigger finger, typically at the thumb. This usually is caused by nodules on the flexor pollicis longus (FPL) and is corrected with surgery.

Nonoperative Treatment

Evans and colleagues[10] described a comprehensive program for conservative management of trigger finger in clients who did not have rheumatoid arthritis. Clients must refrain from all activities that aggravate the symptoms (i.e., gripping activities). A hand-based, volar orthosis is fabricated to support the involved MCP joint or joints at 0 degrees (neutral position). The orthosis must allow full IP flexion (Fig. 28-11). The client is taught to perform a hook fist (complete flexion and extension of IPs with MCP neutral) with the orthosis on, 20 repetitions every 2 hours while awake. After hook exercise, the orthosis is removed for gentle place and hold, full fist motions avoiding locking. The client is instructed to massage the flexor tendon sheath and palm area. If a flexion contracture is present, a night gutter orthosis is used to correct the contracture.

The client follows this program for 3 weeks and then is re-evaluated. If no improvement is seen, the physician decides whether corticosteroid injection or surgery should be done. If improvement is noted, the program is continued for a total of 6 weeks. It is extremely important that clients avoid all possibility of triggering throughout the program.

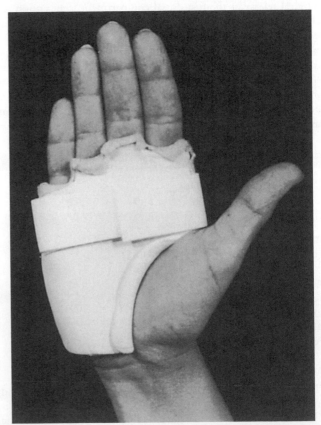

FIGURE 28-11 Hand-based volar orthosis for treatment of trigger finger. (From Evans RB, Hunter JM, Burkhalter WE: Conservative management of the trigger finger: a new approach, *J Hand Ther* 1:60, 1988.)

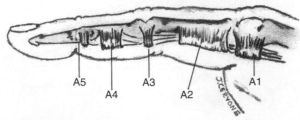

FIGURE 28-10 Finger annular pulleys. (From Falkenstein N, Weiss-Lessard S: *Hand rehabilitation: A quick reference guide and review,* St. Louis, 1999, Mosby.)

Operative Treatment

Operative treatment involves surgical release of the A1 pulley. Surgical and percutaneous techniques can be used for this purpose. After surgery, clients may be sent to hand therapy for edema control, scar management, ROM, or orthosis if needed. Most clients do not need postoperative therapy.

? Question to Discuss with the Physician

Has the client had any corticosteroid injections?

() What to Say to Clients

About Orthoses and Exercise

"Your orthotic prevents your finger from triggering. Along with the proper exercises, this will better nourish the tendon and help it to heal. It is very important to perform the exercises gently and to accomplish full motions in bending and straightening to recover flexibility and function of the tendon."

About Activities of Daily Living

"Please think about any activities you are doing that may apply repeated pressure to your palm at the painful area. For example, using the palm of your hand like a hammer or repeated use of a staple gun can contribute to trigger finger symptoms. Sometimes scissors rub the area inside the affected thumb. Gardening may contribute to the symptoms if you grip the tools tightly for a long period. It will help to change these activities, to frequently change hand and upper extremity positions, to take a break regularly to stretch and reposition yourself, and to try padded gloves. We want you to be able to do the activities you enjoy, but initially some changes must be made so that the symptoms can improve."

Evaluation Tips

- Assess for flexion contractures and treat accordingly.
- Distinguish between possible extrinsic flexor tightness and joint contracture.
- Document pain at the A1 pulley.
- Document crepitus with composite active digital flexion.
- Monitor edema.
- Check that the symptom occurs at the A1 pulley (symptoms sometimes can occur at a different pulley).

Diagnosis-Specific Information That Affects Clinical Reasoning

Composite digital flexion is very difficult to avoid in daily life, and certain tasks are difficult to perform with the MCP orthosis. In some cases an alternative orthosis can be helpful for maximizing function while preventing triggering. For example, a small proximal interphalangeal (PIP) or distal interphalangeal (DIP) volar gutter orthosis can be used as long as it prevents triggering. The orthosis must prevent composite digital flexion, and this is achieved by splinting one of the digital joints. Use of a PIP or DIP volar gutter orthosis may enhance clients' ability to perform

some of their daily activities. It also may minimize the risk of maceration by varying the areas of orthotic contact and coverage.

♡ Tips from the Field

- Trigger finger orthoses should be worn at night to prevent locking. For the thumb, the orthosis can limit either MCP or IP motion. A volar IP gutter orthosis is very easy to use and can be taped in place if necessary. The distal volar end should be trimmed to allow volar thumb pad exposure for sensory input and improved function. The hand-based MCP orthosis can be similar to that used for thumb CMC osteoarthritis (see Chapter 33).
- As with the other diagnoses, teach your clients not to test their symptoms, because this can interfere with their recovery. Sometimes treating the edema is the most important step in resolving trigger finger symptoms.

➢ Precautions and Concerns

- *Warn the client to avoid any activities that could result in triggering for 6 weeks.*
- *Modify place and hold exercises so that no triggering occurs; this may mean limiting these exercises to less than full composite digital flexion initially.*
- *Watch for and manage skin maceration related to orthotic use.*

Other Forms of Tendinopathy

Table 28-1 presents a summary of the involved structures, provocative tests, differential diagnoses, and orthotic considerations for the common forms of tendinitis/tendinosis described in this chapter. It also provides an overview of other UE diagnoses seen by hand therapists.

CASE STUDIES

CASE STUDY 28-1 ▪

D.L., a 30-year-old, left-dominant male, was referred to hand therapy with a diagnosis of left wrist pain. He reported that he was unemployed, was receiving disability payments, and that he was taking medication for obsessive-compulsive disorder. He had a history of substance abuse. The client had left ulnar wrist pain that worsened with wrist ulnar deviation and flexion. He had swelling at the ulnar wrist and pain over the pisiform. The therapist asked him if he had been doing any activities recently that might have aggravated his symptoms. He stated that his favorite pastime was to twirl scarves and that he was working on a scarf twirling routine that he hoped would become an entertainment skit for future employment. He was twirling scarves with repetitive extreme wrist flexion/ulnar deviation motions for 6 hours daily. He rarely took rest breaks. He stated that he liked the repetition of the activity, that it helped pass the time, and that he found it comforting to do.

D.L. was fitted with a custom forearm ulnar gutter orthosis and was instructed to wear it for pain relief. He was started on proximal and postural exercises. Heat and ultrasound were used

TABLE 28-1   Overview of Tendinopathies of the Upper Extremity

Diagnosis	Structures Most Involved	Provocative Tests	Differential Diagnoses	Orthotic Considerations
Lateral epicondylosis	ECRB, EDC	• Cozen's test • Mill's test • Palpation of lateral epicondyle • Resisted wrist extension • Gripping with elbow extended	• Cervical radiculopathy • Proximal neurovascular entrapment • Radial tunnel syndrome	• Volar wrist cock-up orthosis at 35 degrees wrist extension • Counterforce brace on extensor wad • Soft four-finger buddy strap
Radial tunnel syndrome	Superficial radial nerve	• Middle finger test • Percussion of superficial radial nerve (distal to proximal)	• Lateral epicondylitis	• *No counterforce brace*
Medial epicondylosis	Pronator teres, FCR, PL	• Palpation of medial epicondyle • Resisted elbow extension with supination and wrist extension • Repetitive or forceful pronation • Resisted wrist flexion • Passive composite extension(elbow, wrist, digits)	• Cervical radiculopathy • Proximal neurovascular entrapment • Ulnar neuropathy • Elbow ulnar collateral ligament problem	• Volar wrist cock-up orthosis with wrist in neutral • Counterforce brace on flexor wad • Soft four-finger buddy strap
de Quervain's disease	APL and EPB at first dorsal compartment	• Finkelstein's test • Resisted thumb extension or abduction • Pain/thickening at first dorsal compartment	• Osteoarthritis of thumb CMC joint or wrist • Scaphoid fracture • Intersection syndrome • Radial nerve neuritis	• Forearm-based thumb spica cast with IP joint free
Digital stenosing tenosynovitis	Digital flexor tendon at the A1 pulley	• Tenderness at A1 pulley • Possible palpable nodule • Crepitus with active digital flexion • Snapping or locking with active composite digital flexion	• Flexor tendon tumors, ganglia, lipoma	• Hand-based orthosis with MCP joint in neutral • Digital volar gutter orthosis with PIP joint in neutral, MCP and DIP joints free
Intersection syndrome	APL and EPB muscle bellies, approximately 4 cm proximal to wrist where they intersect with ECRB and ECRL	• Swelling locally at muscle bellies • Pain with resisted wrist extension • Similar provocative tests as for de Quervain's tenosynovitis	• de Quervain's tenosynovitis	• Same as for de Quervain's tenosynovitis
EPL tendinitis	EPL at Lister's tubercle	• Pain at Lister's tubercle • Resisted composite thumb extension • Passive composite thumb flexion	• De Quervain's tenosynovitis • Intersection syndrome	• Forearm-based thumb spica cast with composite thumb extension, IP joint included
ECU tendinitis	ECU	• Forearm supination with wrist ulnar deviation • Pain at ulnar wrist	• DRUJ instability • TFCC tear • Ulnocarpal abutment	• Forearm-based ulnar gutter orthosis • *Ulnar head padded as needed for comfort*
FCR tendinitis	FCR	• Resisted wrist flexion and radial deviation • Pain with passive wrist extension • Pain over proximal wrist crease and at scaphoid tubercle	• Ganglion cysts • Thumb CMC osteoarthritis • Scaphoid fracture • de Quervain's tenosynovitis	• Volar wrist cock-up orthosis with wrist in neutral or position of comfort
FCU tendinitis	FCU	• Pain with palpation over pisiform • Resisted wrist flexion and ulnar deviation • Passive wrist extension and radial deviation	• Pisiform fracture • Pisotriquetral arthritis	• Forearm-based ulnar gutter orthosis

APL, Abductor pollicis longus; *CMC,* carpometacarpal; *DIP,* distal interphalangeal; *DRUJ,* distal radioulnar joint; *ECRB,* extensor carpi radialis brevis; *ECRL,* extensor carpi radialis longus; *ECU,* extensor carpi ulnaris; *EDC,* extensor digitorum communis; *EPB,* extensor pollicis brevis; *EPL,* extensor pollicis longus; *FCR,* flexor carpi radialis; *FCU,* flexor carpi ulnaris; *IP,* interphalangeal; *MCP,* metacarpophalangeal; *PIP,* proximal interphalangeal; *PL,* palmaris longus; *TFCC,* triangulofibrocartilage complex.
Modified from Lee MP, Biafora SJ, Zelouf DS: Management of hand and wrist tendinopathies. In Skirven TM et al, editors: *Rehabilitation of the hand and upper extremity,* ed 6, Philadelphia, 2011, Mosby; Evans RB, Hunter JM, Burkhalter WE: Conservative management of the trigger finger: a new approach, *J Hand Ther* 1:59-68, 1988; Trumble TE: Tendinitis and epicondylitis. In Trumble TE, editor: *Principles of hand surgery,* Philadelphia, 2000, WB Saunders; Lindner-Tons S, Ingell K: An alternative splint design for trigger finger, *J Hand Ther* 11:206-208, 1998; and Verdon ME: Overuse syndromes of the hand and wrist, *Prim Care* 23:305-319, 1996.

for pain relief (he had tried ice but did not like it). Gentle AROM for wrist flexion and extension, differential flexor tendon gliding, and light digital strengthening were started when his pain had subsided. These routines were presented as a temporary replacement for twirling with the explanation that they would help his tissue condition improve so that he could resume twirling. D.L. was eager to resume twirling scarves and found it difficult to refrain from performing this activity. In the clinic he practiced modified scarf twirling with short arcs of wrist motion that did not cause pain. This activity was incorporated into his exercise program; he was cautioned not to exceed 5 minutes per hour initially. D.L. followed this guideline carefully and gradually was able to increase the twirling time and to wean off the wrist orthosis. He learned that if he monitored his posture, performed home exercises, and took frequent, brief rest breaks, he could perform longer sessions of scarf twirling once again.

CASE STUDY 28-2 ■

A 45-year-old veterinarian was referred to hand therapy with trigger thumb. She had considerable pain in the area of the A1 pulley of the thumb, which was locking in flexion at night. She would awaken with pain when this occurred. She was seen for fabrication of a hand-based thumb orthosis that supported the MP joint, which was to be used at night, and a very thin (⅛ inch) thumb IP volar gutter orthosis, to be used during the day. Care was taken to ensure that the day orthosis would fit inside her sterile gloves for animal surgery. In discussing her biomechanics and contributing activities, she realized that she used surgical tools that often pressed against the thumb A1 pulley, provoking symptoms. Simulation in the therapy clinic led to alternative tool positions that protected the A1 pulley area. She was seen only once, but she reported 1 week later by phone that she was doing very well clinically.

References

1. Fedorczyk JM: Tendinopathies of the elbow, wrist, and hand: histopathology and clinical considerations, *J Hand Ther* 25:191–201, 2012.
2. Nordin M, Frankel VH: *Basic biomechanics of the musculoskeletal system,* ed 3, Baltimore, 2001, Lippincott Williams & Wilkins.
3. Ashe MC, McCauley T, Khan KM: Tendinopathies in the upper extremity: a paradigm shift, *J Hand Ther* 17:329–334, 2004.
4. McAuliffe JA: Tendon disorders of the hand and wrist, *J Hand Surg Am* 35:846–853, 2010.
5. Fedorczyk JM: Elbow tendinopathies: clinical presentation and therapist's management of tennis elbow. In Skirven TM, Osterman AL, Fedorczyk JM, et al: *Rehabilitation of the hand and upper extremity*, ed 6, Philadelphia, 2011, Mosby, pp 1098–1108.
6. Khan KM, Cook JL, Taunton JE, et al: Overuse tendinosis, not tendinitis: part 1: a new paradigm for a difficult clinical problem, *Phys Sportsmed* 28(5):38–48, 2000.
7. Bozentka DJ, Lopez F: Elbow tendinopathies: medical, surgical, and postoperative management. In Skirven TM, Osterman AL, Fedorczyk JM, et al: *Rehabilitation of the hand and upper extremity*, ed 6, Philadelphia, 2011, Mosby, pp 1109–1114.
8. Fedorczyk JM: Therapist's management of elbow tendinitis. In Mackin EJ, Callinan N, Skirven TM, et al, editors: *Rehabilitation of the hand and upper extremity*, ed 5, St Louis, 2002, Mosby, pp 1271–1281.
9. Lee MP, Biafora SJ, Zelouf DS: Management of hand and wrist tendinopathies. In Skirven TM, Osterman AL, Fedorczyk JM, et al, editors: *Rehabilitation of the hand and upper extremity*, ed 6, Philadelphia, 2011, Mosby, pp 569–588.
10. Evans RB, Hunter JM, Burkhalter WE: conservative management of the trigger finger: a new approach, *J Hand Ther* 1(2):59–68, 1988.
11. Saldana MJ: Trigger digits: diagnosis and treatment, *J Am Acad Orthop Surg* 9(4):246–252, 2001.

29 Finger Sprains and Deformities

Gary Solomon

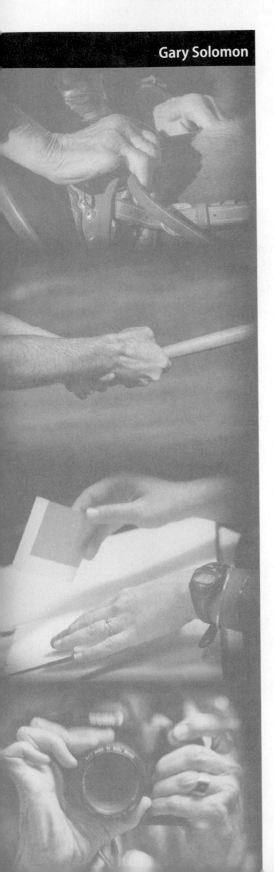

Digital injuries and deformities are common reasons why patients are referred to therapy for treatment. Many patients expect digital injuries to heal on their own, and sometimes do not recognize that the injury can lead to permanent deformity.

Patients may be referred to therapy with the diagnosis of "sprain / strain" for a finger or thumb but may actually have unidentified serious injuries, such as gamekeeper's thumb or a **volar plate (VP)** injury. This may be especially likely when the referral comes from a physician who is not a hand surgeon. In this situation, the therapist has an opportunity to identify the clinical findings and facilitate appropriate treatment.

Injuries to the digits occur often in sports. Football players have a high incidence of proximal interphalangeal (PIP) joint injuries. In these sports-related injuries, dorsal dislocations are more common than volar dislocations. Boutonniere deformities frequently occur in basketball players. Mallet injuries occur when the player's fingertip strikes a helmet or ball.[1] Therapists whose clients participate in sports can expect to see these common sprains and finger injuries as part of their caseload.

Many non-athletes enjoy sports activities after work, and these "weekend warriors" often sustain finger injuries that initially go untreated. Clients who later seek medical attention may have chronic pain, edema, and stiffness. More long-term problems, such as persistent residual pain and swelling, can be very challenging to treat.

Mallet fingers, boutonniere deformities, and swan neck deformities are common finger injuries that can be recognized by a hand therapist. They can be treated successfully by precise management. The trauma and disease processes that cause these deformities vary, but regardless of the cause, the therapist's detailed knowledge of pathomechanics and therapy guidelines helps to manage and direct the course of treatment.

Mallet Finger

A finger with drooping of the distal interphalangeal (DIP) joint is called a **mallet finger** (Fig. 29-1).[2] Typically the DIP can be passively corrected to neutral, but the client is unable to actively extend it; this condition is called a **DIP extensor lag.** If the DIP joint cannot be passively extended to neutral, the condition is called a **DIP flexion contracture.** A DIP flexion contracture seldom is present early after injury; however, if the injury goes untreated, this problem may develop.

Anatomy

The DIP joint of the finger is a **ginglymus joint,** or hinge joint. It is **bicondylar** (it has two condyles) and is similar to the PIP joint in its capsular ligaments. The terminal extensor tendon and terminal flexor tendon attach to the most proximal edge of the distal phalanx. This insertion contributes to the joint's dynamic stability.[3]

Diagnosis and Pathology

A mallet injury frequently is caused by a blow to the fingertip with flexion force or by axial loading while the DIP is extended.[4] The terminal tendon is avulsed. An avulsion fracture also may occur and should be ruled out. Laceration injuries (extensor zone I) are another cause of this deformity. Anterior/posterior (A/P) and true lateral x-rays typically are obtained. In addition, the PIP joint should be examined for possible injury.[5]

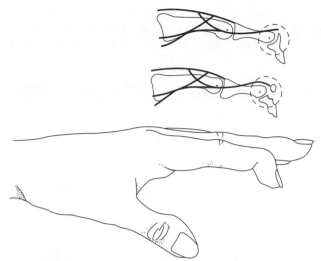

FIGURE 29-1 Mallet finger deformity. A fracture may also occur with this injury. (From American Society for Surgery of the Hand: *The hand: examination and diagnosis,* ed 2, Edinburgh, 1983, Churchill Livingstone.)

Timelines and Healing

The DIP joint is immobilized by an orthosis in full extension for approximately 6 weeks to allow the delicate terminal tendon to heal. The joint should not be allowed to flex even briefly during this period of immobilization. After 6 weeks, the client is weaned off the orthosis while the therapist observes for DIP extensor lag.

Non-Operative Treatment

An orthosis is fabricated to hold the DIP joint in extension to slight hyperextension, depending on the physician's preference. If hyperextension is recommended, the therapist should make sure the position of hyperextension is less than that which causes skin blanching. Exceeding tissue tolerance in DIP hyperextension can compromise circulation and nutrition to the healing tissues.[6]

Many types of DIP orthosis designs are available, and clients sometimes need more than one type (Fig. 29-2). They may also need an orthosis designated for showering; the client can carefully remove it after showering, according to the therapist's instructions, and replace it with a dry orthosis. In this way, the skin is protected against maceration, which occurs if a wet splint is left on a digit. Casting also can be used when client compliance is a concern.

Perforated material is recommended to allow airflow. The PIP should be allowed to fully flex without disturbing the position of DIP extension. If multiple orthoses are provided, consider one dorsal and one volar so that the patient may switch to protect skin integrity.

If the DIP joint cannot be passively extended to neutral, serial adjustments of the orthosis may be done. If necessary, a small static progressive DIP extension orthosis can be used.[7] Edema is treated as appropriate, and normal PIP active range of motion (AROM) with the DIP immobilized is promoted. Dorsal edema and tenderness over the DIP are common and can interfere with full DIP extension.

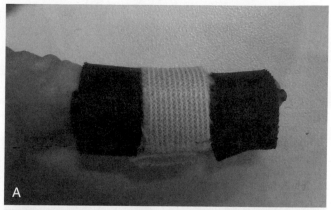

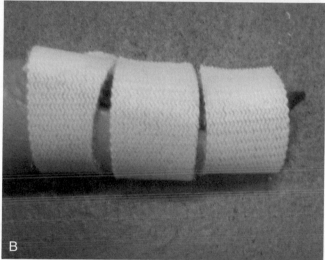

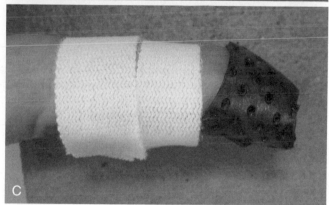

FIGURE 29-2 Mallet orthoses. A, Custom thermoplastic volar. **B,** Dorsal. **C,** Combination dorsal/volar. (Reproduced with permission, Gary Solomon, MS, OTR/L, CHT.)

After 6 weeks of continuous orthosis use, if no DIP extensor lag is present and the physician approves, gentle AROM can be started. A template may be provided (Fig. 29-3) to allow the patient to actively flex and extend the DIP joint from 0° to 25° for 1 week, and then adjusted to allow 35° of flexion the next week. If no lag is present, gentle composite AROM should then be permitted. The therapist should instruct the client to avoid forceful or quick grasping or forceful DIP flexion in the early phase of AROM therapy, and emphasis during exercise should be

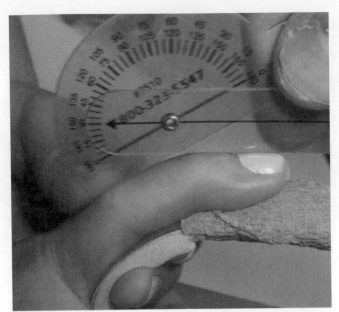

FIGURE 29-3 Exercise template for initial protected AROM. (Reproduced with permission, Gary Solomon, MS, OTR/L, CHT.)

on DIP extension. It is very important to watch for DIP extensor lag. If DIP extensor lag occurs, the orthosis use and exercise progression must be adjusted. Passive motion to restore DIP flexion should not be used except in cases of extreme stiffness with limited progress with AROM only. Passive flexion will significantly increase the risk of extensor lag especially early in the rehabilitation process.

The use of the DIP extension orthosis is typically continued between gentle AROM sessions initially, and then gradually weaned over a 2 to 3 week period. Night orthosis use typically continues for an additional 2 to 3 weeks. If DIP extensor lag recurs, daytime use should be reinstituted. If orthosis use does not correct the DIP extensor lag, surgery may be needed to correct the problem.

If there is a mild extensor lag, the therapist should monitor closely for the development of a secondary swan neck deformity. If PIP hyperextension is noted, then an orthosis that blocks end range PIP extension while allowing full flexion is recommended.

Although the use of an orthosis is best initiated as soon as possible after injury, even a delayed regimen can be effective.[8] Operative intervention can produce complications; therefore, non-operative solutions often are well worth the effort.

Operative Treatment

If the mallet injury has associated large fracture fragments (greater than 30% of the joint surface) or the patient asserts that they cannot be compliant with orthosis use, surgery may be necessary. A variety of procedures can be performed to treat this injury.[4,9,10] Surgical complications include the possibility of infection and nail deformities.

The client may be sent to therapy with the DIP pinned for edema control as needed, instruction in pin site care if the Kirschner wire protrudes through the skin, and a protective orthosis. When the pins are removed, AROM is initiated. The

DIP extension orthosis is continued when the pins are removed and then use is gradually weaned. As with non-operative treatment, the therapist should observe for DIP extensor lag.

? Questions to Discuss with the Physician

- Is there a fracture (bony mallet)?
- Are you anticipating approximately 6 weeks continuous immobilization?
- Does the physician prefer the DIP in neutral position or in hyperextension?
- If the DIP is pinned, how long will the pin remain in place?
- Will an orthosis be needed after pin removal?

( ) What to Say to Clients

About the Injury

"Here is a diagram of the anatomy of the distal digit and the terminal tendon. The terminal tendon is very delicate, and in order to heal, it needs continuous, uninterrupted DIP support for about 6 weeks." Reiterate this concept as necessary until the client appears to understand the importance of continuous DIP extension.

About the Orthosis

"It is important for us to practice techniques for putting the orthosis on and taking it off while maintaining DIP extension. One technique is to keep the hand palm down on the table and carefully slide the orthosis forward. A second technique is to use your thumb to provide support under the fingertip while using your other hand to remove the orthosis, sliding it forward. To reapply, maintain DIP extension with your other hand as you put the orthosis back on."

Work with the client to devise a schedule for removing the orthosis one or two times daily to clean the orthosis and check the skin. Make sure the client knows the proper techniques for keeping the DIP always supported in extension.

Emphasize the importance of skin care: "Moisture that is trapped inside may lead to skin problems such as maceration, which must be avoided." Teach the client what skin maceration looks like.

About Exercise

"Initially, I am going to have you remove the orthosis four to six times a day and gently bend the tip down to the template. In 1 week, I will increase the amount of bending permitted, and the following week, you will begin making a full fist."

"Avoiding resistive or powerful gripping or forceful bending or flexion of the injured fingers and of the entire hand is important to prevent any strain on the healing terminal tendon."

Instruct the client in AROM for the uninvolved digits and especially PIP flexion of the injured digit: "Achieving full PIP active flexion is very important. The injured finger could stiffen at the PIP if it is not exercised gently. It is very important to prevent the uninjured digits from stiffening." Demonstrate and practice gentle PIP blocking exercises, isolated flexor digitorum superficialis (FDS) and "straight ist" motions with the DIP orthosis in place (Fig. 29-4).

Evaluation Tips

- The client's finger is likely to be tender and swollen over the dorsal DIP area. Use a gentle touch around this area.
- Circumferential measurements may be best deferred to avoid causing pain by applying or cinching a tape measure or similar measurement device. Also, measuring the DIP joint is difficult while maintaining and supporting the digit in full DIP extension.
- Assess the client for digital hypermobility. Observe for DIP extensor lag or PIP hyperextension of other digits and treat accordingly (see description of swan neck deformity).
- Check isolated DIP flexion of other digits gently while the injured DIP is immobilized if the client can isolate this without stressing the terminal tendon of the injured digit. This helps prevent the development of a quadriga effect.

Precaution. *Avoid volumetric measurement, because this would leave the DIP unsupported, which is contraindicated.*

Diagnosis-Specific Information that Affects Clinical Reasoning

Individualize the treatment based on your observation and evaluation. If DIP hyperextension has been ordered but the client cannot tolerate it, support the DIP in a tolerable position, and see the client every few days for splint modification until the desired position is achieved. Notify the physician if full DIP extension or hyperextension cannot be achieved in the orthosis.

If edema is significant, assume that you will need to readjust the orthosis as edema resolves, and schedule recheck visits accordingly. Upgrade the interventions as appropriate for edema management.

A client who is hypermobile and has laxity of the uninjured digits is at greater risk of developing a secondary swan neck deformity.

This client needs an orthosis that prevents PIP hyperextension and supports the DIP in extension. Teach clients the isolated FDS exercise with the DIP orthosis in place.

Make sure your client is well trained in monitoring skin tolerances to the orthosis. Using more than one style of orthosis can help prevent skin problems.

Precaution. *Clients should call for a recheck if any skin problems occur.*

♡ Tips from the Field

Orthoses

- Show the client pictures or samples of DIP orthoses. Explain your recommendation in terms of comfort, effectiveness, and adjustability. Ask clients about their preferences. Advise the client to tape (or use Coban) the orthosis in place at night to decrease the risk of the orthosis sliding off during sleep.
- Ask the client about their daily activities. If they perform a lot of fine motor tasks, consider a dorsal mallet orthosis.
- While fabricating the orthosis, keeping the PIP joint in flexion decreases the flexion tension on the FDP and makes it easier to fully extend the DIP joint.
- For a volar orthosis, it is critical that the lateral and medial borders are not greater than half of the width of the digit in order for the straps to contour and hold securely.
- Use a softer strap directly over the DIP joint where the skin is typically sensitive.
- Small orthoses are not always the quickest to make. Allow time to fine-tune the splint and re-adjust it as needed.
- Clients often appreciate having a separate orthosis to use in the shower. Also, they can change into the dry orthosis after the shower, which helps prevent maceration.
- When beginning active flexion of the DIP, trace the DIP in full extension from a lateral view onto a business card. This allows the patient to self-monitor for any developing extensor lag between therapy sessions (Fig. 29-5).

Exercise Template

Alumifoam makes an excellent template to use as a guide when patients begin active DIP flexion. The alumifoam template is also easy to adjust on subsequent visits as increased flexion is permitted.

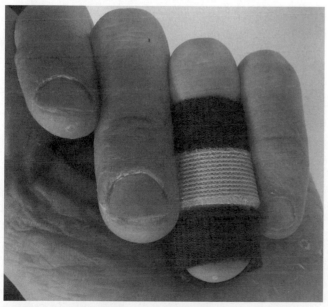

FIGURE 29-4 Straight fist with mallet orthosis permitting full PIP flexion. (Reproduced with permission, Gary Solomon, MS, OTR/L, CHT.)

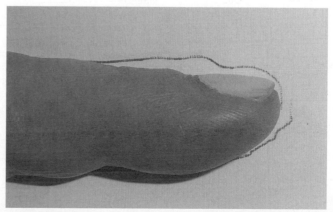

FIGURE 29-5 Tracing lateral view of distal interphalangeal (DIP) position on card for patient to use as reference during home exercise program (HEP). (Reproduced with permission, Gary Solomon, MS, OTR/L, CHT.)

Client Compliance

Some clients need more supervision and follow-up than others. Reasons to recheck the client more often include 1) resolving or fluctuating edema, 2) wound care, 3) PIP stiffness, 4) risk of swan neck deformity developing, and 5) questionable technique for putting on and taking off the orthosis. The therapy note should document whether the client demonstrates good technique in therapy and at follow-up.

> **Precautions and Concerns**
>
> - *Check for skin maceration.*
> - *Emphasize the importance of avoiding forceful or resistive gripping or quick flexion motions.*
> - *Monitor for the development of PIP hyperextension, especially if the client demonstrates laxity of the digits.*
> - *If the orthosis is taped on at night, caution the client to avoid circumferential taping, because this could produce a tourniquet effect.*

Boutonniere Deformity

Anatomy

With a **boutonniere deformity,** the finger postures in PIP flexion and DIP hyperextension (Fig. 29-6). The injury may be open or closed. With a closed injury, the boutonniere deformity may not develop immediately but may become noticeable within 2 or 3 weeks after the injury.[8] The client may have a PIP extensor lag or, with an older injury, a PIP flexion contracture. This distinction affects the therapy choices.

Diagnosis and Pathology

A boutonniere deformity involves disruption of the central slip of the extensor tendon, which normally inserts into the dorsal base

of the middle phalanx. The disruption of the central slip causes the **lateral bands** to slip volar to the PIP joint axis of motion, creating flexor forces on the PIP joint.[11] The imbalance results in hyperextension of the DIP joint.[12] With this DIP posture, the **oblique retinacular ligament (ORL)** of Landsmeer, which is located at the dorsal DIP joint, is at risk of becoming tight. A **pseudoboutonniere deformity** is actually an injury to the PIP VP and is usually the result of a PIP hyperextension injury.

> ◎ **Clinical Pearl**
>
> With a pseudoboutonniere deformity, the damage occurs at the volar surface. With a boutonniere deformity, the damage occurs at the dorsal surface.[1]

Timelines and Healing

A PIP extension thermoplastic orthosis or circumferential cast[13] is typically used day and night for up to 6 weeks (Fig. 29-7). When ROM of the PIP is initiated, flexion to 30° to 45° is typically permitted and advanced 15° per week as long as no lag is present (Fig. 29-8). This is followed by 3 weeks of nighttime and intermittent daytime orthosis use. The orthosis is used during the time needed for the central slip to re-establish tissue continuity and for correction of the deformity.[8]

A variation from complete immobilization for 6 weeks is a short arc motion[6] protocol that combines immobilization with intermittent controlled PIP motion to 30° to 40° of flexion during therapy sessions. After 3 weeks, the patient is provided a template for PIP ROM at home, and the template is advanced 10° to 15° per week if no lag is present.

Non-Operative Treatment

The ability to passively extend the PIP is a common indicator for non-operative treatment with PIP immobilization in extension. The MP and DIP are not included in the orthosis. Serial

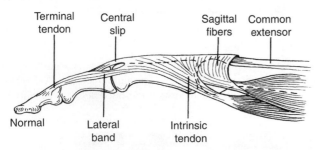

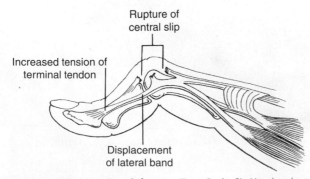

FIGURE 29-6 Boutonniere deformity. (From Burke SL: *Hand and upper extremity rehabilitation: a practical guide,* ed 3, St Louis, 2005, Churchill Livingstone.)

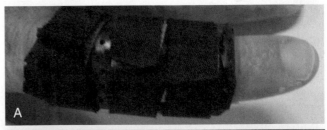

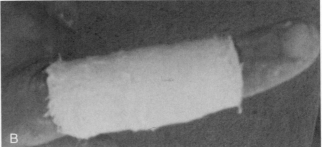

FIGURE 29-7 A, Circumferential boutonnierre orthosis. **B,** Circumferential cast for boutonniere deformity. (Reproduced with permission, Gary Solomon, MS, OTR/L, CHT.)

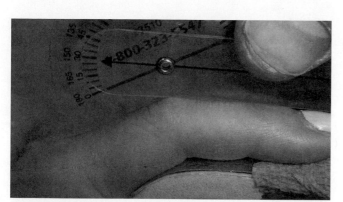

FIGURE 29-8 Initiation of proximal interphalangeal (PIP) protected flexion to 30° using an alumifoam template. (Reproduced with permission, Gary Solomon, MS, OTR/L, CHT.)

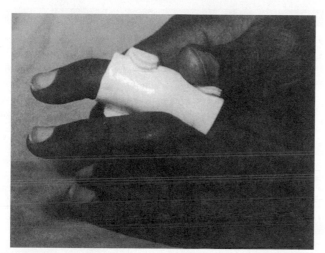

FIGURE 29-9 Oblique retinacular ligament (ORL) stretch entails isolated DIP flexion with PIP supported in extension. This is done actively and passively. (From Clark GL: *Hand rehabilitation: a practical guide,* ed 2, New York, 1998, Churchill Livingstone.)

adjustments may have to be made to achieve full passive PIP extension. Different types of orthoses can be used for this purpose.

While the PIP is immobilized, it is very important that the therapist instruct the client in isolated DIP flexion exercises to recover normal length of the ORL. These exercises are done actively and passively in a gentle fashion (Fig. 29-9). The therapist should watch for normal MP AROM and should exercise this as needed.

Precaution. *After the client has been medically cleared to begin PIP active flexion, initiate restricted amounts of flexion at first and watch for PIP extensor lag.*

It is important to emphasize PIP active extension, which is facilitated by positioning the digit in MP flexion. Continuous orthosis use is reinstituted as needed if a PIP extensor lag develops.

If exercise fails to recover DIP flexion with the PIP extended, **ORL tightness** (limited passive DIP flexion with the PIP extended) may need to be addressed with an orthosis. Various small, custom-made orthoses can be used for dynamic or static progressive DIP flexion with the PIP in full extension.[14]

Operative Treatment

Boutonniere deformity is caused by injury to zone III of the extensor tendons. Various surgical techniques are used to treat

these injuries.[8] The therapy protocol is determined in collaboration with the hand surgeon. The short arc of motion protocol for zone III extensor tendon repairs is appropriate if the client is considered a good candidate for this treatment (see Chapter 31).

Non-Operative Clients
- Is the patient a candidate for early controlled active motion, or would continuous immobilization be preferred?
- Six weeks of immobilization is typical, is that when active PIP flexion should be started?

Operative Clients
- Was a strong repair achieved? (Ask to see the operative report.)
- Would this particular patient benefit from an early active motion protocol or more conservative therapy, such as immobilization?
- Are there any additional precautions?

( ) **What to Say to Clients**

About the Injury

"Here is a diagram of the area of your finger that is injured. Notice how, as a result of injury to the central slip, the lateral bands have slipped forward (volar) and how they now contribute to the bent posture of the PIP joint. The PIP joint needs to be supported in extension for the injured tendon to heal in proper alignment. Also note how the end of the finger is tipped upward (hyperextended). As the injury at the PIP is corrected, the position at tip of the finger will also improve. In addition, specific exercises can help correct this."

About Exercises

"With this diagnosis, improving DIP flexion while the PIP is extended actually helps improve PIP extension. Therefore, flexing just the DIP helps correct the lack of extension at the PIP. It is very important to exercise by bending the tip gently while the PIP is immobilized because this is corrective for your injury."

Evaluation Tips

- Check for hypermobility of the other digits. Do the uninjured digits have a boutonniere-like posture?
- Determine whether the PIP joint can be passively corrected to neutral and whether the DIP joint can be passively corrected to normal flexion with the PIP in extension (that is, check for ORL tightness).
- Check and practice isolated DIP flexion of the other digits. Think ahead about preventing a quadriga effect.
- Check composite flexion of the other digits as you are able.

Diagnosis-Specific Information that Affects Clinical Reasoning

In nonoperative clients, determine whether the injury involves a PIP extensor lag (the PIP can be passively extended to neutral position, but the client cannot actively extend it) or a PIP flexion contracture (the PIP cannot be passively extended to neutral position). This distinction affects orthosis decisions (see later).

Determine whether the client has ORL tightness. With this condition, both active and passive DIP flexion with PIP extension are limited.

♡ Tips from the Field

Clinical Picture

- Edema over the area of injury (dorsal PIP) worsens the deforming forces of a boutonniere position. Treat the edema as a high priority, because this helps recover PIP joint passive extension and promotes normalization throughout. Light compression wrapping can help reduce the edema.
- Isolating and exercising DIP active flexion of the uninjured digits while protecting the injured finger is a good measure for preventing a quadriga effect.
- PIP cylindrical thermoplastic or plaster orthoses may be helpful for performing isolated blocking exercises for DIP flexion. These can be used on all digits to isolate DIP active flexion with varying MP positions.

Orthosis

- If the client has a PIP flexion contracture, a corrective serial cast or orthosis is necessary. Choices for recovering PIP extension include serial static orthoses, serial casts, static progressive orthoses, and dynamic orthoses. These may be prefabricated or custom-made and digit-based or hand-based. The goal of the orthosis is to maximize the total end range time (TERT) in extension and achieve contracture correction without causing increased inflammation of the soft tissues around the PIP joint. Flowers proposes using a Modified Weeks Test to determine the best orthosis to address PIP joint stiffness.[15] The orthosis selection process is based on how much contracture resolution is achieved after the joint is heated and stretched. PROM measurement is initially taken cold and prior to intervention. After ROM in a thermal modality and 10 minutes of end range stretch, a comparative measurement is taken:
  - If there is a 20° change, no orthosis is recommended.
  - If there is a 15° change, an end range static orthosis should be effective.
  - If there is a 10° change, a dynamic orthosis is recommended.
  - If change is less than 5°, a static progressive orthosis is recommended.
- The client should also participate in the orthosis selection process, because activities of daily living (ADLs) and work needs can influence compliance. Comfort, fit, and skin tolerance also all influence these choices.
- If full passive PIP extension is possible, a small PIP extension gutter or cast may be used. Adjust it as needed to accommodate resolution of edema and the client's comfort. It is very important to keep the DIP free and to perform frequent exercises for DIP active and passive flexion while the PIP is splinted in extension.
- If ORL tightness is present, a gentle DIP flexion static progressive or dynamic orthosis may be appropriate. Ease of application and adjustability are criteria that help determine which type should be used.
- If the client has been cleared for active PIP extension and flexion exercises and if ORL tightness is present, try using a dorsal DIP gutter orthosis that maintains DIP flexion while actively exercising PIP extension.

Precaution. *If ORL tightness is present, the client may be at risk of losing flexor digitorum profundus (FDP) excursion, and a quadriga effect could develop.*

◎ Clinical Pearls

After the client has been medically cleared for active PIP extension exercises, position the MP in flexion for the exercises. This can help isolate and achieve active PIP extension.

Check for intrinsic versus extrinsic tightness if composite flexion is limited, and prioritize the MP position accordingly for PIP exercise.

Precaution. *As PIP flexion improves, watch closely for PIP extensor lag.*

➢ Precautions and Concerns

- *Avoid PIP flexion during the protective immobilization phase.*
- *If the client has had surgery, follow the guidelines presented in Chapter 31. Instruct the client in techniques for supporting the digit while putting on and taking off the orthosis for skin care needs. If surgery was not required, instruct the client in ways to manage orthosis and skin care while avoiding PIP flexion. If a cast has been applied, change it at least weekly.*
- *ORL tightness contributes to the boutonniere deforming forces. Monitor this condition throughout the program, and continue exercising active and passive DIP flexion with the PIP extended.*
- *Monitor for loss of FDP excursion and difficulty isolating the FDS, particularly in the involved digit.*
- *If the client has had surgery, adhesions may occur at the incision sites.*

Swan Neck Deformity

Anatomy

In a **swan neck deformity**, the finger postures with PIP hyperextension and DIP flexion (Fig. 29-10).[5] The MP tends to be flexed, and the finger appears to zigzag when observed from the side. The IP joints may be passively correctable, or they may be fixed in their deformity positions. The IP positions in the swan neck deformity are the opposite of their positions in the boutonniere deformity.

Diagnosis and Pathology

The swan neck deformity can be caused by injuries at the level of the DIP, PIP, or MP joint. At the DIP level, a mallet injury can lead to swan neck deformity. In this case, the terminal extensor tendon is disrupted (that is, stretched or ruptured). This allows the extensor force to be more powerful proximally at the PIP joint, leading to PIP hyperextension.[12,16]

If the cause is primarily at the PIP level, the VP/capsule is involved with hyperextension at the PIP joint. The lateral bands are dorsally displaced, contributing to PIP hyperextension; this minimizes the pull on the terminal extensor tendon; therefore, the DIP joint assumes a flexed position. Normally the FDS helps deter PIP hyperextension. However, if the FDS has been ruptured or lengthened, PIP hyperextension forces are less restricted or controlled. Intrinsic muscle tightness compounds the problem.[12]

Painful snapping may be noticed with active flexion. This snapping is caused by the lateral bands at the proximal phalanx condyles.[17]

If the cause of the swan neck deformity is primarily at the MP level, MP volar subluxation and ulnar drift may be the initiating factors, as is seen in rheumatoid arthritis (RA). The MP joint disturbance leads to intrinsic muscle imbalance and tightness with resulting PIP hyperextension forces.[12]

Timelines and Healing

Swan neck deformity is a challenging diagnosis. In conservative management of this condition, an orthosis may be used

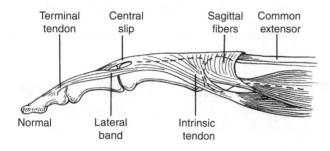
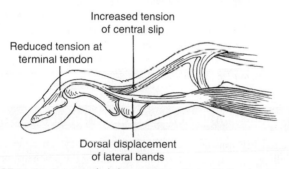

FIGURE 29-10 Swan neck deformity. (From Burke SL: *Hand and upper extremity rehabilitation: a practical guide,* ed 3, St Louis, 2005, Churchill Livingstone.)

indefinitely if it promotes improved function and eliminates painful snapping with active flexion.

Non-Operative Treatment

An orthosis that positions the PIP in slight flexion may be very helpful functionally. Many different kinds of orthoses can be used for this type of deformity, including dorsal blocking (see Fig 29-14 and commercially-available splints, such as the SIRIS (that is, silver ring) splint (Fig. 29-11). The purpose of the orthosis is to prevent hyperextension at the PIP joint and to promote active PIP flexion.

Operative Treatment

Surgery to correct swan neck deformity may be done in conjunction with other reconstructive procedures for clients with RA. Surgical techniques include FDS tenodesis or VP advancement procedures.[16,17] Some researchers have found that capsulodesis and tenodesis techniques for restoring balance lose effectiveness as a result of attenuation if these issues are stressed over time.[18]

After the surgery, clients may be referred to therapy for protective dorsal PIP extension block orthoses (in approximately 30° flexion) or for pin site care, wound care, or edema control. After they have been medically cleared, active DIP extension exercises may be advised. Positioning the digit in PIP flexion helps promote DIP active extension excursion.

Pins/Kirschner wires are often used postoperatively to maintain PIP flexion. When the pins are removed, digit based, dorsal PIP orthoses are used, typically fabricated in approximately 20° to 30° of flexion. This is done to prevent recurrence of PIP hyperextension and imbalance. Active PIP flexion exercises are started when ordered by the surgeon. The PIP dorsal orthosis can remain in place during PIP AROM. The Velcro straps are removed distally to allow PIP flexion while full extension is blocked.

The therapist should focus on balancing digit and hand function while avoiding stress or PIP hyperextension. DIP orthoses may be helpful exercise tools to promote ease of PIP flexion. As a result of the imbalance associated with swan neck deformities, clients habitually have initiated flexion motions with the PIP in hyperextension; visibly

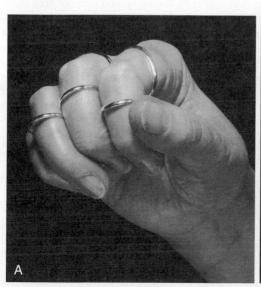
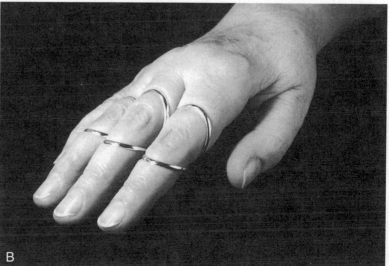

FIGURE 29-11 A SIRIS (silver ring) orthosis prevents PIP hyperextension and allows PIP flexion. (Courtesy of Silver Ring Splint Co., Charlottesville, VA.)

initiating motion with DIP flexion while the PIP is hyperextended. Their flexion motions look awkward and difficult to achieve. The therapist should try practicing gentle arcs of motion with smooth congruent flexion of the PIP and DIP joints. It may be helpful to use a hand-over-hand technique, facilitating flexion with gentle input from the therapist to facilitate normal functional movement mechanics.

? Questions to discuss with the Physician

Non-Operative Clients
- What do you believe was the primary cause of the deformity (RA, VP laxity, untreated mallet)?
- Is surgery a possibility?

Operative Clients
- What structures were repaired? (Ask to see the operative report.)
- When will the pins be removed?
- When can active PIP flexion be started?
- What specific precautions are in order?

( ) What to Say to Clients

About the Injury

"Here is a diagram of the deforming forces associated with swan neck deformity. Notice how the lateral bands have slipped upward (dorsally) and how they now contribute to the overextended posture of the PIP joint. The PIP joint needs to be supported in flexion for balance and proper alignment to be restored."

About Exercises

"With this diagnosis, it is very important to avoid extending the PIP joint beyond its newly pinned or corrected position until the physician upgrades the program. For this reason, we will use a protective dorsal orthosis. When the physician gives the okay for exercise, it is important to practice gentle bending movements at the PIP joint in a comfortable range."

Evaluation Tips

- Check for hypermobility or swan neck posture of uninjured digits. Document this condition if present.
- Determine whether PIP hyperextension is passively correctable or fixed. Does it affect function?
- In a non-operative client, distinguish between primary injury to the DIP or the PIP:
- Stabilize the PIP in neutral position. If the client cannot actively extend the DIP, the injury is primarily a DIP extensor injury. If the client can actively extend the DIP, the injury is primarily a volar PIP injury.
- When exercise therapy has been medically cleared, observe the quality of active flexion and promote practice of motions that do not elicit snapping.

Diagnosis-Specific Information that Affects Clinical Reasoning

Focus treatment on the primary cause of the deformity. If the client has RA, are other digits involved or at risk? Have any tendons ruptured? Consider anti-deformity orthoses for other digits as appropriate. Is MP involvement present? Is intrinsic tightness of

other digits a factor? Nighttime orthosis use or intrinsic stretching (or both) to counteract deforming forces may be valuable.

Is PIP flexion orthosis use likely to be long term? If so, consider a low-profile, long-lasting style, such as a silver ring splint.

♥ Tips from the Field

- Observe the balance of the digit and the hand, and address uninvolved digits unless this is contraindicated. Promote normal range of motion (ROM) throughout the extremity as appropriate.
- If the client's joints are hypermobile, instruct the person in hand use patterns for ADLs that do not encourage PIP hyperextension. For example, teach the client not to put stress on the digits in PIP hyperextension.
- Avoid "intrinsic plus" exercises or positioning during ADL tasks.

➢ Precautions and Concerns

- *If you are treating a mallet injury, watch closely for signs of PIP hyperextension that occur due to DIP splinting (see the "Mallet Finger" section).*
- *Clients do not need to be hypermobile to develop a swan neck deformity after distal digital injury.*
- *Mallet injury is not the only diagnosis that can lead to PIP hyperextension. A distal crush or fracture requiring DIP splinting may also result in PIP hyperextension. Be alert for this, and treat it accordingly with PIP splinting in slight flexion to normalize the balance of the digit.*

Proximal Interphalangeal Joint Injuries

Digital PIP injuries occur frequently, yet they can be extremely challenging to treat. Proper management of therapy helps prevent the situation from becoming frustrating.

PIP joint dislocation is a common injury.[18,19,20] A client initially may ignore a sprain of the small joints of the hand, not realizing the significance of the injury, and may not seek medical attention for days or weeks after the injury. *By this time, significant edema, fibrosis, and stiffness may be established.* Joint enlargement and flexion contractures are common residual problems.[3,16]

◎ Clinical Pearl

Therapists are likely to see clients with digital sprains or dislocations quite often. Because clients may not understand the serious clinical implications of this seemingly simple diagnosis, they can become frustrated with the progression of treatment. Early communication with the client about the nature of the PIP joint injury and the likelihood of a prolonged recovery are important.

Anatomy

Proximal Interphalangeal Joint Architecture

The PIP joint is a hinge joint with 100° to 110° of motion. At the proximal phalanx are two condyles, and between the condyles is the intercondylar notch. Because of the slight asymmetry of the condyles, about 9° of supination occurs with PIP flexion.[3] At the base of the middle phalanx are two concave fossae and a ridge that separates the phalanx's flat, broad base. Stability is enhanced by the amount of congruence of this joint and by its tongue-and-groove contour. The IP joint of the thumb is architecturally similar to the PIP joint of the other digits.[18]

Proximal Interphalangeal Joint Stability

The architecture of the PIP joint, along with its ligamentous support, provides joint stability. The **collateral ligaments** are the main restraints on deviation forces at the PIP joint. These ligaments are 2 to 3 mm thick and are extremely important to the joint's stability. The collateral ligaments have two components: the **proper collateral ligament (PCL)** and the **accessory collateral ligament (ACL),** which are differentiated by their areas of insertion.

The PCL originates on the lateral aspect of the proximal phalanx. The fibers of this ligament insert volarly and distally, on the lateral tubercles of the middle phalanx. The fibers of the ACL insert in a more volar direction on the VP. The VP is fibrocartilaginous and is situated between the collateral ligaments on the volar aspect of the PIP joint. The convergence of the PCL, ACL, and VP at the middle phalanx is known as the *critical corner,* a term that reflects its importance to PIP joint stability.[3]

The anatomic arrangement of the VP functions to prevent PIP hyperextension. The VP also acts as a secondary PIP joint stabilizer laterally when the collateral ligaments have been injured.[3,18]

The dynamic stability of the PIP joint is enhanced by the tendons and ligaments that cross the joint. These are the **central extensor tendon** (central slip), the lateral bands, the **transverse retinacular ligament (TRL),** and the ORL. The central slip is part of the dorsal capsule of the PIP joint and attaches to the middle phalanx at the dorsal tubercle. The lateral bands have intrinsic muscle contributions and lie volar to the MP joint axis; they join dorsal to the PIP joint axis to form the terminal extensor tendon. The TRL originates from the volar surface of the lateral bands and envelops the collateral ligaments and PIP joint, thereby preventing dorsal displacement of the lateral bands. The ORL originates from the flexor sheath, progresses volar to the PIP joint axis, and inserts at the terminal extensor tendon dorsally. The ORL tightens when the PIP joint extends. It provides concomitant PIP and DIP extension and helps prevent hyperextension of the PIP joint (Fig. 29-12).[3]

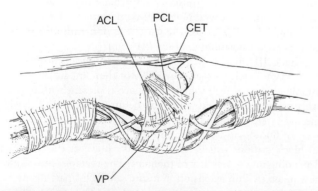

FIGURE 29-12 Structures that provide PIP joint stability include the accessory collateral ligament (ACL), the proper collateral ligament (PCL), the dorsal capsule with the central extensor tendon, and the volar plate (VP). (From Mackin EJ. Callinan N, Skirven TM, et al: *Rehabilitation of the hand and upper extremity,* ed 5, St Louis, 2002, Mosby.)

Diagnosis and Pathology

Physical examination of ligament injuries at the PIP joint requires assessment of joint stability. A/P and true lateral x-rays can identify articular involvement, but x-rays alone may not reveal subtle injuries. The critical issue is whether joint stability exists with active motion.[18]

The **functional stability** of the PIP joint is tested actively and passively. If the client demonstrates normal AROM with no PIP joint displacement, joint stability is adequate despite the injury. A brief period of immobilization can be followed by protected ROM exercises. If the joint is displaced with AROM, major disruption of the ligaments probably has occurred. In these cases the position of immobilization is determined by the physician, partly by identifying the range at which the displacement occurs (Box 29-1). In grade I and mild grade II injuries, the joints are swollen; they also are painful on palpation and with lateral stress.

Direction of Proximal Interphalangeal Joint Dislocation

The direction of dislocation is determined by the position of the middle phalanx at the time of joint injury (Box 29-2). The direction of dislocation typically determines the type of orthosis needed as well as the progression of treatment.[13,16,19,20] Dorsal dislocations involve injury to the distal portion of the VP, and so PIP extension should be limited to prevent further stress on that structure. Volar dislocations involve injury to the central slip, and so PIP flexion should be limited. Lateral dislocations involve the collateral ligaments, and so stress must be avoided on those structures during healing.

BOX 29-1   Grades of Ligament Sprain Injuries

Mild Grade I Sprain
- Definition: No instability with AROM or PROM; macroscopic continuity with microscopic tears. The ligament is intact, but individual fibers are damaged.
- Treatment: Immobilize the joint in full extension if comfortable and available; otherwise, immobilize in a small amount of flexion. When pain has subsided, begin AROM and protect with buddy taping.

Grade II Sprain
- Definition: Abnormal laxity with stress; the collateral ligament is disrupted. AROM is stable, but passive testing reveals instability.
- Treatment: Splint for 2 to 4 weeks. The physician may recommend early ROM, but avoid any lateral stress.

Grade III Sprain
- Definition: Complete tearing of the collateral ligament, along with injury to the dorsal capsule or VP. The finger usually is dislocated by the injury.
- Treatment: Early surgical intervention often is recommended.

AROM, Active range of motion; *PROM,* passive range of motion: *ROM,* range of motion; *VP,* volar plate.
Modified from Campbell PJ, Wilson RL: Management of joint injuries and intraarticular fractures. In Mackin EJ, Callahan AD, Skirven TM, et al, editors: *Rehabilitation of the hand and upper extremity,* ed 5, St Louis, 2002, Mosby; and Glickel SZ, Barron A, Eaton RG: Dislocations and ligament injuries in the digits. In Green DP, Hotchkiss RN, Pederson WC, editors: *Green's operative hand surgery,* ed 4, Philadelphia, 1999, Churchill Livingstone.

BOX 29-2   Directional Types of Proximal Interphalangeal Joint Dislocation

Dorsal PIP Dislocations

Dorsal PIP dislocations are classified according to three subcategories:

- Type I (hyperextension): Volar plate (VP) avulsion and minor split in collateral ligaments longitudinally; if left untreated, this type of dislocation can lead to a swan neck deformity.
- Type II (dorsal dislocation): Dorsal dislocation of PIP joint and VP avulsion with major split in collateral ligaments bilaterally.
- Type III (fracture-dislocation): Dorsal dislocation of the PIP with fracture of the volar articular surface of the middle phalanx. Stability:
  - Fracture less than 30% of middle phalanx articular surface = Stable/non-surgical
  - 30% to 50% = Tenuous; surgical stabilization typically indicated
  - More than 50% = Unstable

Lateral PIP Dislocations

Lateral stability is tested with the PIP joint in extension so that the collateral ligaments and secondary stabilizers, including the VP, can be assessed. Complete collateral ligament disruption is suggested by deformity that exceeds 20° of deformity with gentle stress.

Volar PIP Dislocations

Volar PIP dislocations are rare. The injury may have a rotational component, and the central slip may be ruptured.

Modified from Glickel SZ, Barron A, Eaton RG: Dislocations and ligament injuries in the digits. In Green DP, Hotchkiss RN, Pederson WC, editors: *Green's operative hand surgery*, ed 4, Philadelphia, 1999, Churchill Livingstone.

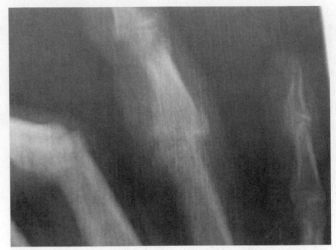

FIGURE 29-13 X-ray of dorsal dislocation. The direction of dislocation is determined by the position of the middle phalanx. (Reproduced with permission, Gary Solomon, MS, OTR/L, CHT.)

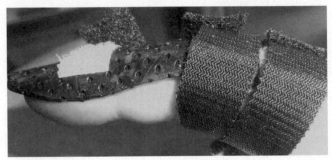

FIGURE 29-14 PIP dorsal block orthosis used to treat dorsal dislocation. The distal strap may be released to allow patient to perform flexion exercises with extension limited to the orthosis level. (Reproduced with permission, Gary Solomon, MS, OTR/L, CHT.)

Timelines and Healing

> ### Clinical Pearl
>
> PIP joint sprains often require immobilization or restricted motion to heal, and clients are at risk for long-standing edema. Permanent limitations in ROM and function are not uncommon.

PIP joint sprains initially have **fusiform swelling** (swelling that is fuller at the PIP joint and tapers at both ends), and ligament fibrosis can progress for over a year after injury, resulting in limitations in ROM and function. *Uninjured digits may become stiff, and a quadriga effect can occur.*

Non-Operative Treatment

Dorsal Dislocation[19,20,21,22]

Dorsal dislocation of a pip joint is typically caused by trauma from a force which pushes the PIP joint into hyper extension causing failure of the volar plate. (Fig. 29-13)[1] Grade I injuries are treated with edema control and PIP immobilization in slight flexion while acute pain is present, which may be for approximately 1 week.

Grade II injuries are treated with a PIP dorsal block orthosis for approximately 6 weeks (Fig. 29-14). PIP extension is typically blocked at 30° for the first 3 weeks, then extension is increased 10° per week for 4 to 6 weeks. If early AROM is prescribed, the therapist instructs the patient to perform gentle flexion exercises but extend only to the orthosis level. Edema is treated as possible. Gentle compression wrapping may be performed. Compressive sleeves may be difficult for the patient to don without compromising the safe positioning of the PIP joint.

Grade III injuries frequently require surgical correction if the fracture involves more than 30% of the joint surface of the middle phalanx.[21,22] If joint congruence is present within a safe range, conservative treatment may be attempted. AROM with specific extension limitations should be provided and based on x-ray or fluoroscopy. The amount of PIP flexion in this PIP dorsal block orthosis usually is 20° to 30°, however this can vary depending on the stability of the joint. The therapist must know how much to limit extension to insure safe ROM parameters.

Operative Treatment

When 30% to 50% of the articular surface of the middle phalanx is involved in the fracture, Kirschner wire PIP extension

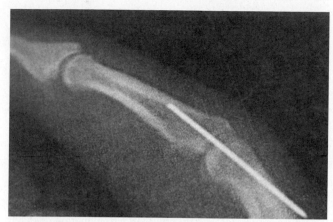

FIGURE 29-15 Kirschner wire fixation of PIP joint for treatment of dorsal dislocation. (Reproduced with permission, Gary Solomon, MS, OTR/L, CHT.)

block (Fig. 29-15), ORIF, external fixation, traction splinting, or VP arthroplasty may be performed for grade III dorsal dislocations.[19,20,21,22] For Fractures of more than 50%, a Hemi-Hamate[22] arthroplasty procedure may be indicated, which involves using a portion of the hamate bone to recreate the shape of the articular surface. In general, motion is initiated in flexion with extension permitted to a designated point of stability, typically determined intra-operatively.

A PIP dorsal block orthosis should be fabricated postoperatively, typically at approximately 30° flexion. Active flexion exercises are permitted with extension limited to the orthosis level. At 3 weeks postoperative, it is usually appropriate to begin to gradually advance extension with unrestricted ROM typically allowed by 6 weeks post-surgery.

Aggressive extension interventions that cannot be tolerated over long periods of time will lead to increased inflammation, edema, and thickening/fibrosis of the joint capsule.[23] A combination of low-tension dynamic or static progressive orthoses as well as static nighttime orthoses can be used to successfully overcome flexion contractures and are well tolerated by patients[24]. Serial casting should also be considered for patients with good PIP flexion but limited extension[25].

? Questions to Discuss with the Physician

Non-Operative Clients
- Does extension need to be blocked, and at what degree is the joint stable?
- It is typical to allow the patient to perform flexion/extension exercises to the orthotic level. Is that appropriate in this case?
- Would you like to gradually increase permitted extension 10° to 15° per week after 3 weeks, or wait until after the patient is re-examined?

Operative Clients
- What structures were repaired? (Ask to see operative report.)
- Is PIP extension to be restricted? If so, to what degree?
- Typical advancement of extension is 10° to 15° per week after 3 weeks. Is that progression appropriate in this case?
- What ROM does the physician expect the client ultimately to achieve?

( ) What to Say to Clients

About the Injury

"This diagnosis is associated with a long timeline for slow healing, and swelling typically persists for a much longer time than you might expect. It helps to be aware of this so that you won't be discouraged by the persistent swelling or stiffness. Sometimes clients have had to have their rings resized, but time will tell whether this will be necessary. It may be helpful to use sleeves or wraps for the swelling for a considerable time."

"Because the injury involved tearing the tissue on the palm side of your finger, we need to protect that tissue by avoiding overstretching it while it heals. You can safely bend your finger, but you need to avoid straightening the injured joint all the way.

"While the tissue is healing over weeks and months, it is very important not to stress the finger with force or high-demand gripping activity. If you do something with your hand and the finger swells or becomes painful, this is a sign that your tissues are not tolerating that much stress. It is best to avoid this response so that the swelling and flexibility can continue to improve."

About the Orthosis

Information might be provided as follows: "The purpose of the orthosis is to stop you from straightening your finger past the level that could cause you to re-dislocate, re-injure, or delay the healing of the finger. Focus on frequently bending the finger, but straightening only up to the orthotic limit.

About Dynamic or Static Progressive Extension Orthoses

"Now that it is safe to work on straightening the finger, the purpose of the orthosis is to position your joint at the end of the range and add light tension to help increase your motion. It is extremely important to understand that more force will not result in a better outcome; however more time at the end of the range is what will help."

Lateral Dislocation

Lateral Dislocation involves failure of either the Medial or Lateral Collateral ligaments of the PIP joint. This is often caused by the finger sustaining a trauma pushing the joint in a sideways direction (Fig. 29-16).

Non-Operative Treatment

Grade I injuries may be managed by edema control and a brief period of resting orthotic use during the acute phase followed by AROM. Buddy straps or a hinged PIP orthosis may be used to support the PIP joint to avoid lateral stress during motion and functional use (Fig. 29-17). Exercises should include DIP blocking and gentle ORL stretches to keep the lateral bands gliding properly.

During the acute phase of grade II injuries, a digital gutter orthosis is typically used and compression wrapping is recommended for edema control. The PIP joint may be in slight flexion,

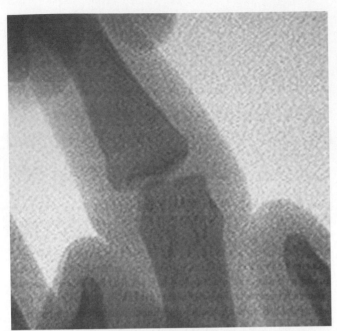

FIGURE 29-16 X-ray of lateral PIP dislocation. (Reproduced with permission, Gary Solomon, MS, OTR/L, CHT.)

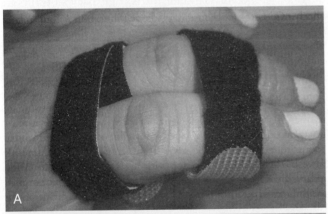

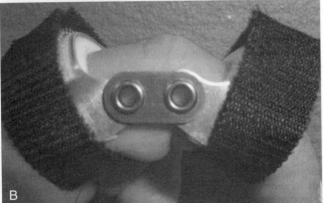

FIGURE 29-17 A, Buddy straps support the injured digit to facilitate motion. **B,** Hinged PIP orthosis supporting PIP during motion. A hinged orthosis is especially useful for index radial collateral ligament (RCL) injury and Small Finger injury. (Reproduced with permission, Gary Solomon, MS, OTR/L, CHT.)

because grade II tears can extend down to the VP. Orthosis use may continue for up to 2 weeks, however gentle early active motion may be initiated with the ligament supported by buddy straps to the adjacent digit on the injured side. For an index finger radial collateral ligament (RCL) injury or small finger collateral ligament injury, the hinged PIP orthosis is recommended. (The small finger PIP joint often does not line up well with the adjacent finger for use of a buddy strap.)

If the joint can be reduced with closed treatment in a grade III injury, the PIP is typically protected with a digital dorsal block orthosis, and short arc motion may be initiated within a stable range. Grade III injuries may require open surgical reduction. While the variety and complexity of surgical interventions is beyond the scope of this discussion, treatment progression is dependent on the stability of fixation and the ability to restore motion gradually without causing further stress to repaired structures.

( ) *What to Say to Clients*

About the Orthoses

"As you begin moving your finger, wearing either a buddy strap or protective hinge will allow you to support the injured ligament as you begin to regain motion in your finger."

About Exercise

"Each time your tissue is stimulated by pain-free movement, favorable clinical responses occur, including lubrication and circulation to promote healing. The more this happens, the better the finger will be. However, exercises that result in swelling or pain are not helpful and are actually detrimental."

Evaluation Tips

- Ask about previous injuries to this or other digits, because pre-existing stiffness may affect the client's prognosis.
- Be very gentle when evaluating the digit; the client's finger may be quite sore.
- Distinguish between fusiform swelling (swelling localized around the PIP joint) and edema throughout the digit.
- When the client is cleared for AROM exercises, check isolated FDS and FDP function. Also check for ORL tightness (that is, check for DIP flexion with PIP extension).
- Distinguish between intrinsic, extrinsic, and joint tightness.
- Inquire about ADLs to determine whether some of them may be detrimental to the healing process.

Diagnosis-Specific Information that Affects Clinical Reasoning

The mechanics of the injury and whether the VP is involved are important pieces of information. If the VP was involved, the PIP should be protected in 20° to 30° of flexion to promote VP healing. Also, keep in mind that collateral ligaments are at risk of tightening if full extension is not achieved in a timely fashion.

Edema management is paramount with PIP joint injuries, which are notorious for persistent swelling. Swelling contributes to pain, shortening or tightening of the collateral ligaments, and loss of joint motion and tendon excursion. Therefore the treatment of swelling should be a clinical priority. Compounding the problem, AROM and all exercises should be limited to the amount of stimulation that does not cause increased swelling.

> ### ◎ Clinical Pearl
>
> Aggressive interventions resulting in a temporary increase in motion, but causing an increase in pain and edema are contra-indicated. The temporary gains are lost, and it becomes more difficult to achieve a long term change.

Devise exercises that are tissue specific. Distinguish between intrinsic and extrinsic tightness and position the finger for exercises accordingly. Check FDS and FDP excursion in the uninjured digits and perform isolated FDS exercises, because these promote PIP flexion and prevent the insidious development of limitations.

♡ Tips from the Field

Tissue Tolerances and Client Education

Monitor tissue tolerances, which dictate the hand therapy intervention. Explain to clients that with this type of injury, they cannot force motion to improve, and strenuous hand movements will only worsen the clinical condition. Despite this instruction, clients may be inclined to perform forceful place and hold exercises to recover flexion, and this is actually injurious to the tissues. Reinforce the concept of tissue tolerances with clients and teach them how to perform pain-free exercises. Friends may have recommended forceful gripping exercises (such as, squeezing a tennis ball or a resistive gripper); explain that the tissues need to be ready for this much stimulation, that negative tissue responses are manifested by swelling and pain after exercise, and that these responses can set back the progression toward recovery.

Buddy Taping

Normally, the finger that supports the injured side is selected. If the middle finger sustained an injury to the PIP RCL, it needs protection to avoid ulnar stress. In this instance, buddy tape the middle finger to the index finger to promote neutral alignment.

Buddy tapes may be most helpful when used at two levels (for example, proximal phalanx and middle phalanx). The important features are support, comfort, and ease of use. Monitor the tightness of the buddy tapes, because tapes that are too tight can worsen the edema by creating a tourniquet effect.

Volar Dislocation[17,19,20,21]

Volar dislocation (Fig. 29-18) is significantly less common than other PIP dislocations.[21] Central slip avulsion, collateral ligament injury, and fracture of the dorsal lip of the middle phalanx may be involved.

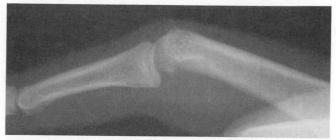

FIGURE 29-18 X-ray of volar PIP dislocation. (Reproduced with permission, Gary Solomon, MS, OTR/L, CHT.)

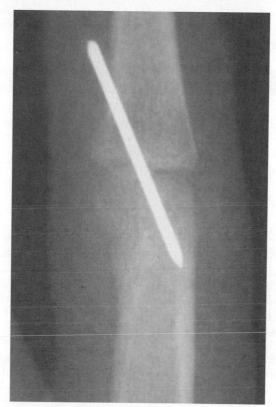

FIGURE 29-19 PIP joint with Kirschner wire/pin to reduce maintain reduction of volar dislocation. (Reproduced with permission, Gary Solomon, MS, OTR/L, CHT.)

Conservative Treatment

If the joint is stable after reduction, and the central slip is intact, gentle ROM may be initiated.

If the central slip is avulsed, the PIP is immobilized in a gutter orthosis with the DIP joint free for approximately 4 to 6 weeks. The patient is instructed to perform isolated DIP blocking exercises to maintain the positioning and integrity of the lateral bands and spiral ORL.

When the patient is clear to begin AROM, short arc motion is initiated. It is also important to support any associated collateral ligament injury with either buddy straps or a hinged PIP orthosis as described in the previous section.

Operative Treatment

If the PIP joint remains unstable after reduction, the joint may be pinned with a Kirschner wire in extension (Fig. 29-19).

Exercise Guidelines

Brief, frequent, pain-free exercises are more effective than infrequent sessions. Explain to the client that tissue tolerance dictates the exercise regimen.

> ### Precautions and Concerns
>
> - *Avoid exercises that cause increased pain or stiffness.*
> - *With PIP joint injuries, the importance of tissue tolerance cannot be overstated.*
> - *Persistent edema that is avoidable can lead to serious clinical and functional consequences.*
> - *The long healing timeline for this type of injury makes therapy a challenge. Therapists must be very creative in providing factual information about steady progress while preventing the client from becoming disappointed or discouraged.*

Thumb Metacarpophalangeal Joint Injury

Clients with injuries of the thumb MP joint, particularly ulnar collateral ligament (UCL) injuries, frequently are referred for hand therapy. Proper hand therapy can favorably affect the recovery of stable, pain-free function in such cases.

Injury to the thumb MP joint may involve either the UCL or the RCL. The UCL is injured ten times as often as the RCL. The treatment guidelines described for UCL injury also apply to the RCL.

Anatomy

The MP joint of the thumb is primarily a hinge joint. Flexion and extension comprise the primary arc of motion. Pronation-supination and abduction-adduction are considered secondary arcs of motion at this joint. Pronation occurs as the thumb MP joint flexes because the radial condyle of the metacarpal head is wider than the ulnar condyle.[3,18]

The thumb MP joint's ROM is unique; it has the most variation in the amount of movement of all the body's joints. ROM at the thumb MP joint ranges from 55° to 85° of flexion. People with flatter metacarpal heads tend to have less motion, and individuals with more spherical metacarpal heads have more motion. Lateral motion at the thumb MP joint ranges from 0° to 20° when the MP is in extension. The stability of this joint comes primarily from ligamentous, capsular, and musculotendinous support.[15]

Laterally, the thumb MP joint displays strong PCLs that arise from the metacarpal lateral condyles and progress volarly and obliquely to their insertion on the proximal phalanx. The ACL originates volar to the PCL and inserts on the VP and the sesamoid bones.[17] The sesamoid bones have been described as the convergence point of the thumb MP joint's periarticular structures.[26,27] The PCLs are tightest with MP flexion.

The thumb MP joint receives stability from thenar intrinsic muscles, specifically the adductor pollicis (AP), the flexor pollicis brevis (FPB), and the abductor pollicis brevis (APB). The FPB and the APB insert on the radial sesamoid, and the adductor pollicis inserts on the ulnar sesamoid.[18,26]

Diagnosis and Pathology

A UCL injury is called **skier's thumb,** because a fall on outstretched hand (FOOSH) with the thumb in abduction is a common skiing injury. The ski pole handle may cause the thumb to abduct. Historically, this injury has also been called **gamekeeper's thumb,** because the term describes an injury that occurred as a result of killing rabbits with a technique that stressed the thumb MP joint radially. Nowadays the term, *gamekeeper's thumb,* refers to chronic UCL instability at the thumb MP joint.[3]

Acute UCL injuries of the thumb MP joint usually involve detachment of the ligament from its proximal phalanx insertion. Concomitant injury of the ACL, the VP, or the dorsal capsule also may occur. If complete disruption occurs along with forceful radial deviation at the thumb MP joint, displacement of the ligament superficially with interposition of the adductor aponeurosis may result; this condition is called **Stener's lesion** (Fig. 29-20).

RCL injuries to the MP of the thumb are less common. The mechanism of injury is usually trauma causing forced adduction of the thumb. Treatment progression follows a similar course to UCL injury with care to avoid lateral stress ulnarly.

Precaution. *Stener's lesion requires surgical correction because the interposition prevents healing of the ligament.*[3]

The thumb MP joint is clinically assessed for MP instability injury by providing gentle stress in radial deviation (to assess UCL) or ulnar deviation (to assess RCL) to the thumb with the MP joint in both extension and flexion at 30°. This result is compared with that on the contralateral side. Physicians may use an injection of anesthetic if pain prohibits testing. Varying criteria are used to describe a complete ligament tear: 1) instability greater than 35°, or 2) instability 15° greater than on the uninjured side.

> ### Clinical Pearl
>
> Stress testing may be more painful on a partial tear than on a complete tear.

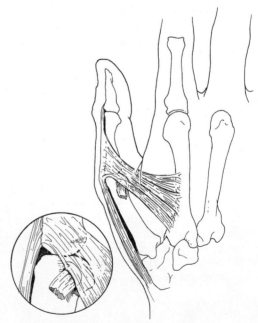

FIGURE 29-20 Stener's lesion. The ulnar collateral ligament (UCL) is displaced with interposition of the adductor aponeurosis. Surgery is required for this type of injury, because interposition of the adductor aponeurosis prevents healing. (From Mackin EJ, Callinan N, Skirven TM, et al: *Rehabilitation of the hand and upper extremity,* ed 5, St Louis, 2002, Mosby.)

X-rays in the A/P, lateral, and oblique views are taken to rule out the possibility of an avulsion fracture. Stress x-rays may also be helpful[27]. Additional imaging techniques, such as ultrasound studies, magnetic resonance imaging (MRI), and arthrograms, may be ordered as necessary. An overlooked and untreated injury can lead to pain and instability.

Timelines and Healing

The thumb MP joint is immobilized for approximately 4 to 6 weeks to allow healing. Thumb IP joint ROM should be encouraged throughout the immobilization stage. It can take a few months after injury for resistive pinch or axial loading of the thumb to be comfortable and safe to perform.

Non-Operative Treatment

If the ligament injury is a partial tear, the thumb is immobilized in a hand-based thumb spica orthosis (with the IP joint left free) for 2 to 4 weeks. After this, AROM exercises are initiated with medical clearance, with the orthosis continued between exercises.[28,29] For UCL injury, typically flexion, extension, and radial abduction are initiated, and AROM is then progressed to gentle palmar abduction and opposition. Progression to active assistive range of motion (AAROM) occurs at approximately 6 weeks. Light key pinch exercises may be started early, but tip pinch and thumb tip loading exercises are not performed until medically approved, which may be 8 weeks or longer after injury. This restriction is necessary in preventing stress on the ligament.[3] For a RCL injury, the progression of treatment is similar however *lateral pinch is avoided for up to 8 weeks.*

Operative Treatment

Surgical procedures may include open reduction and internal fixation (ORIF) to reduce fracture fragments. The UCL may be reattached to its insertion. The MP joint may be pinned, and this often may be done with a slight overcorrection ulnarly to prevent stress on the repaired ligament. A thumb spica cast or thermoplastic orthosis is used for 4 weeks, at which time the pin usually is removed.[3]

AROM of the thumb carpometacarpal (CMC) and MP joints is initiated after pin removal. Scar management and edema control are helpful for minimizing the possibility of adherence of the extensor pollicis longus (EPL) at the incision scar. As in the non-operative program, lateral pinch may be initiated sooner than tip pinch, which should be avoided for about 8 weeks after surgery to prevent stress on the repair. Protective splinting with a hand-based thumb spica orthosis may be used for up to 6 to 8 weeks after the repair. The therapist should inform the client that some tenderness at the ulnar MP joint is normal for a few months after this surgery.[3]

? Questions to Discuss with the Physician

Non-Operative Clients
- We typically begin motion for the thumb for flexion/extension and radial abduction. Is this patient also clear for palmar abduction and opposition?
- Does it appear that we should wait about 8 weeks before allowing resistive tip prehension with this patient?

Operative Clients
- Was there a Stener's lesion?
- How much ROM does the physician expect the client to achieve at the MP joint?
- Should activities requiring resistive tip pinch or axial loading be avoided for 8 weeks?
- Should any other precautions be taken?
- How long should the protective orthosis be used?

( ) What to Say to Clients

About the Injury

"With this diagnosis, it is more important to achieve a pain-free, stable thumb MP joint than it is to achieve full MP motion. You may not recover full MP motion, but achieving functional, pain-free motion for pinching and resistive hand use usually is considered a successful result."

About the Orthosis

"You may need to wear your protective orthosis (Fig. 29-21) to prevent forceful use of or stress on the injured thumb. It may also help signal others to be careful when shaking your hand or interacting with you in public."

About Exercises

"It is important to focus on the motion at the last joint (the IP joint) and to prevent stiffness at this site. However, be careful not to put pressure on the end of the thumb tip or to use a powerful pinching motion against the tip of the thumb until the doctor permits this."

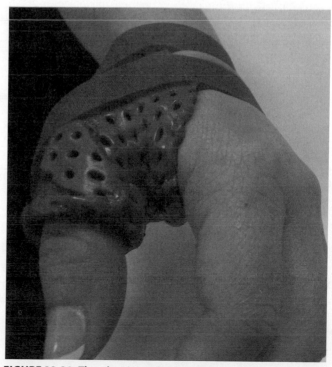

FIGURE 29-21 Thumb spica orthosis with IP joint free. Care is taken to provide good lateral support to MP joint. (Reproduced with permission, Gary Solomon, MS, OTR/L, CHT.)

Evaluation Tips

- Observe the client's contralateral thumb for laxity (including laterally).
- Assess the contralateral thumb for MP and IP AROM.
- Is tightness of the injured thumb's web space present?
- In clients who have had surgery, observe for scar adherence and test for full excursion of the EPL, which also may be adherent.
- Is full IP active extension present with MP extension? If not, is IP active extension present with the MP in some flexion?
- Is IP extensor lag present?
- Explore the client's ADL needs and discuss any adaptations needed to protect the injured tissue.

Diagnosis-Specific Information that Affects Clinical Reasoning

Fabricate the orthosis with a good web space opening and with the thumb positioned to prevent loading of the tip. Placing the thumb CMC in abduction/extension may be more protective for preventing loading than placing it in opposition.

Adjust the orthosis as edema decreases to maintain good lateral stability.

♥ Tips from the Field

- The location of the incision scar can put the EPL at risk for developing adherence at that point. If EPL adherence is present, splinting the IP joint in extension at night or when not exercising may help. Work on scar management and, at that site, position the MP or other proximal joints in some flexion to promote active IP extension.
- The flexor pollicis longus (FPL) is easier to isolate than the FPB. Because of this and because immobilization contributes to MP stiffness, clients often have difficulty isolating active flexion at the thumb MP. If they override with IP flexion, try using a volar IP extension gutter to isolate for MP flexion active exercises. Simultaneous proximal support of the metacarpal also may help.

➢ Precautions and Concerns

- *Be alert for and take steps to prevent the development of a thumb web space contracture. Although a typical approach is to splint in overcorrection (slight ulnar deviation), don't allow tightness of the thumb web space to occur.*
- *Avoid tip loading and resistive pinching.*
- *Assess and problem-solve ADLs to protect injured structures. Try building up the girth of implements (for example, construct padded pens) to reduce the load on the thumb MP joint.*
- *Instruct clients to avoid painful use of the thumb.*

CASE STUDIES

CASE STUDY 29-1 ■

O.D. was a 34-year-old airport transportation van driver, jammed his right small finger while lifting a passenger's suitcase. He was treated initially at an urgent care center and placed in an alumifoam full-finger orthosis, which he was removing for hygiene.

O.D. was referred for a mallet orthosis for his small finger. Options of volar, dorsal, and combination styles were discussed, and it was determined that the combination of a dorsal base with volar support under the distal phalanx would provide the best support and protection for work tasks. The patient was instructed also in isolated PIP ROM in the orthosis.

At 6 weeks, he was referred to begin therapy and demonstrated DIP ROM from 0° to 20°. A template was made from alumifoam at a 25° angle, and the patient was assigned a home exercise program (HEP) to gradually work toward DIP flexion to the template while emphasizing DIP extension.

At follow up the next week (7 weeks post injury), he had achieved his 0° to 25° goal. The template was then adjusted to 40°, and the patient was again instructed to gradually work toward that goal. He was also instructed to remove the mallet orthosis for 1 to 2 hours two times per day during sedentary activity.

At 8 weeks post injury, O.D. was permitted to perform composite fist, hook, and unrestricted DIP active blocking exercises. The orthosis was to be used for 2 hours in the middle of the day and at night. He was permitted to return to work with restrictions of no forceful gripping/heavy lifting, and at 10 weeks post-injury had achieved ROM of 0° to 55°, at which time activity restrictions were lifted.

CASE STUDY 29-2 ■

T.R., a 14-year-old female, came to therapy with a right ring finger PIP dorsal dislocation.

The joint was examined under flouroscan by her hand surgeon who determined that the joint became unstable when extended more than 50°. Surgical options were explained; however the patient and parents opted to attempt conservative treatment.

After joint reduction and several attempts of thermoplastic orthosis fabrication under the flouroscan, the joint reduction could not be maintained adequately. At that time, a digital plaster cast was attempted, and the joint was able to be immobilized and reduced at 60° flexion.

After 3 weeks, the joint was re-examined and was stable enough to increase extension to 45° and was re-casted for one additional week.

Beginning at 4 weeks, a thermoplastic dorsal block was fabricated at 30° flexion, and the patient initiated active flexion and extension to the orthosis level. The orthosis was serially adjusted to allow 10° additional extension per week.

At 8 weeks post reduction, her PIP motion was 15° to 90°, and a low tension PIP extension orthosis was initiated as well as a night gutter for PIP extension.

By 10 weeks post reduction, she had achieved full PIP ROM and resumed unrestricted activities including sports.

CASE STUDY 29-3 ■

S.R., a 38-year-old male, injured his left ring finger playing 16-inch softball, which is a Chicago tradition (no glove is used) and provides a wealth of patients for hand therapy practices. When the finger was injured, he reported pulling it back into place; however, after 4 weeks of pain and swelling, he saw a hand surgeon. The x-ray revealed an intra-articular fracture and VP avulsion.

S.R. had surgical reduction, and his PIP joint was pinned. A hand-based thermoplastic orthosis was fabricated, and the patient was instructed to remove it only for hygiene. Upon arrival to the clinic for follow up 1 week later, the patient had "forgotten" his orthosis and his affected hand was dirty from doing manual work that he reported he could not perform with the orthosis on. The x-ray revealed the pin had bent; however, it was decided to leave the pin in place, and a new protective orthosis was fabricated. Upon pin removal at 5 weeks postoperative, PIP ROM was 30° to 65°; however, the joint was clicking with motion, and the joint surfaces were not congruent. The patient was provided with options for secondary procedures including hemi-hamate and joint replacement, but he decided he would not pursue other options and would be able to work and return to activities with the existing outcome.

References

1. Wright HH, Rettig AC: Management of common sports injuries. In Mackin EJ, Callahan AD, Skirven TM, et al, editors: *Rehabilitation of the hand and upper extremity,* ed 5, St Louis, 2002, Mosby.
2. Brzezienski MA, Schneider LH: Extensor tendon injuries at the distal interphalangeal joint, *Hand Clin* 11:373–386, 1995.
3. Campbell PJ, Wilson RL: Management of joint injuries and intraarticular fractures. In Mackin EJ, Callahan AD, Skirven TM, et al, editors: *Rehabilitation of the hand and upper extremity,* ed 5, St Louis, 2002, Mosby.
4. Hofmeister EP, Mazurek MT, Shin AY, et al: Extension block pinning for large mallet fractures, *J Hand Surg Am* 28:453–459, 2003.
5. American Society for Surgery of the Hand: *The hand: examination and diagnosis,* ed 2, Edinburgh, 1983, Churchill Livingstone.
6. Evans RB: Clinical management of extensor tendon injuries: the therapist's perspective. In Skirvin TM, Osterman AL, Fedorczyk JM, et al, editors: *Rehabilitation of the hand and upper extremity,* ed 6, Philadelphia, 2011, Elsevier Mosby.
7. Biernacki SD: A flexion contracture splint for the distal interphalangeal joint, *J Hand Ther* 14:302–303, 2001.
8. Doyle JR: Extensor tendons: acute injuries. In Green DP, Hotchkiss RN, Pederson WC, editors: *Green's operative hand surgery,* ed 4, Philadelphia, 1999, Churchill Livingstone.
9. Tetik C, Gudemez E: Modification of the extension block Kirschner wire technique for mallet fractures, *Clin Orthop Relat Res* 404:284–290, 2002.
10. Takami H, Takahashi S, Ando M: Operative treatment of mallet finger due to intraarticular fracture of the distal phalanx, *Arch Orthop Trauma Surg* 20:9–13, 2000.
11. Coons MS, Green SM: Boutonniere deformity, *Hand Clin* 11:387–402, 1995.
12. Alter S, Feldon P, Terrono AL: Pathomechanics of deformities in the arthritic hand and wrist. In Mackin EJ, Callahan AD, Skirven TM, et al: *Rehabilitation of the hand and upper extremity,* ed 5, St Louis, 2002, Mosby.
13. Saleeba EC: Dynamic flexion splint for the distal interphalangeal joint, *J Hand Ther* 16:249–250, 2003.
14. Catalano LW, Skarparis AC, Glickel SZ, et al: Treatment of chronic, traumatic hyperextension deformities of the proximal interphalangeal joint with flexor digitorum superficialis tenodesis, *J Hand Surg Am* 28:448–452, 2003.
15. Glickel SZ, Barron A, Eaton RG: Dislocations and ligament injuries in the digits. In Green DP, Hotchkiss RN, Pederson WC, editors: *Green's operative hand surgery,* ed 4, Philadelphia, 1999, Churchill Livingstone.
16. Chinchalkar SJ, Gan BS: Management of proximal interphalangeal joint fractures and dislocations, *J Hand Ther* 16:117–128, 2003.
17. Colditz J: Plaster of Paris: The forgotten hand splinting material, *J Hand Ther* 15:144–157, 2002.
18. Katsoulis E, Rees K, Warwick DJ: Hand therapist led management of mallet finger, *Br J Hand Ther* 10:10–17, 2005.
19. Dennerllein J: finger flexor tendon forces are a complex function of finger joint motions and fingertip fores, *J Hand Ther* 18:120–127, 2005.
20. Chinchalker S, Lanting B, Ross D: Swan neck deformity after distal interphalangeal joint flexion contractures: a biomechanical analysis, *J Hand Ther* 19:420–425, 2009.
21. Calfee RP, Keifhaber R, Sommercamp TG, et al: Hemi-hamate arthroplasty provides functional reconstruction of acute and chronic proximal interphalangeal fracture-dislocations, *J Hand Surg Am* 34(7):1232–1241, 2009.
22. Little K, Jacoby S: Intra-articular hand fractures and joint injuries: part I surgeon's management. In Skirvin TM, Osterman AL, Fedorczyk JM, et al: *Rehabilitation of the hand and upper extremity,* ed 6, Philadelphia, 2011, Elsevier Mosby.
23. Gaffney Gallagher K, Blackmore S: Intra-articular hand fractures and joint injuries: part II therapist's management. In Skirvin TM, Osterman AL, Fedorczyk JM, et al, editors: *Rehabilitation of the hand and upper extremity,* ed 6, Philadelphia, 2011, Elsevier Mosby.
24. Flowers KR: A proposed decision hierarchy for splinting the stiff joint, with an emphasis on force application parameters, *J Hand Ther* 15:158–162, 2002.
25. Glasgow C, Tooth LR, Fleming J: Mobilizing the stiff hand: combining theory and evidence to improve clinical outcomes, *J Hand Ther* 23:392–401, 2010.
26. Mohler LR, Trumble TE: Disorders of the thumb sesamoids, *Hand Clin* 17:291–301, 2001.
27. Rotella JM, Urpi J: A new method of diagnosing metacarpophalangeal instabilities of the thumb, *Hand Clin* 17:45–60, 2001.
28. Galindo A, Suet L: A metacarpophalangeal joint stabilization splint, *J Hand Ther* 15:83–84, 2002.
29. Ford M, McKee P, Szilagyi M: Protecting the ulnar collateral ligament and metacarpophalangeal joint of the thumb, *J Hand Ther* 17:64–68, 2004.

30 Flexor Tendon Injury

Linda J. Klein

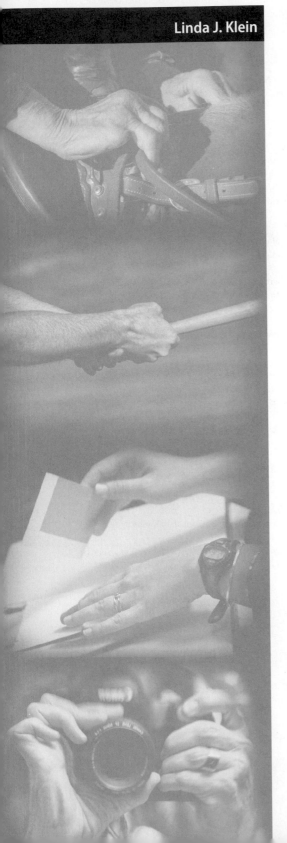

Flexor tendon repair and rehabilitation have posed challenges to surgeons and therapists for decades. Flexor tendons are required to glide large distances to allow the digits full composite flexion and extension, running within a tight pulley system to maximize their efficiency (Fig. 30-1). Following repair, **flexor tendon adhesions** develop quickly, because the tendon becomes adherent to surrounding tissue due to scar formation, especially when repaired within the pulley system. Once adherent, the flexor tendon does not glide as needed to perform active flexion, resulting in functionally limiting deficits in range of motion (ROM) with active range of motion (AROM) more limited than passive range of motion (PROM). Prevention of adhesions to the repaired flexor tendon would be possible if the tendon were allowed to glide immediately after surgery, but this approach historically resulted in rupture of the tendon repair. For this reason, a large number of solutions have been attempted over the past 50 years, resulting in numerous approaches to repair and rehabilitation. The goal of the evolving approaches has been to improve flexor tendon gliding by minimizing adhesion formation to the tendon while avoiding rupture of the repaired tendon.

This chapter helps the therapist gain an understanding of the rationale behind the various approaches to flexor tendon management. Physician and therapist communication is necessary to determine the most appropriate approach for each client. Close supervision by a hand therapist is essential.

Anatomy

The flexor tendons to the digits enter the hand through the carpal tunnel. They are comprised of the flexor digitorum superficialis (FDS) for each finger, flexor digitorum profundus (FDP) for each finger, and flexor pollicis longus (FPL) to the thumb. The FDP tendons are deep to the FDS tendons in the forearm, wrist, and hand. At the level of the proximal phalanx, the FDS tendon separates, becoming two separate slips, which then re-converge just before attachment on the middle phalanx (Fig. 30-2). The FDS flexes the metacarpophalangeal (MP) and proximal interphalangeal (PIP) joints. The FDP tendon emerges through the separation of the FDS tendon at the level of the proximal phalanx and continues distally to insert on the distal phalanx. The FDP tendon is the sole tendon responsible for distal interphalangeal (DIP) flexion of the finger. In the thumb, the FPL tendon inserts on the distal phalanx and is the sole flexor of the thumb interphalangeal (IP) joint.

As the flexor tendons run under the retinaculum and transverse carpal ligament at the wrist and palm, they are surrounded by a **synovial bursa,** which is a sheath filled with synovial fluid that allows tendon gliding without excess friction (see Fig. 30-1). A synovial sheath also surrounds the flexor tendons in the digit, where they run under a series of pulleys that prevent the flexors from bowstringing as active flexion occurs (see Fig. 30-1). Bowstringing describes the manner in which, when the pulleys are not intact, a flexor tendon is pulled away from the bone with a muscle contraction, rather than being efficiently pulled proximally. The pulleys that hold the flexor tendon snugly to the bone result in an efficient proximal glide of the flexor tendon with muscle contraction.

Diagnosis and Pathology

Pathology of the flexor tendon occurs most often by traumatic injury, either by open laceration or closed rupture. The open laceration may be complete or partial, it may include loss of length of the tendon, and it may be a clean laceration, jagged tear, or cut with frayed ends. The wound may be clean or dirty. Associated pulley injuries and ligament, nerve, bone, or vessel injuries may have occurred, increasing the complexity of repair. Repair of the tendon and associated structures is performed as soon after the

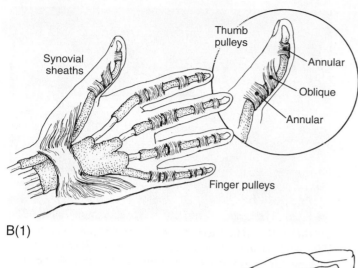

Synovial sheaths

Thumb pulleys

Annular

Oblique

Annular

Finger pulleys

B(1)

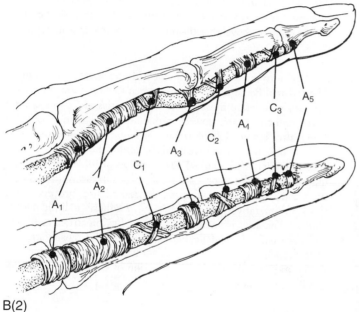

A_1

A_2

C_1

A_3

C_2

A_4

C_3

A_5

B(2)

FIGURE 30-1 Flexor tendon anatomy illustrating the synovial lining around the tendons within the pulley systems at the wrist and within the digits. (From Chase RA: *Atlas of hand surgery*, vol 2, Philadelphia, 1984, WB Saunders.)

injury as possible, often in the emergency room. Occasionally a client may come to the physician's office either acutely or with an old injury, indicating that their "finger doesn't work" due to a previous injury in which the flexor tendon injury may have been missed or because the client did not seek medical care at the time of the injury. Flexor tendon injuries that are seen late are often treated with a flexor tendon graft, or with a salvage procedure.

Closed traumatic injuries of the flexor tendon occur most often to the FDP tendon, due to a rupture from its attachment on the volar surface of the distal phalanx. This injury occurs as the flexed fingertip is extended forcefully, causing rupture of the FDP from the bone or an avulsion fracture. It is also known as **"jersey finger,"** because it is seen in football players holding the jersey of a player attempting to break the grasp by pulling away.

To diagnose if the FDP tendon is intact, hold the finger below the DIP joint and ask the client to bend the tip of the finger (Fig. 30-3). Because the FDP is the only flexor tendon to cross the DIP joint, active DIP flexion indicates that the FDP tendon is intact.

To diagnose whether the FDS tendon is intact, blocking the action of the FDP is necessary, because the FDP assists flexion at the PIP joint. To block the action of the FDP at the PIP joint and

isolate the FDS to determine if it is intact, manually hold all the other fingers completely straight and ask the client to flex the PIP joint of the finger being tested (Fig. 30-4). The DIP joint of the finger being tested should be without tension if the FDP is being blocked successfully by holding the FDP of the other fingers at length.

Timelines and Healing

Flexor tendons retract after laceration or rupture, and surgical repair is necessary to allow healing to regain active motion. The tendon gradually heals after repair by both intrinsic and extrinsic means. The blood supply to the tendon enters from the dorsal surface of the tendon through vinculae supplied by the digital arteries (see Fig. 30-2). Flexor tendons are relatively avascular between these vinculae as well as on the volar surface of the tendon. The vinculae may be damaged during the injury or repair. Lacerated flexor tendons in the digit were initially thought to require blood supply from adhesions to heal following repair (extrinsic healing). Research has since shown that repaired flexor tendons have the

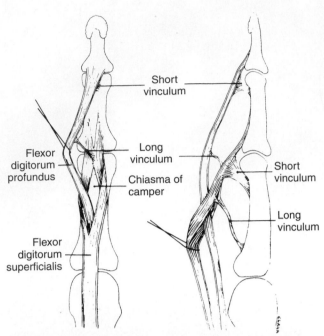

FIGURE 30-2 Flexor digitorum profundus (FDP) and flexor digitorum superficialis (FDS) anatomy in the digit illustrating the split in the superficialis tendon that allows the profundus tendon to continue distally to its insertion on the distal phalanx. (From Schneider LH: *Flexor tendon injuries,* Boston, 1985, Little Brown.)

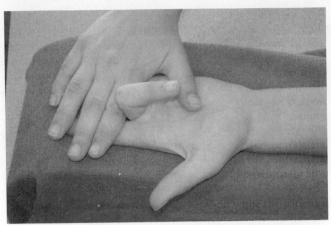

FIGURE 30-4 Test to determine if the flexor digitorum superficialis (FDS) tendon is intact: Hold all other fingers in complete extension to prevent the flexor digitorum profundus (FDP) from assisting, and ask the client to actively flex the proximal interphalangeal (PIP) joint.

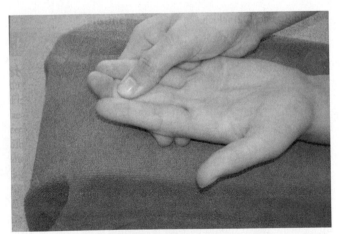

FIGURE 30-3 Test to determine if flexor digitorum profundus (FDP) is intact: Hold below the distal interphalangeal (DIP) joint, and ask the client to actively flex the DIP joint.

ability to heal by nutrition from direct blood supply and from diffusion of nutrients in the synovial fluid that surrounds the tendons as they run within the pulley system (intrinsic healing).[1]

Tendon phases of healing include the **inflammatory phase** (0 to 2 weeks following repair), the **fibroplasia phase,** or reparative phase, (approximately 2 to 6 weeks following repair), and the remodeling phase (more than 6 weeks following repair).[2] During the inflammatory phase, the tendon is at its weakest, and collagen is just beginning to be laid down at the repair site. The intermediate phase of tendon healing is when the tendon repair gains tensile strength. **Tensile strength** describes the amount of force the tendon will tolerate before rupture. During the late phase of tendon healing, the tendon repair continues to gain tensile strength

and begins to remodel in alignment with the tension placed on it. The repaired flexor tendon is considered to have adequate tensile strength to tolerate most functional activities at 12 weeks after repair, and clients are allowed normal use of the hand at 12 to 14 weeks after repair. Rehabilitation following flexor tendon repair is, therefore, most protective of the repair for the first 3 to 4 weeks postoperatively with gradual advancement of force during active motion during the second month if active motion is limited, and use of specific exercises to assist the remodeling process in the third postoperative month of healing if adhesions limit tendon gliding. The advancement from passive flexion to active flexion and eventually resisted flexion depends on the tensile strength of the repair technique and each individual's tissue response to injury and surgery. See the "Progression of Exercises" section for specific guidelines.

Operative Treatment

Flexor tendon repair techniques have been changing for the past decade. Historically, outcomes of flexor tendon repairs in the digit had been plagued by poor results because of adhesions or, if early active motion were attempted, rupture. Numerous studies have investigated suture materials and techniques to determine the best way to create a repair strong enough to tolerate immediate stress on the flexor tendon and obtain gliding while minimizing adhesions, without rupture.[3-10] When lacerated, the flexor tendon ends are approximated and sutured with the technique of choice while attempting to maintain as much of the pulley system as possible. The A2 and A4 pulleys are the most important to preserve to prevent bowstringing. When the FDP has ruptured from its distal phalanx attachment or is lacerated within 1 cm of its distal attachment, the surgeon performs advancement and reinsertion of the tendon.[9] In this situation, the FDP tendon is sewn back to the bone using a suture that extends through the tendon into the distal phalanx and is either attached to the bone with an anchor, or the suture is brought dorsally all the way through the bone and nail, where it is knotted over a button placed on the nail (Fig. 30-5). Repair of the FPL to the thumb is approached in a similar manner as finger flexor tendon repairs.

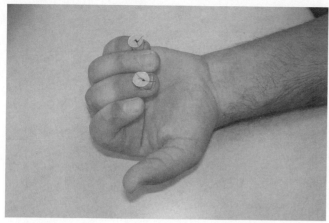

FIGURE 30-5 Suture over a button placed on the nail of a client that has undergone advancement and reinsertion of the flexor digitorum profundus (FDP) to the bone in multiple fingers.

Digital nerve injuries occur frequently when a flexor tendon is lacerated. When a digital nerve repair has been performed, talk to the referring physician about the possible need to block the IP joint in slight flexion within the orthosis for the first 2 to 3 weeks postoperatively to prevent tension on the nerve repair.

Research shows that, in general, the more strands of suture material that cross the tendon repair, the stronger the repair.[3,10] The traditional suture repair technique consists of a two-strand repair, meaning that two strands of suture material cross the repair site. This type of repair tolerates application of an immobilization protocol or **immediate passive motion protocol** in the early phase of tendon healing, but it is not shown to be sufficiently strong enough to consistently tolerate **immediate active motion protocols** following a flexor tendon repair. A four-strand repair has been shown to tolerate gentle active motion.[3] Repairs of six or more strands certainly will tolerate gentle active motion; however, these repairs are technically demanding and may become so bulky as to prevent gliding under the pulleys, create friction, possible wearing, and potential rupture. Thus a four-strand suture technique is commonly used for flexor tendon repair in which an immediate active motion protocol is applied, although some surgeons are electing to perform repairs with six or more strands.[11]

Precaution. *The therapist must know the number of strands used in the repair of a flexor tendon before determining what type of motion protocol may be appropriate.*

Postoperatively, flexor tendon rehabilitation poses a challenge to rehabilitation due to dense flexor tendon adhesions that occur within the flexor pulley system of the digit in zones 1 and 2. Flexor tendon zones of the hand are reviewed in Fig. 30-6. Three basic approaches to rehabilitation of the repaired flexor tendon in the hand are 1) immobilization, 2) immediate passive motion in the direction of the repaired tendon, and 3) immediate active motion in the direction of the repaired tendon. The main difference in these approaches is within the early phase, or first month, of tendon rehabilitation. All flexor tendon approaches protect the flexor tendon repair with some version of a dorsal blocking orthosis that flexes the wrist and/or MP joints to protect the repaired tendon from excessive stretch through approximately 6 weeks postoperatively. Box 30-1 summarizes the orthoses used in the early phase of rehabilitation within the various approaches following flexor tendon repair. The orthoses and exercises for each phase of healing are located in Tables 30-1 through 30-3.

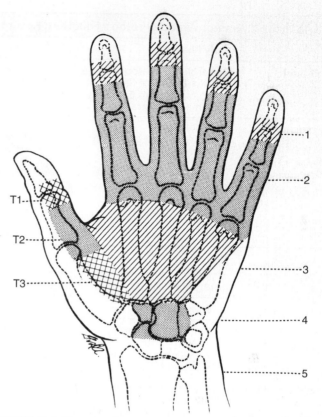

FIGURE 30-6 Flexor tendon zones in the hand. (From Kleinert HE, Schepel S, Gill T: Flexor tendon injuries. *Surg Clin North Am* 61:267, 1981.)

BOX 30-1 **Overview of Orthoses Used for Flexor Tendon Repairs in the Early Phase of Tendon Healing**

Immobilization
- Dorsal blocking orthosis or cast

Immediate Passive Flexion
- Dorsal blocking orthosis with static interphalangeal (IP) positioning (see Fig. 30-8)
- Dorsal blocking orthosis with elastic traction (see Fig. 30-9)

Immediate Active Flexion
- Dorsal blocking orthosis with MP and wrist flexion, static for protection at rest (see Fig. 30-10, *B*)
- Wrist hinge orthosis for exercise (Indiana protocol, see Fig. 30-10, *A*)
- Dorsal blocking orthosis with elastic traction, wrist neutral, for protection and home exercises (Klein protocol, see Fig. 30-11)
- Dorsal blocking orthosis with MP and wrist flexion, with elastic traction, removed in therapy only for active component of exercise (Evans protocol)

TABLE 30-1 Immobilization Protocol Following Flexor Tendon Repair

	Early Phase	Intermediate Phase	Late Phase
Orthosis	Dorsal blocking cast or orthosis • Wrist 20° to 30° flexion • MP joints 50° to 60° flexion with IP joints straight	• Adjust dorsal blocking orthosis to wrist neutral • Remove for exercises	• No protective orthosis • Orthosis for extension at night, if needed

Exercises	• Immobilized
	• Passive flexion by therapist if referred early
		• Passive flexion
		• Duran passive exercises (see Fig. 30-7)
		• Active digital extension with wrist flexed
		• Wrist tenodesis exercise
		• Gentle active digital flexion
		• Assess tendon gliding at 3 weeks; if adherent, add:
		  • Tendon gliding with straight and hook fist (see Fig. 30-13)
		  • Blocking exercises
			Add the following:
			• Full active flexion and extension
			• Blocking
			• Light resistance

TABLE 30-2 Immediate Passive Flexion Protocols Following Flexor Tendon Repair

	Early Phase	Intermediate Phase	Late Phase
Static positioning orthosis	Dorsal blocking orthosis (see Fig. 30-8): • Wrist 20° to 30° flexion • MP joints 50° to 60° flexion • IP joints straight	• Remove orthosis for bathing and exercises	• No protective orthosis • Add night extension orthotic if loss of extension
Elastic traction orthosis	• Same as static positioning orthosis, but add the following: • Elastic traction to fingertips during day (see Fig. 30-9)	• Remove elastic traction from fingertips • Remove orthosis for bathing and exercises	• No protective orthosis • Add night extension orthosis if loss of extension
Exercises	• Passive flexion • Duran passive exercises (see Fig. 30-7) • Active IP extension in orthosis	Remove orthosis, and add the following: • Wrist tenodesis • Place and active hold digital flexion • Gentle active digital flexion • Finger extension with wrist flexed, gradually bring wrist to neutral • Assess tendon gliding • If adherent, add gentle blocking and tendon gliding	Add the following: • Finger extension with wrist neutral, gradually extend wrist • Light resistance if adherent; if minimal adhesions, delay resistance until 8 to 12 weeks • Passive IP extension if needed

TABLE 30-3 Immediate Active Flexion Protocols Following Flexor Tendon Repair

	Early Phase	Intermediate Phase	Late Phase
Orthosis options	• Wrist tenodesis orthosis and static dorsal blocking orthosis (see Fig. 30-10) • Dorsal blocking orthosis wrist neutral, with or without elastic traction (see Fig. 30-11)	• Continue orthosis wear to 6 weeks; if elastic traction was used, discontinue at 4 weeks	• No orthosis, or hand-based dorsal blocking orthosis during heavy activities, work • Dynamic IP extension orthosis after 8 to 10 weeks if IP flexion contracture exists
Exercises	• Wrist tenodesis • Passive digital flexion • Active IP extension with MP joints flexed • Place and active hold in flexion	• Continue with early phase exercises, add the following: • Gentle active flexion • Straight fist (see Fig. 30-13) • Composite fist • Blocking if adhesions present • Passive IP extension if needed	• Continue with intermediate phase exercises, and add the following: • Hook fist (see Fig. 30-13) • Light gripping at 8 weeks if adhesions present, delay if good to excellent tendon gliding

Approaches of Rehabilitation in the Early Phase of Flexor Tendon Healing

An immobilization approach[12,13] is rarely applied following repair of the flexor tendon in the digit, but there are certain situations for which it is appropriate. Children younger than age 12 are most often placed in immobilization for the first 3 to 4 weeks, but evaluate each child related to their maturity level and ability to comply with the exercises and precautions of other approaches. Other individuals who may be placed in immobilization after a flexor tendon repair are those who have cognitive limitations, such as Alzheimer's and noncompliant clients.

When there is a concomitant fracture or significant loss of skin requiring a skin graft, a period of immobilization may be necessary to allow the bone or skin graft to heal adequately before beginning motion.

> ### ◎ *Clinical Pearl*
>
> No active contraction of the repaired flexor musculotendinous unit occurs, and therefore limited, if any, gliding of the flexor tendon occurs in the early phase of rehabilitation in an immobilization approach.

Flexor tendon adhesions and joint stiffness are common complications following immobilization in the early phase of flexor tendon rehabilitation. General guidelines for orthoses and exercises within an immobilization approach are summarized in Table 30-1.

Immediate passive flexion protocols[13-16], developed in the 1960s and 1970s, were the treatment of choice for decades in an attempt to minimize dense adhesions that develop within zone 2. In a study of practice patterns published in 2005,[17] 74% of therapists utilized some type of immediate passive flexion approach for flexor tendon rehabilitation. The therapist should initiate an immediate passive flexion protocol within 3 to 4 days following a traditional two-strand flexor tendon repair or a stronger repair if healing factors or client compliance prohibit placement in an immediate active flexion approach. Fabricate an orthosis that holds the wrist and MP joints in flexion and IP joints in extension to prevent excessive stretch of the repaired tissue. Instruct the client in passive flexion of the fingers using Duran and Houser's technique designed to improve tendon gliding (Fig. 30-7) and active IP extension within a dorsal blocking orthosis. Orthotics and exercise guidelines for immediate passive flexion protocols are summarized in Table 30-2.

The benefits of an immediate passive flexion approach over immobilization are improved circulation for tendon healing, decreased joint stiffness, partial distal gliding of the flexor tendon, and in some cases, a limited amount of proximal gliding of the repaired tendon.

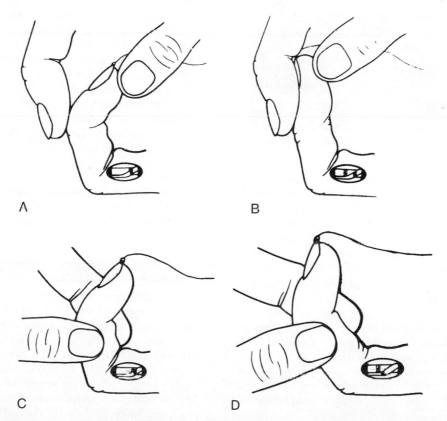

A

B

C

D

FIGURE 30-7 Duran and Houser's exercises for passive flexor tendon gliding. **A** and **B,** With the metacarpophalangeal (MP) and proximal interphalangeal (PIP) joints flexed, the distal interphalangeal (DIP) joint is passively extended. This moves the flexor digitorum profundus (FDP) repair distally, away from the flexor digitorum superficialis (FDS) repair. **C** and **D,** Then, with the DIP and MP flexed, the PIP joint is extended passively. This moves both repairs distally away from the site of repair and any surrounding tissues to which they might otherwise form adhesions. (From Duran RJ, Coleman CR, Nappi JF, et al: Management of flexor tendon lacerations in zone 2 using controlled passive motion postoperatively. In Hunter JM, Schneider LH, Mackin EJ, et al, editors: *Rehabilitation of the hand*, ed 3, St Louis, 1990, Mosby.)

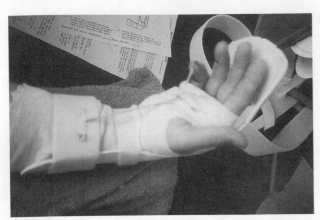

FIGURE 30-8 Dorsal blocking orthosis with static interphalangeal (IP) positioning.

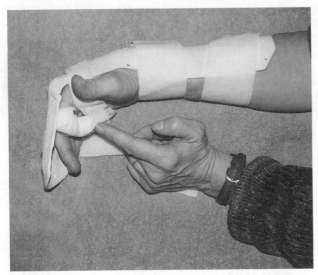

FIGURE 30-9 Dorsal blocking orthosis with elastic traction

While many variations of immediate passive flexion protocols exist, they currently fall into two main categories. These two categories include 1) approaches that use an orthosis that holds the IP joints statically between exercises (Fig. 30-8) during the early phase of tendon healing, or 2) an orthosis with elastic traction to hold the fingers in flexion dynamically between exercises (Fig. 30-9). The rationale for holding the IP joints in flexion between exercises in the early phase of tendon healing is to potentially increase proximal tendon gliding, in part by allowing more time for the tendon to be resting proximally in relation to the repair site and to the pulley system. Holding the digits in flexion decreases stiffness of the digits by applying passive flexion for a greater portion of time. Placement in passive flexion with elastic traction to the fingers between exercises also decreases the potential for inadvertent active flexion of the fingers in the early phase of flexor tendon healing, protecting the tendon from rupture. A frequent complication of holding the fingers in flexion with elastic traction is the increased potential to develop IP flexion contractures and the increased complexity perceived by the client in having a dynamic orthosis on the hand as opposed to a less complicated static orthosis. For those clients using a dynamic flexion orthosis during the day, the elastic traction is detached at night, and the fingers are usually strapped to the hood of the dorsal blocking orthosis. Immediate passive flexion

protocols with elastic traction are an option for those clients who are not showing signs of IP flexion contracture, who can be compliant with the rehabilitation program, and who have no soft tissue healing complications.

Reports indicate a wide variety of results with use of the immediate passive flexion approaches. Limited gliding of the FDP with passive flexion of the digit[18] has been demonstrated, and research continues to develop improved surgical techniques to improve outcomes.

Immediate active flexion approaches following flexor tendon repair began in the 1990s and are the result of surgical advancements with stronger repair techniques (four or more strand repairs), as described earlier. The benefit of an immediate active flexion approach following repair is to achieve flexor tendon gliding prior to the formation of dense flexor tendon adhesions. Numerous researchers[7,19-22] have found significantly improved outcomes with better flexor tendon gliding with use of immediate active flexion rehabilitation approach in the early phase of flexor tendon healing. There are multiple protocols in literature that apply an immediate active flexion component following an adequately strong flexor tendon repair. Orthoses and exercise guidelines for some of the commonly-applied immediate active flexion protocols are outlined in Table 30-3.

Protect the client in a dorsal blocking orthosis at rest, but instruct in **place and active hold** of the fingers in flexion within an appropriate orthosis at home or when in therapy without an orthosis while you assist with the appropriate wrist tenodesis positioning.

- Exercises consist of preparing the digit with slow gradual passive flexion to decrease edema and stiffness, followed by the same passive flexion and active IP extension exercises used for immediate passive motion approaches described in the previous section, and the addition of **wrist tenodesis exercises** and place and active hold flexion as follows:
  - Gently, passively place the fingers in flexion and bring the wrist into 30° extension.
  - Ask the client to hold the fingers in flexion and then release the fingers while the client holds them in place actively. This active component of the exercise, if performed successfully, results in a proximal glide of the flexor tendon that prevents dense adhesions. Watch for trapping of the digit with adjacent digits.
  - Relax the fingers, allow the wrist to relax into flexion with reciprocal finger extension occurring due to wrist tenodesis.

Orthoses

- Wrist hinge orthosis (Fig. 30-10, *A*): Used in the Indiana protocol[19] for exercise. Fabricate forearm and hand portions of the orthosis, with the edges that meet at the wrist formed to block wrist extension at 30°. The MPs of the hand portion are flexed 60° with full IP extension. Also fabricate a dorsal blocking orthosis (see Fig. 30-10, *B*) with the wrist and MPs flexed and the IP's in extension for use between exercises. Benefits include optimal wrist positioning to decrease tension on the repair during active flexion in the early phase of tendon rehabilitation. The client must be trusted to change the orthosis for exercises without using or positioning the injured hand in any other way during changes.
- Dorsal blocking orthosis with wrist neutral (Fig. 30-11): Used in the Klein protocol[20] for both protection and place and active hold exercises at home, removed in therapy for wrist tenodesis

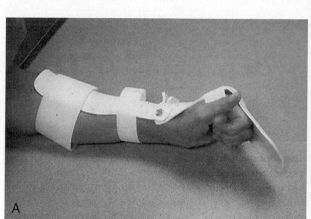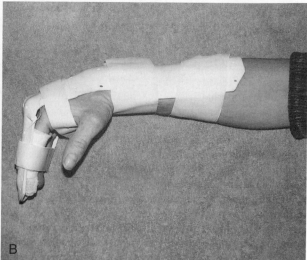

FIGURE 30-10 A, Wrist hinge orthosis for exercise in an immediate active flexion approach to rehabilitation. **B,** Dorsal blocking orthosis with static positioning for protection.

with the active hold component of exercise. In this protocol, orthosis wrist position is based on work by Silfverskiold and May,[7] which used a wrist neutral cast following repair with no increase in rupture rate and had 95% good and excellent results. A wrist neutral position results in significantly less tension during active digital flexion than wrist flexion, but it is not as ideal of a position as partial wrist extension. Current application is used either with or without four-finger elastic traction, depending on the client's tissue response and surgeon preference. Benefits include simple orthotic fabrication and the ability to wear the orthosis at all times, which enables use with clients who are not reliable enough to safely change the orthosis between exercises.

- Dorsal blocking orthosis with wrist and MPs flexed and IP's extended (see Fig. 30-8): Used in the Evans protocol[21] with elastic traction to all four fingers, this traditional dorsal blocking orthosis is removed for wrist tenodesis and place and active hold exercises *in therapy only*. The client performs exercises as in the passive flexion approach described in the previous section at home with no active component except in therapy in the early phase of rehabilitation.

Considerations for placing a client into an immediate active flexion protocol include the following:

- The type of suture repair: When a four or more strand flexor tendon repair has been performed, it is appropriate to consider use of an immediate controlled active flexion protocol with surgeon approval. Although a protocol exists[21] for use of active flexion following a two strand repair, it is applied in therapy only and was originally designed and applied by a very experienced therapist.
- The level of swelling and joint stiffness should be considered, as these factors increase the work of flexion and, if excessive, may prevent a client from being placed into an immediate active flexion approach. **Work of flexion** is a term that describes the amount of tension created within the tendon during active flexion to overcome resistive forces including joint stiffness, edema, friction caused by bulk of repair, tight pulleys, or swelling of the tendon.[23]
- Patient healing factors: The presence of disease, such as diabetes, may result in slower healing.
- The client's compliance level: Low compliance increases the probability that the client will do more than prescribed, or remove the orthosis, increasing potential for rupture. Low compliance should

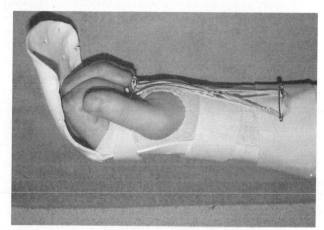

FIGURE 30-11 Dorsal blocking orthosis with elastic traction, wrist neutral. Used in an immediate active flexion approach to rehabilitation.

prevent a client from being placed into an immediate active flexion approach, and if the client is noncompliant, an immobilization approach may be necessary to protect the tendon from rupture.

- The therapist's level of experience: It is recommended that the therapist have a good understanding of flexor tendon healing, suture technique strengths, risks, and precautions before applying an immediate active flexion protocol.

◎ Clinical Pearl

It may be difficult to know the client's compliance level at the first therapy session. When a client demonstrates inability to comply appropriately with the precautions and exercises within a certain approach, changing the rehabilitation approach to one allowing less motion may become necessary, or a cast may be needed instead of a removable orthosis in the first 3 to 4 weeks postoperatively.

Diagnosis-Specific Information that Affects Clinical Reasoning in an Immediate Active Flexion Approach to Rehabilitation

Minimize stress on the tendon during active flexion, especially in the early phase of tendon healing, to prevent rupture. Edema, stiffness, and any internal friction encountered by the tendon because of bulk of repair, tight pulleys, or swelling of the tendon increases work of flexion with active flexion. Our goal as therapists is to minimize the work of flexion, thereby minimizing stress on the repaired tendon, especially when active motion is initiated immediately following repair. This is achieved by minimizing edema and joint stiffness and by using optimal joint positions that minimize the amount of tension developed within the tendon during active flexion.

Optimal Wrist Position

Research has shown that the wrist position that results in the least tension within the flexor tendon during active flexion is that of partial wrist extension and MP flexion.[24] When the wrist is flexed, a significantly increased amount of work is required by the flexor muscles to flex the fingers as compared to when the wrist is slightly extended. By placing the wrist in slight extension, the extensor tendons are given slack at the wrist, allowing the fingers to relax into partial flexion. It requires only a slight pull by the muscle to flex the digits further and actively into a light fist. Thus, most immediate active flexion protocols use a position of wrist neutral to slightly extended during the active flexion exercises and avoid active digit flexion with the wrist flexed.

Avoid tight end-ranges of active flexion in the early phase of flexor tendon healing because this significantly increases tension within the flexor tendon.[21]

Precaution. *Our goal in the early phase of flexor tendon healing in an active flexion protocol is to attain a light fist that includes DIP flexion (to ensure FDP gliding), not a tight fist that is made with force. Education of the client in using this approach is important, for those clients who attempt to do more than allowed are much more likely rupture the repair.*

Initiating Active Flexion

While an *active* flexion component is initiated right after surgery in the immediate active flexion approach, the immobilization and immediate passive flexion approaches do not begin *active* flexion until 3 to 4 weeks postoperatively, or the intermediate phase of tendon healing. Adjust the dorsal blocking orthosis to bring the wrist to neutral at this time, and allow the client to perform active flexion with or without the orthosis. At the first session that active flexion is being performed, follow these steps:

- Loosen the joints with passive flexion and while holding the wrist and MPs in flexion, perform active IP extension.
- Perform passive wrist tenodesis exercises:
  - Passively flex the fingers, and bring the wrist into approximately 30° extension.
  - Bring the wrist to neutral, relax the fingers.
  - Flex the wrist, and actively extend the fingers.
- Perform place and active hold of fingers in flexion with the wrist in partial extension.
- Perform active flexion of the fingers with the wrist in partial extension.
- Assess flexor tendon gliding by comparing passive flexion to active flexion.

When active flexion is significantly more limited than passive flexion, it indicates the presence of adhesions preventing proximal gliding of the flexor tendon. In this situation it is appropriate to consider advancing the client to exercises that add more tension on the tendon in a proximal direction if not improved by the next therapy session.

> ## ◎ Clinical Pearl
>
> When initiating active motion, do it gently with a gradual increase in tension applied to the tendon as healing advances. Grasp or pinch of objects greatly increases tension within the flexor tendons and is, therefore, to be avoided in the early phase of flexor tendon rehabilitation and in the intermediate phase unless adhesions limit gliding.

Progression of Exercises

Progression of exercises following flexor tendon repair should begin with the exercises that result in the least force to the tendon repair, and should increase to those exercises that gradually introduce more tension when gliding is limited. Groth[25] has researched the amount of force created by typical flexor tendon exercises and has provided a "pyramid of progressive forces" to guide therapists in the advancement of exercises when adhesions limit active flexion. The force in exercises advances in this order, from lease force to most force: Passive flexion and protected extension, place and active hold in flexion, active composite fist, hook and straight fist (Fig. 30-12, isolated joint motion (blocking), resisted composite fist, resisted blocking. When adhesions limit active flexion more than passive flexion, advance to the next level of exercises. Allow the client to perform these at home for one to two sessions, and advance to the next level only when there is no improvement within the current level of exercise. Consider the following points when advancing a client in the force of exercise:

- The level of adhesions that would justify increasing tension on the flexor tendon repair is not clearly identified in literature; therefore, this decision relies on judgment, experience, and communication with experienced therapists and the referring surgeon. While one reference in the literature suggests that a 50° difference between passive and active flexion justifies advancing the client,[12] another[26] suggests 15°, and yet another defines an active lag as more than 5° difference between active and passive flexion.[25] I consider a 10° to 15° difference or more between passive and active flexion at the PIP *and/or* DIP joint an indication of the presence of adhesions limiting active flexion. I am most concerned about active DIP flexion, as the FDP tendon tends to become the most densely adherent, limiting composite flexion, fine dexterity and grip strength. Placing an appropriate amount of tension on adhesions facilitates remodeling over time in the direction of the tension, allowing improved gliding of the tendon.

Precaution: *Adding too much force can overpower the adhesions and repair and result in rupture of the repaired flexor tendon.*

- If a client has good early active motion, delay resistive exercises because there are fewer adhesions. If a client lacks motion due to adhesions, resistive exercises can be initiated sooner. Resistance is introduced appropriately when adhesions limit active motion more than passive motion, in an effort to place tension on the scar to improve proximal gliding of the tendon. *This same resistance, however, may overpower the tensile strength of the*

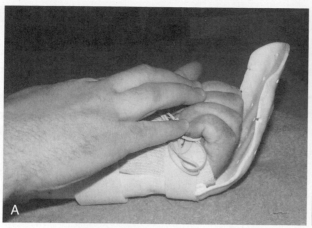
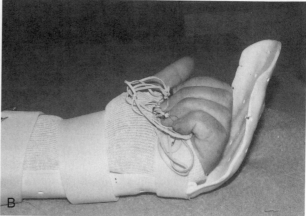

FIGURE 30-12 Place and active hold in flexion following a four-strand flexor tendon repair begins with gentle passive placement of the fingers in flexion using the client's other hand **(A),** followed by release of the fingers while they are held in place actively **(B).**

There are three ways of making a fist:

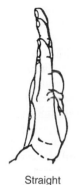

Straight

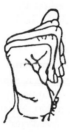

Hook

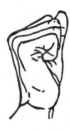

Straight

Fist

FIGURE 30-13 The three different positions of tendon gliding exercises: hook fist, straight fist, and full fist. (From Stewart Pettengill K, van Strien G: Postoperative management of flexor tendon injuries. In Mackin EJ, Callahan AD, Skirven TM, et al, editors: *Rehabilitation of the hand and upper extremity,* ed 5, St Louis, 2002, Mosby.)

repair and result in a rupture. Good active motion of the repaired tendon indicates lack of adhesions that would prevent proximal gliding of the repaired tendon. Tension develops in the flexor tendon when the muscle pulls against added resistance. Without the support and restriction of surrounding adhesions, all this tension is transferred directly through the repaired tendon, and the risk of tendon rupture greatly increases when resistance is introduced. Thus all timelines in this chapter must be individualized, and progression to resistance of the repaired flexor tendon that is showing good to excellent gliding is done at the later of the timelines discussed or is deferred until the referring surgeon determines the tendon is near or at full tensile strength.

Precaution. *Resistance is initiated in the intermediate phase of healing only in the presence of significant flexor tendon adhesions that prevent active flexion more than passive flexion. If active flexion is not limited significantly, resistance is deferred until the late phase of tendon healing or until the surgeon has determined the tendon is near or at full tensile strength. Tendon repairs are never at their full strength when motion is initiated. The risk exists for gapping or potential rupture of a tendon throughout the healing process.*

Knowledge of tendon healing and the relative strength of the tendon repair as time progresses, as well as the restricting effect of tendon adhesions is the basis for determining safe upgrades to resistive exercises of the repaired tendon.

Interphalangeal Flexion Contractures

A frequent complication following flexor tendon repair is development of **PIP flexion contracture,** where the PIP joint is unable to be passively extended due to joint capsule and ligament tightening. To minimize flexion contractures, the dorsal blocking orthosis should be properly fabricated initially with the IPs strapped in extension at night. It is important to attempt to attain full active IP extension as soon as possible after repair to prevent this from occurring. There are safe and appropriate techniques to prevent/correct IP flexion contractures. These should be done only with the supervision of an experienced hand therapist, very gently, with maximal MP flexion of the involved digit to minimize stress on the repaired tendon. This is potentially dangerous and caution must be high.

⊚ Clinical Pearl

The protected position of a flexor tendon is with all other joints that the tendon crosses supported passively in flexion to provide slack to the tendon.

For instance, following a flexor tendon repair, when a PIP joint flexion contracture exists at 4 weeks after repair, support the wrist and MP joint in flexion while applying gentle joint mobilization or passive PIP extension. This will prevent excessive stretch of the repaired flexor tendon while providing assistance to improve extension of the joint. Perform the passive extension slowly and respect any guarding, because this may indicate end range, and the client may protect by engaging the flexor tendon, eliciting resistance which is unsafe to the repair.

A volar extension gutter to improve PIP extension may be used at night beginning at approximately 5 to 6 weeks postoperatively or as approved by the surgeon.

Regardless of the goals, especially following use of an immobilization or an immediate passive flexion protocol, active flexion of a repaired flexor tendon may be limited because of adhesion formation. Limited active flexion of the repaired digit, especially the DIP joint, frequently occurs due to adhesions, and there may be difficulty actively flexing the adjacent digits because of the common muscle belly of the FDP (**quadriga effect**). Grip strength is diminished because of loss of active flexion. Flexor tendons with adhesions commonly require a more prolonged time of rehabilitation with a strong emphasis on a home exercise program (HEP) of blocking exercises and resistance even longer than the 12-week healing period to continue to facilitate tendon gliding during the long remodeling process. Further surgical procedures are available for the repaired flexor tendon with significant adhesions that limit functional use of the hand. If needed, these procedures most often are performed between 4 to 6 months after repair.[2]

Outcomes for the flexor tendon that is allowed immediate passive flexion are improved over those that have been immobilized.[14-16] Outcomes for the flexor tendon following immediate active flexion protocols are even better,[7,19-21] but application of this type of protocol is limited to the strong repair, preferably an experienced therapist, and a compliant and responsible client.

Approaches in Other Zones of the Hand and the Thumb

There are numerous protocols in the literature for flexor tendon repairs in zone 2. Repairs in other areas of the hand receive less attention. Evans[27] has designed a specific protocol for flexor tendon repairs in zone 1. Flexor tendon repairs proximal to zone 2 result in less limiting adhesions and respond better to exercises to improve gliding. The author uses the same orthoses and general time guidelines for repairs in all zones of the repaired flexor tendon unless the surgeon decides to advance the exercises earlier for a client with a strong repair proximal to zone 2.

FPL repair requires a dorsal blocking orthosis for the thumb, holding the CMC in a relaxed position avoiding extension, MP approximately 30° flexed, and full IP extension unless a digital nerve has been repaired and needs protection. The wrist can be positioned in 20° to 30° flexion for a passive flexion protocol, or neutral for immediate active flexion protocol. While some include the fingers in the orthosis,[28] The author allows the fingers to be free. A specific exercise recommended to attain FPL tendon gliding is to stabilize the MP joint while passively flexing and extending the IP joint. A study by Brown and McGrouther[29] showed that gliding of the FPL occurred at the level of the proximal phalanx with the MP joint stabilized while performing passive IP flexion and extension, but no gliding occurred if the MP was flexed during the passive IP motion.

♡ **Tips from the Field**

Orthotic Tips

When applying an orthosis within a few days following a tendon repair, therapists often need to remove postsurgical dressings and apply a light dressing to the surgical incision.

During orthotic fabrication, place the hand in the tendon-protected position. For a flexor tendon repair, this is one of being relaxed in flexion that is attained easily by relaxing the wrist and fingers over the edge of a bolster.

Precaution. *The client may want to stretch or move the hand when the postoperative dressings and orthosis are removed, and it is essential to instruct the client to stay in the position in which he or she is placed during orthotic fabrication.*

Precaution. *As you fabricate the orthosis, it is essential that you avoid placing a stretch on the repaired tendon, because this could cause tendon rupture.*

Evaluation Tips

The first therapy session for a client with a repaired tendon includes removal of dressings and postoperative splint, fabrication of the orthosis described within the protocol chosen, instruction in a HEP, and an abbreviated evaluation. The evaluation portion of the session consists of observation of the wound or surgical incision for drainage, bleeding, or signs of infection, and observation of the amount of swelling in the digits and upper extremity. A verbal description of pain is obtained. Sensation is discussed, and because of the need to fabricate an orthosis at the first appointment, specific sensory testing may be deferred to a later session.

Precaution. *When sensory testing is done, it is important that the hand and digits be maintained in a tendon-protected position.*

ROM is not assessed in the usual manner immediately following a tendon repair. The healing tendon cannot safely be moved through its full excursion in the early phase without rupture. Limited evaluation of ROM is appropriate as indicated in Box 30-2. Box 30-3 describes the method of final assessment of motion following a flexor tendon repair using the Strickland-Glogovac formula.[30]

No strength assessment is appropriate during an evaluation immediately following a tendon potential repair. Assessment of grip and pinch strength is deferred until after the full 12 to 14 week healing period following surgery. Because it is a maximal force activity, The author recommends that grip and pinch strength testing be done with approval of the referring surgeon.

Treatment of tendon repairs in the hand is challenging, requiring us to stay abreast of current changes and gain the experience necessary to understand the process of tendon healing. Box 30-4 summarizes the important concepts to remember when treating a client with a repaired tendon.

Precaution. *It is strongly recommended that you have supervision when beginning to treat tendon repairs to ensure proper hands-on management and an understanding of these important concepts related to the treatment of a client with a flexor tendon repair in the hand.*

BOX 30-2 Evaluation of Range of Motion Following Flexor Tendon Repair

1. In the early phase following a flexor tendon repair, immediately assess passive flexion of all finger joints without disrupting healing tissue, within pain limits.
2. With the wrist and MP joints flexed, assess active IP extension to 0° if no digital nerve injuries are present. *Do not assess composite extension until the intermediate phase of flexor tendon healing, because this could cause tendon rupture.*
3. When using an immediate active flexion protocol, assess the amount of composite finger flexion attained in a place and active hold position with the wrist slightly extended.
4. In the intermediate phase following a flexor tendon repair, evaluate active flexion within all types of protocols. Assess composite finger extension with the wrist flexed and, 1 to 2 weeks later, with the wrist in neutral. *Do not assess grip and pinch strength until after the full 12 week tendon healing process, because this creates significant tension in the repaired tendon.*
5. When healing of the flexor tendon and rehabilitation is complete, calculate the end result of the motion of the injured finger(s) by adding active flexion of the IP joints and subtracting any loss of extension. MP joint motion is not used in this calculation. The formula designed by Strickland and Glogovac[30] commonly is used and can be found in Box 30-3.

BOX 30-3 Classification of Motion Results Following Flexor Tendon Repair[30]

Formula

$$[(PIP + DIP \text{ flexion}) - (\text{loss of PIP extension} + \text{loss of DIP extension})] \div 175 \times 100 = \% \text{ of normal}$$

Classification

Excellent: 85% to 100%

Good: 70% to 84%

Fair: 50% to 69%

Poor: Less than 50%

DIP, Distal interphalangeal; *PIP,* proximal interphalangeal.

? Questions to Discuss with the Physician

Because of the large number of variables that exist in the type and complexity of injuries to tendons, having a good understanding of the injury and surgery before beginning treatment is important. Questions to ask the doctor may include the following:

- Which tendons were lacerated? (This is not always obvious from the laceration.)
- What other structures were included in the injury (nerve, ligament, vessel, bone)?
- Were all structures able to be repaired strongly, or are there concerns with strength or healing of certain structures?
- What type of repair was done (that is, how many strands were used in the flexor tendon repair)?

BOX 30-4 Concepts to Remember When Treating the Repaired Flexor Tendon in the Hand

- Initial orthoses are designed to protect the repaired tendon by preventing tension of the tendon.
- Repaired flexor tendons rupture from stretch into extension or from active flexion that is too strong for the repair to withstand.
- Three types of protocols are designed for postoperative flexor tendon rehabilitation. These are, from the most conservative to least conservative, immobilization, immediate passive flexion, and immediate active flexion protocols.
- Initiate active flexion gently. Active flexion is begun immediately if the surgeon determines the tensile strength of the repair can withstand active flexion, in the intermediate phase of tendon healing for weaker repairs, or when adhesions limit active flexion more than passive.
- The better the active motion in the early to intermediate phase of tendon healing, the fewer adhesions are present. The fewer adhesions present, the longer resistance to the repaired tendon is delayed.
- When performing passive extension to decrease a flexion contracture, have the flexor tendon in a protected position (all other joints held in flexion to give slack to the tendon).
- Advancement from one phase of exercises to the next is done with the awareness of the referring surgeon.
- Resistance to the repaired tendon is deferred unless active motion is limited by adhesions in the intermediate to late phase of tendon healing.

- If referred immediately after repair, is the client being placed into an immobilization protocol or immediate passive or immediate active motion protocol? Clarify the approach you are planning to use for this client.

( ) What to Say to Clients

"A tendon connects the muscle to the bone and is what makes your finger/thumb move in this direction" (illustrate with your hand)." Use a picture or diagram to show the client how the flexor muscle becomes tendon, and how the tendon must be pulled or glide proximally to result in active flexion.

"When your tendon was injured, it could no longer bend your finger/thumb. Now that the surgeon has repaired it, it needs time to heal. A flexor tendon takes 12 weeks to heal. We will increase what you do with your repaired tendon gradually, but if you do too much too soon, it will tear apart. The two things that will cause your tendon to tear apart, or rupture, are a stretch that pulls the repair apart (illustrate on your hand how a stretch into extension would place excessive stretch on a repaired flexor tendon), or a pull from the muscle on the inside that is too strong for the tendon repair to tolerate. For this reason, you must keep your orthosis on at all times for the first month. It will prevent the tendon from overstretching. We will take the orthosis off only in therapy to clean your hand and the orthosis, and to do some additional exercises. If you follow the directions carefully, you also will avoid having the muscle pull too hard on the tendon."

"Under no circumstances should you do more than we instruct you to do with your hand through this healing process, or the tendon may rupture. If it ruptures, it may not be able to be repaired again, or if further surgery is done, the results are not likely to be as good."

CASE STUDIES

CASE STUDY 30-1 ■

J.P. is a 23-year-old man employed as a bartender. He suffered an injury to the volar surface of the small finger, lacerating the FDP and FDS tendons in zone 2 when a glass that he was washing broke in his hand. The surgeon performed a four-strand repair to the tendons and requested an immediate active flexion protocol.

Three days after repair, a dorsal blocking orthosis with the wrist in neutral, MP joints flexed, and IP joints in full extension was fabricated with elastic traction to all four fingers (see Fig. 30-11). J.P. was instructed in a HEP of passive flexion, place and active hold in flexion (Fig. 30-12), and IP extension within the orthosis. He was instructed to keep the orthosis on at all times at home. The orthosis was removed in therapy for cleansing of skin and the orthosis, dressing changes, and wrist tenodesis exercises of 30° wrist extension with gentle passive flexion and wrist flexion as tolerated with fingers relaxed. Passive flexion and place and active hold finger flexion with the wrist in 20° to 30° extension were performed in therapy, and the client did the same at home within the orthosis, keeping the wrist in neutral. IP extension was performed to 0° with the MP joints supported in flexion.

Initial evaluation revealed moderate swelling in the small finger, mild swelling in the hand, and no drainage from the incisional line. Pain was moderate with ROM on the date the orthosis was fabricated. ROM was evaluated for passive finger flexion, IP extension, and place and active hold in flexion gently. Passive small finger flexion was 70° for the MP joint, 70° for the PIP joint, and 50° for the DIP joint. Place and active hold in flexion was evaluated with 70° for the MP joint, 65° for the PIP joint, and 45° for the DIP joint. IP extension was evaluated as −10° for the PIP joint and −5° for the DIP joint with

the MP joints supported in flexion. The client attended therapy two times per week. Gradual gains were made in passive and place and active hold flexion.

At 4 weeks after surgery J.P. was able to attain equal passive and place and hold flexion of 75° for the MP joint, 85° for the PIP joint, and 55° for the DIP joint with IP extension to −5° for the PIP joint and −5° for the DIP joint. At 5 weeks postoperative, the elastic traction was removed from the orthosis. J.P. was allowed to remove the orthosis for active flexion and extension of the fingers with wrist tenodesis and for bathing. At 8 weeks, the orthosis was modified to a hand-based orthosis to allow wrist motion, and J.P. was instructed to use the orthosis at work or during heavy activities to prevent resistance to DIP flexion. Small finger ROM at 12 weeks after surgery was 0° to 90° for the MP joint, 0° to 90° for the PIP joint, and 0° to 70° for the DIP joint (Fig. 30-14). J.P. returned to regular duty and unrestricted use of the hand at 12 weeks after repair with instructions to avoid resisted fingertip resistance (such as, a hook grasp with weight) for another 1 to 2 weeks. The motion results were calculated as $[(90 + 70) − 0] ÷ 175 = 92\%$, which falls into the excellent result category according to the Strickland-Glogovac formula.[30]

This case study is an example of a client with minimal flexor tendon adhesions and good tendon gliding in the early phase of rehabilitation that did not require advancement beyond the place and active hold and active exercises through the entire course of rehabilitation.

CASE STUDY 30-2 ■

S.P. a 28-year-old female, lacerated the FDP and FDS tendons of the left ring finger when attempting to separate frozen meat patties with a knife. She came to therapy 3 days after four strand repairs to the tendons with a request for immediate active flexion approach without elastic traction. A dorsal blocking orthosis with wrist neutral, MPs flexed to 50°, IPs straight is fabricated. Initial evaluation shows mild to moderate edema, minimal drainage from the incisional site with pain reported as 8/10, and significant anxiety verbalized about her injury and the need to move her finger so soon after surgery. Passive flexion is attained to 70° for the MP, 70° for the PIP, and 30° for the DIP. Place and active hold in flexion is 60° for the MP, 45° for the PIP, and 20° for the DIP. Extension of the IP joints with the MPs supported in flexion is −15° for the PIP and −10° for the DIP. Extensive time is spent in client education and reassurance that the pain level will decrease from the current level by performing the exercises

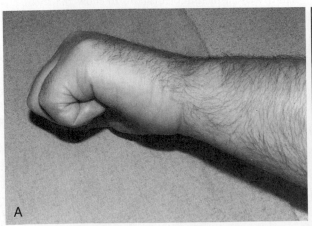
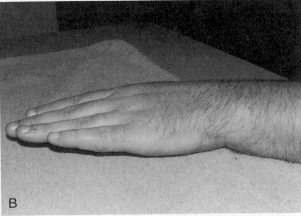

FIGURE 30-14 Case study results at 8 weeks after flexor tendon repair for **(A)** flexion and **(B)** extension.

prescribed and that she is in control of the effort and pain level that results from her exercises.

S.P. is scheduled to attend therapy two time per week, but she missed two sessions in the first 3 weeks. At 2 weeks postoperatively, passive flexion is 75° for the MP, 75° for the PIP, and 35° for the DIP at the end of the session with place and active hold in flexion of 70° for the MP, 55° for the PIP, and 20° for the DIP. The difference between place and active hold and passive flexion is 40°, and the patient is advanced to active flexion. At 3 weeks postoperatively, S.P. has made slight gains to 70° for the MP, 65° for the PIP, and 25° for the DIP; however, there is a 50° difference between passive and active flexion, and gentle blocking exercises are initiated after discussion with the referring surgeon.

The following week, a hook and straight fist is added to the exercise program (see Fig. 30-13). At 6 weeks, gentle gripping with light putty is initiated. Gains are made very gradually, and the result at 12 weeks postoperatively are 0° to 80° for the MP, −10° to 90° for the PIP, and −10° to 30° for the DIP motion. The results according to the Strickland-Glogovac formula[30] are [(90 + 30) − (10 + 10)] ÷ 175 = .57 × 100% = 57% of normal, which falls into a fair result category (see Box 30-3).

This case study demonstrates the advancement of exercises for a client with significant flexor tendon adhesions that limit active flexion more than passive flexion throughout the rehabilitation process.

References

1. Lundborg G, Rank F: Experimental intrinsic healing of flexor tendons based upon synovial fluid nutrition, *J Hand Surg* 3(1):21, 1978.
2. Seiler JG III: Flexor tendon repair, *J Am Soc Surg Hand* 1(3):177–191, 2001.
3. Strickland JW: The scientific basis for advances in flexor tendon surgery, *J Hand Ther* 18(2):94, 2005.
4. Tang J, Gu YT, Rice K, et al: Evaluation of four methods of flexor tendon repair for postoperative active mobilization, *Plast Reconstr Surg* 107:742–749, 2001.
5. Taras JS, Raphael JS, Marczyk S, et al: Evaluation of suture caliber in flexor tendon repair, *J Hand Surg Am* 26A:1100–1104, 2001.
6. Shaeib MD, Singer DI: Tensile strengths of various suture techniques, *J Hand Surg Br* 22(6):764, 1997.
7. Silfverskiold KL, May EJ: Flexor tendon repair in zone II with a new suture technique and an early mobilization program combining passive and active flexion, *J Hand Surg Am* 19:53, 1994.
8. Trail IA, Powell ES, Noble J: The mechanical strength of various suture techniques, *J Hand Surg Br* 17:89–91, 1992.
9. Seiler JG III: Flexor tendon injury. In Wolfe SW, Hotchkiss RN, Pederson WC, et al, editors: *Green's operative hand surgery*, ed 6, Philadelphia, 2011, Elsevier.
10. Momose T, Amadio PC, Zhao C, et al: Suture techniques with high breaking strength and low gliding resistance: experiments in the dog flexor digitorum profundus tendon, *Acta Orthop Scand* 72(6):635–641, 2001.
11. Taras JS, Martyak GG, Steelman PJ: Primary care of flexor tendon injuries. In Skirven TM, Osterman AL, Fedorczyk J, et al, editors: *Rehabilitation of the hand and upper extremity*, ed 6, St Louis, 2011, Elsevier.
12. Cifaldi Collins D, Schwarze L: Early progressive resistance following immobilization of flexor tendon repairs, *J Hand Ther* 4:111, 1991.
13. Pettengill KM, van Strien G: Postoperative management of flexor tendon injuries. In Skirven TM, Osterman AL, Fedorczyk J, et al, editors: *rehabilitation of the hand and upper extremity*, ed 6, St Louis, 2011, Elsevier.
14. Duran RJ, Coleman CR, Nappi JF, et al: Management of flexor tendon lacerations in zone 2 using controlled passive motion postoperatively. In Hunter JM, Mackin EJ, Callahan AD, editors: *Rehabilitation of the hand*, ed 3, St Louis, 1990, Mosby.
15. Kleinert HE, Ashbell TS, Martinez T: Primary repair of lacerated flexor tendons in "no man's land," *J Bone Joint Surg* 49-577, 1967.
16. Dovelle S, Kulis Heeter P: The Washington regimen: rehabilitation of the hand following flexor tendon injuries, *Phys Ther* 69:1034, 1989.
17. Groth GN: Current practice patterns of flexor tendon rehabilitation, *J Hand Ther* 18(2):169–174, 2005.
18. Silfverskiold KL, May EJ, Tornvall AH: Flexor digitorum profundus tendon excursions during controlled motion after flexor tendon repair in zone II: a prospective clinical study, *J Hand Surg Am* 17:122–133, 1992.
19. Strickland JW, Gettle KH: Flexor tendon repair. In Hunter JM, Schneider LH, Mackin EJ, editors: *Tendon and nerve surgery in the hand— a third decade*, St Louis, 1997, Mosby.
20. Klein L: Early active motion flexor tendon protocol using one splint, *J Hand Ther* 16(3):199, 2003.
21. Evans RE, Thompson DE: The application of force to the healing tendon, *J Hand Ther* 6:262, 1993.
22. Trumble TF, Vedder NB, Seiler JG, et al: Zone II flexor tendon repair: a randomized prospective trial of active place-and-hold therapy compared with passive motion therapy, *J Bone Joint Surg* 92(6):1381–1389, 2010.
23. Halikis MN, Manske PR, Kubota H, et al: Effect of immobilization, immediate mobilization, and delayed mobilization on the resistance to digital flexion using a tendon injury model, *J Hand Surg Am* 22:464, 1997.
24. Savage R: The influence of wrist position on the minimum force required for active movement of the interphalangeal joints, *J Hand Surg Br* 13:262, 1988.
25. Groth GN: Pyramid of progressive force exercises to the injured flexor tendon, *J Hand Ther* 17(1):31–42, 2004.
26. Sueoka SS, Lastayo PC: Zone II flexor tendon rehabilitation: a proposed algorithm, *J Hand Ther* 21(4):410–413, 2008.
27. Evans RB: Zone I flexor tendon rehabilitation with limited extension and active flexion, *J Hand Ther* 18(2):128, 2005.
28. Elliot D, Southgate C: New concepts in managing the long tendons of the thumb after primary repair, *J Hand Ther* 18(2):141–156, 2005.
29. Brown C, McGrouther D: The excursion of the tendon of flexor pollicis longus and its relation to dynamic splintage, *J Hand Surg Am* 9:787–791, 1984.
30. Strickland JW, Glogovac SV: Digital function following flexor tendon repair in zone II: a comparison of immobilization and controlled passive motion techniques, *J Hand Surg* 5:537, 1980.

31

Extensor Tendon Injury

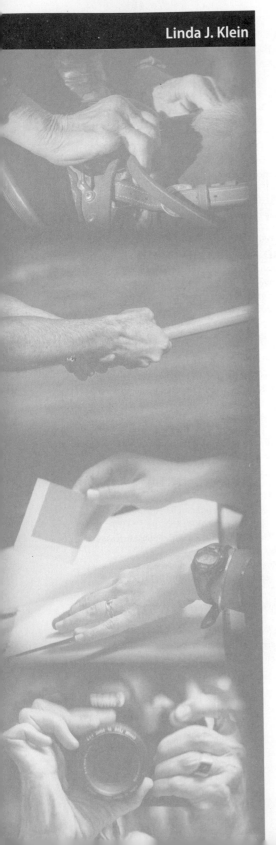

Linda J. Klein

Extensor tendon injuries have long been considered to be less complex than flexor tendon injuries with fewer complications and better results. Numerous authors reflect that complications caused by extensor tendon injuries can be just as frustrating and result in significant loss of motion and function of the injured digit and hand.[1-3] According to Rosenthal and Elhassan, "The extensor muscles to the digits are weaker, their capacity for work and their amplitude of glide are less than their flexor antagonists, yet they require a latitude of motion that is not necessary for flexor function".[1] Extensor tendons are more thin and broad than flexor tendons. They are superficial in comparison with the flexor tendons, allowing adhesion to the fascial layers and skin. Over the proximal phalanx, the extensor tendon has a broad tendon to bone interface that can result in dense adhesions. Shortening of the extensor tendon as a result of surgery may result in difficulty regaining full flexion. Dorsal swelling may prevent the tendons from gliding. Recreating the normal balance between the intrinsic and extrinsic muscle/tendon units can be a difficult task for the surgeon and therapist following extensor tendon injury. Common functional complications include loss of flexion, extensor lag, and decreased grip strength.[2] To prevent these complications, extensor tendon approaches, similar to flexor tendon approaches, have evolved to include controlled passive and active mobilization immediately following surgery. Results, especially in the first 12 weeks, show improved outcome over immobilization.[3-11] The goal of this chapter is for the reader to understand the anatomy, pathology, healing process, and rehabilitation approaches for the differing zones of the extensor tendon to achieve maximal function with minimal complications for the client following extensor tendon repair.

Diagnosis and Pathology

Traumatic injury to the extensor tendons may be by open or closed means. Open lacerations most often occur from a sharp object lacerating the extensor tendon. Open injuries are diagnosed at the time of injury as the wound is explored for tendon, nerve, and ligament damage. Injury to the tendon can vary from a partial to complete laceration or loss of tendon length, from clean to dirty, or from a straight cut made by a sharp edge to a jagged, rough surface. Associated injury to the extensor retinaculum, sagittal bands, bone, ligament, nerve, or vessel may have occurred, or a crushing force may increase the complexity of injury. Repair of the tendon and associated structures is performed as soon after the injury as possible, often in the emergency room.

Closed traumatic injuries of the extensor tendon may occur as a rupture of the tendon from its attachment, from friction of the tendon across a rough bony prominence, or from disease that weakens the tendon, such as rheumatoid arthritis. Closed extensor tendon injuries in the digit include mallet and boutonniere injuries. Rheumatoid arthritis can cause synovial invasion of an extensor tendon, often at the level of the wrist, eventually resulting in its rupture. Closed extensor tendon ruptures also occur at the wrist by friction of the tendon over a bony prominence, such as an extensor pollicis longus (EPL) rupture over Lister's tubercle, or extensor digiti minimi (EDM) rupture over a rough edge of the distal ulna.

This chapter focuses on surgical repair, postoperative healing, and rehabilitation approaches following extensor tendon repair. Closed injuries to the tendon that do not require surgical repair (such as, mallet and boutonniere injuries) are discussed in Chapter 29.

Surgical Repair of Extensor Tendons

Less attention has been given to the types of surgical repair for extensor tendons than flexor tendons. However, the strength of repair of an extensor tendon is important in preventing gapping or rupture when motion is initiated. A number of suture techniques for extensor tendons exists.[1,2,12,13] Newport notes that because extensor tendons are smaller and flatter than flexor tendons and have less cross linking, performing a stronger, multi-strand repair in the extensor tendon is more difficult. The same repair technique performed in an extensor tendon is approximately 50% as strong as if it was performed in a flexor tendon due to the smaller size of the tendon and lack of collagen cross linking.[1,13] The type of suture performed on the lacerated extensor tendon is largely dependent on the area the tendon was injured. The thinner area of extensor tendon (such as, in the digit) will not tolerate multiple strands required for stronger repair.[1] The therapy protocols discussed in this chapter for extensor tendon injury are not dependent on the type of surgical technique used.

Precaution. *The therapist must know, however, whether the surgeon considers the repair to be sufficiently strong to tolerate immediate motion protocols before considering their use.*

Timelines and Healing

Healing of tendons occurs from direct blood supply and synovial diffusion. The blood supply to the extensor tendons is through vascular mesenteries, which travel through the fascia to the tendons from the radial and ulnar arteries and deep palmar arch. Nutrition from synovial diffusion to the extensor tendons occurs from the deep fascial layer in the dorsum of the hand and the extensor retinaculum.[1]

Three basic approaches to rehabilitation of the repaired tendon in the hand are 1) immobilization, 2) immediate passive motion in the direction of the repaired tendon, and 3) immediate active motion in the direction of the repaired tendon. The main difference in these approaches is within the early phase, or first month, of tendon healing.

The early phase of tendon healing consists of the **inflammatory phase** and early **fibroplasia phase** of tendon healing when the tendon is at its weakest and collagen is just beginning to be laid down at the repair site. This phase is also the time when adhesions begin to occur. The intermediate phase of tendon healing includes the period from 3 to 4 weeks to approximately 7 to 8 weeks after repair, during which time the tendon repair gains tensile strength. The late phase of tendon healing includes the period from 7 or 8 weeks to 12 weeks after repair. During this period, the tendon repair continues to gain tensile strength and begins to remodel in alignment with the tension placed on it. The repaired tendon is considered to have nearly full tensile strength at 12 weeks after the repair. Tissue remodeling continues for a number of months.

Most clients who have had an extensor tendon injury and repair are allowed to use their hands functionally by 6 to 8 weeks following repair. The reason for this is that although normal use of the hands consistently offers resistance to the flexor tendons, it rarely offers resistance to the extensor tendons.

Precaution. *Although allowed to use the hand functionally, exercises designed to offer resistance to the extensor tendon should be deferred until the tendon is fully healed to prevent rupture.*

Knowledge of tendon healing is the basis for determining safe advancement to resistive exercises of the repaired tendon. This is an important concept to understand. This guideline affects clinical decisions about strengthening of grip or pinch following a flexor tendon repair or applying resistance to digital extension,

following an extensor tendon repair. Resistance is introduced appropriately to motion of a tendon when adhesions limit active motion more than passive motion in an effort to place tension on the scar to improve proximal gliding of the tendon. *This same resistance, however, may overcome the tensile strength of the repair and result in a rupture.* Good active motion of the repaired tendon indicates lack of adhesions that would prevent proximal gliding of the repaired tendon. Tension develops in the tendon when the muscle pulls again added resistance. Without the support and restriction of surrounding adhesions, all this tension is transferred directly through the tendon, and the risk of tendon rupture greatly increases when resistance is introduced. Thus all timelines in this chapter must be individualized, and progression to resistance of the repaired tendon that is showing good to excellent gliding is done at the later of the timelines discussed or is deferred until the referring surgeon determines the tendon is near or at full tensile strength.

Precautions for Minimizing Tension on a Repaired Extensor Tendon

Tendon repairs are never at their full strength when motion is initiated. The precaution always exists regarding gapping or potential rupture of a tendon until 12 weeks after repair. Two things cause gapping or rupture of a repaired tendon. The first of these is overstretching of the extensor tendon repair by moving too far into flexion (pulling the tendon repair apart) before the tendon is strong enough to tolerate the amount of tension placed on it. The second is an excessive internal pull on the tendon by the muscle during active or resisted motion in the same direction as the repaired tendon. This would include active or resisted extension following an extensor tendon repair before the tendon is strong enough to tolerate that amount of internal tension on the tendon.

Precaution. *When initiating active motion, do it gently with a gradual increase in tension applied to the tendon as healing advances.*

As we encourage tendon gliding for active motion, we must consider the amount of tension the muscle is placing on the repaired tendon to achieve the active motion. Our goal in tendon rehabilitation is to achieve tendon gliding while minimizing tension on the repair during the healing process. We can minimize resistance or tension on the tendon when mobilizing the tendon by decreasing edema and joint stiffness, performing motion slowly and gently, and using optimal positions of proximal joints during active motion. When we mobilize stiff joints associated with the tendon repair in the first 6 weeks after repair, we must do it with the tendon in a protected position.

◎ Clinical Pearl

The protected position of an extensor tendon is with all other joints, especially proximal to the joint being moved, supported in extension to provide slack to the tendon.

For instance, if the PIP joint is stiff following an extensor tendon injury over the dorsum of the hand at 3 weeks after repair, support the wrist and metacarpophalangeal (MP) joint in extension while applying gentle joint mobilization or passive proximal interphalangeal (PIP) flexion. This will prevent overstretch of the repaired extensor tendon while improving flexion of the individual joint.

Because of the large number of variables that exist in the type and complexity of injuries to tendons, having a good understanding of the injury and surgery before beginning treatment is important. Questions to discuss with the physician may include the following:

- Which tendons were lacerated? (This is not always obvious from the laceration.)
- What other structures were included in the injury (sagittal band, ligament, vessel, nerve, bone)?
- Were all structures able to be repaired strongly, or are there concerns with strength or healing of certain structures?
- If referred immediately after repair, is the client being placed into an immobilization protocol or immediate passive or immediate active motion protocol? Clarify the approach you are planning to use for this client.
- For an extensor tendon repair, if not immediately apparent, in which zone is the injury?
- Which joints should be included in the orthosis?
- Is a separate night resting orthosis indicated?
- If not referred immediately following the repair, how was the client positioned following surgery? Was any motion allowed before the time of therapy referral?
- If not referred immediately following surgery, clarify the exercise and activity level that is currently allowed. Is passive flexion and/or resisted flexion or extension contraindicated at the time of referral? Or is the client to be advanced gradually as tolerated?

( ) **What to Say to Clients**

"An extensor tendon connects the muscle to the bone and is what makes your finger/thumb straighten" (illustrate with your hand)." Use a picture or diagram to show the client how the injured extensor muscle becomes tendon, and how the tendon must be pulled by the muscle to glide proximally to result in active extension, and glide distally to allow flexion.

"When your extensor tendon was injured, it could no longer straighten at this (these) joint(s) (illustrate with your hand). Now that the surgeon has repaired it, it needs time to heal. A tendon takes 12 weeks to fully heal, but you will be allowed to use your hand after 6 to 8 weeks for light activities. We will increase what you do with your repaired tendon gradually, but if you do too much too soon, it will tear apart. The two things that will cause your tendon to tear apart, or rupture, are a stretch on the tendon into a bent position (illustrate on your hand how a stretch into flexion would place excessive stretch on a repaired extensor tendon) or a pull from the muscle on the inside that is too strong for the tendon repair to tolerate. For this reason, you must follow the directions for use of your protective brace (orthosis) closely. It will prevent the tendon from overstretching or overuse. Under no circumstances should you do more than we instruct you to do with your hand through this healing process, or the tendon may rupture. If it ruptures, it may not be able to be repaired again, or if further surgery is done, the results are not likely to be as good."

Anatomy

Extrinsic extensor tendons to the digits include the extensor digitorum communis (EDC), extensor indicis proprius (EIP), EDM, EPL, extensor pollicis brevis (EPB), and abductor pollicis longus (APL). Each of these tendons crosses the wrist dorsally, passing under the extensor retinaculum, which is separated into six compartments to maximize mechanical efficiency of the extensor tendons as they cross the wrist, preventing **bowstringing** (Fig. 31-1).

Proximal to the MP joints, the **juncturae tendinum** fibers separate from the EDC tendon, providing a cross-connection to the adjacent EDC tendon. This cross-connection of fibers exists to a variable extent in each individual but most consistently occurs between the EDC to the ring finger and the EDC tendons to the small and middle fingers. The juncturae tendinum fibers assist in extension of the neighboring finger and help maintain the EDC in midline over the metacarpal head during finger flexion.

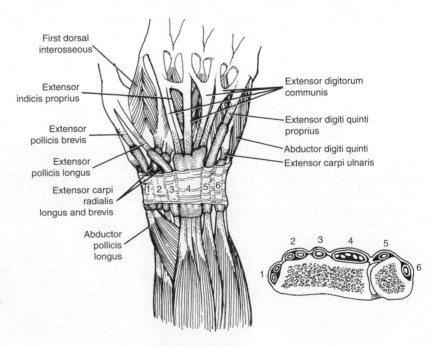

FIGURE 31-1 Extensor tendon anatomy in zones VI and VII. The extensor retinaculum acts as a pulley to maintain the mechanical efficiency of the extrinsic extensor tendons and prevent bowstringing. It also assists in extensor tendon nutrition via synovial diffusion. (From Fess EE: *Hand and upper extremity splinting: principles and methods,* ed 3, St Louis, 2005, Mosby.)

The extrinsic extensor tendons serve the primary purpose of extending the MP joints of the fingers and the thumb MP and IP joints. The EDC also assists in extension of the finger IP joints by its anatomic contribution to the lateral bands and weakly by its attachment on the proximal portion of the middle phalanx.

Extension of the finger PIP and distal interphalangeal (DIP) joints is performed primarily by the lateral bands, which consist of portions of the lumbrical and interossei tendons with contributions from the EDC (Fig. 31-2). The lateral bands on both sides of the fingers pass dorsal to the axis of motion at the PIP and DIP joints and merge over the DIP joint to form the terminal extensor tendon. Extension at the PIP and DIP joints is

delicately balanced by a combination of tendon fibers and ligamentous support in an uninjured finger to prevent excessive dorsal or volar migration (subluxation) of the lateral bands. The transverse retinacular ligament (TRL) supports the lateral bands volarly, and the triangular ligament supports the lateral bands dorsally. The oblique retinacular ligaments (ORLs) run along the sides of the finger and cross the PIP and DIP joints volar to the PIP axis of motion and dorsal to the DIP axis of motion. Thus when the PIP joint extends, it places tension on, or stretches, the ORL. This causes the ligament to tighten across the DIP joint, placing a passive extension assist on the DIP joint by this tenodesis effect.

The IP joint of the thumb is extended primarily by the EPL tendon, and the MP joint is extended by a combination of the EPL and the EPB. The APL, EPB, and EPL tendons extend the carpometacarpal (CMC) joint.

Injuries to the extensor tendon are discussed in relation to the zone of injury, for there are different protocols following repair of the extensor tendon for each set of zones. Extensor tendon zones are reviewed in Fig. 31-3. Orthoses used for extensor tendon repairs in the early phase of tendon healing are reviewed in Table 31-1.

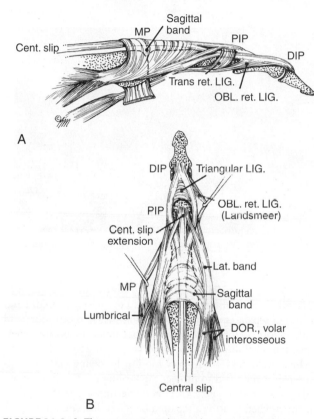

FIGURE 31-2 A, The extensor tendon at the metacarpophalangeal (MP) joint level is held in place by the transverse lamina or sagittal band, which tethers and centers the extensor tendons over the joint. This sagittal band arises from the volar plate and the intermetacarpal ligaments at the neck of the metacarpals. Any injury to this extensor hood or expansion may result in subluxation or dislocation of the extensor tendon. **B,** The intrinsic tendons from the lumbrical and interosseous muscles join the extensor mechanism at about the level of the proximal and midportion of the proximal phalanx and continue distally to the distal interphalangeal (DIP) joint of the finger. The extensor mechanism at the proximal interphalangeal (PIP) joint is best described as a trifurcation of the extensor tendon into the central slip, which attaches to the dorsal base of the middle phalanx, and two lateral bands. The lateral bands continue distally to insert at the dorsal base of the distal phalanx. The extensor mechanism is maintained in place over the PIP joint by the transverse retinacular ligaments (TRLs). (From Doyle JR: Extensor tendons: acute injuries. In Green DP, Hotchkiss RN, Pederson WC, editors: *Green's operative hand surgery,* ed 4, New York, 1999, Churchill Livingstone.)

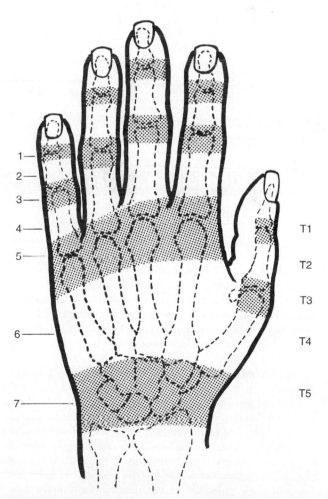

FIGURE 31-3 Extensor tendon zones as defined by the Committee on Tendon Injuries for the International Federation of the Society for Surgery of the Hand. (From Kleinert HE, Schepel S, Gill T: Flexor tendon injuries, *Surg Clin North Am* 61:267, 1981.)

TABLE 31-1	Overview of Orthoses Used for Extensor Tendon Repairs in the Early Phase of Tendon Healing		
Zone of Injury	Immobilization	Immediate Passive Extension	Immediate Active Extension
I and II	DIP extension orthosis (see Fig. 31-4)	None available	None available
III and IV	Finger gutter, full IP extension, taped in place (see Fig. 31-5)	Hand-based outrigger allowing 30° of PIP flexion (see Fig. 31-6)	Finger gutter, taped in place between exercises (see Fig. 31-5) Exercise template with 30° of PIP flexion, 20° of DIP flexion (see Fig. 31-7)
V, VI, and VII	Full-length resting pan in partial wrist extension and full digit extension or slight MP flexion (see Fig. 31-8)	Dynamic MP extension outrigger allowing 30° of MP flexion (see Fig. 31-9, *A* and *B*)	Immediate active extension orthosis using wrist support and yoke (see Fig. 31-10) *Or* dynamic outrigger removed for active extension component

DIP, Distal interphalangeal; *IP*, interphalangeal; *MP*, metacarpophalangeal; *PIP*, proximal interphalangeal.

Zones I and II Extensor Tendon Injuries

Diagnosis and Pathology

Injuries to the extensor tendon in zones I and II result in a mallet finger. Closed injuries may be caused by a tendon rupture or avulsion, resulting in a drooped (flexed) distal phalanx of the digit. Treatment of the closed mallet finger is covered in Chapter 29. Management of an open laceration of an extensor tendon in zones I and II is managed by surgical repair, often with additional support of a pin to hold the DIP joint in extension. Therapy following surgical repair of an extensor tendon in zones I and II is similar to that for closed treatment, which includes immobilization (Fig. 31-4) for a number of weeks as determined by the referring surgeon, followed by a gradual increase in flexion of the DIP joint. Details regarding treatment of the mallet finger are covered in Chapter 29.

Zones III and IV Extensor Tendon Injuries

Diagnosis and Pathology

Injuries in this region may result from closed ruptures or open lacerations. Closed ruptures are often caused by a direct blunt force to the dorsal PIP joint, resulting in rupture of the EDC tendon from its attachment on the middle phalanx. Closed ruptures result in weakened active PIP extension with a limited amount of active PIP extension still present from the intact lateral bands. Over time, development of a larger PIP extension lag results in a boutonniere deformity. Treatment of this injury is covered in detail in Chapter 29.

Open lacerations of the extensor tendon in zones III and IV are common from sharp objects of any kind at the level of the PIP joint and proximal phalanx. Following primary repair of the extensor tendon in this zone, three types of protocols are available in the early phase of tendon healing: immobilization, immediate passive extension, and immediate active extension. Immobilization is often applied, but as advances in surgical management progress, immediate passive, and active motion are being used more commonly, especially in the presence of a complex injury. The three types of protocols vary in application of orthoses and exercises in the early phase of tendon healing for the first 4 weeks following repair. After that time the client is advanced according to the amount of limitation present. Usually, the physician

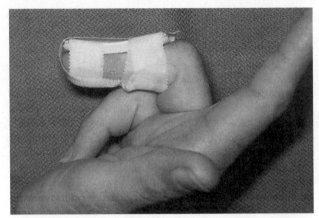

FIGURE 31-4 Distal interphalangeal (DIP) extension orthosis.

determines the protocol and guides the advancement. Determining factors include the type, level, and complexity of injury and strength of repair, as well as patient compliance, motivation, and health factors. Before reviewing the specific protocols for extensor tendon rehabilitation, it is important to understand the ways in which evaluation of range of motion following extensor tendon repair is modified to protect the healing tendon throughout its stages of healing (Box 31-1) and the important concepts to remember when treating a repaired hand tendon (Box 31-2).

Rehabilitation: Early Phase

The early phase of tendon healing begins immediately after repair through the first 3 to 4 weeks following repair.

Immobilization Protocol

- Orthosis: When the repaired extensor tendon is treated with immobilization in the initial phase of tendon healing, a postoperative splint applied by the physician, a finger length cast, or a thermoplastic orthosis made in therapy is applied to hold the PIP joint in full extension. If the lateral bands were injured in addition to the EDC tendon, the DIP is held in full extension as well. The orthosis is worn full time until 3 to 4 weeks postoperatively (Fig. 31-5).
- Exercises: In an immobilization protocol in the early phase of tendon healing, the client moves only the joints that are not restricted within the orthosis. The repaired tendon is protected in extension at all times during the first 3 to 4 weeks.

BOX 31-1 Evaluation of Range of Motion Following Extensor Tendon Repair

Extensor Tendon Repair

1. When initiating therapy in the early phase of healing after an extensor tendon repair, assess passive extension to 0° at all finger joints and wrist extension passively as tolerated.
2. Do not assess active extension immediately following an extensor tendon repair unless an immediate active extension protocol is being used.
3. Do not assess finger flexion in the early phase of tendon healing, with the exception of 30° flexion when an immediate passive or active extension protocol is used. Awareness of the position that protects the tendon is essential when allowing controlled motion in the direction that will place tension on the repair.
4. In the intermediate phase of tendon healing, first evaluate the extensor tendon for flexion at each individual finger joint while supporting the other joints in extension. One to 2 weeks later, evaluate composite flexion of the fingers with the wrist in extension, and evaluate the wrist for flexion with the fingers relaxed.
5. At the completion of treatment, composite flexion of the fingers, subtracting any loss of active extension, gives the total active motion results for the injured digits.

BOX 31-2 Concepts to Remember When Treating the Repaired Tendon in the Hand

- Initial orthoses are designed to protect the repaired tendon by preventing tension of the tendon.
- Repaired tendons rupture from stretch or from active motion by the muscle of the repaired tendon that is too strong for the repair to withstand.
- Three types of protocols are designed for all tendon repairs with the exception of extensor tendon zones I and II. These are, from the most conservative to least conservative, immobilization, immediate passive motion, and immediate active motion protocols.
- Motion, when initiated, is done gently. Motion is begun when the surgeon determines the repair and tensile strength of the tendon can withstand gentle motion.
- The better the active motion in the early to intermediate phase of tendon healing, the fewer adhesions are present. The fewer adhesions present, the longer resistance to the repaired tendon is delayed.
- Passive motion in the direction that would stretch the tendon repair is done for joint stiffness only with the tendon supported on slack in a protected position.
- Advancement from one phase of exercises to the next is done with the awareness of the referring surgeon.
- Resistance to the repaired tendon is deferred unless active motion is limited by adhesions in the intermediate phase of tendon healing.

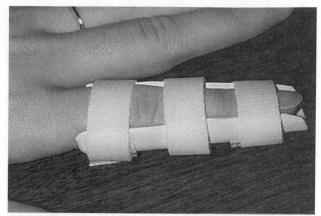

FIGURE 31-5 Finger gutter, taped in place, used for immobilization following zone III to IV extensor tendon repairs, or between exercises in an immediate controlled active motion program.

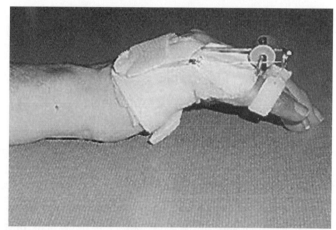

FIGURE 31-6 Hand-based outrigger allowing 30° of proximal interphalangeal (PIP) flexion used in immediate controlled passive program for zone III to IV extensor tendon repairs.

Immediate Passive Extension Protocol

- Indications: When dense adhesions are expected to limit gliding of the tendon, or at the discretion of the referring surgeon, an immediate passive extension approach to rehabilitation to achieve 5 mm of extensor tendon glide distally may be prescribed.
- Orthosis: Within the first 3 days following repair, fabricate a hand-based **extension outrigger orthosis** that supports the MP joint and provides passive extension of the PIP joint (Fig. 31-6). The PIP joint is allowed to flex 30°, with an elastic extension sling bringing the PIP joint back to 0° following the limited amount of flexion.[7] The outrigger holds the finger in full PIP extension at rest, between exercises. The wrist is not included in this orthosis.
- Exercises: Instruct the client to exercise hourly with the orthosis on at all times with ten repetitions of 30° PIP flexion followed by passive extension provided by the sling attachment. Flexion is limited at 30° by an attachment on the outrigger line that blocks further distal migration of the outrigger line at that point. The outrigger orthosis is left in place for the first 3 to 4 weeks. Some protocols allow a gradual increase in the number

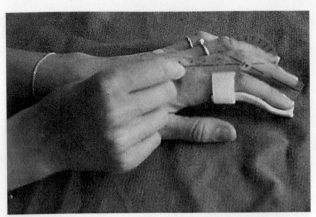

FIGURE 31-7 Exercise template with 30° of proximal interphalangeal (PIP) flexion and 20° of distal interphalangeal (DIP) flexion used in an immediate controlled active motion program for zone III to IV repaired extensor tendon.

of degrees that the PIP is flexed during the 3 to 4 week period.[8] At that time, the orthosis is removed, and the client is allowed to flex to tolerance as discussed in the intermediate phase exercises that follow.

Precaution. *It is important to educate the client not to flex further than instructed to avoid rupture of the repair.*

Immediate Active Extension Protocol

- Indications: An immediate active extension protocol is appropriate for the same situations as an immediate passive extension protocol and has the added benefit of more definitive proximal tendon gliding, as well as the distal tendon gliding that the passive extension exercises provide. Begin the protocol within the first 3 days after repair. An immediate controlled active extension approach entitled the short arc motion protocol or **SAM protocol,** described by Evans,[3,9] is described in the following paragraph.
- Orthosis: The SAM protocol orthosis supports the finger in full IP extension (0° PIP and DIP thermoplastic gutter orthosis or cast) at all times except exercise. Fabricate a second orthosis with 30° of PIP and 20° of DIP flexion that is used as an exercise template (Fig. 31-7). Fabricate a third, shorter finger gutter orthosis that holds the PIP joint in full extension and allows the DIP to flex to tolerance. If the lateral bands also were injured and repaired, the DIP joint is limited to 30° flexion during this exercise, which the client visually monitors.
- Exercises: Hourly, the exercise template is placed on the finger that allows 30° PIP and 20° DIP flexion. The wrist is placed in 30° flexion to give slack to the flexor tendons, resulting in less resistance to active extension of the IP joints. With the finger gutter exercise template in place, the finger is allowed to flex to the exercise template and then perform active extension of the IP joints. If the lateral bands are uninjured, the third exercise orthosis is applied, and while holding the PIP joint in full extension, the DIP is flexed to tolerance. Brief but frequent exercises (ten to twenty repetitions hourly) are performed. At 2 weeks after repair, the exercise template is increased to 40° PIP flexion. At 3 weeks after repair, the exercise template is increased to allow 50° PIP flexion, and at 4 weeks, 70° PIP flexion. The exercises then progress into the intermediate phase of exercises.

Rehabilitation: Intermediate Phase

At 4 weeks, discontinue use of orthosis, and begin active flexion with individual joint flexion. Active flexion is likely to be most limited in the client who has been immobilized in the early phase of tendon healing, as described before. At 5 weeks, advance to gentle composite flexion. Heat may be used to warm the tissues before active exercises.

Precaution. *Client education is important, because early overaggressive flexion of the PIP joint may result in re-injury of the extensor tendon.*

> ### ◎ Clinical Pearl
>
> The tendon that has not been moved in the early phase of tendon healing often is limited by adhesions, and the temptation is immediately to apply force to help it move. The immobilized tendon, however, is not stronger than the mobilized tendon, and motion must be initiated gradually.

> ### ( ) What to Say to Clients
>
> "We are now going to be moving the finger in a way that places a limited amount of stress on the repaired tendon. Because the tendon is not at full strength yet, it is important to do the motions slowly and to aim for a gradual increase in ability to bend the middle and tip joints. You don't want to force the finger down using an outside force (such as, your other hand), or you may reinjure your tendon. We hope to see about 30° of improvement each week, and make sure that you can keep straightening your finger. It is easier to get better at bending the finger, but harder to regain the ability to straighten the finger once it is lost."

At 6 weeks, if active flexion is not showing steady, gradual progress, therapy may advance to use of passive flexion. Heat with support in flexion may assist in regaining composite flexion. Initiate grip strengthening at this time. A gentle dynamic or static progressive flexion orthosis may be used after 6 weeks after repair if flexion remains significantly limited. It is important to consult with the referring surgeon before applying an orthosis that applies force to the repair.

Diagnosis-Specific Information that Affects Clinical Reasoning

When an immediate passive or active extension protocol is used in the initial phase of healing, less limitation in flexion is expected in the intermediate phase of tendon healing.

Precaution. *If steady, gradual progress is being made into flexion, passive flexion or use of dynamic orthoses to increase flexion is deferred until a plateau occurs.*

Limited extension of the IP joints caused by **extensor tendon adhesion** (passive extension is better than active extension) is treated with use of a night extension orthosis, an emphasis on active extension exercises during the day, and less emphasis on strong flexion.

Because IP joint extension is performed most strongly by the lateral bands, it increases efficiency of the extensors to hold the MP joint in flexion while performing active IP extension. This is called *reverse blocking.* MP hyperextension is to be avoided when performing IP extension, because MP hyperextension limits the ability of the EDC to assist in IP extension and decreases efficiency of the lateral bands.

The individual with an extensor tendon repair often is allowed to return to full use of the hand without restriction after 6 weeks and may be discharged from therapy at this time if motion is functional and the client is advancing with a home exercise program (HEP). However, the finger may not achieve a functional level of motion within the intermediate phase of healing when strong adhesions are present, requiring further therapy.

Rehabilitation: Late Phase

From 8 to 12 weeks following extensor tendon repair, the client is allowed full normal use of the injured hand. In therapy, limited flexion continues to be treated with heat that may be combined with stretch, passive and active flexion, blocking exercises, composite flexion exercises, and grip strengthening. Static progressive or dynamic flexion orthoses can be used to supplement the HEP to increase flexion. Limited active IP extension continues to be treated with **reverse blocking exercises,** night IP extension gutter, and the addition of resistance to the repaired tendon. Resistance to extension facilitates a stronger proximal pull on the adherent extensor tendon to improve active extension. This is performed by applying reverse blocking with manual resistance, or the client may extend the fingers against a loop of putty, resistive band strip, or rubber band. However, these exercises are only effective in improving gliding of the extensor tendon in zones III and IV if MP hyperextension is blocked during the exercise. If passive IP extension is limited, use of a dynamic IP extension orthosis intermittently during the day and night static extension orthosis is indicated.

Zones V, VI, and VII Extensor Tendon Injuries

Diagnosis and Pathology

Injuries in zones V, VI, and VII are most often due to lacerations. Another cause of injury to the extensor tendons in zone VII is rupture from disease (such as, rheumatoid arthritis) or bony abnormality resulting in fraying and rupture. Tendon injuries in these zones require surgical repair for healing. Following surgical repair in these extensor tendon zones, there are protocols for all three approaches of immobilization, immediate passive extension, and immediate active extension from which to choose in the early phase of tendon healing.

Rehabilitation: Early Phase

Immobilization Protocol

Immobilization of extensor tendon repairs at the MP joints and proximally is in the form of a full-length resting cast or thermoplastic orthosis (Fig. 31-8). Some surgeons keep the client in a postoperative slab for the full 4 weeks; others have a thermoplastic orthosis fabricated in therapy. The position of the orthosis is in partial wrist extension and full digit extension. Some surgeons prefer slight MP flexion (20°) in the orthosis; however, this may result in an MP extension lag.[3] If the repair is proximal to the juncturae tendinum in the dorsum of the hand, the tendons on

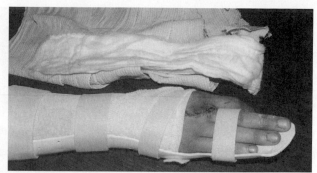

FIGURE 31-8 Full-length resting pan extension orthosis used in an immobilization approach following repair in zone V to VII.

either side of the injured tendons must be supported in extension along with the injured tendon. If the repair is over the MP joint, distal to the juncturae tendinum, the injured finger with the repaired tendon may be held in full extension with the adjacent fingers placed in 30° MP flexion or allowed to flex to tolerance. Flexion of the adjacent fingers, when the repair is distal to the juncturae tendinum, pulls the proximal portion of the repaired tendon distally, relieving tension from the repair. Exercises begin in the intermediate phase of tendon healing in the immobilization protocol, at approximately 4 weeks after repair.

Immediate Passive Extension Protocol

- Indications: Immediate passive extension may be used for complex injuries, multiple tendon injuries, injuries under the extensor retinaculum at the wrist, or by surgeon preference. The most frequently used immediate controlled passive extension program was developed by Evans[3,10] and is described here. In her most recent publication, Evans[3] recommends immediate motion for all extensor tendon repairs proximal to zones I and II. Injuries in zone VII of the finger extensor tendons or zone V of the thumb are in the area of the extensor retinaculum. Evans notes that repairs in this area result in adhesion formation, and recommends treatment by immediate passive or active motion to minimize adhesions. Initiation of this protocol is within the first 3 days following repair.[3,10]
- Orthosis: The orthosis for immediate passive extension consists of an extension outrigger that supports the wrist in extension and the injured fingers in full extension at rest, allowing 30°of MP flexion at the index and long, and up to 40° for the ring and small finger MP joints during exercise (Fig. 31-9). The MP flexion may be blocked at the correct amount of flexion by a volar orthosis or by a stop bead placed on the outrigger line that stops the flexion at the appropriate level. The orthosis is worn full time for the first 3 weeks after repair and is removed in therapy only for exercises and cleansing of the orthosis and skin. When necessary, a night extension orthosis may also be fabricated, and if needed the dorsal component of the orthosis can be removed to simplify dressing when a separate volar support is in place.[3] The client must understand the potential risk of rupture if the orthosis is removed and the finger is allowed to flex too far.
- Exercises: Instruct the client to flex the fingers using only MP flexion, to the orthosis stop (30° to 40°), and then to relax the fingers. When the fingers are relaxed, the outrigger and sling attachments move the fingers passively back to 0° extension.

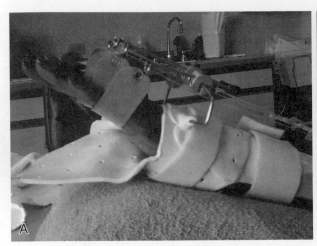
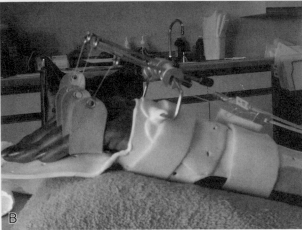

FIGURE 31-9 A, Dynamic metacarpophalangeal (MP) extension outrigger allowing 30° MP flexion. **B,** Active flexion within the immediate passive extension orthosis is blocked at 30° by a volar portion of the orthosis base. Used in an immediate passive program following extensor tendon repair in zones V to VII.

Flexion of 30° to 40° at the MP joint results in 5 mm of distal glide of the extensor tendon, which decreases the dense adhesions that occur with immobilization. The IP joints of the fingers can be flexed gently through their full available range with the MP and wrist joints supported in full extension. The exercises are performed for ten to twenty repetitions hourly. At 3 weeks after repair, remove the flexion block from the orthosis, and allow the client to flex the fingers to tolerance with extension continuing to be assisted by the dynamic slings for another 2 to 3 weeks.

- Passive wrist tenodesis exercises are performed in therapy only, as follows: Full passive wrist extension, allow the MPs to relax to 40° flexion (support the fingers manually to prevent too much flexion); then passively lift the fingers to full extension while allowing the wrist to flex to 20°.
- This protocol can be applied to the repaired EPL tendon of the thumb following repair in zone TV.[3] The orthosis holds the wrist and the thumb MP and CMC joints in extension and applies an outrigger and sling support to the IP joint. The IP joint is allowed to flex 60° to attain 5 mm of tendon gliding in zone TV (under the retinaculum). The passive wrist tenodesis exercise following thumb extensor tendon repair in Zone V is performed by the therapist as follows: Support the wrist at 0°, and hold all joints of the thumb in full extension. Then relax the thumb, and passively extend the wrist to full extension.
- At 3 to 4 weeks exercises are advanced to remove the orthosis to allow gradual active flexion at each individual joint of the thumb and wrist while all other joints are held in extension. The orthosis can be removed for showering and exercises, but worn at all other times until 5 to 6 weeks post repair.

Immediate Active Extension Protocol

- Indications: Evans[3,10] has described a program performed only in therapy only that includes an active motion component for repairs in zones V to VII in the early phase of tendon healing. She suggests its use for any extensor tendon repair, especially repairs that are considered complex, and those under the extensor retinaculum at the wrist. Howell, Merritt, and Robinson[11] describe another immediate controlled active extension protocol that is applied for zones IV to VII extensor tendon repairs.

- Orthoses and Exercise: The following describes these two protocols:
  - Immediate Controlled Active Motion Program designed by Evans: The immediate active rehabilitation approach described by Evans and Thompson[3,10] uses an outrigger orthosis as described in the immediate passive extension program for the client to wear at all times except therapy. In therapy only, the orthosis is removed for the active motion portion of the exercises, as follows: Perform slow, repetitive wrist/MP tenodesis motion as described in the passive motion protocol until the passive motion offers minimal resistance (decreases stiffness and effects of edema). The active hold portion of the exercise is then performed by supporting the fingers in full extension and allowing the wrist to 20° flexion. The client is then asked to hold the fingers actively in this position of extension for a few seconds. The MP joints are then allowed to flex to 30° and actively extend back to 0° with the wrist supported in 20° flexion. This is performed for twenty repetitions in therapy only. Results described by Evans that compare immobilization to the immediate passive and active extension approaches show a significant improvement in tendon gliding using the immediate motion programs.[3,10]
  - Relative Motion Orthotic Positioning for immediate controlled active motion (ICAM) of the repaired extensor tendon in zones IV to VII by Howell, Merritt, and Robinson:[3,11] Within the first 10 days, preferably within the first 3 days after repair, a two-piece orthosis is fabricated. One component of the orthosis is a volar wrist support that holds the wrist in 20° to 25° extension. The second component of the orthosis is a yoke that is made from a long, thin piece of thermoplastic material, which is the width of the proximal phalanx and 1.5 times the length of the dorsum of the hand across the metacarpals. This yoke is wrapped under the injured fingers and over the uninjured fingers to support the injured fingers in 15° to 20° of relative MP hyperextension compared with the adjacent fingers (Fig. 31-10).
- Full active composite flexion and extension as available within the orthosis are performed day 1 to 3 weeks following

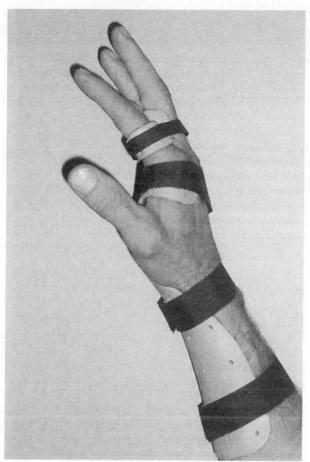

FIGURE 31-10 Immediate controlled active motion (ICAM) orthosis using wrist support and yoke. Also referred to as *relative motion orthosis.* (From Howell JW, Merritt WH, Robinson SJ: Immediate controlled active motion following zone 4-7 extensor tendon repair, *J Hand Ther* 18[2]:182, 2005.)

extensor tendon repair. The client wears the orthosis full time during these 3 weeks. At 3 weeks, the therapist removes the wrist orthosis to allow wrist range of motion (ROM) with the yoke orthosis in place. The client continues to wear the wrist and yoke combination for moderate to heavy activities until 5 weeks after repair. Between 5 and 7 weeks, the client wears only the yoke portion of the orthosis. Most clients were discharged from therapy at 7 weeks postoperatively with better than 90% excellent and good results.[3,10,11]

Rehabilitation: Intermediate Phase

Orthosis

At 4 weeks after repair followed by immobilization, use of protective orthoses is decreased to intermittent use during work and heavy or risky activities and gradually is discontinued. If extension is limited, a night resting pan orthosis in full extension is indicated. With use of an immediate active or passive extension protocol, the orthosis described under those protocols may be continued until 6 to 7 weeks after repair (as described earlier).

Exercises

At 4 weeks after repair of extensor tendons in zones V, VI, and VII, a gradual increase in active flexion for individual joints is allowed as follows:
- MP flexion with IP joints extended
- IP flexion with MP joints extended
- Wrist flexion with fingers extended

Modalities may include heat of choice to decrease stiffness if not otherwise contraindicated.

At week 5 or 6, begin composite flexion of fingers. Gentle passive flexion may be added if flexion is significantly limited. Support the fingers in a flexion wrap to tolerance, and apply heat as appropriate. At 6 to 7 weeks, composite flexion of wrist/fingers may be added.

Diagnosis-Specific Information that Affects Clinical Reasoning

When active MP extension is limited because of adhesions in zone V, VI, or VII, an extensor lag results in which passive extension is better than active extension. In addition to an extension orthosis at night, active extension exercises are important to place proximal tension on the adhesion to improve proximal gliding of the adherent tendon.

Regaining full composite extension, which is a balance of EDC and intrinsic muscle function, may be even more challenging. Supporting the finger in full passive extension, such as on a table, and attempting to lift the limited finger up from the table can facilitate this motion. When the repaired EDC is adherent, although clients are unsuccessful in lifting the finger up from the table, they often can feel the proximal tugging of the extensor tendon on the dorsal hand. This is necessary to facilitate proximal gliding of the tendon and provides feedback to clients that they are using the correct muscle/tendon. If clients flex the MP joints during this exercise, rather than using the EDC to attempt to lift the MP joint, they will feel increased pressure on the table from the fingertip, providing feedback that they are using the wrong muscles. It may be helpful to have the client use the uninjured hand to hold the injured hand gently flat on the table while performing the composite extension lift with the injured hand. This allows them to feel and possibly see the tug on the adherent extensor tendon.

Precaution. *This exercise should be done only 6 weeks or more after repair because the uninjured hand may be offering resistance to the repaired extensor tendon while supporting the hand downward on the table.*

Ⓒ Clinical Pearl

The most effective way to improve active MP extension is with the IP joints flexed or relaxed. When the MP joint is limited in active extension and the client attempts to lift the unsupported finger actively, the intrinsic muscles often work first, for they are not limited by adhesions. Because the intrinsic muscles perform IP extension with MP flexion, when they work to extend the finger without effective EDC gliding, strong IP extension and MP flexion result, defeating the purpose of the exercise. Isolated MP extension is achieved with the IP joints relaxed in flexion and is the most successful way to begin to attain proximal gliding of the adherent EDC proximal to the MP joint.

Rehabilitation: Late Phase

Continue with exercises to maximize proximal and distal gliding of the extensor tendon as described for the intermediate phase exercises. Add grip strengthening and gradual increase in functional upper extremity exercise beginning at 6 weeks after repair. For deficits in flexion, add dynamic or static progressive flexion orthotic use intermittently during the day beginning at 6 to 8 weeks after repair, as approved by the referring surgeon.

CASE STUDY 31-1 ■

E.E., a 53-year-old meat cutter, sustained a work-related saw injury of the dorsal right small finger while cutting meat. He was seen at an emergency room at a workmen's compensation clinic associated with the workplace. He developed an infection, was treated with intravenously administered antibiotics, and was referred to the hand surgeon 8 days after injury. Surgery was performed 9 days after injury, and exploration showed a ragged laceration extending into the extensor mechanism, including the central slip. The saw also had removed part of the dorsal condyle and articular surface of the PIP joint. The central slip was repaired, and the PIP joint was pinned in almost full extension (Fig. 31-11).

E.E. was referred to therapy 10 days after repair for fabrication of a thermoplastic orthosis to support the wrist in neutral and the ring and small fingers in extension and to protect the pin (Fig. 31-12). The surgeon chose full support and immobilization because of the combination of bone and tendon injury, history of infection, and questionable level of understanding and compliance by the client.

The pin was removed 4 weeks after surgery, and active therapy was initiated three times per week. For the first week, use of the orthosis was continued between bathing and exercises. Beginning the second week (5 weeks postoperatively), the orthosis was used only when E.E. was out of the house until 6 weeks after surgery. Initial ROM of individual joints was 0° to 50° for MP joints, −15° to 20° for PIP joints, and 0° to 5° for DIP joints. Wrist motion was present through 75% of normal range. E.E. was instructed in a HEP for active individual joint flexion, reverse blocking extension exercises, and passive extension. Because of extreme limitations in motion, exercises were advanced to include active composite flexion and gentle passive flexion of individual joints within a week of starting therapy. After 1 week, AROM was 0° to 60° for MP joints, −25° to 40° for PIP joints, and 0° to 10° for DIP joints. Passive extension was to −5° at the PIP joint.

The client returned to light duty wrapping meat at 5 weeks after surgery while wearing the protective orthosis. Therapy consisted of wrapping the fingers in flexion to tolerance with a heat application, followed by active and passive flexion and extension exercises, reverse blocking exercises, and functional grasp and release activities. Buddy straps from small to ring finger were provided in an attempt to improve motion of the small finger. ROM at 6 weeks after repair was 0° to 75° for MP joints, −30° to 55° for PIP joints, and 0° to 10° for DIP joints. Passive extension was available to −5° at the PIP joint, indicating extensor tendon adhesions. Active motion improvements stalled at this time. Improvements of 10° of flexion at each joint would be made in therapy; however, the client would arrive in therapy with the same limitations in motion as the previous session. At 8 weeks after injury, functional strengthening was initiated, and

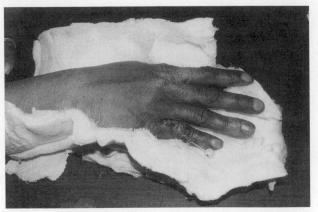

FIGURE 31-11 Complex extensor tendon injury in zones III and IV requiring repair and pin support.

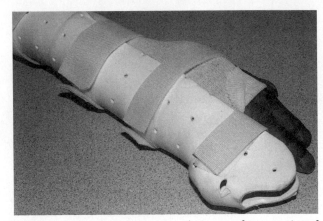

FIGURE 31-12 Full-length extension ulnar gutter for protection of pin and tendon repair.

putty was provided for resistance exercises at home in addition to active and passive home exercises.

The diagnosis of post-traumatic arthritis of the PIP joint was made by radiographic evaluation 11 weeks after surgery. Therapy was discontinued at this time with ROM of 0° to 90° for MP joints, −25° to 60° for PIP joints, and 0° to 25° for DIP joints at the end of a session. The surgeon will continue to follow the client for motion and function of the small finger and hand and will make a determination in the future regarding potential benefit of further surgery, including extensor tenolysis to remove tendinous adhesions.

This case demonstrates the difficulty of regaining flexion and extension of the IP joints with a complex injury when dense adhesions form between the extensor tendon, surrounding tissue, and bone in zones III and IV. An immediate motion protocol, which may have prevented the limiting adhesions, was not considered because of the involvement of injury to the bone at the articular surface and because of client understanding and compliance issues. This case shows that when this combination of factors exists, it may be necessary to immobilize the digit and accept an intact tendon with adhesions, recognizing the potential need for further surgery to improve motion and function.

References

1. Rosenthal EA, Elhassan BT: The extensor tendons: evaluation and surgical management. In Skirven TM, Osterman AL, Fedorczyk JM, et al: *Rehabilitation of the hand and upper extremity*, ed 6, Philadelphia, 2011, Elsevier Mosby, pp 487–520.

2. Newport ML, Tucker RL: New perspectives on extensor tendon repair and implications for rehabilitation, *J Hand Ther* 18(2):175–181, 2005.

3. Evans RB: Clinical management of extensor tendon injuries: the therapist's perspective. In Skirven TM, Osterman AL, Fedorczyk JM, et al: *Rehabilitation of the hand and upper extremity*, ed 6, Philadelphia, 2011, Elsevier Mosby, pp 521–554.

4. Mowlavi A, Burns M, Brown RE: Dynamic vs. static splinting of simple zone V and zone VI extensor tendon repairs: a prospective, randomized, controlled study, *Plast and Recon Surg* 115(2):482–487, 2005.

5. Talsma E, de Haart M, Beelen A, et al: The effect of mobilization on repaired extensor tendon injuries of the hand: a systematic review, *Arch Phys Med Rehabil* 89:2366–2372, 2008.

6. Hall B, Lee H, Page R, et al: Comparing three postoperative treatment protocols for extensor tendon repairs in zones V and VI of the hand, *Am J Occup Ther* 64(5):682–688, 2010.

7. Walsh MT, Rinehimer W, Muntzer E, et al: Early controlled motion with dynamic splinting versus static splinting for zones III and IV extensor tendon lacerations: a preliminary report, *J Hand Ther* 7(4):232–236, 1994.

8. Thomes LJ: Early mobilization method for surgically repaired zone III extensor tendons, *J Hand Ther* 8(3):195–198, 1995.

9. Evans RE: An analysis of factors that support early active short arc motion of the repaired central slip, *J Hand Ther* 5(4):187–201, 1992.

10. Evans RE, Thompson DE: The application of force to the healing tendon, *J Hand Ther* 6(4):266–284, 1993.

11. Howell JW, Merritt WH, Robinson SJ: Immediate controlled active motion following zone 4-7 extensor tendon repair, *J Hand Ther* 18(2):182–190, 2005.

12. Lee SK, Dubey A, Kim BY, et al: A biomechanical study of extensor tendon repair methods: introduction to the running-interlocking horizontal mattress extensor tendon repair technique, *J Hand Surg Am* 35:19–23, 2010.

13. Newport ML, Williams CD: Biomechanical characteristics of extensor tendon suture techniques, *J Hand Surg Am* 17(6):1117–1123, 1992.

32

Tendon Transfers

Deborah A. Schwartz

Working with clients undergoing tendon transfer surgery is an incredibly exciting and rewarding process. As a therapist, you most likely will be working with individuals who sustained trauma or injuries resulting in compromised functional abilities. This trauma may have been a life-changing event and will require tremendous support and understanding on your part. Their progress from the initial incident toward independent function has plateaued. Or perhaps your client has never experienced great hand function due to congenital deformities. Tendon transfer surgery offers the possibility of improved or enhanced function for the client and, perhaps, a more independent lifestyle. The approach to tendon transfer surgery should be that of a team effort, involving the surgeon, client, you as therapist, and psychological support from social workers or psychologists as needed. You have an important role to play from the beginning and throughout the entire course of rehabilitation. During the pre-surgery assessment, you evaluate and record accurately all of the client's functional abilities and progress. Only you can report to the team the details on what the client can and cannot do and what he clearly hopes to accomplish via the surgery. You also work as an educator to the client and his family, and you explain the entire process of the planned surgical procedures, including what to expect from every stage. You serve as active advocate as well, working with the surgeon to help clarify what is most important to your client in terms of recovery of functional activities. You can arrange for counseling as needed with the social worker or psychologist and help prepare the client for support services and postoperative employment opportunities. Do not hesitate to refer the client to their case manager (if this is a workman's compensation case) or to their health insurance company to seek out these additional support services. Preoperative therapy sessions are devoted to conditioning, stretching the tissues and tight joints, and strengthening of the selected donor muscles. Postoperatively, you are the key rehabilitation specialist, having the most one-on-one contact with your client. Consider your work together as a partnership with your client to maximize progress and advance him toward his functional goals.

Indications

Tendon transfer surgery involves the operative repositioning of a tendon of a working muscle to take over the function of an absent or nonfunctioning muscle.[1] Tendon transfer surgery is, above all, an attempt to rebalance an imbalanced hand (Fig. 32-1).

Indications for tendon transfer surgery include imbalance in the hand caused by central neurologic deficits, such as seen in spinal cord injuries or cerebral palsy, or trauma to the upper extremity where nerves and tendons are lacerated or crushed and cannot be repaired.[2] Prolonged nerve compression can also lead to irreversible damage of muscle. Other causes for muscle imbalance are disease processes, such as poliomyelitis, rheumatoid arthritis, or Charcot Marie Tooth syndrome (which affects the intrinsic muscles of the hand causing wasting of the muscle fibers), and congenital deformities, such as those occurring with brachial plexus palsy or thumb hypoplasia.[2-5]

Additional procedures might include a **free muscle transfer**[6] where the entire muscle-tendon unit is transferred with intact nerve and blood supply preserved; **neurotization,** or nerve transfer,[2] which involves the implantation of a donor motor nerve into denervated vascularized muscle; or **tenodesis,**[7] which is an automatic movement of a joint produced by a more proximal joint. A commonly cited example of tenodesis is demonstrated during active wrist extension when the digits and thumb fall naturally into flexion. Surgery can create or enhance a tenodesis effect by rerouting the transected tendon across a more proximal joint and attaching it there.

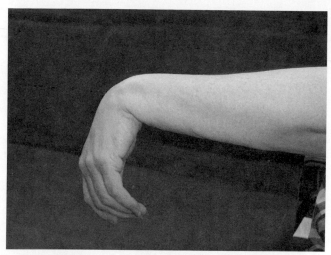

FIGURE 32-1 Imbalanced hand due to radial nerve palsy.

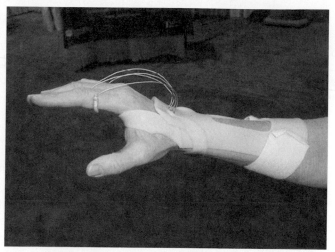

FIGURE 32-2 Dynamic orthosis for radial nerve palsy.

General Considerations

Alternative procedures may have been performed prior to tendon transfer surgery, such as nerve decompression, nerve repair, and muscle or tendon repair.[1] Tendon transfers may be considered as a restorative option when there is no further recovery or nerve regeneration from the precipitating event. Surgeons typically wait 3 to 4 months for this plateau to occur.[2-5]

The prerequisites for this surgery are:[1,2-5]

- Analysis of client's needs
- Bony stability
- Edema or inflammation have subsided
- Adequate soft tissue bed
- Mobile joints
- **Expendable donor muscles** (Muscles perform a certain function, but alternate muscles also perform the same function. The transfer of the expendable muscle does not in itself cause another deficit of motor function.)
- Functional sensation in the affected extremity

Additionally, although it is implied, it should be stated openly that a key component for the success of this elective surgery lies in the motivation and understanding of the client. Without clearly-defined functional goals and a willingness to work toward the outcome, the surgical procedure by itself will not lead to improved outcomes. The client must demonstrate active participation in the process.[8,9]

◎ Clinical Pearl

The client needs to have an appreciation of the surgical expectations and limitations offered by tendon transfer surgery. Carefully explain to your client that the concept of "normal" hand function and/or appearance is unrealistic. Reinforce the key point that the goals of this surgery are to improve functional outcomes and independence.

The selection of the donor tendons must take into consideration the following:[1,2-5,9]

- A muscle that has sufficient strength to overcome the strength and passive tension of the antagonist muscle
- A muscle that lies in an appropriate direction of the desired action

- A muscle that travels a straight route and performs a single function
- Potential excursion of the muscle once it is freed from all connective tissue attachments

The muscle should contract through a distance about equal to the resting length of individual muscle fibers. The required **excursion** is the excursion needed to move a joint through its full range of motion (ROM), but the available excursion is limited by the surrounding connective tissue.[1]

Additional considerations that come into play are the staging of multiple procedures on both the flexor and the extensor sides of the extremity, and the selection of alternative procedures, such as **arthrodesis** (joint fusion) and/or tenodesis. The rehabilitation plan typically immobilizes and protects the transfer during the first 3 to 4 weeks post-surgery.[1,2,4,8,9]

Preoperative Treatment

Clients with peripheral nerve injuries can benefit from therapeutic intervention while awaiting either nerve regeneration or restorative surgery. The fabrication of well-designed orthoses can greatly increase the functional capabilities of clients diagnosed with radial, median, and/or ulnar nerve palsies. Left unsupported, these nerve injuries can lead to significant joint contractures and overstretching of muscle tendon units.[8-12] At a minimum, peripheral nerve injuries cause joint stiffness and discomfort, as well as awkward posturing. A variety of immobilization or mobilization orthoses can be fabricated for this purpose:

- Clients with radial nerve palsy require support of the wrist and metacarpophalangeal (MP) joints in extension (Fig. 32-2).
- Clients with median nerve palsy require support and positioning of the thumb in opposition and abduction for fine motor tasks (Fig. 32-3 and Fig. 32-4).
- Clients with ulnar nerve palsy require that the MP joints be positioned in flexion to prevent clawing of the ulnar digits and to substitute for lack of intrinsic function. If the median nerve is also involved, clients may require additional support for the thumb in abduction (Fig. 32-5 and Fig. 32-6).

If the client has elected to proceed with tendon transfer surgery, therapeutic management includes the preoperative evaluation, conditioning, and client education.[9,13] Unfortunately, many of the

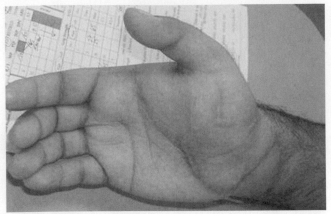

FIGURE 32-3 Client with adducted thumb due to median nerve palsy.

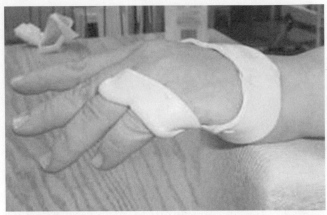

FIGURE 32-5 Static anti-claw orthosis (figure-eight) for ulnar nerve palsy.

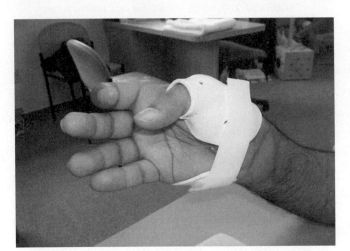

FIGURE 32-4 Functional orthosis for median nerve palsy.

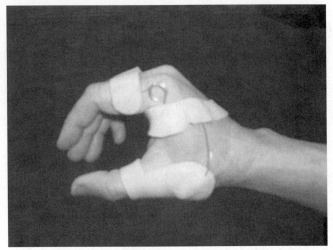

FIGURE 32-6 Dynamic orthosis for ulnar nerve palsy/median nerve palsy.

clients requiring hand therapy may not have been seen by you prior to their surgery. If this is the case with your client, you must work quickly and effectively to gain the client's confidence and trust. But ideally, the entire process includes your contributions as the therapist, starting with the preoperative evaluation and coursing also through preoperative conditioning and education as well as postoperative rehabilitation. Working together for this extended time period reinforces the rapport between you and your client.

The Evaluation

Begin your evaluation with an interview to determine the client's expectations of the outcomes from the planned surgery. When working with a child, meet and discuss this with the family as well. The evaluation should also include the following:

- Assess the client's ability to comply with the postoperative rehabilitative protocol. It is helpful if you have already worked with the client through their post trauma rehabilitation, but you can still develop a rapport with the client at any point by explaining concepts; developing a working relationship as coach, educator, and partner; and forming a treatment plan geared toward function.
- Record a detailed history of the injury, all of the surgical procedures, and all of the therapy that has taken place up to this point, leading to the decision for tendon transfer surgery.

- Examine the affected extremity; observe and record the skin appearance and the placement of scars, adhesions, atrophy of muscles, prominent bony landmarks, and skin coloring.
- Determine sensory status using the Semmes-Weinstein monofilament test, two-point discrimination testing, and/or stereognosis testing.[9,14] When working with children, you will need to closely observe how they integrate the use of their involved hand into play. You can incorporate a game of stereognosis to determine their ability to interpret sensory input in their involved hand. **Stereognosis** refers to the ability to perceive and recognize the form of an object using cues from its size and texture. Evaluating a child may be a bit more challenging, but it is possible through creative and interactive play and by discussing your observations of the use of the affected extremity with the parents.[9,13]
- Take active range of motion (AROM) and passive range of motion (PROM) measurements. Evaluate each joint carefully to ascertain whether it has a hard or soft end feel, and note whether a contracture is present or if there is ligament laxity in the joint. If a contracture is present, you need to address this prior to surgery. If the joint is extremely lax, you should mention this to the surgeon so that the proper amount of tension can be applied during the surgery.
- Evaluate the current use of the hand through functional testing, such as the Jebsen Hand Function Test (JHFT),

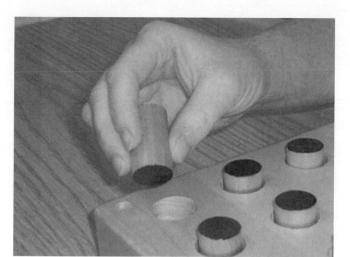

FIGURE 32-7 Functional dexterity test.

TABLE 32-1	Manual Muscle Testing	
Grade	Terminology	Description
5	Normal	Full ROM and full strength
4	Good	Full ROM against gravity with some resistance
3	Fair	Full ROM against gravity
2	Poor	Full ROM with gravity eliminated
1	Trace	Slight contraction without joint movement
0	None	No evidence of contraction

ROM, Range of motion.

the functional dexterity test (FDT) (See Fig. 32-7), or the Moberg's pickup test[9,15].

In addition to the above assessments, observe the client's movement patterns, and note all of the **compensatory movement patterns.**[11,14] These are patterns of movement that your client may have begun to use to make up for the lack of normally functioning muscles. These movement patterns can lead to overstretching and weakening of muscles that are not yet injured. You will need to retrain your client not to use these patterns of movement after surgery. It is best to point these patterns out early and teach your client to recognize them. Instruct your client to avoid these movement patterns in preparation for the surgery.

Include one of the following client self-report outcome measures: the Canadian Occupational Performance Measure (COPM), Disabilities of the Arm, Shoulder, and Hand (DASH) or QuickDASH, or the Michigan Hand Outcomes Questionnaire (MHQ).[13-17] These self-assessments contribute crucial information to an overall picture of how the client rates their own independent functioning, and theyhelp determine how your client views progress toward achievement of functional goals throughout the rehabilitation process.

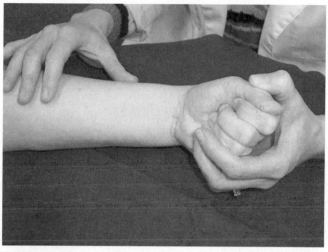

FIGURE 32-8 Figure of manual muscle testing flexor carpi ulnaris (FCU).

Perform manual muscle testing (Table 32-1) to determine what muscles are indeed paralyzed and what muscles may act as donor muscles. It is important to ensure that all possible donor muscles are strong enough to be transferred to new positions.[2,4,13,18] Donor muscles should function at a grade of full ROM against gravity or higher.[1,9] Selecting the muscles that are typically described as donor muscles in textbooks as being available without verifying that they are present and active is not enough. Not everyone may have a palmaris longus (PL) tendon available for transfer![3]

ⓘ *Tips from the Field*

A video recording and/or clinical pictures can greatly assist you in recording the preoperative functional level. You can even use your own cell phone or the client's cell phone to do this. Just make sure to ask permission first. This is a great tool for assessing compensatory movement patterns, checking progress, and comparing how the client was functioning prior to surgery and after surgery in the course of rehabilitation.

At the conclusion of the assessments, record a list of the greatest functional needs of the client in their own words. Ask what they would most like to do with their involved hand. Hold a hairbrush? Drink from a soda bottle? Hold a water bottle so that they can open the cap independently? Do not make the mistake of telling the client what these goals should be. Let the client define in their own words what would they would like to accomplish. In the case of young children, let the parents step in and describe what they would like to see.

ⓘ *Clinical Pearl*

It is helpful to create a list of four muscle groups as follows:
- What muscles are working? All muscles detected by manual muscle testing.
- What muscles are not working? All muscles not detected by manual muscle testing.
- What functions are needed? All motions needed to improve function.
- What muscles are available? All expendable muscles with full ROM against gravity and some resistance[13] (Fig. 32-8).

During the course of your evaluation, you can utilize an orthosis to simulate the proposed function of the tendon transfer. This can help a client see right away if changing the position of a specific joint can indeed improve function. For example, prior to **opponens-plasty** (tendon transfers to restore thumb opposition), fabricate a short opponens thumb orthosis and observe the client's ability to hold and/or pinch while wearing this orthosis.[9-12] You may note that your client displays an improved pinch or an increased ability to hold a tool. Or you might try fabricating a wrist orthosis for a client contemplating tendon transfers for wrist extension. The ability to keep the wrist in extension greatly improves grasp and release patterns of the digits. Wearing a wrist orthosis might enable your client to demonstrate improved hand functioning. In addition, wrist support helps prevent shortening of the wrist flexors.[9-12]

◎ Clinical Pearl

- Help your client create realistic expectations and functional goals. Make sure they understand what the possible outcomes may be.
- Explain terms and procedures so that your client can really understand you.

Once the donor muscles have been selected and a plan for surgical intervention is set, help the client prepare for the procedure both physically and emotionally.

Ask the surgeon if you, as the consulting therapist, can attend the tendon transfer surgery. This is a unique opportunity to gather information and make observations. It also allows you to see firsthand the status of the involved tendons, the strength of the repair, and what specific tendons were used (which might not be what was planned in advance).

( ) What to Say to Clients

"The surgeon is going to reroute one of your working muscles to the joint where the muscle does not work. The therapy before the surgery is very important to get you ready and help make the surgery more successful. We need to make sure that your joints are nice and loose with passive motion exercises and stretching. We need to stretch the joint to full range of motion. In addition, I might have you wear an orthosis to maintain the stretch over time. I might have you wear the orthosis at night so that it doesn't affect your ability to use your hand during the day. If your joint is tight, the donor tendon will not be able to move your joint through the full range of motion. We are going to try and exercise the donor muscle before the surgery to help it get stronger so that it will be ready to work in its new position."

Donor muscle strengthening can be performed through progressive resistive exercises and/or through biofeedback and/or neuromuscular electrical stimulation[9] (Fig. 32-9). An example of this would be strengthening of the pronator teres (PT) muscle prior to transferring this tendon to the insertion of extensor carpi radialis brevis (ECRB) for wrist extension after radial nerve palsy.

◎ Clinical Pearl

It is extremely beneficial to enable your client to gain awareness of the donor muscle contraction and learn how to recruit it independently prior to surgery. Have your client place their noninvolved hand on the donor muscle belly during activity

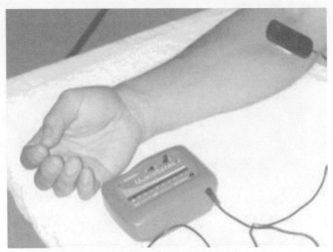

FIGURE 32-9 Neuromuscular electrical stimulation.

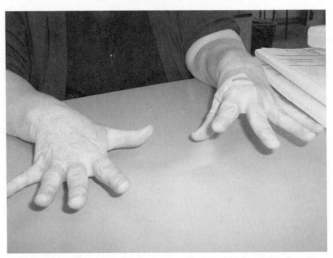

FIGURE 32-10 Client after tendon transfers for radial nerve palsy.

to feel the contraction. For example, let your client feel the PT muscle contracting during active pronation. If they cannot feel it easily, you can make their contraction stronger and more palpable by offering some resistance to their forearm in the direction of supination, and ask them not to let go. Let your client practice contracting this muscle first with self-applied resistance and gradually learn how to contract independently without resistance.

Make sure to inform clients of the loss of sensory input along the distribution of the injured peripheral nerve and the potential for burns and/or skin breakdown. It may be very obvious to your client when they have no feeling in the fingertips due to a median nerve or ulnar nerve injury. However, even the radial nerve has a sensory terminal branch, the dorsal sensory branch of the radial nerve. This area of insensate skin can be injured when the client begins to use their hand in activities of daily living (ADLs). Note bandage over dorsal first web in Fig. 32-10 where client burned herself removing items from a hot oven.

Throughout the course of the preoperative therapy program, engage your client in a discussion of realistic functional outcomes.

BOX 32-1 Common Tendon Transfer Procedures for Median Nerve Palsy[2-5,20]

Camitz: Palmaris longus is transferred for palmar abduction (not true opposition)

Royle, Bunnell, and Thompson: Flexor digitorum superficialis of the ring finger transferred for opposition with different distal attachment techniques

Huber: Abductor digiti minimi transferred to abductor pollicis brevis for opposition

Richter and Peimer: Transfer of the flexor digitorum superficialis of the ring or little to abductor pollicis brevis for opposition

---

BOX 32-2 Common Tendon Transfer for Radial Nerve Palsy[2-5,20]

PT to ECRB for wrist extension

Boyes: FDS (middle) to EDC for MP extension and FDS (ring) to EPL and EIP

Brand: FCR to EDC for MP extension and PL for thumb extension

Jones: FCU to EDC for MP extension

In addition, FCR to APL and EPB for thumb radial abduction

APL, Abductor pollicis longus; *ECRB*, extensor carpi radialis brevis; *EDC*, extensor digitorum communis; *EIP*, extensor indicis proprius; *EPB*, extensor pollicis brevis; *EPL*, extensor pollicis longus; *FCU*, flexor carpi ulnaris; *FCR*, flexor carpi radialis; *FDS*, flexor digitorum superficialis; *MP*, metacarpophalangeal; *PL*, palmaris longus; *PT*, pronator teres.

BOX 32-3 Common Tendon Transfer Procedures for Ulnar Nerve Palsy[2-5,20]

Brand: ECRB with a graft to the intrinsic muscles via the lateral bands

Burkhalter: FDS of the middle is inserted onto the proximal phalanx, not the lateral band

Modified Stiles-Bunnel: FDS of the ring and middle is split into slips and inserted into the lateral band of each finger or the lateral part of P1

Zancolli Lasso: FDS is passed through the pulley and sutured back onto itself to improve MP flexion

Additional procedures described to restore power pinch and thumb adduction:

Boyes: Brachioradialis is extended with a free graft and passed between the third and fourth metacarpals to insert on the adductor tubercle of the thumb

Smith-Hastings: ECRB is transferred to ADP at the first metacarpal for restoration of power pinch

ADP, adductor pollicis; *ECRB*, extensor carpi radialis brevis; *FDS*, flexor digitorum superficialis; *MP*, metacarpophalangeal.

---

the literature—nearly fifty for radial nerve palsy alone.[3] Make sure you confer with the surgeon to specify exactly which donor muscles were utilized (Fig. 32-11 through Fig. 32-13).

? Questions To Discuss with the Physician

Whenever possible, ask to see the operative report. Make sure you and the surgeon share a realistic understanding of the expected outcomes. In addition, you should ask the surgeon the following questions:

- What specific muscles were transferred to what insertion sites?
- Were pulleys created to alter the course of the pull?
- What was the quality of the transferred muscle tendon?
- Were grafts needed (to increase the length)?
- What type of suturing technique was utilized?
- How long should the tendons be immobilized?
- How was the tension of the transferred muscles determined?

Postoperative Treatment: General Guidelines

Postoperative treatment can be divided into three phases for easy reference: early, intermediate, and late. The general guidelines for therapeutic intervention are described first. Examples of different tendon transfers and specific therapeutic interventions are addressed afterward and again in several case examples at the end of this chapter.

The Early Phase (Weeks 1 to 4)

Postoperative treatment begins with the positioning of the involved extremity in a protective cast, avoiding any tension on the transferred tendons. This allows healing to take place without overstretching or ruptures of the transfers.[9,13,14]

Include the perspective of the surgeon in this dialog and the perspective of the parents if young children are involved. Discuss the time frame of surgery, postoperative immobilization, and postoperative course of therapy visits. Avoid surprises regarding the time and commitment expected afterward. Outline the schedule of follow-up visits with the surgeon as well, because many clients and their parents expect to see the surgeon at every therapy visit if therapy occurs in the physician's office. Always strive to establish a genuine rapport with your client and create a solid working and trusting relationship.

Operative Treatment: General Guidelines

Based on the requirements of each client and the results of the manual muscle testing, the surgeon selects the donor muscles for transfer. Various names have been assigned to specific sets of transferred tendons for each of the three main nerve palsies of the upper extremity. It is a good idea to be familiar with these classic procedural names, such as the Royle, Camitz, or Huber transfers for thumb abduction or opposition in median nerve palsy[3,19-21] (Box 32-1); the Brand, Jones, and modified Boyes transfer for radial nerve palsy[2-5,19] (Box 32-2); or the Brand, Stiles-Bunnel, or Zancolli Lasso procedures used in the treatment of ulnar nerve palsy[8,18,21] (Box 32-3). There are many more names, procedures, and modifications described in

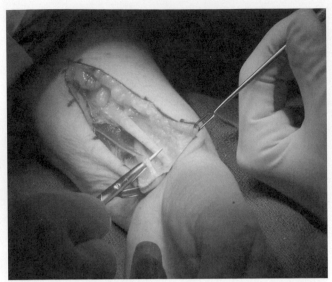

FIGURE 32-11 Surgical pictures identifying the palmaris longus (PL) and the flexor carpi radialis (FCR).

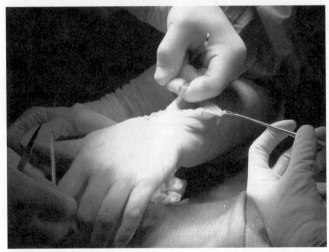

FIGURE 32-12 Surgical pictures identifying the extensor pollicis longus (EPL).

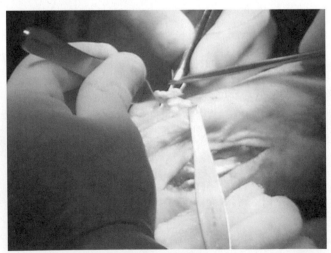

FIGURE 32-13 Surgical pictures identifying Pulvertaft weave of tendons.

During the early phase of rehabilitation:

- Create an exercise program for the noninvolved digits and joints.
- Monitor your client's extremity for edema.
- Make sure the cast is secure and fits well.
- Educate your client on the time required for adequate healing.
- Review the time frame and anticipated course of therapy.

The client may be anxious to already see the results of the surgery and learn what the functional outcomes might be. Educate your client on the different phases of the rehabilitative course. Explain that the transferred tendons require adequate time for healing. At each session, it may be beneficial to review the functional goals, the time frame, and the anticipated course of therapy.

( ) *What to Say to Clients*

"Move all of your uninvolved joints outside of the postoperative dressings while the tendon transfers heal. Perform regular active exercises of everything not in the cast. Periodically elevate your arm to reduce swelling. You must inform the surgeon immediately if the cast seems loose."

If the cast becomes loose, offer to fabricate a thermoplastic orthosis as an alternative to a new cast, because this will be a bit more comfortable for your client.

The Intermediate Phase (Weeks 4 to 6)

During the intermediate phase of postoperative rehabilitation, therapeutic intervention is much more involved and hands on. The postoperative cast is removed. Replace it with a thermoplastic orthosis, maintaining the same protected positioning as the cast.[9,13]

As you examine your client's extremity, note the placement of volar and dorsal incisions. The amount of scarring can be quite extensive on both sides of the extremity, because the surgery requires a great deal of exposure to locate and secure the donor tendons in their new insertion sites. You can now initiate scar management techniques. Be sure to include friction massage, desensitization, ultrasound, and perhaps elastomer and silicone gel products. Silicone gel products also work to hydrate the scar tissue as well as compress it[9,22] (Fig. 32-14).

Utilize therapeutic heat in the form of heat packs, whirlpool, and/or fluidotherapy to improve the elasticity of your client's tissue, as well as to reduce joint stiffness and increase the blood flow to the involved area.[3,14] Begin AROM to isolated joints. Perform gentle active and active-assisted motions for short sessions several times a day to reduce joint stiffness. For example, isolated joint motions might be thumb interphalangeal (IP) joint flexion and extension, or MP joint flexion and extension following tendon transfers for extensor pollicis longus (EPL) and extensor digitorum communis (EDC) (Fig. 32-15).

Precaution: *Remember to avoid composite motion and overstretching of the transferred muscles.*

Now you can begin facilitation of the transferred muscle tendons in earnest. This is the core of the rehabilitation program.[14] The advantage of preoperative conditioning and education becomes apparent here. Clients who are able to recruit previously conditioned muscles learn to quickly activate these muscles with their new functions. Introduce **facilitation techniques** for those clients who show signs of difficulty initiating

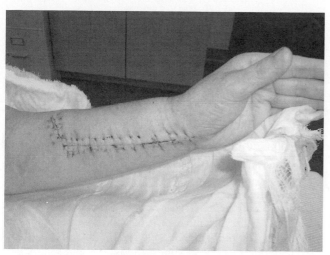

FIGURE 32-14 Scarring after tendon transfer surgery.

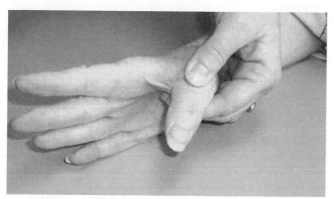

FIGURE 32-15 Picture of isolated motion at the thumb interphalangeal (IP) joint.

BOX 32-4   Facilitation Techniques

Place and hold: Place your client's wrist or finger in the desired position, and ask them to maintain this position. Count to 10. Educate your client to perform this on their own.

Using both hands simultaneously: Have your client perform the desired motion with both hands at the same time.

Using the donor muscle action: Have your client try to perform the donor muscle's original action, and monitor for the new muscle action to occur.

Resistance to the donor muscle: Offer gentle resistance to the donor muscle (its original action).

Verbal cues: Encourage the desired motion through words and description.

Tapping, vibration: Gently tap over the donor muscle, or use a small vibrator on this area to initiate stimulation of the donor muscle.

Visual and functional cues: Ask your client to imagine holding an object or performing a task with the involved hand. Look for small muscle activity in the desired motion.

Mirror training: Place the affected hand behind the mirror, and have your client perform the desired function with both hands. However, your client will be able to see only the noninvolved hand and its reflection in the mirror. Monitor the involved hand for motor activity.

Neuromuscular electrical stimulation (NMES): Use NMES to recruit the donor muscle activity. Place the smaller electrodes over the motor points for the donor muscles and place the larger dispersive pad over a non-contractile area.

---

the desired motion. Facilitation techniques (Box 32-4) are specific strategies utilized to recruit the donor tendon to function in its new capacity (Fig. 32-16 through Fig. 32-18).

> ### ◎ Clinical Pearl
>
> The use of mirrors in hand therapy is growing rapidly. To facilitate a donor muscle, the mirror is placed vertically in front of the client to reflect the non-injured hand in the place of the injured hand. The client moves the non-injured hand in the desired motion and receives visual feedback that both hands are moving together. It is recommended to perform this activity twice a day in a quiet environment and concentrate on the hand in the mirror, while moving both hands at the same time.[23]

> ### ◎ Clinical Pearl
>
> Transferred muscles are easily fatigued. Perform slow and controlled repetitions to promote good patterns of use. Thirty minutes or less may actually be all that is tolerated in a session. Do not overdo the exercise sessions!

> ### ( ) What to Say to Clients
>
> "As you begin to use your newly transferred muscles, make sure your motion is accurate and precise. Make sure it goes in the

desired motion. If you notice a slight change of direction, your muscle is tired, and you must take a break. Try ten repetitions as a starting point. Do several short sessions throughout the day, and afterward put your orthosis on to rest. The orthosis helps to maintain the best position of the transferred muscle until it is strong enough to do this on its own. Do not be alarmed at how quickly this new muscle gets fatigued! It takes time for it to adjust to its new role. You will see it getting stronger slowly but surely. Every day it will be a bit stronger than the previous day."

➢ Precautions and Concerns

- *No PROM against the transferred muscle*
- *No resistance to the desired motion*
- *No composite motion that puts tension on the transferred muscle*
- *Do not overwork the transferred muscle*

Now is the time to make the therapeutic process more interesting and more personal for your client. Move beyond standard and rote exercises. Introduce functional activities into the rehabilitative program once the firing of the transferred muscle is consistent and AROM is within functional limits. Do not forget to include functional activities that were outlined during preoperative goal setting. Provide many opportunities to practice activities that have personal meaning for your client.

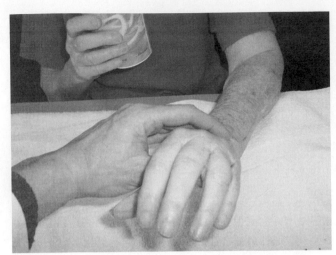

FIGURE 32-16 Place and hold facilitation technique for wrist extension.

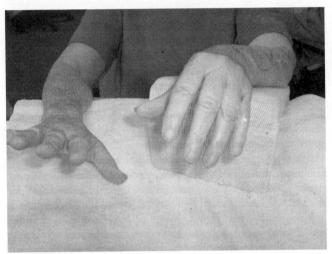

FIGURE 32-17 Place and hold facilitation technique for both hands simultaneously.

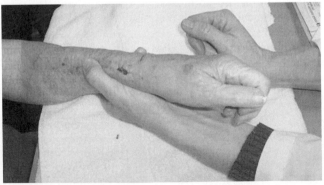

FIGURE 32-18 Providing resistance to donor muscle.

The Late Phase (Weeks 6 to 12)

At 6 weeks post-surgery, you can begin to add strengthening exercises to your client's therapeutic sessions, including motion against gravity. The emphasis remains on good quality ROM. You can encourage your client to gradually discontinue

use of their orthosis, except when their extremity shows fatigue. Encourage the incorporation of the hand into your client's ADLs, including bathing, dressing, leisure, and work activities. Do not rush to add PROM in the opposite direction of the transferred muscles. These passive exercises are to be added only if necessary, because they continue to put strain and tension on the transferred muscles.[9,13]

"Now your muscle has healed in its new position and has enough strength for you to use every day in your regular routines and actions. Try to use your hand normally for all of your activities of daily living. Try to eat and get dressed using both hands. Make sure your movements are correct and do not substitute with your other muscles. Do not overdo it! If your hand feels tired, rest it, and wear your orthosis"

Diagnosis-Specific Information that Affects Clinical Reasoning

The Median Nerve

The median nerve (see Fig 24-10) receives contributions from the lateral and medial cords of the brachial plexus. There are no terminal branches in the upper arm. The anterior interosseous branch begins about 5 cm above the medial epicondyle, and innervates the flexor pollicis longus (FPL), the flexor digitorum profundus (FDP) to the index, and the pronator quadratus (PQ).[3-5,9] The median nerve proper innervates the PT, flexor carpi radialis (FCR), flexor digitorum superficialis (FDS), PL, and the FDP of the middle finger. A recurrent motor branch originates off the median nerve in the carpal tunnel and innervates the thenar muscles opponens pollicis (OP), flexor pollicis brevis (FPB), abductor pollicis brevis (APB), and lumbricals of the index and middle.[3-5,20] One anatomical variation is the Martin Gruber anastomosis that has a motor component connected to the ulnar nerve in the forearm. This may alter the client's presentation of muscle function during your evaluation.[20]

High injury to the median nerve may result in deficits in pronation (loss of PT and PQ), loss of wrist flexion in radial direction (loss of FCR), and weak finger flexion (FDS and FDP to the index and middle). More common are injuries or trauma to the lower portion of the median nerve affecting deficits of MP flexion (median innervated lumbrical muscles), and loss of thumb opposition (APB, OP, and FBP).[3-5,12,20]

Operative Treatment: Restoration of Opposition/Opponensplasty

The most disabling functional loss after injury to the median nerve is the loss of thumb opposition. Opposition refers to the complex action of bringing the thumb up and out of the palm. Indications that this function may need restorative care are median nerve palsy, a congenital deformity (such as, thumb hypoplasia), trauma to tendons and nerves, and/or a disease process (such as, Charcot Marie Tooth syndrome).[3-5,12,19,20] During the preoperative evaluation, look for tightness of the first web space. Begin with gentle stretching of this passively. You can also

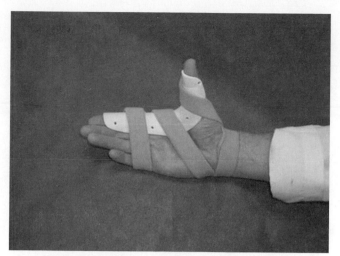

FIGURE 32-19 Orthosis to stretch the first web space.

address a tight first web space by initiating activities that promote wide abduction. Fabricate a static progressive web spacer orthosis to maintain the stretch at night (Fig. 32-19).[9-12]

The primary muscles for opposition are the APB, OP, and FPB.[19] A variety of procedures involve different donor muscles to restore the loss of these muscle's actions (see Box 32-1).

The therapist must know which muscle was used as the donor tendon, because this directly affects the choice of postoperative protective orthosis, the correct facilitation techniques, and activity selection.

Following the 3 to 4 weeks of immobilization in a postoperative cast, fabricate a long opponens orthosis for your client to protect the transferred tendon if it crosses the wrist. Make sure to place the thumb in wide abduction. Instruct your client to wear the orthosis day and night initially and to remove it only for exercises.

♡ Tips from the Field

The easiest facilitation technique is the place and hold exercise. Using this technique, place the client's wrist or finger in the desired position (of the transferred muscle), and ask him to hold the wrist or finger in place against gravity. For example, if the FDS to the ring has been used as a donor muscle to restore thumb abduction, place the client's thumb in abduction, and ask the client to hold it there while flexing the ring finger simultaneously. Count aloud as the client maintains the thumb position. Try to hold for 5 seconds, and increase gradually to 10 seconds. Do this for several repetitions. Do not be discouraged by the lack of full motion or the inability to sustain the position for more than a few seconds. This weakness and fatigue will gradually improve, and your client will start to see progress shortly. He will soon be able to recruit the donor muscle more quickly and sustain the contraction for longer periods. As soon as your client can facilitate the transferred muscle independently and without much effort, encourage the use of the thumb during ADLs. Facilitate wide thumb abduction and opposition by creating activities that incorporate the use of large diameter objects for grasp. Progress your client gradually to activities that require holding smaller diameter objects.

As you note improved control over the thumb's AROM, instruct your client to reduce orthotic wear during the day.

Make sure your client is comfortable using the thumb in all ADLs. Do this gradually over time. Have your client continue to wear their orthosis during the nighttime and for protection when around crowds and in unfamiliar settings until 12 weeks post-surgery.[9]

The Radial Nerve

The radial nerve (see Fig 24-5) is the continuation of the posterior cord of the brachial plexus.[3] It lies on the posterior side of the upper arm and winds around the humerus from medial to lateral under the triceps muscle.[11] The radial nerve may be injured along with humeral fractures at the level of the spiral groove, usually sparing the triceps muscle insertion. The radial nerve can also be injured by trauma or surgeries of the elbow and humerus.[3] Many injuries will recover spontaneously. However, serious injuries to the radial nerve cause loss of wrist extension from the functions of the ECRB, extensor carpi radialis longus (ECRL), and extensor carpi ulnaris (ECU); loss of finger extension from EDC, extensor indicis proprius (EIP), and extensor digiti minimi (EDM); and loss of thumb extension and abduction from EPL, extensor pollicis brevis (EPB), and abductor pollicis longus (APL).[3-5] This injury is often called "wrist drop deformity" due to the classic wrist flexion or dropped wrist posture (see Fig. 32-1).[11]

◎ Clinical Pearl

The brachioradialis (BR) muscle is the first to be innervated by the radial nerve in the arm. Although there are minimal functional deficits associated with the loss of this muscle, it is important to monitor this muscle while awaiting nerve reinnervation. Recovering motor function of the BR muscle implies that wrist and MP joint extension will soon be recovered as well.[4,5]

There may be a sensory deficit in the dorsal first web space if the level of injury occurs proximal to the branching of the radial nerve into its two terminal branches: the radial sensory nerve and the posterior interosseous nerve.[12] Although this area has minimum functional impact, your client may still be susceptible to burns in this area without being aware of them.

◎ Clinical Pearl

Always educate your client regarding the potential for burns and injuries to insensate areas of skin (see Fig 32-10). Note the bandage over dorsal first web where the client burned herself removing items from a hot oven.

Preoperative Treatment

Preoperative treatment is always geared toward maintenance of function and prevention of, or correction of joint contractures. A loss of grip strength may be present due to the lack of wrist stabilizers. It is difficult for your client to extend their digits and release objects. They may allow the wrist to drop into flexion and pronation to achieve digital release (Fig. 32-20 and Fig. 32-21). Over time, this can cause overstretching of the paralyzed muscles and become a fixed deformity.[12] Address contractures or joint tightness of the wrist by stretching and the use of static, static progressive, and/or functional orthoses.[8-12]

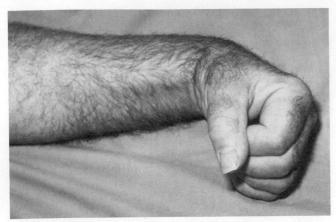

FIGURE 32-20 Client with radial nerve palsy.

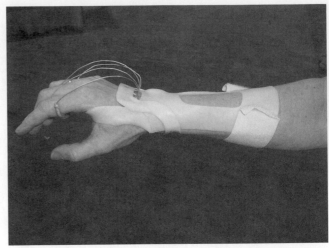

FIGURE 32-23 Dynamic orthosis for radial nerve palsy with wires for MP extension.

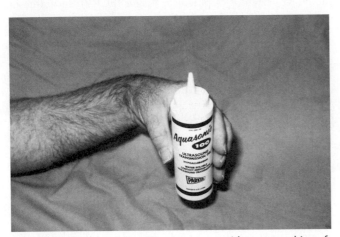

FIGURE 32-21 Compensatory grasp pattern with overstretching of wrist extensors.

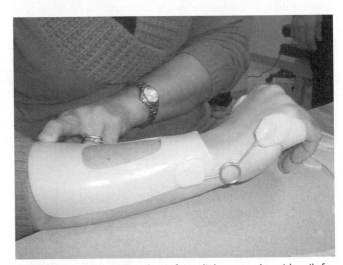

FIGURE 32-24 Dynamic orthosis for radial nerve palsy with coils for wrist extension.

> **Clinical Pearl**
>
> There are many different orthotic designs and many different thermoplastic materials to choose from; each one provides a different functional solution. Remember to keep your design simple. Involve your client in the fabrication process. Make sure your completed orthosis is easy to don and doff and improves or enhances your client's function. Otherwise, it will not be utilized.

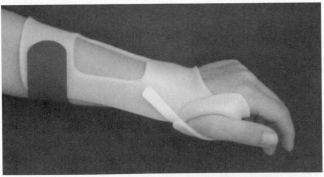

FIGURE 32-22 Dorsal wrist cock up orthosis.

Operative Treatment: Restoration of Wrist Extension

Tendon transfers following radial nerve palsy are performed with the combined goals of restoring wrist extension, finger extension at the MP joint level, and thumb extension and abduction.[3-5] The PT muscle is typically selected as a donor tendon for wrist extension (leaving the PQ available for active pronation) and additional donor muscles are included to power and restore digital and thumb extension. Typical donor muscles may include FCR or FDS of the middle to EDC, and PL to EPL. However, there are many variations to these procedures.

Preoperative treatment addresses the lack of functional wrist and digital extension through creative orthotic fabrication. Clients who require a forceful grip may benefit most from a static wrist orthosis, either dorsal or volar based. Consider the benefits of a dorsal based wrist orthosis that does not block the sensory input from the palm (Fig. 32-22).

Clients needing more wrist or finger mobility may prefer a dynamic wrist or finger orthosis (Fig. 32-23 and Fig. 32-24).[12]

The indications for restoration of wrist extension may also include cases of cerebral palsy where there is unbalanced wrist posturing in flexion due to increased flexor tone.[14] This posture makes hand function difficult, because it places the wrist extensors in an overstretched position while causing shortening of the wrist and digital flexors.[24] The donor muscle typically utilized in cases of cerebral palsy to enhance wrist extension is the flexor carpi ulnaris (FCU), which is surgically repositioned to assist the ECRL in active wrist extension.[14,24] Assessing the client for voluntary control of the digits with the wrist placed in extension is critical.[24] Do this by holding the wrist in extension, have the client make a fist with his digits, and then open them. If the client does not exhibit voluntary control of the digits in this position, he may use the tenodesis motion to allow his digits to open and release objects. Enhancing wrist extension hampers his ability to use his digits in this method and may not be beneficial.[13]

Early Phase

Following tendon transfer surgery for wrist extension, the upper extremity is typically placed in a long arm cast with the elbow positioned in 90° of flexion (to protect the origin of the PT muscle), the forearm is positioned in pronation, the wrist is positioned in 30° to 40° of wrist extension, and the MP joints are positioned in 0°extension. The IP joints can be left free.[3-5,9,14] Cast immobilization usually lasts 3 to 4 weeks.

At 4 weeks, the cast is replaced with a long arm thermoplastic orthosis fabricated to maintain the arm in the same position as previously described. Instruct your client to remove this orthosis during the day for AROM exercises. As your client gains ROM and demonstrates good control over the transferred tendons, orthotic wear is reduced to nighttime protection only—up and through 12 weeks.[9]

Intermediate Phase

Introduce the facilitation techniques previously described to activate the transferred muscles (see Box 32-4).

Begin activation of the donor tendon with a simple place and hold in wrist extension. Place your client's wrist in extension, and have your client try to hold the wrist in this position for 5 to 10 seconds initially. Gradually increase the length of this muscle contraction. Or try having your client extend their wrist actively with both hands simultaneously. If no response can be elicited, offer some resistance to the transferred muscle's original function. For example, if PT was used as a donor muscle for wrist extension, give some resistance to pronation while the client attempts to supinate the forearm. You should see some indication of active wrist extension with this maneuver. Do not expect full wrist ROM or even 50% of wrist ROM! The transferred tendon is very weak and still needs time to heal and strengthen. Approach these facilitation techniques very slowly and carefully.

If multiple tendon transfers have been performed in the same surgery, approach each one as a separate entity with facilitation strategies for each motion. For example, following the wrist extension exercises described earlier, you can attend to the digital and thumb transfers and facilitate these in a similar fashion with place and hold exercises for MP joints in extension and for the thumb in extension. If a muscle transfer was utilized that includes both of these functions together, such as the Boyes transfer[2,21] that incorporates the FDS (ring) to both the EPL and the EIP, you must work with these two motions as a single function (see Box 32-2).

Make sure your client is able to demonstrate active wrist and finger extension and maintain an isometric contraction. Gradually introduce more activities into therapy sessions that require these motions.

Late Phase

At 8 to 12 weeks after surgery, your therapeutic intervention should focus on your client's ability to move through functional if not full ROM in all affected joints. You can add strengthening exercises to the routine. Sustained grip activities and progressive resistance exercises for wrist and finger extension are good choices. By now, your client should demonstrate using their involved extremity for all ADLs. Discuss any areas of concern or weakness. If it is not necessary for your client to regain full wrist flexion for functional activities, do not perform passive stretches into wrist flexion. You do not want to stretch out the tendon transfer.

Operative Treatment: Restoration of Thumb Extension

Thumb extension may be lost either due to radial nerve injury, or due to muscle and tendon trauma independent of other muscle involvement. Clients may experience a closed rupture of the EPL tendon after a distal radius fracture.[25] Tendon rupture is also common in clients with rheumatoid arthritis.[26] The EIP is typically chosen as a donor muscle for the thumb extensor.[26] Following tendon transfer surgery, the wrist and thumb are placed in full extension, including the IP joint of the thumb. After 3 to 4 weeks of postoperative immobilization, fabricate a long opponens orthosis, including the IP joint of the thumb in full extension.

Orthoses as Aids to Movement

To facilitate active thumb extension at the thumb MP joint, fabricate a small thumb IP extension orthosis. This allows the client to generate force specifically at the thumb MP joint and not involve the IP joint in the exercise (Fig. 32-25).

Similarly, to facilitate digital MP flexion and extension without IP flexion, fabricate a circular digital extension orthosis for all four digits that helps to generate force specifically at the MP joints and block the force going distally. Your client can practice active MP flexion and extension exercises wearing the orthosis and will later be able to recruit this motion without the orthosis (Figs. 32-26 and 32-27).

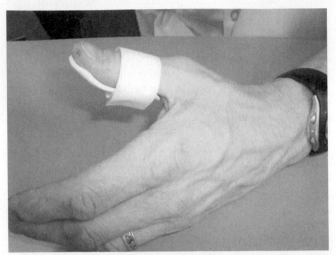

FIGURE 32-25 Facilitation of thumb MP extension.

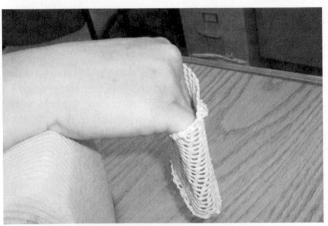

FIGURE 32-26 Blocking orthosis to facilitate MP flexion.

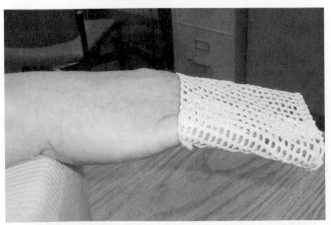

FIGURE 32-27 Blocking orthosis to facilitate MP extension.

The Ulnar Nerve

The ulnar nerve (see Fig 24-16) is the largest branch of the medial cord and carries fibers from C8 and T1.[4,5,11,20] In the forearm, it provides innervation to FCU and to FDP of the ring and little digits. In the hand, it innervates the hypothenar muscles and palmaris brevis, adductor pollicis (AP), the third and fourth lumbrical muscles, the dorsal and palmar interossei and FPB.[4,5,12,20] Clients with injury to the ulnar nerve palsy present with weak wrist flexion, deficits in power grip, a flattened metacarpal arch, the loss of lumbrical function and MP flexion, and decreased pinch strength. High ulnar nerve injury is defined as proximal to the insertion of the flexor group, and low ulnar nerve injury is defined as distal to innervation of FDP. Low ulnar nerve injuries typically demonstrate clawing of the ulnar digits due to hyperextension of the MPs from unopposed extrinsic extensors and strong over pull of the unopposed FDP.[4,5,20] In high level ulnar nerve injuries, the FDP is also affected, and therefore there is no clawing deformity. Ulnar nerve palsy causes difficulty in grasping objects as the digits begin rolling into flexion starting with the IP joints followed by late MP joint flexion. The normal MP joint flexion pattern powered by the intrinsic muscles is lost, and it is extremely difficult to hold objects in the hand.[12] In fact, as your client attempts to grasp an object, you will note that his digital flexion begins at the fingertips that roll into flexion, closing up the hand before it actually encounters the object.[7] The sensory deficit of ulnar nerve involvement also contributes to the functional loss.

© **Clinical Pearl**

Two additional signs of ulnar nerve involvement are as follows:[4,5]
1. Wartenberg's sign: Eccentric abduction of the little finger due to unopposed EDQ and paralysis of palmar adductors (Fig. 32-28)
2. Froment's paper sign: Substitution of FPL for AP and first dorsal interosseous; the sign is positive if the client flexes the IP joint with key pinch (Fig. 32-29).

Be sure to look for these signs in your evaluation, and record your tests as positive if present.

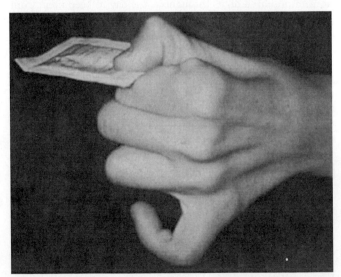

FIGURE 32-28 Wartenberg's sign. (From Burke SL: *Hand and upper extremity rehabilitation: a practical guide*, ed 3, Philadelphia, 2005, Churchill Livingstone.)

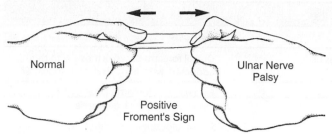

FIGURE 32-29 Froment's paper sign. (From Burke SL: *Hand and upper extremity rehabilitation: a practical guide*, ed 3, Philadelphia, 2005, Churchill Livingstone.)

Preoperative Treatment

Goals of preoperative treatment for ulnar nerve palsy include preventing contractures of the MP and PIP joints and maintaining the normal length of the extrinsic flexor muscles.[12] Provide your client with an anti-claw orthosis. This simple orthosis supports the metacarpal arch and holds the ulnar digits in flexion at the MP joint, preventing overstretching of the intrinsic muscles. It can be either a static or dynamic orthosis (see Fig. 32-5 and Fig. 32-6).

> ### ◎ Clinical Pearl
>
> Bouvier's test is a method used to determine which type of tendon transfer procedure should be selected for correction of ulnar nerve deficits in the hand.[4,20] Your client is asked to extend the digits while blocking extension of the MP joints. If your client is able to recruit the extrinsic extensors to do this task, the test is a positive one, and the goal of the tendon transfer surgery is to provide MP flexion via insertion of the donor muscle into the proximal phalanx. If the test is negative, then the tendon transfer surgery must not only provide MP flexion but also add a component of IP extension via insertion into the lateral bands. Discuss the results of your findings with the surgeon.

Operative Treatment: Restoration of Intrinsic Function

The surgeon may select from a variety of surgical procedures to correct the deformities associated with ulnar nerve paralysis[4,5,7,20] (see Box 32-3).

Postoperative Treatment

Following surgery and the normal immobilization period of 3 to 4 weeks, fabricate an immobilization orthosis to maintain the MP joints in flexion. This can be either a forearm based dorsal blocking orthosis, or a volar wrist orthosis with MPs in flexion and IPs in extension. After 4 weeks of immobilization, instruct your client to begin gentle AROM exercises. Be sure to include isolated motions at the elbow, wrist, and MP joints.[20] It is important to mobilize one joint at a time to avoid increased tension on the transfer. Instruct the client to gently flex and extend the MP joints from their resting posture in full flexion.

> ### ➢ Precautions and Concerns
>
> - *Avoid full MP extension. (This will overstretch the transfer.)*
> - *Avoid passive flexion and extension of the IP joints.*

Initiate facilitation techniques to the transferred muscles. Use the facilitation techniques described earlier. As your client progresses to full control of digital motion, include functional activities of meaning into therapy. Encourage active use of the involved hand during all ADLs. Modify the original forearm based orthosis to a hand based orthosis. Tell your client to practice but not to overstress composite flexion of the digits. Avoid heavy resistance toward full extension, because this may cause overstretching of the transfer.[7,20] Begin gentle strengthening exercises at 8 weeks after surgery. Monitor your client for good quality motion. Full activity can be resumed by 12 to 14 weeks, depending on each individual. Gradually wean your client from orthotic wear.

Additional Tendon Transfer Protocols

The most commonly performed tendon transfer protocols have been described here. Tendon transfers are also routinely performed for clients following spinal cord injuries and for clients suffering from traumatic injuries of the brachial plexus, as well as for clients with birth brachial plexus palsy (Table 32-2).[6,13,27] Preoperative and postoperative rehabilitation follows the same guidelines outlined here. Carefully evaluate the client for functional deficits, and create functional goals for the surgery. Protect the transferred muscles in a tension-free position for 3 to 4 weeks. Begin activation of the transferred muscles in their new positions of function. Utilize facilitation techniques as needed to activate the transfers. Always incorporate functional activities into the treatment. It is crucial to understand the anatomical deficits involved in each specific procedure.

What's New in the Field?

Recent studies have compared immediate active mobilization of tendon transfers in clients to the conventional postoperative immobilization of 3 to 4 weeks, which is typically prescribed.[4,28] The benefits of a reduced course of rehabilitation are significant with less time away from work being an important consideration. Early active motion was also compared with a dynamic orthosis protocol.[29] Early mobilization protocols appear to be safe and cost effective. Clients report less pain and regain function and motion more quickly. Additional studies indicate that the use of "wide awake" procedures in the absence of general anesthesia may also benefit tendon transfer clients. Adjustments for tension on the transferred muscle can be performed prior to skin closure.[30] The client is also able to make an immediate association and perform the desired motion in the operating room.

Strategies for Success

Tendon transfer surgery can offer clients greatly improved functional outcomes. A team approach, including surgeon, client, and therapist along with other health care individuals if needed, benefits everyone involved. Careful preoperative evaluation, appropriate client selection, and thorough observation and planning must be done prior to surgery. Clients with limited sensory function are not good surgical candidates.[24] Defining the most critical functional goals of the client is imperative, as well as assessing

TABLE 32-2   Not So Common Tendon Transfer Procedures

Condition	Indications	Procedure	Orthosis
Spinal cord injury	Lack of key pinch and pronation	Brachioradialis to FPL	Dorsal forearm based orthosis with thumb adducted, wrist in neutral, and elbow free
Spinal cord injury	Lack of elbow extension	Biceps to triceps	Elbow extension orthosis at night Elbow flexion block during day
Spinal cord injury	Lack of palmar grasp	ECRL to FDP	Dorsal blocking orthosis with wrist in neutral, MP joints in flexion, and IP joints in extension
Brachial plexus birth palsy	Lack of shoulder external rotation/abduction	Latissimus dorsi and teres tendons to posterior shoulder cuff	Airplane orthosis with arm in 30° to 40° of external rotation and 120° of abduction
Brachial plexus birth palsy	Lack of elbow flexion	Steindler (Flexor-Pronator transfer)	Elbow flexion orthosis in 100° to 110° of elbow flexion

ECRL, Extensor carpi radialis longus; *FDP,* flexor digitorum profundus; *FPL,* flexor pollicis longus; *MP,* metacarpophalangeal.
Modified from Ashworth S, Kozin SH: Brachial plexus palsy reconstruction: tendon transfers, osteotomies, capsular release and arthrodesis. In Skirven TM, Osterman AL, Fedorczyk JF, et al, editors: *Rehabilitation of the hand and upper extremity,* ed 6, Philadelphia, 2011, Mosby, pp. 792-812; Hammert WC, Heest AEV, James MA, et al: Tendon transfers. In Hammert WC, Calfee RP, Bozentka DJ, et al, editors: *ASSH manual of hand surgery,* Philadelphia, 2010, Wolters Kluwer/Lippincott Williams & Wilkins, pp. 145-169; and Peliovich AE, Bryden AM, Malone KJ, et al: Rehabilitation of the hand and upper extremity in tetraplegia. In Skirven TM, Osterman AL, Fedorczyk JF, et al, editors: *Rehabilitation of the hand and upper extremity,* ed 6, Philadelphia, 2011, Mosby, pp.1684-1705.

the available musculature to achieve these goals. Client education regarding every aspect of the surgery and rehabilitation process enhances cooperation and outcomes. Judicious use of orthoses and activities of meaning enhances therapeutic interventions. Pay careful attention to the anatomy and the timetable of healing to help make the rehabilitation process successful.

CASE STUDIES

CASE STUDY 32-1 ■ Radial Nerve Palsy and Restoration of Wrist, Finger, and Thumb Extension

S.K. is a 74-year-old, right-hand dominant female living alone in an assisted living facility. She sustained a humeral fracture on her left side after a fall on the pavement. The arm was placed in a long arm cast for about 5 weeks. It was only after the cast was removed that she reported the inability to extend her wrist and her digits. A diagnosis of radial nerve palsy was made, and she was referred to hand therapy for ROM exercises and orthotic fabrication.

A dynamic MP extension orthosis was provided for the client to use during functional activities throughout the day. In addition, a wrist cock up orthosis was provided for nighttime wear. After 3 to 4 months with no discernible nerve regeneration, the surgeon began plans to perform tendon transfer surgery.

The therapist performed a detailed client interview and determined that the client was having trouble with basic ADLs, including the ability to feed and dress herself unassisted. Her hobbies at the assisted living facility included playing cards, typing a community newsletter for the group, and participating in communal activities. She was unable to type or hold cards in her involved left hand and therefore was no longer participating in any of the group activities at the home. The therapist performed a full preoperative evaluation, including manual muscle testing to determine which muscles could be used as possible donor muscles. S.K. demonstrated above fair muscle grades in all median nerve and ulnar nerve innervated muscles.

The surgeon performed the following tendon transfers:
• PT to ECRL

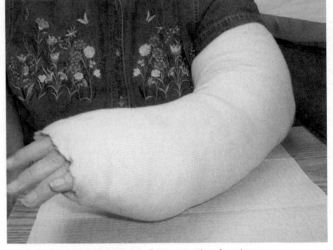

FIGURE 32-30 Postoperative dressings.

• FCR to EDC
• PL to EPL

After surgery, S.K. was placed in a long arm cast for 4 weeks with the elbow positioned in 90° of flexion, the forearm in pronation, the wrist in 30° of extension, and the MP joints in 0° degrees of extension (Fig. 32-30 and Fig. 32-31).

S.K. was instructed to mobilize her shoulder and digits throughout the period of immobilization. At 4 weeks post-surgery, the postoperative dressings were removed, and the therapist fabricated a long arm orthosis, maintaining this same positioning of the arm. Gentle isolated motions were initiated for wrist, digits, and thumb (Fig. 32-32 through Fig. 32-35).

At this time, facilitation techniques were initiated to activate the transferred muscles. Place and hold exercises were introduced for all of the transferred muscles, and resistance to supination was utilized to recruit the PT (donor muscle to the wrist extensors). These two facilitation techniques proved to be extremely successful and helped to activate the transferred muscles. Before long, S.K. could do these by herself (Fig. 32-36).

Therapy sessions were kept short, because the transferred muscles showed fatigue quickly. As the muscles gained strength, S.K. the

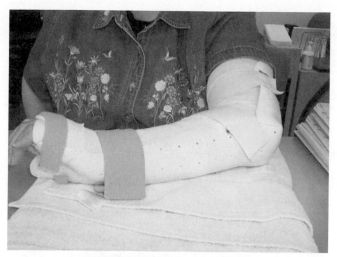

FIGURE 32-31 Long arm orthosis.

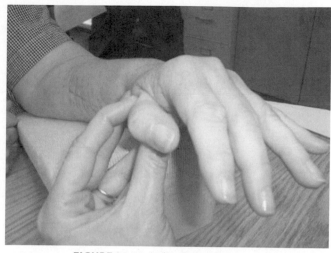

FIGURE 32-32 Isolated thumb flexion.

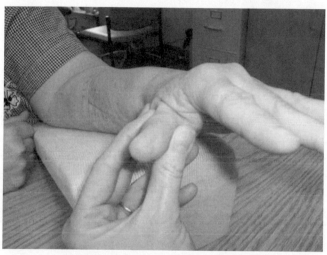

FIGURE 32-33 Isolated thumb extension.

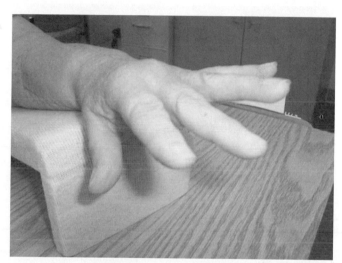

FIGURE 32-34 Isolated MP extension.

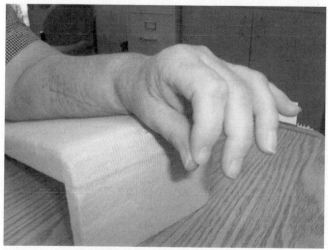

FIGURE 32-35 Isolated MP flexion.

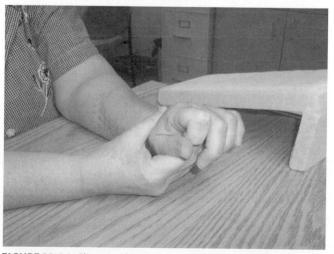

FIGURE 32-36 Client performing place and hold independently to recruit wrist extension.

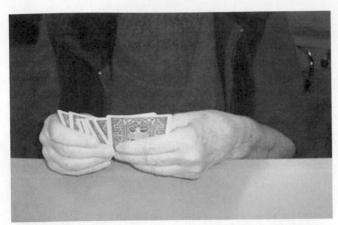

FIGURE 32-37 Including activities of meaning into therapy sessions—holding cards.

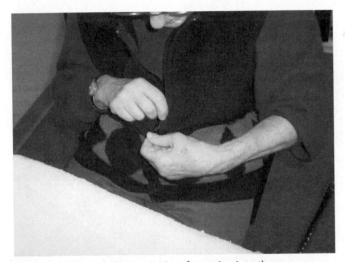

FIGURE 32-38 Including activities of meaning into therapy sessions—self dressing.

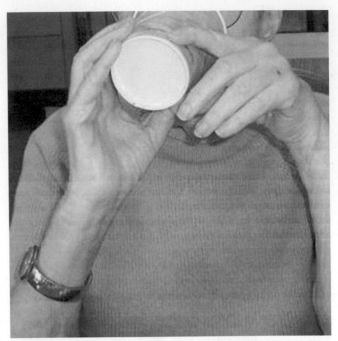

FIGURE 32-39 Including activities of meaning into therapy sessions—self feeding.

client was able to sustain the contraction for longer periods of time and more frequently throughout the session. Along with the facilitation techniques, therapy sessions included activities of meaning to the client, such as holding playing cards, simulated typing, and drinking with the involved hand (Fig. 32-37 through Fig. 32-39).

At 6 weeks post-surgery, the long arm orthosis was modified to a wrist cock up orthosis for nighttime use only. S.K. was encouraged to incorporate the left upper extremity in all ADLs. She progressed through strengthening exercises for wrist extension and was discharged to a home program at 11 weeks post-surgery. It is important to note that while S.K. never achieved full wrist extension against gravity, she did realize adequate wrist extension for all ADLs.

CASE STUDY 32-2 ■ Median Nerve Palsy and Abductorplasty

C.B. is a 62-year-old, right-handed female with severe carpal tunnel syndrome, which has been progressively worsening over

time and has resulted in thenar muscle wasting and weak opposition. She reports pain, numbness, and difficulty manipulating objects. The surgeon performed carpal tunnel release surgery and at the same time, performed an abductorplasty to restore thumb abduction. In this case, the FDS of the ring finger was selected as a donor muscle and inserted into the APB muscle.[21] C.B. was referred to therapy at 2 weeks post-surgery for fabrication of a long opponens orthosis, protecting both the surgical site and maintaining wide thumb abduction. Initially, exercises were performed for the uninvolved digits, and shoulder and elbow ROM was encouraged to reduce swelling and prevent joint stiffness. Scar management of the volar forearm scars was also begun along with desensitization techniques. At 4 weeks post-surgery, the orthosis was taken off for daily active exercise sessions. The place and hold facilitation technique was initiated with the thumb placed in wide abduction, and the client was asked to maintain the position. In addition, she was asked to oppose the thumb to the ring finger. C.B. learned to actively recruit the motion of the FDS via some resistance to the ring finger in flexion.

Activities progressed from those incorporating a wide grasp, such as holding small balls, to those that demanded a smaller and stronger pinch, like placing Chinese checkers in a tray. ADLs were introduced to the therapeutic regiment, such as buttoning, writing, and computer typing. Slowly the client was able to return to her previous level of full independent functioning. Tendon transfer surgery paired with carpal tunnel release surgery was successful at eliminating the client's complaints of numbness and tingling in her median nerve innervated digits, as well as restoring stronger and more functional thumb motion (Fig. 32-40 through Fig. 32-42).

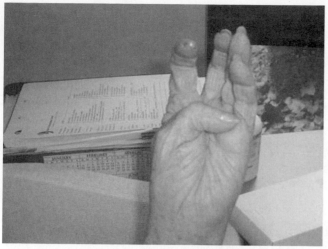

FIGURE 32-40 Thumb abduction.

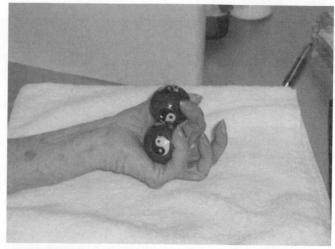

FIGURE 32-42 Thumb activity holding and manipulating chime balls.

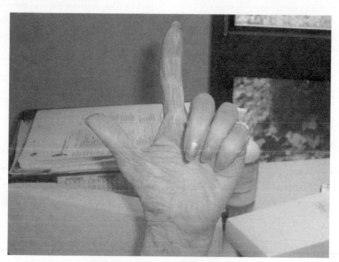

FIGURE 32-41 Thumb extension.

References

1. Botte MJ, Pacelli LL: Basic principles in tendon transfer surgery. In Fridén J, editor: *Tendon transfers in reconstructive hand surgery*, London and New York, 2005, Taylor and Francis, pp 29–49.
2. Sammer DM, Chung KC: Tendon transfers: part I. principles of transfer and transfers for radial nerve palsy, *Plast Reconstr Surg* 123(5):169e–177e, 2009.
3. Kozin SH: Tendon transfers for radial and median nerve palsies, *J Hand Ther* 18:208–215, 2005.
4. Ratner JA, Pelijovich A, Kozin SH: Update on tendon transfers for peripheral nerve injuries, *J Hand Surg Am* 35(8):1371–1381, 2010.
5. Ratner JA, Kozin SH: Tendon transfers for upper extremity peripheral nerve injuries. In Skirven TM, Osterman AL, Fedorczyk JF, et al, editors: *Rehabilitation of the hand and upper extremity*, ed 6, Philadelphia, 2011, Mosby, pp 771–780.
6. Kang L, Wolfe S: Traumatic brachial plexus injuries. In Skirven TM, Osterman AL, Fedorczyk JF, et al, editors: *Rehabilitation of the hand and upper extremity*, ed 6, Philadelphia, 2011, Mosby, pp 749–759.
7. Leclercq C: Tenodeses in reconstructive hand surgery. In Fridén J, editor: *Tendon transfers in reconstructive hand surgery*, London and New York, 2005, Taylor and Francis, pp 69–83.
8. Birch R, Carlstedt T: Musculotendinous unit transfers after nerve injury. In Fridén J, editor: *Tendon transfers in reconstructive hand surgery*, London and New York, 2005, Taylor and Francis, pp 51–68.
9. Duff SV, Humpl D: Therapist's management of tendon transfers. In Skirven TM, Osterman AL, Fedorczyk JF, et al, editors: *Rehabilitation of the hand and upper extremity*, ed 6, Philadelphia, 2011, Mosby, pp 781–791.
10. Lohman H, Coppard BM: Splinting for nerve injuries. In Coppard BM, Lohman H, editors: *Introduction to splinting: a clinical reasoning and problem solving approach*, St Louis, 2008, Mosby Elsevier, pp 279–307.
11. Moscony AMB: Common peripheral nerve problems. In Cooper C, editor: *Fundamentals of hand therapy: clinical reasoning and treatment guidelines for common diagnoses of the upper extremity*, St Louis, 2007, Mosby Elsevier, pp 201–250.
12. Van Lede P, van Veldhoven G: *Therapeutic hand splints: a rational approach*, ed 2, Asker, Norway, 2006, van Veldhoven.
13. Ashworth S, Kozin SH: Brachial plexus palsy reconstruction: tendon transfers, osteotomies, capsular release and arthrodesis. In Skirven TM, Osterman AL, Fedorczyk JF, et al, editors: *Rehabilitation of the hand and upper extremity*, ed 6, Philadelphia, 2011, Mosby, pp 792–812.
14. Schwartz DA: Strategies for facilitation of tendon transfers for enhanced wrist extension in cerebral palsy: a case report, *Br J Hand Ther* 10:10–16, 2005.
15. Yancosek KE, Howell D: A narrative review of dexterity assessments, *J Hand Ther* 22:258–270, 2009.
16. Schoeneveld K, Wittink H, Takken T: Clinimetric evaluation of measurement tools used in hand therapy to assess activity and participation, *J Hand Ther* 22:221–236, 2009.

17. MacDermid JC, Tottenham V: Responsiveness of the disability of the arm, shoulder, and hand (DASH) and patient-rated wrist/hand evaluation (PRWHE) in evaluating change after hand therapy, *J Hand Ther* 17(1):18–23, 2004.

18. Lieber RL: Muscle architectural and biomechanical considerations in tendon transfer. In Fridén J, editor: *Tendon transfers in reconstructive hand surgery*, London and New York, 2005, Taylor and Francis, pp 1–19.

19. Richer RJ, Peimer CA: Flexor superficialis abductor transfer with carpal tunnel release for thenar palsy, *J Hand Surg Am* 30:506–512, 2005.

20. Sammer DM, Chung KC: Tendon transfers: part II. transfers for ulnar nerve palsy and median nerve palsy, *Plast Reconstr Surg* 124(3):212e–221e, 2009.

21. Hammert WC, Heest AEV, James MA, et al: Tendon transfers. In Hammert WC, Calfee RP, Bozentka DJ, et al, editors: *ASSH manual of hand surgery*, Philadelphia, 2010, Wolters Kluwer/Lippincott Williams & Wilkins, pp 145–169.

22. Pettengill K: Therapist management of the complex injury. In Skirven TM, Osterman AL, Fedorczyk JF, et al, editors: *Rehabilitation of the hand and upper extremity*, ed 6, Philadelphia, 2011, Mosby, pp 1238–1251.

23. McCabe C: Mirror visual feedback therapy: a practical approach, *J Hand Ther* 24:170–179, 2011.

24. Koman LA, Li Z, Patterson Smith B, et al: Upper extremity musculoskeletal surgery in the child with cerebral palsy: surgical options and rehabilitation. In Skirven TM, Osterman AL, Fedorczyk JF, et al, editors: *Rehabilitation of the hand and upper extremity*, ed 6, Philadelphia, 2011, Mosby, pp 1651–1658.

25. Rosenthal EA, Elhassan BT: The extensor tendons: evaluation and surgical management. In Skirven TM, Osterman AL, Fedorczyk JF, et al, editors: *Rehabilitation of the hand and upper extremity*, ed 6, Philadelphia, 2011, Mosby, pp 487–520.

26. Lubahn J, Wolfe TL: Surgical treatment and rehabilitation of tendon ruptures and imbalances in the rheumatoid hand. In Skirven TM, Osterman AL, Fedorczyk JF, et al, editors: *Rehabilitation of the hand and upper extremity*, ed 6, Philadelphia, 2011, Mosby, pp 1399–1407.

27. Peliovich AE, Bryden AM, Malone KJ, et al: Rehabilitation of the hand and upper extremity in tetraplegia. In Skirven TM, Osterman AL, Fedorczyk JF, et al, editors: *Rehabilitation of the hand and upper extremity*, ed 6, Philadelphia, 2011, Mosby, pp 1684–1705.

28. Rath S: A randomized clinical trial comparing immediate active motion with immobilization after tendon transfer for claw deformity, *J Hand Surg Am* 34:488–494, 2009.

29. Giessler GA, Przybilski M, Germann G, et al: Early free active versus dynamic extension splinting after extensor indicis proprius tendon transfer to restore thumb extension: a prospective randomized study, *J Hand Surg Am* 33:864–868, 2008.

30. Bezuhly M, Sparkes GL, Higgins A, et al: Immediate thumb extension following extensor indicis proprius to extensor pollicis longus tendon transfer using the wide awake approach, *Plast Reconstr Surg* 119:1507–1512, 2007.

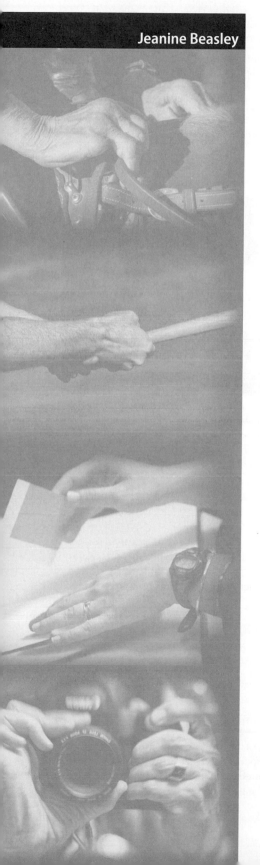

33

Arthritis

Jeanine Beasley

Arthritis is the leading cause of disability in the United States.[1] More than 100 diseases and conditions fall into the category of rheumatic diseases.[2] The most common, **osteoarthritis (OA),** affects nearly 27 million Americans over the age of 25[3] and is the most common joint disorder throughout the world.[4] OA is associated with a defective integrity of the articular cartilage and changes in the underlying bone.[5] **Rheumatoid arthritis (RA)** affects more than 1.5 million Americans[6] and is a chronic, systemic, inflammatory, autoimmune disorder.[7] The inflammatory process associated with RA manifests itself primarily in the **synovial** tissue.[8] In addition to RA and OA, the therapist also may treat other rheumatic diseases, such as **systemic lupus erythematosus** (a systemic autoimmune disease characterized by inflammation and blood vessel abnormalities), **gout** (a disorder caused by uric acid or urate crystal deposition), **bursitis** (inflammation of the bursa), and **fibromyalgia** (diffuse widespread pain often with specific tender points). [2, 3, 7, 8] In the United States nearly 50 million adults over the age of 18 report being told by a physician that they have some form of arthritis, and over 21 million adults have activity limitations attributed to arthritis.[9] Clearly, with this level of prevalence, many therapists at some time will find these clients on their caseload, or be questioned about arthritis by colleagues and family. The therapist must have an understanding of the disease process, potential deformities, and how it can affect the clients' activities of daily living (ADLs). Client education about the disease and awareness of treatment options are also critical aspects of the treatment process.

Osteoarthritis

Pathology

OA is often called the *wear-and-tear disease,* but research demonstrates that the breakdown in the articular cartilage is due to both mechanical and chemical factors.[10] Changes in the articular cartilage and the subchondral bone result from the chondrocytes failing to maintain the necessary balance of the extra cellular matrix.[11-13] Complex biomechanical factors appear to activate the chondrocytes to produce degradative enzymes.[14, 15] This degradation then corresponds to failure of the articular cartilage to act as a shock absorber, resulting in progression of the disease. Mechanical factors, such as abnormal loading of the joint from trauma, heavy labor, joint instability, and obesity, can increase the risk of OA.[16] Aging is also a risk factor, because aging cartilage contains less water and fewer chondrocytes, decreasing the capacity of the cells to restore and maintain the cartilage.[13] Clients from all corners of the world report similar patterns of joint involvement[12] including the distal interphalangeal (DIP) joints (35%) and the carpometacarpal (CMC) joint of the thumb (21%).[9, 17-19] In addition, 50% of patients with DIP involvement also have proximal interphalangeal (PIP) joint involvement.[20] Affected persons have a genetic susceptibility, and OA occurs more frequently in women over age 50 than in men of the same age. [13,18]

In addition to the cartilage breakdown, new bone formation (or **osteophytosis**) can occur, resulting in pain and limitations of joint movement. **Osteophytes,** or bone spurs, occurring at the metacarpophalangeal (MP) joints can contribute to **triggering** (limited digital range of motion [ROM] caused by dragging of the tendon as it passes through a pulley) of the flexor tendons,[4] or **locking** (the digit locks into flexion as the tendon fails to pass through a pulley). **Nodules** can occur with OA at the PIP joint and are called **Bouchard's nodes,** and at the DIP joint they are called **Heberden's nodes.**[13] Deformities as a result of this arthritic process include a mallet finger deformity at the DIP joint and lateral deviation or boutonniére deformities at the PIP joint.[18] The client may also demonstrate reduced ROM, pain, **crepitus** (**grating** or popping as the digit flexes and extends), and signs of inflammation.[9] In the lower extremity, the knees and hips commonly are affected.

Precaution. *If the client needs to use a walker or crutches because of lower extremity pain, this can put additional stress on the joints of the hands.*

Timelines and Healing

Currently, no cure is available for OA. Treatment is based on the specific needs of each patient and the stage of the disease. In the early stage, radiology reveals a reduction in the joint-spaces and swelling of the periarticular tissues; the moderate stage demonstrates osteophytes, subchondral sclerosis, and cysts. In the late stage, bone erosion, subluxation, and fibrotic ankylosis are common.[18] Regarding postoperative care, the timelines follow the phases of wound healing. This includes the inflammatory phase during the first few days after surgery. Healing continues to the proliferative phase or fibroplasia, which often lasts from 4 days to approximately 3 weeks after surgery and is when the fibroblasts lay beds of collagen. During this stage, many of the postoperative protocols incorporate a balance between specific orthoses and gentle exercise. Finally, the remodeling phase or maturation phase occurs, which often begins 3 weeks after surgery and can last several years with gradual increase in the tensile strength of the collagen fibers.[21]

Evaluation

The evaluation should include an assessment of pain, active range of motion (AROM), joint stability, joint inflammation, palpation, and ability to do ADLs. Pain can be measured at rest and with activities with a 10 cm visual analog scale (VAS), with 0 being no pain and 10 being severe pain.[22] I have observed clinically that many clients with arthritis tend to underestimate their pain. Document areas of inflammation by specifying which joints are involved. If the joint is warm and red, it may be in an acute inflammatory stage, and this should be noted. The evaluation of ADLs should include home, work, and leisure activities, because clients often seek help when their meaningful activities are threatened. Standardized tests, such as the Canadian Occupational Performance Measure (COPM)[23] and Arthritis Impact Measurement Scales (AIMS) health status questionnaire,[24] can be helpful in determining areas of ADL limitations and setting goals in collaboration with the patient. In regards to the evaluation of the basal joint of the thumb with OA, the Eaton classification has been widely used to define severity as well as guide treatment.[25] The stages are highlighted in Table 33-1. It is important to note that treatment should be based on the severity of the symptoms reported by the patient and not simply on the radiographic stage.[26]

Precaution. *Passive range of motion (PROM) measurements usually are not recommended, especially if there is a lack of joint stability. Do not apply passive stretch to an OA joint that lacks stability, because this can be injurious.*

Evaluate thumb joint stability by having the client attempt a tip pinch. Ligament stability may be questioned if the thumb MP and interphalangeal (IP) joints are unable to maintain a near-neutral position during pinch. Assessing lateral joint stability of the digits is important at the PIP and DIP joints. Test the involved joint by stabilizing the proximal phalanx and gently moving the distal phalanx laterally in each direction. A greater degree of joint play is evident when joint stability is decreased. Lateral deviation of the IP at rest should also be

TABLE 33-1	Eaton Radiographic Classification for Staging Basal Joint Arthritis
Eaton Stage	**Radiograph**
Stage I	Normal appearance of articular surface and slight joint space widening.
Stage II	Minimal sclerotic changes of subchondral bone with osteophytes and loose bodies less than 2 mm.
Stage III	Trapeziometacarpal joint space markedly narrowed and cystic changes present. Subluxation of the metacarpal may have occurred. Osteophytes and loose bodies greater than 2 mm.
Stage IV	Presence of scaphotrapezial joint disease with narrowing.

From Eaton RG, Glickel SZ: Trapeziometacarpal osteoarthritis. Staging as a rationale for treatment, *Hand Clin* 3(4):455-471, 1987.

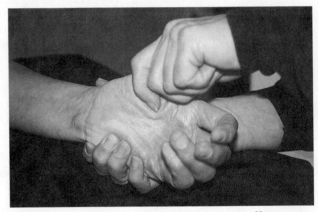

FIGURE 33-1 The grind test as described by Swanson[27] for crepitus at the carpometacarpal (CMC) joint involves compressing the joint while gently rotating the metacarpal at the CMC joint. (From Beasley J: Therapist's examination and conservative management of arthritis of the upper extremity. In Skirven TM, Osterman AL, Fedorczyk JM, et al, editors: *Rehabilitation of the hand and upper extremity*, ed 6, St Louis, 2011, Elsevier, p. 1332.)

noted if evident. Document fixed deformities that cannot be corrected passively when gently positioned by the therapist. Fixed joint deformities in OA can include DIP flexion or angulation, CMC adduction, and thumb MP joint extension or flexion.

Grating or crepitus evident at a joint can indicate damaged cartilage. The **grind test** for degenerative joint disease at the CMC joint involves compressing the joint while gently rotating the head of the metacarpal on the trapezium[27] (Fig. 33-1). Pain and crepitus at the CMC joint generally are considered positive findings.

Non-Operative Treatment

Non-operative treatment begins with a complete evaluation to determine the client's specific needs. Treatment can include joint protection principles, modalities, exercise, orthoses, and adaptive equipment as outlined subsequently.

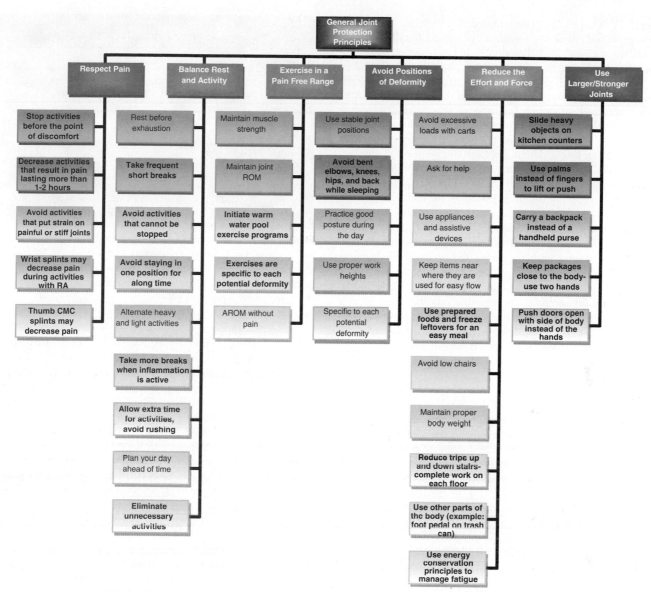

FIGURE 33-2 Overview of joint protection principles. (Based on concepts by Cordery;[29] Melvin;[39] Meenan, et al.;[24] and Hammond, et al.[85] The concepts have been grouped into themes by this author. Chart is used with permission from Beasley J: Osteoarthritis and rheumatoid arthritis, *J Hand Ther.* 25(2):163-172, 2012.)

General Joint Protection Principles

Joint protection principles ideally are initiated early in the disease process in hope of decreasing stress and damage to the involved joints.[28-30] This is completed through altered work methods to educate the client on proper joint alignment and the use of adaptive equipment. Joint protection for OA should also take into account the specific deformity or potential deformity, which may include instability of the CMC joint and the deformities of the involved IP joints.[29, 30] Common joint protection principles for both OA and RA are categorized by themes in Fig. 33-2. Because excessive pinching during ADL imparts large forces to the unstable thumb CMC joint, educating patients in techniques that decrease pressure and force applied to the thumb CMC joint is important.[31] There is moderate evidence to support joint protection education and adaptive equipment for increased hand function and pain reduction in patients with OA.[32] The European League Against Rheumatism (EULAR)[33] in their systematic

review recommended joint protection education combined with an exercise regimen for all patients with hand OA. Another systematic review found moderate evidence to support combining joint protection with adaptive device provision for increased hand function and pain reduction.[32] Adaptive equipment used in one study included enlarged writing grips, Dycem, an angled knife, a book holder, and other equipment based on the client's ADL[34] and resulted in improvements in grip strength and global hand function. Adaptive equipment that can help to increase leverage and also distribute the pressure in the hand includes larger-diameter pens, broad key holders, large plastic tabs on medicine bottles, and car door openers. As handle diameter increases, reduced digit force on a tool is needed. Basic science in tool design has developed in the engineering fields to accurately measure these forces. It is reported that in normal hands, the most comfortable handle is 19.7% of the user's hand length[35] and that the ideal tool handle design is a cylinder with a 33-mm diameter.[36] It has also been determined that to decrease the maximum push pull force on a tool, a cylindrical handle must be parallel to the push/pull direction.[37] It has also been reported that a handle design that reduces wrist ulnar deviation requires the least amount of grip force.[38] Additional joint protection techniques include moving objects out of the hand (for example, using a shoulder strap tote bag instead of a brief case with a handle) to help distribute the pressure to larger joints when carried closer to the body. [28] Clients often place strong forces on the hands when lifting themselves from one position to another. In some cases, adaptive equipment can reduce the effort on the lower extremities (such as, a lift chair, a shower chair, or elevated toilet seat) by reducing the stress placed on the hands.

The therapist should also take into consideration the client's sociocultural context. The client may or may not have insurance coverage or finances for adaptive equipment or orthoses. Carefully discuss options with the client and weigh them in terms of cost versus value in meeting the client's specific needs. The therapist should be aware of community resources, including civic, community, or religious organizations that may provide adaptive equipment (for example, grab bars and elevated toilet seats) for specific socioeconomic situations. For further information on joint protection, the reader is encouraged to review the work *Adult Rheumatic Diseases* (2000), by Melvin and Ferrel.[39]

Modalities

Modalities have a long history of use in the treatment of arthritis. Many patients with OA report beginning their day with a warm shower or bath as increased tissue temperatures result in temporary neuromuscular effects that decrease pain and muscle tension.[40] Types of superficial heating agents include paraffin, Fluidotherapy, hot packs, microwave packs, hydrotherapy, and electric mitts. Decreasing pain and maintaining or improving ROM is a primary goal in the application of these agents. Research continues to add to the body of knowledge concerning heat and other modalities for OA, including non-thermal ultrasound, electrotherapy, cryotherapy, and low level laser therapy. [41] A systematic review by Zwang, et al.[33] examined the benefits of heat and ultrasound and found predominantly only level IV evidence (expert opinion). According to the review by Valdes and Marik,[32] there is weak to moderate level evidence supporting the use of heat modalities in decreasing pain and improving grip strength in patients with OA, and low level laser therapy was no better than the placebo.

Precaution. *When clients benefit from superficial heat modalities and use them in their home exercise program (HEP), the therapist must instruct them carefully to avoid the possibility of burns.*

Exercise

General principles of exercise include avoiding painful AROM and PROM by working within the client's comfort level. General AROM exercises for the hand include wrist flexion and extension, gentle digit flexion and extension, and thumb opposition. There is moderate evidence to support hand exercises in OA for increasing grip strength, improving function, improving ROM, and pain reduction.[32] Combining joint protection and pain-free hand home exercises were found to be an effective means to increase hand function, as measured by grip strength and self-reported global functioning in persons with hand OA.[42] Exercise programs that utilize AROM as opposed to pinch strengthening [32,43] were found to be more effective. One study that used

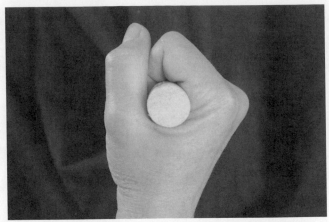

FIGURE 33-3 Stretching and massage of the first web space may help prevent the adduction contracture and subsequent MP hyperextension deformity.[45] Thumb web space stretching or widening can be done by having the client grasp a 1-inch wooden dowel as part of the home exercise program (HEP).

resistive pinch strengthening resulted in some of the participants leaving the study due to increased hand symptoms.[44] For example, even light putty-pinching exercises impart large forces[31] to an unstable CMC joint that may aggravate a potential deformity. Stability must not be sacrificed for a possible increase in strength. A stable pain-free thumb provides a post against which the digits can grip and pinch effectively. Stretching and massage of the first web space may help prevent the adduction contracture and subsequent MP hyperextension deformity.[45] Thumb web space stretching or widening can be done by having the client grasp a one inch wooden dowel (Fig. 33-3) as part of the HEP, as well as techniques to relax the adductor pollicis (AP). Anatomically, strengthening the first dorsal interosseous may help provide stability to the base of the CMC, because it originates at the base of the first metacarpal.[45] In regards to the tendons, grip strengthening is a common example of an exercise that can aggravate inflamed flexor tendons. A digit that is triggering or locking will not be improved with grip strengthening exercises, which can increase these symptoms.

Precaution. *Therapy exercises should never create deforming forces or cause pain in the osteoarthritic client.*

Research on overall body conditioning has been reported to result in decreased pain and increased static and dynamic grip strength.[46] A study on low impact general conditioning demonstrated increased aerobic capacity, decreased depression, and decreased anxiety in patients with arthritis.[47]

Precaution. *Keep ROM exercises pain-free to prevent stretching of joint structures. Use strengthening programs for the osteoarthritic hand with caution to avoid aggravation of deformities.*

The Thumb

OA can affect all of the joints of the thumb with a swan neck deformity as one of the most common. It is often characterized at the CMC joint by metacarpal adduction and subluxation from the trapezium, MP joint hyperextension, and IP joint flexion (Fig. 33-4). Pinch is often painful because the CMC subluxation becomes more pronounced during heavy pinch activities.

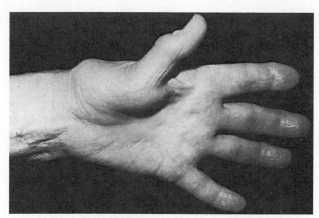

FIGURE 33-4 The type III thumb deformity involves subluxation of the carpometacarpal (CMC) joint, metacarpophalangeal (MP) joint hyperextension, and distal joint flexion. (From Terrono AL, Nalebuff EA, Phillips CA: The rheumatoid thumb. In Skirven TM, Osterman AL, Fedorczyk JM, et al, editors: *Rehabilitation of the hand and upper extremity*, ed 6, St Louis, 2011, Elsevier, p. 1347.)

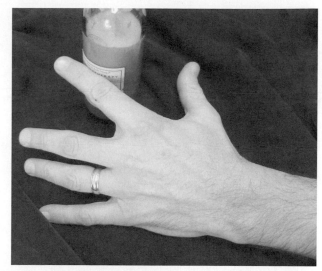

FIGURE 33-5 Having the patient push a glass with the index digit while the rest of the hand is stabilized can help strengthen the first dorsal interosseous muscle.

The thumb IP joint sometimes assumes a flexed position. The Eaton classification has been widely used to define severity and guide treatment of this deformity through radiographs.[25] The Eaton stages are highlighted in Table 33-1. When evaluating the thumb, determine the specific pattern of deformity so that treatment can be more specific in terms of orthotic support and therapeutic management.

? Questions to Discuss with the Physician

• What joints of the thumb are involved (as seen on the radiographs)?
• Is there also joint involvement of the wrist?
• Is the client using any medications for this condition?

( ) What to Say to Clients

About the Condition

"Here is a picture (radiograph) of a thumb with osteoarthritis. The problem often starts at this joint (the carpometacarpal). With wearing down of the cartilage and weakening of the joint ligaments and capsule, this joint has a tendency to dislocate or slide out of place. Over time, this results in a thumb that has difficulty abducting or moving away from the palm of the hand (at the carpometacarpal). The next joint of the thumb (metacarpophalangeal) then has to do extra work, and it often stretches out and hyperextends."

About Orthoses

"We are going to try a couple of splints that may help to give the thumb some stability. We have several options, but we need to see what works best for you and your activities of daily living. Some people like one type of splint for night wear and a less restrictive splint for day wear."

About Exercise

"Heavy pinch activities and exercises put a lot of stress on this (the carpometacarpal) joint and can decrease joint stability. It is important that your hand exercises be pain-free. Exercises

that can be helpful include a gentle stretching of the first web space (adductor pollicis) with massage, as well grasping a 1-inch dowel to gently wedge the web space. Strengthening the muscle (the first dorsal interossius) on the side of your index finger may help stabilize the base of your thumb. Pushing a glass sideways with your index finger (Fig. 33-5) with your hand stabilized is a nice way to activate this muscle. For your general conditioning, warm-water pool exercises may be helpful in managing your osteoarthritis."

Evaluation Tips

• Determine whether the thumb deformity is passively correctable. This involves gentle positioning opposite of the deformity; gently stabilize the base of the metacarpal on the trapezium, place the CMC in abduction and the MP in flexion (Fig. 33-6). This is the proper position for the orthosis.
• Determine how the disease process is affecting the client's ADL and what the client is seeking regarding therapy. This allows you to determine whether the client will be compliant with the program.

Diagnosis-Specific Information that Affects Clinical Reasoning

If the orthosis fits well, the client will report decreased pain with pinch activities, because it is stabilizing the CMC joint in the proper position. Radiographs during active pinch can verify that the orthosis is properly maintaining the metacarpal on the trapezium.[49]

◎ Clinical Pearl

If the thumb deformity is not passively correctable, the orthosis can help provide support but cannot change the deformity.

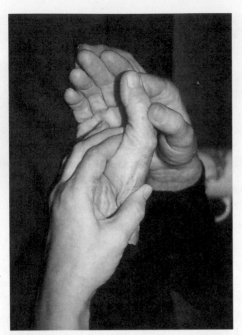

FIGURE 33-6 When the thumb deformity is passively correctable, the placement of the therapist's hands often determines the forces that are needed to apply the orthosis correctly. (Concept courtesy of Judy Leonard, OTR, CHT. From Beasley J: Soft orthoses: indications and techniques. In Skirven TM, Osterman AL, Fedorczyk JM, et al, editors: *Rehabilitation of the hand and upper extremity*, ed 6, St Louis, 2011, Elsevier, p. 1614.)

♡ *Tips from the Field*

The therapist has several choices when selecting the proper orthosis for the client. The orthosis can be custom fabricated of lightweight thermoplastics, or in some cases a soft material (for example, Neoprene) can be used, if the strapping is applied properly, to counteract the deforming forces (Fig. 33-7 through Fig. 33-9). There are also several prefabricated options available. This author has had good client acceptance and reported pain reduction with both the neoprene Comfort Cool Thumb CMC Restriction Splints (see Fig. 33-8) (available from North Coast Medical) and The Push MetaGrip (see Fig. 33-9) (available from HandLab). This acceptance is due to decreased pain and increased joint stability when using their properly fitted orthoses during pinching activities. Clients often misinterpret this as an increase in strength. A stable, pain-free thumb is important to hand function and provides a post to which the digits can grip and pinch effectively.

In some cases, the client has a large thumb IP joint that makes donning and removing the orthosis difficult. The orthosis must be large enough to fit over this joint while providing support to the proximal phalanx. One easy way to enlarge the orthosis thumbhole when it is nearly cool is to remove the orthosis from the client and then insert a closed scissors into the thumb portion of the splint and gently open the scissors (Fig. 33-10). Another technique is to pry open the seam that would be supporting the proximal phalanx after the orthosis has cooled. The unsecured seam then can be expanded partially when the orthosis is applied and secured with a Velcro® strap. An additional solution is an orthosis that does not include the MP or has a dorsal proximal phalanx flap (Fig. 33-11) to help

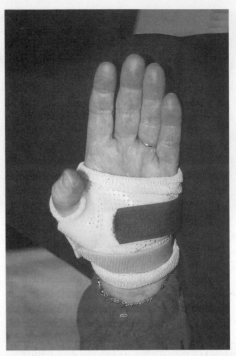

FIGURE 33-7 The hand-based thumb spica orthosis for deformities that are passively correctable can help decrease pain. The orthosis places the metacarpal in gentle palmar abduction and the metacarpophalangeal (MP) joint in slight flexion. The wrist strap gives the splint additional stability to stabilize the carpometacarpal (CMC) joint. (From Beasley J: Therapist's examination and conservative management of arthritis of the upper extremity. In Skirven TM, Osterman AL, Fedorczyk JM, et al, editors: *Rehabilitation of the hand and upper extremity*, ed 6, St Louis, 2011, Elsevier, p. 1339.)

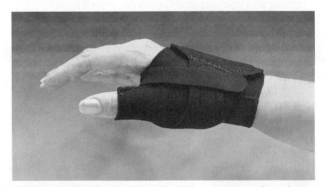

FIGURE 33-8 Comfort Cool Thumb CMC restriction orthosis has an additional strap to support and gently compress the CMC joint. The splint also gently positions the metacarpal in abduction. (Photo and splint courtesy of North Coast Medical, Inc., Morgan Hill, CA. From Beasley J: Soft orthoses: indications and techniques. In Skirven TM, Osterman AL, Fedorczyk JM, et al, editors: *Rehabilitation of the hand and upper extremity*, ed 6, St Louis, 2011, Elsevier, p. 1614.)

position the MP joint in flexion as described by Colditz.[50] If the joints proximal to the trapezium are also involved, such as the scaphoid and trapezoid (this is referred to as **pantrapezial arthritis**), the orthosis may need to incorporate the wrist,[51] requiring a forearm-based thumb spica orthosis (Fig. 33-12).

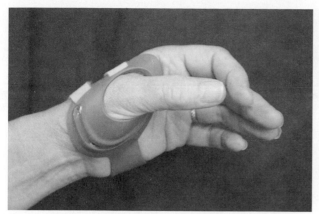

FIGURE 33-9 The Push MetaGrip from HandLab supports the carpometacarpal (CMC) with an imbedded contoured metal insert that assists in stabilizing the metacarpal on the trapezium.

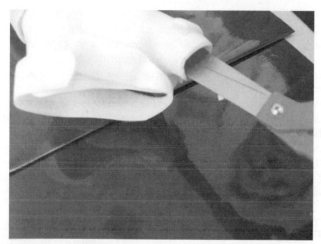

FIGURE 33-10 One easy way to enlarge the orthotic thumbhole, when it is nearly cool, is to insert a closed scissors into the thumb portion of the orthosis and gently open the scissors.

The client usually responds favorably to wearing the orthosis if it is comfortable and fits correctly. Many clients wear the soft orthosis during the day and the more rigid orthosis at night.[49] Other clients feel that the rigid splint supports the thumb more completely, reporting decreased pain and rejecting the soft orthosis. In cases of bilateral involvement, only one rigid orthosis should be fabricated at the first visit to determine how the client responds. This assists the therapist in the decision making process. Once the client has decided on an orthosis for one hand, the client will have a preference for the other hand.

> **▷ Precautions and Concerns**

- *The most troubling possible problem with any orthosis is the development of pressure areas. The client should return for at least one follow-up visit to make any necessary orthotic adjustments.*
- *Remember, an orthosis that is clean is not being worn. Usually, a clean orthosis is one that is uncomfortable to wear and needs adjustment. Some clients hesitate to ask for orthotic adjustment for fear of offending their therapist.*

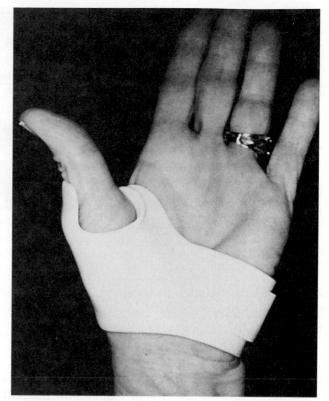

FIGURE 33-11 This orthosis designed by Judy Colditz for carpometacarpal (CMC) joint subluxation has a metacarpophalangeal (MP) block to prevent MP hyperextension. This orthosis makes donning and doffing easier when there is a large thumb interphalangeal (IP) joint. (From Colditz J: Anatomic considerations for splinting the thumb. In Mackin EJ, Callahan AD, Skirven TM, et al, editors: *Rehabilitation of the hand and upper extremity*, ed 5, St Louis, 2002, Mosby, p.1870.)

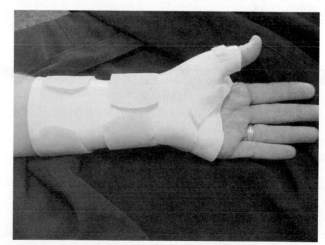

FIGURE 33-12 A thumb spica orthosis for use when the arthritic process also involves the wrist.

Operative Treatment

Therapy after Carpometacarpal Interposition Arthroplasty

CMC interposition arthroplasty involves resection of CMC joint that then allows the metacarpal to return to an abducted position.[48] A donor tendon is rolled up and inter-positioned in

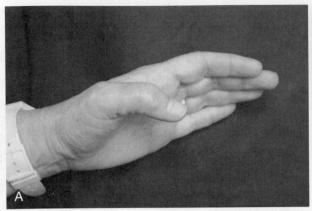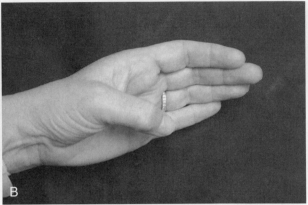

FIGURE 33-13 Clients with carpometacarpal (CMC) osteoarthritis (OA) have often been compensating before surgery by only moving their thumb IP and MP joints. One exercise technique for this is to have the client flex the thumb IP and MP joints **(A)** (and try to keep them flexed) while moving the CMC joint in gentle flexion and extension **(B).**

the joint space. The ligaments are usually reconstructed and help to provide the CMC joint stability. Hyperextension of the MP joint may be corrected as well. In most cases the client is in a cast for 4 to 6 weeks and then is referred for an orthosis. The postoperative course varies from surgeon to surgeon. When the surgeon allows CMC AROM, it is important to help the client learn how to move it properly. Frequently, these clients have been compensating before surgery by only moving their thumb IP and MP joints. One exercise technique for this is to have the client flex the thumb IP and MP joints (and try to keep them flexed) while moving the CMC joint in gentle flexion and extension (Fig. 33-13). Techniques to restore the thumb web space and strengthen the first dorsal interosseous (see Fig. 33-5) may also be helpful in the promotion of CMC stability.[45] The postoperative orthosis may be worn anywhere from 6 to 12 weeks from the date of surgery depending on the preferences and protocols of individual surgeons.

Precaution. *Many surgeons recommend waiting at least 3 months before any heavy pinching activities are allowed.*

<table>
<tr><td>**?**</td><td>**Questions to Discuss with the Physician**</td></tr>
</table>

- May we see the client while they are still in the cast for thumb IP, digit, elbow, and shoulder AROM, as well as edema management?
- When will the cast be removed?
- At the time of cast removal, should we apply a hand-based or forearm-based orthosis?
- At what point may we begin gentle AROM of the CMC joint?
- At what point may we discontinue the orthosis?
- How long would you prefer that we have the client wait before doing heavy pinch ADL?

<table>
<tr><td>**( )**</td><td>**What to Say to Clients**</td></tr>
</table>

About the Condition

"The surgery helped to correct the joint deformities you were having as a result of your osteoarthritis. The two little scars on your arm (or leg) are due to the retrieval of the donor tendon graft. The tendon was rolled up and placed in the joint between the trimmed bones."

About the Orthosis

"Now that your cast has been removed (4 to 6 weeks after surgery), we need to make you an orthosis to maintain the proper position and stability of the joint that has been reconstructed. To get the best result, we need to maintain a good balance between mobility and stability. You will need to wear your new orthosis between exercise sessions and at night until discontinued by your surgeon. It is important that your orthosis be comfortable and not cause any pressure areas."

About Exercise

"When it is approved by your surgeon, we will start gentle exercises of your new carpometacarpal joint. It is a joint that you have not moved in a long time. Before the surgery, you mainly moved the end and middle joints of your thumb. We will begin by gently trying to touch the tip of each finger and move your thumb in a small circle. I will show you an exercise where you try to keep your thumb end (interphalangeal) and middle joint (metacarpophalangeal) bent while you try to move the base of your thumb in and then away from your hand (carpometacarpal flexion, extension, and abduction) (see Fig. 33-13). We will also show you how to relax and massage the muscle at your thumb web (adductor pollicis). In addition, strengthening the muscle (the first dorsal interosseous) that moves your index finger toward the thumb can be helpful (see Fig. 33-5). We may have you doing grip-strengthening exercises that do not involve the thumb. The thumb is a stable post for the digits. We usually do not do pinch-strengthening exercises because they put too much stress on a repair that we want to be stable. Doing pinch activities too soon can compromise the surgical repair."

<table>
<tr><td>**Evaluation Tips**</td></tr>
</table>

- Many clients who arrive for therapy are surprised at how long the recovery is for this surgical procedure.
- Most clients are usually not in much pain. Those that have pain may have had a tight cast or an irritation of the superficial branch of the radial nerve. These clients complain of burning pain and should be sent immediately to the physician for a cast adjustment.

Continued

Evaluation Tips—cont'd

- Movement of the CMC joint is often difficult. Many clients moved only the MP and IP joints before surgery. Therapy involves muscle reeducation to move the CMC into abduction without the MP and IP joints hyperextending.
  Precaution. *When making the orthosis, take care to avoid any pressure to the base of the thumb, which can irritate the sensitive superficial branch of the radial nerve.*
- After being in a cast for several weeks, the skin will be very dry, and the scars may be sensitive. The client will appreciate a gentle cleaning of the skin and an application of lotion. If the scars can tolerate it, initiate gentle scar massage. Show the client how to do scar massage a couple of times each day as part of their HEP.
- Be aware and look for signs of complex regional pain syndrome with this population (see Chapter 12).

Diagnosis-Specific Information that Affects Clinical Reasoning

Most clients gain AROM quickly and want to resume activities as soon as possible. Many ADLs require a strong pinch and must be delayed until approved by the physician. Decisions to return to work depend on the type of activities that are done at work.

Tips from the Field

Orthoses

The orthotic tips previously outlined for the thumb spica orthosis apply after surgery for CMC interposition arthroplasty. An additional area of concern following this surgery is that special attention should be paid to avoid pressure from the orthosis at the incision site and at the base of the thumb near the superficial branch of the radial nerve. This area can be very sensitive in some clients. In some cases the client may progress from a forearm-based to a hand-based orthosis during the postoperative program. Some clients after being cleared to return to work prefer a soft neoprene orthosis (see Fig. 33-8) to help make the transition. This orthosis supplies gentle support while allowing ROM after the rigid splint is discontinued. In clients with persistent pain from the superficial branch of the radial nerve, the same neoprene orthosis (see Fig. 33-8) can provide gentle padding and protection to the hand.[52] This padding helps to prevent accidental bumping or irritation as the client's activity level gradually increases.

Client Compliance

Client compliance is usually not an issue because this is an elective surgery. A more common problem is that clients may do too much too soon after surgery. The therapist must stress the need for CMC joint stability to maximize the postoperative outcome.

Precautions and Concerns

- *Avoid heavy pinch activities for up to 3 months after this surgery.*
- *Avoid pressure areas from the orthosis especially over the base of the thumb and incision sites.*

- *The orthosis should position the thumb opposite of the preoperative deformity but should not force the thumb into position.*
- *Be alert for signs of complex regional pain syndrome, including persistent pain and heightened sympathetic nervous system responses.*
- *If the superficial branch of the radial nerve is irritated, some clients report relief with a transcutaneous electrical nerve stimulation unit. A silicone gel pad also may be helpful.*

Therapy after Carpometacarpal Fusion

See the Evolve website for information regarding therapy after CMC fusion.

Distal Interphalangeal Joint

Anatomy and Pathology

Clients with OA at the DIP joints often have enlargements called *Heberden's nodes.*[13] These nodes appear because of osteophytes or bony outgrowths near where the extensor tendon inserts on to the distal phalanx. When these nodes are present at the PIP joints, they are called *Bouchard's nodes.*[13]

Timelines and Healing

OA at the DIP joints can be painful initially, but pain usually decreases over time as they progress through the stages of OA.

Non-Operative Treatment

Some clients are referred for DIP joint orthoses during this painful time. The orthoses can help support the joints and are helpful in decreasing pain.[55] The client may also be referred for joint protection and modalities. Other clients are referred to therapy for an orthosis that may help mimic a DIP fusion before a possible surgery. This can assist the client to determine whether they would like to undergo a surgical fusion of the DIP joint. Another option is the application of various elastic tapes to the DIP joints, because this technique has been reported by some clients to be helpful in decreasing pain.

Questions to Discuss With the Physician

- Is the client a candidate for a DIP fusion?
- Are the DIP orthoses for pain management?

What to Say to Clients

About the Condition

- "The end joints of the fingers (distal interphalangeal) are one of the most common sites of osteoarthritis."
- "These joints (distal interphalangeal) can be painful for a time, but usually the pain gradually goes away."

About the Orthoses

- "If you are having pain, orthoses or elastic tape on the end joints of the fingers (distal interphalangeal joints) can give some relief (Fig. 33-14). Most clients do not have pain for an extended period, but the orthoses or tape can be helpful during this temporary painful time."

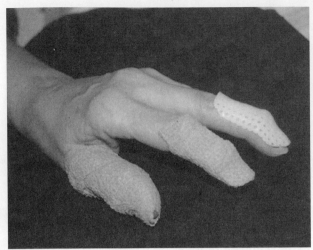

FIGURE 33-14 Orthoses to the distal interphalangeal (DIP) joints usually only are used with patients who are demonstrating a painful flare-up, those patients who are considering a surgical fusion, or following surgical fusion.

- "If you are considering a surgery to fuse your DIP joints, the orthoses may help you decide on this elective surgery."

About Exercise

- "Many clients with morning stiffness use heat to increase mobility before exercise or before starting their day. They usually apply it for about 20 minutes when stiffness is a problem."
- "It is helpful to avoid holding objects tightly with the fingers for a long time. This position keeps the joint bent, under stress, in a position of possible deformity, and can increase pain."

Evaluation Tips

Determination of the client's specific needs before providing treatment is important. Some clients do not wish to wear an orthosis, whereas others are at the clinic only for an orthosis. Be aware of the client's ADL and the specific joint protection principles that may need to be recommended (see Table 33-1).

Diagnosis-Specific Information that Affects Clinical Reasoning

Orthoses are usually used only with clients who are in a painful acute inflammatory stage or those who are considering surgical fusion.

♡ Tips from the Field

Orthoses

Because of the presence of Heberden's nodes and joint inflammation, orthoses to the DIP joints need to conform well and provide even pressure distribution. Thin or "light" orthotic materials are recommended, and the material should have excellent drape characteristics, such as Polyform light or Orfit.

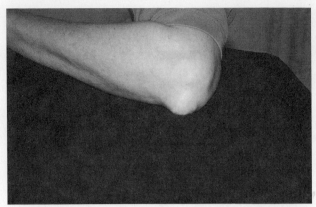

FIGURE 33-15 Rheumatoid nodules near the elbow joint. (From Beasley J: Therapist's examination and conservative management of arthritis of the upper extremity. In Skirven TM, Osterman AL, Fedorczyk JM, et al, editors: *Rehabilitation of the hand and upper extremity*, ed 6, St Louis, 2011, Elsevier, p. 1333.)

These orthoses usually are made on the dorsal surface to allow for tactile input of the volar surface for ADLs (Fig. 33-14). To hold these splints in place, a non-adhesive wrap, such as Coban or Co-Wrap is recommended.

Client Compliance

Client compliance is good if the orthoses fits well and decreases pain during the acute inflammatory flare-up. Many clients reject the orthoses after the flare-up. Clients, who report they have no pain at the DIP joints but demonstrate joint inflammation during the evaluation, are less likely to wear the orthoses.

⟩ Precautions and Concerns

During an acute flare-up, the skin is very sensitive at the dorsal DIP level. Orthoses should conform well to prevent any pressure areas. Comfort is the key to splinting the DIP joints.

The orthoses should fit snugly so that they do not slide on the digit but should not be so snug as to feel constricting. The dorsal design allows the client to feel objects (meals, phones, keyboards, and so on) more easily on the volar surface.

Edema changes may necessitate orthotic modifications as the swelling decreases.

Rheumatoid Arthritis

RA is an inflammatory, systemic, autoimmune disorder.[57] The inflammatory process associated with RA manifests itself primarily in the synovial tissue.[58] Joint destruction occurs when the synovial **pannus** expresses enzymes allowing cartilage penetration, cartilage damage, and joint erosion.[57] RA is evident worldwide with prevalence rates at approximately 1% and varying among ethnic groups.[59,60] The evaluation and treatment of the client with RA can be challenging for even the most experienced therapist. The disease can affect the intricate balance of the hand when joints and soft tissue structures become compromised.

Therapeutic treatment is individualized and specific to the client's deformity or potential deformity, stage of the disease, and ADL needs. Only after a complete evaluation are goals and treatment methods selected to meet the needs and expectations of these clients. Client education about the disease and treatment options is critical in the treatment process.

Diagnosis and Pathology

RA typically affects the joints symmetrically[61] and hand involvement most commonly includes the MP, PIP, thumb, and wrist joints.[58] Early symptoms include morning stiffness lasting more than an hour and fusiform swelling of the PIP joints.[61] Flexor tendon **tenosynovitis** can reduce digit motion, strength, and in some cases result in a trigger finger if nodular thickening occurs.[58] Deformities of the hand include MP joint ulnar deviation with palmar subluxation and radial deviation of the metacarpals or the zigzag deformity.[58, 61] Other deformities include PIP swan neck and boutonnière deformities,[58, 61] and a variety of thumb deformities.[48] **Rheumatoid nodules** commonly occur over pressure areas at the elbows and digits.[58, 61] Onset of symptoms can be abrupt, but more commonly a slower progression occurs over several weeks.

> ### Clinical Pearl
>
> With RA, the joint involvement is often symmetrical and bilateral.[61]

The therapist must have an understanding of the stages of the disease process, as well as potential deformities. This knowledge will assist in determining the appropriate treatment options. Recent medications for RA have altered the course of this chronic condition. The therapist also must note that the client may return to earlier stages during the clinical course and will have remissions and exacerbations as the disease progresses.

During the acute phase, or stage I, as classified by Steinbrocker, et al.,[62] the client demonstrates joint swelling and inflammation that is warm when palpated. This is the most painful phase, and it is also when most clients seek medical care.

The subacute, or stage II, phase often is marked by a decrease in symptoms. The inflammatory synovium forms a pannus that extends beyond the cartilage and invades ligament attachments and tendons.[63] Nodules (small rounded lumps) may be evident at the joint **bursa** (a fluid-filled sac that decreases friction) or along the tendons. Joint ROM is usually less painful, and there are no obvious deformities. In the destructive, chronic active stage III, the client often reports less pain, but irreversible joint deformities have progressed.[62,63] Stage IV has been referred to as *chronic inactive* or *skeletal collapse and deformity*. The joint deformities are considerable and may include instability, dislocation, spontaneous fusion, and bony or fibrous **ankylosis** (stiffening of a joint).[62,63]

Timelines and Healing

Unfortunately, there is no cure for RA at this time. During the last decade, there has been significant progress understanding the molecular pathogenesis[64] and role of the immune system in the arthritic process. The medical intervention of arthritis now includes early and aggressive treatments for greater control of inflammation and joint erosion.[65] Despite these medical advances, it is important to understand that arthritis is still a chronic condition,[66] and these medical advances do not permanently change

the destructive behavior of the immune system.[64] The therapist can help manage the symptoms as the disease progresses with client education, modalities, orthoses, joint protection, and adaptive equipment. The postoperative timelines and protocols for specific surgeries follow.

Non-Operative Treatment

Evaluation

A complete evaluation of the client is necessary and includes ROM, ADL, joint deformities, stage of the disease process, previous surgeries, expectations of therapy, and pain.

Range of Motion

Measurements of AROM of the rheumatic hand varies daily with increased stiffness often noted in the morning.[67] Goniometric measurement should be done when possible, but deformities make this difficult in the later stages. Measurements of composite digit flexion, active digit extension, and thumb opposition often give more functional information. Some clients are unable to perform palmar pinch and instead use a lateral pinch because of a pronation deformity of the index digit.[68] The degree of ulnar deviation at the MP joints can provide helpful information for measuring progression of joint deformities. This measurement should be done with the digits in active available extension to avoid friction from a table, which can change the degree of ulnar deviation.

> ### Clinical Pearl
>
> Ulnar deviation often varies in MP flexion and extension because of ligament laxity, and therefore the position of the MP joint should be reported in combination with the ulnar drift measurements.

Loss of AROM can also be caused by tendon rupture. Rupture occurs as the tendon glides over roughened and irregular bone areas.

Precaution. *The extensor pollicis longus and the extensor digitorum communis tendons of the third, fourth, and fifth digits are particularly vulnerable to rupture.*

The tendon, which may be weakened by the inflammatory synovium, can fray and eventually rupture, resulting in loss of motion.[69] The extensor tendons are more vulnerable to rupture than the flexor tendons because of their proximity to the distal radius, ulna, and carpal bones. Extensor tendon rupture at the wrist level most often is seen with extensor pollicis longus at **Lister's tubercle** (a boney prominence) and with extensor digitorum communis at the distal end of the ulna. The extensor digiti quinti is often the first extensor to rupture and may signal the potential rupture of the other extensor tendons.[70]

Strength

Adams, et al.[71] reported that hand grip strength acts as a reliable indicator of upper extremity functional ability. The Jamar dynamometer has demonstrated good reliability,[72] and measurements should be completed following the clinical recommendations of the American Society of Hand Therapists (ASHT).[73] In addition the B&L Engineering pinch gauge is considered the "gold standard" when measuring pinch strength. [74] Joint instability, rather than weakness, is usually more problematic during ADLs. Even with adequate muscle strength, clients will be unable to maintain a grip on an object if their joints collapse into deformities.

Activities of Daily Living

Evaluation of the client's functional level begins as the client enters the clinic. Observation as the client removes a coat and sits at a table can be invaluable in understanding their ability to pinch and grasp, complete simple functional activities, and even use the hand for mobility (such as, using crutches). Joint deformities can be observed and may be accentuated with simple activities. The speed by which the client enters the clinic often provides qualitative information as to the level of pain and the involvement of the lower extremities. The therapist must gain an understanding of the client's home and support system when planning the HEP and potential orthotic designs. For example, if the client is unable to don an orthosis independently, a caregiver will be needed. The therapist needs to evaluate the client's goals for therapy carefully to make sure that they are realistic. A client diary, as described by Devore,[70] can give insight into the needs of the client and make the client an active participant in the treatment process. The diary helps the client to determine problem areas with ADLs, including which joints are involved and also whether the joint difficulties are because of pain, power, or position. The diary can also assist with client "ownership" of the therapy program. This self-determination of problem areas facilitates client goal setting and client follow through.

Pain

Pain caused by acute inflammation is usually greater in the early stages of the disease than in the end stages when severe deformities are evident. Pain analog scales can be used to determine the effectiveness of treatment, but clinical observation suggests that these clients, in the later stages, rate their pain much lower than anticipated by the therapist. Orthoses may be helpful in decreasing pain but should be balanced with the ADL requirements of each client. Rheumatoid nodules can be painful when palpated and should be noted in the evaluation, because they may affect orthotic design or strap placement (see Fig. 33-15). Pain and/ or numbness from nerve compressions caused by **synovitis** also may be evident. Compression of the median nerve, or carpal tunnel syndrome, is one of the most commonly seen conditions at the wrist. The ulnar nerve can be compressed at Guyon's canal (a canal adjacent to the hook of the hamate) at the wrist and at the **cubital tunnel** (the groove between the medial epicondyle and the olecranon of the ulna) at the elbow.

Diagnosis-Specific Information that Affects Clinical Reasoning

Joint Deformities

Palpate joint deformities to help determine whether they are fixed or passively correctable, dislocated, or partially dislocated. Note this information in your evaluation. Common wrist and hand deformities are discussed as follows with orthotic and other treatment options in the non-operative section.

Swan Neck Deformity

The **swan neck deformity** is characterized by flexion of the DIP joint and hyperextension of the PIP joint (see Fig. 29-10). Synovitis of the flexor tendons can erode the PIP joint volar plate,

which normally helps prevent PIP joint hyperextension. The flexor tendon synovitis also limits PIP joint flexion and causes the client primarily to use the MP joints for digit flexion.[63] This results in an **intrinsic plus position** (MP flexion with IP joints extended) during grasping activities, causing an altered pull of the intrinsic muscles. This altered pull tends to facilitate dorsal subluxation of the lateral extensor tendons and PIP joint hyperextension. The DIP joint then flexes reciprocally by action of the flexor digitorum profundus tendon. The action of the extensor mechanism thus is concentrated at the PIP joint, resulting in PIP hyperextension, if the PIP **volar plate** (a thick fibrocartilaginous structure on the volar aspect of the PIP joint) is lax or disrupted. Studies that looked at orthoses for swan neck deformities at the PIP joint reported greater acceptance and tolerance with prefabricated orthoses[75] than custom-made orthoses and also reported that Silver Ring Splints(orthoses) improved dexterity in selected patients with RA. [76]

Boutonnière Deformity

The **boutonnière deformity** is characterized by PIP joint flexion and DIP joint hyperextension. Synovitis causes the central tendon to become weakened, lengthened, or disrupted from the bony and capsular attachments allowing the PIP joint to rest in flexion. The lateral bands then rest volar to the axis of the PIP joint, resulting in PIP joint flexion and DIP joint hyperextension (see Fig. 29-6). Orthotic techniques for the boutonnière deformity are outlined in Chapter 29.

Metacarpophalangeal Joint Ulnar Deviation and Palmar Subluxation

The MP joints, unlike the PIP hinge joints, have more planes of movement in that they also can abduct, adduct, pronate, and supinate. With this degree of mobility, the hand collapses into deformities if the restraining system of tendons, ligaments, or bony structures is disrupted by synovitis. Additional factors that can contribute to the development of the ulnar deviation deformity include an anatomic susceptibility and ulnar and volar forces applied during ADLs.[63] The flexor tendons exert strong ulnar and volar forces at the MP joint. Lateral pinch activities, gripping an object, writing, and even gravity, tend to place ulnar and volar deviating forces at the MP joints (Table 33-2). The deformity also may include radial deviation of the wrist[77] (Fig. 33-16). With ligament instability, the carpal bones can shift into a variety of deformities. Ulnar displacement of the proximal carpal row results in radial deviation of the hand.[51] An orthosis can be used in the treatment of this condition. Steultjens, et al.[78] reported in their systematic review that orthoses can decrease pain and improve grip strength but may decrease hand AROM. Another study compared groups of RA patients wearing soft and hard night resting orthoses and found that both groups had decreased pain.[79] RA deformities can make proper fitting of an orthoses challenging. When fitting the RA hand with MP ulnar deviation and palmar subluxation, consider the position of the metacarpals, which are often in radial deviation. Aligning the MP joints in an anti-ulnar deviation position may contribute to the digit CMC radial deviation deformity. The orthosis should be designed to address all of the issues involved in the zigzag deformity.[80]

◎ **Clinical Pearl**

Ulnar deviation and palmer subluxation of the MP joints is the most common deformity seen in RA.

TABLE 33-2   Joint Protection Principles for the Metacarpophalangeal Joints with Rheumatoid Arthritis

Activities That Aggravate Metacarpophalangeal Ulnar Deviation	Joint Protection Techniques
Closing a jar with the right hand	Use the heel of the hand to close the jar or use a jar opener with two hands.
Smoothing a sheet with shoulder adduction	Use shoulder abduction to smooth the sheet.
Stirring with a spoon using forearm pronation and lateral pinch on spoon	Stir with the forearm in neutral with the spoon head held on the ulnar side of the hand using a cylindrical grasp.
Resting the hand on the chin, with ulnar forces to the digits	Avoid resting the hand on the chin or place the chin in the palm.
Lifting a cup of coffee	Use two hands and a lightweight cup.
Cutting foods	Use a knife with a 90° handle, a pizza cutter, or electric knife.
Lateral pinch to turn the key in the car door or ignition	Use a built-up key turner.
Carrying a purse strap with a lateral pinch	Use a fanny pack, back pack, or shoulder bag.

From Haviland N, Kamil-Miller L, Sliwa J: *A workbook for consumers with rheumatoid arthritis,* Rockville, MD, 1978, American Occupational Therapy Association; Cordery JC: Joint protection: a responsibility of the occupational therapist, *Am J Occup Ther* 19(5):285-294, 1965; Cordery, J, Rocchi M: Joint protection and fatigue management. In Melvin J, Jensen G, editors: *Rheumatologic rehabilitation: assessment and management,* vol 1, Bethesda, MD, 1998, American Occupational Therapy Association, pp. 279-322; Cooney WP, Chao EYS: Biomechanical analysis of static forces in the thumb during hand function, *J Bone Joint Surg* 59(1):27-36, 1977; Valdes K, Marik T: A systemic review of conservative interventions for osteoarthritis of the hand, *J Hand Ther* 23:334-349, 2010; Zhang W, Doherty M, Leeb BF, et al: EULAR evidence based recommendations for the management of hand osteoarthritis: report of a Task Force of the EULAR Standing Committee for International Clinical Studies Including Therapeutics (ESCISIT), *Ann Rheum Dis* 66(3):377–388, 2007; Melvin JL, Ferrel KM, editors: *Adult rheumatic diseases,* vol 2, Bethesda, MD, 2000, The American Occupational Therapy Association.

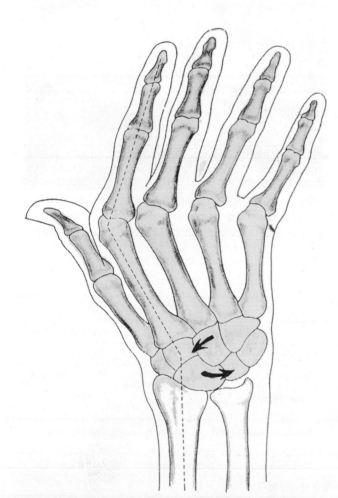

FIGURE 33-16 The zigzag deformity with wrist radial deviation and metacarpophalangeal (MP) joint ulnar deviation. (Redrawn with permission from Melvin JL: *Rheumatoid disease: occupational therapy and rehabilitation,* ed 3, Philadelphia, 1989, FA Davis, p. 281.)

Volar Subluxation of the Carpus on the Radius

Ligament laxity caused by chronic synovitis at the wrist and the natural volar tilt of the distal articular surface of the radius can result in volar subluxation of the carpus on the radius (Fig. 33-17). An orthosis for this condition usually includes a volar component to support the wrist.[81] The research on wrist orthoses is inconclusive at this time although one systematic review found that patients who wore wrist and resting hand orthoses preferred to use them.[82]

Distal Ulna Dorsal Subluxation

Instability of the distal ulna is common in RA. The distal ulna is normally less prominent in supination and more prominent in pronation. The RA disease process often weakens the ligamentous structures causing dorsal prominence of the distal ulna, pain, and crepitation with pronation and supination.[63] This instability and dorsal prominence of the ulna also may lead to extensor tendon disruption at the wrist level. Orthoses to provide stability to the distal ulna can be helpful in decreasing pain with pronation and supination (Fig. 33-18).[52]

Thumb Deformities

Terrono, et al.[48] have identified common patterns of thumb deformity in the rheumatoid thumb (Table 33-3). Type I is common with MP joint flexion and distal joint hyperextension (Fig. 33-19). **Type III** is also common with CMC subluxation, metacarpal adduction, MP joint hyperextension, and distal joint flexion (see Fig. 33-4). With the type III deformity the orthotic recommendations are comparable to the previously described osteoarthritic thumb deformity. The reader is referred to Terrono, et al.[48] for further information on RA thumb deformities.

Crepitus

Grating or crepitation during AROM may be palpated or heard. It sounds like a crunching or popping sound. Volar inspection

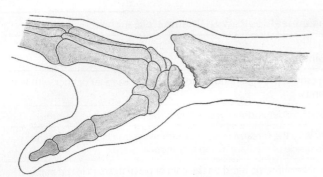

FIGURE 33-17 The natural volar tilt for chronic synovitis can result in volar subluxation of the carpus on the radius. (Redrawn with permission from Melvin JL: *Rheumatoid disease: occupational therapy and rehabilitation*, ed 3, Philadelphia, 1989, FA Davis, p. 280.)

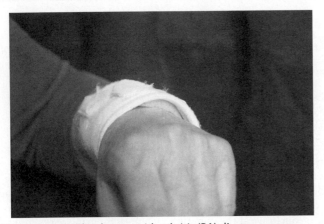

FIGURE 33-18 The rheumatoid arthritis (RA) disease process often weakens the ligamentous structures causing dorsal prominence of the distal ulna, pain, and crepitation with pronation and supination.[63] This instability and dorsal prominence of the ulna also may lead to extensor tendon disruption at the wrist level. This orthosis (Count'R-Force Radial Ulnar Wrist Support, North Coast Medical) is padded at the dorsal distal ulna and volar distal radius to support and stabilize the ulna. Orthoses that provide stability to the distal ulna can be helpful in decreasing pain with pronation and supination.[52]

of the hand should include palpation of the **first annular (A1) pulleys** (at the volar aspect of the MP joints) as the client flexes and extends the digits. A thickening of the flexor tendons, triggering, or periodic locking of the digit in flexion indicates flexor tenosynovitis (inflammation of the synovial lining of the tendon sheaths).

Skin Condition

An evaluation of the skin condition should include color, temperature, and areas of swelling. In the initial stage, the skin often is red and warm. In the later stages the skin may be very thin and bruise easily, which may be due to the long-term use of steroids and/or anti-inflammatory medications. Fragile skin characteristics can affect postoperative healing and reduce tolerance to an orthosis.

Precaution. *Skin tears may occur with only minimal shearing, such as rubbing from dressings or from the edge of a table.*

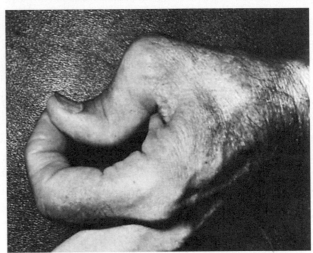

FIGURE 33-19 The type I deformity with metacarpophalangeal (MP) joint flexion and distal joint hyperextension. (From Terrono AL, Nalebuff EA, Phillips CA: The rheumatoid thumb. In Skirven TM, Osterman AL, Fedorczyk JM, et al, editors: *Rehabilitation of the hand and upper extremity*, ed 6, St Louis, 2011, Elsevier p. 1345.)

Type	Also Called	Carpometacarpal	Metacarpophalangeal	Interphalangeal
I	Boutonnière deformity	Not involved	Flexion	Hyperextension
II	(Uncommon)	Flexion and adduction	Flexion	Hyperextension
III	Swan neck deformity	Flexion, adduction, and subluxation	Hyperextension	Flexion
IV		Adduction and flexion as it progresses	Radially deviated and UCL unstable	Not involved
V		May or may not be involved	Unstable volar plate, hyperextension	Not involved
VI	Arthritis mutilans	Collapse resulting from bone loss at any level		

TABLE 33-3 Rheumatoid Arthritis Thumb Deformities

UCL, Ulnar collateral ligament.
Based on categories by: Terrono AL, Nalebuff EA, Phillips CA: The rheumatoid thumb. In Skirven TM, Osterman AL, Fedorczyk JM, et al, editors: *Rehabilitation of the hand and upper extremity*, ed 6, St Louis, 2011, Elsevier, p.1345.

Non-Operative Treatment

Joint Protection

The purpose of initiating joint protection principles early in the OA and RA disease process is to decrease joint stress and damage through altered work methods and to educate patients on proper joint alignment, and the use of adaptive equipment.[29,30] Common general joint protection principles for both OA and RA are categorized by themes in Table 33-2. For more complete information on specific principles and techniques as applied to specific deformities, the reader is referred to works by Cordery, Rocchi, and Melvin.[29,30,39] A systematic review found joint protection education beneficial for patients with RA.[83] A randomized controlled trial of patients with early RA demonstrated that 8 hours of instruction in joint protection decreased pain, morning stiffness, and doctor visits, as well as improved grip strength and self-efficacy, and maintained function.[84] Educational-behavioral joint protection programs that involve skill practice, goal-setting and HEPs were more effective than short instruction and/or information booklets. This was demonstrated by fewer deformities, less morning stiffness, improved ADL scores, and joint protection adherence.[85] Additionally, a small study sample (n = 28) demonstrated that instruction in energy conservation with cognitive-behavioral strategies decreased pain and fatigue and increased physical activity.[86]

Joint protection principles for RA should address the specific deformity or potential deformity. For example, joint protection for a patient with a tendency to develop a swan neck deformity should avoid activities that place the PIP joints in full extension, such as holding a book. In contrast, if the patient has a tendency toward a boutonnière deformity, PIP flexion activities (such as, using a hook grasp to carry a bag) should be discouraged. Patients with MP joint ulnar deviation tendencies should be aware of activities that place ulnar deviating forces on the MP joints and use alternative grasping techniques (see Table 33-2). With the thumb, joint protection principles focus on decreasing the amount of force used for pinching activities. The joint protection principles outlined previously for the osteoarthritic client also apply to the RA client. In addition, a systematic review found moderate evidence that combining joint protection with adaptive device provision resulted in increased hand function and pain reduction.[32]

Modalities

A variety of modalities have been used for the RA patient with unclear results.[87-89] A systematic review found improved ROM, improved grip and pinch strength, and reduced pain and stiffness with paraffin wax baths.[87] One review found that ultrasound was effective in increasing grip strength, decreasing morning stiffness, and reducing the number of swollen and painful joints.[89] Transcutaneous electrical nerve stimulation (TENS) has been found to help decrease pain in RA.[88] Another review found evidence that low-level laser therapy decreased pain and morning stiffness.[90] Decreasing pain and maintaining or improving ROM are primary goals in the application of these agents. The stage of the arthritic process is also a determining factor.

Precaution. *During the acute inflammatory phase when joint temperatures are elevated, heat is contraindicated, because it can promote inflammation.*

Cryotherapy, which lowers joint temperatures, reduces pain, and decreases inflammation, is more appropriate during the acute phase but many clients cannot tolerate cooling treatments.

During the subacute and chronic phases, heat may be more applicable to decrease pain, encourage relaxation, improve ROM, and increase functional use of the hand.

Exercise

General principles of exercise include avoiding painful AROM and PROM and working within the client's comfortable ROM. General exercises for the hand include AROM of the wrist, gentle digit flexion and extension, and thumb opposition. Keep ROM exercises pain-free to prevent overstretching of joint structures that may be vulnerable or distended by the inflammatory process. Shoulder and elbow AROM in the supine position is also beneficial for preventing stiffness. Clients often obtain increased shoulder motion in the supine position, because the effects of gravity are reduced in this position. Generalized conditioning for the patient with RA has been found to improve stamina and muscle strength and is recommended as routine practice in patients with RA.[91] One study found low impact general conditioning utilizing walking or aquatics increased endurance and aerobic capacity in patients with RA.[92] Clinically the psychosocial benefits of group exercise in a warm pool, tai chi, and other pain-free exercise programs have been reported by patients to this author as very beneficial.[80]

Strengthening

Precaution. *Strengthening programs for the rheumatic hand should be used with caution to avoid aggravation of deformities.*

Stability must not be sacrificed for a possible increase in strength. Grip strengthening is a common example of an exercise that can place the digits in increased ulnar deviation during flexion if the position of the digits is left unchecked. A systematic review reported that there was not strong research evidence for or against hand exercises in the treatment of persons with RA.[93]

Precaution. *Therapy exercises should never create deforming forces or cause pain.*

Remedies

Most therapists treating the client with RA are approached for advice on a variety of home remedies. These can include copper bracelets, magnets, nutritional supplements, diets, homeopathy, topical preparations, and many others. It is important that the therapist use care in addressing these questions. The therapist should scrutinize research on nontraditional treatments carefully. As therapists, we cannot act as advocates, working outside our scope of practice, nor can we refuse to review nontraditional methods of treatment. When evaluating the effectiveness of any treatment, we should remember that RA is a disease of remissions and exacerbations. Many clients report improvement with a variety of home treatments. Asking oneself whether the client might have improved even without the treatment is always reasonable. Of course, the therapist should advise the client against any nontraditional therapy that has the potential for harm.

Wrist and Metacarpophalangeal Joint Deformities

With ligament instability, the carpal bones can shift into a variety of deformities. Ulnar displacement of the proximal carpal row results in radial deviation of the hand.[94,95] The MP joints may be affected secondarily and demonstrate ulnar deviation (Fig. 33-20).

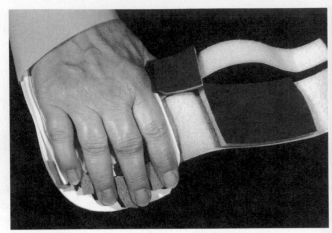

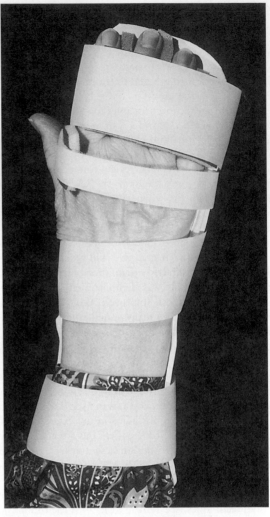

FIGURE 33-20 When splinting the zigzag deformity, the therapist needs to avoid forcing digits into alignment with an orthosis that leaves the wrist positions unchecked. The long lever arm involved in placing the digits into alignment can cause the wrist to go into additional radial deviation. This night orthosis helps to guide the wrist into gentle ulnar alignment and the metacarpophalangeal (MP) joints into radial alignment. This orthosis also is used at night following MP implant resection arthroplasty. (From Boozer JA: Splinting the arthritic hand, *J Hand Ther* 6:46, 1993.)

? Questions to Discuss with the Physician

- Is the orthosis primarily for nightwear?
- Are there any tendon ruptures?
- Is surgery an option for this client in the future?

( ) What to Say to Clients

About the Condition

"Your hand is demonstrating a deformity in which the fingers go in one direction and the wrist goes in another. This can look like a zigzag deformity."

"When you have rheumatoid arthritis, the lining of the joint becomes active and moves outside of the joints. This can damage the structures around the joint and including the cartilage, ligaments, joint capsule, tendons, and boney structures."

About the Orthosis

"The orthosis is designed to be worn at night to keep your fingers and wrist in good alignment. It should be comfortable and can help decrease your pain."

"Some clients like to wear soft orthoses during the day for heavier activities. This keeps your fingers in position but lets you do some activities."

About Exercise and Joint Protection

"Learning ways that you can protect your joints and avoid positions of deformity can be helpful."

"Sometimes adaptive equipment can be helpful to decrease the stress on the joints as you do some activities. I can help you determine the best options for you."

"Any exercise that you do should be pain-free and should avoid positions of deformity."

"It is important to be gentle with the exercises and not force the hand into uncomfortable positions."

Evaluation Tips

Even with severe deformities, clients are able to somehow do a great deal with their hands during their ADLs. Be sure to find

Continued

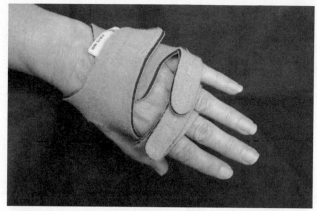

FIGURE 33-21 A soft neoprene anti-ulnar deviation orthosis is often helpful for day wear when a client with RA demonstrates MP ulnar deviation. (Rolyan Hand-Based In-Line Splint from Sammons Preston.)

♡ *Tips from the Field*

Orthoses

If the digits alone are aligned radially in the orthosis without supportive correction of the wrist position, the wrist can be pulled into further radial deviation. This is undesirable because the goal is to gently to position all involved joints. In the orthosis, a strap at the head of the metacarpals provides a necessary stop to counterbalance the long lever arm alignment pull of the digital straps or spacers (see Fig. 33-20). The resting pan orthosis also places the MP joints in gentle extension to decrease palmar subluxation of the proximal phalanx. The hand should never be forced into a position, because you cannot correct a severe deformity. Small foam spacers provide a soft but forgiving alignment to the MP joints and yield to changes in digit size caused by edema or inflammation. The spacers are cut from a sheet of self-adhesive Temper Foam. A second method for applying ulnar pull to the wrist metacarpals is to secure a Beta Pile II or some other double-sided Velcro loop strap to the inside of the orthosis at the head of the metacarpals. The gentle pull of this strap helps keep the wrist from its tendency to follow the digits into radial positioning when aligned in the orthosis. Some clients also wear soft neoprene digit alignment orthoses during the day to protect their hands during more active ADLs. The gentle pull of the radial alignment strips can help to keep the digits in proper position, counteracting the ulnar deviation forces (Fig. 33-21).

Client Compliance

A client will wear an orthosis that fits well and is comfortable for an extended time. Some clients return for new orthoses every year because of wear and tear. If the client returns with a clean orthosis, it is most likely not being worn. Most clients need orthoses for both hands, which can make nighttime trips to the bathroom difficult. Alternating an orthosis on the right hand and the left hand every other night can be helpful in managing this situation.

▷ *Precautions and Concerns*

The digits and wrist should never be forced into an aligned position.

According to Brand, et al.,[18] it is important to avoid the use of the long lever arm of the digit to extend the MP joint. If the proximal phalanx tilts rather than glides into position, it can wear away at the dorsal lip of the phalanx. This results in an orthosis that actually increases pain and absorption of the joint surface.

Clients who are fitted with night orthoses should be made aware of proper application techniques to avoid this joint tilting, and the orthosis should be formed properly, allowing the joint to glide into position.

Swan Neck Deformity

Swan neck deformity is characterized by flexion of the distal DIP joint and hyperextension of the PIP joint.

❓ *Questions to Discuss with the Physician*

- Is surgery an option for this client in the future?
- What is the condition of the joints as observed on the radiographs?

( ) *What to Say to Clients*

About the Condition

"Rheumatoid arthritis can loosen the stability of your joints, ligaments, and tendons resulting in the fingers going into a swan neck deformity."

"As you use your hand, the middle (proximal interphalangeal) joints of your fingers tend to buckle backward and your end (distal interphalangeal) joints bend. This makes it difficult to grasp objects."

About Orthoses

"Orthoses can help keep the middle (proximal interphalangeal) joints flexed. This has a secondary effect on the end (distal interphalangeal) joints, helping them to straighten. This is the position opposite your deformity."

"There are several styles of orthoses that can work for you. These orthoses allow your fingers to bend but prevent your middle joints (proximal interphalangeal) from buckling backward."

"Some of the orthoses are made out of plastic, and some are made out of metal to look like special rings on your fingers."

About Exercise

"It is important that you maintain the bending ability (proximal interphalangeal flexion) of the middle joints. This is done by taking your other hand and gently bending it toward the palm."

"Activities like holding a book or an electronic tablet can keep your middle joints straight while bending your knuckles (metacarpophalangeal). This can aggravate this deformity. You should avoid activities that keep your middle joints straight for a long time."

Evaluation Tips

Take care to measure the AROM and PROM of the PIP joints and DIP joints. If the joints are passively correctable, the client is usually a good candidate for the swan neck orthosis.

♡ *Tips from the Field*

Orthoses

In clients demonstrating a swan neck deformity, orthotic techniques that prevent PIP joint hyperextension, yet allow flexion, are often effective. These orthoses are needed long term and

therefore should be durable. Many of the low-temperature plastic splints can wear out and need to be replaced frequently. There is research evidence of greater client acceptance and tolerance for prefabricated swan neck orthoses.[75] A high-temperature plastic option, the Oval-8 splint, is available in a variety of sizes and can be obtained from 3-Point Products, Inc. (Stevensville, Maryland). This is a prefabricated splint (Fig. 33-22, *A*) is available in many sizes and is fitted in the clinic. Minor one-time changes can be made to this high-temperature plastic using a heat gun at the lateral central joint of the orthoses (see Fig. 33-22, *B*). For clients who are between sizes, the ring orthosis can be worn with the smaller ring placed proximally. Many clients may use this fit option with digit swelling fluctuations from day to day. A metal custom-sized splint, the SIRIS splint (Fig. 33-23, *A*), is available from the Silver Ring Splint Co. (Charlottesville, Virginia). The therapist measures these splints with a special tool, the EZ-Sizer (see Fig. 33-23, *B*), which is available from the company. These orthoses are

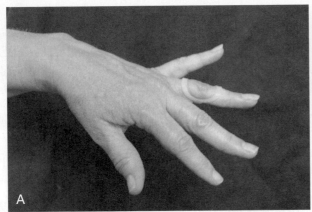
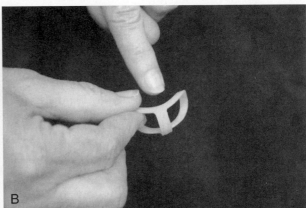

FIGURE 33-22 A, A high-temperature plastic option, the Oval-8 splint, is available in a variety of sizes and can be obtained from 3-Point Products, Inc. (Stevensville, MA). This prefabricated orthosis is available in many sizes and is fitted in the clinic. **B,** Minor one-time changes can be made to this high-temperature plastic using a heat gun at the lateral central joint of the orthosis. For clients who are between sizes, the ring orthosis can be worn with the smaller ring placed proximally.

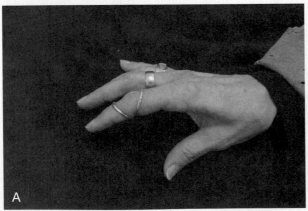
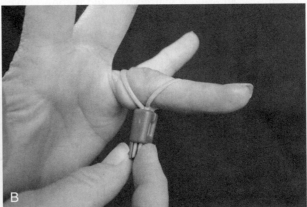

FIGURE 33-23 A, Metal custom-sized splint, the SIRIS splint, is available from the Silver Ring Splint Co. (Charlottesville, VA). These orthoses are well tolerated by clients because they allow most activities of daily living (ADLs) and do not need to be removed for hand washing. In one study, dexterity was improved with selected clients with rheumatoid arthritis (RA) using the orthosis.[76] The Silver Ring orthoses have solder that is designed to tolerate multiple adjustments to account for digit swelling. If the rings are opened, it is tighter on the finger. Conversely, if the two rings are brought closer together, the orthoses is looser on the finger. **B,** The therapist measures for the SIRIS splint with a special tool, the EZ-Sizer that is available from the company.

well tolerated by clients, because they allow most ADLs and do not need to be removed for hand washing. In one study, dexterity was improved with selected RA clients using the orthosis.[76] The Silver Ring orthoses have solder that is designed to tolerate multiple adjustments to account for digit swelling. If the rings are opened, the orthosis is tighter on the finger. Conversely, if the two rings are brought closer together, the orthosis is looser on the finger.

Client Compliance

Client compliance with both of the aforementioned swan neck orthoses is typically excellent if the orthosis fits well, because it allows most ADLs.

▷ *Precautions and Concerns*

Take care to ensure that the orthoses are not too tight or too loose. If they are too loose, the client often loses them; if they are too tight, they can cause pressure areas.

In the case of the Silver Ring splints, the client should have a good understanding of how to adjust the orthosis to account for changes in finger size from day to day.

Some clients with sensitive skin may react to the metal; if need be, a special coating is available from the manufacturer.

Operative Treatment

See the Evolve website for detailed information on postoperative care of MP implant resection arthroplasty.

CASE STUDIES

CASE STUDY 33-1 ▪ Non-Operative Treatment of Rheumatoid Arthritis

B.L. is a 53-year-old nurse with RA. She works 40 hours a week on the cardiac care unit of a local hospital and reports that her pain is largely under control with medication. She has two children in college and likes to play the organ at church. She reports that with some activities, such as playing the organ, her right PIP joints hyperextend at her right index and ring digits. This requires her to push even harder on the organ keys, which is sometimes painful. She would like some support that would give her index and ring finger (PIP) joints stability yet allow her to do her activities.

B.L. was fit with size 5 and 6 Oval 8 splints (from 3-Point Products, Inc.) because there is evidence of greater acceptance and tolerance with prefabricated orthoses[75] than custom-made orthoses for this condition. She was shown the proper way to apply the orthoses to prevent PIP joint hyperextension yet to allow full PIP joint flexion. She was instructed that the orthoses would be tighter when applied in the opposite direction and that this might be useful if her swelling were to decrease. She was instructed in joint protection principles including avoiding the intrinsic plus position as she held a book or electronic tablet. She was shown PROM to the PIP joints to help maintain PIP flexion.

B.L. returned to the clinic 1 week later with her husband. She reported increased stability as she played the organ. She felt the orthoses increased the stability of her PIP joints at work and during various other ADLs. Her husband had heard about the Silver Ring

splints and wanted to purchase a Silver Ring SIRIS orthosis for her ring finger with her birthstone for their anniversary. The therapist was aware of a study that found Silver Ring splints improved dexterity in selected patients with RA.[76]

She was measured for the Silver Ring splint using the EZ-Sizer. The correct size was determined and the form was completed. Her husband had purchased the birthstone previously, and this was included for placement on the ring with the order. The couple mailed in the form and the stone. The form stated the ring was to be delivered to the hand clinic for fitting by the therapist.

The Silver Ring SIRIS orthosis arrived 8 days later and was fit to the client. She was instructed in how to make adjustments to the orthosis fit by bending the rings together (for a looser fit) or apart (for a tighter fit). This would help the ring fit appropriately when there were edema fluctuations. B.L. continued to wear her Oval 8 orthosis on her index finger.

B.L. stopped by the clinic 2 weeks later. She had lost her Oval 8 splint. She reported decreased pain and increased stability with her orthosis and was wearing them day and night. They allowed full PIP joint flexion but prevented PIP hyperextension. She also felt she needed less pain medicine with the orthoses in place during activities. Her lost Oval 8 splint was replaced, and she was encouraged to contact the therapist if further assistance was needed.

CASE STUDY 33-2 ▪ Operative Treatment of Rheumatoid Arthritis

See the MP IRA case on the Evolve website.

CASE STUDY 33-3 ▪ Operative Treatment of Osteoarthritis

N. B. is a 70-year-old female with CMC OA. She has been seeing the hand therapist for several years and has managed her pain with a hand-based thumb spica orthosis at night and a soft neoprene orthosis during the day as needed. The orthoses have worked well in the past, but the pain has been increasing. She arrived in the hand clinic today in a cast and is 10 days post CMC interposition arthroplasty. Her stiches had been removed that day by the physician's office staff, and a cast had been applied. The client was referred to therapy for AROM of uninvolved joints and postoperative care.

N. B. is demonstrating significant pain at her wrist near the incision site. She also has limited shoulder (80° flexion and abduction) and elbow (30°/100°) AROM. The client described her pain as burning and radiating down to her thumb tip. She was immediately taken back to the physician's office (located next door) where the cast was cut, spread, and rewrapped. This relieved pressure on the superficial branch of the radial nerve, and the client was comfortable in her cast. Returning back to therapy the client was instructed in AROM for the shoulder, elbow, and thumb IP joint (which was not supported in the cast). She was also instructed in elevation techniques and given suggestions for completing ADLs with one hand. She lives at home with her husband who attended the therapy session. Her husband reported that he could begin some simple cooking for N. B., but he would need her verbal guidance.

N. B. returned the following week for hand therapy reporting no pain. She now had full AROM of the shoulder, elbow, and thumb IP joint. Some edema was still evident and elevation techniques were reviewed, as well as gentle edema massage to the digits. An appointment was made for 4-weeks post-surgery for application of her thumb spica forearm-based orthosis. This was the same day as her physician's appointment for cast removal. She was instructed to contact the therapist if there were any concerns prior to that time.

N. B. returned after her physician's appointment at the 4-week point and was fit with a forearm-based thumb spica orthosis. Her skin was cleaned due to post cast dryness, and lotion was applied. She was independent in donning and doffing the orthosis. Gentle AROM was initiated to the thumb including gentle opposition and flexion. N. B. had a tendency to move her MP and IP joints during the exercises and not her CMC joint. She was shown how to keep these joints slightly flexed during the CMC exercise to facilitate gentle movement and muscle reeducation. Gentle massage was completed to the thumb web space to decrease thumb metacarpal adduction. Her husband was shown how to assist with this as well. Scar massage with the lotion of N. B.'s choice was initiated to the incision twice daily in her HEP after demonstration by the therapist.

N. B. returned to the hand clinic at 5 weeks post-surgery. She had 45° of CMC palmar abduction and could oppose all of the digit tips with her thumb. She was cautioned to wait one more week before removing her orthosis for ADLs and to avoid heavy pinch activities for at least 3 months post-surgery.

At 6 weeks post-surgery the thumb spica orthosis was discontinued. A soft neoprene Comfort Cool orthosis was applied for wear during some activities that N. B. felt might be problematic until her strength returned, such as cooking and making beds. She demonstrated 30 lbs of grip strength at this visit. She was shown simple grip strengthening exercises with putty to be done two times a day, avoiding thumb pinch. Thumb pinch should be avoided for the first 3 months post-surgery.

Vendor Information

Available from North Coast Medical (www.ncmedical.com)
- Comfort Cool Thumb CMC Restriction Splints
- Count'R-Force Radial Ulnar Wrist Support
- Orfit
  Available from Patterson Medical (www.pattersonmedical.com)
- Rolyan Hand-Based In-Line Splint
- Coban
- Co-Wrap
- Velcro
- Polyform light
- Temper Foam
- Beta Pile II
  Available from HandLab (www.Handlab.com)
- The Push MetaGrip
  Available from 3-Point Products (www.3pointproducts.com)
- Oval-8 splint
  Available from Silver Ring Splints Co. (www.silverringsplint.com)
- SIRIS
- EZ-Sizer

References

1. Bureau of Census: US Department of Commerce, Centers for Disease Control and Prevention: Prevalence of disabilities and associated health conditions among adults—United States, *Morb Mortal Wkly Rep* 50(7):120–125, 1999. 2001.
2. Callahan LF, Yelin EH: The social and economic consequences of rheumatic disease. In Kippel JH, Crofford LJ, Stone JH, et al: *Primer on the rheumatic diseases*, ed 12, Atlanta, GA, 2001, Arthritis Foundation, pp 1–4.
3. Lawrence RC, Felson DT, Helmick CG, et al: Estimate of the prevalence of arthritis and other rheumatic conditions in the United States, *Arthritis Rheum* 58(1):26–35, 2008.
4. Brandt KD, Doherty M, Lohmander S, editors: *Osteoarthritis*, New York, NY, 1998, Oxford University Press.
5. Roach HI, Tilley S: The pathogenesis of osteoarthritis. In Bronner F, Farach-Carson MC, editors: *Bone and osteoarthritis: topics in bone biology*, London, 2008, Springer Verlag, pp 1–8.
6. Myasoedova E, Crowson CS, Kremers HM, et al: Is the incidence of rheumatoid arthritis rising? Results from Olmsted County, Minnesota, 1955-2007, *Arthritis Rheum* 62(6):1576–1582, 2010.
7. Klareskog L, Catrina AI, Paget S: Rheumatoid arthritis, *The Lancet* 373:659–672, 2009.
8. Oegema TR, Lewis JL, Mikecz K, et al: Osteoarthritis and rheumatoid arthritis. In Einhorn TA, O'Keefe RJ, Buckwalter JA, editors: *Orthopaedic basic science*, ed 3, Rosemont, IL, 2007, American Academy of Orthopaedic Surgeons, pp 395–413.
9. Cheng YJ, Hootman JM, Murphy LB, et al: Prevalence of doctor-diagnosed arthritis and arthritis-attributable activity limitation—United States, 2007-2009, *Morb Mortal Wkly Rep* 59(39):1261–1265, 2010.
10. Keuttner KE, Goldberg V, editors: *Osteoarthritic disorders*, Rosemont, IL, 1995, American Academy of Orthopedic Surgeons.
11. Brinker MR, O'Conner DP: Basic sciences. In Miller MD, Brinker MR, editors: *Review of orthopedics*, ed 3, Philadelphia, 2008, WB Saunders, pp 1–153.
12. Berenbaum F: Osteoarthritis: pathology and pathogenesis. In Klippel JH, editor: *Primer on the rheumatic diseases*, ed 13, New York, 2008, Springer, pp 229–234.
13. Dieppe P: Osteoarthritis: clinical features. In Klippel JH, editor: *Primer on the rheumatic diseases*, ed 13, New York, 2008, Springer, pp 224–228.
14. Mankin HJ, Grodzinsky AJ, Buckwalter JA: Articular cartilage and osteoarthritis. In Einhorn TA, O'Keefe RJ, Buckwalter JA, editors: *Orthopaedic basic science: foundations of clinical practice*, ed 3, Rosemont, IL, 2007, American Academy of Orthopedic Surgeons, pp 161–174.
15. Erggelet C, Mandelbaum BR: *Principles of cartilage repair*, Wurzburg, Germany, 2008, Springer.
16. Roach HI, Tilley S: The pathogenesis of osteoarthritis. In Bronner F, Farach-Carson MC, editors: *Bone and osteoarthritis: topics in bone biology*, vol. 4, London, 2008, Springer Verlag, pp 1–18.
17. Kalichman L: Hernández-Molina G: Hand osteoarthritis: an epidemiological perspective, *Semin Arthritis Rheum* 39(6):465–476, 2010.
18. Fumagalli M, Sarzi-Puttini P, Atzeni F: Hand osteoarthritis, *Semin Arthritis Rheum* 34(6 Suppl 2):47–52, 2005.
19. Wilder FV, Barrett JP, Farina EJ: Joint-specific prevalence of osteoarthritis of the hand, *Osteoarthr Cartil* 14:953–957, 2006.
20. Kaufmann MD, Logters TT, Verbruggen G, et al: Osteoarthritis of the distal interphalangeal joint, *J Hand Surg Am* 35:2117–2125, 2010.
21. Cooper C: Fundamentals of clinical reasoning: hand therapy concepts and treatment techniques. In Cooper C, editor: *Fundamentals of hand therapy*, St Louis, 2007, Mosby, pp 3–21.
22. US Department of Health and Human Services: *Acute Pain Management Guideline Panel: Acute pain management in adults: operative procedures* Quick reference guide for clinicians, AHCPR Pub No. Rockville, MD, 1995, US Government Printing Office. 92–0019.
23. Law M, Baptiste S, McColl M, et al: The Canadian occupational performance measure: an outcome measure for occupational therapy, *Can J Occup Ther* 57(2):82–87, 1990.
24. Meenan RF, Mason JH, Anderson JJ, et al: AIMS2. The content and properties of a revised and expanded Arthritis Impact Measurement Scales Health Status Questionnaire, *Arthritis Rheum* 35(1):1–10, 1992.
25. Eaton RG, Glickel SZ: Trapeziometacarpal osteoarthritis. Staging as a rationale for treatment, *Hand Clin* 3(4):455–471, 1987.
26. Van Heest AE, Kallemeier P: Thumb carpal metacarpal arthritis, *J Am Acad Orthop Surg* 16:140–151, 2008.
27. Swanson A: Disabling arthritis at the base of the thumb: treatment by resection of the trapezium and flexible (silicon) implant arthroplasty, *J Bone Joint Surg* 54(3):456–471, 1972.
28. Haviland N, Kamil-Miller L, Sliwa J: *A workbook for consumers with rheumatoid arthritis*, Rockville, MD, 1978, American Occupational Therapy Association.
29. Cordery JC: Joint protection: a responsibility of the occupational therapist, *Am J Occup Ther* 19(5):285–294, 1965.
30. Cordery J: Rocchi M: Joint protection and fatigue management. In Melvin J, Jensen G, editors: *Rheumatologic rehabilitation: assessment and management*, vol. 1, Bethesda, MD, 1998, American Occupational Therapy Association, pp 279–322.

31. Cooney WP, Chao EYS: Biomechanical analysis of static forces in the thumb during hand function, *J Bone Joint Surg* 59(1):27–36, 1977.

32. Valdes K, Marik T: A systemic review of conservative interventions for osteoarthritis of the hand, *J Hand Ther* 23:334–349, 2010.

33. Zhang W, Doherty M, Leeb BF, et al: EULAR evidence based recommendations for the management of hand osteoarthritis: report of a Task Force of the EULAR Standing Committee for International Clinical Studies Including Therapeutics (ESCISIT), *Ann Rheum Dis* 66(3):377–388, 2007.

34. Stamm TA, Machold KP, Smolen JS, et al: Joint protection and home hand exercises improve hand function in patients with hand osteoarthritis: a randomized controlled trial, *Arthritis Rheum* 47(1):44–49, 2002.

35. Kong YK, Lowe BD: Optimal cylindrical handle diameter for grip force tasks, *Int J Ind Ergon* 35:495–507, 2005.

36. Sancho-Bru J, Giurintano DJ, Perez-Gonzalez A, et al: Optimum tool handle diameter for a cylinder grip, *J Hand Ther* 16:337–342, 2003.

37. Seo NJ, Armstrong TJ, Young JG: Effects of handle orientation, gloves, handle friction and elbow posture on maximum horizontal pull and push forces, *Ergonomics* 53(1):92–101, 2010.

38. Hallbeck MS, Cochran DJ, Stonecipher BL, et al: Hand-handle orientation and maximum force, *Industrial Ergonomics* 5:800–804, 1990.

39. Melvin JL, Ferrel KM, editors: *Adult rheumatic diseases, vol. 2 of Rheumatologic Rehabilitation Series*, Bethesda, MD, 2000, The American Occupational Therapy Association.

40. Fedorczyk JM: The use of physical agents in hand rehabilitation. In Skirven TM, Osterman AL, Fedorczyk JM, et al: *Rehabilitation of the hand and upper extremity*, ed 6, Philadelphia, 2011, Elsevier, pp 1495–1511.

41. Bracciano AG: *Physical agent modalities*, ed 2, Thorofare, NJ, 2008, Slack.

42. Boustedt C, Nordenskiöld U, Lundgren Nilsson A: Effects of a hand-joint protection program with an addition of splinting and exercise: one year follow-up, *Clin Rheumatol* 28(7):793–799, 2009.

43. Stamm TA, Machold KP, Smolen JS, et al: Joint protection and home hand exercises improve hand function in patients with hand osteoarthritis: a randomized controlled trial, *Arthritis Rheum* 47(1):44–49, 2002.

44. Rogers MW, Wilder FV: Exercise and hand osteoarthritis symptomatology: a controlled crossover trial, *J Hand Ther* 22:10–18, 2009.

45. O'Brien VH, Russell Giveanu M: Effects of a dynamic stability approach in conservative intervention of the carpometacarpal joint of the thumb: A retrospective study, *J Hand Ther* 26:44–52, 2013.

46. Rogers MW, Wilder FV: The effects of strength training among persons with hand osteoarthritis: a two-year follow up study, *J Hand Ther* 20:244–250, 2007.

47. Minor MA, Hewitt JE, Webel RR, et al: Efficacy of physical conditioning exercise in patients with rheumatoid arthritis and osteoarthritis, *Arthritis Rheum* 32(11):1396–1405, 1989.

48. Terrono AL, Nalebuff EA, Philips CA: The rheumatoid thumb. In Skirven TM, Osterman AL, Fedorczyk JM, et al: *Rehabilitation of the hand and upper extremity*, ed 6, Philadelphia, 2011, Elsevier, pp 1344–1355.

49. Beasley J: Therapist's examination and conservative management of arthritis of the upper extremity. In Skirven TM, Osterman AL, Fedorczyk JM, et al: *Rehabilitation of the hand and upper extremity*, ed 6, Philadelphia, 2011, Elsevier, pp 1330–1343.

50. Colditz J: Anatomic considerations for splinting the thumb. ed 5, In Mackin EJ, Callahan AD, Skirven TM, et al: *Rehabilitation of the hand and upper extremity*, vol. 2, St Louis, 2002, Mosby, pp 1858–1874.

51. Melvin JL: *Rheumatic disease in the adult and child: occupational therapy and rehabilitation*, ed 3, Philadelphia, 1989, FA Davis.

52. Beasley J: Soft splints: indications and techniques. ed 6, In Skirven TM, Osterman AL, Fedorczyk JM, et al: *Rehabilitation of the hand and upper extremity*, vol. 2, Philadelphia, 2011, Elsevier, pp 1610–1619.

53. Ryan GM, Young BT: Ligament reconstruction arthroplasty for trapeziometacarpal arthrosis, *J Hand Surg* 22:1067–1076, 1997.

54. Hartigan BJ, Stern PJ, Kiefhaber TR: Thumb carpometacarpal osteoarthritis: arthrodesis compared with ligament reconstruction and tendon interposition, *J Bone Joint Surg Am* 83(10):1470–1478, 2001.

55. Ikeda M, Ishii T, Kobayashi Y, et al: Custom-made splint treatment for osteoarthritis of the distal interphalangeal joints, *J Hand Surg* 35(4):589–593, 2010.

56. Stern PJ, Fulton DB: Distal interphalangeal joint arthrodesis: an analysis of complications, *J Hand Surg* 17(6):1139–1145, 1992.

57. Scott DL, Kingsley GH: *Inflammatory arthritis in clinical practice*, London, 2008, Springer.

58. Oegema TR, Lewis JL, Mikecz K, et al: Osteoarthritis and rheumatoid arthritis. In Einhorn TA, O'Keefe RJ, Buckwalter JA, editors: *Orthopaedic basic science*, ed 3, Rosemont, IL, 2007, American Academy of Orthopaedic Surgeons, pp 395–413.

59. Lawrence RC, Felson DT, Helmick CG, et al: Estimates of the prevalence of arthritis and other rheumatic conditions in the United States. Part II, *Arthritis Rheum* 58:26–35, 2008.

60. Waldburger JM, Firestein GS: Rheumatoid arthritis: epidemiology, pathology, and pathogenesis. In Klippel JH, editor: *Primer on the rheumatic diseases*, ed 13, New York, 2008, Springer, pp 122–132.

61. Tehlirian CV, Bathon JM: Rheumatoid arthritis: clinical and laboratory manifestations. In Klippel JH, editor: *Primer on the rheumatic diseases*, ed 13, New York, 2008, Springer, pp 114–121.

62. Steinbrocker O, Traeger CH, Batterman RC: Therapeutic criteria in rheumatoid arthritis, *J Am Med Assoc* 140(8):659–662, 1949.

63. Swanson AB: Pathomechanics of deformities in hand and wrist. In Hunter JM, Schneider LH, Mackin EJ, et al: *Rehabilitation of the hand: surgery and therapy*, ed 3, Philadelphia, 1990, Mosby, pp 891–902.

64. Klareskog L, Catrina AI, Paget S: Rheumatoid arthritis, *The Lancet* 373:659–672, 2009.

65. Hafstrom I, Albertsson K, Boonen A, et al: Remission achieved after 2 years treatment with low-dose prednisone in addition to disease-modifying antirheumatic drugs in early rheumatoid arthritis is associated with reduced joint destruction still present after 4 years: an open 2-year continuation study, *Ann Rheum Disease* 68:508–513, 2009.

66. VanTuyl LHD, Felson DT, Wells G, et al: Evidence for predictive validity of remission on long-term outcome in rheumatoid arthritis: a systematic review, *Arthritis Care Res* 62(1):108–117, 2009.

67. Anderson RJ: Rheumatoid arthritis: clinical and laboratory features. In Kippel JH, Crofford LJ, Stone JH, et al: *Primer on the rheumatic diseases*, ed 12, Atlanta, GA, 2001, Arthritis Foundation, pp 218–225.

68. Devore GL, Muhleman CA, Sasarita SG: Management of pronation deformity in metacarpophalangeal implant arthroplasty, *J Hand Surg* 11(6):859–861, 1986.

69. Melvin JL: Therapist's management of osteoarthritis in the hand. ed 5, In Mackin EJ, Callahan AD, Skirven TM, et al: *Rehabilitation of the hand and upper extremity*, vol. 2, St Louis, 2002, Mosby, pp 1646–1665.

70. Devore GL: Preoperative assessment and postoperative therapy and splinting in rheumatoid arthritis. In Hunter JM, Schneider LH, Mackin EJ, et al: *Rehabilitation of the hand: surgery and therapy*, ed 3, Philadelphia, 1990, Mosby, pp 942–952.

71. Adams J, Burridge J, Mullee M, et al: Correlation between upper limb functional ability and structural hand impairment in an early rheumatoid population, *Clin Rehabil* 18(4):405, 2004.

72. Fess EE: The need for reliability and validity in hand assessment instruments, *J Hand Surg* 11(5):621–623, 1986.

73. Fess EE: *Clinical assessment recommendations*, Moran, CA, 1981, American Society of Hand Therapists.

74. Mathiowetz V, Vizenor L, Melander D: Comparison of baseline instruments to the Jamar dynamometer and the B&L engineering pinch gauge, *The OTJR* 20(3):147–161, 2000.

75. Schegget M, Knipping A: A study comparing use and effects of custommade versus prefabricated splints for swan neck deformity in patients with rheumatoid arthritis, *J Hand Surg Br* 5(4):101–107, 2000.

76. Spicka C, Macleod C, Adams J, et al: Effect of silver ring splint on hand dexterity and grip strength in patients with rheumatoid arthritis: an observational pilot study, *Hand Ther* 14(2):53–57, 2009.

77. Flatt A: *Care of the arthritic hand*, ed 4, St Louis, 1983, Mosby.

78. Steultjens EM, Dekker J, Bouter LM, et al: Occupational therapy for rheumatoid arthritis, *Cochrane Database Syst Rev*(1)CD003114, 2004.

79. Callinan NJ, Mathiowetz V: Soft versus hard resting hand splints in RA: pain relief preference and compliance, *Am J Occup Ther* 50:347–353, 1996.

80. Biese (Beasley) J; Arthritis. In Cooper C, editor: *Fundamentals of hand therapy: clinical reasoning and treatment guidelines for common diagnoses of the upper extremity*, St Louis, 2007, Elsevier, pp 348–375.

81. Colditz JC: Arthritis. In Malick MH, Kasch MC, editors: *Manual on management of specific hand problems*, Pittsburgh, 1984, AREN Publications, pp 112–136.

82. Egan M, Brosseau L, Farmer M, et al: Splints and orthosis for treating rheumatoid arthritis, *Cochrane Database Syst Rev*(4)CD004018, 2001.

83. Christie A, Jamtvedt G, ThuveDahm K, et al: Effect of nonpharmacological and nonsurgical interventions for patients with rheumatoid arthritis: an overview of systematic reviews, *Phys Ther* 87(12):1697–1715, 2007.

84. Freeman K, Hammond A, Lincoln NB: Use of cognitive behavioral arthritis education programs in newly diagnosed rheumatoid arthritis, *Clin Rehabil* 16:828–836, 2002.

85. Hammond A, Freeman K: The long term outcomes from a randomized controlled trial of an educational behavioral joint protection programme for people with rheumatoid arthritis, *Clin Rehabil* 18:520–528, 2004.

86. Furst GP, Gerber LH, Smith CC, et al: A program for improving energy conservation behaviors in adults with rheumatoid arthritis, *Am J Occup Ther* 41:102–111, 1987.

87. Welch V, Brosseau L, Casimiro L, et al: Thermotherapy for treating rheumatoid arthritis, *Cochrane Database Syst Rev*(2)CD002826, 2002.

88. Brosseau L, Yonge KA, Welch V, et al: Transcutaneous electrical nerve stimulation (TENS) for the treatment of rheumatoid arthritis in the hand, *Cochrane Database Syst Rev*(2)CD004377, 2003.

89. Casimiro L, Brosseau L, Welch V, et al: Therapeutic ultrasound for the treatment of rheumatoid arthritis, *Cochrane Database Syst Rev*(3)CD003787, 2002.

90. Brosseau L, Welch V, Wells GA, et al: Low level laser therapy (classes I, II and III) for treating rheumatoid arthritis, *Cochrane Database Syst Rev*(4)CD002049, 2005.

91. Hurkmans E, van der Giesen FJ, VlietVlieland TP, et al: Dynamic exercise programs (aerobic capacity and/or muscle strength training) in patients with rheumatoid arthritis, *Cochrane Database Syst Rev*(4)CD006853, 2009.

92. Minor MA, Hewitt JE, Webel RR, et al: Efficacy of physical conditioning exercise in patients with rheumatoid arthritis and osteoarthritis, *Arthritis Rheum* 32(11):1396–1405, 1989.

93. Wessel J: The effectiveness of hand exercises for persons with rheumatoid arthritis: a systematic review, *J Hand Ther* 17:174–180, 2004.

94. Shapiro JS, Heijna W, Nasatir S, et al: The relationship of wrist motion to ulnar phalangeal drift in the rheumatoid patient, *Hand* 3:68–75, 1971.

95. Shapiro JS: The wrist in rheumatoid arthritis, *Hand Clin* 12(3):477–498, 1996.

96. Brand P, Hollister AM, Agee JM: Transmission. ed 3, In Brand PW, Hollister AM, editors: *Clinical mechanics of the hand*, vol. 3, St Louis, 1999, Mosby, pp 61–99.

97. Biese J, Goudzwaard P: Postoperative management of metacarpophalangeal implant resection arthroplasty, *Orthopedic Physical Therapy Clinics of North America* 10(4):595–616, 2001.

98. Madden MD, Devore G, Arem MD: A rational postoperative management program for metacarpophalangeal joint implant arthroplasty, *J Hand Surg* 2(5), 1977. 385–366.

99. Kirkpatrick WH, Kozin SH, Uhl RL: Early motion after arthroplasty, *Hand Clin* 12(1):73–86, 1996.

100. Swanson AB, deGroot Swanson G, Leonard J: Postoperative rehabilitation programs in flexible implant arthroplasty of the digits. In Hunter JM, Schneider LH, Mackin EJ, et al: *Rehabilitation of the hand: surgery and therapy*, ed 4, St Louis, 1995, Mosby, pp 1351–1376.

101. Beckenbaugh RD: The development of an implant for the metacarpophalangeal joint of the fingers, *Acta Orthop Scand* 70(2):107–108, 1999.

102. Cannon N, et al: MP implant arthroplasties: postoperative management (for rheumatoid arthritis). In Cannon N, et al: *Diagnosis and treatment manual for physicians and therapists*, ed 3, Indianapolis, IN, 1991, Hand Rehabilitation Center of Indiana, pp 13–15.

103. Massy-Westropp N, Krishnan J: Postoperative therapy after metacarpophalangeal arthroplasty, *J Hand Ther* 16:311–314, 2003.

104. Massy-Westropp N, Massy-Westropp M, Rankin W, et al: Metacarpophalangeal arthroplasty from the patient's perspective, *J Hand Ther* 16:315–319, 2003.

105. Phillips CA: The management of patients with rheumatoid arthritis. In Hunter JM, Schneider LH, Mackin EJ, et al: *Rehabilitation of the hand: surgery and therapy*, ed 3, Philadelphia, 1990, Mosby, pp 903–907.

106. Boozer JA, Sanson MS, Soutas-Little RW, et al: Comparison of the biomechanical motions and forces involved in high profile versus low profile dynamic splinting, *J Hand Ther* 7(3):171–182, 1994.

107. Ascension MCP: *PyroCarbon Total Joint Arthroplasty, post-operative protocol*, Austin, TX, 2003, Ascension Orthopedics, Inc.

108. Beckenbaugh RD: The development of an implant for the metacarpophalangeal joint of the fingers, *Acta Orthop Scand* 70(2):107–108, 1993.

109. Boozer JA: Splinting the arthritic hand, *J Hand Ther* 6:46–48, 1993.

34

Burns

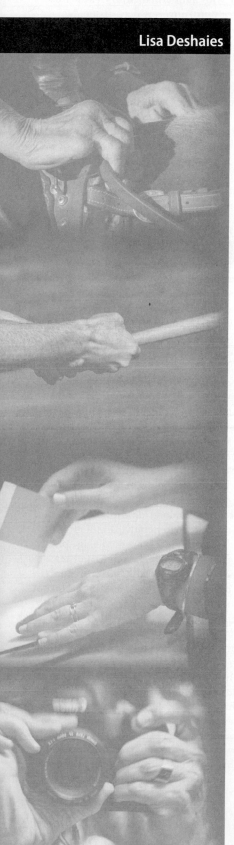

Lisa Deshaies

According to the American Burn Association, a burn of any depth to the hand is classified as a major injury that requires treatment at a specialized burn center. However, therapists may see clients with burns in a variety of clinical settings after acute management of the injuries. Burn injuries are caused by thermal, chemical, or electrical action. The causes are numerous and include house fires, motor vehicle accidents, and contact with an electrical current or hot objects or liquids at home or at work.[1,2]

> ◎ **Clinical Pearl**
>
> Dorsal hand burns are most often flame or explosion injuries; palmar burns occur more frequently from chemicals, friction, or hi-voltage contact.[3]

Along with their effect on hand function, burns can have a significant impact on a person's social and psychologic functioning.[4] Scarring, perceived disfigurement, and loss of control over the body and the environment may lead to significant body image changes, social avoidance, anxiety about the future, and hopelessness.[5] Reduced income and reluctance to discuss emotions may also be contributing factors.[6] Other psychologic symptoms that commonly develop after a burn injury are sleep disturbances, depression, anxiety disorders, and posttraumatic stress.[7]

Related cognitive, emotional, and physiologic problems (such as, lack of concentration, apathy, pain, and low energy) can influence the client's recovery, making it difficult for the client to comply fully with treatment. Significant others are also affected and have concerns of their own.[8]

To plan the appropriate intervention, therapists who treat burn injuries must thoroughly understand the related anatomy and the wound healing and scar maturation processes. Emotional support for the client as well as significant others is crucial to a positive outcome.

Anatomy

The skin is the largest organ of the human body. Its essential functions include providing protection against bacterial invasion, preventing excessive loss of body fluids, regulating body temperature through perspiration, shielding deep structures from injury, absorbing certain substances (for example, vitamin D), and receiving sensory feedback from the environment.[9-11] Without the protection skin affords, exposed underlying tissues (for example, muscle and tendon) become desiccated, and nerve endings are exposed. An important nonphysiologic function of the skin is to provide a cosmetic covering of the body that is unique to each individual.

Normal skin is composed of two basic layers, the epidermis and the dermis. The **epidermis** is the thin, avascular, outermost layer, which accounts for only about 5% of the skin's thickness. The **dermis,** which is much thicker, contains blood vessels, nerves, hair follicles, sweat and sebaceous glands, and the epithelial bed from which the skin regenerates. The thickness of the skin varies according to its location.

> ◎ **Clinical Pearl**
>
> On the hand, the dorsal skin is much thinner than the palmar skin.

> ◎ **Clinical Pearl**
>
> For the hand to function fully, the dorsal skin must be non-adherent and elastic, allowing hand closure, and the palmar skin must be thick enough to withstand forces arising from daily use.[3,12]

The structure and function of the skin also vary. Dorsal hand skin contains hair follicles and sebaceous glands, whereas palmar skin does not. Palmar skin contains a greater number of sensory end organs.

The delicate balance of the intrinsic and extrinsic musculotendinous systems also can be affected by a burn injury.[3]

Diagnosis and Pathology

The temperature and duration of exposure to heat and the characteristics of the skin burned determine the amount of tissue destruction. Burn injuries are classified by both depth and extent. The larger and deeper the burn, the worse the prognosis.[13,14] Other factors include premorbid diseases and associated trauma.[13] Burn depth is assessed by visual examination to determine the extent of damage to or the destruction of anatomic structures. Depth can be described by degree (that is, first, second, third, or fourth) or by thickness (superficial partial thickness, deep partial thickness, full thickness, and full thickness burn with subdermal injury); thickness is the more descriptive and contemporary method (Fig. 34-1). Because skin thickness varies, a burn to the hand may involve tissues at different depths.

A **superficial partial thickness burn** (which corresponds to first and second degree burns) involves the epidermis and possibly portions of the upper dermis. This type of burn is red or bright pink, blistered, soft, and wet. Sensation is intact, and the exposure of nerve endings results in pain and sensitivity to temperature, air, and light touch. Because the epithelial bed is intact, this type of burn can re-epithelialize spontaneously in 2 weeks or earlier, therefore skin grafting is not necessary.

A **deep partial thickness burn** (which corresponds to a deep second-degree burn) involves the epidermis and a deeper portion of the dermis. Hair follicles, sebaceous glands, and epithelial elements remain intact. This type of burn is mottled red or waxy white, soft, wet, and elastic. Sensation may or may not be present, depending on the extent to which nerve endings have been exposed or damaged. Re-epithelialization can occur in approximately 3 to 6 weeks, but skin grafting may be done to expedite wound closure.

Precaution. *A deep partial thickness burn may convert to a full thickness burn.*

A **full thickness burn** (which corresponds to a third-degree burn) involves the epidermis and the entire dermis, including hair

follicles, nerve endings, and the epithelial bed. Sebaceous glands may be involved if the burn extends to the subcutaneous fat layer. Sensation is absent because nerve endings have been destroyed. This type of burn is white or tan, waxy, dry or leathery, and rigid. Spontaneous re-epithelialization is impossible, and skin grafting is required.

A **full thickness burn with subdermal injury** (which corresponds to a fourth-degree burn) involves deep tissue damage to fat, muscle, or possibly bone. Electrical burns often cause this type of injury. These burns require extensive debridement of necrotic tissue, followed by skin grafting. Amputation may be necessary if the damage is too extensive and severe.[10,14]

The extent of a burn is determined by estimating the percentage of the body surface burned. The two methods used for this are the rule of nines and the Lund-Browder chart. The extent of injury is described as the percentage of the **total body surface area (TBSA)** burned. A rough estimation is that the palm of the client's hand represents approximately 1% of the client's body surface. Each side of the hand is considered 1.5% of the body surface; therefore a person with circumferential burns to both hands would have a 6% TBSA burn.[15]

Timelines and Healing

The objective with any wound, including a burn, is to obtain quick healing to minimize scar formation and associated sequelae. The length of time required for wound closure is the most important determinant of scar development. Age, genetics, and burn depth and location are other variables.[16]

Wound healing is a dynamic cellular process that consists of three overlapping phases. Phase 1, the inflammatory (or exudative) phase, is characterized by inflammation and the presence of neutrophils and macrophages, which are responsible for clearing debris and preparing the wound for repair. This phase begins when the wound occurs and lasts 3 to 5 days. Phase 2, the fibroblastic (or proliferative or reparative) phase, lasts 2 to 6 weeks. It is characterized by the presence of fibroblasts, which lay down collagen and myofibroblasts, which cause **wound contraction.** The newly formed epithelium is very thin and fragile, and the tensile strength of the wound increases with collagen proliferation. Collagen is deposited in a random, disorganized fashion. Wound contraction continues even after epithelialization but to a lesser degree. Phase 3, the maturation (or remodeling) phase, may last for years. Collagen continues to cross-link, and tensile strength increases progressively.[17,18] Typically, 50% of normal tensile strength has been regained by 6 weeks, and the ultimate tensile strength is only about 80% of that of normal skin.[17,19] As scars mature, collagen deposition slows, and the breakdown of excessive collagen proceeds until scar maturity is reached.

Hypertrophic scars may develop after burns, with a reported prevalence rate of 32% to 72%.[7] Risk factors include dark skin, burns to the upper limb, burn severity, time to heal (longer than 3 weeks), and multiple surgical procedures. Hypertrophic scars are raised, thick, red, tight, and itchy. They also contract, often with deforming force. Scars that cross joints are the most problematic, because **scar contraction** can lead to loss of functional joint mobility. Scar hypertrophy and contraction are most active for the first 4 to 6 months.[20] Clients with full range of motion (ROM) early on may lose motion in the ensuing months; therefore long-term follow-up therapy is needed. Scars that soften over

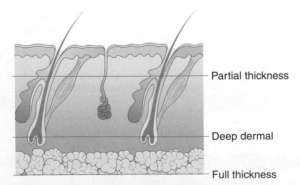

FIGURE 34-1 Classification of burns by thickness. (From Leveridge JE: Burns. In Prosser R, Conolly WB, editors: *Rehabilitation of the hand and upper limb,* Edinburgh, 2003, Butterworth Heinemann.)

the first 6 to 12 months have an improved prognosis for full joint function.[14] As long as scars are active, they may be responsive to intervention with conservative therapy. Once scars have matured, surgical intervention is required to improve ROM or cosmetic appearance.

Phases of Burn Recovery

Four overlapping phases of recovery have been described for burn injuries: (1) emergent, (2) acute, (3) skin grafting, and (4) rehabilitation.[20] The emergent phase comprises the first 2 to 3 days after injury. The acute phase is considered to be the interval from day 2 or 3 to wound closure, which can occur by spontaneous healing or surgical intervention. The skin grafting phase is the period during which grafting is performed to cover wounds in the acute phase or as a component of reconstructive surgery in the rehabilitation phase. The rehabilitation phase lasts from wound closure to scar maturity.

> **◎ Clinical Pearl**
>
> Edema and poor positioning are the primary deforming forces in the emergent and acute phases. After the wound has been closed in the skin grafting and rehabilitation phases, scar contraction becomes the major deforming force.

Non-Operative Treatment

The course of treatment is influenced by the depth and extent of the burn injury, the client's medical status, the stage of wound healing, and the physician's plan of care. Nonsurgical management is an option for partial thickness burns, because they are able to regenerate epithelium.[3,10,20] Treatment is aimed at preventing infection, promoting healing, and minimizing complications.

Dressings

Dressings are used to protect the wound and provide an optimum environment for healing. Dressings may be the adherent or non-adherent type, and they can serve a number of purposes, including infection control, comfort, wound immobilization, fluid absorption, debridement, and early pressure.[13,17] Numerous dressing products and wound care/dressing change schedules are available. The selection of dressings and topical agents depends on the type and status of the wound; it also is often influenced by the physician's preference. Therapists must work closely with the physician so that they fully understand the dressing program and the rationale for it.

Positioning

Positioning is important in the early phases of burn recovery to minimize edema, because edema can cause ischemia, intrinsic muscle tightness, deforming positions, loss of motion, adhesions, and fibrosis. Edema is a natural component of the wound healing process, and burns create local and systemic responses.[21] Postburn edema develops rapidly within the first hour, peaks up to 36 hours after injury, and usually resolves within 7 to 10 days.[20] Edema still present in later stages is a matter of great concern.

Precaution. *To prevent a decrease in arterial flow to the hand, elevate the hand to heart level only in the emergent phase.*[20]

In addition to elevation, use pressure techniques (for example, compression wraps, sleeves, or gloves) as needed, taking care to monitor circulation and skin integrity, because fragile wounds and scars break down easily.

Positioning is also used to prevent loss of motion from soft tissue shortening. The position of comfort typically is that of shoulder adduction and internal rotation, elbow flexion, wrist flexion, and thumb adduction. Loss of motion can occur in joints not even involved in the burn injury. Facilitate proper positioning out of the expected pattern using pillows, bulky dressings, foam wedges, or orthoses.

> **◎ Clinical Pearl**
>
> Remember a burn treatment adage: the position of comfort is the position of deformity.

Orthoses

Orthoses can be used to facilitate wound healing by immobilizing the wound and protecting key structures in the hand. It is important to note that not all hand burns require orthotic intervention. The decision to use an orthosis or not depends on the depth and extent of the burn and the client's ability to tolerate positioning, exercise, and function. Most superficial partial thickness burns do not require an orthosis, because healing is completed within 3 weeks. An orthosis should be considered if healing is compromised, or there is a significant limitation in active extension or flexion of hand joints.[20] In some cases an orthosis may be indicated for a client who is unable to actively move the hand or for a client who may move too aggressively. Orthoses are used more often with deeper burns. Despite static orthotic intervention in the early phases of wound healing to prevent burn scar contracture, the incidence of contracture has been reported as 5% to 40% with weak evidence supporting their effectiveness.[22]

> **◎ Clinical Pearl**
>
> In the emergent and early acute phases, edema can lead to poor positioning and the classic burn deformity of wrist flexion, MP hyperextension, IP flexion, thumb adduction, and a flattened palmar arch.

Unless otherwise indicated, immobilize the hand with the wrist in extension, the metacarpophalangeal (MP) joints in flexion, the interphalangeal (IP) joints in extension, and the thumb in abduction. Slight wrist extension encourages MP flexion by means of a tenodesic effect, and MP flexion in turn puts tension on the collateral ligaments to prevent shortening. Proximal interphalangeal (PIP) joint extension protects the vulnerable extensor mechanism, and thumb abduction maintains the first web space. Considerable variation in ideal joint angles can be found in the literature.[23] A consensus calls for wrist extension of 15° to 30°, MP flexion of 50° to 80°, full IP extension or slight flexion, thumb abduction midway between radial and palmar abduction, MP flexion of 10°, and full thumb IP extension (Fig. 34-2).[10,16,20] For isolated burns to the palmar surface, position the wrist in neutral to slight extension, the IP joints in full extension and abduction, and the thumb in radial abduction and extension.[20] *Never*

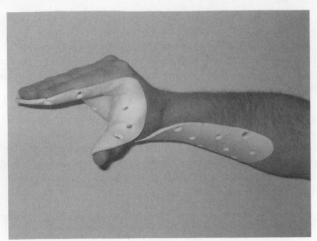

FIGURE 34-2 Positioning orthosis for an acute hand burn.

force joints into the ideal position. Although prefabricated orthoses are available, custom orthoses made from perforated material are preferable because they allow a more precise fit and can be adjusted to accommodate changes in edema and joint mobility. Orthoses can be secured by gauze wraps, elastic bandages, or straps.

Precaution. *Carefully monitor and adjust how the orthosis is secured to ensure there is no vascular compromise.*[20]

For clients with significant involvement of the IP joints, the surgeon may opt to place Kirschner wires across the joints to obtain complete immobilization and protection of the extensor mechanism.[3]

Orthoses may also be used in the later phases of recovery to prevent or correct **scar contracture.** To prevent contracture, use static orthoses, placing joints in positions opposite the direction the scar will pull. Common burn scar contractures in the hand are wrist flexion from volar burns, wrist extension or flexion from dorsal burns, thumb adduction from a burn to the first web space, MP and IP extension from dorsal hand burns, and MP and IP flexion from volar hand burns. Have the client wear the static orthosis at night only, if possible, to avoid compromising functional hand use during the day. Use serial static dynamic orthoses (also known as *elastic mobilization*) or static progressive orthoses (also known as *inelastic mobilization*) to regain ROM with joint and/or scar contracture. Place scars under tension in an elongated position to promote new cell growth, collagen remodeling, and tissue lengthening.[11,24]

Circumferential burns may require alternating use of different orthoses to address all scars.[16]

Exercise

Exercise is important in the early phases of burn recovery to control edema, promote tendon gliding, and help maintain ROM and strength. Have the client perform active motion with the dressings removed while you carefully monitor the status of the wound. Muscle pumping exercises with a low number of repetitions can help with edema. Include lumbrical position exercises and adduction/adduction of the fingers to contract intrinsic muscles. If the client is unable to move effectively through full ROM, perform *gentle* active assistive or passive motion. It is important to stay within wound and pain tolerance; take care to put your hands on the most stable and least painful areas of the wound.

Precaution. *Aggressive motion at this stage is harmful to fragile tissue and results in more scarring.*[20] *To prevent tendon rupture, do not perform IP motion if extensor tendon involvement is known or suspected.*

In the later phases of recovery, emphasize exercises to achieve full active and passive wrist and hand motion. Include gentle passive exercises for individual joint tightness. Composite wrist and finger flexion or extension exercises may also be needed for scars that cross several joints (commonly seen with dorsal hand burns). Look for the scar to blanch, which indicates it is being effectively stressed.[20] Resistive exercises can help with regaining strength and muscle endurance. Stronger muscles are better able to move against tightening scars. Have the client perform resistive exercises in both directions to address scar and tendon adhesions. Use exercises and therapeutic activity to promote strength, dexterity, coordination, and hand function.

Joint mobilization for stiff joints can begin during the scar maturation phase once the scar has adequate tensile strength to tolerate the friction caused by mobilization techniques.

Continuous passive motion (CPM) has been reported to be an effective adjunct to therapy in the treatment of hand burns for clients who show little active motion because of pain, anxiety, or edema.[25]

Precaution. *Be very careful using CPM if extensor tendon injury is involved or suspected, because this technique might be too forceful for the delicate extensor mechanism.*

Functional Hand Use

Functional hand use in daily activities should be encouraged as much as possible throughout all phases of recovery. Assistive devices, such as built-up handles, can facilitate functional use if limitations exist. Using the hand has important physical and psychologic benefits; it facilitates motion, strength, endurance, tendon glide, and edema reduction, and it gives the client a sense of self-control and sufficiency. However, keep in mind that improvement in pain, healing, motion, and strength does not always lead to spontaneous reintegration of the hand into tasks. Clients may be fearful of pain or of injuring fragile tissues. Acknowledge these concerns and provide support to help the client overcome them.

Scar Management

The goal of scar management is to modulate scars as much as possible to achieve a flat, smooth, supple, and cosmetically acceptable scar. Because scar formation is an unavoidable component of wound healing, the best we can hope to accomplish is to minimize scarring by altering its physical and mechanical properties through interventions, such as compression, silicone products, massage, and physical agent modalities. The exact mechanisms by which these interventions work are not well understood, and objective support of their efficacy is less than adequate, but they have produced positive clinical effects.[26,27]

Compression can be provided through a variety of means, including orthoses, compression wraps, and pressure garments. The processes of hypertrophic scarring and scar contraction begin shortly after injury; therefore early application of pressure is advised (that is, within 2 weeks of wound closure).[16,20,28] As a rule of thumb, use interim compression bandages and gloves until the hand is ready to be measured for a custom-fitted pressure garment. Pressure from self-adherent elastic wraps is effective in both

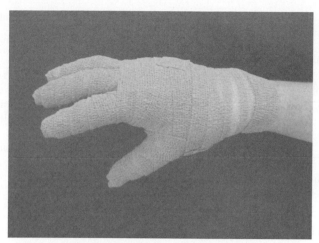

FIGURE 34-3 Self-adherent compression wrap.

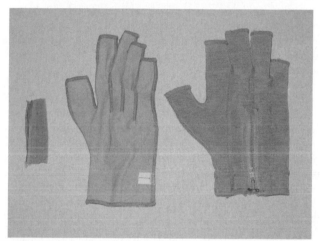

FIGURE 34-4 Prefabricated digital sleeve, prefabricated glove, and custom pressure glove.

edema and scar management, and these wraps can be used over light dressings as needed (Fig. 34-3).[16,28] Grade the amount of pressure to make sure it is tolerable. Prefabricated digital sleeves and gloves are an option once the scar is able to tolerate the shear forces created by putting them on, taking them off, and motion while wearing them. Measure for a custom glove only after edema has plateaued, wounds are smaller than a quarter, and the scar is ready to tolerate the heavier pressure and friction custom gloves impose (Fig. 34-4).[20] To be most effective, compression devices should be worn continually except during skin hygiene routines and exercise. It may take time for clients to tolerate full-time wear.

Silicone products are available in many forms, including sheets and putty. Some silicone gel sheets are self-adherent, whereas others must be held in place. Silicone can be used alone, but is often combined with pressure although the effectiveness of using both together has been mixed.[29,30] Some manufacturers make pressure garments with a thin silicone lining, but these may be more difficult for a client to put on and remove because of increased friction from the silicone. The recommended wearing time for silicone is a minimum of 12 to 24 hours a day; close monitoring is required since its occlusive nature may cause maceration.[16,20]

Precaution. *Do not apply silicone over open wounds or fragile skin.*

Massage, delivered manually or with a vibrator, may be helpful for freeing restrictive fibers, reducing itching, and relieving pain.[31,32] Begin with gentle massage of newly healed skin to avoid blister formation and skin breakdown. As tensile strength improves, progress to greater pressure causing scar blanching and massage with circular motions to work the scar in all directions. Lubricate the scar before massage to precondition the tissue. Massage should be performed at least twice a day.[16,20]

Physical agent modalities (for example, hot packs, paraffin, fluidotherapy, and ultrasound) have been used for burn scars to precondition tissues for exercise and activity.[16,20] Heat can reduce pain and improve elasticity of collagen fibers making the scar easier to mobilize. Paraffin combines the benefits of heat and skin lubrication, both of which are useful before motion. Fluidotherapy can also help with desensitization of hypersensitive scars. Dense burn scars are best heated by ultrasound.

Precaution. *Care must be taken with heat modalities, because scars may have diminished sensation and heat tolerance. Never use heat on open wounds or broken skin.*

Operative Treatment

Full thickness burns require surgical intervention because reepithelialization is not possible. Deep partial thickness burns that would require prolonged spontaneous healing (generally longer than 2 to 3 weeks) may be treated surgically to improve functional and cosmetic results.[3,14]

Early excision of nonviable burned skin (known as *escharotomy* or *fasciotomy*) may be needed to establish a healthy wound bed and to maintain blood perfusion.[3,16] The wound then can be covered with tissue transfers, cultured epithelial skin, or skin substitutes. A **heterograft (xenograft)** is skin taken from another species, such as a pig. A **homograft (allograft)** is human skin, most often taken from a cadaver. Heterografts and homografts are used as a temporary wound covering until the client's own skin can be used. An **autograft** is the client's own skin, taken as a graft harvested from a **donor site** and placed on the recipient wound site.[12,33] It may be a **split thickness skin graft (STSG)** or a **full thickness skin graft (FTSG)**. The thicker the graft, the more dermal appendages it will contain. Thinner STSGs typically are used to cover the dorsal hand. Thicker STSGs or FTSGs commonly are used for the palmar surface, because they provide better sensibility and durability.[12] STSGs may be applied as is (known as a *sheet graft*), perforated to allow drainage of fluid (known as a *meshed graft*), or meshed and expanded to cover more surface area. A **flap,** which includes fascial and/or muscle layers, may be needed for deep wounds with exposed tendon or bone.[33,34] Grafts and flaps require time to heal and leave scars at both the recipient and donor sites.

ⓞ *Clinical Pearl*

Scar contraction of grafts occurs; the thinner the graft, the more it will shrink.[33]

Grafts that are meshed and expanded tend to produce more scarring and contraction than sheet or unexpanded mesh grafts.[12,14] Cultured epithelial grafts are composed of sheets of epidermal cells grown in a laboratory. These very thin, fragile grafts are used for clients who do not have adequate donor sites; they afford poor coverage for hands.[12,20]

Postoperative therapy for burn wounds treated surgically is crucial for maximizing functional outcomes. Postoperative protocols vary according to the surgical procedure and the surgeon's preference. STSGs and FTSGs typically are immobilized for several days after surgery to allow establishment of vascularity and graft adherence. Cultured skin grafts are progressed more slowly than standard STSGs because of their fragile nature. Flaps usually are immobilized for slightly longer than grafts because they do not take as readily. Grafts and flaps are like any other healing wound in that time is required for collagen deposition and improvement of tensile strength. Initiate and cautiously progress positioning, orthotic intervention, exercise, and scar management as soon as graft or flap stability allows.

Precaution. *Healing tissues are very susceptible to injury in the first 3 weeks, especially from shearing forces.[3,12] Monitor carefully for signs of blistering or breakdown. Discuss with the surgeon whether therapy can proceed or should be discontinued temporarily.*

Surgery is an integral part of the rehabilitation phase for contracture release and reconstruction. Surgical intervention also may be used after the scar has reached maturity. In children, surgery may be needed periodically until growth is complete because of a discrepancy between the rapid rate of bony growth relative to the slower rate of scar tissue growth. Scar contracture release involves introducing more skin in areas where tight scarring has caused ROM limitations. Tissue transfers as described above are common, as are local rotational and advancement flaps (for example, Z-plasties).[12,14,33] Postoperative treatment follows guidelines and timelines similar to those for wound coverage.

? Questions to Discuss with the Physician

Non-Operative Clients

- What are the wound care and dressing guidelines?
- Will an orthotic be needed?
- Are there any known or suspected problems with tendon or joint integrity?
- Are any precautions necessary with regard to elevation, motion, or compression?

Operative Clients

- What surgery was performed? (Obtain a copy of the operative report if possible.)
- What type of graft or flap was used?
- What was the intraoperative ROM?
- How well had the graft or flap taken when postoperative dressings were removed?
- What are the wound care and dressing guidelines?
- Are there any problems with tendon or joint integrity?
- Will an orthosis be needed?
- Are any precautions required with regard to elevation, motion, or compression?
- What postoperative protocol would you like followed?

( ) What to Say to Clients

About the Injury

"A burn causes serious injury to the skin. Skin is important for preventing infection and for protecting deeper structures in our hands. Here is a diagram showing the layers of the skin and key anatomic features, such as hair follicles, sweat glands, oil glands, and nerve endings. The burn you sustained injured your skin to this depth, and this is how your skin will be affected."

Customize your information according to the client's level of injury and the symptoms related to pain and sensation.

About Wound Care and Healing

"The primary concern is to help you heal as quickly as possible to prevent infection and to minimize scarring. This is the wound care and dressing program that has been designed for you. It is important that you understand it, feel comfortable with it, and follow it closely."

Clients may have less pain and anxiety if they perform or assist with their wound care. Educate and practice with the client and significant others as often as needed to increase their comfort level. If a tissue transfer will be or was used, explain the purpose of it and what the client can expect at the recipient and donor sites.

About Scar Management

"Wounds heal with a process of scar formation. It may take several months or years for your active scars to complete the process of becoming mature. Active scars are red and may become thick, raised, and firm. Active scars also tend to become tight and may get very itchy, especially in the first 2 or 3 months. As the scars mature, you'll see the redness fade to your more normal skin color, and the scars will be flatter, softer, and less itchy. Scars are more sensitive to sunlight; therefore you should use sunscreen or gloves to protect them. You should wash your hands with mild soap; don't use anything with a strong detergent, which can dry your skin. Dry scars crack or injure more easily, and they may itch more. Over time your scars will become more durable, but they will never be quite as resilient as your normal skin. Because the feeling in your scars may not be normal, you'll have to rely more closely on visually inspecting them for signs of injury. Scars also don't have the natural ability to stay moist; therefore you will need to lubricate your skin frequently throughout the day to keep it healthy. Avoid moisturizers with a high perfume or alcohol content, which can cause dryness. Although we can't prevent scarring, we can try to keep your scars as flat, soft, and mobile as possible using interventions, such as massage, pressure, and silicone."

Educate the client and significant others so that they understand the scar management program, how to monitor for skin problems, and how to care for pressure and silicone devices properly.

About Orthoses

"Orthoses are used to help keep your active scars from becoming tight and causing loss of joint motion. They can also be used to regain motion you may have lost since your burn injury. It is important to follow the wearing schedule we set and to watch out for any problems with your skin that orthoses may cause."

Make sure that the client and significant others understand the purpose of each orthotic, the wearing schedule, and how to care for the orthotic.

About Exercise

"Exercise is important to keep your joints and scars mobile. The exercises designed for you include some for stretching your scars, some to help your tendons glide, and some to make your hand stronger. Always make sure to moisturize your scars well before you start your exercises so that they don't crack."

Educate the client and significant others about the purpose of each exercise and when and how each should be performed.

About Function

"One of the best ways to keep your hand moving is to use it as much as possible during all your normal daily activities. Although it may be a little awkward at first, using your hand will help your scars to stay supple, your joints to remain loose, and your muscles to become strong. You may have to be a little more careful to protect your scars from injury by monitoring for signs of pressure or blistering."

If assistive devices are used, explain, "These devices will help you use your hand better right now until it becomes easier for you to hold things or to do more with your hand."

Evaluation Tips

- Be careful and gentle when placing your hands or tools (for example, a goniometer) over healing wounds, fragile scars, and insensate or hypersensitive areas.
- Contractures may be caused by scar tightness, joint tightness, or both. Differentiate between a scar contracture and a joint contracture by watching for blanching and by palpating for tension of the scar.
- Scars that cross several joints need to be assessed closely. Assess individual joint active range of motion (AROM) and passive range of motion (PROM) with the scar in a relaxed position to measure the true joint motion. Tension on the scar may limit motion and make it appear that joint mobility is affected. For example, in a client with dorsal hand burns, place the wrist and MP in full extension while measuring PIP flexion. Once you have determined individual joint mobility, assess composite active and passive motion to determine if and how the scar is limiting motion.
- Use photographic images to help track wound healing and scar appearance. Quantify open wounds by measuring their size in centimeters and by describing their features (for example, color, integrity, drainage, and odor).[17] Quantify scars using scar assessment tools, such the Vancouver Burn Scar Scale, which rates pigmentation, vascularity, pliability, and height.[35,36] Assessing the client's subjective rating of the scars through visual analog scales is also beneficial, because the client's perception may not match yours. Despite the objective improvement you see, the client may not share your opinion that the scars are better.[37] Remember also to evaluate donor sites.
- Use hand tracings to evaluate and track changes in web spaces. You can obtain the most accurate representation by using a thin ballpoint refill without the pen body.
- Do not use volumetric measurement if open wounds are present without first obtaining the physician's permission. *Always disinfect the volumeter after use.*
- Watch for signs and patterns of peripheral nerve involvement. Nerve damage can be caused by direct injury, infection, or neurotoxicities. Localized compression caused by tight scars, poor positioning, or edema is also common.[20]
- Discuss how the burn is affecting the client's overall ability to function. Ascertain which activities are most important for the client to resume, and determine the factors that are most interfering with the client's ability to function.

Diagnosis-Specific Information that Affects Clinical Reasoning

Each client has unique clinical, functional, psychologic, social, and cultural needs. Individualize treatment based on your evaluation results and an understanding and appreciation of each person. Empower the client and significant others to be involved throughout therapy through education and an open approach that fosters active participation. Provide the client with a sense of control by presenting choices whenever possible. Because the scar maturation process may take several years, make sure you give clients all the tools they need to manage their own care. Teach clients how to perform interventions for themselves at every possible opportunity rather than doing the treatment for them; this facilitates better long-term outcomes. Treatment needs also are dictated by the depth and location of the burn, the timing of injury and surgical procedures, the stage of wound healing, and the phase of burn recovery. Anticipate potential scar contractures and direct treatment at preventing or correcting them. The principles of hand burn treatment can be applied to burns on any area of the body.

Precaution. *Work closely with the physician on the plan of care and report any new problems promptly.*

Dorsal burns to the hand commonly result in a thumb web space contracture that limits functional positioning of the thumb and finger web space contractures that limit digital abduction and possibly MP flexion. Loss of MP, IP, and composite finger flexion is also typical. In some cases the hand may have assumed an intrinsic minus position from poor early positioning, edema, or scar contraction (Fig. 34-5). A boutonnière deformity also may be present if the extensor mechanism was damaged. Palmar burns often cause limited thumb, finger, and composite extension.

Keep in mind that every scar is unique, and clients will have a variety of clinical problems; therefore perform a thorough

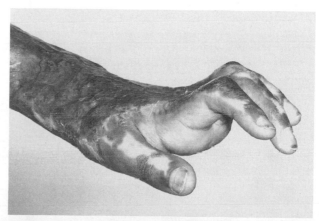

FIGURE 34-5 Dorsal hand burn resulting in the intrinsic minus deformity position. (From Thornes N: Therapy for the burn patient. In Prosser R, Conolly WB, editors: *Rehabilitation of the hand and upper limb*, Edinburgh, 2003, Butterworth Heinemann.)

evaluation to identify needs. The treatment of burn injuries is a dynamic process. Prioritize treatment based on the scars that are most active and the most functionally limiting. Re-evaluate often and shift treatment in response to changing needs. Circumferential scars are especially challenging, because they involve scars that pull in both directions possibly limiting joint flexion and extension.

Edema

If open wounds or fresh grafts are present, obtain the physician's permission before taking volumetric measurements. When elevating the hand, keep the elbow as straight as possible to aid flow. To provide more even pressure, use foam inserts placed in the palm, between the fingers, or on the dorsum of the hand under compressive wraps and prefabricated gloves.

Wound Care

When applying a dressing to the hand, make sure to wrap the digits individually and separately from the hand so as not to restrict motion unnecessarily and impede hand function (Fig. 34-6). If the thumb is involved in the dressing, pay attention to thumb positioning, and wrap it to facilitate functional palmar abduction. Wrap dressings over gauze pads in finger web spaces to provide early pressure. Keep the thickness of dressings consistent if an orthosis or interim garment is to be worn over them.

Scar Management

Scar hypersensitivity is a common problem that often must be addressed before the client is able to tolerate other interventions, such as orthoses, pressure, or massage. Hypersensitive scars on the palmar surface can also significantly impede hand function. Use graded stimuli to lessen sensitivity, taking care to stay within the scar's pressure and shear force tolerances to avoid injury.

Use inserts under compression devices to augment pressure in difficult areas, such as the web spaces and the palmar arch. Inserts can be made from products such as thermoplastics, silicone or foam (Fig. 34-7).[16,20,28] Grade pressure to the tolerance of the scar. A graded sequence may be compressive wraps using self-adherent elastic materials, progressing to a prefabricated glove made from soft material, progressing to a custom-fitted pressure glove. Order custom garments with the client's specific needs in mind. Zippers or Velcro closures make it easier for the client to put on and remove gloves with less trauma to fragile skin. Open tips allow for better finger sensation and hand function. Most manufacturers offer different grades of fabric from which the glove can be made. Select the material based on scar tolerance and functional demands. Very fragile scars may need a glove made of soft material; scars with good tolerance in a very active client may require a more durable material. Panels of soft material can be strategically placed in areas prone to discomfort or scar breakdown, such as bony prominences and the thumb web space (Fig. 34-8). Suede or other fabric patches and strips can be sewn onto the palmar surface to increase the glove's durability and prevent objects from slipping on slick fabric.[20]

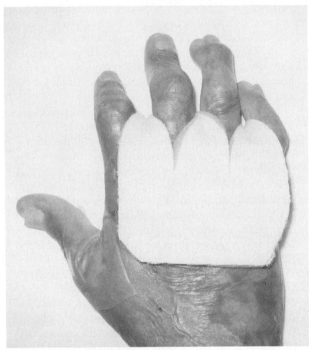

FIGURE 34-7 Silicone gel sheet in the thumb web space and foam inserts in the finger web spaces to augment pressure under the glove.

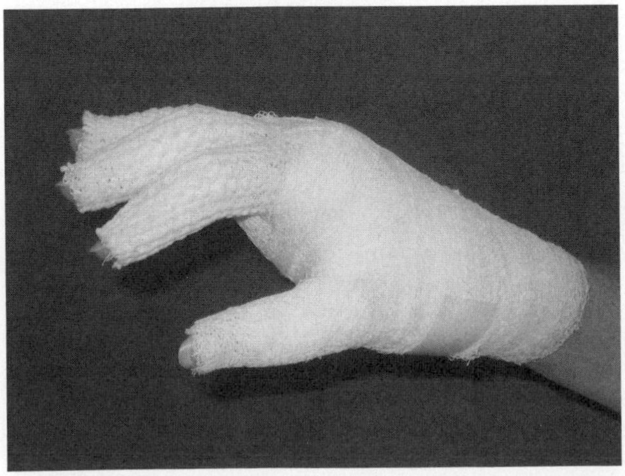

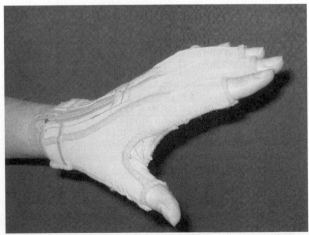

FIGURE 34-8 Custom pressure glove with dorsal zipper, open tips, and a soft panel in the thumb web space.

FIGURE 34-6 Hand dressing that allows unimpeded motion.

Compression materials stretch as the client wears them throughout the day. Laundering the garments helps materials return to their original state. Provide the client with two sets of all garments so that each day a clean one can be put on that provides the appropriate amount of pressure. Custom garments generally last 2 to 4 months under normal wearing conditions. Some clients struggle to keep to the wearing schedule because these garments are tight, they can be uncomfortably hot to wear, and they may limit dexterity and functional sensation. To improve follow-through, provide clients with a choice of design and color and teach them the purpose of the garments.[38]

Precaution. *Watch for allergic reactions, skin maceration or breakdown, and circulation or sensory impairments caused by compression garments, silicone, and inserts.*

Orthoses

Make sure to fabricate orthoses over any dressings, inserts, or garments the client will be wearing underneath them to ensure optimal fit. If you are molding an orthosis directly over scars that may be hypersensitive or heat sensitive, apply a thin cotton sleeve or a light dressing before placing warm material on the client. Relieve pressure over bony prominences or other areas of concern by temporarily placing padding over them before molding the orthosis; this will "bubble out" the material. Avoid lining or padding the orthosis itself unless absolutely necessary, because this makes the orthosis very difficult to keep clean. If lining or padding is used, place it on the orthotic material before molding.

Because wounds and scars are fragile, it is critical to smooth all edges completely. Select thermoplastic material based on the type of orthosis and its intended purpose. A material with full memory is well suited for a serial static orthosis that will be remolded numerous times. A material with excellent conformability is appropriate for an orthosis designed to apply pressure to uneven scars. A material with good rigidity is desirable for an orthosis that must withstand the force of a strongly contracting scar. The choice and placement of strapping also must be carefully considered to prevent the creation of pressure or shear forces.

To prevent unnecessary stiffness or disuse, design wearing schedules that leave the hand free for function and motion as much as possible.

Precaution. *With very active scars, just a few hours without an orthosis may result in significant loss of motion.*

As scars become more mature, wearing time can gradually be reduced, especially if the client's activity level or pressure devices are sufficient to control scar shortening.

Serial casts, serial static orthoses, dynamic orthoses, and static progressive orthoses all can be used to treat the wrist and hand. The type of orthosis used depends on the location of the scar, the direction of scar contraction, and the therapist's preference. Orthotic intervention to apply stress to burn scars often involves placing joints in positions not commonly used for other hand conditions, such as the wrist in flexion, the MP joints in extension, the thumb in radial abduction, or all joints in composite extension. Think creatively to design an orthosis that provides the most benefit. Leave uninvolved joints free whenever possible. Consider using a less restrictive orthosis during the day and a more restrictive orthosis at night. Orthoses may require frequent remolding or modification as edema

diminishes, the shape of the scar changes, or scar tightness improves or worsens.

Thumb web space contractures respond well to serial static orthoses. An orthosis that conforms completely to the web space often is most effective. Position the thumb in the plane of abduction where you can achieve maximal stretch (as noted by scar blanching). Strapping can be anchored around the wrist to apply pressure in the desired direction and to keep the orthosis firmly in place (Fig. 34-9).

Serial casts or gutter orthoses can be used for IP flexion contractures. Casting may be a better choice for severe contractures, because plaster conforms better than thermoplastics. Gutter orthoses can be secured with self-adherent compression wrap for a more secure and conforming fit.

MP extension contractures can be treated with serial static, dynamic, or static progressive MP flexion orthoses. In some cases, use of a simple wrist extension orthosis or a hand-based lumbrical bar orthosis during the day combined with functional use of the hand can encourage MP flexion. This can be complemented by use at night of a more restrictive orthosis designed to apply sustained stress to the scar. A full contact palmar orthosis can be effective for flexion contractures caused by palmar hand burns (Fig. 34-10).

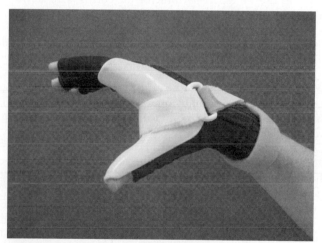

FIGURE 34-9 Thumb abduction orthosis for scar contracture of the first web space.

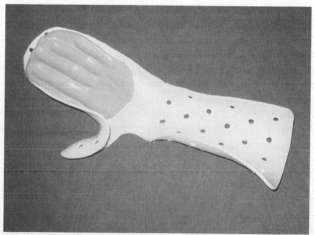

FIGURE 34-10 Full contact orthosis with silicone elastomer putty insert for palmar scar contracture.

Exercise

Include exercises for scar stretching, ROM, and tendon gliding as appropriate. Strengthening exercises are also useful, because strong muscles are better able to pull against tight scars. Gripping and putty exercises are effective for encouraging composite flexion of the hand. Scars should be well lubricated before exercising. Exercises for non-burned areas may be needed to regain motion or strength lost through immobilization or disuse.

Promoting Function

Use assistive devices to help promote functional use through all phases of burn recovery. Build up handles on utensils or use universal cuffs to assist with grasp. Tight scars can limit dexterity and slow speed of performance. Improvement in skin integrity, pain, motion, and strength does not automatically equate with spontaneous return to functional hand use. Integrate therapeutic activities (for example, woodworking or leather crafts) and meaningful functional tasks into the therapy program to help clients see their functional potential and gain confidence in their hand use. Discuss self-care, home, community, leisure, or vocational demands with each client and address specific interfering factors. Reintegrating into social activities can be especially difficult for clients with scarring. Work with the client to figure out ways to return to activities as independently, safely, and comfortably as possible. Keep in mind that the ultimate goal is a return to the client's prior level of function.

Psychosocial Adjustment

Recovery from a burn injury goes beyond the healing of anatomic structures. Be aware of factors that may interfere with treatment and recovery, such as pain, anxiety, and depression. Take time to establish rapport and trust with your client. Provide encouragement, understanding, and emotional support throughout therapy. Facilitate client involvement and a sense of self-control during the therapeutic process to the fullest extent possible. Refer the client to other health care providers as appropriate to help address problems. Educate the client and significant others about resources for support. Many national and local organizations offer information, peer counseling, support groups, and recreational activities for burn survivors and their significant others. Find information through the American Burn Association and the Phoenix Society for Burn Survivors.

Reassessment

Reassess scar activity and ROM frequently, because the scar's status can change quickly for the better or worse. Adjust the treatment program, goals, and priorities accordingly. Share the results with the client and significant others, to serve as positive reinforcement if improvements are noted or to motivate them to more closely follow therapy recommendations if no gains are seen or the scar's status has deteriorated. Collaborate closely to problem solve issues as soon as they arise.

◎ Clinical Pearl

To be effective, compression must conform to the scar.

➤ Precautions and Concerns

- *Facilitate wound healing and control edema to reduce the extent of scarring.*
- *Follow appropriate infection control procedures during wound care and dressing changes.*
- *When using orthoses on an edematous hand, never force joints into the ideal position. Instead, position the joints as close to the ideal as possible, and modify the orthosis gradually over time as edema diminishes.*
- *Be especially careful with PIP joints when extensor tendon injury is known or suspected; mobilize these joints only with permission from the physician.*
- *When orthoses and pressure devices are used, monitor closely for signs of skin breakdown.*
- *Be cautious with the use of thermal treatments over newly healed wounds or scars.*
- *Carefully assess the client's work environment. Clients with a large-percentage body burn have a decreased tolerance for hot temperatures. Chemicals also may pose an increased risk to scars.*

CASE STUDY 34-1 ▪

DL is a 24-year-old, right-hand dominant auto mechanic who sustained 8% TBSA circumferential burns to his right hand in a small explosion at work. The palmar wound was a mix of superficial and deep partial thickness burns that crossed the wrist into the forearm; the dorsal injury involved deep partial thickness burns. The client was admitted to a local burn unit, where he underwent early excision and grafting of the dorsal hand injury with STSGs from his right thigh. The palmar burn was treated with nonsurgical management. DL was referred to the outpatient hand clinic for therapy 3 weeks after surgery.

Treatment

DL arrived at the therapy clinic with his hand wrapped in a bulky dressing, even though he had no open wounds. He stated that it was "too painful" to leave his hand uncovered. He had mild edema, most notably on the dorsum of the hand. The following values were recorded for the right hand:

	AROM (degrees)	PROM (degrees)
Index finger MP	30/55	25/60
PIP	35/65	30/85
DIP	5/40	0/50
Middle finger MP	25/40	15/50
PIP	40/70	40/80
DIP	10/50	5/60
Ring finger MP	25-55	20-65
PIP	40/75	35/80
DIP	15/35	10/35
Small finger MP	10/30	10/40
PIP	55/70	35/75
DIP	20/55	10/60
Thumb MP	20/45	20/55
IP	0/5	0/15
Abduction	0-30	0-35

The scars were not hypertrophic but were very red, dry, and tight, as noted by blanching at end-ranges of motion. The hand did not appear to have been recently washed. Grip strength measured 15 lbs. All motor function was intact. Touch-pressure sensation was normal with monofilament testing, but hypersensitivity of the palmar surface was noted throughout the evaluation. DL lived with his girlfriend, who accompanied him to therapy. He was able to perform his basic activities of daily living (ADLs) using his left hand only.

The immediate treatment priorities were determined to be reducing hypersensitivity, resolving edema, and improving ROM for both hand opening and closing. Hypersensitivity and a fear of pain or damage to his skin were limiting DL's ability to care for his hand and to want to move it or use it. This issue initially was addressed by having him gently wash his hand and apply lotion to scars at the beginning of therapy sessions. DL was reluctant to do this for the first few sessions, and he needed a lot of encouragement to do a thorough job. After the third session, his hand consistently appeared clean upon his arrival for therapy. He also was able to tolerate having the therapist massage his scars after he performed massage for the first few minutes.

DL felt unable to leave his hand unbandaged, but he did agree to try a self-adherent compressive wrap to help manage edema and provide some light pressure to his scars. Foam inserts were placed in the palm and web spaces and on the dorsum of the hand. The wrap was applied with very light pressure at first, and DL was able to tolerate a little more pressure each time as hypersensitivity diminished and his trust of his therapist increased. Two weeks into therapy, the edema had almost resolved, and the hypersensitivity had improved enough that DL felt he could wear a soft, prefabricated pressure glove. This allowed him to move more freely and to remove the glove often for skin hygiene, massage, and progressive desensitization with textures. When the edema had resolved completely, DL began wearing a custom-fitted pressure glove.

Increasing ROM was addressed through a combination of orthoses, exercise, and functional use. DL lacked motion in both flexion and extension, and the therapist had to prioritize which joints and motions to focus on first. Gaining MP flexion and PIP extension were selected as priority concerns. Gutter orthoses were made for each finger and worn over the compression wrap. The aim was to serially gain IP extension ROM and transfer flexor forces to the MP joints to improve active MP flexion ROM. A volar wrist orthosis with the wrist in extension was also fabricated for use during the day to encourage MP flexion and prevent contraction of the volar forearm scar that crossed the wrist. Orthoses worn at night were geared toward improving composite extension ROM. A volar wrist-hand orthosis was fabricated with the wrist and fingers in maximum extension and the thumb in maximum abduction. Because each finger IP needed to be positioned at a different angle, the wrist-hand orthosis was fabricated over the existing gutter orthoses for a more precise fit. Once IP extension had improved, lacking only about 15° to neutral, and active MP flexion also had improved (in about 2 weeks), gutter orthoses were weaned off during the day to facilitate IP flexion and

functional use of the hand. The daytime wrist orthosis was discontinued shortly thereafter.

Active and gentle passive exercises for all joints were initiated and had to be progressed slowly. As DL's hypersensitivity and edema improved, so did his ability to tolerate more vigorous exercises. Strengthening exercises were graded from squeezing a large, soft foam ball to putty. Later in the program, DL was able to perform weight well exercises with progressive resistance.

To help DL begin to integrate functional use of his hand at the beginning of therapy, soft, large-diameter tubing was used on his eating utensils and toothbrush. Because he was able to do tasks easily using his left hand, he was reluctant to consider trying with his right hand "until it got better." Once he understood the therapeutic value of active daily use for reducing the edema, hypersensitivity, and scar tightness, he was willing to integrate functional use as part of his home exercise program (HEP). When he saw that his hand looked and felt better after he began using it, he became eager to do more at home. DL shared with the therapist that he was a drummer who occasionally performed with a band made up of friends. The therapist was able to tap into this interest as a means to motivate DL by making drumming a focus of his HEP. He was asked to bring in a small drum and his drumsticks, and together DL and the therapist were able to devise modifications for his right drumstick. Soft padding was wrapped around the proximal end of the stick to a diameter large enough to allow him to hold it. As composite finger flexion improved, the diameter of the padding was reduced. Therapeutic activities were performed in the therapy clinic to improve fisting and strength. These included leather stamping and a woodworking project in which he fabricated a weight well for himself to use at home. The final activities involved tool use simulating work tasks. DL was concerned about being able to wear his pressure glove at work without getting it dirty. He brought in vinyl gloves that he typically wore on his hands at work and found that a larger size fit well over his pressure glove. He began doing some work on his car at home.

Result

Throughout the therapy program, DL was educated in all aspects of his injury and care. Building trust, fostering his sense of control over his care, providing him with choices, allowing him to see his progress by continually sharing re-evaluation results, and tapping into motivating interests were keys to his successful rehabilitation. Upon discharge from therapy, DL had regained full AROM, and hypersensitivity had resolved. Grip strength was 75 lbs. He was wearing his pressure glove full time. He returned to using his right hand as dominant for all activities, which was enough to maintain full composite flexion without requiring orthoses. He continued to wear a night orthosis that positioned his wrist and hand in composite extension whenever he felt his volar scars were tightening. He felt confident about managing his scars long term and knew how to progress his hand strengthening exercises at home. His physician cleared him to return to work shortly after therapy ended.

References

1. Pruitt BA, Wolf SE, Mason AD: Epidemiological, demographic, and outcome characteristics of burn injury. In Herndon D, editor: *Total burn care*, ed 4, New York, 2012, Elsevier, pp 15–45.
2. Chen X, Huang T, Nugent N, et al: Care of a burned hand and reconstruction of the deformities. In Herndon D, editor: *Total burn care*, ed 4, New York, 2012, Elsevier, pp 645–659.
3. Germann G, Weigel G: The burned hand. In Wolf SW, Hotchkiss RN, Pederson WC, et al: *Green's operative hand surgery*, ed 6, Philadelphia, 2011, Elsevier, pp 2089–2120.
4. Rosenberg L, Lawrence JW, Rosenberg M, et al: Psychosocial recovery and reintegration of patients with burn injuries. In Herndon D, editor: *Total burn care*, ed 4, New York, 2012, Elsevier, pp 743–753.

5. Low FA, Meyer WJ, Willebrand M, et al: Psychiatric disorders associated with burn injury. In Herndon D, editor: *Total burn care*, ed 4, New York, 2012, Elsevier, pp 733–741.

6. Reeve J, Frances J, McNeill R, et al: Functional and psychological outcomes following burn injury: reduced income and hidden emotions are predictors of greater distress, *J Burn Care Res* 32:468–474, 2011.

7. Lawrence JW, Mason ST, Schomer K, et al: Epidemiology and impact of scarring after burn injury: a systematic review of the literature, *J Burn Care Res* 33:136–146, 2012.

8. Sundara DC: A review of issues and concerns of family members of adult burn survivors, *J Burn Care Res* 32:349–357, 2011.

9. Lewis GM, Heimbach DM, Gibran NS: Evaluation of the burn wound: management decisions. In Herndon D, editor: *Total burn care*, ed 4, New York, 2012, Elsevier, pp 125–130.

10. Malick MH, Carr JA: *Manual on management of the burn patient*, Pittsburgh, 1982, Harmarville Rehabilitation Center Educational Resource Division.

11. Richard RL, Staley MJ: Biophysical aspects of normal skin and burn scar. In Richard RL, Staley MJ, editors: *Burn care and rehabilitation: principles and practice*, Philadelphia, 1994, FA Davis, pp 49–69.

12. Pedersen WC: Nonmicrosurgical coverage of the upper extremity. In Wolf SW, Hotchkiss RN, Pederson WC, et al, editors: *Green's operative hand surgery*, ed 6, Philadelphia, 2011, Elsevier, pp 1645–1720.

13. Hartford CE: Care of outpatient burns. In Herndon D, editor: *Total burn care*, ed 4, New York, 2012, Elsevier, pp 81–92.

14. Simpson RL: Management of burns of the upper extremity. In Skirven TM, Osterman AL, Fedorczyk JM, et al, editors: *Rehabilitation of the hand and upper extremity*, ed 6, Philadelphia, 2011, Elsevier, pp 302–316.

15. Mlcak RP, Buffalo MC, Jiminez CJ: Prehospital management, transportation, and emergency care. In Herndon D, editor: *Total burn care*, ed 4, New York, 2012, Elsevier, pp 93–102.

16. Serghiou MA, Ott S, Whitehead C, et al: Comprehensive rehabilitation of the burn patient. In Herndon D, editor: *Total burn care*, ed 4, New York, 2012, Elsevier, pp 517–549.

17. von der Heyde RL, Evans RB: Wound classification and management. In Skirven TM, Osterman AL, Fedorczyk JM, et al, editors: *Rehabilitation of the hand and upper extremity*, ed 6, Philadelphia, 2011, Elsevier, pp 219–232.

18. Hawkins HK, Finnerty CC: Pathophysiology of the burn scar. In Herndon D, editor: *Total burn care*, ed 4, New York, 2012, Elsevier, pp 507–516.

19. Peacock EE: *Wound repair*, ed 3, Philadelphia, 1984, WB Saunders.

20. Tufaro PA, Bondoc SL: Therapist's management of the burned hand. In Skirven TM, Osterman AL, Fedorczyk JM, et al, editors: *Rehabilitation of the hand and upper extremity*, ed 6, Philadelphia, 2011, Elsevier, pp 317–341.

21. Edgar DW, Fish J, Gomez M, et al: Local and systemic treatments for acute edema after burn injury: a systematic review of the literature, *J Burn Care Res* 32:334–347, 2011.

22. Schouten HJ, Nieuwenhuis MK, van Zuiljen PPM: A review on static splinting therapy to prevent burn scar contracture: do clinical and experimental data warrant its clinical application? *Burns* 38:19–25, 2012.

23. Richard R, Staley M, Daugherty MB, et al: The wide variety of designs for dorsal hand burn splints, *J Burn Care Rehabil* 15:275–280, 1994.

24. Brand PW, Hollister AM: *Clinical mechanics of the hand*, ed 3, St Louis, 1999, Mosby.

25. Covey MH, Dutcher K, Marvin JA, et al: Efficacy of continuous passive motion devices with hand burns, *J Burn Care Rehabil* 9:397–400, 1988.

26. Anzarut A, Olson J, Singh P, et al: The effectiveness of pressure garment therapy for the prevention of abnormal scarring after burn injury: a meta-analysis, *J Plast Reconstr Aesthet Surg* 62:77–84, 2009.

27. O'Brien L, Pandit A: Silicone gel sheeting for preventing and treating hypertrophic and keloid scars, *Cochrane Database Syst Rev* (1): CD003826, 2006.

28. Staley MJ, Richard RL: Scar management. In Richard RL, Staley MJ, editors: *Burn care and rehabilitation: principles and practice*, Philadelphia, 1994, FA Davis, pp 380–418.

29. Steinstraesser L, Flak E, Witte B, et al: Pressure garment therapy alone and in combination with silicone for the prevention of hypertrophic scarring: randomized controlled trial with individual comparison, *Plast Reconstr Surg* 128:306e–313e, 2011.

30. Li-Tsang CWP, Zheng YP, Lau JCM: A randomized clinical trial to study the effect of silicone gel dressing and pressure therapy on posttraumatic hypertrophic scars, *J Burn Care Res* 31:448–457, 2010.

31. Bell PL, Gabriel V: Evidence based review for the treatment of post-burn pruritus, *J Burn Care Res* 30:55–61, 2009.

32. Field T, Peck M, Hernandez-Reif M, et al: Postburn itching, pain, and psychological symptoms are reduced with massage therapy, *J Burn Care Rehabil* 21:189–193, 2000.

33. Levin LS: Management of skin grafts and flaps. In Skirven TM, Osterman AL, Fedorczyk JM, et al, editors: *Rehabilitation of the hand and upper extremity*, ed 6, Philadelphia, 2011, Elsevier, pp 244–254.

34. Jones NF, Lister GD: Free skin and composite flaps. In Wolf SW, Hotchkiss RN, Pederson WC, et al, editors: *Green's operative hand surgery*, ed 6, Philadelphia, 2011, Elsevier, pp 1721–1756.

35. Sullivan T, Smith J, Kermode J, et al: Rating the burn scar, *J Burn Care Rehabil* 11:256–260, 1990.

36. Tyack Z, Simons M, Spinks A, et al: A systematic review of the quality of burn scar rating scales for clinical and research use, *Burns* 38:6–18, 2012.

37. Martin D, Umraw N, Gomez M, et al: Changes in subjective versus objective burn scar assessment over time: does the patient agree with what we think? *J Burn Care Rehabil* 24:239–244, 2003.

38. Stewart R, Bhagwanjee AM, Mbakaza Y, et al: Pressure garment adherence in adult patients with burn injuries: an analysis of patient and clinician perceptions, *Am J Occup Ther* 54:598–606, 2000.

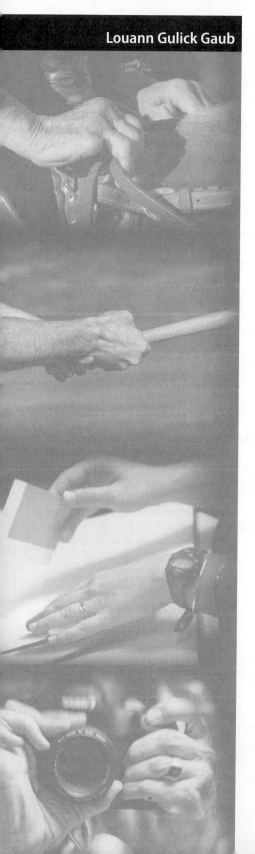

35

Infections

Louann Gulick Gaub

Hand therapists are often the first persons to identify early signs of inflammation or infection in their clients, such as redness (**rubor** or **erythema**), edema (**tumor**), heat (**calor**), and pain (**dolor**). By knowing suspicious signs of infection, the therapist can promptly communicate problems with the physician, leading to earlier diagnosis and treatment. Prompt attention may make the difference between a nonsurgical solution and a surgical one.

In a 2008 practice analysis by the Hand Therapy Certification Commission, in consultation with Professional Examination Service, most therapists who responded reported treating clients who had infection as part of their diagnosis. Fifty-six percent of respondents reported infections in 1% to 10% of their patients, and 26% reported infections in 11% to 25% of their patient population.[1]

The terms *inflammation* and *infection* differ in that **inflammation** is, "a localized protective reaction of tissue to irritation, injury, or infection, characterized by pain, redness, swelling, and sometimes loss of function."[2] **Infection** is the "invasion of the body by pathogenic microorganisms."[3] Infection can lead to loss of tissue and even death in some cases if left untreated. It can occur with a minor scratch or with a major trauma. Since the initial use of penicillin in 1942,[4,5] the incidence of hand infections and complications have greatly decreased. However, bacteria evolves, and the sensitivity of bacteria to antibiotics can change. Many infected wounds contain more than one type of offending organism, and some bacteria have adapted to a point that available antibiotics may not affect them. One such resistant organism is **methicillin-resistant *Staphylococcus aureus* (MRSA).**[4] There has been an increased incidence of MRSA in hospitals and the community. By 2003, more than 50% of *Staphylococcus aureus* isolates in US hospitals were MRSA.[4]

General Principles

When the skin is broken, bacteria contaminates the wound. This bacteria will either be fought off by the host or develop into an infection. The susceptibility of the host to infection depends upon many factors, such as the severity of injury and whether multisystems are involved. Certain conditions increase the susceptibility to infections, such as diabetes mellitus,[6,7,8] AIDS, Raynaud's disease,[7] malnutrition, obesity,[6,7] renal failure, burns, immunosuppression seen with cancer or transplantation recipients,[6] alcoholism, drug abuse, and others.[7]

Many types of microorganisms can cause infection in the hand, but the most common is *Staphylococcus aureus,* which may comprise from 50% to 80% of all hand infections.[7] The second most common pathogen found in hand infections is β-*hemolytic Streptococcus.* Many wounds contain more than one pathogen, such as in bite injuries.[7,9,10]

Infections may start out as **cellulitis,** a superficial infection of the skin and subcutaneous tissue that normally does not produce an **abscess** (a localized collection of pus). The involved area is tender, warm, and marked by erythema. Incision and drainage are not routinely performed for cellulitis, but the procedure is done if an abscess develops.[7,10]

A trivial injury left untreated may lead to a very serious hand infection that progresses rapidly, called **lymphangitis.** Lymphangitis can involve the superficial lymphatic vessels that arise from the skin, but can also lead to the deep lymphatic vessels following the course of the arterial system. Some signs of lymphangitis could include fever, nausea, tachycardia, or red streaking up the hand and forearm along the lymphatic pathways. An abscess may form at the elbow or axilla if the infection is left untreated. The most common cause of lymphangitis is a *Streptococcus* organism[5] (Fig. 35-1).

Cellulitis and lymphangitis are considered superficial spreading infections. There are other types of infections found in the hand, such as subcutaneous abscesses, synovial sheath, and fascial space infections. Subcutaneous abscesses include paronychias, felons, and subepidermal abscesses. With any infection of the hand, even if located on the palmar surface, more edema may be present dorsally on the hand because of the anatomy and direction of flow of the lymphatic system.[7]

Anatomy and Pathology

Perionychium

The **perionychium** comprises the whole nail structure consisting of the nail bed (germinal and sterile matrix), nail plate, nail fold, eponychium, hyponychium, and paronychium (Fig. 35-2). The nail fold is the proximal depression into which the proximal nail fits. The nail fold has a dorsal roof (eponychium).[11,12] The **lunula** is the white arc seen at the base of the nail just distal to the eponychium. The highly vacularized nail bed shows through the nail normally appearing pink in color.[12] The **hyponychium,** between the nail bed and the distal nail, helps in protection against fungal and bacterial contamination. The hyponychium

contains leukocytes and lymphocytes that provide defense against invasion of the subungual area (under the nail). The paronychium is the lateral skin on the edge of the nail plate and bed.[11,12]

The fingernail is not only important aesthetically but is also needed functionally. The nail provides counter-pressure against the finger when pinching or holding onto an object, which improves the sensitivity. The fingernail is important for protection, can help regulate temperature, and promotes dexterity.[11,12]

In a traumatic fingertip injury, a **subungual hematoma** (confined mass of blood under the nail) may develop from bleeding underneath the nail plate. Bleeding separates the nail bed from the nail plate and can cause throbbing pain due to pressure. The hematoma can be evacuated by forming a hole in the nail. This procedure is performed by the physician.[11]

Paronychia

Paronychia refers to an infection of the soft tissue around the nail or nail plate (Fig. 35-3). It is the most common infection in the hand.[13] A hangnail, nail biting, or manicure are often the cause and can start on the lateral border of the nail.[13,14] In children, paronychia is associated with thumb or finger sucking. Erythema, swelling, and pain may occur at the lateral fold or base of the fingernail.[14] The most common causative organism of an acute paronychia is *Staphylococcus aureus*.[9,10,15]

> ◎ **Clinical Pearl**
>
> Paronychia is the most common hand infection. It may be acute or chronic.

Chronic paronychia is more common in people who immerse their hands in water or detergents frequently. Middle-aged women are most commonly affected, as are people who work in jobs that require frequent cleaning. Finger suckers and individuals with diabetes are more susceptible to chronic paronychias.[13] Normally, the hyponychium protects the subungual space from invading organisms. When the finger is repeatedly immersed in water and exposed to alkaline, the protective barrier is violated and bacterial or fungal organisms more easily enter.[11] The most common offender is *Candida albacans* and other fungal organisms.[7,13] Individuals with chronic paronychias suffer with repeated erythema and drainage. A decrease in vascularity of the nail fold due to frequent infections may increase the chance of more invading organisms causing new episodes. If not adequately treated, the nail may exhibit permanent nail deformity (Fig. 35-4).

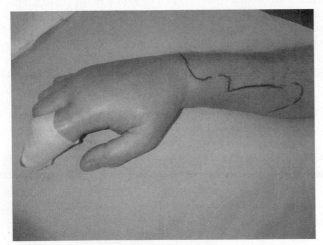

FIGURE 35-1 Lymphangitis and purulent flexor tenosynovitis. Markings on forearm indicate progressing erythema and edema. (Courtesy of Dr. James Nappi, Hand & Microsurgery Associates, Columbus, OH.)

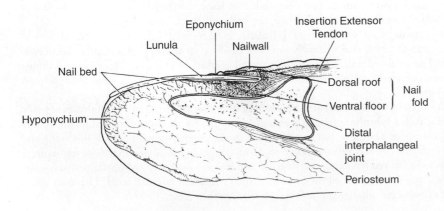

FIGURE 35-2 Anatomy of the nail bed. (From Sommer NZ, Brown RE: The perionychium. In Wolfe SW, Hotchkiss RN, Pederson WC, et al, editors: *Green's operative hand surgery,* ed 6, Philadelphia, 2011, Churchill Livingstone.)

Eponychia

When the infection involves the tissue overlying the base of the nail in addition to one lateral fold beside the nail, it is more accurately called an **eponychia.** In an eponychia, pus can develop near the lunula, the white arch visable at the base of some fingernails.[13] An infection can begin on one side of the nail as a paronychia, then less commonly extend around the base to the opposite side of the nail, called a *run-around infection.*[7,10] Therefore, an eponychia can develop from an extension of an untreated paronychia.

Felon

An infection involving the distal finger pad is called a **felon.** The finger pad or pulp is divided into multiple compartments by fibrous septa that connect to skin and extend to bone. A subcutaneous abscess (pus) in these tiny compartments causes pressure with swelling and can create redness and an intense pain. A penetrating trauma, such as with splinters or finger-stick blood tests, can be the mechanism of injury.[10,14] If left untreated, the abscess from the felon can extend into the distal phalanx and lead to osteomyelitis (inflammation of bone and marrow) or **osteitis** (inflammation of bone). The tip of the finger holds the highest concentration of sensory receptors in the hand,[13] so when pressure develops in the finger pulp, pain is usually severe. The longer the felon is untreated, the greater is the chance that increased tension in the septal compartments causes shut off of blood supply to the distal phalanx.[9]

Flexor Sheath Infection

The flexor tendons in the hand move within synovial sheaths. Within these sheaths, there is poor vascularization, but the tendons receive much of their nutrition by diffusion from the synovial fluid.[13] This synovial fluid environment is enticing for bacterial growth. When infection occurs within the enclosed sheath, a **purulent flexor tenosynovitis** (or pyogenic flexor tenosynovitis) develops.[7,14] Increased pressure from bacterial proliferation within the sheath leads to even less blood supply (through the vincular system) and can cause tendon necrosis and rupture. Flexor sheath infections are most commonly caused by *Staphylococcus aureus* and β*-hemolytic Streptococcus.*[13,14]

Dr. Allen Kanavel, a pioneer in the treatment of hand infections in the early twentieth century, described four signs (**Kanavel's cardinal signs**) to identify purulent flexor tenosynovitis. These are 1) a semi-flexed finger position, 2) uniform volar swelling of the finger, 3) tenderness along the tendon sheath, and 4) excruciating pain with passive extension of the finger.[7,13,14]

Even if treated early, purulent flexor tenosynovitis can lead to permanent tendon scarring and lack of function. Tendon necrosis or the spread of infection to deep fascial spaces can occur if the infection advances. Although more uncommon, radial and ulnar bursal infections may occur in association with flexor tendon sheath infections of the thumb or small fingers. There may be tenderness and swelling at the distal wrist crease, along the hypothenar or thenar eminence, in addition to the cardinal signs of Kanavel in either the small finger or thumb.[13]

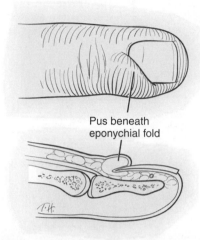

A

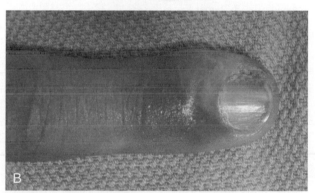

B

FIGURE 35-3 Inflamed paronychium and eponychium with pus below the eponychial fold. (From Stevanovic MV, Sharpe F: Acute infections. In Wolfe SW, Hotchkiss RN, Pederson WC, et al, editors: *Green's operative hand surgery,* ed 6, Philadelphia, 2011, Elsevier Churchill Livingstone.)

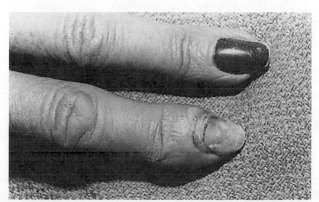

FIGURE 35-4 Chronic paronychia. (From Mackin EJ, Callahan AD, Skirven TM, et al, editors: *Rehabilitation of the hand and upper extremity,* ed 5, St Louis, 2002, Mosby.)

> ### ◎ *Clinical Pearl*
>
> Flexor tenosynovitis is recognized by the presence of four Kanavel cardinal signs: 1) semi-flexed finger position, 2) uniform volar swelling of the finger, 3) tenderness along the tendon sheath, and 4) excruciating pain with passive extension of the finger.[7,13,14]

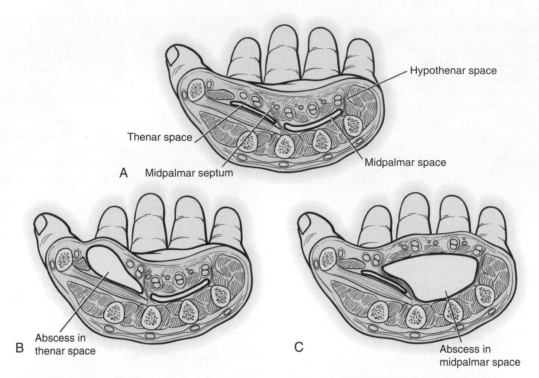

FIGURE 35-5 **Deep palmar spaces.** **A,** Potential spaces of the mid palm. **B,** Thenar space abscess. **C,** Midpalmar space abscess. (From Stevanovic MV, Sharpe F: Acute infections. In Wolfe SW, Hotchkiss RN, Pederson WC, et al, editors: *Green's operative hand surgery*, ed 6, Philadelphia, 2011, Elsevier Churchill Livingstone.)

Fascial Space Infection

Infection can develop or pus may accumulate in a number of potential spaces in the hand (Fig. 35-5). Potential spaces are the 1) thenar, 2) hypothenar, 3) midpalmar spaces in the hand, and 4) Parona's space in the forearm. More superficial spaces are the 5) dorsal subcutaneous space, 6) dorsal subaponeurotic space, and the 7) interdigital web spaces (collar-button abscesses occur here).[13] Infection may be caused by a penetrating injury or by spread from an adjacent flexor tendon sheath infection. These clients may present with tenderness and swelling over the palmar spaces. Dorsal hand swelling is also present, as in most other hand infections, since the palm consists of tight fascia that limits the accumulation of swelling. The dorsal hand anatomy consists of a more loosely organized connective tissue that allows greater expansion of edema in the soft tissue.[13] The presence of infection in the fascial spaces is treated as a medical emergency and usually requires surgical drainage.[7,13]

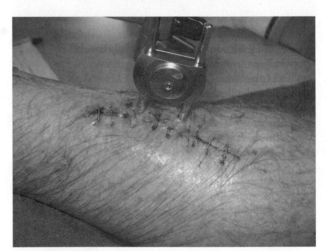

FIGURE 35-6 Infection around the proximal screw site of an external fixator in the forearm. (Courtesy of Louann Gulick Gaub.)

Osteomyelitis

Infection in the bone, or **osteomyelitis,** can result when an infection is not eradicated in nearby soft tissue or if there is a penetrating trauma.[13,16] A felon or bite injury can lead to osteomyelitis, and *Staphylococcus* is the most common pathogen. Intact bone cortex provides a good barrier to penetration of pathogens, but trauma to the bone allows a pathway for infection. If local inflammation causes necrosis of the bone, called a **sequestrum,** pathogens can more easily live there due to the deficient vascularity. Antibiotics are less effective in areas of necrotic bone.[16]

When hardware (such as, pins, screws, and plates) are required for fixation of a bone fracture, pathogens can enter the bone and cause infection. Infection can develop around a pin or screw site (Fig. 35-6). Most pin tract infections are minor if treated appropriately with antibiotics and good wound care around the hardware.[13] Incidence of pin tract infections is considered to be infrequent, ranging from 0.5% to 21%.[13-19] External fixation may have a higher rate of infection than internal fixation.[19] Most infections from pins and screws are minor and do not lead to significant osteomyelitis if treated early. However, this infection can necessitate the early removal of hardware and can result in necrosis of the bone if the infection cannot be controlled.[13,16]

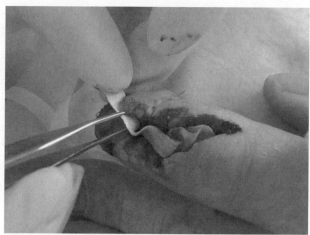

FIGURE 35-7 Wound packing with strip gauze. Wound left open to heal by secondary intention. (Courtesy of Louann Gulick Gaub.)

Common Mechanisms of Injury and Infection

Human Bite

Human saliva can contain a number of bacterial and viral organisms causing infection. The hand can become contaminated with human saliva by several means: a fist striking the tooth, nail biting, a dental instrument, or a bite. A **fight bite** or **clenched-fist injury** can result if a client strikes a person's face. A tooth may lacerate the skin over the dorsal third, fourth, or fifth metacarpals. This relatively thinly protected area may be vulnerable to a fracture of the metacarpal or phalanx, an infection in the joint capsule, and a laceration of the extensor tendon.[7,9,10,14] The client may not seek medical attention initially because the wound may seem unimportant. A delay in treatment may increase the chance of a more severe infection, including osteomyelitis.[7,9,14] After surgical drainage and antibiotics, the wound is usually healed by **secondary intention** (left open, not closed with suturing).

Animal Bite

Contrary to what some people believe, the saliva of dogs and cats contains a number of disease-causing organisms with the most common offender being *Pasteurella multicida*.[7,10,20-22] Even a cut or scratch can become infected if an animal licks it.[21] Dog bites are more common than cat bites; however, cat bites are more likely to result in infection. A cat's teeth are sharper and thinner, causing a puncture wound. These wounds close quickly, are difficult to clean, and may introduce bacteria deep into the tissue. Dog bites are more likely to cause soft tissue damage due to the crushing or lacerating effect of their teeth. If bitten, immediately washing with soap and warm water is recommended. The client should seek immediate medical attention, especially if they have a compromised immune system (such as, diabetes, liver disease, HIV/AIDS, has had their spleen removed, and so on).[21] Most animal bite wounds are left open to heal by secondary intention.

Intravenous Drug Abuse

Drug abusers attempt venous access with typically dirty needles. They may inject the chemical into the soft tissue causing necrosis and infection. Infections acquired by injections of drugs may begin as a subcutaneous abscess or progress into an infection involving the tendon sheaths, joints, or fascial spaces. A drug abuser may not seek prompt medical attention and may have poor compliance with treatment. Additionally, intravenous (IV) drug abusers tend to have a deficient immune response with a higher rate of malnutrition, hepatitis, and HIV/AIDS.[7,20] Forearm infections due to IV drug abuse may create increased pressure in the deep tissues. This compression may lead to deoxygenation of the muscles, nerves, and blood vessels. Severe edema, pain in the forearm with finger flexion, and pain with passive extension may be an indication of **Volkmann's contracture.** This is a serious emergency, as the muscles are dying. A fasciotomy (surgical opening of skin and fascia) may then be required to drain infection from the tissue and lower the tissue pressure.[20]

Mycobacteria

The most common mycobacterial infection in the hand is *Mycobacterium marinum*. It is often difficult to diagnose since the symptoms can be diverse, and the appearance of symptoms may not occur for weeks or months after innoculation.[23] The infection often begins when the client has a puncture wound or skin abrasion and has contact with fish fins or fish tanks. They can also get the mycobacterial infection while at a beach, lake, or pool. The presentation may be of skin lesions or nodules along lines of lymphatic drainage, or localized tenosynovitis of the flexors or extensors.[7] Since the infection may be prolonged but relatively unpainful, the client may not receive appropriate treatment. This delay can allow the synovial structures to be destroyed.[7,10,23]

Fungal Infections

Fungal infections occur in the hand, but rarely require surgery. Contamination with soil, thorns, or splinters may start an infection, such as sporotrichosis. The presentation is of painless papules that can eventually spread along paths of lymphatic drainage.[23] Fungal infections can also attack the nail and lead to thickening and discoloration. *Candida,* one species of pathogen, can produce a nail deformity that is most frequently seen in those with peripheral vascular disease, Raynaud's disease, or Cushing's syndrome.[22] *Candida* infections can occur when the client places their hands frequently in wet or alkaline conditions, because the hyponychium has lost its protective ability to fend off infections.[11] Most fungal organisms can be treated with systemic or topical antifungal medications.[10,11]

Viruses

The two most common viral infections of the hand are herpetic whitlow and periungual warts.[11] Periungual warts, caused by the human papillomavirus, is usually more of a cosmetic problem. There are various treatments, both surgical and nonsurgical, but most warts resolve within two years. However, eradication of the wart is the optimal treatment since surrounding tissue may be invaded during this time.[23]

Herpetic whitlow is caused by the herpes simplex virus and can be contacted directly through the mucous membranes or through broken skin. It can be spread by touching the fingers (with open skin) to herpes lesions in the mouth or genital areas.[14,23] Herpes whitlow is most often seen in health care workers who are exposed to secretions in the mouth if not using universal precautions. One or more fluid-filled vesicles on the finger, swelling, discomfort, or redness are characteristics of herpetic whitlow. It can be confused with a felon or paronychia since some symptoms are similar.[14,22] The virus usually resolves on its own in 10 to 14 days, so medical management does not involve surgery. In fact, incision is contraindicated because drainage may result in developing a bacterial infection.[7,11,14,22]

Timelines and Healing

The longer the client takes to seek appropriate medical treatment after the initiation of infection, the higher the severity of tissue damage. Healing and timelines also depend on the location of infection, the client's medical status, extent of injury, and structures involved. Delayed treatment or complexity of infection may lead to the need for incision and drainage, compartment release, secondary reconstructive surgeries, or even amputation.

Non-Operative Treatment

After an injury, prompt wound care can help to prevent infection. When possible, immediately washing or flushing out the wound with soap and warm water may remove dirt, saliva, or a foreign body that contains bacteria.[21] If the injury is more severe, prompt medical attention is important. Often the injury may seem trivial, such as a small bite wound over the metacarpal obtained during a fight, and the client may not seek medical attention. Remind your clients: *when in doubt, it is safest to consult a medical expert early on.*

> ## ◎ *Clinical Pearl*
>
> If infection and acute inflammation are present, the involved area should be immobilized to help prevent the spread of the infection and to reduce pain and edema. The area should be immobilized in a position that prevents deformity or stiffness, such as the **safe position (intrinsic plus position),** with the wrist in slight extension, the MP joints in flexion, and the IP joints in extension (unless not appropriate for injured structures).

Non-operative treatment for the acute paronychia consists of oral antibiotics (usually anti-staphylococcal), warm soaks, and resting of the digit. Surgical drainage is performed if an abscess (pus) develops. Chronic paronychia may be more difficult to treat, especially if the client works in moist environments with substances that impair the hyponychium's natural barrier against fungi and bacteria. Chronic paronychia can be treated with antifungal or antimicrobial agents along with avoidance of prolonged immersion of hands in water and alkalines.[12]

Felons, infections in the pulp of the tip of the finger, should be treated with appropriate oral antibiotics (usually anti-staphylococcal) promptly. Otherwise, surgical drainage is inevitable to prevent further spread to other tissue and necrosis of the distal phalanx.[7,9] Purulent (or pyogenic) flexor tenosynovitis is also best treated immediately, certainly within 12 to 24 hours of onset. Non-operative treatment includes oral or IV antibiotics (usually fighting *Staphylococcus aureus* or β-*hemolytic Streptococcus*), immobilization in a splint, warm soaks, and elevation.[12,14] Infection within the sheath can spread rapidly and can impair the function of the tendon, spread to other fascial spaces, and can ultimately lead to necrosis of the tendon. These infections are closely monitored since non-operative treatment may not be sufficient. Surgical intervention is often needed.[12,14]

It is important to understand that therapists do not make the diagnosis of any infection or condition in this chapter. The therapist's role is to describe the clinical appearance of the hand to the physician or physician's staff if possible infection signs are observed, such as erythema, an increase in drainage, purulent drainage, increase in pain, or increase in edema. The physician will make the diagnosis.

Operative Treatment

Post-surgical therapy may include wound care, edema control, splinting for rest and protection, and range of motion (ROM) exercises depending on the involved structures. Infections that involve only the tip of the finger and are less serious often do not require a referral to hand therapy.

Surgical intervention for acute paronychia involves evacuation of pus around the nail fold. The surgeon may remove part or all of the nail.[15] If non-operative treatment does not work for the chronic paronychia, a procedure called *eponychial marsupialization* is performed. This procedure removes an elliptic area of skin in the proximal nail fold to encourage improved drainage.[7,22]

Other infections, such as felons, animal or human bites, or purulent flexor tenosynovitis, may be treated surgically by incision and drainage if conservative treatment does not resolve the infection within 48 hours.[7,13-15] Therapists are more likely to treat these more complicated cases postoperatively. Treatment is individualized according to the structures involved and extent of injury.

Hand therapists often treat clients who require internal or external hardware fixation for their fracture (for example, pins, screws, or plates). Infection rates with Kirschner wire fixation are considered to be relatively uncommon. Hsu, et al.[17] found superficial pin track infection in 6% of all pins in their study. Pins placed in the metacarpals or phalanges had a higher incidence of infection complications than pins in the wrist and forearm (distal radius and ulna).[17] Others found 3% to 8.3% rate of pin track infections.[18,19] Exposed pins may increase the incidence of infection compared to pins that are buried beneath the skin.[19,24]

? *Questions to Discuss with the Physician*

- What structures were involved in the infection?
- What are the precautions or guidelines for active or passive range of motion (AROM, PROM)?
- What are the wound care guidelines (for example, soaking, frequency of dressing changes, dressing technique, packing an open wound)?
- Do you want the client to do home dressing changes?
- Is splinting desired? If so, what structures should be immobilized and in what position? Should the wrist be included in the orthotic?

What to Say to Clients

If Infection is Suspected

"Check your hand for an increase in redness, swelling, heat, and pain. Call your physician's office if you develop a fever, if you feel sick, or if you suspect your symptoms are worsening. Identifying early signs of infection can make a big difference in the speed of your recovery."

Postoperative Clients

"It is very important always to keep your hand elevated above your heart to minimize swelling. Swelling can lead to stiffness and pain. Managing swelling early promotes better recovery of function in your hand. It is also important to adhere to the wound care guidelines to decrease chances of infection."

Evaluation Tips

- If infection is suspected, describe and measure the symptomatic area (for example, the area of erythema) so that you can later compare it with observations during subsequent visits.
- If an infection is suspected, do not cause unnecessary pain by taking measurements of ROM or proceeding with therapeutic exercise. Contact the physician's office right away to describe your observations while the client is in your clinic. You may find that doing ROM or activities were contraindicated.
- Find out if any treatment is contraindicated, such as PROM or resistive exercise.
- Check dressings to document amount of drainage, color, quality of the wound, or odor (see the "Evaluation" section in Chapter 5).
- Watch for and document skin maceration.
- Monitor and document appearance around pin or screw sites. Slight erythema may be present postoperatively but should be closely monitored for increase in erythema or other infection signs. Pin tract infections can lead to osteomyelitis.[13,17] Pin care should be done according to the physician's preference.

Diagnosis-Specific Information that Affects Clinical Reasoning

Prompt treatment is important when infection begins. If you observe possible signs of infection, the physician should be called while the client is present in the clinic. If you are not sure because the signs are very mild, try to determine the client's ability to monitor worsening symptoms while at home. Instruct in signs to look for and how to contact the physician's office if symptoms persist or worsen. If the client feels uncomfortable with the decision-making or is unable to accurately make that decision, recommend more frequent therapy visits so that you can monitor the situation more closely.

Precaution. *If infection is suspected, it is better to have it documented that the physician's office was contacted than to wish later that this had been done.*

Wound care guidelines are determined by the treating physician. If the status of the wound changes (for example, increase in drainage that is soaking through the dressing, or wound is changing in color), the dressing guidelines may need to be changed. Therapists who work closely with hand surgeons may often make many of these decisions due to their close working relationship and training. Therapists who do not have this understanding and relationship with a particular referring physician should discuss any wound care changes before proceeding with another treatment plan.

Tips from the Field

Orthotics

Orthotic needs are determined by the structures involved. It may be necessary to immobilize more joints due to pain or protection of healing tissues. Discuss orthotic options with the physician. The client with purulent flexor tenosynovitis, for example, may initially benefit from an orthotic that includes the wrist and positions the hand in intrinsic plus position. Stiffness may develop as a result of their tenosynovitis and disuse, so a proximal interphalangeal (PIP) extension orthotic is beneficial after the infection is controlled.

Wound Care

Instruct clients in signs of inflammation, such as redness, swelling, pain, and heat. Therapists should understand that a degree of these signs accompany the normal early inflammatory stage of a healing wound. Purulence does not always indicate infection.[24] It is best to have the physician assess the wound if there is a suspicion of infection. Postoperatively, the wound may be left open to heal by secondary intention so that purulent material can easily drain. The physician may request that you and/or the client lightly pack the open wound with strip gauze to keep the superficial wound open to allow the deeper portion to contract first (Fig. 35-7).

Wound care may also include debridement of slough (dead skin) or eschar (black wound) since these nonviable tissues impede the normal cellular response. This dead tissue forms a mechanical block and can increase the growth of bacteria in the wound.[24] If you do not feel comfortable in performing any of these wound care techniques, you should discuss this with the physician.

The therapist can have an important role in the wound healing and infection control processes. Appropriate techniques that may prevent or control infection are protection of the wound with a dressing (barrier to the environment), cleaning the wound per physician's preference (mild soap and water or other cleansing solutions), removal of necrotic tissue, and removal of excess drainage. Topical antiseptics may or may not be recommended by your physician since they are cytotoxic and may not only harm bacteria but also destroy cell walls in healthy tissue.[21,24] With infection, warm water soaks between two to four times per day may be prescribed by the physician to promote drainage.[9,15]

An important role for the therapist is to instruct the client in dressing changes. Include a family member in the instruction if that person plans to help at home. Instruct the client not to change the wound care process unless advised to do so by the therapist or physician.

Edema Control

After injury or surgery, all wounds have some edema. It is a component of the normal inflammatory response to injury and is a result of excess fluid in the intercellular spaces.[25] If edema is excessive, nutrients and waste have difficulty diffusing between cells and capillaries. Excessive swelling can increase chances for infection, delay the healing process, and increase stiffness and scarring.[24,25] It is best to prevent excessive edema than to treat it after it is a significant problem. Managing edema may include elevation, compression with external wraps, gentle AROM if approved by the physician, and use of cold modalities if not contraindicated (for example, patients with circulatory compromise).[24-26]

Therapeutic Modalities

Use of therapeutic modalities can be helpful in treating edema, pain, and stiffness. However, therapists should be cautious when choosing modalities to treat those with an active infection. Some modalities may be contraindicated, such as ultrasound, contrast baths, intermittent pneumatic compression pumps, kinesiotaping, or iontophoresis.[26]

Client Expectations

Infection can make a minor injury become a permanent disability in the use of the hand. Explain the importance of early management of infection with timely communication with the physician and adherence to treatment guidelines recommended by the therapist and physician. Explain the implications realistically, but try to emphasize the positive. The therapist has an important role guiding the client through a potentially life-changing event in order to achieve a more functional, pain-free upper extremity.

> ### ➤ Precautions and Concerns

- *Watch for redness, swelling, heat, pain, or fever. Instruct clients to check for these signs at home and to contact their physician immediately if infection is suspected.*
- *If the client is not complying with restrictions or dressing guidelines, note this in your documentation.*

CASE STUDIES

CASE STUDY 35-1 ■

F.P., a retired gentleman, lacerated his dominant index finger with a machete while sharpening it during a television program. He was initially seen in the emergency room (ER), and his wounds were closed. After referral to a hand surgeon, F.P.'s flexor digitorum profundus (FDP) was repaired 10 days later.

At his postoperative joint visit with therapist and physician, he had some erythema, swelling, and tenderness around the proximal incision. His breath had a strong odor of alcohol. Two sutures were removed to express purulent-looking drainage. The physician prescribed antibiotics and soaks in warm water and liquid soap twice daily. The therapist began only gentle limited passive flexion within a dorsal blocking splint due to pain. The physician recommended seeing him the following day.

The next day, the client presented with an increase in erythema along the volar wrist with moderate edema in the wrist, index finger, and dorsum of his hand. He refused to be admitted to the hospital. He stated that he had not started the antibiotics until an hour before his appointment. F.P. also admitted to having difficulty with depression and hoarding.

The following day, he did not wear his splint. He had worsening symptoms and was admitted for IV antibiotics and incision and drainage of purulent flexor tenosynovitis and deep space infection.

In proceeding weeks, the client's compliance was questionable. He required a static progressive extension orthosis for all of the flexor tendons due to tendon adherence not only of his index finger but also the other fingers as a result of his deep space infection and compartment syndrome. Active motion of all digits continue to be problematic, but F.P. was ultimately able to achieve a functional gross grasp. He did not opt for tenolysis to gain more AROM. F.P.'s case is an example of how a noncompliant client can add complexity to treating infection appropriately.

CASE STUDY 35-2 ■

G.P., a 40-year-old housewife, sustained a cat bite in her home. She washed her finger, applied a Band-Aid, and continued her daily routine without concern. About 12 hours later, significant pain and edema developed rapidly. In the ER, the hand surgeon observed signs consistent with developing purulent flexor tenosynovitis of her dominant index finger and opted for incision and drainage. The flexor tendon sheath was incised, decompressed, irrigated, and first annular (A1) pulley released. Serous fluid and purulence were drained. The client stayed overnight for monitoring and IV antibiotics.

Two days postoperatively, the client came to hand therapy. Her bulky dressing was removed, her hand was soaked in warm water and liquid soap, and wound packing was removed. The wound was open and left to heal by secondary intention. There were no visual signs of infection. The wound was loosely repacked with narrow strip packing gauze and a dry dressing was applied. The client and husband were instructed in twice daily soaking and wound packing at home. She was able to perform tendon-gliding exercise with minimal difficulty. Three weeks later, G.P.'s wound was nearly fully closed and she had full ROM. Prompt appropriate medical attention averted lasting tendon dysfunction.

CASE STUDY 35-3 ■

H.D. crushed his non-dominant middle finger at work in a trash dumpster. The hand surgeon performed an open reduction and internal fixation (ORIF) to his distal interphalangeal (DIP) joint, a radial collateral ligament repair, a zone I extensor tendon repair, and nail bed repair. At his postoperative visit with the therapist and physician, H.D. had moderate erythema confined to the finger, moderate to severe pain, and swelling. The physician removed all sutures and the nail while in the office in order to allow removal of any purulent drainage. The wound was soaked and packed. The therapist instructed the client in how to soak and pack the wound at home, but H.D. did not feel comfortable performing his own dressing changes initially. He opted to come to therapy every day to have the therapist do the wound packing. The therapist made a digit-based orthotic including the PIP and DIP.

After 1 week of daily therapy visits, H.D. felt more comfortable performing soaking and dressing changes at home. He then attended therapy twice weekly for wound and infection monitoring, ROM, and other therapeutic activities. At 3 weeks and the time of this writing, his wound is nearly fully closed, he has a functional ROM, and he is back to work doing restricted duty until he is able to do his regular job.

Acknowledgment

The author would like to thank Cynthia Cooper for the use of portions of her text from the previous edition of this chapter.

References

1. Dimick MP, Caro CM, Kasch MC, et al: 2008 practice analysis study of hand therapy, *J Hand Ther* 22(4):361–375, 2009.
2. *The American Heritage Dictionary of the English Language*, ed 4, 2009, Houghton Mifflin Company.
3. *Collins English Dictionary—Complete and unabridged*, 2003, HarperCollins Publishers.
4. Arias CA, Murray BE: Antibiotic-resistant bugs in the 21st century—a clinical super-challenge, *N Engl J Med* 360:439–443, 2009.
5. Flynn JE: Severe infections of the hand: a historical perspective. In Jupiter JB, editor: *Flynn's hand surgery*, ed 4, Baltimore, 1991, Williams & Wilkins.
6. Pruitt BA, et al: Infections: bacteriology, antibiotics, and chemotherapy. In Jupiter JB, editor: *Flynn's hand surgery*, ed 4, Baltimore, 1991, Williams & Wilkins.
7. Taras JS, et al: Common infections of the hand. In Skirven TM, Osterman AL, Fedorczyk JM, et al, editors: *Rehabilitation of the hand and upper extremity*, ed 6, Philadelphia, 2011, Elsevier Mosby.
8. Fitzgibbons PG: Hand manifestations of diabetes mellitus, *J Hand Surg Am* 33:771–775, 2008.
9. Crandon JH: Common infections of the hand. In Jupiter JB, editor: *Flynn's hand surgery*, ed 4, Baltimore, 1991, Williams & Wilkins.
10. Neviaser RJ: Infections. In Green DP, editor: *Operative hand surgery*, ed 2, New York, 1988, Churchill Livingstone.
11. Wegener EE: Identification of common nail and skin disorders, *J Hand Ther* 23:187–197, 2010.
12. Zook EG: Anatomy and physiology of the perionychium, *Hand Clin* 18:553–559, 2002.
13. Stevanovic MV, Sharpe F: Acute infections. In Wolfe SW, Hotchkiss RN, Pederson WC, et al, editors: *Green's operative hand surgery*, ed 6, Philadelphia, 2011, Elsevier Churchill Livingstone.
14. Clark DC: Common acute hand infections, *Am Fam Physician* 68(11):2167–2176, 2003.
15. Ritting AW, O'Malley MP, Rodner CM: Acute paronychia, *J Hand Surg Am* 37(5):1068–1070, 2012.
16. Honda H, McDonald JR: Current recommendations in the management of osteomyelitis of the hand and wrist, *J Hand Surg Am* 34:1135–1136, 2009.
17. Hsu LP, Schwartz EG, Kalainov DM, et al: Complications of K-wire fixation in procedures involving the hand and wrist, *J Hand Surg Am* 36(4):610–616, 2011.
18. Rizvi M, Bille B, Holtom P, et al: The role of prophylactic antibiotics in elective hand surgery, *J Hand Surg Am* 33(3):413–420, 2008.
19. Richard MJ, Wartinbee DA, Riboh J, et al: Analysis of the complications of palmar plating versus external fixation for fractures of the distal radius, *J Hand Surg Am* 36(10):1614–1620, 2011.
20. Cahill JM: Special infections of the hand. In Jupiter JB, editor: *Flynn's hand surgery*, ed 4, Baltimore, 1991, Williams & Wilkins.
21. LSU School of Veterinary Medicine: What you should know about animal bites, Official Web Page of Louisiana State University (website): *http://www.vetmed.lsu.edu/animal_bites.htm*. Accessed June 17, 2013.
22. Keyser JJ, Littler JW, Eaton RG: Surgical treatment of infections and lesions of the perionychium, *Hand Clin* 6(1):137–153, 1990.
23. Abzug JM, Cappel MA: Benign acquired superficial skin lesions of the hand, *J Hand Surg Am* 37:378–393, 2012.
24. Von Der Heyde R, Evans RB: Wound classification and management. In Skirven TM, Osterman AL, Fedorczyk JM, et al, editors: *Rehabilitation of the hand and upper extremity*, ed 6, Philadelphia, 2011, Elsevier Mosby.
25. Villeco JP: Edema: a silent but important factor, *J Hand Ther* 25:153–160, 2012.
26. Hartzell TL, Rubinstein R, Herman M: Therapeutic modalities—an updated review for the hand surgeon, *J Hand Surg Am* 37(3):597–621, 2012.

36

Ganglions and Tumors of the Hand and Wrist

Julie Pal and Jackie Wallman

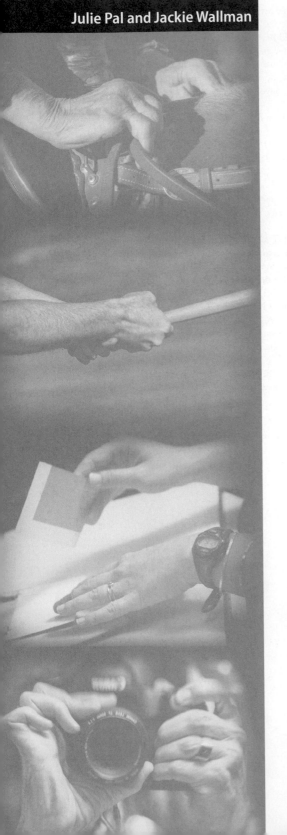

Tumors of the forearm and hand can arise from any tissue in the upper extremity including synovium, fat, skin, lymphatics, nerves, blood vessels, or bone. Tumors are classified into three categories: tumor mimicking lesions, benign tumors, and malignant tumors.[1] A therapist is likely to see these clients on their caseload because of the prevalence with which these clients come to our referring physicians. For this reason, it is important to know the common sequence of diagnosis and treatment, to have an appreciation for the tissues involved, and to know how to manage both the physical care and psychological implications of an upper extremity tumor.

Ganglion Cysts

Ganglion cysts are the most common tumors, accounting for 15% to 60% of all cases of the hand and wrist.[1] The presentation and diagnosis can be confusing, and treatment is variable. A thorough medical history of related trauma or repetitive use of the extremity and reports of rapid changes in growth and pain are vital for providing appropriate client care. Although malignancy is unlikely, significant changes in growth, size, and appearance warrant prompt referral to the primary care provider or surgeon.

Diagnosis and Epidemiology

A **ganglion** is a mucin-filled soft tissue cyst, formed from the synovial lining of a joint or tendon sheath.[2] Theories on formation of ganglions include mucoid degeneration, synovial herniation, and trauma to the joint capsule or ligaments.[2] Ganglions are generally painless. They tend to fluctuate in size with time and activity, and they may or may not resolve without intervention. Ganglions can appear gradually over time, or suddenly. They usually occur singly and in very specific locations, but they have been reported from almost every joint in the wrist and hand.[2] If enlarged, the ganglion can produce pain secondary to pressure on the nearby tissues and structures. Clients tend to report pain in positions of extreme wrist flexion, extension, or with weight bearing activities through the wrist.[1] The **posterior interosseous nerve (PIN)** in the dorsal wrist capsule, the **median nerve** as it passes through the carpal tunnel, and the **ulnar nerve** within Guyon's canal at the wrist have all been known to be symptomatic when there is a ganglion within these structures.[2] Usually, ganglion cysts arise from the **scapholunate joint** and ligament in the wrist. The main cyst is connected by a mucin-filled cleft interconnecting the cyst to the underlying joint (Fig. 36-1).[2]

Demographics

Ganglions can occur at any age in either gender, and they can resolve spontaneously or require therapeutic or surgical intervention. Ganglions occur more frequently in women, between the teenage years through middle adulthood. They are found more often in clients with ligamentous laxity. A recent history of trauma or injury is present in 10% of cases, or there may be a history of repetitive use of the hand or extremity.[2] Ganglions have been diagnosed in children, but spontaneous healing almost always occurs within 2 years of diagnosis. A pediatric client is seldom a surgical candidate for ganglion excision.[1]

Anatomic Sites

Dorsal wrist ganglions are the most common, comprising 60% to 70% of all hand and wrist ganglions.[2] They are seen over the dorsum of the wrist, usually between the extensor

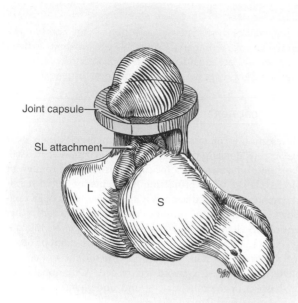

FIGURE 36-1 The ganglion and scapholunate *(SL)* attachments are shown with connection to the joint via mucin clefts through capsule. *L,* Lunate; *S,* scaphoid. (From Athanasian EA: Bone and soft tissue tumors. In Wolfe SW, Hotchkiss RN, Pederson WC, et al, editors: *Green's operative hand surgery,* ed 6, Philadelphia, 2011, Churchill Livingstone.)

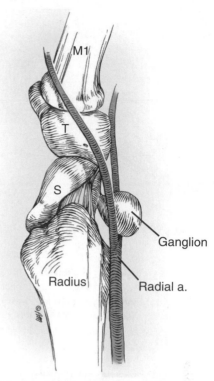

FIGURE 36-3 The usual relationship of the ganglion to the radial artery and the volar capsule. *M1,* First metacarpal; *S,* scaphoid; *T,* trapezium. (From Athanasian EA: Bone and soft tissue tumors. In Wolfe SW, Hotchkiss RN, Pederson WC, et al, editors: *Green's operative hand surgery,* ed 6, Philadelphia, 2011, Churchill Livingstone.)

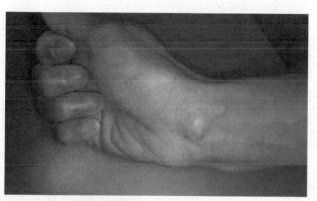

FIGURE 36-2 Volar wrist ganglion.

pollicus longus and extensor digitorum communis, at the level of the scapholunate ligament. **Volar wrist ganglions** are the second most common type of ganglions, comprising 15% to 20% of cases. They are usually associated with the underlying scapholunate ligament and less often over the scaphotrapezial joint. A volar wrist ganglion is commonly seen on the radial aspect of the wrist (over the flexor carpi radialis tendon) (Fig. 36-2). When evaluating a volar wrist ganglion, the therapist should palpate the cyst, and perform an **Allen's vascular test** (described in Chapter 5). A mass that is pulsatile in nature or obstructs blood flow to the hand is indicative of a vascular tumor, but it can easily be misidentified as a volar wrist ganglion because of the proximity to the radial artery and the scapholunate joint (Fig. 36-3).

Retinacular cysts are a type of ganglion that develops from a tendon sheath, rather than a joint. A **volar retinacular ganglion** is palpable and symptomatic near the proximal inter phalangeal (PIP) joint or the metacarpophalangeal (MP) joint. An

extensor retinacular ganglion is uncommon but, if detected, usually involves the first extensor compartment (abductor pollicis longus and extensor pollicis brevis) and can be associated with **de Quervain tenosynovitis** (inflammation of the synovial lining surrounding the extensors within the first dorsal compartment). Retinacular cysts form on the tendon sheath itself, not the tendon within (Fig. 36-4).

Hidden or **occult ganglions** can be a source of unexplained wrist pain and disproportionate tenderness.[2] Due to the deep location in the wrist, this type of ganglion is a common source of pressure on the PIN within the dorsal capsule, causing dorsal wrist pain.[2] The ganglion may be detected by placing the client's wrist in marked volar flexion.[2] An **intraosseus ganglion** is rare and usually is detected with involvement of the scaphoid or lunate. computed tomography (CT) scan or magnetic resonance imaging (MRI) may be indicated for these clients, who have ongoing wrist pain of unclear etiology and without a visible cyst.

Mucous cysts are a type of ganglion that is seen on the dorsal joints of the digits, most often the base of the middle phalanx and/or the distal phalanx (Fig. 36-5). There is close association between mucous cysts and osteoarthritis of the DIP and PIP joints.[2] The mucous cyst typically forms over an osteophyte on the DIP joint known as a **Heberden's node.** Longitudinal grooving of the nail secondary to pressure on the nail matrix may be seen with this.[2] A **carpal boss** is an osteoarthritic spur that forms over the carpal metacarpal joint of either the index or long fingers where the extensor carpi radialis longus and brevis insert. A carpal boss is firm, non-mobile, tender to palpation, and can be observed with the wrist placed in flexion.

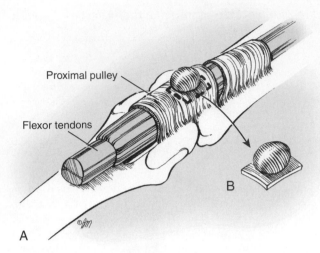

FIGURE 36-4 A, Volar retinacular ganglion in situ on the proximal annular ligament (A1 pulley) of the flexor tendon sheath. **B,** Excised specimen with a surrounding margin of tendon sheath. (From Athanasian EA: Bone and soft tissue tumors. In Wolfe SW, Hotchkiss RN, Pederson WC, et al, editors: *Green's operative hand surgery,* ed 6, Philadelphia, 2011, Churchill Livingstone.)

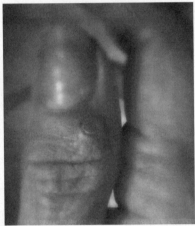

FIGURE 36-5 Mucous cyst. (From Sweet S, Kroonen L, Weiss L: Soft tissue tumors of the forearm and hand. In Skirven TM, Osterman AL, Fedorczyk JM, et al, editors: *Rehabilitation of the hand and upper extremity,* ed 6, St Louis, 2011, Mosby.)

Timelines and Healing

Clients seek a physician because they are worried about potential malignancy, impaired function, weakness, or pain.[2] The course of treatment is dependent on the approach that the client and surgeon agree upon. Indications for treatment of ganglia include pain, interference with activity, nerve compression, and ulceration of overlying skin.[3]

Non-Operative Treatment

Watchful waiting is indicated for clients who do not have persistent pain or limitation of function.[2] The surgeon may also choose to aspirate the cyst with or without a corticosteroid. Studies have shown 60% recurrence of ganglions with this approach, although resolution can occur with repeated aspiration.[1]

> **⊙ Clinical Pearl**
>
> Aspiration and/or corticosteroid injection is not commonly performed for volar wrist ganglions because of proximity to the radial artery and potential for complications.[1] Surgery is best reserved for clients with persistently symptomatic ganglions.

Operative Treatment

Surgical resection is the most effective treatment, classically used after exhausting nonsurgical options.[4] The ganglion is excised, and a portion of the attached joint capsule is removed to prevent ganglion recurrence while protecting ligaments for carpal stability. If the tumor is solid or diagnosis is questionable, an open excision allows for biopsy of the tumor to assist with plans for further interventions. A client who chooses to have an operative mucous cyst excision usually does so for aesthetic reasons, pain, or ulceration of the overlying skin. It is important for the underlying osteophyte to be excised to avoid recurrence.[1] Occasionally the excisional aspect of the mucous cyst and underlying osteophyte requires a skin graft or flap.[5]

> **⊙ Clinical Pearl**
>
> Newer techniques in arthroscopic surgery have been shown to minimize postoperative complications with scar formation in dorsal wrist ganglions. The procedure is most suitable if the ganglion is on the dorsal aspect of the wrist in association with the scapholunate ligament. These procedures can be performed with minimal tissue trauma and better evaluation of the radioscaphoid and midcarpal joints of the wrist. This also ensures that a ganglion with multiple clefts is excised entirely.[5]

Timeline for Therapy

Non-Operative

Therapeutic timelines vary considerably, depending on whether the client has joint stiffness, functional impairment, and pain. Therapeutic approaches aim to preserve and improve function without pain. Goals should include:

1. Symptom management: Allowing tissue support with the use of a resting orthotic
2. Gentle home exercise programs (HEPs): Aimed at maintaining range of motion (ROM) and function
3. Instruction in heat and cold modalities as well as contraindications and precautions of both: For example, the client should not use heat if pain and swelling have increased; in this case, a cold pack would be appropriate for acute symptoms

Postoperative

If the client has had an open tumor excision, a bulky dressing is in place for approximately 5 days. ROM is usually initiated within the first 2 weeks postoperatively. Initially, avoid heat modalities, passive range of motion (PROM), passive stretching, or aggressive ROM. The client should be instructed in active range of motion (AROM) exercises to reduce scar formation and decrease stiffness and swelling in the wrist and digits. These activities may be painful initially; clients are instructed to perform exercises slowly. With dorsal wrist ganglion excision, volar wrist flexion *must* be emphasized.

If a skin graft or local flap is used for coverage of a DIP mucous cyst excision, the DIP joint will be immobilized, and the graft will be protected for approximately 2 weeks prior to beginning motion. Another reason to immobilize following a mucous cyst excision would be if the extensor tendon has to be detached and reattached to excise the cyst.

Precaution: *Following mucous cyst excisions, be cautious when considering passive joint stretching to avoid exacerbation of the underlying osteoarthritic joint changes.*

? Questions to Discuss with the Physician

- What structures were involved?
- If the ganglion was at the wrist, is wrist stability a concern?
- What are the medical expectations for recovery of ROM?
- When is AROM to be initiated?
- Should PROM be avoided?
- Are there any precautions?
- Is an orthotic indicated? If so, in what position? Should it be used for stability or for symptom management?[6]

() What to Say to Clients

Non-Operative Approach

"You may notice a fluctuation in size of your ganglion from time to time. You may also notice a fluctuation in size when you change the position of your hand and wrist. With heavy or repetitive use, pain and symptoms may increase but will subside with tissue rest. Wearing a forearm-based wrist orthotic may be helpful."

Operative Approach

"You might experience stiffness and pain with the use of your hand following surgery. Be careful to allow yourself time to heal. It is important to use your wrist, but your symptoms will increase with heavy use or activity. The goal is to have decreased pain. To achieve this, avoid the 'no pain, no gain' approach to rehabilitation."

Evaluation Tips

- Postoperative stiffness is best avoided with early and gentle wrist and digit ROM.
- Begin with AROM, especially volar wrist flexion. Avoid aggressive motion or passive stretching initially.
- Pinch and grip strength testing should not be performed initially as part of the evaluation if the client has been referred to therapy following an operative excision.
- History of acute trauma, activity with resultant wrist pain, or onset of a ganglion may be indicative of an underlying scapholunate sprain or other ligament sprain. Avoid aggressive ROM and strengthening if the ganglion is a result of trauma. If pain and functional limitations persist, the client should be re-evaluated by the physician or referred to a hand surgeon.
- Dorsal wrist ganglions can be easily confused with extensor tendon synovitis or a carpometacarpal boss . If the client has diffuse dorsal wrist swelling and/or pain with wrist and/or digit extension, the client more likely has extensor tenosynovitis. A carpometacarpal boss can be distinguished by the bony landmark of at the base of the second or third metacarpal.

Diagnosis-Specific Information that Affects Clinical Reasoning

Addressing the client's initial concerns when they are diagnosed with a ganglion is important. Typically, improved use of their hand without pain or improved cosmesis is their primary goal. "Perfect" ROM and strength does not take precedence over pain reduction and stability of the wrist.

♡ Tips from the Field

Orthotics

In a client who is treated non-operatively, a forearm-based wrist orthotic can help support tissue and joints of the wrist. The orthotic should be functional so that the client is able to perform activity with minimal pain. The orthotic is used as needed by the client.

On occasion, a DIP protection orthotic may be indicated for a client who has had a mucous cyst excision.

Client Expectations

Communication is vital between therapist and client for a successful outcome. The therapist must be clear about realistic goals for therapy and the importance of controlled progression of therapy, exercise, and activity. Likewise, the therapist should pay close attention to the client's goals and concerns in order to tailor a treatment plan that achieves these requirements.

Flare-Ups

It is inevitable that the client will aggravate their symptoms from time to time. A flare of pain or swelling is best treated with rest, orthotic management, and activity modifications. Symptoms will resolve as long as they are not continually aggravated.

Scar Maturation

A client with a ganglion excision should be taught scar management techniques as soon as the sutures are removed and the skin is healed enough to tolerate pressure. The client should be instructed in scar massage with pressure and stretch in order to limit excessive scar formation and adhesions to underlying structures. Silicone gel sheeting or paper tape can be issued for the client to wear on incisional sites, when healed, to assist with proper scar formation.

Complications

The most common postoperative complication is early ganglion recurrence following surgical excision. If a ganglion has not been excised completely, there is a high likelihood that it will return. Repeat excision can be performed; scar formation and adherence to underlying structures are of utmost concern and importance with repeat surgical excision in the same area. Neuroma formation can also be a complication following a surgical procedure if there is damage to a branch of a nearby sensory nerve.

Stiffness of the wrist or digits can be expected following a ganglion excision or with prolonged orthotic use. If volar wrist flexion limitations persist following dorsal wrist ganglion excision, very gentle static progressive wrist flexion orthotics are indicated, or treatment techniques, such as "heat and stretch" with the wrist placed in flexion to tolerance during heat application. If the client has underlying osteoarthritis of the digit or wrist, care and caution should be given before initiating passive stretches to avoid a flare reaction and increased pain.

- *With an excised dorsal wrist ganglion, the therapist should address and monitor wrist flexion, because this is most difficult for the client to regain.*
- *Monitor postoperative wound healing. Exercises that put stress on a wound site or incision with sutures delay healing and increase scar formation.*
- *If a skin graft or flap is required for a mucous cyst excision, avoid tension on the graft. Heat and cold modalities and DIP motion are contraindicated until approved by the physician. The client may require a DIP protective orthotic.*
- *Digital and thumb AROM are important postoperatively to avoid digital stiffness, to prevent and improve edema in the hand, and maintain soft tissue mobility. Provide HEPs for digital ROM early in therapy.*

Other Tumors of the Hand and Wrist

Most of the soft tissue masses that occur in the forearm and hand are benign. Of those that are benign, many can be diagnosed clinically, require no treatment, and are asymptomatic.[2] Most of the soft tissue tumors in the forearm and hand are not painful. The exceptions are glomus tumors, which are known to be very painful, or tumors that cause compression on a nerve. A small percentage of the tumors are malignant and may require aggressive medical treatment.

Diagnosis and Epidemiology

Diagnosis of the tumor relies on a thorough history and physical examination by the physician. Plain radiographs are often indicated to look for involvement of bone or presence of calcification within soft tissues. During the initial examination, if malignancy is a possibility, a MRI is currently the test of choice to further delineate the anatomy of the tumor.[1] Ultrasound, bone scans, and CT scans may also be used to further study the tumor. If malignancy is suspected, a **biopsy** (a sample taken surgically from the tumor) with possible excision is often indicated to determine the best course of action.

Types of Tumors

Giant-cell tumors are the second most common soft tissue tumors seen in the upper extremity. Other names for this benign tumor are **fibrous xanthoma, localized nodular tenosynovitis,** and **pigmented villonodular tenosynovitis.**[2] Although their various names indicate otherwise, the tumor does not uniformly contain giant cells and is not typically associated with the tendon sheath.[2] This tumor can be located on the volar or dorsal surface of the hand or finger. The most common location is on the volar surface of the proximal phalanx.[1]

Lipomas are common soft tissue tumors comprised of mature fat cells and characterized by their soft consistency. Typically, these tumors are not painful unless their slow growth causes compression on a nerve. Their size and location can vary widely in the upper extremity. The most common location within the hand is the deep palmar space.[1]

Vascular tumors in the forearm and hand can be either congenital or acquired. These tumors are typically a blue, red, or

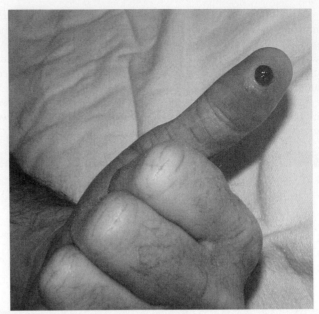

FIGURE 36-6 Pyogenic granuloma of the tip of the thumb. (From Haase SC, Chug KC: Skin tumors. In Wolfe SW, Hotchkiss RN, Pederson WC, et al, editors: *Green's operative hand surgery*, ed 6, Philadelphia, 2011, Churchill Livingstone.)

purple lesion. They may or may not be painful, or **pulsatile** (pulse is palpable).[1] Failure of congenital differentiation results in **hemangiomas** (benign tumors of dilated blood vessels), **congenital arteriovenous malformations** (abnormal connection between arteries and veins), and **lymphangiomas** (tumors of lymphatic vessels).[1] Common acquired vascular tumors are pyogenic granulomas and glomus tumors. A **pyogenic granuloma** presents as a red mass that bleeds easily (Fig. 36-6). It is generally accepted that this tumor is caused by trauma and subsequent infection. **Glomus tumors** are benign tumors comprised of all tissues contained in a glomus body. A glomus body is a normal structure, comprised of an arteriovenous anastomosis within the retinacular layer of the skin that functions as a thermoregulator. Glomus tumors are most commonly seen in the subungual region of the finger.[7] The triad of symptoms that often accompany these tumors are cold hypersensitivity, paroxysmal pain, and pinpoint pain.[7] Occasionally, these tumors will erode into bone.[7]

An **epidermal inclusion cyst** develops following a penetrating injury, in which a fragment of keratinizing epithelium is pushed into the subcutaneous tissue. This tissue proliferates, forming keratin that over the course of several years produces a tumor. They most commonly occur in males from 30 to 40 years of age, and the most common location is the left long finger or thumb.[2]

The two most common types of nerve tumors are **neurilemomas (schwannomas)** and **neurofibromas.** These benign tumors are rare, accounting for only 1% of tumors of the hand.[1] Neurilemomas are slow growing tumors that arise from the Schwann cells. They are most commonly located in the flexor surface of the forearm or hand. These tumors present in clients from 40 to 60 years of age and can be misdiagnosed as ganglion cysts.[2] Neurofibromas also arise from the Schwann cells but also involve the nerve tissue, which may cause neurological symptoms.[1]

Benign tumors of the epithelium include the common wart, or **verruca vulgaris,** caused by an infection with human papillomavirus. These tumors may involve any part of the hand, and are commonly found at sites of trauma. **Dermatofibroma,** also known as **cutaneous fibrous histiocytoma,** and **keratoacanthoma,** are benign epithelial tumors. These lesions are significant, because they can be confused with malignant epithelial lesions on the forearm and hand due to their appearance and coloration.[1]

The most common primary bone tumor in the hand is an **enchondroma,** accounting for 90% of hand bone tumors. Approximately 35% of these tumors occur in the hand. These benign cartilaginous tumors are most commonly found in the proximal phalanx, followed by the metacarpal, and middle phalanx.[2] These tumors are often diagnosed when the client presents with a fracture caused by a minor trauma or with an area of localized, likely painless edema.[2] These lesions may also be an incidental finding on plain radiographs.[2]

There are three types of malignant epithelial tumors, which are listed in the order of most to least rate of incidence in the forearm and hand: **squamous cell carcinoma,** which may spread to deeper tissues; **melanoma,** potentially life-threatening due to rapid spread to lymph nodes; and **basal cell carcinoma,** which tends to stay localized.[1] All of these tumors seem to have a direct link with sun exposure.

Soft tissue sarcomas are malignant tumors that originate in muscle and connective tissues. They are rarely seen in the forearm and hand. They can be aggressive and metastasize; therefore they may be medically managed aggressively with amputation, chemotherapy, and radiation therapy.[1]

Timelines and Healing

Timelines and healing for tumors vary widely. The medical management and general health of the client will determine the rate of wound closure. The type and extent of damage to tissues caused by the tumor and the course of treatment will certainly be a factor in functional outcome. A complex case involving a client with multiple comorbidities and treated with radiation therapy may have poor tissue quality and slower healing.

Non-Operative Treatment

- Since many spontaneously resolve, delayed treatment is the conventional treatment for hemangiomas that appear soon after birth.
- Warts are treated non-surgically (for example, cryotherapy or topical salicylate).
- Congenital arteriovenous malformations are initially treated with compression gloves, elevation, and medication.[1]

Operative Treatment

- Treatment for giant-cell tumors is surgical excision (Fig. 36-7). Recurrence rates for these tumors are high—up to 50%.[8]
- Large lipomas can be difficult to excise. Recurrence rates are low.[1]
- If surgery is deemed necessary for hemangiomas, it can be complex due to separating normal and abnormal tissues and risk of vascular compromise. Both feeder vessels are ligated, and the tumor is excised.[1] Surgery for a lymphangioma is equally as challenging but poses less risk to distal vascularity.

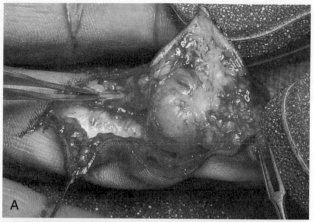
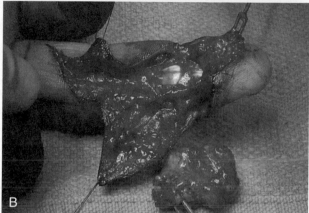

FIGURE 36-7 Surgical resection of giant-cell tumor of the tendon sheath. (From Sweet S, Kroonen L, Weiss L: Soft tissue tumors of the forearm and hand. In Skirven TM, Osterman AL, Fedorczyk JM, et al, editors: *Rehabilitation of the hand and upper extremity,* ed 6, St Louis, 2011, Mosby.)

- Excision of congenital arteriovenous malformations is reserved for painful lesions or those that have failed conservative management.[1]
- Surgical excision is the commonly accepted treatment of pyogenic granulomas; however, the use of electrocautery, silver nitrate, and laser has been attempted with some success.[1]
- The treatment of symptomatic glomus tumors includes excision of the tumor after first removing the nail plate and is followed by repair of the nail bed.[1]
- Inclusion cysts are excised with the goal of removing the entire wall of the cyst, as well as its contents, in order to minimize recurrence.[1]
- Neurilemomas can typically be excised without damage to the nerve fibers. Postoperative neurologic deficits following excision of neurofibromas are not uncommon, due to the involvement of underlying nerve tissue. Ten percent of clients have multiple neurofibromas, which is known as **von Recklinghausen's disease** or *neurofibromatosis.*[1]
- Usually, dermatofibromas are excised for differential diagnosis and to rule out malignancy.
- Medical management of malignant tumors depends on the clinical findings. Extensive surgery and reconstruction may be required to restore function. Chemotherapy and radiation therapy may also be utilized.

? **Questions to Discuss with the Physician**

- What structures were involved?
- What are the guidelines for wound care?
- What are the precautions and guidelines for AROM?
- What type of orthotic, if any, is desired?
- What is the long-term prognosis?
- If reconstruction for aesthetics or function is warranted, what other surgeries are planned?

( ) **What to Say to Clients**

"It will take time to heal from the surgery to remove your tumor. The surgery will leave a scar on your skin and below the surface. It will be important that you understand the correct exercises to do but also give your hand time to rest between exercises. Our main goals for therapy are to manage your scar tissue and swelling and regain the motion in your hand, in order to help you to return to everyday activities without pain. The tumor that you had removed may reoccur and require additional treatment in the future."

In addition, to prepare for discussions with clients, gather information from the physician and surgical reports. Be prepared to answer questions about the anatomy that is involved. Anatomy books are often helpful. Set timelines and realistic expectations to regain functional use of their hand. Clients will often ask if you have seen a similar case before; answer honestly.

Evaluation Tips

- First and most importantly, listen to your clients. You may be the first person they have been able to confide in about their concerns. Be gentle and supportive. They are most likely worrying about malignancy of their tumor and may be dealing with the impact of serious medical findings.
- Prioritize wound healing.
- Screen or assess sensory perception so that the client can be instructed regarding precautions as needed.
- Try to avoid any aspects of evaluation that cause pain.

◎ **Clinical Pearl**

Be aware that dressing changes, especially during the initial visit, may bother some clients more than others. Reactions can vary widely, so be prepared to assist clients with symptoms of nausea or being "light-headed." This may be especially true for clients who are concurrently undergoing radiation or chemotherapy treatment with hand therapy.

Diagnosis-Specific Information that Affects Clinical Reasoning

The therapist must communicate with the physician in order to have a clear picture of the medical diagnosis and treatment plan for each client. As discussed, there is variability for each type of tumor in presentation, location, functional implications, and medical management. This can make treating these clients challenging but rewarding.

♡ **Tips from the Field**

Orthotics

When an orthosis is needed, keep in mind the purpose of the orthosis, the anatomy that is involved, and the functional demands of the client. Tissues may be fragile and care should be taken to assure that the orthosis is comfortable. It is important to support the tissues adequately while preventing future deformities, especially if a nerve has been compromised.

Client Expectations

Be positive, and reassure clients about their functional use and hand appearance. Help them to set realistic expectations and to see gains they have made with review of measurements and/ or documentation of return to activities of daily living (ADLs).

Activities of Daily Living

Assisting the client to recover functional use of their upper extremity is an important part of the therapist's role. Find out what ADLs are important to the client, and incorporate these into the treatment. Also, consider use of adaptive equipment or task modification to allow the client to participate in home or work activities.

➢ **Precautions and Concerns**

- *Be aware that some physical agent modalities are contraindicated for a client who has had a malignant tumor excised.*
- *Instruct the client in ROM exercises for proximal uninvolved joints to prevent stiffness and reduce edema.*

CASE STUDIES

CASE STUDY 36-1 ■ Mucous Cyst

A 66-year-old, retired, right hand dominant female came to therapy 8 days following a right carpal tunnel release and right thumb IP mucous cyst excision. She stated that the majority of her trouble before surgery was numbness in her digits secondary to carpal tunnel syndrome. She elected to have the mucous cyst excised since "the doctor was already going to be operating on my right hand anyway." During the initial evaluation the client stated that her finger numbness was already improving, and she was independent with all HEPs related to the carpal tunnel release. She admitted that the majority of her pain and discomfort following surgery was with her thumb, and it bothered her that she was not able to bend her thumb well for functional activity and opposition. Her thumb IP motion was significantly limited and painful compared to the opposite hand, and her ADL function was limited due to inability to use her thumb. At 12 days post-surgery, the client was given gentle thumb AROM exercises, instructed in scar massage techniques, and provided with a thumb compressive sleeve to provide support and help decrease edema.

After 6 weeks of therapy the client confided that all of her symptoms with the carpal tunnel release were resolved, although she continued to have residual pain and stiffness in her thumb IP joint. She was now able to use her right thumb for most activities and was instructed in long-term HEPs for maintenance of thumb function, including AROM, use of heat agents as needed for comfort with use and exercise, and a resting static IP extension orthotic to help support and rest the joint and avoid an IP extensor lag. The client was pleased with the improvements in therapy and following her surgery, but was disappointed to have had "new" pain following the mucous cyst excision. When the patient was discharged, she was comfortable with self-management of her symptoms and use of long-term HEPs.

CASE STUDY 36-2 ■ Ganglion

A 37-year-old, right hand dominant, female came to therapy following an office visit with the hand surgeon. She explained to the therapist that she detected a volar wrist ganglion years ago that resolved spontaneously. However, with the recent birth of her third child, the ganglion reappeared and became painful with most activities. After electing to see a physician, she was referred to therapy for fabrication of a forearm-based wrist orthotic to assist with symptom management and rest to surrounding tissues. The client explained that she was not interested in surgery and stated that the physician had explained that she was not a candidate for an injection or aspiration of the cyst due to the proximity of the ganglion to the radial artery and potential of injury with steroid injection.

A forearm-based wrist orthotic was fabricated in a neutral wrist position and education was provided regarding the importance of wrist and digit ROM to avoid stiffness and how to wean from the orthosis if the symptoms subside. It is also explained to the client that she may need to wear the orthosis more often at first to help alleviate her acute symptoms, but that orthotic wear can be modified and reduced as symptoms of pain resolve. The client planned to use the orthosis during homemaking tasks and cooking, but will leave it

off while caring for her infant. She assured you that the therapeutic plan is great was glad to carry out her treatment plan independently, and planned to call and schedule a follow-up appointment only if pain and limitations of function persist. The patient called 1 month later and stated that her symptoms have nearly resolved and that the ganglion was not even visible most days. She had no further questions and was discharged from therapy.

CASE STUDY 36-3 ■ Soft Tissue Sarcoma

A 16-year-old male client came to the clinic with a diagnosis of a recently excised rare sarcoma in his right dominant wrist. The sarcoma was situated around and within the nerve fibers of his median nerve. After a biopsy, approximately 4 cm of his median nerve was completely excised at the wrist and distal forearm. The client was very apprehensive during the first few sessions about ROM of the wrist and forearm and had difficulty looking at his incision. The client had complete sensory loss in the median nerve distribution distal to the surgical site as expected. What was not expected was that motor function remained in the thenar eminence, which allowed very good fine motor skill, including writing and using eating utensils. The client apparently had an anatomical anomaly that provided motor innervation to most of his intrinsic thumb muscles. A volar forearm-based wrist orthotic was fabricated to support the healing tissues. Other treatment included wound care, gentle AROM and PROM, scar management, fine motor coordination tasks, and instruction regarding protection and compensation for the permanent sensory loss in his hand. When the client was discharged, he had weaned from the orthotic and resumed his normal ADLs. There were no plans for further surgery or medical treatment except monitoring.

References

1. Sweet S, Kroonen L, Weiss L: Soft tissue tumors of the forearm and hand. In Skirven TM, Osterman AL, Fedorczyk JM, et al, editors: *Rehabilitation of the hand and upper extremity*, ed 6, St Louis, 2011, Mosby, pp 289–301.
2. Athanasian EA: Bone and soft tissue tumors. In Wolfe SW, Hotchkiss RN, Pederson WC, et al, editors: *Green's operative hand surgery*, ed 6, Philadelphia, 2011, Churchill Livingstone, pp 2141–2195.
3. Teh J, Vlychou M: Ultrasound guided interventional procedures of the wrist and hand, *Eur Radiol* 19:1002–1010, 2009.
4. Gallego S, Mathoulin C: Arthroscopic resection of dorsal wrist ganglia: 114 cases with minimum follow-up of 2 years, *Arthroscopy* 26:1675–1682, 2010.
5. Edwards SG, Johansen JA: Prospective outcomes and associations of wrist ganglion cysts resected arthroscopically, *J Hand Surg Am* 34:395–400, 2009.
6. Cooper C: Ganglion cysts and other common tumors of the hand and wrist. In Cooper C, editor: *Fundamentals of hand therapy*, St Louis, 2007, Mosby, pp 412–420.
7. Koman LA, Paterson Smith B, Smith TL, et al: Vascular Disorders. In Wolfe SW, Hotchkiss RN, Pederson WC, et al, editors: *Green's operative hand surgery*, ed 6, Philadelphia, 2011, Churchill Livingstone, pp 2197–2240.
8. Plate AM, Lee SJ, Steiner G, et al: Tumorlike lesions and benign tumors of the hand and wrist, *J Am Acad Orthop Surg* 11:129–141, 2003.

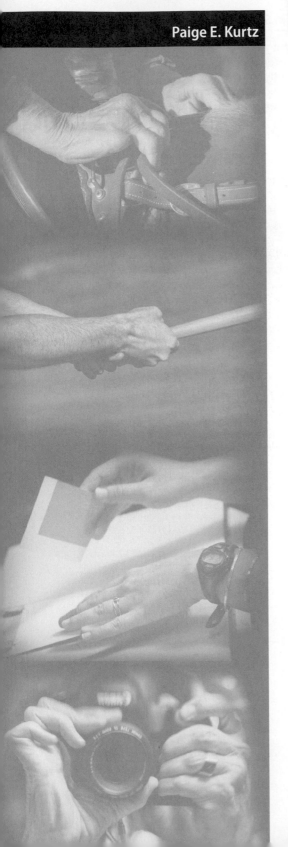

37 Traumatic Hand Injury Involving Multiple Structures

Paige E. Kurtz

Traumatic hand injuries can be both the most daunting and the most rewarding conditions that hand therapists treat. Deciding where to start with a new evaluation can be intimidating for a therapist; however, once therapy is underway, and throughout the rehabilitation process, the experience of participating in a client's recovery can be remarkable and rewarding. Being part of the progress from initial evaluation to final status and good function is truly gratifying.

The systems approach is the easiest way to evaluate, prioritize, and treat traumatic and complex injuries. Consider each individual system involved; then, for each system, determine the stage of the injury and how it can best be treated in light of necessary precautions. This approach makes it much easier to choose the correct interventions for each system according to its stage. Systems that should be considered include the skin (wound/graft), tendons (flexors, extensors, or both), nerves, blood vessels (veins and arteries), and bones (fractures, fusions, and joint surfaces). Pain and edema are additional considerations.

Plan ahead throughout the course of therapy. If future surgery is to be expected, incorporate that fact into the goals of therapy and treatment planning. For example, if tenolysis or tendon grafting is likely, maximize passive range of motion (PROM); if tendon transfer is expected, maximize the strength of potential donor muscles. During the process, continually educate your clients about what may be coming next and how current treatments will benefit them in the long run.

Most traumatic hand injuries involve many different structures and systems. The most extreme and complex injuries require a **replant;** that is, an amputated finger, hand, or arm is reattached surgically to re-establish viability and function. Not all traumatic hand injuries involve a replant or **revascularization** (a surgical procedure to repair severed arteries or veins to restore blood supply to a limb). However, the precautions and the decision-making and treatment processes are similar across the spectrum of these injuries.

> **◎ Clinical Pearl**
>
> Keep in mind that the goal of rehabilitation after a traumatic injury is not to regain a completely normal hand, but rather to regain maximal function with minimal pain.

As soon as possible, determine the reasonable functional outcome, given the extent and location of the injury; keep in mind that a client can be functional with less than "normal" range of motion (ROM). At this point, work with your client to set reasonable goals and expectations for both of you. Often, one of the most important parts of therapy is managing expectations and providing psychosocial support.

Precaution. *Achieving a pain-free hand with functional prehension, grip, and grasp is better than pushing to gain a few more degrees of ROM while jeopardizing stability. It usually is not worth risking the possibility of increasing pain and edema and reducing the chance of long-term success.*

Clients' satisfaction with their outcome is related to their expectations, as explained by the surgeon before surgery and reinforced by the therapist after surgery.[1]

Anatomy

Traumatic, multisystem injuries can involve many different structures from the surface of the skin through to the bone. Complex injuries, including replants and revascularizations, may occur at any level of the extremity, from the upper arm to the fingertips. To treat these injuries successfully, therapists must have a thorough working knowledge of the anatomy involved. They must know the locations and workings of veins and arteries; the stages of wound healing; the anatomy and healing processes of tendons, ligaments, and bone; and the biomechanics and interrelationships of these tissues and structures during functional movement.

The therapist first must understand the mechanics of a "normal" (that is, uninjured) hand, because this provides the basis for maximizing the client's hand function after surgery. If you understand the implications of the injury and the surgery, you will be better able to set realistic goals and formulate a good treatment plan. Decision making is related to healing times and sequences and may depend on the surgery performed. Some structures may need to be protected while others must be mobilized early in therapy; this can be difficult to manage. Treatment of the traumatic hand injury can become a balancing act, requiring you to determine which joints to move and which structures to protect, and when stability is more important than mobility. Some stress on healing structures is good because it stimulates healing, but too much stress can cause a loss of stability. How aggressively to push the therapy depends on the skills and knowledge of the physician and therapist, as well as the ultimate goals and expectations.

The therapist must know what tissues were disrupted and to what extent, the effect of different types of injuries on different tissues, and what surgical procedures were performed to repair those tissues. The position of the hand at the time of injury may affect which structures were injured and at which level (that is, the anatomic location of injury). The therapist must take into account the effect of the injury on surrounding, uninjured structures and attend to those uninjured structures throughout the extremity (for example, the shoulder or elbow) to prevent additional loss of function.

Anatomically, consider the functional implications of the anatomy and the injury. Moran and Berger[2] have described seven basic maneuvers that constitute basic hand function; these include three types of pinch and four types of grasp. These can be further categorized into two primary functional uses of the hand: pinch between the thumb and finger (or fingers) and grip. Pinch is affected by a radial side hand injury, which influences prehension and fine motor coordination. Grip is affected by an ulnar side hand injury, which diminishes composite grip and stability. Keep these functional movements in mind when planning treatment and devising exercises and activities.[3]

Clinical Pearl

Finger flexors offer more function than extensors. However, in ADLs, wrist extension generally is more useful than wrist flexion. The importance of the thumb's contribution to overall hand function cannot be ignored; thus, maintaining a good web space and opposition is critical. It is imperative to work for a strong, stable wrist; without it, finger function and grip strength will be impaired. Keep in mind also that regaining functional use of the hand is very difficult without functional sensibility.

Diagnosis and Pathology

Traumatic hand injuries can be caused by many types of force, from sharp lacerations to crush injuries. The mechanism of injury (for example, tearing, crushing, cutting, or twisting forces) and

---

BOX 37-1   Surgical Procedures Used To Treat Complex Hand Injuries

Skin
- Skin may be sutured in primary repair.
- Graft or flap may be placed for wound coverage.
- Skin may be left open for secondary closure to allow further debridement and to prevent constriction over vascular structures.

Tendons
- Flexors and extensors are repaired.
- Tendon grafts or transfers or tendon removal is performed in preparation for a future graft, often with insertion of a temporary spacer.

Nerves
- Nerves are repaired with or without grafting.

Blood vessels
- Veins and arteries are repaired with or without grafting.

Bone fixation
- Bone fixation is performed using bone grafts, fixators, wires, pins, plates, screws, or other devices.
- Joint arthroplasty implant may be inserted where joint surfaces cannot be repaired.
- Joint fusion may be performed.

---

the cleanliness of the wound are important pathologic factors. A closed crush injury may show little visible damage but may involve fractures or **ischemia** as a result of extensive damage to internal structures.

Primary treatment typically is performed in the emergency department, ideally with immediate referral to a hand specialist and replant team. The hand surgeon evaluates the injury with regard to what can and cannot be salvaged and restored to good function. Many systems and algorithms are available to aid problem solving and prioritization in the emergency department and operating room. Generally, the thumb, if salvageable, is always replanted as a priority. With multiple-digit amputations, the surgeon tries to replant as many as practical. Replants are nearly always attempted at any level in children. Incomplete amputations are also treated with maximum aggressiveness.[3] Box 37-1 lists surgical procedures used to treat complex hand injuries.

Timelines and Healing

Operative Treatment

Most or all involved structures are repaired surgically, depending on the timing of surgery and the extent of injury. The hand surgeon evaluates which structures can be repaired and which cannot be salvaged and therefore must be amputated or considered for later surgical interventions. Irrigation and debridement are performed first to remove contaminants and nonviable tissue.

The order of repair generally begins with stabilization of the injury. Blood flow and fracture stabilization are most critical, and these guide the surgeon's planning. Typically, bony injuries are fixed first, using techniques that are expedient but that also allow early ROM. Bone shortening may be done to allow for easier end-to-end repair of other structures. This ultimately can affect biomechanics, possibly resulting in compromised ROM and strength.

Tendon repairs often are performed next, unless the vascular status is severely compromised. When both flexors and extensors are involved, the surgeon tries to restore balance between the two, giving priority to functional flexion. Generally, vascular and nerve repairs are performed next, and then skin coverage is addressed.

The initial goal of the surgeon is to restore the framework that allows the client and therapist to work toward a good functional outcome with a reasonably strong structure, optimal skeletal alignment and joint mobility, vascular flow, and the potential for functional tendon balance and glide. If the injury is extremely complex, scar, tendon and nerve grafts, joint contractures, and other deficits may be addressed by further surgeries.

Many of the involved systems may be in different stages of healing after surgery. For example, a finger fracture may have good stability because of stable internal fixation, but an overlying skin graft or infection may delay wound healing. The systems approach can be very helpful for such cases.

Prioritize the systems during the initial evaluation. There is no specific hierarchy of systems; however, without healing in some systems, no further healing occurs in any of the others. The general order of importance is as follows:

1. Surgical repairs in arteries and veins (critical for providing nutrients for healing and survival of the repaired structures)
2. Bone injury, ligament injury, and fracture fixation (ROM exercises require a stable support structure)
3. Prioritize flexor tendons over extensor tendons (functional use favors flexors, although balance should be maintained as much as possible)
4. Nerves and sensibility (nerve recovery is a slow process; nerve injuries tend to be protected when nearby blood vessels and tendons are protected)
5. Edema (must be controlled and minimized, because it may contribute to stiffness and fibrosis)
6. Wound, scar, and soft tissue (prevent and minimize contractures)
7. Pain (if pain is not managed, clients cannot perform exercises)

The goals and priorities early in therapy (0 to about 3 weeks after surgery, the acute phase) are to manage and protect repairs, prevent joint stiffness in all uninvolved joints, control edema, manage the wound, manage pain, educate the client, and provide psychosocial support. As the client progresses into the intermediate phase (3 to 6 weeks after surgery), therapy focuses more on increasing ROM of involved structures, managing scarring, continuing wound care and protection, and initiating functional use of the involved extremity. Later phases focus on building and maximizing ROM, endurance, strength, and function.

? Questions to Discuss with the Physician

Whenever possible, obtain a copy of the operative report. Make sure you and the physician have the same understanding of treatment goals and expectations; do not hesitate to ask for clarification when needed (Box 37-2). Other important questions include the following:

- What types of repairs were done, and how strong are the repairs?
- What is the most appropriate orthotic position to protect the repairs?[4]
- What limits and restrictions were created by the surgical procedures?

BOX 37-2   Information Needed From the Physician

Therapists should make sure they obtain the following information from the client's physician or surgeon:

1. What do I need to hold (that is, protect) and what can I move?
2. What was injured, at what (anatomic) level, and what was repaired?
3. What type of injury was this (that is, crush, tear, blade/laceration, type of blade, clean or dirty injury)?
4. What are your expected outcomes and goals?

With Surgical Repairs

1. What structures were repaired and how?
2. What is the quality of the repairs?
3. What is the strength of the repairs?
4. Is there tension on any repairs?
5. What is the tendon quality; what is the relationship of the repair site to the pulleys?
6. How strong is any fracture fixation? Is anything fused? How is joint mobility? Was bone shortening performed?
7. Are any skin graft or flap precautions required?
8. Are any tissues or ROM to be protected?
9. Are there any tissues with questionable viability that should be watched closely?
10. What are your anticipated time frames for progression?
11. Were any structures not repaired? What is the plan for them?

Therapists spend considerable time developing a rapport with their clients, which means that clients sometimes are more likely to report problems and concerns to the therapist than to the physician. Also, therapists see clients more regularly and often are more likely to notice subtle changes that indicate potential problems.

◎ Clinical Pearl

Do not be afraid to confer with the physician in a timely manner on any information that appears to be important regarding the client's status, complaints, or problems.

( ) What to Say to Clients

About the Injury

Try to give clients perspective about their injury and realistic goals for the outcome. Teach them that a good outcome is about getting enough movement to use the hand to regain independence in normal everyday tasks but will not necessarily mean "normal" ROM. "I am not going to worry about getting your hand back to normal, we are going to focus on you being able to use your hand for as many normal things as possible." Work to develop a partnership: "I'm the coach, but you have to do the practices. We will work together to get you the best use of your hand. If you do not do your exercises consistently at home, there is nothing we can do a few times a week here in therapy that will make up for it."

Discuss the ramifications of not complying with contraindications and precautions: "If you are not careful about doing the exercises as I show you or you do not wear your orthosis, it could mean your hand will not heal as it should. If something goes wrong, it could even mean you'll need another surgery to fix your hand again."

Clients come to rely on their therapists for information, and they often ask questions they are afraid to ask the physician. Do not hesitate to refer the client to the physician for questions you cannot answer.

Clients often are more compliant with therapy and achieve better outcomes when the underlying anatomy and the healing process are explained to them in common terms. Try to explain what the client is attempting to achieve with specific exercises, using terms the client can understand. Provide basic information on how the flexors and extensors work and explain that many of the muscles that move the fingers originate near the elbow. When possible, use models, pictures, or drawings to show specific anatomic features. Explain how the normal anatomy was affected by the injury and what outcome the client should expect. If future surgery is likely, make sure the client understands that and incorporate it into the goals of therapy.

About Orthoses

The splint or orthosis is a critical component of protection and stability with traumatic injuries of the hand. Clients must understand that the orthosis may serve both protective and corrective functions; therefore it is essential that they wear it as directed by their therapist.

Help them understand the importance of the orthosis and why the hand is positioned a certain way: "This orthosis is important for protecting the injured structures in your hand so that they can heal correctly. If you take it off and move out of the position in which it holds your hand, some of the repairs may not be able to handle the stress of the new position."

About Exercises

Most clients are afraid to move any part of the hand immediately after surgery, especially if they feel pain, have swelling or open wounds, or if they can see pins sticking out of the hand. The therapist must stress the importance of movement despite these problems: "You will not hurt your hand if you do the exercises just as I showed you. If you do not do the exercises, getting good movement back will be more difficult. We cannot wait for the swelling to go away, the pins to come out, or the wound to heal before we start moving your fingers. By that time, your fingers will be really stiff, and it will hurt more to move them." Make sure the client understands that "more" exercises are not necessarily better, and that they should follow your directions on how often to exercise and how many repetitions to perform as closely as possible.

Evaluation Tips

- The initial evaluation may be mostly "hands off" because of the client's pain and fear and, often, the need to establish trust and rapport at this time. Before seeing the client, gather all information available on the type of injury and the treatment to this point, especially the operative reports. The initial evaluation may be a time to gain trust and establish ground rules, to do an overview assessment of the status of various systems, and

to perform necessary aspects of therapy (for example, wound care and orthosis fabrication).
- When you begin an evaluation, consider comorbidities and overall health status. Ask whether the client is a smoker or diabetic or has any other health problems. These can delay healing in all systems.
- Make sure to ask about support systems, including friends and family. Monitor clients' behavior toward the injured hand: Are they able to look at the hand, or do they treat it as if it belonged to someone else or as if they would like to get rid of it? To achieve a good outcome, the client must develop "ownership" of the injured hand and take some responsibility for recovery.
- Visually inspect the following:
  - Vascular status (check skin color)
  - Wound status (use wound color system: black, yellow, red) (see Chapter 5)
  - Finger stiffness (at the initial evaluation, measure full active range of motion [AROM] and PROM as appropriate, given precautions, and only if essential)
  - Edema (for example, minimal, moderate, or severe)
- Check ROM at uninvolved joints (for example, shoulder and elbow)

See Chapters 5 and 13 for more detailed information.

Clinical Pearl

At the initial evaluation, obtaining specific measurements is not as important as making a global assessment of the client's status, and establishing a baseline for treatment planning.

Diagnosis-Specific Information that Affects Clinical Reasoning

The following sections present a general discussion of the critical areas to evaluate for each system, precautions and contraindications, and healing guidelines and timelines. More detailed information on specific systems is available in the relevant chapter in this text.

Bone Injury: Fracture

With a complex injury, all surrounding and unaffected joints should be moved immediately, if possible, depending on the type and location of fracture and the type of fixation. Beginning ROM exercises as soon as the physician permits helps enhance fracture healing. During the evaluation, consider precautions, the type of fixation, and the expected stability of structures. The surgeon may have elected to shorten bony structures at the time of fixation. This may allow for a cleaner, more stable fixation, and it facilitates end-to-end repair of tendons, nerves, and blood vessels in the area; however, it also may greatly alter the mechanics of musculotendinous units in the arm and hand.

Surgical fixation may be achieved with pins and Kirschner wires, joint implants, plates and screws, interosseous wiring, or even joint fusion (Fig. 37-1). An important goal of surgery is to achieve as much stability as possible, creating the framework for movement in rehabilitation.[6,7]

Precaution. *Avoid excess stress at the fracture or fusion site or pin site and watch for signs of infection.*

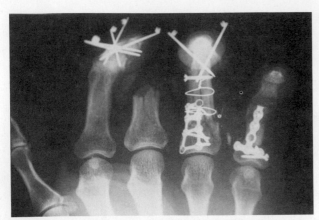

FIGURE 37-1 X-ray film showing amputation and internal fixation.

If revascularizations were done in conjunction with fracture fixation, the chance of delayed healing or nonunion is greater because of a decrease in the delivery of nutrients to the area.

Precaution. *A joint next to a fracture may need to be moved to begin ROM protocols. If this is the case, be aware of the location and type of fracture and the fixation and stability. Manually stabilize the bone during movement, and do not torque across the fracture site.*

If the surgeon has established sufficient fracture fixation, ROM around a fracture site may be initiated immediately, starting from the midrange and progressing to full ROM as appropriate, observing precautions for tendons, nerves, and vascular structures.[8]

See Chapters 25 and 27 for further indications, contraindications, and typical timelines for healing.

Revascularization: Arteries and Veins

Revascularizations and replants often are categorized together as the most complex injuries because injury to an artery or vein (or both) with revascularization affects peripheral blood flow, which in turn affects the potential for survival of nearly every other structure in the hand. In complicated cases, surgeons may not repair both arteries into a digit; the digit therefore has decreased vascularity because of the repair and because it has only one functioning artery.[4,7] After surgery, these clients are placed in a "hot" (for example, 75° F to 80° F) room in the hospital to help increase peripheral circulation. Keep in mind that the decreased circulation after arterial repair affects the healing rate of the wound, tendon, and fracture in an extremity because of the decrease in peripheral circulation and delivery of nutrients to the area.

If possible, have the client exercise with the dressing off so that you can observe the vascular status. Ideally, therapy should be performed in a comfortable, warm room, away from air conditioner vents. While working with the client, monitor the color, capillary refill, and temperature in the injured hand.

Precaution. *A dusky (grayish) finger or hand indicates severely diminished vascularity caused by arterial compromise; a purple color suggests venous congestion. Alert the referring physician if you note either a dusky or purple appearance. Either of these could signify distress for the finger, which could lead to failure of the replant.[10]*

A major precaution with revascularizations is to avoid anything that challenges the weakened peripheral vascular system. The client must not eat or drink anything vasoconstrictive, such as caffeine and chocolate. Smoking is prohibited, because it causes

severe vasoconstriction, reduces peripheral circulation, and affects the blood's ability to carry oxygen.[9] Compressive bandages (for example, elastic stockinette, tape, or gloves) should not be used for 3 to 8 weeks, until the vascular status has stabilized. Monitor for compression caused by orthotic material and straps. Constantly check the color of the fingers with regard to capillary refill.

Another precaution to keep in mind is to avoid using cold treatments in the acute phase (3 to 6 weeks or longer after surgery). If the injury occurs during the winter, advise the client to keep the hand warm with a mitten, an oven mitt, or a scarf for both comfort and safety. Many experts recommend avoiding the use of a whirlpool, because it puts the hand in a dependent position; if a whirlpool is used, it must be run at neutral temperature.[5,11] Contrast baths should also be avoided, because they may cause vasospasm followed by vasoconstriction. Mild heat may be used 4 to 8 weeks after surgery, once vascularity has stabilized. However, keep in mind that the insensate hand does not have a warning system to let the client know when a substance is too hot; it also cannot dissipate heat as well (that is, the tissue burns more easily). Although elevation is a good way to reduce edema, excessive elevation challenges the vascular system. The hand therefore should not be held significantly above the level of the heart, because this puts stress on the newly repaired arteries and can cause failure.[5]

Specific treatment considerations require positional protection of artery and vein repairs similar to that for flexor tendons (that is, an orthosis with the wrist and fingers flexed, such as a flexor tendon dorsal protective orthosis), because neurovascular bundles generally are volarly located (see Chapter 30). If the bone was not shortened, the physician may need to use vein grafts to ensure adequate circulation without putting tension on the system. If tension is unavoidable, precautions must be observed, such as more flexed positioning in the orthosis and in therapy. If no other injuries or complications are involved, vascular structures can be moved soon after surgery. If tendon injuries or fractures occur in the same digit, follow the highest level of precautions to protect these structures appropriately.

Nerve Injury: Laceration and Repair

Like vascular injuries, nerve injuries often occur with flexor tendon injuries. In such cases, treat according to the appropriate flexor tendon protocol. Tension on the nerve guides decision making on protocols. As with tendon injuries, establishing early gliding is essential.

A nerve injury leaves part of the hand insensate. This is not a significant problem in the early phase of therapy, while the client is continually wearing the orthosis. However, it becomes a concern when the client begins to perform activities of daily living (ADLs) out of the orthosis.

Precaution. *The client must be taught to take care with ADLs (for example, heat, sharp objects); the eyes must be used as a sensory guide for the nerves. The therapist must use caution with use of a dynamic or static progressive orthosis and any other external compression, as well as heat and ice, because of the lack of a warning system for ischemia.*

A client with decreased sensibility may be unable to tell whether the temperature of a substance is excessively hot or cold.

A full sensibility evaluation is not necessary immediately after a traumatic hand injury. Because it takes some time for the repaired nerves to reinnervate an area, a cursory screening is practical at the initial evaluation to detect areas of sensory deficit. A full sensibility evaluation rarely is worthwhile earlier than 1 month after surgery. Follow-up re-evaluations should be performed approximately once a month thereafter, because nerves regrow slowly from the injury site to the distal fingertips

After the client has regained protective sensation, begin sensory reeducation to teach the brain to recognize signals from the peripheral nerves.[5] Start with constant pressure and moving touch. Begin with the client's eyes open and progress to eyes closed; vary between the involved and uninvolved side or area. Desensitization exercises should be performed for hypersensitivity.

◎ Clinical Pearl

Remember that sensitivity to and intolerance of cold are common for up to 2 years after a nerve injury and sometimes longer.[9,19]

See Chapter 24 for more specific information.

Flexor and Extensor Tendons: Tendon Repair

Most hand therapists are familiar with the treatment of either flexor tendon injuries or extensor tendon injuries, but prioritizing becomes more difficult when the two must be treated at the same time. With a replant or if both flexors and extensors have been lacerated, priority almost always is given to the flexors over the extensors, because flexion is more important for function. However, the ideal is to maintain a normal balance between the two systems **(tenodesis).** A replanted hand or finger usually is immobilized in a position similar to that for a flexor tendon injury, because the *safe position* is relatively balanced, slightly favoring the flexors and neurovascular bundles over the extensors. Gliding of involved structures should be increased as soon as possible to increase the delivery of nutrients, enhance healing, reduce edema, and reduce the potential for adhesions.

Treatment rules generally are the same as those for typical hand therapy protocols with regard to healing phases. Therapy after replantation should follow a version of the referring physician's preferred flexor tendon protocol, modified to protect the extensors. Generally, begin metacarpophalangeal (MP) joint ROM, along with limited ROM of the proximal interphalangeal (PIP) and distal interphalangeal (DIP) joints, to prevent extensor lag and increase ROM via tenodesis. Major precautions are similar to those for flexor and extensor tendon protocols: protect against a full active fist or full extension of the fingers, and avoid resistance until the structures have healed. If bone shortening was performed, the normal biomechanics of both the flexors and extensors will have been modified, therefore completely normal ROM is not a practical expectation.

For more specific information, guidelines, and protocols, see the description of early protective motion (EPM) later in this chapter; also see Chapters 30 and 31.

Edema

Increased edema causes increased resistance with AROM. This is a very important consideration in the introduction of early ROM for a complex traumatic injury. Longstanding, significant edema leads to increased fibrosis and scar formation. Edema can be evaluated by means of circumferential measurement, volumetric measurement (after wound closure), or visual, subjective assessment of the edema as minimal, moderate, or severe.

Treatment for edema begins with elevation of the hand to the level of the heart and not significantly higher. Excessive elevation challenges the damaged and repaired arterial system in the hand or arm.[11,17] It is important to avoid compression after revascularization until a stable, strong vascular flow has been re-established; this can take 6 to 8 weeks. AROM exercises can be performed as appropriate in the treatment protocol to create a pumping mechanism. Longstanding edema and the fibrosis that often occurs after a traumatic hand injury usually result in larger digits, and the client probably will have to have rings resized. To determine the most stable size, the client should wait 6 to 12 months after the last surgery to have jewelry resized.

Compression may be used after the vascular system has stabilized. Such devices and techniques include elastic bandages, compressive gloves, elastic stockinette, manual edema mobilization, or retrograde massage. See Chapter 3 for more specific management protocols.

Wound Healing and Scar Management

The presence of an open wound can change treatment priorities. Complex wounds often accompany complex injuries. Wound evaluation should include assessment and documentation of location, size, color (red/yellow/black), and drainage (type, color, and amount). Watch for signs of infection, which include redness that extends beyond the area of the wound, warmth, increased edema, increased pain, drainage, and unusual colors and odors (see Chapter 21).

Skin grafts must be treated with special care until they have stabilized. The precautions are similar to those for a typical wound with special attention paid to avoiding friction and excessive compression over the graft site. Good nutrition is critical for wound healing, including an adequate intake of protein and vitamins. Encourage the client to discuss nutrition questions with the physician or other experts as appropriate.

Treat all wounds with care to avoid shear or mechanical stress from dressings and to prevent maceration while maintaining a moist wound bed.

Precaution. *Do not use cytotoxic chemicals, such as peroxide and povidone-iodine, on granulating wound tissue.*

Although agents, such as povidone-iodine and peroxide, are helpful for reducing contaminants in a wound, they also can affect the viability of new tissues.

In the early stages, wound care focuses on promoting healing and wound closure, preventing infection, and protecting healing structures.[11] In later stages, wound management involves efforts to modify and manage scarring through the use of scar massage, gel sheets, Otoform, elastomer, and so on. Therapy attempts to manage and control scarring while preventing future problems, such as the formation of adhesions and contractures. Keep in mind that scar heals all injured structures. Scar is essential for healing, but it must be managed to minimize adhesions, which limit tendon glide, and scar contractures, which occur as the scar matures. It is important to control these two side effects of scarring because they limit ROM.

Scar tissue is different from normal skin tissue. It has less tensile strength and therefore may be more susceptible to abrasions and tearing. Scar tissue also sunburns easily and should be protected from sun exposure for approximately 6 months or until the scar is pale, soft, and supple. An easy way to protect scars on the hand is to cover them with a lip balm that has a high sun protection factor (SPF). The heavy, waxy balm stays on the scar, and the tube is portable and inexpensive.

See Chapters 21 and 34 for further information on wounds and scar management.

Pain

Pain affects the client's ability to deal with an injury and to follow a home exercise program (HEP). Pain is normal with a complex injury. However, when the pain is out of proportion to the injury for some time, a psychologic consultation may be beneficial.

Orthoses

Appropriate orthosis use and fabrication is important for supporting the injured hand, maintaining a position of balance, protecting the injured and repaired structures, and preventing future deformity. The orthosis typically used for a replant is similar to that for flexor tendon lacerations: a forearm-based dorsal block orthosis with the MP joints in flexion and the interphalangeal (IP) joints in extension. The exact wrist position depends on the structures involved and the surgeon's preference.

> ### ◎ Clinical Pearl
>
> When fabricating an orthosis consider the locations of pins, the vascular supply with regard to strapping and pressure areas, and tension on nerve or tendon repairs. Avoid placing straps directly over repair sites. Use wide straps to spread pressure over the hand.

> ### ◎ Clinical Pearl
>
> Prioritize the problems and orthosis design to support and protect the most significant concerns while maintaining a balance between the flexors and extensors.

Protocols for Mobilization

No true protocols exist for mobilization because injuries vary so widely. However, general guidelines are based on two approaches, delayed mobilization and early mobilization.

Delayed Mobilization

In some cases delaying mobilization is appropriate, because it allows the initial inflammatory response to decline while structures heal in a balanced position. As a result, fewer precautions are necessary after the immobilization period. Delayed mobilization may be used for young children or for any client who may not be fully cooperative.

If the MD prescribes this protocol, immobilize the hand in protected position (flexed wrist and finger, similar to the position used in a dorsal protective flexor tendon orthosis and keep it wrapped in a bulky compressive dressing for 3 weeks. At 3 weeks after surgery, fit the client with a removable dorsal block orthosis (wrist flexion of 15°, MP flexed 50° to 70°, and PIP/DIP joints fully extended to 0°, unless different positioning is prescribed by the surgeon), and begin gentle AROM exercise of the replanted

TABLE 37-1	Delayed Mobilization Protocol for Replants
Postoperative	**Exercise or Intervention Timeline**
0 to 3 weeks	No ROM
3 weeks	AROM of involved structures PROM of uninvolved structures
4 weeks	NMES
6 weeks	Dynamic orthosis PROM of involved structures Initiate use of hand for ADLs
8 to 10 weeks	Strengthening exercises

ADL, Activity of daily living; *AROM,* active range of motion; *NMES,* neuromuscular electrical stimulation; *PROM,* passive range of motion; *ROM,* range of motion.

digit or digits, along with full AROM and PROM of uninvolved digits. Initiate light manipulation activities as soon as practical, to enhance ROM exercises. At 4 weeks after surgery, add neuromuscular electrical stimulation (NMES) to assist with tendon glide. With medical clearance, at 6 weeks, initiate PROM in the replanted digit 6 weeks after surgery if fractures have healed sufficiently. If the fracture is clinically healed, add a dynamic or static progressive orthosis as needed. Have the client begin using the hand out of the orthosis for light ADLs after 6 weeks, making sure precautions for the insensate parts of the hand are observed. Begin with use of the hand in eating meals and slowly incorporate more ADLs. Add strengthening exercises at 8 to 10 weeks after surgery after verifying solid fracture healing (Table 37-1).[13]

Early Mobilization

EPM is a suggested replant treatment guideline that has been described in the hand therapy literature.[14,15] EPM is based on the premise that it allows for differential tendon glide and early movement while maintaining a balance between the flexors and extensors and minimizing the tension on repaired structures by means of tenodesis (in therapy this refers to mobilization of one or more joints by using the tendinous connections that run past those joints and the relationship between flexors and extensors). Tenodesis is seen with the natural flexion of the fingers that occurs when the wrist is extended and the natural extension of the fingers that occurs when the wrist is flexed. This protocol can be used for digital or hand replants characterized by stable fixation and a clean injury.

Early Protective Motion I. The first treatment phase is EPM I. This phase begins 4 to 10 days after surgery (or 24 hours after discontinuation of anticoagulants), once viability of the replanted part has been established. Fit the client in a dorsal block orthosis with the wrist in neutral to slight flexion and the fingers in maximum practical MP flexion and IP extension. The orthosis may be refitted as tolerated to increase MP flexion and IP extension later in the program. Initiate clinical and home exercises at this time.

Focus on using a gentle, passive tenodesis motion to proportionally move the MPs, IPs, and wrist. Help the client passively extend the MP and IP joints (naturally and with gentle assist) while the wrist is gently flexed (actively, if appropriate) (Fig. 37-2). Then help the client actively extend the wrist to neutral (with passive assist as needed) while you and gravity assist the fingers into MP flexion (Fig. 37-3). Ideally, PIP and DIP extension are

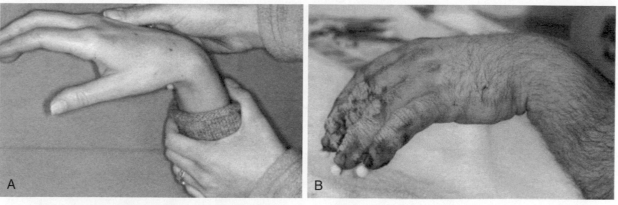

FIGURE 37-2 A and **B,** Early protective motion (EPM) I wrist flexion and MP/IP extension.

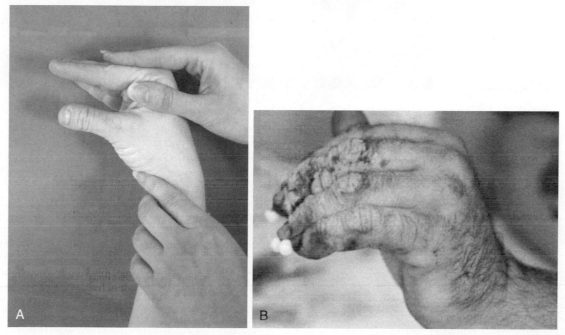

FIGURE 37-3 A and **B,** EPM I wrist extension with MP flexion.

increased at the same time through viscoelastic forces in the hand. This movement must be proportional and balanced between flexors and extensors. The goal of EPM I is to establish gliding of the intrinsic and extrinsic flexors and extensors and the wrist and MP joints to minimize stiffness while protecting involved structures.

Precaution. *EPM I should be modified if the MPs are tight or severely limited by edema or joint stiffness, if bony fixation is not stable enough to tolerate ROM in nearby joints, or if related structures were repaired under tension.*

AROM should be performed regularly for all uninvolved and proximal joints throughout the day. Exercises may be used to strengthen proximal musculature if the client is compliant. Contralateral strengthening, by means of motor neuron retraining, may be used to minimize loss of strength.

Early Protective Motion II. The EPM protocol is advanced to passive EPM II 7 to 14 days after surgery, after a few days of EPM I movement. The goals of this phase are to reduce tendon adhesions, prevent/minimize PIP joint stiffness, provide differential tendon gliding, and improve tendon tensile strength. The client should continue EPM I while adding the intrinsic plus "table"

and intrinsic minus "hook" exercises to enhance differential gliding and gentle contraction of the long flexors and extensors and intrinsics; the wrist remains neutral throughout the hook position. To create the hook position, passively extend the MP joints and gently assist the PIP and DIP joints into slight flexion (Fig. 37-4).

Precaution. *Limit PIP flexion to less than 60° until 4 to 6 weeks after surgery to protect the central slip. If resistance is felt, do not progress ROM further.*

From the hook position, move to the table position, using gravity to assist flexion of the MP joints while assisting extension of the PIP and DIP joints into neutral (intrinsic plus) (Fig. 37-5). Interestingly, in the intrinsic plus position, the flexor digitorum superficialis (FDS) and flexor digitorum profundus (FDP) tendons are virtually inactive, because MP flexion and PIP extension in this position are primarily achieved with contraction of the interossei and lumbrical muscles. Therefore a strong contraction in this position should not overly stress the repairs to the long flexors or extensors.

Significant edema or extensor tendon damage limits PIP joint ROM in this protocol and should alert you to progress slowly.

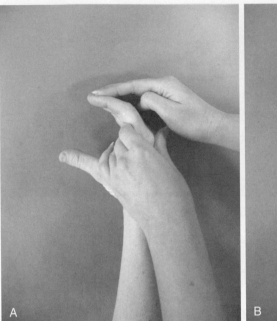
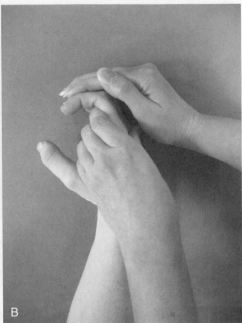

FIGURE 37-4 EPM II hook position.

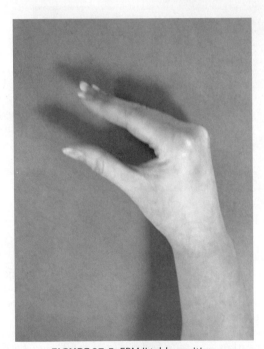

FIGURE 37-5 EPM II table position.

⊚ **Clinical Pearl**

Slow, gentle movement helps reduce edema, gentle stress on healing tissues can help stimulate healing, and some gliding in the extensors can reduce extension-limiting adhesions. According to Silverman,[14,15] the hook to table movement is the most effective and safest movement that allows ROM at all three joints of the fingers, along with gliding of both long flexors (the FDS and the FDP) and all components of the dorsal mechanism and the extrinsic extensor (extensor digitorum communis).

Active EPM II is initiated 14 to 21 days after surgery. Progress to place and hold exercises by assisting the hand into the intrinsic minus hook position. Ask the client to hold the position with a gentle active contraction, then move the hand to the intrinsic plus table position and again ask for an active contraction. At this point, as appropriate and tolerated, add active gliding and isolated FDS gliding exercises and strengthen the interossei in the intrinsic plus position. This upgrade allows initiation of active gliding in non-composite range, continuing use of tenodesis and relying on balance to move the intrinsic and extrinsic flexors and extensors without overstressing any system. Initiate use of functional exercises as soon as able. These may include picking up large beads and putting them into a container using modified prehension (Fig. 37-6). Returning to "normal" activities as soon as possible helps the client to regain a more functional, positive connection between the brain and the hand.

At 4 weeks after surgery, the client may begin gradually to increase wrist extension past neutral with the digits loosely flexed, increasing overall tenodesis-related ROM. The client also should slowly progress toward full composite active flexion and extension at this time (depending on tightness). Continue to reassess the orthosis to ensure correct fit and positioning.

Six weeks or later after surgery, add gentle passive stretching, NMES as indicated for adhesions, and more aggressive blocking exercises and upgrade functional exercises. Continue to progress with caution, given the likelihood that replanted or revascularized structures will heal more slowly than expected because of their diminished vascular and nutritional status. Introduce use of a dynamic or static progressive orthosis as appropriate for stiffness, but in this area, also, keep in mind that circulation will not be normal. Spread out pressure across as wide an area as possible with wide straps and cuffs and good orthosis contour and by keeping traction light. A serial static extension orthosis worn at night can provide gentle stretch over many hours and does not interfere with functional use during the daytime.

If the physician has assessed and verified fracture consolidation, add pinch and grip strengthening as early as 8 weeks after

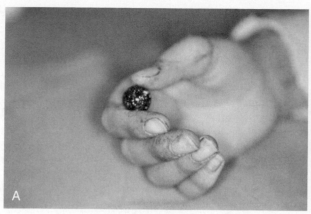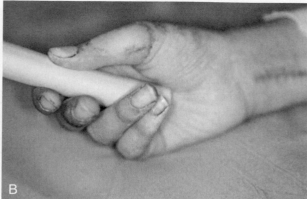

FIGURE 37-6 A, Functional prehension exercises. **B,** Functional grasp exercise.

TABLE 37-2	Highlights of Early Protective Motion Protocol
Postoperative Timeline	**Exercise or Intervention**
4 to 10 days	EPM I MP extension with wrist flexion MP flexion with wrist extension
7 to 14 days	EPM II passive Continue EPM I Passively move client's fingers between "table" MP flexion with IP extension (intrinsic plus) and "hook" MP extension with IP flexion (< 60°) (intrinsic minus)
14 to 21 days	EPM II active Continue EPM I and EPM II passive Place and hold hook and table positions Progress to active hook and table Isolated FDS tendon exercises Interossei strengthening (intrinsic plus) Light functional activities
28 days	Increase wrist extension to full with flexed fingers Progress to full AROM and finger PROM Begin gentle blocking exercises
6 weeks	NMES Passive stretching of involved structures Full nonresistive use for ADLs (precautions for insensate hand) Dynamic orthosis use
8 weeks	Light strengthening exercises

ADL, Activity of daily living; *EPM,* early protective motion; *FDS,* flexor digitorum superficialis; *IP,* interphalangeal; *MP,* metacarpophalangeal; *NMES,* neuromuscular electrical stimulation; *ROM,* range of motion.

surgery. Continue to upgrade the program, emphasizing reconditioning of the entire upper extremity. Table 37-2 presents highlights of the timelines and interventions for EPM. (See Silverman and colleagues[14,15] and Chan and LaStayo[5] for a more specific description of this protocol.)

Amputation

The hand surgeon generally makes every effort to salvage viable tissues in the hand. However, amputation is preferable to spending time and energy trying to save a finger that ultimately would remain stiff, insensate, and nonfunctional. This is especially true if the stiff finger would interfere with the functioning of the remaining digits.[8]

From a therapy standpoint, amputations are simple to treat because relatively few precautions are required. The primary focus is on promoting uncomplicated wound healing and desensitizing sensitive tissues. Neuroma formation is a possibility, and this may be addressed through desensitization and use of a variety of gel sheeting products.

The most serious problem with amputations may be the psychologic effect on the client. Although any traumatic injury may result in a malformed hand, the loss of a digit often causes the greatest stress and concern to the client. By emphasizing the positive effects of the amputation on overall functional recovery, the therapist can aid the client in coping with this loss. Functional or cosmetic prostheses may be helpful later, and showing the client pictures of these early on also can be helpful. If the client continues to greatly mourn the loss, referral to a psychiatric professional may be appropriate.[18]

Secondary Procedures

Despite the hard work of both the client and the therapist, secondary procedures are common after therapy is completed and when a clinical plateau has been reached. During the last phase of therapy, as you head toward discharge, consider the remaining issues that might be addressed with a secondary surgery. Assess for and address tightness of the joint capsule, intrinsic and extrinsic tightness, tendon and scar adhesions, and scar contracture; and plan ahead for future surgeries, which may include tenolysis, capsulectomy, joint contracture release, web space revision, tendon graft, and tendon transfers.[16] Maximizing PROM and strength is important before tenolysis and many other follow up procedures. Communicate with the physician so that you understand the surgical procedures and objectives in advance; then, explain the next surgery to the client, in addition to the probable course of therapy so that you can help them develop reasonable time and commitment expectations before undertaking another procedure.

Summary

Treatment of a traumatic hand injury requires simultaneous evaluation and management of many different types of injuries and the results of surgical procedures. An organized, logical systems approach allows you to assess each system individually and then prioritize the systems for treatment. Taking care to follow precautions is the guiding principle for treatment.

In traumatic hand injuries, the therapist can help produce significant improvements in appearance and function while working with a client over many months from initial evaluation to discharge. For this reason, treating these clients can be a very rewarding experience for a hand therapist.

Additional Thoughts on Diagnosis-Specific Information

- Determine which systems are involved, and then prioritize them.
- Determine the stage of each system, and decide how to treat this stage appropriately.
- Fracture fixation affects the appropriateness of early AROM and PROM.
- Healing varies with age, health, nutritional status, and smoking status. Vascular repairs can delay healing.
- Edema affects tendon glide and ROM by increasing resistance to movement, creating adhesions and fibrosis, and increasing pain.
- There is a fine line between being as aggressive as possible to improve the condition and being too aggressive. Some stress on healing systems encourages healing but being too aggressive can lead to fracture nonunion or tendon rupture or other problems. The ideal is to move everything as early as possible without compromising the surgical repair. *Monitor tissue responses and adjust the therapeutic regimen accordingly if a flare reaction occurs.*
- Incorporate functional exercises into therapy as soon as possible. Clients who are medically cleared to perform AROM can work on picking up, holding, and turning objects in their hands or on passing items from hand to hand.

> ◎ **Clinical Pearl**
>
> Clients tend to respond better to short frequent exercise sessions of fewer repetitions performed more often than to lengthy sessions performed infrequently.

Precaution. *Respect pain; modify exercises for limitations.*
- Work within a reasonable pain tolerance; ask clients to get to their end-range and then hold.
- Make therapy interesting, creative, functional, and purposeful.
- Consider functional outcomes and goals—strength needs versus endurance needs for work and ADLs.
- Strengthen every joint through the maximum available range. If you notice the client is "cheating" or cannot move a weight through full ROM, consider reducing the resistance.
- Strengthen proximal joints and the contralateral side as soon as possible after therapy. Use bilateral exercises and activities to demonstrate and "retrain" the involved hand.
  See Chapter 4 for more information on strengthening.

> ➤ **Precautions and Concerns**

Revascularizations (Arterial and Venous Flow)

- *Decreased circulation after arterial repair affects the rate of healing for wounds, tendons, and fractures because of the decrease in peripheral circulation and delivery of nutrients to*

the area. Typical protocol timelines generally must be extended by a few weeks.
- *Keep the hand warm and avoid exposure to cold or sudden/extreme temperature changed by using a mitten, an oven mitt, or a scarf.*
- *In the early phase of healing, be very gentle when changing dressings; avoid changing them in cold, drafty areas (for example, under an air conditioning vent).*
- *Emphasize to clients that they must not eat or drink anything vasoconstrictive, such as caffeine or chocolate. Smoking is prohibited. Appropriate hydration and nutrition are imperative for healing.*
- *Do not use compressive bandages (elastic tape, gloves, sleeves) until vascular status has stabilized.*
- *Prevent compression from orthosis material and straps.*
- *Constantly monitor the color of the fingers with regard to capillary refill.*
- *Do not use cold treatments in the acute phase.*
- *Do not use a whirlpool, because it puts the hand in a dependent position.*
- *Do not use contrast baths, because they may cause vasospasm followed by vasoconstriction.*
- *Mild heat may be used once vascularity has stabilized. However, the insensate hand does not have a warning system to let the client know when a substance is too hot; also, it cannot dissipate heat as well (that is, it burns more easily).*
- *Although elevation is a good way to reduce edema, excessive elevation challenges the vascular system; the hand should not be held significantly above the level of the heart.*

Tendon Repairs

- *Protect against a full active fist or full extension of the fingers.*
- *Avoid resistance from excessive co-contraction in early stages.*
- *Edema increases resistance during early ROM exercises; modify your approach if you encounter resistance.*

Fractures

- *Avoid excess stress at fracture, fusion, or pin sites while mobilizing a complex injury.*
- *If revascularization has been done in conjunction with fracture fixation, expect delayed healing or nonunion as a result of a decrease in the delivery of nutrients to the area.*

Nerve Injury and Repair

- *Nerve injuries leave part of the hand insensate. Teach the client to use caution with ADLs (that is, avoid injury from exposure to heat or use of sharp objects).*
- *Use caution with use of dynamic or static progressive orthoses and any other external compression because of the lack of a warning system for ischemia.*
- *Also use heat and ice treatments cautiously.*
- *Remind the client that cold intolerance and pain after a nerve injury is common for 2 or more years.[19]*

Incisions, Wounds, and Grafts

- *Make sure that dressings do not exert shear or mechanical stress on healing wounds.*
- *Prevent maceration while maintaining a moist wound bed.*
- *Avoid using cytotoxic chemicals (for example, peroxide, povidone-iodine) on granulating wound tissue.*

CASE STUDY 37-1 ◾

M.H., a 15-year-old, right hand dominant, male high school student sustained a complex laceration of his right hand while cutting a piece of wood with a saw blade during shop class. Because he was cutting wood, the wound was relatively clean. However, because the saw blade was an old one, it did a moderate amount of tearing damage. The following injuries were noted:
- Thumb: Amputation at the MP joint
- Index finger: Laceration of FDS and FDP, radial and ulnar neurovascular bundles
- Middle finger: FDS and FDP laceration, open fracture of the metacarpal neck, lacerations of the radial and ulnar digital arteries and veins in the digit (radial digital nerve [RDN], ulnar digital nerve [UDN], radial digital artery [RDA], and ulnar digital artery [UDA])
- Ring finger: Laceration of FDS and FDP, RDN, UDN, UDA
- Small finger: Extensor tendon laceration

The following procedures were performed:
- Thumb: Replant with MP arthrodesis, vein graft, flexor pollicis longus (FPL) tendon repair, extensor repair, nerve repair, artery repair
- Index finger: Revascularization, repair of common digital artery to ulnar digital artery, FDS/FDP repair in zone II, repair of RDN/UDN
- Middle finger: Debridement of metacarpal head and neck (intra-articular fracture), volar plate repair, repair of common digital artery to ulnar digital artery, FDS/FDP repair in zone II, nerve repair
- Ring finger: RDN/UDN repair, FDS repair in zone II, excision of FDP, insertion of Hunter rod
- Small finger: Debridement, repair of 50% extensor laceration just proximal to PIP joint

M.H. had his first outpatient appointment with the hand surgeon 6 days after surgery. The physician changed his dressing, and he was referred for an orthosis and hand therapy. The orthotic order stated: "Orthoplast to tips, thumb spica, wrist 10° flexion, MPs at 90° in digits." The therapy referral requested "modified Duran protocol, no movement of thumb, ignore ext in small finger (only partial injury)."

At his first hand therapy visit, M.H.'s hand was rebandaged with the lightest possible dressing, and he was fitted with a dorsal protective orthosis with slight wrist flexion and maximum reasonable MP flexion. The thumb was positioned in mid-abduction for protection in a safe position and to minimize the potential for web space contracture (Fig. 37-7).

Although this had the elements of a complex injury, problem solving using the systems approach highlighted some exceptions worth considering in the treatment planning:
- The replant injury occurred in the thumb. Because of the importance of this digit, the surgeon opted for a delayed mobilization protocol to protect the revascularization and fusion. Also, because the thumb is relatively independent, it could be considered and treated separately from the other digits. While the thumb was primarily immobilized, tenodesis exercises to the fingers would have some effect on gliding of some of the structures in and near the thumb.
- Most of the tendon injuries occurred in the flexors; therefore they could be treated as simple tendon lacerations with revascularization and nerve repair. According to the surgeon's orders, the small finger extensor tendon injury was not treated as a precaution, and this led to implementation of a modified version of the Duran protocol.
- Precautions for revascularization were followed throughout therapy for the vascular repairs.
- The fracture at the thumb MP joint was fused and was treated therapeutically as a fusion. The fracture at the middle finger MP joint did not significantly affect any protocols.

Initial Evaluation

At the initial evaluation, the following findings were noted:
- Pain: 3 to 5 on a scale of 1 to 10 (3-5/10)
- Edema: Moderate in digits and palm
- Sensibility: Not tested (NT), anticipated loss secondary to nerve injuries
- Wounds: Slight serosanguineous drainage
- ROM: Passive flexion to within 1 inch of palm; extension of middle finger, ring finger, small finger to orthosis; index finger has 30° flexion contracture at PIP; ROM to thumb and wrist not attempted

The therapist kept the initial evaluation brief and cursory to get a good overview of the situation.

Therapy Goals
Short-Term Goals
1. Protect injury and surgical repair through use of protective orthosis and education.
2. Increase passive flexion to the palm to enhance tendon glide, joint mobility, and prepare for AROM.
3. Promote wound healing and closure.
4. Initiate scar management program as indicated to minimize scarring and adhesions to maximize potential ROM.

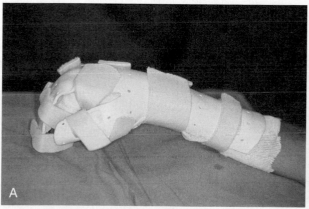
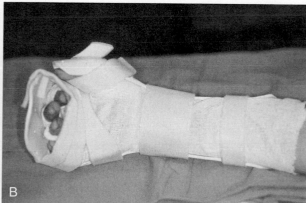

FIGURE 37-7 A and **B,** Dorsal protective orthosis with slight wrist flexion and maximum reasonable MP flexion. The thumb is positioned in mid-abduction.

Long-Term Goals

1. Increase PROM of fingers to within normal limits (WNL) for potential AROM and function.
2. Increase AROM of index finger, middle finger, and small finger to greater than 60% of normal limits for grasp/release of a 1-inch diameter object.
3. Client to use hand in more than 50% of ADLs.
4. In cases in which the therapist does not know specifically what to expect in terms of outcome, the best course is to predict a basic level of function and ROM. PROM must be maximized if there is to be any hope of regaining full AROM and to obtain the best results after secondary surgery.

Home Exercise Program

Both the client and his mother were educated extensively about the surgical procedures performed, the expectations of surgery, and the necessity of a second surgery for replacement of the Silastic rod with an active tendon graft. They also were taught how to perform wound care, dressing changes, and ROM exercises. They were given the following initial HEP.

Home Exercise Program to be Done Every Other Hour

- Push the big knuckles down all together, hold 5 seconds each (passive MP flexion).
- Push the big knuckle down, push the fingertip in, on each finger, one at a time; hold 5 seconds each; do three to five times per finger (passive composite flexion).
- Push the big knuckles in as far as able, straighten fingers (one at a time), relax, repeat five times (passive MP flexion with active IP extension; enhances long flexor glide and intrinsic action).

Note that the HEP was written in common terms that the client and his mother would understand.

At the client's second visit for therapy, tenodesis was added. The client was taught to combine wrist extension with a passive fist and then to flex the wrist and allow the fingers to extend naturally. The therapist was hopeful that some minimal gliding would occur in the thumb tendons without disrupting the healing and fusion there (Fig. 37-8).

Three to Four Weeks after Surgery

At approximately 3 weeks after surgery, the physician gave approval to begin performance of a place and hold fist to try to mitigate the heavy scarring that was forming. Heavy scarring that

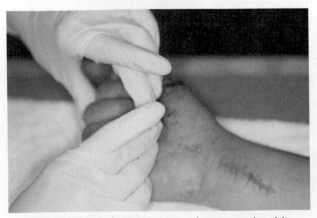

FIGURE 37-8 Early PROM at second postoperative visit.

limits ROM suggests that the client is forming good scar to heal the wounds and that the protocol may be progressed more rapidly. Whirlpool treatment was added, at a neutral temperature (approximately 94º F) and with the hand in a neutral position, to clean the wound and help manage pain, which had increased slightly with the upgrades in therapeutic exercises. Transcutaneous electrical nerve stimulation (TENS) was also tried for pain management but was not helpful. About 4 weeks after surgery, active finger flexion, extension exercises, and blocked finger flexion exercises were added.

The physician was consulted about beginning thumb AROM. He approved initiation of IP blocking exercises with the still-healing MP fusion protected, as well as abduction/adduction exercises. Because active finger and thumb ROM were now safe and acceptable, M.H. began to use his hand for light prehension exercises in the clinic and at home. He was not yet allowed to use the hand for ADLs at home because of the concern that he might overdo it, especially with the thumb. He began functional prehension, picking up beads and grasping a foam tube (see Fig. 37-6). Because scarring was becoming more of a problem, scar massage was increased at the volar MP scars. M.H. was an exception to the typical delays in healing after a replant or revascularization, because he was young and still growing. His body was able to produce new tissue, especially scar tissue, faster than most adults. His program therefore could be speeded up when it became apparent that scar formation was becoming an issue.

Five to Six Weeks after Surgery

Five weeks after surgery, M.H.'s ROM evaluation showed that active MP flexion was WNL, PIP flexion averaged about 55° to 60°, and DIP flexion was about 17°. MP extension lag averaged 15°, but the PIPs of the index, middle, and ring fingers were very limited in extension, at about −45°. The client had full passive flexion of all fingers. The thumb web space showed tightness in both radial abduction (35°) and palmar abduction (27°), and he had only 10° of thumb IP flexion. He had very good wrist ROM with wrist extension at 55° and flexion to 73°. Sensibility was functional with diminished protective sensation; the Semmes-Weinstein evaluation showed the thumb, index finger, middle finger, and ring finger at 4.31 and the small finger at 3.61.

A note was sent to the physician at this time stating that M.H.'s tissue was "adherent, but gaining ROM" and that the web scar/contracture were a concern. The physician was asked when thumb PROM would be permitted, whether ultrasound treatment could be used for the scars, and whether the tolerable stretch for full passive extension of the fingers could be increased. The physician approved discontinuation of the protective orthosis, recommended the orthosis be modified to try to increase the thumb web space, and approved ultrasound treatment for the scars. He allowed use of a passive extension orthosis "as per normal protocol." He told the therapist, "I doubt he'll get much thumb IP motion, but it's okay to begin PROM." Discontinuing protective orthosis at 5 weeks after surgery is a bit unusual, but this young client apparently was forming a significant amount of scar and healing more rapidly than a full grown adult with the same injury. Sensibility, although diminished, was sufficient to protect him from additional injury and to allow use of the hand functionally in light ADLs.

Changes in therapy included conversion of the dorsal block orthosis to a volar design with Otoform to scar for PIP extension. A thumb web stretch also was built into the orthosis (Fig. 37-9). M.H. began writing practice using a foam pen grip; he also practiced picking up marbles and in-hand manipulation skills. Moist heat was added at 6 weeks after surgery, and ultrasound treatment with extension stretch to the volar scars was added to increase passive extension of the fingers.

Seven Weeks after Surgery

At 7 weeks after surgery, the HEP consisted of the following:
- Web spacer orthosis with Otoform, 4 hours a day and at night
- AROM and PROM exercises, including blocking, opposition, place and hold, and wrist ROM, ten repetitions, four to six times a day
- Scar massage

- Light to moderate use of the hand for ADLs, including writing and eating (Fig. 37-10)

In the clinic M.H. continued with moist heat, ultrasound treatment of scars, and one-on-one ROM exercises with emphasis on blocking. Mildly resistive activities were initiated, including use of a gripper with light tension (Fig. 37-11). The client used it in the normal position, gripping with the fingers, and also reversed it in his hand to pull down with the thumb. Putty rolling was done to stretch the fingers and elicit co-contraction of the finger and wrist flexors and extensors. The client also continued to practice writing and picking up pegs and marbles.

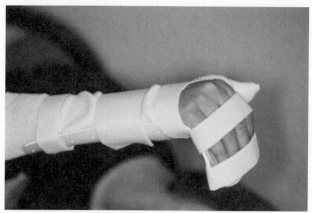

FIGURE 37-9 At 6 weeks after surgery, the dorsal block orthosis was converted to a volar design with a thumb web stretch.

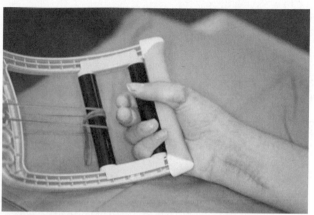

FIGURE 37-11 Client using a gripper at 7 weeks after surgery.

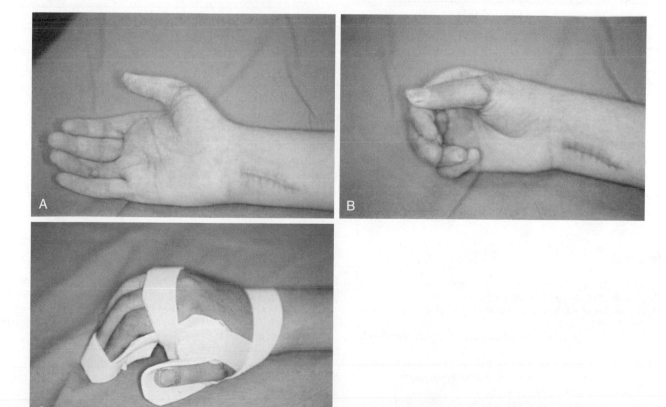

FIGURE 37-10 A to C, At 7 weeks after surgery, the client's home exercise program (HEP) consisted of ROM exercises. He also started using a web spacer orthosis.

Eight Weeks after Surgery

At 8 weeks after surgery, a baseline grip evaluation was performed. The right grip strength average was 10 lbs and the left was 43 lbs. The physician approved gentle strengthening, including the addition of putty exercises to the HEP, gripping, pinching, and rolling. One of M.H.'s goals was to be able to carry a bucket of water or feed so that he could return to his summer job working on a farm. He therefore began a graded program of picking up and carrying weights in the clinic and at home with the goal of working up to 20 lbs. A Baltimore Therapeutic Equipment (BTE) work simulator was added in the clinic to help improve strength and endurance. By 12 weeks after surgery, the client primarily was performing a HEP with upgrades for strengthening.

Four to Six Months after Surgery

M.H.'s final evaluation was done approximately 4 months after surgery. Referring to his injured right hand, he said, "I can do anything with it," and he demonstrated lifting a 20-lb weight. Grip strength in the right hand had increased to 42 lbs. The findings at this evaluation are shown as follows:

Measurements at Four Months after Surgery

RANGE OF MOTION

	Thumb	Index Finger	Middle Finger	Ring Finger	Small Finger
MP		0/88	0/100	0/105	0/95
PIP			−40/95	0/80	0/77	0/95
DIP		0/20	0/15	0/0	0/82
Semmes-Weinstein monofilament test	3.22	3.22	3.22	2.83	2.83

DIP, Distal interphalangeal; *MP,* metacarpophalangeal; *PIP,* proximal interphalangeal.

	Right Hand	Left Hand
Grip strength	42 lbs	59 lbs
Lateral pinch	14 lbs	17 lbs
Three-jaw pinch	14 lbs	18 lbs

M.H. returned to the surgeon 6 months after surgery. He had decided that he did not want a tendon graft to the FDP of the ring finger; he felt that he was functional, and he did not want to go through rehabilitation again. At this time several other surgical procedures were performed, including release of a thumb web space contracture (by Z-plasty); release of a volar skin contracture on the index finger (Z-plasty); and removal of the Hunter rod in the ring finger, which left the client with a superficialis finger (that is, he had no flexion force at the DIP, which meant he could end up with a boutonnière deformity).

M.H. returned to therapy 9 days after surgery, and an orthosis was fabricated to maintain the web space and hold the index finger in full extension. He had minimal pain (0-2/10) and edema. Index finger extension was −30°, thumb radial abduction was 65°, and thumb palmar abduction was 60°. The client was instructed in wound care and in full ROM exercises with emphasis on index finger PIP extension blocking and web space stretching. Because he was already familiar with therapy, he was seen only once a week for program and orthotic modifications and upgrades, which included the addition of strengthening exercises and a gel sheet.

M.H. was seen for the last time in therapy 6 weeks after surgery. He reported full functional use of the hand in all ADLs and was prepared to return to his summer job soon thereafter. The final outcome measurements for this client are shown here:

Final Measurements

RANGE OF MOTION

	Index Finger	Middle Finger	Ring Finger	Small Finger
MP	0/90	0/99	0/95	0/90
PIP	−20/95	0/85	0/88	0/95
DIP	0/24	0/22	0/0	0/82

DIP, Distal interphalangeal; *MP,* metacarpophalangeal; *PIP,* proximal interphalangeal.

Grip strength:
Right hand: 44 lbs
Left hand: 62 lbs
Thumb radial abduction: 60°
Thumb palmar abduction: 60°

References

1. Wilhelmi BJ, Lee WP, Pagensteert GI, et al: Replantation in the mutilated hand, *Hand Clin* 19:89–120, 2003.
2. Moran SL, Berger RA: Biomechanics and hand trauma: what you need, *Hand Clin* 19:17–31, 2003.
3. Morrison WA, McCombe D: Digital replantation, *Hand Clin* 23:1–12, 2007.
4. Walsh JM: Replantation. In Burke SL, Higgins J, McClinton MA, et al, editor: *Hand and upper extremity rehabilitation: a practical guide,* ed 3, New York, 2006, Churchill Livingstone.
5. Chan SW, LaStayo P: Hand therapy management following mutilating hand injuries, *Hand Clin* 19:133–148, 2003.
6. Huish SB, Hartigan BJ, Stern PJ: Combined injuries of the hand. In Mackin EJ, Callahan AD, Skirven TM, et al, editor: *Rehabilitation of the hand and upper extremity,* ed 5, St Louis, 2002, Mosby.
7. Rizzo M: Complex injuries of the hand. In Skirven TM, Osterman AL, Fedorczyk J, et al, editor: *Rehabilitation of the hand and upper extremity,* ed 6, Philadelphia, 2011, Mosby, pp 1227–1238.
8. Freeland AE, Lineaweaver WC, Lindley SG: Fracture fixation in the mutilated hand, *Hand Clin* 19:51–61, 2003.
9. Jones NF, Chang J, Kashani P: The surgical and rehabilitative aspects of replantation and revascularization of the hand. In Skirven TM, Osterman AL, Fedorczyk J, et al, editor: *Rehabilitation of the hand and upper extremity,* ed 6, Philadelphia, 2011, Mosby, pp 1252–1272.
10. Maricevich A, Carlsen B, Mardini S, et al: Upper extremity and digital replantation, *Hand* 6:356–363, 2011.
11. Pettengill KM: Therapist's management of the complex injury. In Skirven TM, Osterman AL, Fedorczyk J, et al, editor: *Rehabilitation of the hand and upper extremity,* ed 6, Philadelphia, 2011, Mosby, pp 1238–1252.

12. Sherman R, Pederson WC, LaVia AC: Replantation. In Berger RA, Weiss AP, editors: *Hand surgery*, vol 2, Philadelphia, 2004, Lippincott Williams & Wilkins, pp 1521–1543.

13. Cannon NM: *Diagnosis and treatment manual for physicians and therapists*, ed 4, Indianapolis, 2001, Hand Rehabilitation Center of Indiana. 196–200.

14. Silverman PM, Willette-Green V, Petrilli J: Early protected motion in digital revascularization and replantation, *J Hand Ther* 2:84–101, 1989.

15. Silverman PM, Gordon L: Early motion after replantation, *Hand Clin* 12:97–107, 1996.

16. Neumeister MW, Brown RE: Mutilating hand injuries: principles and management, *Hand Clin* 19:1–15, 2003.

17. Beris AE, Lykissas MG, Korompilias AV, et al: Digit and hand replantation, *Arch Orthop Trauma Surg* 130:1141–1147, 2010.

18. Grob M, Papadopulos NA, Zimmerman A, et al: The psychological impact of severe hand injury, *J Hand Surg Eur* 33(3):358–362, 2008.

19. Gustafson M, Hagberg L, Holmefur M: Ten years follow-up of health and disability in people with acute traumatic hand injury: pain and cold sensitivity are long-standing problems, *J Hand Surg Eur* 36(7):590–598, 2011.

38 Preventing and Treating Stiffness

Corey Weston McGee

The inflexible distal upper extremity occurs in many client populations in a variety of rehabilitative settings. The rehabilitation therapist working with clients who are prone to or experiencing distal upper extremity stiffness should be armed with background knowledge in anatomy, soft tissue mechanics, soft tissue healing, the etiology and pathomechanics of conditions predisposing to or resulting in distal upper extremity stiffness, and the medical-surgical management of such conditions. Additionally, the novice therapist should have a fundamental understanding of how to differentially identify the type/location of stiffness. Without a well-executed evaluation, the therapist's approach toward preventing or remediating stiffness may be misguided and ineffective. Likewise, the therapist must be capable of applying the evaluation results by appropriate planning and administering of interventions that are appropriate to the client, the client's condition, and, when applicable, their phase of healing. Additionally, in the case of the occupational therapist, his or her intervention planning and interventions should be true to their discipline and be occupation-focused.

Diagnosis

Broadly speaking, the term *stiffness* implies that there is a mechanical resistance to deformation. In the case of the "stiff" distal upper extremity, this resistance results in a limitation in joint mobility. Let's now focus on some of the most common sources for limitation in joint mobility. Prior to reducing our clients to a diagnosis, however, it is important to recognize all of the other factors, intrinsic or extrinsic to the client, which may be influencing his or her incorporation of an affected upper extremity into daily occupations. The therapist who recognizes the interaction of person, environment, and task will likely be most successful in helping to restore his or her clients' upper extremity function.

There are many sources for limitations in joint mobility. These can be psychosomatic (that is, guarding due to pain or in anticipation of pain) or physical in etiology. Physical restrictions of joint mobility may result from collagenous or muscular changes that arise from metabolic disorders, such as diabetic "cheiroarthopathic" hand, or systemic conditions, such as inflammatory arthritis, or nonuse.

Nonuse resulting from pain, denervation, and immobilization triggers a cascade of problems that further perpetuate stiffness. These include muscle atrophy (and further weakness), edema, muscle collagen fiber cross-linkage, and altered motor programs (Fig. 38-1). All of these must be considered when working to undo the effects of upper extremity nonuse.

Physical limitation in joint mobility may also result from decreased tendon excursion due to scarring or tenosynovial thickening (for example, from trigger finger or de Quervain's tenosynovitis). Movement may also be restricted by changes in more superficial structures, such as skin. Limitations in the excursion of skin due to trophic changes that are proximal, peri, or distal to a joint may result in poor joint mobility (for example, scleroderma and burn scarring).

Edema in the distal upper extremity produces a similar effect by making skin taut or "full" to the point where joint mobility is restricted (that is, passive insufficiency). This creates more work for the flexor tendons attempting to move stiff joints, and when uncontrolled or chronic, can lead to subcutaneous hardening (that is, fibrosis), which further restricts joint mobility and can lead to additional complications.

Other soft tissues that may indirectly restrict joint mobility include adhered or taut muscular fascia and taut peripheral nerves. In both cases, these adhered or taut structures can create painful and restricted joint mobility. See Chapters 12 and 24 for additional information on the cause and treatment of these conditions.

Lastly, a joint may be restricted by changes in the joint's bony architecture. Arthritis; ankylosis (that is, fusion); and bony malalignment resulting from fracture, subluxation, or

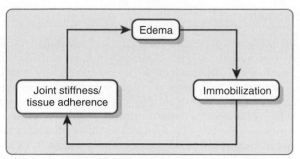

FIGURE 38-1 Cycle of nonuse. (Adapted from Skirven TM, Osterman AL, Fedorczyk JM, et al, editors: *Rehabilitation of the hand and upper extremity*, ed 6, Philadelphia, 2011, Mosby, p. 896.)

dislocation may result in structural "blockades" to joint motion. Chapters 25, 27, and 33 explore these conditions and the treatment of resultant physical and occupational performance limitations.

Timelines and Healing

Before discussing why, when, and how to assess and intervene with those who have upper extremity joint mobility limitations, a review of the process by which healing occurs is necessary. As we move through this review, it is important to consider concerns or processes that are unique to that phase in healing. In addition to reviewing the body's responsiveness to soft-tissue injury, we will identify the primary focus to the therapist working with clients in each of these phases.

After hemostasis has been achieved, our body responds during the first 2 to 12 days after a soft tissue injury through local vasodilatation and infiltration of white blood cells that clean up dead cells and, in the case of a wound, help to fight off infection. This phase is referred to as the **inflammatory stage.** Late in this phase, early bonding of the injured tissue begins via the migration of disorganized collagen fibers. A primary repair (that is, via suture) of injured soft tissue will typically require some amount of immobilization until the end of this phase to help facilitate healing. It is at this time that edema is prevalent and should be treated (see Chapter 3 for interventions). Edema control is often the emphasis at this time. The therapist works to facilitate prompt healing so that mobilization can be initiated. When inflammation is well controlled, the fibroblasts are signaled to begin their job of strengthening the repair of the damaged tissue. This is the **fibroblastic stage** and lasts from 3 days to about 3 weeks post injury in ideal conditions. Evolved fibroblasts soon begin laying down disorganized collagen fibers that cross-link with one another to stabilize the injury. This cross-linkage does not permit these fibers to efficiently move relative to one another and thus are an early source of stiffness.[1] Edema continues throughout much of this phase as the wound environment continues to be **hyperemic.** Additionally, disuse leads to weakness of muscles that are antagonistic to this early stiffness. Stiffness early in this phase typically has a **soft end feel** but can feel firm as healing progresses. During this phase the therapist continues to focus on controlling edema and begins looking for critical opportunities to introduce appropriate controlled-stress to these healing structures to maintain soft tissue elasticity by promoting more functional organization of the collagen fibers.[2] In the **maturation phase,** the process of laying down collagen normalizes and strong cross-linkages between collagen fibers form. Stiffness early in this phase feels firm

in nature; however if pervasive for long periods, may feel hard. By this time, the therapist's options become fewer.

Although stiffness can result from the cascade of processes that occur following traumatic injury, it can also occur in those who have systemic conditions that create inflammatory responses in a number of soft tissues (for example, rheumatoid arthritis, and scleroderma) or in those with conditions of the central nervous system (for example, brain and spinal cord injury), the peripheral nervous system (for example, peripheral nerve injury), muscle (for example, muscular dystrophy) and the neuromuscular junction (for example, myasthenia gravis). In the inflammatory conditions, the role of the therapist, when possible, is to control inflammation and control or prevent stiffness. For those with conditions affecting the nervous system, muscle, or neuromuscular junction, the therapist must focus on preventing stiffness that results from heightened or lessened tone, nonuse, and muscle changes. Remediating or preventing stiffness and subsequent deformity is done to promote occupational performance and participation. The therapist, however, must recognize that these approaches alone will not guarantee such and must consider other barriers, such as inadequate social supports, and conflicting habits, roles, and routines, as well as other approaches that may also enable participation (for example, adaptation, prevention, and health promotion). This top-down approach makes participation and performance central and does not assume that impairments in joint mobility are the only barriers to optimal function. The focus of this chapter is on correcting or preventing stiffness, but as therapists we do not treat stiffness alone; we work with a client to enable engagement in occupations and participation. This perspective deserves attention in the rehabilitation therapies.

Evaluation Tips

The evaluation of the client with a stiff hand begins as it should with any client. This first step involves seeking background information on the client's medical condition(s), date of onset of medical condition or surgery, orders, and precautions. This is accomplished via a chart review, communications with referral sources, and interview of the client. This data will guide the therapist's reasoning through the evaluation and intervention processes.

The therapist then gathers an occupational profile. This is achieved by interview and survey (for example, Canadian Occupational Performance Measure [COPM][3]) and entails seeking information on your client's:

- Areas of occupation
- Routines, habits, and roles
- Perceived and observed performance in occupations
- Importance and satisfaction of problematic areas of occupation
- Perceived barriers to engaging in such occupations

Your interview will also yield information about:

- Your client's chief complaints
- The motivation level of your client

- Whether pain is experienced during movement; if so, where, how bad, and what

Clinical Examination

Generally speaking, the therapist should perform a clinical examination when:
- Stiffness is believed to be responsible for occupational performance deficits.
- Range of motion (ROM) deficits are suspected to lead to deformity and subsequent disability.[4]
- Protocol necessitates interventions aimed at preventing or resolving joint motion limitations.
- Assessing joint mobility is not contraindicated.

Observation of Hand Use in Manual Occupations

When a source of joint stiffness is unknown, it may be beneficial to first observe the client's use of his hand when performing various occupations that are manual in nature.

© **Clinical Pearl**

If MP extension precedes wrist extension during reaching tasks, then your client either has weakness of the prime movers of the wrist (that is, extensor carpi radialis brevis and longus) or altered motor programming. If wrist extension overtly precedes MP and PIP flexion during grasp, then your client is likely experiencing some long finger flexor weakness or impaired differential flexor tendon gliding. Conversely, if wrist flexion precedes MP extension then long finger extensors may be weak or there may be an exaggerated imbalance of wrist stabilizer strength (that is, flexors > extensor).[5]

Signs of Triggering

While inspecting the affected region, the therapist may check for signs of clicking, squeaking (crepitus), or locking (triggering) of thumb or finger joints after moving from flexion into extension to rule in or rule out symptoms of tenosynovitis. This may involve provocative testing to better understand the nature of the joint restriction.

Scarring

The therapist will also inspect for incisional scars, scarring that spans joints, or scarring that is proximal/distal to the stiff joint (see Chapter 34). Along with this, the observation of scar blanching (turning a white hue) or migration of surface scarring during joint movement may indicate that scar tissue is restricting mobility.

© **Clinical Pearl**

In the case of incisional scarring, expect to observe distal movement of an adhered scar when the affixed musculotendinous unit is elongated (for example, a dorsal hand incisional scar moving distally when a fist is made and long finger extensors are put on stretch) and expect to see proximal movement of that same scar when the musculotendinous unit is shortened (for example, the same dorsal hand incisional scar moving proximally when the fingers are brought into extension and the long finger extensors are shortened).

Goniometry

ROM assessment determines the nature and extent of stiffness in a given joint and is the most commonly used measure of change in joint mobility. To determine whether weakness or soft tissue/bony restrictions are sources of limited joint mobility, the therapist will take both active and passive measurements. Generally speaking, a goniometric measurement of the hand is subject to a 5° measurement error,[5] and because of this, goniometric measurements need to have a discrepancy of greater than 5° for there to be a "real difference."[6] This is true for all of the following circumstances:
- When comparing active measurements to normative data
- When comparing active measurements to passive measurements of the same joint
- When comparing baseline goniometric measures to those taken when re-evaluating

The first step is to compare active measurements to normative measures. If a "real difference" exists that is impeding function, then compare the findings to a passive measurement of the same joint. If the passive measurement is 5° more than the active measurement, weakness or adherence is likely contributing to joint motion limitations. If active movement and passive movement are within 5° of one another yet are different from the norms, then a passive restriction is present. To further complicate things, it is possible to have both weakness and passive restrictions affecting the same joint. In these cases you would expect to have passive measures more than 5° below the norm and active measures more than 5° below passive measurements. When a passive limitation has been confirmed, a **firm** or **hard end feel** is experienced. The firm end feel indicates a soft tissue restriction, whereas the hard end feel indicates a boney block to movement.[7] True boney blocks to movement are not responsive to stretching and for clients with such limitations, the focus should shift to an adaptation approach.[8] If soft tissue is impeding joint motion, a series of differential tests will help to further explain the origin of the impediment.

Proximal Interphalangeal Joint Stiffness

These tests are most commonly used when proximal interphalangeal (PIP) joint passive flexion is limited and the therapist wants to determine if **extrinsic** finger extensor, **intrinsic** (lumbrical), or joint **capsule tightness** are responsible. If posturing in metacarpophalangeal (MP) flexion lessens available passive PIP flexion, there is extrinsic extensor tightness (Fig. 38-2) whereas when a posture of MP extension lessens passive PIP flexion, there is intrinsic (lumbrical) tightness.[8] Fig. 38-3 illustrates the testing procedure for this. If the posture of the MP joint does not at all influence passive PIP joint flexion yet passive PIP motion is still limited, a contracted joint capsule is likely the problem. A similar process can be followed when attempting to determine the source of PIP extension contractures. In this case, the therapist measures the available passive PIP extension with MP extension and compares to MP flexion. If the values remain unchanged, capsular tightness is likely responsible;[9] if there is greater than 5° difference in PIP passive extension, extrinsic finger extensor tightness is likely responsible. Extrinsic tightness is commonly experienced by those with spasticity, forearm fractures, or those who have had immobilized wrists or elbows. Intrinsic tightness is commonly experienced by those who have sustained hand crush

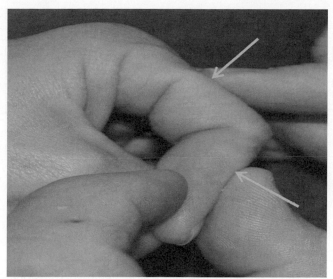

FIGURE 38-2 Test for extrinsic extensor tightness. Position: Place MP joint in maximal flexion. Test: Passively flex the PIP joint. Rule out PIP joint contracture by repeating with the MP joint extended. Interpret: Extrinsic extensor muscle tightness is present if PIP joint motion is greater when MP is extended than when is flexed. PIP joint contracture is present if position of MP does not influence PIP flexion.

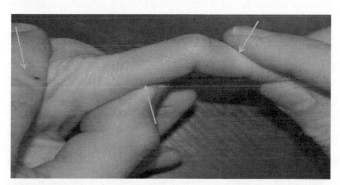

FIGURE 38-3 Test for intrinsic tightness. Position: Place MP joint in full extension. Test: Passively flex the PIP joint. Rule out PIP joint contracture by repeating with the MP joint flexed. Interpret: Intrinsic muscle tightness is present if PIP joint motion is greater when MP is flexed than when is extended. PIP joint contracture is present if position of MP does not influence PIP flexion.

injuries, metacarpal fractures, and those with rheumatoid arthritis. In addition to the reduced grasp associated with intrinsic tightness, there is evidence to support that this tightness may, at times, be partially responsible for the development of carpal tunnel syndrome.[10]

Distal Interphalangeal Joint Stiffness

Extrinsic finger flexor tightness (tested by comparing passive distal interphalangeal [DIP] extension with wrist in flexion to passive DIP flexion with wrist in neutral) or capsular (joint) tightness can restrict DIP passive extension. Conversely, DIP passive flexion is typically hindered by either a contracted joint capsule or **oblique retinacular ligament (ORL) tightness** (Fig. 38-4) An ORL tightness test (Fig. 38-5) determines the source of limited passive flexion. If by placing the PIP in extension

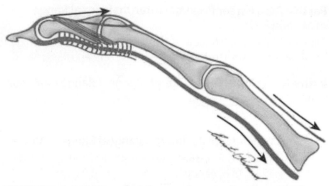

FIGURE 38-4 Anatomy of oblique retinacular ligament (ORL). The ORL originates from the volar surface of the A2/C1 pulleys of the proximal phalanx and travels "obliquely" toward the dorsum of the distal phalanx where it inserts into extensor mechanism. (Adapted from Skirven TM, Osterman AL, Fedorczyk JM, et al, editors: *Rehabilitation of the hand and upper extremity*, ed 6, Philadelphia, 2011, Mosby).

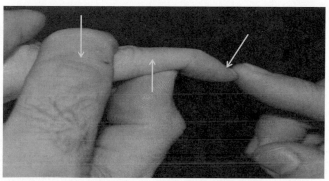

FIGURE 38-5 Test for oblique retinacular ligament (ORL) tightness. Position: Place PIP joint in full extension. Test: Passively flex the DIP joint. Rule out PIP joint contracture by repeating with the PIP joint flexed. Interpret: ORL tightness is present if DIP joint motion is greater when PIP is flexed than when extended. DIP joint contracture is present if position of PIP does not influence DIP flexion.

your client's passive DIP flexion measurements become more impaired, then ORL tightness is present. If changing the posture of the PIP joint does not alter your DIP flexion measurements, then the joint capsule is likely contracted. A tight ORL often accompanies a boutonnière deformity and, along with the management of a PIP flexion contracture, requires therapeutic attention.

In all cases of intrinsic or extrinsic tightness, there may also be capsular and ORL tightness. Case Study 38-1 illustrates this.

CASE STUDY 38-1 ■

Sandy recently sustained a crush injury to her dominant right hand that required pinning of her ring finger PIP joint. She is now 6 weeks out and ready for passive stretching of all affected joints. Your ROM assessment reveals the following:

Active Ring Finger Proximal Interphalangeal Range of Motion

With ring finger in MP flexion: 30° to 60°
With ring finger in MP extension: 30° to 70°

Passive Ring Finger Proximal Interphalangeal Range of Motion

With ring finger in MP flexion: 30° to 60°. Firm end feel is noted.
With ring finger in MP extension: 30° to 70°. Firm end feel is noted.

Active Ring Finger Distal Interphalangeal Range of Motion

With PIP joint in −30° of extension: 0° to 20°
With PIP joint in 70° of flexion: 0° to 45°

Passive Ring Finger Distal Interphalangeal Range of Motion

With PIP joint in −30° of extension: 0° to 24°. Firm end feel noted.
With PIP joint in 70° of flexion: 0° to 65°. Firm end feel noted.

Circumferential Measurements

Right ring finger midshaft proximal phalanx: 7.5 cm
Right ring finger midshaft middle phalanx: 7.0 cm
Left ring finger midshaft proximal phalanx: 5.0 cm
Left ring finger midshaft proximal phalanx: 4.5 cm
Pain: 1/10 on numerical pain scale

Your Interpretation

There is no discrepancy in active and passive PIP measurements; therefore weakness or adherence does not explain the loss of motion. MP posture did not change the available passive PIP extension; therefore capsular tightness is limiting PIP extension. MP posture did, however, alter PIP flexion passive range of motion (PROM); thus, extensor extrinsic tightness (not intrinsic) is in part responsible for passive PIP flexion limitations. But there is still a 40° discrepancy between passive flexion, so capsular tightness is also limiting PIP flexion. In summary, there is likely PIP capsular tightness restricting flexion and extension, as well as extrinsic extensor tightness restricting flexion. Additionally, the DIP joint's flexion limitation is a result of ORL tightness as well as some weakness in or difficulty recruiting the flexor digitorum profundus (FDP). Greater than 2 cm discrepancy in circumferential measures compared to the unaffected extremity, although not empirically validated, is often accepted to indicate clinically significant edema. Fortunately, the firm end feel would indicate that there are no bony blocks to movement. We'll revisit Sandy's case later when we begin discussing intervention planning.

Wrist Stiffness

Extrinsic tightness can also impact wrist motion. Differential testing is useful to determine the origin of wrist stiffness. The follow reasoning can be followed when determining the cause of wrist stiffness:

- Passive wrist extension that is not impaired with fingers in flexion but is impaired when adding finger extension indicates extrinsic finger flexor tightness
- Passive wrist flexion that is not impaired with fingers in extension but is impaired when adding finger flexion indicates extrinsic finger extensor tightness
- Passive wrist movement that is impaired but not impacted by the posture of the digits is likely capsular in origin or due to tightness of the prime movers (for example, extensor carpi radialis brevis, or flexor carpi radialis). If the posture of the elbow (flexed versus extended) influences wrist movement, the prime wrist movers may be tight; if not, capsular tightness is likely responsible
- Passive wrist flexion less than the unaffected side regardless of finger or elbow posturing and further impaired by finger or elbow posturing in extension or flexion indicates both capsular tightness and muscular tightness

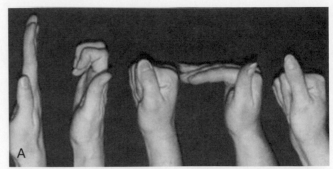

FIGURE 38-6 Differential flexor tendon gliding exercises. (From Skirven TM, Osterman AL, Fedorczyk JM, et al, editors: *Rehabilitation of the hand and upper extremity*, ed 6, Philadelphia, 2011, Mosby.)

Extrinsic Tendon Adherence and Muscular Tightness

Tendon-incisional scar adherence may be a source of passive joint limitations. In such cases, adherence of extrinsic tendons presents slightly differently than does muscular shortening. Extrinsic tightness will likely influence the mobility of all joints crossed by the muscle-tendon unit; however scar adherence impacts only joint mobility distal to the site of adhesion. This is because there is muscular elasticity proximal to the site of adherence yet, because a tendon has little elasticity, there is minimal motion from the point of tendon adherence distally. Likewise, tendon-tendon adherence may occur; particularly in the case of the extrinsic flexors. In this situation, the passive excursion of these tendons would be unaffected yet active composite fisting would be challenging because the adhered FDP and flexor digitorum superficialis (FDS) tendons are less capable of **differentially gliding** relative to one another.[11] Differential gliding may be compromised after flexor tendon repairs, with carpal tunnel syndrome, or following carpal tunnel release surgery. Active tendon gliding exercises (Fig. 38-6) are often prescribed, when not contraindicated, to prevent or remediate problems with differential gliding in such cases. Differential tests for joint motion are very detailed and typically involve modifying the posture of joints that are proximal or distal to the joint of interest. Therapists need to be intentional and consistent in positioning the joints proximal and distal to those that are measured. If therapists are not consistent in their goniometric assessment, interrater reliability suffers and so does our ability to document the effectiveness of our interventions.

> ### ◎ *Clinical Pearl*
>
> Extrinsic tightness will likely impact wrist and digital mobility, whereas with adhesions, joint mobility is limited only distal to the site of adhesion.

Edema Evaluation

With any client who has stiffness resulting from trauma, an inflammatory condition, dependency, weakness, or nonuse, an evaluation for the presence of edema is critical. See Chapter 3 for a more details on the process of edema assessment and intervention. Early attention to edema when present or when expected is crucial.

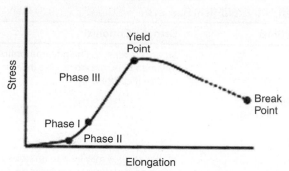

FIGURE 38-7 Phases of the stress-strain relationship. Phase 1 (elastic): Soft tissue elongates due to stress, elastin elongates, collagen uncoils and elongates in the direction of the stretch. Phase 2 (elastic): The stress applied and strain of soft tissue increase together exponentially. Phase 3 (elastic): Continued application of stress produces little more tissue elongation. Yield point (plastic): Changes in the physiological make-up of soft tissue occur. Break point: The point at which soft tissue has exceeded its capacity to elongate and is subject to trauma (leading to an inflammatory response). (From Richard RL, Staley MJ: *Burn care and rehabilitation: principles and practice*, Philadelphia, 1994, FA Davis.)

Neurological Tone

Clients with spasticity or flaccidity may experience stiffness. In nearly all cases, therapists should prevent stereotypical postures that encourage contractures. For more on the client with a "neurological hand," see Chapter 40.

Hand Therapy (Non-Operative) Interventions

The first steps are to work with the client to identify barriers to performance, prioritize which barriers to address, and collaborate to formulate client centered goals. The client's priorities and the therapist's clinical knowledge and reasoning skills allow priorities to be established.

Soft Tissue Mechanics

While each form of soft tissue has its own unique properties, the mechanics of soft tissue are generally applicable to all types. The therapist's ability to stretch or prevent tightness relies heavily on the relationship between stress and strain (Fig. 38-7). **Stress** is the amount of force per unit area (that is, pressure) applied to soft tissue. **Strain** is a result of stress and is expressed mathematically as the change in length of soft tissue/original length × 100. Most biological materials have elastic and plastic properties. Materials that are elastic return to their original form when stress is removed, whereas material that is plastic undergoes a change in composition that remains stable when stress is eliminated. To safely elongate or maintain the length of a soft tissue, *strain must occur only in the elastic range*. Stress that results in elongation of soft tissue into its plastic range will lead to microtearing, inflammation, and fibrosis. It has been suggested that 200 g (1/2 lb) of force[12] is sufficient to adequately stress the PIP joint. However, these types of torque measurements are seldom performed clinically and thus therapists typically rely on subjective report from the client and changes in objective measures (for example,

goniometry) to determine if the "just right" force administered by, for example, an orthotic intervention has been achieved. Ideally, your client should report the sensation of stretching but not pain while wearing a mobilizing orthosis.[8] This brings us to the next important concept, strain rate, or the amount of tissue elongation per unit of time. Although the amount of stress is critical, so is the duration that this stress is longer than the **total end range time (TERT)** or amount of time a contracted joint is placed at its maximal length, the better the results.[13] This combined low stress, long TERT or **low load, long duration (LLLD) approach** is believed to be best practice when attempting to resolve soft tissue contracture, because it promotes reorganization of collagen fibers within their elastic range without undue strain.[13] (Table 38-1) highlights intervention options that are specific to a given impairment as well as a given phase of healing.

Although Table 38-1 provides a descriptive recipe for intervention planning specific to many joint restrictions experienced across the three phases of healing, it fails to illustrate much of the clinical reasoning that either justifies or precludes their administration. The novice hand therapist often becomes preoccupied with becoming technically proficient in administering a plethora of assessments and interventions yet may struggle with reasoning through where to start and why. The following tips have been compiled to aide in decision making.

Early Active Mobilization

When not contraindicated may help to break the edema-disuse-stiffness cycle. If motion contraindications are present, active mobilization of the joints distal and proximal to the immobilized segment(s) should be instituted to avoid undue capsular-ligamentous shortening and pocketing of edema.

What Joint(s) to Treat First

Finger MP flexion and PIP extension, wrist extension, elbow extension, and forearm supination are most difficult to get back. For these reasons, early effort to regain or prevent stiffness in these movements is recommended. Active mobilization of the finger flexors should be initiated as early as possible to prevent tendon adherence and intrinsic tightness. A client-centered approach should be used when appropriate. For example, if your client is a transcriptionist, early focus on forearm pronation may better facilitate her return to paid employment. The therapist must address movements that are physiologically most predisposed to contracture and resistant to intervention, as well as movements that best enable a return to the desired occupations. If your client's distal upper extremity stiffness is pervasive, a discussion with the client, therapist, and surgeon may help to explore how to best balance the needs and goals of the client with clinical priorities.

When an orthotic intervention for joint tightness is warranted, the therapist should design orthoses that act only on the joint(s) with capsular tightness. Conversely, when musculotendinous shortening is present, an orthosis must be constructed to place all joints crossed by that muscle into an antagonistic posture.

How to Isolate the Effects of a Prime Mover on the Target Joint

At times it is necessary to isolate joints that may not receive the full attention of a prime mover. For example, the FDS will

TABLE 38-1   Intervention Highlights across Phases of Healing and Physiological Barriers

Healing Phase	Physiologic Barriers		Therapist Interventions	Orthotic Option(s)

Inflammatory (2 to 5 days post-injury in optimal circumstances)	Edema		• Elevation
			• PAMs
			  • Cryotherapy in most cases
			  • High volt[14]
			  • Pulsed ultrasound
			• Proximal lymphatic decongestion
			• Pumping/proximal motion
			• Light compression
				Static orthoses may help to immobilize inflamed structures to resolve inflammation (Fig. 38-8).

	Pain/anxiety		• Elevation
			• PAMs
			  • Cryotherapy in most cases
			  • High volt
			  • Pulsed ultrasound
			  • TENS
			• Early controlled use of permitted digits/segments
			• Guided imagery/relaxation
				Static orthoses may help to immobilize inflamed structures to control pain.

	Nonuse of affected extremity		• Early controlled use of permitted digits/segments • Imagery/ mirror therapy to unaffected with immobilization • AROM to permitted joints distal and proximal to injury (ideally within 2 days) • Every 2 hours five to ten repetitions for 5 seconds	Use of orthoses that are as "least restrictive" when medically indicated. Be certain to avoid unwarranted restriction of adjacent joints.

	Decreased knowledge		• Education
			  • Protection
			  • Home programming
				Education on orthotic care and wear schedule.

Fibroblastic (5 to 21 days in optimal circumstances)	Edema		• See inflammatory phase
			• Controlled active use of affected extremity during occupations
			  • Must find balance between activity and elevation
			  • Elevate when not engaged in activity
			  • Schedule breaks for elevation	

	Pain/anxiety		• See inflammatory phase • Monitor for CRPS	Static/protective orthoses may control pain and support use during aggravating occupations.
	Forearm tightness (distal and radioulnar joints)	Pronation	• AROM • Gentle passive motion	Rolyan supination/pronation splint (Fig. 38-9).
		Supination	• AROM • Gentle passive motion	Rolyan supination/pronation splint
	Wrist tightness (radiocarpal and ulnocarpal joints)	Extrinsic (due to muscular or skin tightness)	• Moist heat to extensor and flexor wads • AROM to wrist with tenodesis and also in composite manners (wrist flexion/finger flexion, wrist extension and finger extension) • Gentle passive motion (wrist flexion/finger flexion, wrist extension and finger extension)	If immobilization is indicated (unless contraindicated), wrist should posture in 15° of extension to prevent flexion contracture. With volar wrist scarring, wrist should also be positioned in slight wrist extension. With dorsal wrist scarring, a more neutral wrist is preferred to prevent extensor contracture.
	MP/PIP tightness	Intrinsic	• Active "intrinsic minus" stretches	Hand based "intrinsic minus" orthosis with MPs extended to facilitate active stretches. A dynamic outrigger can be added in mid-fibroblastic phase (Fig. 38-10).
		Extrinsic (due to muscular or skin tightness, or adhesions)	• Moist heat to flexor/extensor wads • PIP blocking exercises • Controlled active movement • Gentle passive movement • Controlled active use in daily occupations • Differential tendon glides	Static or serial static orthoses at night and during times of rest. Intrinsic plus position (Fig. 38-11) is best for extensor tightness and a modified resting pan splint best for flexor tightness (Fig. 38-12). In mid-fibroblastic phase, dynamic splinting can be used.

TABLE 38-1   Intervention Highlights across Phases of Healing and Physiological Barriers—cont'd

Healing Phase	Physiologic Barriers		Therapist Interventions	Orthotic Option(s)
	DIP tightness	ORL	• DIP blocking exercises with PIP held in extension	PIP flexion blocking orthotic to isolate DIP flexion (Fig. 38-13).
		FDP (due to muscular or volar skin tightness, or adhesions)	• Differential tendon glides • AROM to wrist and also in composite manners (wrist extension and finger extension) • Gentle passive motion (wrist extension and finger extension)	Static or serial static modified resting pan orthotic (see Fig. 38-12).
	Nonuse of affected extremity/ weakness		• Biofeedback to assist with recruitment/cortical remapping • NMES to difficult to recruit muscles • Early controlled use in daily occupations • Early isolative active motion specific to commonly "forgotten" muscle groups (e.g., ECRB, FDS, etc.) • Active assistive exercises when antigravity strength is limited	Blocking orthotics to assist with isolation of difficult to recruit muscles (Fig. 38-14).

	Decreased knowledge		• Education
			  • Controlled active use/restrictions
			  • Home programming
			  • Splint wear schedule
				Education on orthotic care and wear schedule.

Maturation (3 to 6 weeks up to 2 years with select soft tissue)	Edema		• Manual edema mobilization • Chip bags if fibrotic • Active movement • Compression • Elastic taping techniques	
	Pain		• See inflammatory phase • Imagery and mirror therapy	
	Forearm tightness (distal and radioulnar joints)	Pronation	If no change from thermal modalities and manual therapy, unlikely to respond to passive or active stretching because collagen cross-linking is so pervasive. In this case, an orthotic intervention is required.	JAS Pro/Sup Static Progressive Orthotic (Fig. 38-15)
		Supination	If no change from thermal modalities and manual therapy, unlikely to respond to passive or active stretching because collagen cross-linking is so pervasive. In this case, an orthotic intervention is required.	JAS Pro/Sup Static Progressive Orthosis
	Wrist tightness (radiocarpal and ulnocarpal joints)	Extrinsic (due to muscular or skin tightness)	• Moist heat and lotion to skin scarring • Scar massage	• Serial casting • Static progressive splinting (Fig. 38-16)
		Capsular	Heated ultrasound	• Serial casting • Static progressive splinting
	MP/PIP tightness	Intrinsic		Hand-based intrinsic minus orthosis with static progressive outrigger
		Extrinsic (due to muscular or skin tightness, or adhesions)	• Heated ultrasound to site of adhesion • Moist heat and lotion/massage to skin scarring	• Forearm-based static progressive orthoses • Serial casting • Casting motion to mobilize stiffness[15] (Fig. 38-17)
		Capsular	Heated ultrasound	• Hand or finger based static progressive orthoses (Fig. 38-18) • Serial casting (Fig. 38-19)

Continued

TABLE 38-1   Intervention Highlights across Phases of Healing and Physiological Barriers—cont'd

Healing Phase	Physiologic Barriers		Therapist Interventions	Orthotic Option(s)
	DIP tightness	ORL	Heated ultrasound	PIP flexion blocking orthosis with static-progressive DIP flexion mobilizing outrigger (Fig. 38-20)
		FDP (due to muscular or volar skin tightness, or adhesions)	Heated ultrasound to site of adhesion	Static progressive orthosis
		Capsular		DIP static progressive extension mobilizing outrigger (Fig. 38-21)
	Nonuse of affected extremity/ Weakness		• Biofeedback to assist with recruitment/cortical remapping • NMES to difficult to recruit muscles • Early controlled use in daily occupations • Early isolative active motion specific to commonly "forgotten" muscle groups (e.g., ECRB, FDS, etc.) • Active assistive exercises when antigravity strength is limited	Blocking orthoses to assist with isolation of difficult to recruit muscles
	Decreased knowledge		• Education • Controlled active use/restrictions • Home programming • Splint wear schedule	Education on orthotic care and wear schedule.

AROM, Active range of motion; *CRPS,* complex regional pain syndrome; *DIP,* distal interphalangeal; *ECRB,* extensor carpi radialis brevis; *FDP,* flexor digitorum profundus; *FDS,* flexor digitorum superficialis; *JAS,* Joint Active Systems, Inc.; *NMES,* neuromuscular electrical stimulation; *ORL,* oblique retinacular ligament; *PAM,* physical agent modality; *PIP,* proximal interphalangeal; *TENS,* transcutaneous electrical nerve stimulation.

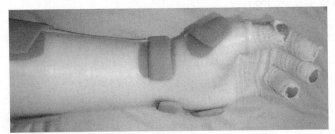

FIGURE 38-8 Volar forearm-based wrist and thumb CMC/MP immobilization orthosis (Courtesy of C. McGee.)

normally first move the MP when contracting. However, when the PIP is stiff, blocking the MP in extension allows for the FDS to be more focused at flexing the PIP joint. Conversely, blocking the MPs into flexion best assists the interossei and lumbrical muscles with extending the PIP. Blocking orthoses or exercises can help these prime movers more effectively mobilize the stiff joint.

When Is an Orthotic Intervention Needed?

When stiffness is present, the goals of orthotic interventions are to remodel collagen fibers, remediate tendinous adhesions, and lengthen tight tissues.[12] However, an orthotic intervention may also be indicated to rest inflamed tissue to allow healing and prevent sclerosis associated with chronic inflammation (for example, insertional biceps tendonitis), or it can be used

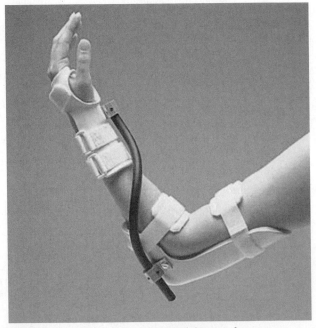

FIGURE 38-9 Posterior upper arm based dynamic forearm supination mobilizing orthosis (From Patterson Medical (website): www.pattersonmedical.com/app.aspx?cmd=searchResults&sk=supination+kit.)

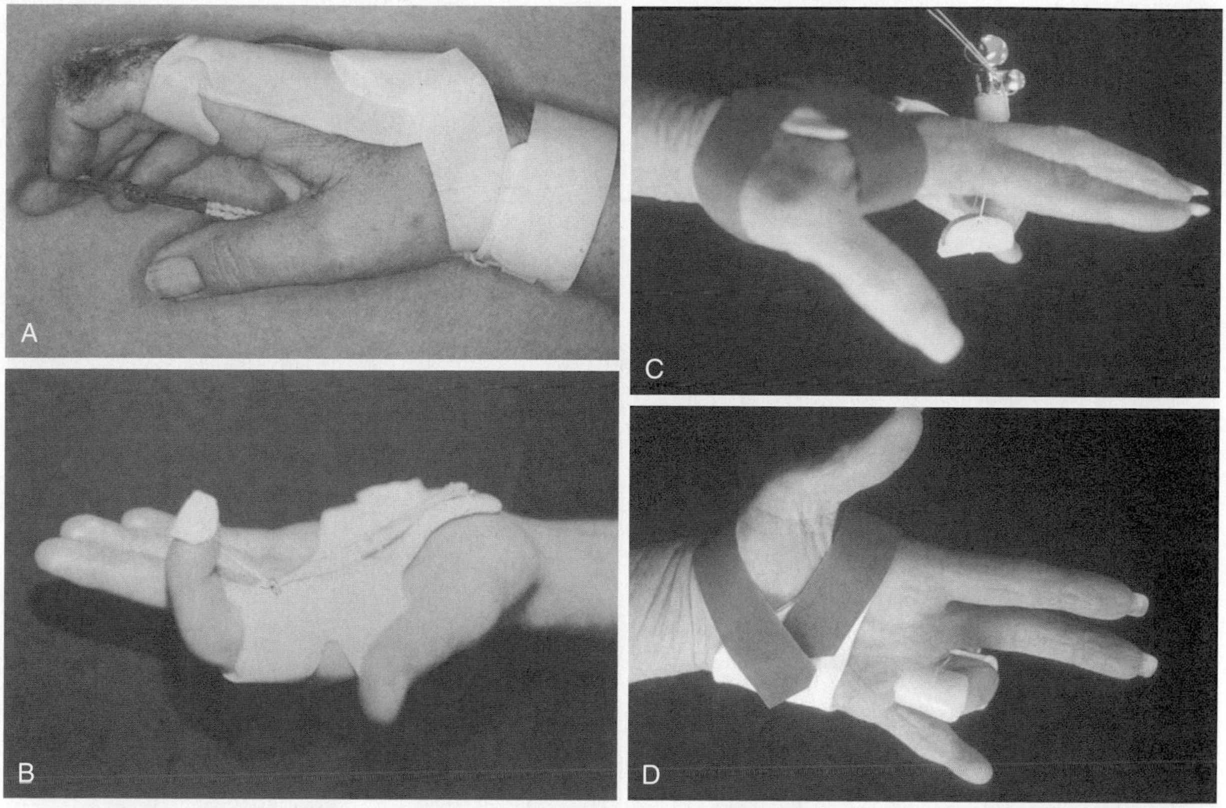

FIGURE 38-10 Volar hand-based static MP flexion blocking and dynamic PIP/DIP flexion mobilization orthosis (From Fess EE, Gettle K, Philips C, et al, editors: *Hand and upper extremity splinting: principles and methods*, ed 3, St Louis, 2005, Mosby.)

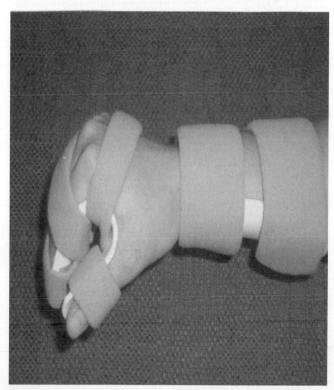

FIGURE 38-11 Volar forearm-based intrinsic plus orthosis (Courtesy of C. McGee.)

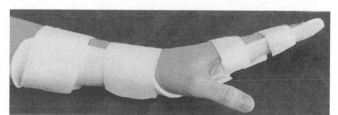

FIGURE 38-12 Volar forearm-based serial static wrist and second to fifth digit extension mobilizing orthosis (From Berger RA, Weiss AC, Weiss AP, editors: *Hand surgery*, Philadelphia, 2003, Lippincott Williams and Wilkins.)

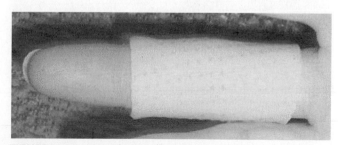

FIGURE 38-13 Circumferential finger-based PIP flexion blocking orthosis (Courtesy of C. McGee.)

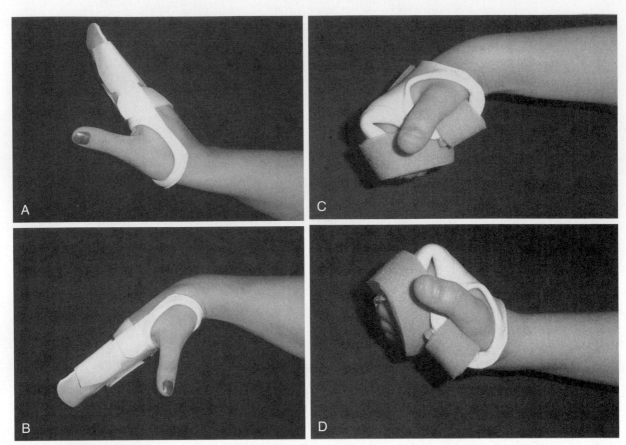

FIGURE 38-14 Dorsal hand based static second to fifth MP extension blocking orthosis (From Fess EE, Gettle K, Philips C, et al, editors: *Hand and upper extremity splinting: principles and methods*, ed 3, St Louis, 2005, Mosby.)

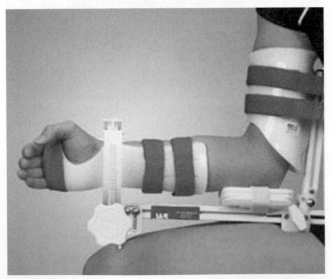

FIGURE 38-15 Circumferential upper arm based static progressive forearm pronation mobilizing orthosis (From Joint Active System (JAS) (website): www.jointactivesystems.com/JAS-Systems/1/3/JAS-ProSup.aspx.)

to provide controlled stress to healing tissue to prevent adherence and promote proper healing (for example, flexor tendon repairs).[16] Moreover, a mobilizing orthotic intervention should be implemented within 2 months of the onset of the stiffness to optimize responsiveness.[17]

Healing Phase Aside, How Do I Choose the Correct Type of Mobilization Orthoses

A screen called the **Modified Week's Test**[18] will help you to determine which type of orthosis is appropriate. The screen first involves taking a goniometric measurement of the affected joint followed by the administration of a thermal modality for 15 to 20 minutes. Then, manual therapies are directed at the joint (for example, mobilizations and therapeutic stretching). If the joint motion improves by10° to 20°, you should fit the patient with a serial-static or dynamic orthosis. If the gain is less than 10°, a static-progressive orthosis should be used.

How and When to Use Occupation-Based Interventions

See website for information on this topic.

How to Ensure Learning and Carry-Over

Most hand therapy intervention requires continuous follow-through by the client/family/caregivers. This can be challenging, especially when relatively complex exercises and orthoses are often used to address complex problems. I recommend the

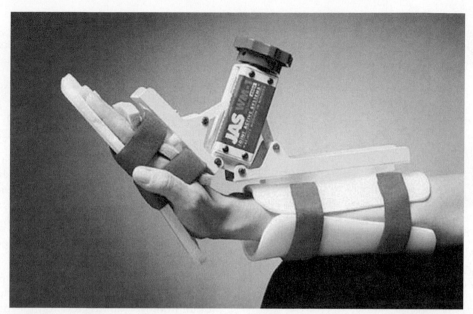

FIGURE 38-16 Circumferential forearm-based static progressive wrist extension mobilizing orthoses (From Fess EE, Gettle K, Philips C, et al, editors: *Hand and upper extremity splinting: principles and methods*, ed 3, St Louis, 2005, Mosby.)

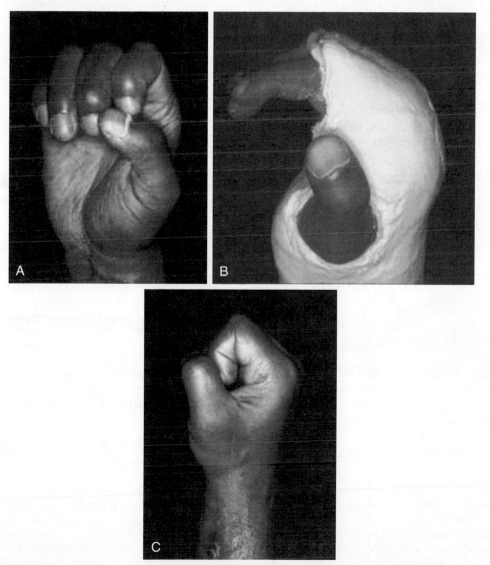

FIGURE 38-17 Casting motion to mobilize stiffness.[4] (From Skirven TM, Osterman AL, Fedorczyk JM, et al, editors: *Rehabilitation of the hand and upper extremity*, ed 6, Philadelphia, 2011, Mosby.)

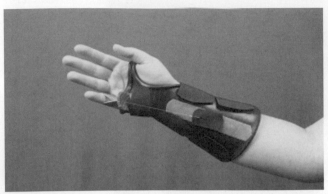

FIGURE 38-18 Volar forearm-based static progressive SF MP flexion mobilizing orthosis (Courtesy of C. McGee.)

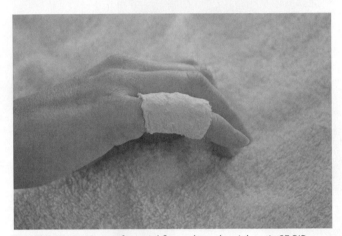

FIGURE 38-19 Circumferential finger-based serial static SF PIP extension mobilizing cast. (Courtesy of C. McGee.)

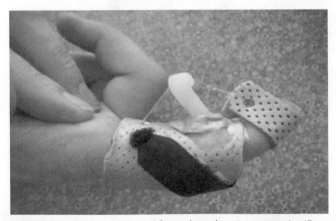

FIGURE 38-20 Circumferential finger-based static progressive IF flexion mobilizing orthosis (With permission from Celine Cantin, OT, CHT, Owner/operator of Coastal Hand Clinic, Surrey, BC.)

following to help foster learning and carry-over when not in therapy:

- Use video phones to record the performance of therapeutic activity or exercise, or orthotic application; digital photography can also be beneficial.
- Verbal instructions should always be accompanied by written/video instructions. Be certain that client education

materials are being written at the sixth-grade level; consider using readability scorecards[20] to assess the readability of your materials.

When Prolonged Protective Positioning Is Necessary

A closed-pack (that is, when joint is most congruent and ligaments most taut) "intrinsic plus" position (see Fig 38-11) that involves postures of the wrist in 20° extension, second-fifth MPs in 60° to 70° of flexion, first to fifth IPs in extension, and thumb MP in extension, and carpometacarpal [CMC] in midposition) is ideal to prevent ligamentous shortening. There are occasions, however, when closed-pack position is not completely possible due to edema or discomfort. In these instances a "functional position" (Fig. 38-22) should be achieved.

How Long Should I Plan to Carry Out an Orthotic Intervention to Mobilize a Stiff Joint?

This ultimately depends upon the type of mobility deficit (that is, flexion vs. extension) and how long the stiffness has been present. Intuitively and as previously mentioned, flexion is typically the quickest to respond to mobilization orthoses and recent evidence supports this. Glascom, Flemming, and Tooth[21] report that PIP extension contractures maximally respond to a dynamic orthotic intervention within 12 weeks, whereas PIP flexion contractures will not maximally respond until 17 weeks or more of dynamic orthotic wear. Similarly, these authors describe that extension contractures respond well to 6 hours of daily TERT, whereas flexion contracture may respond best to 11 hours. Lastly, regardless of the type of mobility deficit, when stiffness has been present for 8 weeks or less, it responds better to an orthotic intervention than stiffness that has been present for 3 months.[17] In these more chronic cases, a longer treatment duration should be expected.

> ### Clinical Pearl
>
> Neuromuscular electrical stimulation (NMES) and biofeedback can be useful tools to help re-establish "lost" motor programs that result from immobilization and disuse. When limited joint mobility appears to be related to your client's difficulty with recruiting prime and secondary movers, try helping your clients refresh their "motor memories" through these techniques.

> ### Clinical Pearl
>
> Capsular pattern tightness (that is, when a joint's AROM = PROM regardless of the posture of joints that are proximal or distal to it) will likely not resolve with active or passive stretching. In these cases, LLLD serial static or static progressive orthoses or serial casting may be your best bet.

CASE STUDY Continued

Sandy (continued)

Let's now revisit Sandy from Case Study 38-1. If you recall, Sandy has ring finger PIP joint capsular and extrinsic tightness, DIP joint ORL tightness, and some difficulty recruiting her FDP. Given this interpretation and the aforementioned guidance on intervention planning and intervening, it's time to plan and prioritize treatment.

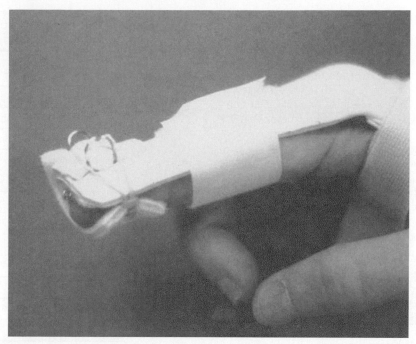

FIGURE 38-21 Dorsal hand-based static progressive index finger DIP extension mobilizing orthosis (From Skirven TM, Osterman AL, Fedorczyk JM, et al, editors: *Rehabilitation of the hand and upper extremity*, ed 6, Philadelphia, 2011, Mosby.)

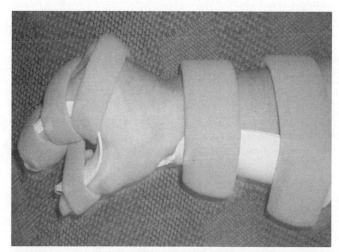

FIGURE 38-22 Volar forearm-based functional hand orthosis (Courtesy of C. McGee.)

Additional Assessment Data

Knowing what you now know about the Modifed Week's Test,[18] at your initial visit with Sandy, you administered superficial moist heat to the flexor/extensor surfaces of the hand and forearm, joint mobilizations, and some passive stretching; then you took follow-up PROM measurements. The PIP extension goniometric measurements of the affected joints were unaffected by this combination, but the passive flexion of the PIP joints (with MP in flexion) improved from 60° to 90°. The passive flexion of the DIP joint with PIP in extension was unaffected by the heat and manual therapies.

Your Interpretation

1. PIP extension deficits respond best to a static progressive orthotic intervention, and given that digital PIP extension can be difficult to recapture, it requires early attention.
2. PIP flexion deficits do not require an orthotic intervention and will likely respond well to preparatory interventions, such as heat and composite wrist and ring finger MP/PIP flexion stretching, as well as purposeful activities that require combined wrist and digital flexion such as:
   • Brushing hair
   • Using a screwdriver to tighten screws
   • Rolling out dough with a rolling pin
3. DIP oblique retinacular deficits respond best to a static progressive orthotic intervention, whereas the apparent weakness of/ difficulty recruiting the FDP is best addressed through biofeedback, NMES, DIP blocking, and strengthening exercises.

Your Prioritized Intervention Plan

1. Address occupational performance through modifications to her occupations, hand-occupation interfaces (equipment, and so on), or environment modifications to support engagement.
2. Address right ring finger edema through modalities, active mobilization, and compression. Remember to remove elastic wraps, such as Coban, for active exercise, because compression may make unnecessary work for the long finger flexors.[22]

3. Address PIP joint extension PROM through a static progressive orthotic intervention.
4. Address limited PIP joint flexion PROM through superficial heat, manual therapies, and composite therapeutic stretching to her extensor wad, and purposeful activity/occupations.
5. Once PIP extension has been regained, a static progressive orthosis to address DIP flexion may help to resolve ORL tightness; however the altered motor program/weakness of the FDP may need NMES/biofeedback and DIP blocking/resistance training via composite fisting with a putty or sponge.
6. Education on home programming and orthotic wear/care are also essential to success.
7. Home programming should include digital edema sleeve wear, manual edema mobilization, PIP extension orthosis wear/care at night, moist heat soaks followed by sustained composite stretching to long finger extensors, and differential tendon glides with emphasis on full-fists to encourage maximal FDP excursion.

Assessing Therapy Outcomes

When and What to Reassess

First and foremost, a client and occupation-centered therapist revisits occupational performance/satisfaction, participation, and progress toward your client's goal-attainment. This author suggests repeating primary outcome measures once a week. The literature does not clearly describe how frequently to reassess the stiff hand; however the recommended dosage or duration of an intervention may assist therapists in planning reassessment. For example, serial casting is most effective when applied for a period of 6 days.[13] For this reason, a reassessment of joint motion should be performed once a week following cast removal. Generally speaking, the frequency of administration and choice of tools depends on your intervention frequency/duration, third-party payer constraints, institutional policy, and so on. Because most interventions for the stiff hand are intended to impact edema, pain, passive/active joint mobility, and strength, the tools used to assess (such as, baseline) should be administered once again (ideally by the same therapist, in the same standardized fashion, and at the same relative time of day) to determine responsiveness. New assessments may be introduced along the way given that some may be contraindicated during early phases of healing (for example, strength testing).

Ideally, weekly goniometric assessments of the targeted areas are suggested and Cummings and Tillman[23] report that a 3° gain in joint ROM per week is an acceptable standard for remodeling connective tissue. Of course, given that hand goniometry is subject to a 5° measurement error, a difference of more than 5° is the most convincing that your interventions are impacting change.

How Much Active Motion Is Enough?

Because each individual's occupational and environmental demands are unique, determining a desired goniometric outcome can be challenging. In the absence of any literature that describes how much joint mobility is required for specific occupations or tasks, a therapist may resort to asking the client to engage in a task with the unaffected hand and then use their

TABLE 38-2	Functional Goniometric Measures of the Distal Upper Extremity	
	Joint	Joint Active Motion (Degrees)
Hand[24]	Second to fifth MP flexion	61
	Second to fifth PIP flexion	60
	Second to fifth DIP flexion	39
	First MP flexion	21
	First IP flexion	18
Wrist[25]	Flexion	54
	Extension	0
	Ulnar deviation	40
	Radial deviation	17
Forearm[26]	Supination	60
	Pronation	40
Elbow[30]	Flexion	130
	Extension	−30

DIP, Distal interphalangeal; *IP,* interphalangeal; *MP,* metacarpophalangeal; *PIP,* proximal interphalangeal.

skills in activity analysis to observe and describe the joint mobility that is likely necessary to perform the given activity with the affected side. This may not always be possible when, for example, your client has bilateral involvement, when a task is bimanual, or when the kinematics of the right hand are quite different from the left when unilaterally performing a given task (for example, twisting a jar or turning a key). Simply put, required joint mobility is occupation- and task-specific, and occupation-specific activity analysis may help to illustrate what is required. The ability to engage is the ultimate outcome measure of your interventions, and if a client is unable to engage after your interventions, it may be that his or joint mobility is the limiting factor. As a rule, however, our limited literature on the topic indicates that clients should be capable of engaging in most daily activities if the following active goniometric measures are achieved (Table 38-2).

What to Do If Progress Is Slow-Going

There will be times where your interventions may not all prove successful. When improvements in joint mobility are not accomplished after more than 2 weeks in active treatment, it may be necessary to re-evaluate your intervention plan. Be certain to check with your client to learn if their habits, roles, and routines are barriers to performing their home exercise programs (HEPs). You may need to help your client to identify how to best incorporate therapeutic occupations, exercises, and orthotic interventions into his or her lifestyle. It may just be that you haven't yet found the right approach, or that the intervention approach you have chosen needs refinement. In either case, turn to your colleagues, and ask for The Health Insurance Portability and Accountability Act of 1996 (HIPAA) compliant advice; turn to the literature to learn more about what is best practice. Be creative yet be scientific when trying new things. Lastly, although it is not in our nature to give up on our clients, a referral back to the physician may be necessary. If this is necessary, you are not giving up or failing your client. Rather, you are advocating on his or her behalf to expedite progress and keep costs down.

Operative Interventions

Surgical interventions or medical procedures may be required when hand rehabilitation is unsuccessful in remediating or preventing stiffness. It may also be that your client comes to you after undergoing surgery to capitalize on the newly acquired joint mobility, prevent regression, and continue toward occupational engagement. Hand rehabilitative clients occasionally undergo the following surgeries when they are either unresponsive to therapy or when therapy is not known to be effective:

- Open capsulectomy: For capsular contracture that does not respond to conservative measures. After surgery, early hand rehabilitation and mobilization is recommended.
- Tenotomy: To release long standing musculotendinous tightness by "lengthening" the tendon through the surgical division of a tendon.
- Tenolysis: The surgical removal of scar tissue impacting slide of tendon. Preoperative hand therapy is important for promoting PROM. Early postoperative hand therapy is recommended after this procedure.
- Surgical decompression of tendon sheaths or pulleys: When stenosing tenosynovitis is the culprit of joint restriction.
- Surgical release and skin grafting: When cutaneous scarring is impeding joint movement.
- Palmar fasciotomy or palmar needle aponeurotomy: This may be used when diseased palmar fascia is restricting digital extension (see Chapter 39).

? Questions to Discuss with the Physician

Unless standing protocols are already in place, seeking clarification on which postoperative protocol is to be employed is important prior to intervening with your client. Ask questions like:
- Is it okay for me to begin active range of motion (AROM) versus blocking exercises, passive motion, or resistance activities/exercises?
- What is the client's activity status? Can he/she begin using her hand in lightly resistive activities, such has oral care or self-feeding?
- If you have concerns about protocol, would you like to progress your client, or try a different intervention? Be diplomatic when approaching the referring physician, convey your clinical reasoning. For example, I have a 17-year-old client who is an instrumentalist and exceptionally responsible. Could we attempt an early passive motion regiment rather than cast immobilization? Convey scientific reasoning and evidenced-base literature to support your requests when necessary.
- When your client is failing to respond to your interventions, ask if additional imaging or testing might assist in better understanding the clinical status. In some cases it may be necessary to inquire whether the client is a candidate for surgery.

( ) What to Say to Clients

About Low Load, Long Duration Orthotic Interventions

"Much of the soft tissue in your arm is like a rubber band. Rubber bands break when stretched too far and too quickly, and just like a rubber band, your muscle and tendons are stretchy but will also tear when stretched too hard or fast. This is why a gentle but long stretch is necessary to loosen things up without hurting you. The old adage, "no pain no gain," does not apply here, and too hard of stretching may set you back."

Nonuse

"Using your affected hand in activities like (list medically-appropriate and client-centered options here) helps to control pain, swelling, and tightness. Movement of this hand helps to trick the brain into perceiving less pain, helps muscles get stronger, and helps muscles pump the swelling away from your arms."

Fostering Ownership

"Therapy is a partnership that involves work in and outside of the clinic. For therapy to benefit you, we need to work together to figure out what works best for you and how to thread therapy into your daily life. Progress depends a great deal on how well you are able to do what you've learned in therapy when outside of therapy. It also depends on how well, how often, and how long we infuse therapy into your daily routine. This can't be accomplished without work on both of our parts."

Diagnosis-Specific Information that Affects Clinical Reasoning

Therapeutic Contracture

In some instances, remediating stiffness may be contraindicated. In the case of a joint fusion, a hard (boney) end feel would indicate that the contracture will not be responsive to mobilization. In the case of a person with C6 tetraplegia, tenodesis formation is requisite for hand function and requires shortening of long finger flexors and extensors to occur. Composite stretching of long wrist and digits into flexion or extension is contraindicated.

Surface Scarring and Tendon Adhesions

When movement of joints beneath, proximal, or distal to surface scarring (for example, following a split-thickness skin graft) is limited, lubricate the area, and apply a gentle "frictionless" massage. Then perform composite stretching to the affected joint, as well as those proximal and distal. This assists in remodeling the contracting scar centrally, as well as on the periphery. If modalities or manual therapies are not successful, then mobilizing orthoses may be required.

◎ Clinical Pearl

Skin scar tissue that is restricting motion responds best to sustained low-load stretching to the point of scar blanching.[28] Paraffin wax, lotion, massage, and silicon sheeting products[29] may assist in preparing scarred skin for stretch. Instructing your clients on self-stretching is important, because therapy sessions typically cannot focus solely on stretching. Additionally, nocturnal serial static orthoses may support new gains in ROM and should be implemented until scar tissue is fully mature.

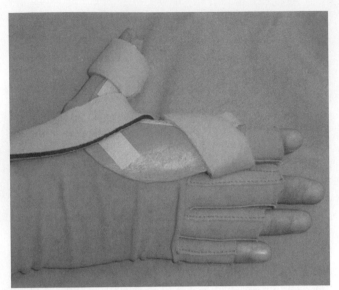

FIGURE 38-23 Radial hand-based static first carpometacarpal (CMC) web spacer orthosis (Courtesy of C. McGee.)

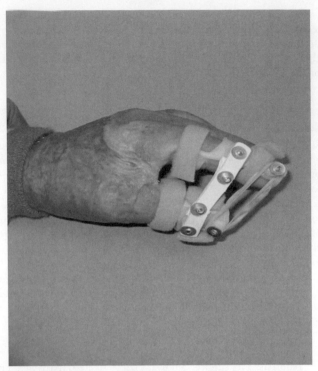

FIGURE 38-24 Bi-surfaced hand-based dynamic first carpometacarpal (CMC) palmar abduction mobilizing orthosis (Courtesy of C. McGee.)

⊙ Clinical Pearl

When surface scarring appears to be restricting the glide of superficial tendons, you may notice that this scarring moves in concert with these tendons. A heated ultrasound to this scar tissue, some massage, and lastly a small piece of Dycem to stabilize the surface scar during "tendon gliding type" exercises may facilitate a nonsurgical "lysis of adhesions."

Pre-Surgical Dupuytren's

There is little evidence to support the use of hand therapy to prevent or remediate stiffness that results from pre-surgical Dupuytren's disease.[30] If a client has been referred to you with this condition, it's likely that the course of the disease is advanced and impeding function. In cases such as this, an adaptive approach can be taken so that the client can engage in as many occupations as possible. However, advise the client to seek consultation with a hand surgeon as soon as possible if there are functional limitations.

Nerve Injuries

Alternating the wear of orthoses that substitute for weak movements with those intended to prevent stereotypical deformities may prevent long-term dysfunctional postures while a nerve is regenerating. For example, a client with a radial nerve palsy may require an dynamic MP extension mobilizing orthosis during daily activities but should use a resting hand orthosis to prevent long finger/thumb and wrist flexor shortening at night.

Web Space Contracture

Certain conditions, such as median nerve palsies, first CMC arthritis, and burns, are predisposed to a first web space contracture. In such cases, orthotic interventions are recommended to prevent adductor pollicis contracture by positioning the joint in a functional yet anti-deformity posture with a hand-based spica or other static orthoses for nighttime wear (Fig. 38-23). At times, however, restoration of the web space requires orthotic interventions (Fig. 38-24). Depending on the results of the Modified Week's Test, deep heat, acupressure, and stretching to the adductor pollicis may also help to remediate web space contracture.

➤ Precautions and Concerns

- *Short duration high strain (force) passive stretching will not promote soft tissue elongation regardless of the phase of healing. It will likely delay healing and cause tissue damage.*
- *Make certain you are adhering to medical/post-surgical protocol by facilitating only the permitted type (for example, active, place and hold, passive) of motion to the permitted joints.*
- *Always be certain to provide training and written materials on care and wear of orthoses designed to prevent or remediate stiffness. Inadequate education may result in skin ulceration as well as other adverse events.*

References

1. Madden JW: Wound healing: the biological basis of hand surgery, *Clin Plast Surg* 3(1):3–11, 1976.
2. Cyr LM, Ross RG: How controlled stress affects healing tissues, *J Hand Ther* 11(2):125–130, 1998.
3. Carswell A, McColl MA, Baptiste S: The Canadian Occupational Performance Measure: a research and clinical literature review, *Can J Occup Ther* 71(4):210–222, 2004.
4. Flinn NA, Jackson J, McLaughlin Gray J, et al: Optimizing abilities and capacities: range of motion, strength, and endurance. In Radomski M, Latham CA. *Occupational therapy for physical dysfunction*, ed 6, Philadelphia, 2008, Wolters Kluwer/Lippincott Williams & Wilkins, pp 81–185.
5. Long C: Intrinsic-extrinsic muscle control of the fingers: electromyographic studies, *J Bone Joint Sur* 50(5):973–984, 1968.
6. Groth GN, VanDeven KM, Phillips EC, et al: Goniometry of the proximal and distal interphalangeal joints, Part II: placement preferences, interrater reliability, and concurrent validity, *J Hand Ther* 14(1):23–29, 2001.
7. Kaltenborn FM: *Mobilization of the extremity joints: examination and basic treatment techniques*, Olso, Norway, 1980, Olaf Noris Bohkandel.
8. Colditz JC: Therapist's management of the stiff hand. In Skirven TM, Osterman AL, Fedorczyk JM, et al: *Rehabilitation of the hand and upper extremity*, ed 6, Philadelphia, 2011, Elsevier Mosby, pp 894–921.
9. Bunell S: *Surgery of the hand*, ed 2, Philadelphia, 1948, JB Lippencott.
10. Cobb TK, An KN, Cooney WP: Effect of lumbrical muscle incursion within the carpal tunnel on carpal tunnel pressure: a cadaveric study, *J Hand Sur Am* 20(2):186–192, 1995.
11. Wehbé MA, Hunter JM: Flexor tendon gliding in the hand. Part II. Differential gliding, *J Hand Sur Am* 10(4):575–579, 1985.
12. Brand PW, Hollister A: *Clinical mechanics of the hand*, ed 3, St Louis, 1999, Mosby.
13. Flowers KR, LaStayo P: Effect of total end range time on improving passive range of motion, *J Hand Ther* 7(3):150–157, 1994.
14. Bettany JA, Fish DR, Mendel FC: Influence of high voltage pulsed direct current on edema formation following impact injury, *Physical Ther* 70(4):219–224, 1990.
15. Colditz JC: Plaster of Paris: the forgotten splinting material, *J Hand Ther* 15:144–157, 2002.
16. Klein L: Early active motion flexor tendon protocol using one splint, *J Hand Ther* 16(3):199–206, 2003.
17. Glascow C, Tooth L, Fleming J, et al: Dynamic splinting for the stiff hand after trauma: predictors of contracture resolution, *J Hand Ther* 24:195–206, 2011.
18. Flowers K: A proposed hierarchy for splinting the stiff joint, with emphasis on force application parameters, *J Hand Ther* 15(2):158–162, 2002.
19. Amini D: Renaissance occupational therapy and occupation based hand therapy, *OT Practice* 9(3):11–15, 2009.
20. Seubert D: Design readability scorecard. 2010, *Health communications* (website), www.healthcommunications.org. Accessed October, 20, 2012.
21. Glascow C, Fleming J, Tooth L: The long-term relationship between duration of treatment and contracture resolution using dynamic orthotic devices for the stiff proximal interphalangeal joint: a prospective cohort study, *J Hand Ther* 25:38–47, 2012.
22. Buonocore S, Sawh Martinez R, Emerson JW, et al: The effects of edema and self-adherent wrap on the work of flexion in a cadaveric hand, *J Hand Surg* 37(7):1349–1355, 2012.
23. Cummings GS, Tillman LI: Remodeling of dense connective tissue in normal adult tissues. In Currier DP, Nelson RM, editors: *Dynamics of human biologic tissues*, Philadelphia, 1992, FA Davis, p 45.
24. Hume MC, Gellman H, McKellop H, et al: Functional range of motion of the joints of the hand, *J Hand Surg* 15(2):240–243, 1990.
25. Ryu JY, Cooney WP, Askew LJ, et al: Functional ranges of motion of the wrist joint, *J Hand Surg* 16(3):409–419, 1991.
26. Safaee-Rad R, Shwedyk E, Quanbury AO, et al: Normal functional range of motion of upper limb joints during performance of three feeding activities, *Arch Phys Med Rehabil* 71(7):505–509, 1990.
27. Morrey BF, Askew LJ, Chao EY: A biomechanical study of normal functional elbow motion, *J Bone Joint Surg Am* 63(6):872–877, 1981.
28. Moore ML, Dewey WS, Richard RL: Rehabilitation of the burned hand, *Hand Clin* 25(4):529–541, 2009.
29. Chan KY, Lau CL, Adeeb SM, et al: A randomized, placebo-controlled, double blind, prospective clinical trial of silicone gel in prevention of hypertrophic scar development in median sternotomy wound, *Plast Reconstr Surg* 116(4):1013–1020, 2005.
30. Hurst L, Starkweather KD, Badalamente MA: Dupuytren's disease. In Peimer C, editor: *Surgery of the hand and upper extremity*, New York, 1996, McGraw-Hill.

39

Dupuytren's Disease

Karen Donahue Pitbladdo and
Vincent R. Hentz

Dupuytren's disease is a benign connective tissue disorder affecting the palmar fascia that can lead to flexion contracture of the metacarpophalangeal (MP) joints and the proximal interphalangeal (PIP) joints. Although surgical treatment continues to be the preferred intervention, recently, **collagenase enzymatic fasciotomy** has proven to be a successful non-surgical alternative. Research on rehabilitation following both surgical and non-surgical approaches for Dupuytren's contracture is limited. Presently, postoperative treatment including splinting, exercise, and scar management is based on principles of wound healing and contracture management. While this chapter provides guidance and recommendations, therapists treating this condition are cautioned to use sound clinical judgment and individualize treatment rather than following a protocol-based approach.

History

Dupuytren's disease is eponymously attributed to Baron Guillaume Dupuytren, a French physician, who first described the condition in a December, 1831, lecture at the Hotel Dieu, as reported by his assistants.[1] At the time of his report, Dupuytren was unaware that others had previously described the condition. The earliest identifiable report was by the Swiss physician, Felix Plater, in 1614. In 1777, Henry Cline from London described the condition and had demonstrated in cadavers that the palmar fascia alone was involved.[2] The condition was briefly mentioned by Kline's pupil, Astley Cooper in his 1822 "Treatise on Dislocations and Fractures of the Joints."[3] Nonetheless, in his "Lecons orales" published in 1832, Dupuytren's description of the condition, the pathoanatomy, and treatment were presented in far greater detail than the previous reports.[4] Since that time, although many surgeons and scientists have contributed to our understanding of the disease and its treatment, the precise etiology of the condition remains unknown.

Epidemiology

Although most commonly seen in older men of northern European descent, Dupuytren's disease is seen globally across nearly all ethnic groups. In Caucasians, the global incidence is said to be 3% to 6% with the incidence increasing with advancing age.[5] The disease appears to be inherited in 10% to 30% of cases with an autosomal dominant inheritance pattern of variable penetrance.[6] Men usually present 10 years earlier with a peak incidence at age 45 to 50 and, compared to women, have higher prevalence of this disease, varying from 10:1 to 2:1 depending on the series reported.[7,8] Age of onset is significant, because those patients with an early onset are more likely to experience a more severe clinical course.

Presentation

Dupuytren's disease frequently appears as an isolated affliction of the fascia of the palm and digits. The thumb and index rays are much less often involved (5% to 7%) than the ulnar digits (50% to 60%).[9] Studies report bilaterality existing between 42 to 98% of cases.[10] In some patients, it occurs in conjunction with fibroproliferative involvement of the plantar fascia, termed Ledderhose disease, or the fibrous tissues of the tunica albuginea of the penis, termed **Peyronie disease,** or within the subcutaneum over the PIP joint, here termed **knuckle pads.** This constellation of fibroproliferative disorders is referred to as **Dupuytren diathesis,** a concept attributed to Hueston[11] who recognized several predisposing or "at risk" factors, including a positive family history, bilaterality, and the lesions outside the hands mentioned earlier. Early age of onset has been previously mentioned.

There is a notable relationship between Dupuytren's disease and several other diseases or conditions including the following:

- Diabetes mellitus[12]: There is a well-established increased incidence of diabetes in patients with Dupuytren's disease; although Dupuytren's disease, when present, is typically more nodular and less cordlike.
- Alcoholism[13]: Some studies have shown a positive correlation.
- Trauma[14]: The role of trauma is also controversial. Some studies show a positive correlation. Dupuytren's disease following trauma usually is non-progressive and may retrogress suggesting that this may be a different pathologic condition.
- Epilepsy[15]: The incidence of Dupuytren's disease in epileptic patients is notably high according to some studies. The role of phenobarbital, commonly prescribed for epilepsy, in the development of Dupuytren's disease is controversial.

Pathoanatomy and Evolution

In the hand, Dupuytren's disease is characterized by the presence of two structures, **nodules** and **cords**.[16] Nodules are comprised of hyper-cellular collagen bundles, whereas cords are less cellular. There is disagreement regarding whether these are distinct aspects of the disease or simply stages in the evolution. A controversy remains regarding whether normal fascia converts to Dupuytren's disease or develops independently. It remains curious as to why some elements (such as, longitudinal fibers) become involved, while anatomically adjacent elements (such as, the transverse and vertical elements) do not.

Disease in the Palm

Nodules, along with skin pits and distortions of the distal palmar crease are often the first visible evidence of Dupuytren's disease (Fig. 39-1). They typically appear near the distal palmar crease on the ulnar side of the hand and may be symptomatic with patients describing itching and burning, or they may be completely asymptomatic. They may appear and rapidly or slowly enlarge, or they may appear and remain stable for decades.

At a later stage, cords may appear. Longitudinal cords, termed *pretendinous cords,* parallel the pretendinous bands and may insert in a fashion similar to the insertions of the normal longitudinal fascia, or they may continue on into the digit as a central cord, inserting into the proximal or middle phalanx (Fig. 39-2). Contracture of the pretendinous cord, under the influence of myofibroblasts, thus, may cause an isolated MP or a combined MP and PIP joint contracture, depending on the distal insertion of the cord. This pretendinous cord, continuing distally into the digit as a central cord, usually does not disturb the anatomical course of the neurovascular bundle (NVB), and its surgical dissection should be relatively easy and safe.

Frequently, the pretendinous cord becomes contiguous with the diseased lateral digital fascia, now termed *lateral digital cord,* to then become what has been termed a *spiral cord* (Fig. 39-3). This pathoanatomic variant, because it causes a contracture of the MP joint, displaces the NVB centrally and superficially, placing it in harm's way of the unskilled and unwary surgeon.

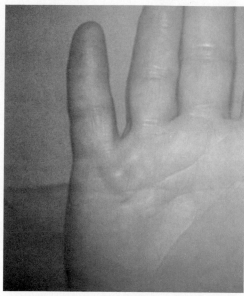

FIGURE 39-1 Dupuytren nodule typically seen in the ulnar side of the hand.

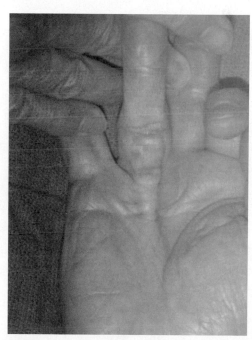

FIGURE 39-2 Pretendinous cord of the ring finger.

In the finger, the pathoanatomy of Dupuytren's disease is more complex than that of the palm, mirroring the more complex normal fascial anatomy of the digit (see Fig. 39-3). McFarlane[17] identified four cords that may cause a contracture of the PIP joint including the following:

- Central cord
- Lateral cord
- Spiral cord
- Retrovascular cord (which may also extend across the distal interphalangeal [DIP] joint causing contracture of this joint.)

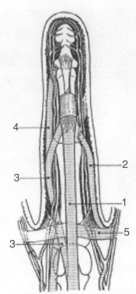

FIGURE 39-3 The fascial elements in the finger. *1,* Central cord; *2,* lateral digital cord; *3,* spiral cord; *4,* retrovascular cord; *5,* natatory cord. (Redrawn from Leclercq C: The management of Dupuytren disease. In Mathes SJ, Hentz VR, editors: *Plastic surgery,* Philadelphia, 2006, Saunders.)

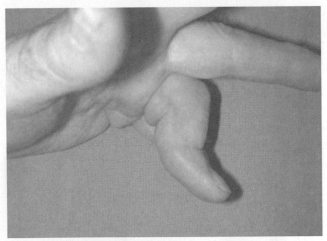

FIGURE 39-4 A boutonnière deformity characterized by flexion of the PIP joint and hyperextension of the DIP joint.

Other Digital Pathology Associated with Dupuytren's Disease—Pseudo-Boutonnière

The DIP joint may become hyperextended in association with more severe PIP joint contractures. This deformity has been attributed to Dupuytren's disease involvement of Landsmeer's oblique retinacular ligament (ORL), but this seems unlikely; the deformity now is thought to be a secondary effect of the PIP contracture that creates an imbalance between flexor and extensor tendons as they act across the DIP joint and progressive overstretching of the DIP joint's volar plate.

The affected digit may assume a posture similar to a so-called "boutonnière" deformity with a flexed PIP joint and a hyperextended DIP joint (Fig. 39-4). Over time, the DIP joint's volar plate becomes ineffective, the central slip of the extensor mechanism becomes elongated and ineffective, and the lateral bands

across the middle phalanx become contracted. Simple excision of cords of Dupuytren's disease will not be successful in restoring function to this digit.

The thumb may become flexed and adducted as a consequence of Dupuytren's disease affecting the fascias of the first web space, thumb, and index finger.

The span of the digits may be compromised as natatory cords appear and contract.

Operative Treatment

Surgery continues to be the gold-standard treatment for progressive Dupuytren's contractures. Typically, intervention is recommended in patients with MP joint contractures of at least 30° and/or any PIP joint contractures with associated functional impairment.[9] A variety of surgical interventions exist and are largely classified by the amount of diseased tissue removed.

Percutaneous Needle Aponeurotomy

The least invasive of surgical interventions, **percutaneous needle aponeurotomy/fasciotomy** may be considered little more than a modification of the original technique performed by Sir Astley Cooper and later known as the *Cooper fasciotomy.*[18] This technique, modified and later revived by the French rheumatologists, Lermusiaux and Debeyre,[19] is ideal for elderly individuals with multiple comorbidities, because it allows for a rapid increase in finger extension with minimal recovery time and can be safely performed under local anesthetic alone. The technique has grown in popularity since its reintroduction, and a number of excellent publications document its initial efficacy and safety when performed by experienced practitioners. The durability in terms of time to recurrence seems to be the major criticism of the technique. Nevertheless, it has become part of many hand surgeons' armamentarium to treat contractures of both MP and PIP joints. As typically described, the surgeon uses a fine-tipped hypodermic needle, stabbed through the skin at multiple locations overlying the contracting cord to make a series of micro-lacerations. The cord, thus weakened, eventually ruptures and the contracted joint extends to various degrees. Multiple involved fingers can be treated at the same operative procedure.

Fasciotomy

Fasciotomy refers to simple division of a cord without resection of tissues. Various techniques have been described and are still performed, including making a stab wound over the cord—termed by some, *percutaneous* or *subcutaneous fasciotomy.* Most have restricted its use to the palmar cords. The technique involves making a stab wound over the pretendinous cord with the blade parallel to the cord, creating a small longitudinal incision. The blade is turned perpendicular to the cord, the cord is divided, and the finger is stretched. If a more extensive incision is made, this is termed *open fasciotomy.* This was Dupuytren's and Cooper's original technique. There are few indications today for this procedure.

Fasciectomy

The more widely-used procedure to treat Dupuytren contractures is regional (subtotal or limited) **fasciectomy,** which remains today the accepted gold-standard for primary contracture release.

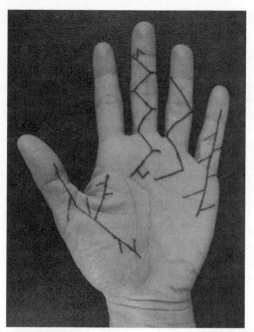

FIGURE 39-5 Some of the common incisions used for surgical exposure of the diseased cords.

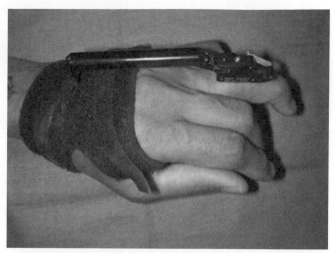

FIGURE 39-6 A Digit Widget attached by pins to the middle phalanx. Rubber bands are used to slowly extend the PIP joint.

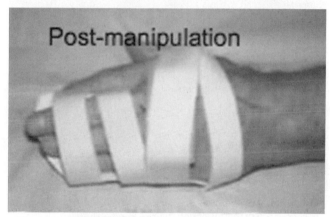

FIGURE 39-7 Volar hand-based orthosis.

This procedure involves generous skin incisions (Fig. 39-5) and careful dissection and excision of just the involved diseased fascia. This is different from radical fasciectomy advocated by McIndoe and Beare,[20] who recommended extensive removal of involved and noninvolved palmar and digital fascia. This treatment has fallen out of favor due to its higher complication rates without convincing evidence of a lower rate of recurrence. There exist many variations of so-called limited, as opposed to radical, fasciectomy. They differ primarily in the extent of exposure (that is, dissection and removal of the contracting fascia). For example, rather than removing all involved fascia, the surgeon may choose to excise only a short segment at a location determined to result in maximum extension of the contracted joint. This has been termed *segmental fasciectomy,*[21] to distinguish this procedure from open fasciotomy.

The incisions are either sutured directly or closed by advancement or rotation/transposition (Z-plasty) flaps, the wounds are covered with skin grafts, or the wound is simply left open to heal by secondary intention (McCash technique[22]). These are not mutually exclusive techniques, and often all three maneuvers may be employed in the same hand. It is yet to be established that one fasciectomy technique yields notably improved results over another. All are associated with a low but consistent incidence of complications, including hematoma formation, nerve and vessel injury, delay in healing, joint stiffness, particularly loss of PIP joint flexion, and complex regional pain syndrome (CRPS).

The surgical treatment of post-surgical recurrent contractures is even more complicated, because the skin is now scarred and the internal anatomy disturbed. The surgeon frequently must modify the technique to avoid disastrous complications, such as digital necrosis. One modification that addresses severely contracted PIP recurrences involves the initial application of gradual soft-tissue distraction devices, such as the Digit Widget, to straighten severely contracted PIP joints (Fig. 39-6). The device is attached to the skeleton of the middle phalanx, and a clever force-couple mechanism powered by rubber bands and monitored by the hand therapist gradually elongates contracted PIP joint capsule, volar plate, and collateral ligaments. At an obligatory second surgery, the scarred skin and pathologic fascia is removed and a full-thickness skin graft inserted.

Therapy Following Operative Treatment

Within the first several days post-surgery the client returns to the clinic to have the operative dressings removed. In the case of surgery involving flaps or grafts, the surgeon may choose to delay some additional days before referring to a therapist. When a graft or flap is not performed, the therapist may be the first person to see the wound post-surgery. In this circumstance, having knowledge of the surgery performed is important, as well as how the surgeon would like the wound managed. Evaluation of the wound, description of active range of motion (AROM), edema, pain, color, and drainage is documented. Apply a light dressing and instruct in gentle exercise and edema management. Fit the client with an orthosis (Fig. 39-7 through Fig. 39-9) at this time. A dorsal orthotic may be preferred to prevent maceration to the surgical wound. If the release was

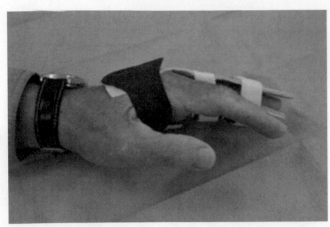

FIGURE 39-8 Dorsal hand-based orthosis.

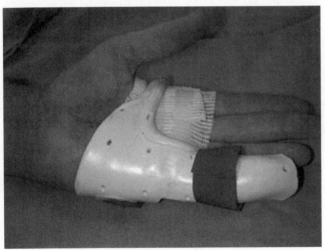

FIGURE 39-9 Volar-based hand orthosis.

performed on the fifth digit, a hand-based orthosis including just the fourth and fifth digit is indicated. With release of the fourth digit, the third and fifth digits are typically included in the orthosis. Clients who have multiple procedures may be best supported by a full resting hand-based orthosis. Patient comfort and the therapist's observation of tissue reaction must guide orthotic fit. Aggressive stretch with the orthosis, especially early in the healing process, can cause flare and compromise healing. Take care not to put stretch on the healing structures to prevent hypoxia to the tissues.[23]

? Questions to Discuss with the Physician

- What was the extent of contracture prior to surgery?
- What was the extent of surgery needed, and was there nerve or vessel injury?
- How was the skin closed? Was a flap or graft used?
- How long should the hand be immobilized if there is a graft or flap?
- Was a McCash procedure used?
- How would you like the wound managed?

( ) What to Say to Clients

Wound Care

Despite discussion of the extent of surgery by the surgeon, the client is often surprised and is sometimes overwhelmed by the appearance of their wound. Before undressing the wound, it is helpful to prepare the client by saying, "Your surgeon has had to make some cuts on your skin to be able to cover a wider area than was there before. You will see zigzags and cuts to prevent the skin from tightening and preventing movement as you heal."

In the case of a McCash procedure, more reassurance is necessary. You may explain by saying, "Your surgeon has chosen to let your body heal on its own and that will take a little time. We will work together to help your hand stay clean and heal faster."

Exercise

"Even though you have stitches and swelling, it is important to begin moving your hand. Your swelling will actually decrease with movement. Written handouts guide you to move at least every other hour. Do your exercises slowly until you feel a stretch, hold that position and repeat."

About the Orthosis

"The purpose of your orthosis is to provide a gentle stretch to the parts of your hand that have become shortened. Another purpose is to resist the effects of the scars that form as a consequence of your surgery, because they try to contract and pull your fingers back into flexion. We will need to make adjustments to the orthosis over the next few weeks to improve the fit as your swelling goes down, your wounds heal, and your movement improves. You should continue to wear the orthosis at night for approximately 4 months."

Evaluation Tips

Evaluation and description of the wound is imperative at each treatment session, because infection can be a significant risk factor to successful management.[24] A therapist who is familiar with the stages of wound healing is better able to consult with a physician if a problem arises. Infection may spread quickly, so any suspected signs or symptoms (such as, increased pain, redness, discharge, and foul odor) should be conveyed immediately to the referring surgeon.

The presence of edema and pain immediately post-surgery often precludes the ability to take accurate joint measurements. A gross description of movement, such as the distance from tip of finger to palmar crease, is helpful. Edema can be monitored using circumferential measurements if this does not contaminate a wound.

Evaluate pain using a visual analog scale (VAS). Because CRPS is a risk factor, awareness of a client's pain response is necessary.[25-27]

Diagnosis-Specific Information that Affects Clinical Reasoning

As with most hand rehabilitation, having the client establish a relationship with a single therapist who guides them throughout the healing is best. It is rare that a client is not anxious about the extent of surgical wounds, pain, edema, and bruising that accompanies the surgical management of Dupuytren's disease. A single therapist has more credibility looking at the wound and assessing its healing than if a variety of therapists remark on its progress. Effective edema management with elevation, movement, and compression prevents excess scar formation. It is often frightening for a client to move while there are stitches and open areas in their hand, especially when bleeding occurs.

♡ *Tips from the Field*

Gentle passive range of motion (PROM) with your hand placed dorsally on theirs, guiding them into flexion is a less painful way to begin movement. Light dressing (possibly with Coban wrap) allays their concern about bleeding and supports their tissue. Placing their hand in an elevated position during treatment conveys the importance of elevation.

Postoperative Treatment

Week One

During the first week of treatment, especially for more complex surgeries, a client should be given the option of attending therapy frequently. Observation and care of wounds, management of edema, and addressing the possibility of a flare prevents some of the risk factors inherent with this surgery.

Typically therapists manage the wound following surgery and provide information to the surgeon during the course of treatment. It is important to discuss the surgeon's preference regarding the use of specific dressings and wound care. At the first postoperative visit, usually after 2 to 4 days, the operative dressing is removed, and the wound is assessed and covered in a light dressing. The dressing typically includes a non-adherent dressing like Adaptic or Xeroform. It is important to use this type of dressing sparingly to prevent maceration.

Exercise

Teach the client gentle exercise, including tendon gliding, blocking, passive and active motion, and tenodesis. Have the client demonstrate these exercises. Clients are often very reticent to move their hand when there are open wounds. Instruct clients to elevate their hand as much as possible during the day and to perform their exercises every other hour.

Orthoses

The orthosis is fabricated as described earlier, paying special attention not to compromise vascular structures with stretch. A dorsal orthosis is preferable when there are open wounds both to prevent maceration, as well as for comfort. Straps are placed to support the fingers and dorsum of the hand comfortably against the orthosis but not with enough stretch to cause blanching or pain. There is no reason to overstretch tissues during the early part of wound healing, because the risk for contracture and scarring is primarily from edematous tissue.

Weeks Two to Three

Time should be set aside during the early part of the second week to more carefully assess both PROM and AROM. Re-evaluate

sensation as well as wounds. Stitches are typically removed in the first 10 to 14 days, allowing for early scar management techniques, such as gentle scar massage and use of silicone gel sheets.

As the edema decreases and dressings are reduced, readjust the orthosis to ensure proper fit. If the client has had a graft or flap, movement is initiated at about 10 days postoperative. Treatment for these clients mimics the early sessions described earlier.

Exercise and Activity

The client continues the exercises with encouragement to progress to end range. Instruct them to use their hand in light activities of daily living (ADLs), minimize dressings, and incorporate their hand in bilateral activity.

➢ *Precautions and Concerns*

The therapist should be very observant of signs of flare or early signs of CRPS. These clients are often reticent to involve their hands in bilateral activity, and they posture their hand protectively. Discussion of their pain management, sleep patterns, and anxiety should alert the therapist to early symptoms of CRPS and indicate the necessity of involvement of their surgeon.[27]

Three Weeks and Later

Scar management, exercise, and orthotic adjustment are the primary aspects of therapy going forward. Reassess their AROM and PROM to pinpoint the specific adjustments in the orthosis as well as tissue-specific guidelines for exercises. Joint stiffness and loss of preoperative flexion may be complications of surgery that can be avoided.[28,29] Scar management includes massage, use of silicone gel sheets[30] or paper tape, and stretching exercises. A palmar orthosis may be considered at this time if a dorsal orthosis had been used. If the client can tolerate the silicone sheet between their skin and their orthosis at night, the firmer support adds compression. Occasionally a client cannot tolerate silicone gel and develops a rash. Trying Otoform may be an alternative, as well as closed cell padding on the orthosis.

◐ *What to Say to Clients*

"It is important that you use your hand in functional activity. You may find that your hand tires with sustained grip or that you notice stiffness or swelling in the morning when you remove your orthosis. Your hand will continue to heal over the next few months. Continue to use the orthosis at night and manage your scar with the silicone gel and scar massage."

CASE STUDY 39-1 ■

B.L. is a 61-year-old, right-hand dominant machinist of Scandinavian descent. The only significant findings in his past medical history are that he is diabetic and a social drinker. He has no memory of a serious injury to his right upper extremity. In the last year, he has noticed that he has lost the ability to straighten the middle and ring fingers of his right hand, and this seems to be getting worse (Fig. 39-10, *A*). He remembers his father having something similar, but the condition was never addressed by a physician. B.L. states that the contracture "annoys" him. Although he can still use tools, he can no longer straighten his fingers enough to get his wallet out of his pocket. He also hesitates to greet people with a handshake, because he cannot clear his palm of his last two fingers. He consulted a hand surgeon, and they decided that surgery was necessary because of the level of contracture and the progression of these changes.

Surgical Procedure

The physician performed a McCash open palm procedure to resect the diseased tissue that caused the contracture at the MPs. Additional dissection was needed to release the PIP of the middle and ring fingers and to remove diseased bands (see Fig. 39-10, *B*). The palmar wound was left open to heal by secondary intention with direct closure of the incisions in the middle and ring fingers. The sutures were to be removed in 2 weeks.

Two Days after Surgery

The physician referred the client back to the hand therapist and prescribed range of motion (ROM) exercise, edema control, wound management instructions, and fabrication of an orthosis. Although the client had no sympathetic signs before surgery, a dorsal extension orthosis was provided that allowed 30° of MP flexion the first 1 to 2 weeks; this prevented compromised delivery of nutrients to the tissue and wound bed, as well as anoxia. The PIPs were placed in extension to the hood of the orthosis. AROM exercises were initiated immediately with ten repetitions of gentle flexion to the palm every 2 to 3 hours and extension. Active flexion to the distal palmar crease was limited, measuring 2.5 cm in the ring finger and 2.8 cm in the small finger. Edema management included elevation and AROM. The client was instructed to wash the palm wound and change the small bandage twice daily. The client was seen for therapy three times a week; at each visit he was given exercises for AROM, tendon gliding, and gentle passive flexion stretch within tolerance.

Eleven Days after Surgery

B.L. had no adverse responses to using the orthosis the granulation bed around his palmar wound was good, and he was ready to

have the PIP stitches removed. He was able to make a full active fist but struggled to maintain extension. His orthosis was modified at 2 weeks to increase the MP position to 0 (neutral); the tissue reaction was watched closely.

Two Weeks after Surgery

With his orthosis adjusted and his stitches removed, B.L. demonstrated good extension and flexion at the MPs and limited discomfort with exercise and splinting. Edema was minimal, but the limitations in PIP extension continued. More isolated exercise was given to the PIPs, and the client was given a gutter orthosis to wear at night with mild tension into PIP extension. This was to be followed by blocking exercise in the morning after removal of the orthosis. The palmar wound had not yet fully closed, and Bart was instructed to keep it clean.

Three and One-Half Weeks after Surgery

The palmar wound was closed, and PIP extension was resolved. The client's only complaint concerned the dense wound and palmar hypersensitivity. A daily desensitization program was added, along with ultrasound treatments in the clinic. B.L. also was given a silicone gel sheet for use at night. His splinting time was reduced to use at night, and he was monitored closely for changes in ROM. The therapist incorporated hand activities, including manipulating money, using the computer keyboard, and grasping and releasing large objects, to address the client's preoperative functional goals.

Five Weeks after Surgery

B.L. began gentle strengthening exercises and lightly resistive tool grasp, along with desensitization.

Twelve Weeks after Surgery

The client returned to his job as a machinist. He was delighted with his outcome (see Fig 39-10, *C*).

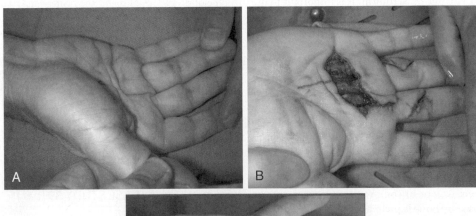

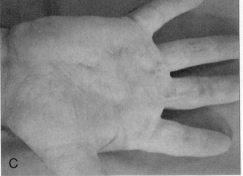

FIGURE 39-10 A, Prior to surgery; **B**, Post-surgery; **C**, After rehabilitation.

Non-Operative Treatment

Although surgery continues to be the most reliable and accepted method to treat progressive Dupuytren's contractures, numerous non-surgical interventions have been tried over the years. These include hand therapy, corticosteriod injections, dimethylsulfoxide injections, topical vitamin A and E, topical verapamil, and antimetabolites, such as 5-fluorouracil. There is some scientific evidence that frequent injections of triamcinolone softens nodules and perhaps alters the natural history of the disease. There are no scientifically valid studies demonstrating efficacy of any other oral or topical agents—only anecdotal reports and profit-driven advertising. In some European countries, soft penetration radiation given during the nodular phase of the disease has been shown to alter the course of disease by retarding or eliminating the progression of nodules to the cord phase.

Recently, enthusiasm for a non-surgical alternative has been heightened by the introduction of an injectable bacterial-derived collagenase as a primary treatment of a contracted digit.[26] A series of carefully performed clinical studies that proved the safety and efficacy of collagenase resulted in Food and Drug Administration (FDA) approval of Xiaflex (Auxilium Pharmaceuticals, PN) in 2010. The FDA and manufacturer have established the following inclusion criteria: a MP or PIP joint contracture of at least 20° associated with a palpable cord. A minute volume of the agent is injected into the cord. Within hours the collagenase has broken down the chemical bonds between the collagen moieties so that 24 hours post-injection, traction on the cord likely results in its rupture and extension of the previously contracted joint.

Therapy after Collagenase Enzymatic Fasciotomy

The client is referred to hand therapy 1 or 2 days after the injected finger has been manipulated into as much extension as possible. This typically takes place 24 hours following injection. A brief evaluation is performed, which includes a description of the appearance of the hand. Color, bruising, and skin tears at the time of manipulation are noted. Measurements are taken of both AROM and PROM. Pain, edema, and sensation are documented. The client is taught to begin moving their hand; exercises including tendon gliding and blocking both for flexion and extension are begun. If the release was performed on the fifth digit a hand-based nighttime orthosis including just the fourth and fifth digit is constructed. With release of the fourth digit, the third and fifth digits are typically included in the orthosis. Patient comfort and the therapist's observation of tissue reaction must guide orthotic fit. Aggressive splinting especially early in the healing process can cause flare and compromise healing.

?   Questions to Discuss with the Physician

- What was the extent of the contracture before the injection?
- Did the cord spontaneously rupture or was significant stretch applied?
- If there is a skin tear, how would you like the wound managed?

( )   *What to Say to Clients*

About the Condition

"The injection was meant to weaken the cord that is causing your finger to bend. Because of the stretch on other structures when your finger was extended, you may feel tenderness in your palm. It is expected that during the first week the bruising will subside. Healing can be helped by gentle movement, elevation, and use of an orthosis."

About the Orthosis

"The orthosis is needed to maintain the fingers in a straight position. The orthosis should be worn at night and you should stretch and do ROM exercises during the day. In the next week you should wear the orthosis less during the day and then only at night. It is important that your orthosis be comfortable and not cause any pressure areas."

About Exercise

"We will begin exercise to decrease swelling and restore movement. It is best to do the exercises every other hour and to do them slowly. I will give you a handout on tendon gliding and blocking exercises" (see Chapter 1). "While you are healing from the injection, it is not advised to do strengthening exercises or to use your hand in forceful gripping activity for the next 2 weeks."

Evaluation Tips

Despite the surgeon preparing the client for bruising or a tear in the skin, clients are sometimes surprised to see discoloration. Clients should be reassured and encouraged to participate in edema management, including local ice for short periods, elevation, and gentle movement.

➢   Precautions and Concerns

- *When making the orthosis take special care not to create excessive tension on the tissue, because this may cause localized hypoxia.[23] A dorsal orthosis is sometimes preferred, because it allows the patient to adjust the tension and keeps the palmar surface exposed for observation.*
- *A hand-based orthosis-volar or dorsal-is made placing the MPs in slight flexion if the release was performed at the PIP joint. For MP release, full extension is indicated.*
- *Be aware to look for signs of CRPS with this population (see Chapter 12).*

Diagnosis-Specific Information that Affects Clinical Reasoning

The extent of contracture prior to injection is somewhat predictive of the course of treatment and results. Because the injection method is performed on mild to moderate disease, typically across a singular joint, and surgical wounds are not present, patients can resume daily activity more quickly. If the MP was involved, reoccurrence rates have shown to be less in long term follow-up as compared to PIP involvement.[26] If the client smokes, is diabetic, is older, or has frail tissues, healing will likely be delayed. There have been few reports of major adverse effects of the collagenase injection. The small finger has a higher risk of pulley injury, tendon rupture, and boutonnière deformity.

♥ Tips from the Field

Regular exercise throughout the day is more beneficial than a singular long session. Encourage clients to return to therapy to manage PIP contractures that have not resolved with the injection. These are typically clients with a more significant contracture of the PIP prior to injection. Close attention to fitting with static progressive splints or adjusting the night splint maybe necessary.

Prefabricated extension-assist orthoses can help provide gentle extension force across the PIP joint for short intervals during the day. This orthosis is not recommended for flexion contractures greater than 30° or if there is a firm contracture.

Teach blocked extension exercises to improve active extension of the PIP joint by having the patient flex the MP joint and place support dorsally against the proximal phalanx. Doing so allows the extensor digitorum to exert more leverage across the PIP and provides a better position for the lumbrical muscles to extend the IPs.

Client compliance for splinting and exercise is varied. Instruct patients to wear their orthosis at night for 3 to 6 months to prevent contracture of tissues that had been shortened prior to the procedure. The orthosis will not prevent recurrence of the disease.

References

1. Dupuytren G: Contracture du petit doigt et de l'annulaire de la main gauche dissipé complètement par le simple débridement de l'aponévrose palmaire, 1831, Gazette Hop.
2. Cline H: Notes of pathology, St Thomas's Hospital Medical School Library London, UK 1777:185.
3. Cooper A: On dislocations of the fingers and toes—dislocation from contraction of the tendon. In Cooper A, editor: *A treatise on dislocations and fractures of the joints*, London, 1822, Longman, Hurst, Rees, Orme, Brown & Cox.
4. Dupuytren G: Leçons orales de Clinique Chirurgicale faites à l'Hotel-Dieu Baillière, 1832, Paris.
5. Early P: Population studies in Dupuytren's contracture, *J Bone Joint Surg Br* 44:602–613, 1962.
6. Ling R: The genetic factor in Dupuytren's disease, *J Bone Joint Surg Br* 45:709–718, 1963.
7. Shaw R, Chong A, Zhang A, et al: Dupuytren's disease: history, diagnosis and treatment, *Plast Reconstr Surg* 120:44e–54e, 2007.
8. Ross D: Epidemiology of Dupuytren's contracture, *Hand Clin* 15:53–62, 1999.
9. Leclercq C: Non-surgical treatment. In Tubiana R, Leclercq C, Hurst L, et al: *Dupuytren's disease*, London, 2000, Martin Dunitz, pp 234–255.
10. Mc Farlane R: Some observations on the epidemiology of Dupuytren's disease. In Hueston J, Tubiana R, editors: *Dupuytren's disease*, ed 2, Edinburgh, 1985, Churchill Livingstone, pp 122–126.
11. Hueston J: *Dupuytren's contracture*, Edinburgh, 1963, E&S Livingstone.
12. Merle M, Merle S: Maladie de Dupuytren et diabète. In Tubiana R, Hueston JT, editors: *La maladie de Dupuytren*, ed 3, Paris, 1986, l'Expansion Scientifique, pp 90–92.
13. Bradlow A, Mowat A: Dupuytren's contracture and alcohol, *Ann Rheum Dis* 45:304–307, 1986.
14. Clarkson P: The aetiology of Dupuytren's disease, *Guy Hosp Rep* 110:52–62, 1963.
15. Brenner P, Mailander P, Berger A: Epidemiology of Dupuytren's disease. In Berger A, Delbruck A, Hinzmann R, editors: *Dupuytren's disease*, Berlin, 1994, Springer Verlag, pp 244–254.
16. Mc Grouther D: The microanatomy of Dupuytren's contracture, *Hand* 13:215–236, 1982.
17. Mc Farlane R: Pattern of the diseased fascia in the fingers in Dupuytren's contracture, *Plast Reconstruct Surg* 54:31–39, 1974.
18. Leclercq C: The management of Dupuytren disease. In Mathes SJ, Hentz VR, editors: *Plastic surgery*, Philadelphia, 2006, WB Saunders, pp 729–758.
19. Lesmusiaux J, Debeyre N: Le traitement medical de la maladie de Dupuytren. L'actualite rhumatologique 1979 presenteeaux praticien. Expansion Scientifique Francaise 1980.
20. McIndoe A, Beare R: The surgical management of Dupuytren's contracture, *Am J Surg* 95:197–203, 1958.
21. Andrews J, Kay H: Segmental aponeurectomy for Dupuytren's disease: a prospective study, *J Hand Surg Br* 16:255–257, 1991.
22. Mc Cash C: The open palm technique in Dupuytren's contracture, *Br J Plast Surg* 17:271–280, 1964.
23. Evans R, Dell P, Fiolkowski P: A clinical report of the effect of mechanical stress on functional results after fasciectomy for Dupuytren's contracture, *J Hand Ther* 15(4):331–339, 2002.
24. Bulstrode N, Jemec B, Smith P: The complications of Dupuytren's contracture surgery, *J Hand Surg* 30(5):1021–1025, 2005.
25. Mullins PA: Postsurgical rehabilitation of Dupuytren's disease, *Hand Clin* 15(1):167–174, 1999.
26. Watt A, Hentz V: Collagenase clostridium histolyticum: a novel nonoperative treatment for Dupuytren's disease, *Int J Clin Rheumatol* 6:123–133, 2011.
27. Reuben SS: Preventing the development of complex regional pain syndrome after surgery, *Anesthesiology* 101(5):1215–1224, 2004.
28. Bayat A, McGrouther DA: Management of Dupuytren's disease—clear advice for an elusive condition, *Annals of the Royal College of Surgeons of England* 88(1):3–8, 2006.
29. Zyluk A, Jagielski W: The effect of the severity of the Dupuytren's contracture on the function of the hand before and after surgery, *J Hand Surg European* 32(3):326–329, 2007.
30. van der Wal MB, van Zuijlen PP, van de Ven P, et al: Topical silicone gel versus placebo in promoting the maturation of burn scars: a randomized controlled trial, *Plas Reconstruct Surg* 126(2):524–531, 2010.

40

The Neurological Hand

Gillian Porter and Lara Taggart

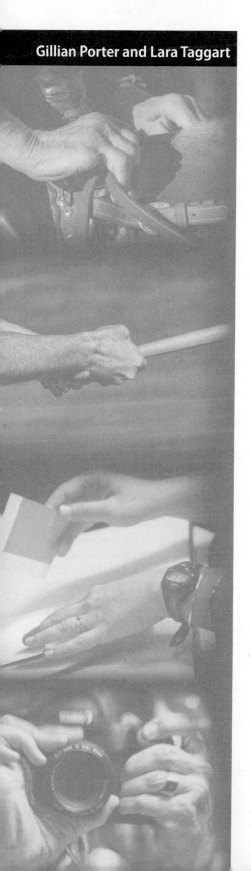

The neurological hand can be complex. Motor and sensory impairments, **spasticity/hypertonicity, learned disuse/nonuse,** and perceptual issues make rehabilitation of this hand a challenge. And since not every neurological injury or impairment has the same symptoms among clients,[1] predicting outcomes in a neurological patient's hand progress can be difficult. However, when a neurological client makes progress in hand skills or experiences an increase in functional use of his hand, the reward is significant. This chapter is designed to assist clinicians in the assessment and treatment of the neurological hand and to offer suggestions for orthotic options to promote optimal positioning at rest and in function.

Common Diagnoses Associated with the Neurological Hand

The most typical diagnoses associated with neurological conditions that are referred for treatment include but are not limited to the following:

- Cerebrovascular accident (CVA)
- Traumatic brain injury (TBI)
- Cerebral palsy (CP)
- Multiple sclerosis (MS)
- Parkinson disease (PD)
- Spinal cord injury (SCI)
- **Dystonia**

- **Hemiplegia/hemiparesis**
- **Edema**
- Spasticity
- Decreased coordination
- Muscle weakness
- Pain
- Joint stiffness/decreased range of motion (ROM)

Timeline of Intervention

Brain injury can lead to a broad spectrum of symptoms and disabilities. Persons with an acquired brain injury from CVA and TBI can exhibit motor disorders in which the UEs often show common clinical symptoms, such as spasticity, decreased muscle strength, incoordination, impaired sensation, and inability to bear weight symmetrically.[2]

The rate of functional recovery after stroke has been reported to be non-linear with the most rapid recovery in the first 3 months. On the other hand, muscle strength in the paretic upper extremity (UE) shows greater recovery in the initial 6 months post-stroke, and some individuals achieve motor recovery years after injury. Currently, there are studies of brain recovery with rats and post induced CVA. Neuroscientists have discovered there are still gains in brain recovery even though changes or improvement in functional behavioral may not be evident. There is no research to show recovery stops at 6 months.

It has been estimated that 3 months after a stroke, only 20% of clients attain full recovery of UE function, and 30% to 66% of these individuals are unable to use their affected UE in meaningful activities.[3] Intervention to increase hand skills is very individualized, and the level of practical return varies between individuals. Therefore, as therapists, it is important to assess not only functional status but also the priorities of the individual's hand use.

There is an absence of consistency between researchers and clinicians in the use of terminology to describe changes in motor ability after stroke. Recovery is a dynamic process that cannot be encapsulated at one point in time. However, use of a descriptive UE functional guideline to assist with goal writing and intervention planning is helpful. This is further addressed later in the chapter.

Using neuroimaging techniques to diagnose acute capsular stroke, Wenzelburger and colleagues[4] found that lesions in the posterior regions of the internal capsule were associated with chronic dexterity deficits in the affected UE. At baseline assessment, muscle strength was the only predictor significantly associated with dextrous hand function at 6 months post-stroke. Duncan and colleagues[5] reported motor and sensory scores on the Fugl-Meyer Assessment (FMA) at day 5 after stroke accounted for 74% of the variance in the composite scores at 6 months post stroke. However, it is not possible to delineate the contribution of UE sensation to the recovery of discrete dextrous hand function from such composite scoring of the **sensorimotor** functions in the UEs.[5]

MS is the most common autoimmune, inflammatory, demyelinating disease of the central nervous system (CNS). MS is characterized by a combination of damage to both gray matter and white matter with an ensuing loss of tissue leading to cortical atrophy. The neurological symptoms with relation to the hand include sensory disturbances, motor impairment, intention tremor, **ataxia,** and impaired motor coordination.[6] The clinical symptoms of MS are highly variable depending on the site and extent of CNS involvement. However, difficulty with object manipulation caused by deterioration of hand dexterity is a common and important clinical feature with mildly involved MS clients.[7] Additionally, UE function seems to be related to a decrease or loss of light touch-pressure and two-point discrimination sensations of the hand, as well as a decrease in elbow flexion strength. UE strengthening and sensorial training of the hand may contribute to increased UE function in clients with MS. Therefore, testing of both static and dynamic manipulation tasks may be needed for a more complete assessment of hand function in various populations. However, an explicit overview of arm-hand training programs is lacking with the MS population.

Hemiparetic CP is a common neurological disorder that affects sensorimotor function and development in children. Functional motor developmental delay or deconditioning of the affected limb is known to contribute to compensatory use of the intact limb rather than attempting to use the involved limb. Subsequently, the impaired limb undergoes reduction in muscle size or atrophy and associated muscle weakness. Recently, neuro-**facilitation** approaches began to integrate weight bearing and muscle strengthening exercise with neuromuscular electrical stimulation (NMES), **biofeedback, forced use,** repetitive training, and **bilateral arm training,** which were based on contemporary motor learning and control theories to maximize motor recovery in individuals with neurological impairments.

Cervical spinal cord injury (cSCI) can lead to devastating impairments, and yet to date, there is no reliable clinical treatment. In humans, cSCI, including complete and incomplete **tetraplegia,** represents about 62% of all spinal cord injuries.[8] This type of injury can cause severe impairments affecting the use of the UEs. Regaining partial or full function of the arm and hand could make significant improvements in client quality of life, and it is considered to be a priority for clients with cSCI.[9] Recently, there has been increasing interest in developing cSCI models in rodents; hence, having sensitive and reliable methods to evaluate forelimb motor functions is of potential importance. Donnelly, et al.[10] identified functional limitations in the SCI population associated with several broad areas. The study surveyed 41 clients with SCI in the early stage of recovery for their perceived level of satisfaction and performance in these areas. The top five identified areas of concern were: functional mobility, including transfers and wheelchair use (19%); dressing (13%); grooming (11%); feeding (8%); and bathing (7%).

Clients recently diagnosed with a neurological condition benefit from having both a physiatrist, who specializes in physical medicine and rehabilitation, and a neurologist, who treats the nervous system, throughout their recovery.[11] Many will have a neurologist assigned at the acute stage of their injury and may need to seek a different physician or neurologist to continue managing their care in the later stages of recovery. A neurologist typically oversees needs, such as routine tests to monitor any changes in recovery. Both neurologists and physiatrists may manage medication specific to a client's neurological injury, such as to address seizures, spasticity, and **neurogenic** pain. Having consistent follow-up with a physician is essential, especially if a client is experiencing some of the most common barriers to progression of the neurological hand: spasticity, pain, and edema.

Spasticity

One of the most common barriers for a neurological hand is spasticity. In a survey of over 500 **stroke** survivors, 58% experience spasticity, and only 51% of those with spasticity have received treatment.[12] Spasticity can be difficult to manage and has the potential to sabotage recovery.

First, it is important to determine whether a client's spasticity is already being managed by oral medication (muscle relaxer or antispasmodic), such as, but not limited to, Baclofen, Zanaflex, Flexeril, Valium, or Dantrium,[13,14] Botoxinjections, or the intrathecal baclofen pump (ITB).[14] Second, it is important to understand the client's routine with oral medication and/or Botoxinjections. In a perfect world, a client has a consistent relationship with the physician (physiatrist or neurologist) managing his spasticity in order to monitor the effectiveness of the intervention(s). However, it is not uncommon for the therapist to encourage a client to seek spasticity management or suggest to a client's physician more comprehensive tone management. Spasticity is known to develop and/or change over weeks, months, or years after a brain injury,[15] which when left undiagnosed or undermanaged can lead to debilitating UE changes. Unmanaged spasticity interferes with successful functional use of the affected UE,[15] increasing the odds of developing patterns of learned non-use that may become extremely difficult to overcome.

In cases where a client's spasticity is being managed by an intervention(s), it is worthwhile to discover the client's dosage amount and routine for oral medication or ITB therapy, when his last series of injections occurred, and when his next series of Botox injections are to occur. Understanding a client's routine with his spasticity intervention promotes optimal results in therapy. Botox injections, for example, are usually received every 3 to 4 months with the first noticeable effects typically occurring within the first 2 weeks of injections.[16] If a client is seeking therapy toward the end of his injection cycle, intervention may result in less desirable outcomes. An oral medication or ITB dose schedule is important to understand, because the best results may be achieved soon after receiving a dose. Some ITB dose schedules can be programmed to correlate with a client's treatment schedule and/or times of the day when he is most functional. Therapy following a dose of oral medication may offer positive results in reducing spasticity to benefit intervention; however, these muscle relaxers may also have the negative side effect of decreasing a client's ability to remain alert and attentive to therapy.

As a therapist, it is good practice to correspond with a client's physician regarding observations made of a client's degree of spasticity, location, and impact on function. It is not uncommon to utilize a measure, such as the Ashworth Scale, Modified Ashworth Scale (MAS), or Tardieu Scale, to assess levels of spasticity in specific UE muscles and provide a client's physician with the findings. Such communication should include remarks about the impact of spasticity on function, particularly during grasp and release demands in various reaching patterns. This may assist in providing a comprehensive picture of the client's ability to utilize the affected UE while under the influence of spasticity. It is also important to communicate with physicians the degree to which a client uses his affected hand in functional activities and/or exercise, because there is the potential to inject a Botox dose in digit flexors that renders grasp too weak to carry objects and/or unable to progress an exercise orthosis, such as the SaeboFlex.

Severe cases of spasticity may cause soft-tissue shortening and decreased joint ROM. In these cases, Botox can be administered prior to orthotic positioning or serial casting to promote the most optimal conditions for increasing soft tissue length and joint ROM.

If clients are not progressing because of spasticity, it may be worthwhile to place their therapy visits on hold in order to resume after more comprehensive spasticity management is achieved. This way, a client has the opportunity to receive the maximal benefit of therapeutic intervention.

It is important to encourage clients to ask their physician questions about the available options to manage spasticity, as well as their potential risks and side effects.

Pain

Pain is an obvious barrier in a client's ability to effectively incorporate his affected hand in meaningful tasks. Referring a client to his neurologist, physiatrist, or pain specialist is critical to managing pain, particularly if the pain is neurogenic. Clients may benefit from asking their physicians the possible side-effects of pharmacological intervention, and discussing a dosage regime that will lead to minimal interference with daily activities and rehabilitation. Clients may also wish to inquire about holistic interventions for pain management.

Edema

Edema reduces passive range of motion (PROM) and active range of motion (AROM), coordination, and effectiveness of grasp and pinch. Edema can result from injury, dependent positioning of the affected UE, a comorbid medical condition, poor positioning habits while seated or lying down, and medications. For persistent cases of edema that do not respond to basic edema management techniques or are suspected to be the result of medication, it is important to refer clients to their physician (neurologist, physiatrist, or cardiologist) to discuss options of how to decrease the edema. In severe cases of edema, a referral to a lymphedema specialist may be in order, not only to address the problem, but also ensure the movement of fluid does not negatively impact a client's cardiac status.

Other Considerations

Therapists may also benefit from asking questions and providing feedback regarding issues, such as blood pressure, oxygen saturation rate, or any medical issue that may interfere with a client's ability to participate in therapy. Therapists working with neurological patients' UEs often request prescriptions from physicians regarding equipment that may benefit in the **neuro-reeducation** and positioning of an affected hand, such as orthoses, transcutaneous electrical nerve stimulation (TENS)/NMES units, and/or compression garments.

What to Say to Clients

Clients often ask, "Will I ever regain 100% function in my (affected) hand?" This is a difficult question to answer, particularly since no two clients with the same neurological condition are the same.[1] Recovery varies based on many factors, starting with the type of diagnosis. Conditions, such as CVA and TBI, depend on location and extent of injury, the number and extent of barriers present (that is, spasticity, edema, pain, cognition, visual-perceptual issues, and so on), compensatory patterns of movement, orthopedic issues, patterns of learned nonuse, and other issues. Understanding the difference in how a neurological hand causes symptoms in the various stages of recovery is also important. For example, the answer to this question for someone with a paralyzed UE within the acute phase of a CVA will be different than the answer for someone who possesses a chronic neurological hand several years post injury. More degenerative conditions, such as MS and PD, require a different approach. Maintenance, prevention, and adaptation, especially in the chronic stages of these conditions, can be a more appropriate focus than recovery of lost function.[1] The following sections give some suggested comments and considerations for treating patients with hemiplegic/hemiparetic hands and for patients with progressive conditions.

The Hemiplegic/Hemiparetic Hand per Stage of Recovery

Acute Stage (Initial Injury up to Discharge from Hospital/Inpatient Rehabilitation)

This is a difficult stage, because many clients in this stage have concomitant concerns (that is, mobility, dependence for activities of daily living (ADLs), speech, vision, cognition, and so on) complicating the recovery of the hemiplegic hand. Areas of focus for therapy in this stage tend to be, but are not limited to: ADL performance, bed mobility, transfers, community mobility, positioning, and UE orthosis needs. The patient's hand's available AROM, fine motor coordination (FMC), and sensation, as well as the presence of barriers, impacts a therapist's approach in how to involve the hand in self-care. A paralyzed, **edematous** hand requires a therapist to teach the client and family positioning, self-PROM exercises, and edema management techniques. An affected hand with emerging movement and the beginning of spasticity will require self-AROM exercises, orthosis, and client/family education regarding functional return. Concomitant visual perceptual and/or cognitive deficits, such as a **visual field hemianopsia/neglect** and decreased cognitive attention, and sensory deficits require the additional challenge of increasing clients' attention to their affected UE. This is not only important for sensory reeducation but also for decreasing the risk of injury during transfers, mobility, sitting, and so on.

Since a primary focus of acute rehabilitation following brain injury is ADL performance, inclusion of the affected hand is dependent on how well it can contribute to function. How to involve the affected UE as an assist in self-care is addressed later in this chapter. The challenge at this level of care is balancing the focus of increasing a client's independence in self-care and addressing the recovery of the affected UE. If paralyzed, inclusion of the affected hand in self-care is limited; training a client to dress, shower, complete toilet hygiene, and so on, will often rely on unilateral techniques. If a neurological hand's deficits are limited to decreased FMC, encouraging a client to continue utilizing his hand as either his dominant hand or as an equal assist during fine motor activities is important. Humans are inclined to find the most efficient and effective method of completing a task to conserve energy.[17] If the less affected hand can complete a task faster with better quality, or if a client has not experienced adequate success in utilizing his affected hand, he may passively accept a unilateral UE existence.[13] And the beginning of learned nonuse could commence as early as this stage in recovery.

Points to consider and comments for clients and family at the acute stage:

1. Encourage functional use and inclusion of the affected UE in daily activities. Neuroscientists have discovered a "use it or lose it" phenomenon in brain cells during development and in adult brains with stroke, Alzheimer's disease, and other motor neuron diseases.[18]

> ◎ **Clinical Pearl**
>
> Brain cells that are not stimulated by activity will self-destruct. Encouraging the affected UE to participate in meaningful, daily tasks (such as, brushing hair) can stimulate better quality of movement as well as an increase relevancy of a task to a client.[13] Increased engagement of an affected UE in purposeful activities at this stage bodes well for maintaining neuronal connections for activities that are deeply embedded within the brain from years of repetition.

2. Develop the mantra: "Repetition, repetition, repetition, *with variety.*" Research on motor learning has revealed repetition in random practice format (that is, repetition of specific tasks with variability in sequence) is better than a blocked practice format (that is, repetition of the same task) within a treatment session.[13] Otherwise known as *motor variability,* or *repetition without repetition,*[19] this concept suggests the movements required for a specific task (such as, tying shoes) need high repetition in a variety of contexts in order to promote more successful conversion of the actual task. In other words, clients need lots of practice to learn/relearn how to use their affected hand in functional tasks.

3. Emerging movement will likely appear different than movement at a client's level of function before the injury. As movement returns, clients may have a difficult time figuring out *how* to use their affected hand,[13] or are deterred from using their affected hand because the emerging movement does not appear familiar. For example, clients knew how to tie their shoes prior to their injury, and likely did so without thinking of the movement required by their hands to complete the task. As they attempt familiar tasks (such as, tying shoes) after their injury, their affected hand may not be able to contribute as expected. Assisting clients in recognizing what they see now is only a

beginning, and though their movements may not appear the same, different movement patterns can be used, albeit short- or long-term, to complete a task.

> ◎ **Clinical Pearl**
>
> It has been proposed that synergistic movement patterns can result as a strategy to allow for the variance in motor performance.[20] These movement patterns have the potential to reflect the beginning of more "normal" movement, returning to PLOF, or result in compensatory movement strategies. And although there are treatment approaches that suggest it is best to avoid abnormal patterns of movement,[1] discouraging such variance may deter movement in the affected hand altogether and lead to learned nonuse.

4. Be cautious when discussing expectations of recovery. Clients have reported hearing comments from health care professionals that caused them to believe there is no hope for recovery. This leaves a lasting impression that can deter clients from working on their hands and contribute to a negative attitude about their hands. We have seen clients who started out with a nonfunctional hand in the acute stage have discharged from outpatient therapy writing and typing with their affected hand.

5. Dispel the theory that recovery plateaus within the first 6 months of injury.

> ◎ **Clinical Pearl**
>
> **Neural plasticity** is recognized as the anatomic and functional changes in the CNS based on: 1) activation of parallel pathways to maintain function within a damaged area, 2) activation of silent pathways, and 3) synaptogenesis, or the formation of new connections.[21]

One study involving brain imaging of chronic stroke survivors revealed improvement in function correlated with increased activity in multiple areas of the brain.[22] Studies such as this support plasticity occurs even in the later stages of recovery. Furthermore, a client's ability to capitalize on returning movement may not occur for a long time post injury. For instance, having the ability to plan and realize variance in movement, such as how to incorporate a lateral pinch in daily activities where a tip-to-tip pinch was formally used, can take time for the client to discover and the brain to problem-solve.

6. ROM, positioning, and orthotic needs can be addressed at this stage with correlating client/family/health care worker education on techniques and how to progress matters, such as an orthotic wearing schedule.[13] Clients and families need to know how to don/doff the orthosis, how to care for an orthosis, and the signs of improper fitting. Posting signs with instructions and pictures to assist health care employees to adhere to a positioning and/or orthotic routine may be necessary.

7. Educate clients and families on spasticity (if applicable) and encourage consistent contact with a physician to manage their tone.

8. Reinforce bilateral UE involvement in self-care.

> ◎ **Clinical Pearl**
>
> Research has shown improvement in affected UE functional performance secondary to bilateral training.[23]

One study involving transcranial magnetic stimulation (TMS) noted subjects experienced increased speed and functional ability to complete tasks with the affected UE after bilateral training.[24] This was accompanied by a significant increase in corticomotor representation of the involved limb within the affected hemisphere. For more details on bilateral training, see the "Tips from the Field" section later in this chapter.

Post-Acute Stage (After Release from Hospital/ Inpatient Rehabilitation, Up To 12 Months Post-Injury)

In many cases, emerging motor and/or sensory return occurs in this stage. Although there may still be lingering associated concerns to address, a more intent focus to rehabilitate the hand can begin. Ideally, a client arrives with an assigned neurologist and/ or physiatrist, in possession of a resting hand orthosis, and with his spasticity managed (if applicable). If not, these areas need to be addressed in addition to functional return of the hand. Clients may arrive to outpatient therapy making statements, "I want my hand back," or "When I get my hand back, I will…" Family members may also press for therapy to "fix [the client's] hand." Providing realistic feedback is a balance between keeping a client motivated while also preparing him for the potential fact his functional return will not likely be at 100% prior level of function (PLOF). Of course, variability in recovery exists depending on the severity of injury.[25] Regardless, it is important to stress that the neurological hand has the potential to continue making improvement. As clients start noticing other clients and the difference between hand presentations, it is important to also remind them that not every injury is the same. As a therapist, comparing clients can be both a benefit and a hazard; it can be beneficial as one prepares for the hand's progression, and it can be a hazard if it limits a therapist's approach at treating the neurological hand. Clients may also wonder why their affected lower extremities (LE) are making greater progress than their hand. It may be a benefit to educate them on the location of their stroke, the motor homunculus, and how the UE is typically more involved than the LE following an injury, such as a CVA.[26]

At this stage, relearning activities that previously required no thinking with a hand that is now more difficult to control often leads to frustration, resulting in a pattern of learned nonuse. Concurrent cognitive and motor planning issues have the potential to confound recovery and increase client frustration.

Additional points to consider and comments for clients and family at the acute stage:

1. No two neurological conditions are alike.[1] This is important to realize, because they may compare themselves to other clients.
2. Recovery of function takes time, practice, and commitment. Remind clients that they did not learn how to tie their shoes from one attempt. Consider timing them to provide realistic feedback of their efforts, because clients will often feel as though a task took "forever," when, in fact, it may have only taken a couple minutes.
3. Promote self-learning with the client and encourage him to try tasks that he may not expect to be able to do. When a client figures out how to accomplish a difficult task on his own, there is greater potential for carryover outside of therapy.
4. Clients need to be successful. Plan activities for that "just right challenge" and grade accordingly in order to promote success. Whichever direction is required to grade an activity for successful results, client engagement is essential in realizing his hand's potential.

5. Encourage realistic short-term goals. When faced with goals such as, "I want to play my classical guitar again," stated by a client with trace digit movement 4 months after a stroke, it is important to avoid dismissing the goal. Instead, return with a comment such as, "That is a good long-term goal. Here is where your hand is now, and in order to achieve your long-term goal, we will need to achieve this short-term goal first."
6. Be positive and supportive when a client incorporates his affected hand in daily activities. Clients can be their own worst critic, because the functional return of their affected hand may not appear the same at PLOF. Providing positive feedback may assist in increasing their confidence to utilize their affected hand with greater consistency.
7. Identify patterns of learned nonuse and tenaciously seek ways to include the affected hand as a functional assist to break these patterns. The earlier learned nonuse habits can be broken, the better. Consider reviewing a constraint protocol if appropriate, or introducing a tool, such as the motor activity log (MAL), without full implementation of a constraint protocol to help clients identify functional activities in which to incorporate their affected UE.
8. Respect the former role of the affected hand. Asking clients to complete activities with their affected, less dominant hand that would otherwise be performed by their dominant hand is not likely to be received well by the client.

Chronic Stage (12 Months or Longer Post-Injury)

Clients at this stage may be seeking an update to their home exercise program (HEP), have experienced a change in status with their hand, or are interested in exploring additional ways in which to incorporate their affected hand in daily activities. Some clients in the chronic stage had very little treatment intervention during the acute and post-acute stages and may be receiving therapy to address their affected hand for the first time. Clients in the chronic stage of recovery should arrive with an assigned neurologist and/or physiatrist, in possession of resting hand orthosis, and with their spasticity managed (if applicable). If not, these areas need to be addressed during therapy. Clients may require an updated orthosis to accommodate orthopedic changes to their hand and/or changes in their spasticity.

Additional points to consider and comments for clients and family at the acute and post-acute stages:

1. It is important to reiterate that clients can regain function several years post injury.
2. Since learned nonuse patterns have the potential to be well-ingrained in chronic survivors, it may be beneficial to focus on bilateral UE tasks, because this may encourage more automatic use of their affected hand during functional tasks.
3. In cases of learned nonuse, encourage a client to identify a specific number of tasks for which his affected hand can complete on a regular basis as a starting point for automatic use in functional activities. For example, have a client agree to use his affected hand to carry objects during mobility or stabilize objects as a support for the less affected UE.

Progressive Conditions

For clients diagnosed with progressive conditions, such as PD, MS, or other conditions that contribute to declining FMC skills or grip and pinch effectiveness, the focus of therapy can differ. This depends on severity of fine motor deficits, length of time from initial diagnosis and/or appearance of first symptom, and comorbid issues, such as arthritis, decreased sensation, fatigue, and decreased cognitive skills. The length of time from initial diagnosis or appearance of first symptom is not necessarily a predictor of fine motor performance or response to techniques involving recovery of function, because these conditions often have variability in presentations. Therefore, it is important to evaluate and treat each client with a progressive condition on an individual basis and focus on his fine motor skills with respect to function (that is, buttoning, writing, typing, meal preparation, feeding, grooming, and so on). One study indicated a positive response to modified Constraint Induced Therapy (mCIT) on behalf of clients with PD in Hoehn and Yahr stages II to III as demonstrated by improvement in action research arm test (ARAT), FMA, and box and block test (BBT) scores.[27] Of particular interest is the finding that **bradykinesia** may be reduced through mCIT activities. However, a significant limitation in this study is the fact the researchers did not assess functional performance in daily activities. Therefore, they could not infer their results lead to increased or more effective use of the affected hand(s) in daily activities that require fine motor skills. In both MS and PD, research has shown that the more chronic and severe the symptoms, the more difficulty a client will have with dexterity.[28,29] This results in clients requiring more assistance and modification to tasks involving dexterity.[28]

Barriers to completing tasks that involve FMC for individuals with PD include, but are not limited to: tremors, decreased initiation of movement or freezing, weakness in pinch and grasp, medication "off-time," and decreased attention to tasks (particularly when out of their visual field).[1] People with PD respond well by completing movement with high amplitude and high effort.[30] Though anecdotal, clients report increased ease in fine motor activities (such as, handwriting or buttoning) when prior to initiating these tasks, they sit with increased trunk extension and "activate" their hand by completing high amplitude "finger flicks."

Barriers for individuals with MS include, but are not limited to: fatigue, weakness in pinch and grasp, decreased sensation, and decreased attention.[1] Research is limited with respect to individuals with MS recovering lost function. Therefore, therapy should focus on preserving existing skills through fine motor exercises and consistent use in meaningful activities while educating clients to avoid fatigue.

Points to consider and comments for clients and family with progressive conditions:

1. Time of day may impact effectiveness of dexterity, because medication regimes, level of alertness, or degree of fatigue may correlate with performance. Try to organize tasks with high dexterity demands with times of the day when performance has its best potential.
2. Though recovery of lost function may not be attainable for clients with more chronic and severe symptoms, modification and adaptation may assist in increasing a client's participation in instrumental activities of daily living (IADL) tasks that require dexterity, while decreasing dependence in caregiver support.
3. Encourage upright posture and "finger flicks" prior to engaging in (and throughout as needed) fine motor tasks for people with PD.
4. Promote tasks that accentuate existing fine motor skills in order to preserve the current level of functional ability. This may

decelerate disease progression and reduce caregiver burden over the long-term.
5. Respect to what degree a client utilizes dexterity skills throughout his daily routine and promote realistic functional goals for the client and family. For example, a client with PD who also possesses concomitant cognitive, FMC, and motor planning deficits can preserve independence in feeding through increased availability of finger-foods. In severe cases involving cognitive and motor planning deficits, utensil management can often be frustrating, and training these clients to use adaptive equipment (AE) may not lead to successful outcomes.

Evaluation Tips

Commonly used assessments for evaluating hand function in the neurological setting are as follows:

- Box and block test (BBT)
- Nine hole peg test (NHPT)
- Action research arm test (ARAT)
- Fugl-Meyer Assessment (FMA)
- Motor activity log (MAL)
- Stroke impact scale (SIS)
- Functional independence measure (FIM)
- Wolf-Motor Function Test (WMFT)
- Functional test for the hemiplegic/paretic upper extremity (FTHUE)
- Jebsen-Taylor Hand Function Test
- Grip and pinch dynamometer testing

Improving motor impairment, increasing daily function, and enhancing quality of life are the primary goals of stroke rehabilitation. The assessments listed earlier represent some of the tools used to evaluate the neurological hand. When choosing an appropriate evaluation tool, it is important to use your clinical observations. Some assessments are more appropriate for a higher functioning hand, whereas other assessments are better for a lower functioning hand.

The BBT assesses gross manual dexterity by counting the number of blocks that can be transported individually from one compartment of a box to another within 1 minute. Higher scores are indicative of better manual dexterity. The reliability, validity, and responsiveness of the BBT have been established in clients with stroke. The NHPT is a timed test of fine manual dexterity. Participants place nine pegs in nine holes and then remove them as quickly as possible. The time needed to complete the task is measured in seconds, and a lower score indicates better dexterity. The NHPT has been demonstrated to have high reliability, validity, and responsiveness in clients with stroke. The ARAT assesses the ability to handle objects based on 19 items that are divided into four subscales of grasp, grip, pinch, and gross movement scored by a four-level ordinal scale ranging from 0 (no movement) to 3 (normal movement). A total scale score maximum of 57 indicates normal performance. The ARAT has established reliability, validity, and responsiveness in clients with stroke.

Three other well-developed outcome measures are widely used to assess UE motor impairment for persons with spasticity and hemiplegia.[31] The FMA assesses motor impairment and is reported to be highly correlated with FTHUE scores,[13] the MAL evaluates daily function, and the SIS determines quality of life; all have adequate reliability and validity. Both the MAL and SIS rely on self-report data.

Adequate validity has been established for the BBT in clients with acute stroke, MS, and TBI, and in elderly clients with UE impairment. The ARAT has good construct validity in measuring UE motor function for clients with chronic stroke. BBT and ARAT had better concurrent validity than the NHPT in clients with chronic stroke at pre- and post-treatment with better correlations to the FMA and MAL. These findings attest to the relationship between motor impairment and daily functions.

The FIM is part of the uniform data system for rehabilitation in the acute phase. The FIM is one of the most widely used methods of assessing functional status in persons with a disability.[32] The FIM includes 18 items, each with a maximum score of 7 and a minimum score of 1. Total possible FIM scores range from 18 to 126. The areas examined by the FIM include: self-care, sphincter control, transfers, locomotion, communication, and social cognition. These areas are further divided into motor and cognitive domains.[33] The FIM is intended to serve as a basic indicator of the severity of disability.

The WMFT was designed to assess functional motor ability of clients with moderate to severe UE motor deficits. It has been found to be useful for characterizing the motor status of higher functioning chronic clients who have experienced a stroke or TBI. The inter-test and interrater reliability is high for both performance time and functional ability rating scales. However, the test has limited usefulness for lower functioning chronic clients. The problem is that such clients are only able to complete less than half of the items on the WMFT, which lends to a sparse sampling of their motor ability. A graded version of the test was developed to address this problem.

The FTHUE is an UE assessment that tests the client's ability to complete ADLs in order of increasing complexity. It consists of seven levels requiring clients to complete 17 tasks based on Brunnstrom's hierarchy of motor return.[34] Task complexity ranges from evidence of an **associated reaction** during resisted elbow flexion of the less affected UE, to the fine motor skills required to remove a rubber band placed on the outside of a client's affected UE digits without using his less affected UE. Activities are timed and graded based on a quality of movement scale. This test was found to be reliable under test-retest conditions.

Lastly, the Jebsen-Taylor Hand Function Test looks at seven subtests to assess hand function. The seven timed sub tests include: handwriting; turning over cards; grasping and releasing small objects (for example, pennies, paper clips); stacking checkers; picking up and releasing beans with a spoon; and grasping and releasing large empty then weighted cans. This test has good test-retest reliability and good concurrent validity compared to other tests of upper limb dexterity.

Choosing an appropriate evaluation tool is one part to assessing a client's involvement of his affected hand in daily tasks. It is also important to obtain additional information, such as the following:
- Chief complaint/reason for referral
- History of present illness; onset of injury
- Past medical history
- History and present use of orthosis
- Prior therapy: Other therapy services received should include type (that is, inpatient or outpatient), when, and duration.
- Social history
- Living situation
- Mobility
  - Use of assistive devices
  - Driving status

- Employment: If a client is considering return to gainful employment or volunteer work, it is important to assess the extent to which he is going to involve his affected hand in activities, such as carrying, stabilizing, writing, typing, and so on.
- Communication; use of assistive technologies, if applicable
- ADLs:
  - Presence of durable medical equipment (DME) and AE
  - Level of independence
- PROM/AROM: Assess presence and cause of limitations, such as pain, edema, soft tissue restriction, **joint contractures,** spasticity, and so on.
- Edema
- Spasticity:
  - Assess using Ashworth Scale, MAS, or Tardieu Scale
  - Past and present use of tone management
- Sensation:
  - Light touch
  - Two-point discrimination
  - Sharp/dull
- **Kinesthesia:**
  - Pain/temperature
  - **Stereognosis**
- Cerebellar testing:
  - **Dysdiadochokinesia**
  - **Dysmetria**
- Cognitive testing
- Visual perception testing: There are many aspects of vision related to hand function, because vision often guides UE engagement. Visual deficits that could interfere with a client's ability to engage his hand in activities include, but are not limited to: visual field neglect/inattention, visual field hemianopsia, and difficulty with tracking/pursuits, **diplopia,** and fixation
- Identify the client's goals.

Diagnostic-Specific Information that Affects Clinical Reasoning

Functional Progression of the Neurological Hand

After assessing a client and his hand using the aforementioned objective measures, it is important to evaluate *how* a client utilizes his affected hand in daily activities. Assessing a hand's performance in measurements, such as the WMFT and the Jebsen-Taylor Hand Function Test, reveals only a portion of movement potential—a therapist needs to understand what a client *does* with his hand throughout the course of his day. Assessing a client's ability to achieve a perfect tip-to-tip pinch between D1-D2 to grasp a paperclip in the WMFT may be irrelevant if his most effective and more commonly used pinch is a lateral pinch to carry papers or fold laundry. A client may also attain test scores that would infer equal, or near-equal, ability to complete functional tasks as compared to his less affected UE but fail to incorporate his affected hand secondary to learned nonuse. The tendency for learned nonuse can occur regardless of whether the affected hand was a client's dominant or non-dominant UE prior to injury.

The influence of hand dominance in stroke recovery has limited research. One study concluded greater reliance on the ipsilateral UE to the lesion when the lesion is in the right hemisphere, demonstrating a strong right hand preference among right hand dominant survivors.[35] Meaning, if a right hand dominant individual has a right hemisphere injury, there is a greater chance he will prefer to utilize his right hand during daily tasks. Conversely, left hand dominant survivors did not demonstrate increased hand preference when their injury was in the ipsilateral hemisphere, and instead demonstrated more bilateral UE involvement in tasks.[35]

Understanding the developmental progression of grasp can be effective at identifying needs in ROM and motor control to achieve basic grasps and progress to more complex grasp skills. Examining the hand in this manner also allows a therapist to set realistic goals in grasp skills, because it would be logical, per developmental progression, for the neurological hand to master a gross grasp prior to a refined pinch. However, the neurological hand may not follow developmental milestones in the recovery of hand skills. Barriers (such as, spasticity, difficulty with motor planning, joint deformities, lack of coordination, and decreased sensation) can interfere with the developmental progression of the neurological hand. Instead of using these parameters to set goals regarding hand function, it may be beneficial to recognize the type of grasp most likely to be achieved by a client, and its potential effectiveness in daily activities. Goals can then be established according to functional potential. The following list is extracted in its entirety from its resource to be offered as a reference from which to derive functional goals

Functional Levels of the Hemiplegic Upper Extremity[36]

I. Classification of Function—Seven Levels
   Level 1—No voluntary motion, no functional use
   Level 2—Beginning active motion, no functional use
   Level 3—Dependent Stabilizer: Minimal voluntary motion, able to do the following types of activities:
   1. Move arm away from side while putting shirt into pants on affected side.
   2. Move arm away from side while adjusting side or back of shirt with less affected UE.
   3. Stabilize shirt at bottom for buttoning in front.
   4. Stabilize wet cloth at lap level while less affected UE applies soap.
   5. Weigh down paper while less affected UE is writing.
   Level 4—Independent Stabilizer: Moderate mass flexion pattern, including some shoulder motion against gravity, and moderate gross grasp are capable of performing the following types of activities:
   1. Hold up trousers while transferring to/from toilet.
   2. Hold toothbrush while less affected UE applies toothpaste.
   3. Hold handle and help open a drawer or refrigerator.
   4. Stabilize a mixing bowl at table level while the less affected UE mixes/stirs.
   5. Stabilize a bottle with a cap while the less affected UE twists the cap open.
   Level 5—Gross Motor Assist: Strong mass flexion pattern, some elbow extension control, moderate gross grasp (some release is helpful but not necessary), and some lateral pinch should be able to perform the following types of activities:
   1. Assist less affected UE in pulling donning/doffing socks/nylons.
   2. Reach and wash less affected UE and armpit.
   3. Hold dish while washing/wiping with less affected UE.
   4. Hold and assist in manipulating a broom for sweeping.
   5. Assist less affected UE in wringing a rag or sponge.
   Level 6—Functional Assist: Ability to combine components of strong mass flexion and extension patterns, including fair plus shoulder control, strong grasp/release, and strong pinch/release are able to perform the following types of activities:
   1. Assist in tying bows.

   2. Assist in fastening a zipper.
   3. Hold a utensil and stabilize food item while less affected UE cuts.
   4. Hold/stabilize pot lid while less affected UE pours out liquid.
   5. Hold pencil and begin to write legibly.
   Level 7—Refined Functional Assist: Fair plus to good isolated control in shoulder, elbow, and wrist, strong grasp/release, lateral and palmar prehension, and ability to manipulate individual digits are able to perform the following types of activities:
   1. Lace shoes
   2. Thread needle
   3. Manage safety pin to secure material
   4. Screw nut onto bolt
   5. Pick up coins
II. Classification of Function—Four Levels
   Level 1—Placement of Arm
   1. No prehension
   2. Move then fix in space (stabilize paper, bear weight)
   Level 2—Use in Relationship to an Object
   1. Shoulder adduction to clamp object under arm
   2. Forearm hook to carry objects
   3. Finger hook to carry objects
   4. Fixed hand to push and pull as weight to stabilize object
   Level 3—Use of Prehension
   1. Supportive—holds handrail
   2. Transports—moves objects
   3. Use of tool—use of object to accomplish a task
   Level 4—Skilled Independent Finger Motion
   1. Typing
   2. Playing piano
   Examples of goals:
1. Client will consistently demonstrate UE wrist/digit control to maintain cylindrical grasp of water bottle to work toward inclusion as a gross assist in daily activities.
2. Client will use his right UE as a functional assist by demonstrating pinch/release skills during 25% or more of dressing both upper and lower body.
3. Client will incorporate his UE as an equal refined functional assist during meal preparation demands (that is, cutting, chopping, dicing, mixing, stirring, and so on).

Assessments to Consider Per Functional Level of the Hemiplegic Upper Extremity

Level 1—Test measurements not likely appropriate
Level 2—FTHUE
Level 3—FTHUE, WMFT (simple tasks), FMA, grip and pinch dynamometer, SIS, MAL
Level 4—FTHUE, WMFT (simple tasks), FMA, grip and pinch dynamometer, SIS, MAL
Level 5—FTHUE, WMFT (simple and complex tasks), FMA, grip and pinch dynamometer, SIS, MAL
Levels 6 and 7—FTHUE, WMFT (simple and complex tasks), FMA, grip and pinch dynamometer, SIS, ARAT, BBT, NHPT, Jebsen-Taylor Hand Function Test, MAL

Some Common Presentations/Physiological Changes that Interfere with Functional Grasp and Release

1. **Intrinsic minus position** or "claw hand" (D2-D5 proximal interphalangeals [PIPs] in flexion with meta-carpophalangeals [MPs] in neutral)
2. **Flexor synergistic pattern** placing wrist/digits/thumb in insufficient position for grasp
3. **Indwelling thumb**
4. Spasticity/hypertonicity pattern, including D2-D5 MP flexion and wrist extension (lumbrical grip with wrist in extension)
5. Spasticity/hypertonicity in thenar eminence (thumb adducted and/or opposed at CMC and MP to insufficient position for grasp)
6. Flexor tendon shortening (active insufficiency) with extensor tendon lengthening (passive insufficiency)
7. Ataxic/dystonic movement leading to difficulty with coordination
8. Decreased sensation
9. Reaching pattern with forearm in supination rendering an ineffective hand position for grasp and release
10. Decreased arch control limiting grasp capability (that is, client only able to complete span grasp secondary to decreased intrinsic control to form arches necessary for cylindrical or lumbrical grasp)
11. Digit-initiated wrist movement limiting position of hand for grasp
12. Composite digit movement or lack of ability to manipulate individual digits making pinch control difficult or non-existent
13. Joint instability/deformities: Subluxations, collateral ligament laxity, shifting **volar plate,** boutonnière, swan neck
14. Contractures

Tips from the Field

The following tips are adapted from approaches developed by clinicians using evidence-based practice:

Tip 1: Addressing Spasticity

For the purpose of this chapter, moderate to severe UE spasticity relates to neurological clients who lack volitional control over wrist and digit flexion or extension secondary to spasticity. One would think removing spasticity immediately and in its entirely would be advantageous. However, some clients have learned to use spasticity to their advantage. Therefore, therapists should be sensitive to the fact he may have adopted movement patterns that depend on spasticity/hypertonicity. For example, clients with spastic hemiplegia may have learned to use the increased muscle tone in their weak LE to support functional transfers and gait. Removing this increased tone by treating the spasticity might unmask the underlying weakness and prevent these functions. Spasticity in the hand may assist a client to achieve a functional grasp, and if reduced/removed, the client's grasp may be too weak to continue its role in functional tasks. It is important to educate clients that spasticity and muscle strength are not synonymous, and with the reduction of spasticity comes opportunity to develop the strength and motor control for improved, volitional involvement in functional activities. Conversely, a client's spasticity can be so severe that it prevents any degree of functional involvement. Regardless of function, spasticity has the potential to lead to other barriers, such as deformities, pain, and inadequate hygiene.

Clients with spasticity experience difficulty inhibiting unwanted tone and facilitating a volitional muscle control; therefore, it is important to educate clients on facilitation and **inhibition techniques.**

Facilitation and Inhibition Techniques

Facilitory Techniques/Suggestions
* Quick stretch
* Vibration
* Kinesiotape
* NMES
* **Overflow** or associated reaction
* Tapping the muscle belly
* Stroking the muscle belly
* Working in synergistic patterns

Inhibitory Techniques/Suggestions
* Weight-bearing
* Fatiguing antagonists of desired movement
* E-stim (quick successive contractions to relax flexors in order to exercise/strengthen extensors), or use of Bioness H200 Hand Rehabilitation System "Fast 3" program
* Kinesiotape
* Mental imagery
* Vibration (stimulation applied to the antagonist of the spastic muscle in order to decrease spasticity)
* Stretching program
* Orthoses
* **Serial casting**
* Referral for medical management of spasticity

Tip 2: Sensory Reeducation

Somatosensory deficit is not uncommon following stroke and can be present with other neurological diseases. Evidence in this area highlights a broad range of interventions to address sensory deficits and is conflicting,[37] because one protocol is not distinctly identified as being superior over another. Anecdotally, significant variability exists in both client sensory presentation and response to intervention, requiring an individualized approach in managing deficits. Variability in presentations and response to intervention is often associated with concurrent motor and/or cognitive deficits. The most notable findings indicate electrical somatosensory stimulation improves hand motor function.[38]

Somatosensory training can include:

- Contrast bathing
- Thermal stimulation
- Intermittent pneumatic compression
- Sensory training using robotics
- Brushing
- Weight-bearing
- TENS/NMES
  - Electrode placement protocols specific to sensory reeducation
  - Conduction glove
- Stereognosis
- Vibration
- Tactile input

Tip 3: Edema

Three different treatment approaches to aid in the reduction of hand edema following stroke have been studied, including passive motion exercises, neuromuscular stimulation, and intermittent pneumatic compression.[39] Findings indicate that continuous passive motion and electrical stimulation are potentially more effective treatments for hand edema than intermittent pneumatic compression. Volumetric assessments of the hand appear to provide the best estimation of changes in edema (a change of 12 mL or more is considered clinically significant). However, measurement comparisons of the circumference of the hand at mid-finger, proximal to the MPs, and wrist can also be used to document changes in the edematous hand.[40] Treatment approaches to address edema may include:

- Medifit glove (compression glove)
- Kinesiotaping
- Contrast-bathing
- Soft-tissue mobilization
- Positioning
- Fist pumps above the heart
- Caregiver education

Tip 4: Increase Attention to the Affected Upper Extremity

- Proprioceptive feedback
- Blend of active assist range of motion(AAROM) and resistance
- Resistance
- Vibration
- Perturbations
- Visual regard
- **Mirror box therapy**

Tip 5: Hand Dominance

Research studies regarding hand dominance and neurological conditions are limited. As illustrated in the "Diagnostic-Specific

Information that Affects Clinical Reasoning" section of this chapter, right hand dominant individuals with an ipsilateral brain injury prefer to use their right UE, whereas left hand dominant individuals with an ipsilateral injury prefer more bilateral UE involvement.[35] There is emerging research linking deficits in hand function to specific hemispheric damage. For example, evidence of hemispheric specialization in the control of automatic reach-to-grasp actions reveals left hemispheric specialization in visual-motor transformation of grasp pre-shaping and right hemispheric specialization in transport-grasp coordination.[41]

Tip 6: Weight-Bearing

The incorporation of UE weight-bearing activities is an important and common practice for normalizing muscle tone in clients following brain injury. Repetitive UE weight-bearing inhibits hypertonicity and facilitates activation of both agonist and antagonist muscle groups. While there is limited information regarding both objective evaluation and intervention for unilateral and bilateral training, one study concluded a strong correlation between UE weight-bearing measures and FIM motor scores. Bilateral UE weight-bearing conditions yielded the highest significant correlation. Based on these findings, therapists should consider utilizing bilateral motor training to increase weight-bearing in an affected UE.[42]

One study examined external and internal factors that can affect weight-bearing. External factors, according to Serrien, et al.,[43] arise from information provided by the environment in which the movement is produced. Therefore, the unilateral or bilateral condition itself is an external factor modifying the UE weight-bearing pressure. Internal factors, on the other hand, refer to the person's related conditions from his CNS. For example, a client's attention can affect movement and symmetrical weight-bearing of the extremity.[43]

In the clinic, it is not uncommon to incorporate the use of a static hand-shaped paddle to support digit MPs and PIPs in a neutral position as the wrist is positioned into extension for weight-bearing throughout the entire UE. Consideration should be given to accommodate changes in digit position, pressure, and/or comfort level as the wrist is moved into extension, because the degree of spasticity and/or flexor tendon shortening may impact the effectiveness and comfort of a hand-paddle.

Tip 7: Constraint Induced Therapy and Modified Constraint Induced Therapy

Constraint induced therapy (CIT) and mCIT protocols (that is, forced use) have been proven effective at improving UE function in CVA clients with benefits lasting longer than 1 year.[44] CIT and mCIT protocols have specific inclusion and exclusion criteria, protocols for practice, and yield the best outcomes when supported by dedicated therapists/caregivers and client motivation. If not supervised properly, poor compliance with the protocol can result, yielding less than desirable outcomes.[45]

Tip 8: Bilateral Training

Research involving imaging has shown improvement in affected UE functional performance secondary to bilateral training.[23] The most effective protocol establishing whether bilateral UEs should move concurrently, with/without synchronicity, and use of rhythmic cuing or visual feedback (such as, mirror imaging) has yet to be identified. Further research is needed to identify how well the movement(s) learned in bilateral training can be translated to other tasks. Theoretically, the use of the intact limb helps to promote functional recovery of the impaired limb through facilitative coupling effects between the upper limbs.[46]

One study noted the importance of intention for simultaneous movement being more significant than simultaneous movement alone.[47,48] On anecdotal experience, bilateral training has been effective in assisting clients initiate and discover movement in their affected UE, as well as problem-solve a movement pattern that they cannot complete unilaterally with their affected UE.

Tip 9: Neuromuscular Electrical Stimulation/ Functional Electrical Stimulation/Transcutaneous Electrical Nerve Stimulation/Electromyogram

Neuromuscular Electrical Stimulation/Functional Electrical Stimulation

NMES/FES is often used with the neurological hand. Functional electrical stimulation (FES) refers to the application of NMES to help achieve a functional task. FES is a technique that uses bursts of short electrical pulses to generate muscle contraction by stimulating motor neurons or reflex pathways. Three forms of NMES are available: 1) cyclic NMES, which contracts paretic muscles on a preset schedule and does not require participation on the part of the client; 2) electromyogram (EMG) triggered NMES, which may be used for clients who are able to partially activate a muscle and may have a greater therapeutic effect; and 3) neuroprosthetic applications of NMES, which can ultimately improve or restore the grasp and manipulation functions required for typical ADLs.[49] However, there are certain factors to consider with use of NMES. One factor is tendon shortening due to spasticity.

> ### Clinical Pearl
>
> If an individual has moderate to severe tone with tendon shortening, use of electrical stimulation can elicit hyperextension of digit joints, which can threaten joint integrity. If this is the case, then reducing intensity and evaluating the position of the wrist and hand to promote the most optimal tendon excursion is important.

Evaluate intensity by how much extension or flexion of digits can be elicited before hyperextension is noted. Alter position to decrease stretch on shortened tendons, or consider blocking proximal digit joints in neutral or slight flexion to allow better tendon excursion distally.

Several reviews and meta-analyses examining the benefit of NMES have been conducted. A meta-analysis of four studies concluded that FES enhanced strength.[50] However, conclusions are limited by the methodology of the trials (small sample size, inadequate blinding), and the difficulty in correlating improved strength with improved function. A systematic review by de Kroon, et al.[51] assessed the effect of therapeutic electrical stimulation of the affected UE in improving motor control and functional abilities after stroke. The authors included six randomized control trials in their review and concluded that there is a positive effect of electrical stimulation on motor control. However, conclusions could not be drawn regarding its effect on functional abilities.

Transcutaneous Electrical Nerve Stimulation

TENS capitalizes on the use of afferent stimulation to increase inflow of sensory signals to enhance plasticity, which in turn, yields better outcomes in rehabilitation.[52] Several trials have examined the use of TENS treatment in the restoration of motor function following stroke. Many of the trials presented assessed motor function, pain, spasticity, and a variety of other outcomes in both the upper and lower extremities.[51] Evidence regarding the efficacy of using TENS to improve motor recovery, spasticity, and ADLs is conflicting.

Electromyogram with Neuromuscular Electrical Stimulation

Some devices combine EMG and electrical stimulation, requiring volitional muscle contraction of a desired movement. One disadvantage with electrical stimulation is the tendency for clients to passively allow the machine to do the work. However, with the addition of EMG capability, the electrical stimulation will not be evoked until there is an EMG reading reflecting trace AROM of the desired movement. EMG biofeedback uses instrumentation applied to the client's muscle(s) with external electrodes to capture motor unit electrical potentials. As the instrumentation converts the potentials into visual or audio information, the client has access to visual pictures and/or auditory indications of the degree to which he is activating his muscle.

Tip 10: Hand/Palmar Shaping

Grasping deficits have been described in terms of altered hand orientation as the hand approaches an object, which may correlate with compensatory movement strategies of the arm and trunk.[53] Compensatory movement in the proximal UE and trunk can occur as a result of deficits in hand configuration or aperture during grasp. Therefore, it is important to consider positioning and shape of the hand when assessing and treating reach-to-grasp movement.

Rehabilitation interventions for clients with grasp deficits should stress anticipatory hand pre-shaping required for objects of varying size and shape. It is important not only to know where there is a deficit (such as, the difference in grip aperture), but it is also necessary to understand its cause (for example, weakness in the thenar or hypothenar muscles causing decreased arch control or uncoordinated grip). In order to address hand shaping, consider the following:

- Open/closed kinetic chain exercises
- Positioning to support distal movement (that is, decreasing proximal excursion to allow increased focus on distal control)
- Grading force of movement
- Closing the sensory loop
- Working in/out of synergistic patterns

Tip 11: Adaptive Movements

As the client attempts to use his affected hand, observe the patterns of muscle weakness, the degree of interjoint coordination, and the lack of joint and muscle flexibility secondary to decreased soft tissue length or spasticity/hypertonicity. Notable adaptive movements include:

- Pre-grasp: No terminal extension of the digits, disproportionate opening of the hand to compensate for muscle imbalance, and/or decreased wrist control for optimal position of the hand for grasp.

- Grasping: If the client has the ability to extend digits, excessive force can be observed due to difficulty gauging the amount of force need to grasp. At times, clients will use the same force to grasp an empty plastic cup as they would to grasp a gallon of milk. Also, decreased palmar thumb abduction with D1 IP in extension can impede the ability to effectively achieve a pad to pad pinch.
- Releasing objects: Clients may attempt to utilize grasp driven by **tenodesis.** Though AROM wrist motion may be limited, wrist flexion may be accomplished through relaxation of hypertonicity instead of AROM in order to allow the digit tendons to lengthen (passively or actively) for release. The disadvantage of this technique causes limitations in ability to grasp and release larger objects particularly in cases with limited AROM digit extension.

Tip 12: Mirror Box Therapy

Mirror box therapy can assist in reducing unilateral neglect, because it brings attention to the affected UE.[54] While mirror box therapy can be an effective modality, it is not for everyone. Subjectively, it requires considerable skill in being able to maintain sustained attention. Clients observe their less affected UE complete motor tasks in the reflection of a mirror as a way to simulate the same movement in their affected UE.[55] Research involving TMS imaging has shown primary motor cortex excitability exists in the ipsilateral hemisphere of unilateral hand movement as subjects watch the mirror image of their unaffected UE complete motor tasks.[56] This activity was completed without any active movement in the affected UE, which was occluded from view.

Tip 13: SaeboFlex and SaeboReach Orthoses

The use of neuro rehabilitation orthoses has gained recent popularity. Saebo's Functional Neurological Dynamic Orthoses, the SaeboFlex and SaeboReach, are devices used to treat clients with limited hand and arm function. For the purpose of this chapter, the most distal orthosis, the SaeboFlex, will be of primary focus. The SaeboFlex allows clients with moderate to severe UE hemiparesis to participate in the latest treatment advances by incorporating their affected hand in highly **repetitive task-specific training.** The concept behind this orthosis challenges the traditional neuro rehabilitative concept of "proximal to distal" recovery by introducing "distal to proximal" recovery. The SaeboFlex is a dynamic custom-fabricated wrist, hand, finger orthosis designed to strengthen grip and assist in release as needed.

Tip 14: Bioness H200 Hand Rehabilitation System

The Bioness H200 Hand Rehabilitation System (or Ness H200) is an advanced FES system intended to provide clients with a mechanism to regain function and movement of their affected UE. The device allows for the precise delivery of patterned FES to selected muscles in the forearm and hand to facilitate various grasp and release patterns.

Tip 15: TheraTogs

TheraTogs are an elasticized orthosis garment and strapping system which can be used to position the hand and wrist for grasp and release. TheraTogs promote the functional alignment of the UE, both proximally and distally, to include the wrist and thumb.

Tip 16: Robotics/Virtual Reality/Telerehabilitation

Robotics

Robotic devices can be used to assist a client in a number of circumstances. Robotic devices can aid with PROM to help maintain ROM and flexibility, temporarily reduce hypertonia, or resist passive movement. Robotic devices can also assist ROM when a client cannot achieve AROM independently. Robotics may be most appropriate for clients with dense hemiplegia, although robotics can benefit higher-level clients by increasing strength through resisted movement.[57]

The Hand Mentor by Kinetic Muscles, Inc., is an exercise therapy robotic device based on motor learning principles to engage the user, provide meaningful feedback during the performance of repetitive activities, and utilize a massed practice training schedule. The consistent, repetitive, and progressive nature of the Hand Mentor may increase the quantity and quality of sensorimotor information provided to the patient, which has been shown to modulate motor cortex function and excitability and promote motor learning. The Hand Mentor requires clients to utilize wrist and digit flexors and extensors, ideally actively, but can assist passively if needed during computerized audiovisual tasks that provide feedback of movement.

Virtual Reality

Virtual reality training is an innovative new treatment approach that may enhance cortical reorganization following stroke. To date, only a few randomized control trials have been conducted. One study involved two trials using popular gaming systems— the Playstation EyeToy and the Nintendo Wii.[58] The authors hypothesized improvement in UE function following stroke could be attributed to the avoidance of learned nonuse behavior or by repeated task practice.

Telerehabilitation

Few examples of formal client testing involving telerehabilitation approaches are available. One study highlighted the feasibility of remote retraining of arm movement in stroke patients through Java Therapy software.[59] A participant trained at home using a computer mouse and keyboard as input devices while interacting with a web-based library of games and progress charts. The programs automatically recorded participant performance, and the information was transmitted to a central database for analysis. The study concluded movement parameters of the participant improved over several training sessions.

Tip 17: Complementary Medicine

Complementary medicine tends to focus on noninvasive and stress-reducing techniques and can supplement or be used in conjunction with more conventional treatment methods. Certain Asian countries, such as China and Korea, have utilized acupuncture in treating stroke; however, scientific study in this area is fairly recent and controversial. Effectiveness of acupuncture in aiding stroke recovery indicates mixed results with questionable research design methods. For instance, several studies did not use a control group and for those including control groups, the participants were not clearly randomized. Yet, some studies indicate when acupuncture is used in conjunction with other therapy, the technique can be effective in improving specific motor function of extremities following stroke. The greatest benefit from this technique results from early intervention post-stroke.[60]

Orthoses

Whether to issue an UE orthosis, at what stage in recovery,[13] and determining the most appropriate type of orthosis are important decisions to be made by a therapist. There are many variables to consider when assessing the type of orthosis to acquire for a client. Design options include: static/immobilization, dynamic/mobilization, static-progressive, hand- or forearm-based, positioned on the volar or dorsum surface, and prefabricated/fabricated. Material properties to consider consist of, but are not limited to: conformability, resistance to stretch, memory, rigidity, bonding, working time, thickness, perforated or nonperforated, and Neoprene.[61] Companies offering prefabrication options include: SaeboStretch, Softpro, Dynasplint Systems, and FREEDOM Omni Progressive, to name a few. The neurological hand will likely change throughout the course of recovery; therefore, choosing the type of orthosis and when to introduce it to the client and caregiver can be critical. For example, a static, forearm-based resting hand orthosis fabricated for a client while he is in inpatient rehabilitation may need to be refitted, replaced, or discontinued months later secondary to changes in the hand. And if an orthosis is introduced without comprehensive education on how to don/doff, progress a wearing schedule, or what signs to watch for that indicate possible harm, the wearing of the orthosis may actually lead to complications, such as deformities, pain, injury, and edema. These complications can arise from improper application and wearing, or changes in the hand may cause the orthosis to no longer achieve or fulfill its original intent.

The aims of an orthosis for a neurological client include: reduction in spasticity and/or pain, lengthening of soft tissue, maintenance of joint alignment, improvement in functional outcome, and prevention of contracture/deformities and edema.[61] There is evidence that the use of orthoses in CVA does not reduce spasticity in the long-term.[62] Conversely, the use of orthoses that provide a low-load, prolonged stretch at end range has proven to reduce spasticity/hypertonicity and contractures.[13] Evidence regarding use of orthoses for the spastic UE is controversial.[61] However, there are anecdotal reports of increased relaxation and reduced tone experienced in the digits and wrist during and after orthotic wear. There is also evidence that hand splinting does not decrease impairment or reduce disability with UE function during recovery after a stroke.[62] However, orthoses can be used to increase flexor tendon length, decrease the potential for passive insufficiency from extensor tendon lengthening, and promote neutral positioning of wrist and digit joints and tendons.[63]

Research suggesting superiority of a particular orthotic design over another with respect to the CVA hand is limited.[13] There is a history of debate over two different concepts to splinting the CVA hand: 1) the biomechanical approach, which emphasizes support of joint alignment, soft tissue length, and prevention of contractures; and 2) the neurophysiologic approach, which considers reflexive response, facilitation/inhibition through sensory input and positioning, and the neurological basis of spasticity.[13] As therapists, it is important to consider a client's biomechanical needs for an orthosis as well as the potential for a neurological response to an orthosis. For example, clients may experience an increase in spasticity/hypertonicity from physical contact with an orthosis or the positioning of their wrist and digits in the orthosis. The former can be addressed by considering different material or location of input (that is., volar or dorsal base of support or the addition of proximal joint support to decrease the stretch on a distal joint), and the latter by modifying the angles of the wrist and digits. This typically means decreasing the amount of stretch to the hypertonic muscles, such as modifying the orthosis to allow for increased digit and wrist flexion, thereby reducing the amount of stretch to the spastic/hypertonic flexors.[61] It is also important to evaluate the impact of an orthosis on a client's daily routine, as some orthoses may be too complicated to manage independently or may overwhelm an already strained caregiver. Either situation has the potential to lead to complications and inappropriate or no use of the orthosis at all.

In addition to these considerations, the following are evaluation tips and management strategies to consider when assessing a client's hand for an orthosis.[13,61]

Potential Presentations Indicating the Need for an Orthosis

1. Soft tissue restrictions into digit flexion or extension (both intrinsic and extrinsic), limited D1-D2 web space, and lack of functional digit excursion secondary to wrist movement (that is, increased digit flexion during neutral to extended wrist position)
2. Joint contractures
3. Decreased joint ROM, muscle weakness, tendon laxity, and decreased coordination causing difficulty with functional grasp
4. Hygiene issues secondary from moderate-severe spasticity or joint contracture
5. Resting hand posture in otherwise neutral position

Points to Consider Prior to Issuing and When Managing an Orthosis

1. Client/caregiver ability to don/doff and manage an orthotic wearing schedule
2. Sensory deficits compromising an accurate reflection of the orthosis fit leading to potential injury
3. Impact on functional use, because orthoses have the potential to block functional movement: Orthotics that impede movement should ideally be worn when the client is least likely going to include his hand during grasp and release demands.
4. The presence of edema
5. Pressure leading to possible injury
6. Instruct maintenance and follow-up care that is realistic for the client and caregiver: Developing an orthotic wearing schedule can be helpful for a client and caregiver, as well as providing sequential photographs of the donning process and end result reflecting the correct positioning of the orthotic for a HEP. Ensuring clients and caregivers can demonstrate the donning/doffing process and following up with their ability to progress a wearing schedule are recommended.

Common Orthoses Used for Addressing Neurological Issues

1. Static or dynamic forearm-based resting hand orthoses—prefabricated options from companies, such as SaeboStretch , Softpro, Dynasplint Systems, and FREE-DOM Omni Progressive, to name a few; and fabricated immobilization varieties with or without finger separation and increased thumb abduction to promote reflex inhibition.[61] These orthoses are typically worn overnight in a supported position, because they have the tendency to restrict participation in grasp and release and cause an unwanted load on proximal joints.

2. Static progressive orthoses with adjustable dial or ratcheting components (for example, orthoses from Joint Active Systems, Inc. [JAS] and Dynasplint Systems), worn to provide prolonged, progressive stretch over specific period(s) of time throughout the day. After wearing a static progressive orthosis. it is recommended the client continues to wear his Dynasplint on a lower load stretch, or don a static or dynamic forearm-based resting hand orthosis to enforce a low-load, prolonged stretch, because this assists in maintaining any gains made in tissue length from the static progressive orthosis. Caveats in maintaining these types of orthoses include: the need for consistent follow-up by a therapist; clients/caregivers to be vigilant in managing a wearing schedule and observing/acting on concerns; and the fact major adjustments and upkeep typically require a company representative or orthotist.

3. Wrist cock-up orthoses (prefabricated options include various over-the-counter brands or brands offered through DME/AE providers with volar, dorsal, or circumferential support, as well as options with extra support to block wrist deviation; and fabricated immobilization or mobilization varieties), worn to support the wrist in a position to promote optimal positioning of digits for grasp and pinch demands. This may involve a neutral or slightly flexed wrist position to promote tenodesis grasp. Wrist orthoses may also protect the wrist during transfers, particularly involving clients with visual neglect/hemianopsia. A wrist orthosis that interferes the least with grasp and pinch demands is recommended.

4. Orthoses to promote neuro-reeducation (that is, blocking of D2-D5 MPs in neutral position to allow the client to focus on increased PIP flexion) or functional positioning of the hand and digits for grasp and release (MP blocking splint, intrinsic minus splint, hand-based anti-claw, Oval 8's or Silver Ring, thumb spica, digit IP and D1 abduction immobilization splints, digit mobilization splints, and so on). Caveats of these orthoses include: frequent donning/doffing; consistent monitoring for redness, swelling, and so on; client vigilance in using the orthosis appropriately and managing an often complicated wearing schedule; and the static nature of these orthoses do not bode well in accommodating changes with spasticity during functional use.

5. Fabric-based orthoses (Neoprene strapping, Comfort Cool Thumb Adductor Strap, Benik thumb strap or hand-based D1 or D1-D2 support, Theratogs, digit buddy straps, and so on) to promote functional positioning of digits via dynamic blocking or facilitation. Caveats of these orthoses include: frequent donning/doffing with the donning process being potentially complex, and the risk of spasticity/hypertonicity overcoming orthotic support.

6. Serial casting can be used to treat contractures and has been proven effective in promoting elongation of tissue length.[61] Progressive casting over a period of days or weeks provides an excellent opportunity to apply a low-load, prolonged stretch to spastic/hypertonic or contracted joints and soft tissue. Another benefit includes the reduction of spasticity secondary to the neutral warmth provided by the casting materials.[61] Casts are typically applied to promote a prolonged stretch just below maximal range and/or prior to activating spasticity.[61] Casts are left on for 3 to 5 days before checking skin integrity and response to treatment, and can be applied weekly up to 3 to 5 weeks.[61] A successful result per cast is noted by a gain in ROM of 10° to 20°.[64] Exclusion criteria can include: edema, digit or wrist subluxation, fracture, heterotrophic ossification, open wounds, or client intolerance. Impaired sensation may also be a concern. Caveats to casting include decreased functional use of the casted UE, issues with skin integrity and pressure, poor tolerance or client agitation, increased edema, circulatory changes, and itching.[13,61] Subjective experience includes the use of batting material to wrap digits to provide a prolonged stretch into extension as a precursor to casting. Not only does this offer a less aggressive approach to stretch, but it also decreases tone via neutral warmth and allows for a therapist to assess a client's response more easily.

Common Barriers in Treating the Neurological Hand

Spasticity	Poor motor planning
UE weakness (proximal and/or distal)	**(apraxia)**
	Edema
Decreased coordination (ataxia, dysmetria)	Pain
Visual-perceptual deficits	Soft tissue limitations
Cognitive deficits	Joint contractures
Sensory impairments	Depression
Decreased caregiver support	Learned nonuse/disuse
Poor case management	Behavioral issues
Socioeconomic issues lending to decreased access to resources	**Aphasia**

References

1. Pedretti L, Early MB: *Occupational therapy: practice skills for physical dysfunction*, ed 5, St Louis, 2001, Mosby.
2. Rosenstein L, Ridgel AL, Thota A, et al: Effects of combined robotic therapy and repetitive-task practice on upper-extremity function in a patient with chronic stroke, *Am J Occup Ther* 62(1):28–35, 2008.
3. van der Lee JH, Beckerman H, Lankhorst GJ: The responsiveness of the Action Research Arm test and the Fugl-Meyer Assessment scale in chronic stroke patients, *J Rehabil Med* 33(3):110–113, 2001.
4. Wenzelburger R, Kopper F, Frenzel A, et al: Hand coordination following capsular stroke, *Brain* 128(1):64–74, 2005.
5. Duncan P, Reker D, Kwon S, et al: Measuring stroke impact with the stroke impact scale: telephone versus mail administration in veterans with stroke, *Med Care* 43(5):507–515, 2005.
6. Reddy H, Narayanan S, Woolrich M, et al: Functional brain reorganization for hand movement in patients with multiple sclerosis: defining distinct effects of injury and disability, *Brain* 125(12):2646–2657, 2002.
7. Verheyden G, Nuyens G, Nieuwboer A, et al: Reliability and validity of trunk assessment for people with multiple sclerosis, *Phys Ther* 86(1): 66–76, 2006.
8. UAB School of Medicine Department of Physical Medicine and Rehabilitation: The UAB-SCIMS information network, *Spinal Cord Injury Model System Information Network* (website): http://www.spinalcord.uab.edu/show.asp?durki=21819. Accessed August 20, 2012.
9. Augutis M, Anderson CJ: Coping strategies recalled by young adults who sustained a spinal cord injury during adolescence, *Spinal Cord* 50(3): 213–219, 2012.
10. Donnelly C, Eng JJ, Hall J, et al: Client-centered assessment and the identification of meaningful treatment goals for individuals with a spinal cord injury, *Spinal Cord* 42(5):302–307, 2004.
11. Health library: rehabilitation for stroke, *John Hopkins Medicine* (website): http://www.hopkinsmedicine.org/healthlibrary/conditions/adult/cardiovascular_diseases/rehabilitation_for_stroke_85,P00805/. Accessed August 19, 2012.
12. National Stroke Association: New survey emphasizes need for more, better care after stroke, *The National Stroke Association* (website): http://www.stroke.org/site/DocServer/NSA_Stroke_Perceptions_Survey_Press_Release__final_.pdf?docID=1943. Accessed August 21, 2012.
13. Gillen G, Burkhardt A: *Stroke rehabilitation: a function-based approach*, ed 2, St Louis, 2004, Mosby.
14. Spasticity skeletal muscle relaxers, eMedExpert (website): www.emedexpert.com/classes/skeletal-muscle-relaxers.shtml. Accessed July 4, 2013.
15. Pharmacologic management of spasticity following stroke, Physical Journal (website): http://ptjournal.apta.org/content/84/10/973. Accessed July 4, 2013.
16. Spasticity management, Stroke Survivors Association of Ottawa (website): http://www.strokesurvivors.ca/new/SpasticityManagement.php. Accessed August 21, 2012.
17. Herzfeld R, Kramer H: Re-wiring the brain, re-shaping the mind: an integral approach to transformation, *Integral New York's Ken Wilber Meetup* (website): http://www.meetup.com/kenwilber-58/events/61658802/. Accessed August 20, 2012.
18. Queensland Brain Institute (QBI): More brain research suggests "use it or lose it," *Science Daily* (website): http://www.sciencedaily.com/releases/2008/02/080207091859.htm. Accessed August 21, 2012.
19. Bernstein NA: *The co-ordination and regulation of movements*, Oxford, 1967, Pergamon Press.
20. Latash L, Scholz JP, Schoener G: Motor control strategies revealed in the structure of motor variability, *Exerc Sport Sci Rev* 30(1):26–31, 2002.
21. Font MA, Arboix A, Krupinski J: Angiogenesis, neurogenesis and neuroplasticity in ischemic stroke, *Curr Cardiol Rev* 6(3):238–244, 2010.
22. Zorowitz R, Brainin M: Advances in brain recovery and rehabilitation 2010, *Stroke* 42:294–297, 2011.
23. Cauraugh J, Summers J: Neural plasticity and bilateral movements: a rehabilitation approach for chronic stroke, *Prog Neurobiol* 75(5): 309–320, 2005.
24. Summers J, Kagerer F, Garry M, et al: Bilateral and unilateral movement training on upper limb function in chronic stroke patients: A TMS study, *J Neurol Sci* 252(1):76–82, 2007.
25. Mayo Clinic staff: Stroke rehabilitation: what to expect as you recover, *Mayo Clinic* (website): http://www.mayoclinic.com/health/stroke-rehabilitation/BN00057. Accessed August 21, 2012.
26. Twitchell TE: The restoration of motor function following hemiplegia in man, *Brain* 74(4):443–480, 1951.
27. Lee K-S, Lee W-H, Hwang S: Modified constraint-induced movement therapy improves fine and gross motor performance of the upper limb in Parkinson disease, *Am J Phys Med Rehabil* 90:380–386, 2011.
28. Poole J, Nakamoto T, Skipper B, et al: Dexterity, visual perception, and activities of daily living in persons with multiple sclerosis, *Occupational Therapy In Health Care* 24(2):159–170, 2010.
29. Pradhan S: Use of sensitive devices to assess the effects of medication on attentional demands of precision and power grips in individuals with Parkinson disease, *Med Biol Eng Comput* 49(10):1195–1199, 2011.
30. Farley BG, Fox CM, Ramig LO, et al: Intensive amplitude-specific therapeutic approaches for Parkinson's disease: toward a neuroplasticity-principled rehabilitation mode, *Top Geriatr Rehabil* 24(2):99–114, 2008.
31. Fugl-Meyer AR, Jääskö L, Leyman I, et al: The post-stroke hemiplegic patient. 1. A method for evaluation of physical performance, *Scand J Rehabil Med* 7(1):13–31, 1975.
32. Berglund K, Fugl-Meyer A: Upper extremity function in hemiplegia, *Scand J Rehabil Med* 18:155–157, 1986.
33. Stineman MG, Shea JA, Jette A, et al: The functional independence measure: tests of scaling assumptions, structure, and reliability across 20 diverse impairment categories, *Arch Phys Med Rehabil* 77:1101–1108, 1996.
34. Winstein CJ, Rose DK, Tan SM, et al: A randomized controlled comparison of upper-extremity rehabilitation strategies in acute stroke: a pilot study of immediate and long-term outcomes, *Arch Phys Med Rehabil* 85:620–628, 2004.
35. Rinehard JK, Singleton RD, Adair JC, et al: Arm use after left or right hemiparesis is influenced by hand preference, *Stroke* 40(2):545–550, 2009.
36. Occupational therapy: functional levels of the hemiplegic upper extremity, *Terapia-Ocupacional.Com* (website): http://www.terapia-ocupacional.com/articulos/LevelsoftheHemiplegic.shtml. Accessed August 8, 2012.
37. Doyle S, Bennett S, Fasoli SE, et al: Interventions for sensory impairment in the upper limb after stroke, *Cochrane Database Syst Rev* (6):CD006331, 2010.
38. Schabrun SM, Hillier S: Evidence for the retraining of sensation after stroke: a systematic review, *Clin Rehabil* 23:27–39, 2009.
39. Leibovitz A, Baumoehl Y, Roginsky Y, et al: Edema of the paretic hand in elderly poststroke nursing patients, *Arch Gerontol Geriatr* 44:37–42, 2007.
40. Post MW, Visser-Meily JM, Boomkamp-Koppen HG, et al: Assessment of edema in stroke patients: comparison of visual inspection by therapists and volumetric assessment, *Disabil Rehabil* 25:1265–1270, 2003.
41. McCombe-Waller S, Whitall J: Hand dominance and side of stroke affect rehabilitation in chronic stroke, *Clin Rehabil* 19:544–551, 2005.
42. Reistetter T, Abreu BC, Bear-Lehman J, et al: UE weight-bearing after brain injuries, *Occup Ther Int* 16(3-4):218–231, 2009.
43. Serrien DJ: Interactions between new and pre-existing dynamics in bimanual movement control, *Exp Brain Res* 197(3):269–278, 2009.
44. Wolf SL, Winstein CJ, Miller J, et al: Effect of constraint-induced movement therapy on upper extremity function 3 to 9 months after stroke: the EXCITE randomized clinical trial, *JAMA* 296(17):2095–2104, 2006.
45. Ploughman M, Shears J, Hutchings L, et al: Constraint-induced movement therapy for severe upper-extremity impairment after stroke in an outpatient rehabilitation setting: a case report, *Physiother Can* 60(2): 161–170, 2008.

46. Latimer CP, Keeling J, Lin B, et al: The impact of bilateral therapy on upper limb function after chronic stroke: a systematic review, *Disabil Rehabil* 32:1221–1231, 2010.

47. McCombe-Walle S, Whitall J: Bilateral arm training: why and who benefits? *NeuroRehabilitation* 23:29–41, 2008.

48. Mudie MH, Matyas TA: Can simultaneous bilateral movement involve the undamaged hemisphere in reconstruction of neural networks damaged by stroke? *Disabil Rehabil* 22:23–37, 2000.

49. Popovic DB, Popovic MB, Sinkjaer T, et al: Therapy of paretic arm in hemiplegic subjects augmented with a neural prosthesis: a cross-over study, *Can J Physiol Pharmacol* 82:749–756, 2004.

50. Glanz M, Klawansky S, Stason W, et al: Functional electrostimulation in poststroke rehabilitation: a meta-analysis of the randomized controlled trials, *Arch Phys Med Rehabil* 77(6):549–553, 1996.

51. de Kroon JR, van der Lee JH, IJzerman MJ, et al: Therapeutic electrical stimulation to improve motor control and functional abilities of the upper extremity after stroke: a systematic review, *Clin Rehabil* 16(4): 350–360, 2002.

52. Sonde L, Kalimo H, Fernaeus SE, et al: Low TENS treatment on post-stroke paretic arm: a three-year follow-up, *Clin Rehabil* 14(1):14–19, 2000.

53. Sangole AP, Levin MF: Palmar arch modulation in patients with hemiparesis after a stroke, *Exp Brain Res* 199:59–70, 2009.

54. Altschuler EL, Wisdom SB, Stone L, et al: Rehabilitation of hemiparesis after stroke with a mirror, *Lancet* 353(9169):2035–2036, 1999.

55. Mirror box therapy/mirror visual feedback:*Research and Hope* (website): http://researchandhope.com/stroke/mirror-box-therapy. Accessed August 21, 2012.

56. Garry MI, Loftus A, Summers JJ: Mirror, mirror on the wall: viewing a mirror reflection of unilateral hand movements facilitates ipsilateral M1 excitability, *Exp Brain Res* 163:118–122, 2005.

57. Burgar CG, Lum PS, Shor PC, et al: Development of robots for rehabilitation therapy: the Palo Alto VA/Stanford experience, *J Rehabil Res Dev* 37:663–673, 2000.

58. Fischer HC, Stubblefield K, Kline T, et al: Hand rehabilitation following stroke: a pilot study of assisted finger extension training in a virtual environment, *Top Stroke Rehabil* 14:1–12, 2007.

59. Piron L, Tonin P, Trivello E, et al: Motor tele-rehabilitation in post-stroke patients, *Med Inform Internet Med* 29(2):119–125, 2004.

60. Laures JS, Shisler RJ: Complementary and alternative medical approaches to treating adult neurogenic communication disorders: a review, *Disabil Rehabil* 26(6):315–325, 2004.

61. Jacobs ML, Austin N: *Splinting the hand and upper extremity: principles and process*, Baltimore, 2003, Lippincott Williams & Wilkins.

62. Lannin NA, Herbert RD: Is hand splinting effective for adults following stroke? A systematic review and methodologic critique of published research, *Clin Rehabil* 17(8):807–816, 2003.

63. Tyson SF, Kent RM: The effect of upper limb orthotics after stroke: a systematic review, *NeuroRehabilitation* 28(1):29–36, 2011.

64. Hill J: Management of abnormal tone through casting and orthotics. In Kovich KM, Bermann DE, editors: *Head injury: a guide to functional outcomes in occupational therapy*, Gaithersburg, MD, 1988, Aspen, pp 107–124.

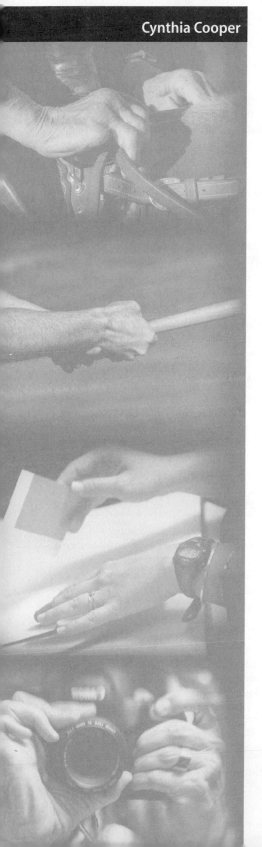

41

Cynthia Cooper

Hand Therapy for Chemotherapy-Induced Peripheral Neuropathy

Many people who have been treated with chemotherapy complain of upper extremity (UE) neuropathy that interferes with their activities of daily living (ADLs) including work and negatively impacts their overall quality of life. Certain chemotherapy agents are known to cause this problem but are necessary for best medical management. However, some patients have to discontinue their medication due to the severity of the neuropathy.[1] For these patients, this difficult choice may shorten their lifespans.

In the oncology literature, there are no descriptions or acknowledgments of the value of hand therapy for patients with chemotherapy-induced UE neuropathy. Articles in oncology journals refer to rehabilitation but appear to define rehabilitation as medication only and do not mention the potential value of hand therapy. Likewise, hand therapy literature has not identified this population as a diagnostic group that could benefit from our services. To make matters more challenging, oncologists are not typically in the habit of referring their patients with neuropathy to hand therapy. For them to do so, we must spark their interest and their availability to learn about our services as hand therapists.

Definition of Chemotherapy-Induced Peripheral Neuropathy

Chemotherapy-induced peripheral neuropathy (CIPN) is defined as somatic or autonomic signs or symptoms resulting from damage to the peripheral nervous system (PNS) or autonomic nervous system (ANS) caused by chemotherapeutic agents.[2] CIPN tends to be worse in patients with pre-existing nerve entrapments or neuropathies.[3] It has been reported that 30% to 40% of patients receiving chemotherapy experience CIPN, and as more aggressive pharmacological agents are developed and survival rates increase in the future, this number is projected to grow.

Quality of life is adversely affected by CIPN, and symptoms can interfere with treatment resulting in a reduction of dosage or even discontinuation of life-sustaining medications.[4] This is called a **dose limiting factor.** Currently there are no proven methods to treat CIPN.

Anatomy and Physiology Related to Chemotherapy-Induced Peripheral Neuropathy

Peripheral nerves are comprised of nerve fibers with varied myelination, morphology, functions, and chemical features. These differing fibers vary in their resistance to and response to the toxicity of chemotherapy drugs. Most nutritional, metabolic, and toxic neuropathies are **axonopathies,** meaning the pathology is axonal. The axon or the **Schwann cell** is typically the site of lesion.[2]

◎ Clinical Pearl

The vulnerability of a nerve to chemotherapy is influenced by its length. Longer nerves are more vulnerable than shorter nerves. In general, sensory fibers tend to be at higher risk to anticancer drug toxic effects than motor fibers.

Any portion of the PNS or the central nervous system (CNS) or even muscle can be injured by anticancer drugs. Symmetrical distal polyneuropathy is the most common pattern of symptoms. Other patterns of peripheral nerve disease in CIPN are radiculopathy, plexopathy, polyradiculoneuropathy, mononeuropathy, and multiple mononeuropathy (also known as mononeuritis multiplex).

Symptoms

> ### Clinical Pearl
>
> While the deficits of CIPN can be sensory or motor or autonomic, most polyneuropathies are purely sensory.[5] Paresthesias initially occur distally in a glove and stocking distribution and are worst on volar surfaces of the hands and plantar surfaces of the feet.

In CIPN, **allodynia** (experiencing pain with stimuli that is not typically painful) occurs especially in response to hot or cold. Motor impairment occurs less frequently and usually has a later onset. Purely autonomic symptoms are uncommon, but some autonomic involvement combined with PNS involvement is common.

Fine motor skills are affected, impairing activities, such as buttoning, donning earrings, doing clasps, and handling or manipulating small objects. **Sensory ataxia** is more severe when the eyes are closed or the lighting is low. Proprioceptive sensory disturbances also occur, as demonstrated by **Romberg sign,** which is a loss of balance that occurs when the patient stands with the eyes closed. Motor neuropathy presents with signs of weakness, cramps, atrophy, and fasciculation. Like sensory symptoms, the onset is typically distal. Findings of proximal weakness may be indicative of another condition, so be sure to mention this finding to the referring provider.

Nociceptive pain is defined as pain that is caused by structural dysfunction, such as a fracture. **Neuropathic pain** is defined as pain that is caused by peripheral nerve dysfunction and is typically sensory pain. This type of pain is difficult for patients to describe in words.

> ### Clinical Pearl
>
> Neuropathic pain has been associated with depression more often than somatic pain. In my clinical experience, many hand therapy patients, not just those with CIPN, experience neuropathic pain; and hand therapists should be addressing this in their clinical reasoning and treatment plans.

Small Fiber Neuropathy

Most CIPNs are described as **mixed fiber neuropathies** because there is involvement of both large and small fibers. Small fiber neuropathy is a result of damage to A-delta and C fibers, which are the smallest unmyelinated fibers. These fibers carry sensations of temperature and dull pain. Patients with small fiber neuropathy have intense neuropathic pain that is worse than those with large fiber neuropathy. They also demonstrate autonomic symptoms because autonomic fibers are small non-myelinated fibers. It is harder to clinically diagnose small fiber neuropathy than large

fiber neuropathy in part because nerve conduction studies examine only large fibers that are myelinated and fast conducting.

Chemotherapy-Induced Peripheral Neuropathy Symptom Timeline

Symptoms of CIPN may disappear when the chemotherapeutic agents are discontinued, but some symptoms may persist even after the medications have been stopped. This is called the **coasting phenomenon,** which is a result of slow physiopathology or slow drug clearance.

Chemotherapeutic Agents Involved in Chemotherapy-Induced Peripheral Neuropathy

Certain chemotherapeutic agents have been identified as drugs that contribute to CIPN. At the time of this writing, they include microtubule-stabilizing agents (MTSAs), platinum compounds, cisplatin, oxaliplatin, carboplatin, vinca alkaloids, proteasome inhibitors, thalidomide, and lenalidomide.

Diagnosis of Chemotherapy-Induced Peripheral Neuropathy

Simple clinical assessments are usually sufficient to diagnose CIPN. As noted earlier, nerve conduction studies are useful in identifying large myelinated fast conduction nerve involvement, but they do not identify small fiber dysfunction. In the oncology literature, scales of symptom severity describe levels of impact on ADLs. One such scale is the National Cancer Institute Grading: Common Terminology Criteria for Adverse Events (CTCAE) version 3.0 that scores neuropathic pain with grades 1-4.[6] Another scale is the Total Neuropathy Scores (TNS) that reflects sensory, motor, autonomic, and strength symptoms with grades 1-4.[2] The National Cancer Institute Common Toxicity Criteria–Version 3 scores motor and sensory symptoms with grades 1-5.[1]

Neuroplasticity

Hand therapists are experts on sensory reeducation and desensitization. These treatment programs are based on concepts of **neuroplasticity,** which refers to the fact that our brains can be reorganized neuronally in response to stimuli. Neuroplasticity involves learning, habituation, memory, and cellular recovery.[7,8] Key concepts of neuroplasticity are:

- Sensory perception is experienced by the CNS and is a dynamic process.
- Hand use affects receptor morphology. In other words, use it or lose it. Disuse of a hand leads to deteriorative and regressive changes in sensory receptors, whereas promoting hand use is thought to stimulate new receptors.[9]
- One single stimulus can excite multiple receptors because of the overlap of receptive fields of certain nerve fibers.

> ### Clinical Pearl
>
> When we touch our patients, are we remapping their brains?

( ) *What to Say to Clients*

"Our perception of sensation is very complex and is affected by many variables, including posture, swelling, movement, and stimulation, such as touching different materials. It has been shown that avoiding use of the hand worsens the sensory symptoms, and light use, visual imagery, or tactile stimulation can help it improve."

Hand Therapy Treatment for Patients with Chemotherapy-Induced Peripheral Neuropathy

My work treating patients with CIPN has been based on extrapolation of hand therapy's traditional sensory interventions with modifications in order to target the unique characteristics of the CIPN population. I encourage readers to add to this program with additional interventions based on their clinical reasoning and their patients' presentation. The program that I currently use is described in the following section.

Evaluation Tips

Begin with conversation and rapport-building. Ask about the patient's medical history, medications, surgeries, and past medical history, including prior injuries or nerve entrapments of the UEs. Learn whether any nodes have been removed. Inquire about the patient's social support system. Assess the impact of symptoms on ADLs. Consider using the Canadian Occupational Performance Measure (COPM) so that your treatment goals and plan are personalized and relevant to the patient.

Ask about the patient's pain. Discern whether it is neuropathic or nociceptive or both. Is it constant or intermittent? If it is intermittent, what are the provokers, if any? Is fatigue a factor influencing the pain experience?

If there are sensory symptoms, is the presentation one of sensory pain (burning or sharp shooting pain) or sensory impairment (numbness or tingling) or both? Map the areas of sensory complaints. Are there paresthesias? If so, are they positional? I have not found pressure threshold testing or moving or static two-point testing to be very meaningful clinically with this population, and in my experience, these tests are often too painful to justify using.

Screen range of motion (ROM). Look for extrinsic or intrinsic tightness and excursion of flexor digitorum profundus (FDP) and flexor digitorum superficialis (FDS). Measure the patient's edema. Observe the patient's posture. Patients who have had surgery have often developed postural accommodations for pain relief and these accommodations may contribute to nerve entrapment or vulnerability. Perform appropriate gentle provocative maneuvers using your clinical judgment. These may include, but are not limited to: cervical screening, palpation of epicondyles, middle finger test, elevated arm stress test, elbow flexion test, Phalen's test, tests for Tinel's sign at the cubital tunnel and the volar wrist, thumb carpometacarpal (CMC) grind test, and Finkelstein's test. Be careful about using upper limb tension testing, because this may be provoking.

Treatment

There appear to be three categories of hand therapy treatment that are effective in treating patients with CIPN: 1) manual therapy, 2) active range of motion (AROM) and nerve and tendon glides, and 3) desensitization/sensory reeducation. Each patient will respond uniquely, so explore and determine which of these categories seem to be the most effective. Begin with patient education regarding neuroplasticity. Welcome the patient's significant other(s) to participate.

◎ *Clinical Pearl*

Significant others of patients with CIPN often feel helpless and want to be able to assist in the therapy and home exercise program (HEP). Include them as much as possible so that they can be involved in providing symptom relief to their loved one.

Manual Therapy

Emphasize edema control. Try light, non-adherent compressive wraps, but be sure that these are not applied tightly. Do not perform manual edema mobilization or retrograde massage if the patient has had any nodes removed. If the lymphatic system has been disrupted by surgery, refer the patient to a trained lymphedema therapist and instead perform other interventions described later.

Instruct the patient in breathing, as appropriate; particularly if the patient is breathing shallowly from the chest (see Chapter 20). Gentle manual therapy can be very effective with sensory symptoms. Try a comfortable carpal tunnel stretch while the patient actively extends the digits, and ask whether this is helpful for sensory pain and/or sensory normalization. Consider teaching the patient's significant other how to do a gentle carpal tunnel stretch on them. Perform gentle palmar fascial stretches and gentle mobilizations, such as intermetacarpal sweeps. If the interphalangeal (IP) joints are painful, lightly stroke up the sides along the ulnar collateral ligaments and radial collateral ligaments, moving volar to dorsal. Myofascial techniques can also be very normalizing, especially over the volar and dorsal forearms. Be gentle with all manual techniques.

Active Range of Motion/Nerve and Tendon Gliding

Explain and emphasize the relevance of proximal motion for distal sensory symptomatology. Instruct in AROM in pain-free ranges, including trunk motion and shoulder circles, as appropriate, for shoulder, elbow, wrist, and hand AROM. Perform tendon gliding exercises and nerve glides/slides bilaterally and gently, as appropriate. Include FDP and FDS glides. Try soft isometric contractions of wrist flexors and extensors in neutral positions.

Desensitization/Sensory Reeducation

Explain that disuse due to sensory pain or impairment contributes to and reinforces the sensory symptoms. Explore strategies to maximize well-tolerated use of the hand. If sensory pain is reported, try applying paper tape over the areas of sensory pain (Fig. 41-1). I have found this to be surprisingly effective on sensory pain. Some patients report painful fingernails. If this is the case, try paper tape over the nails (Fig. 41-2). I have seen this simple strategy help patients use the computer again without pain.

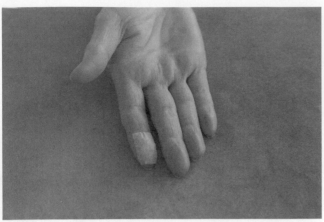

FIGURE 41-1 Paper tape applied over areas of sensory pain. (Photo by Cynthia Cooper. Used with permission.)

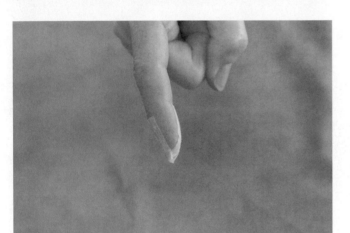

FIGURE 41-2 Paper tape applied over painful fingernail. (Photo by Cynthia Cooper. Used with permission.)

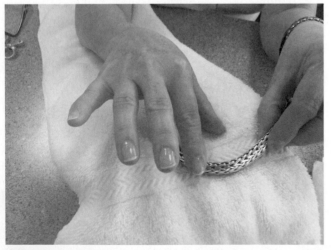

FIGURE 41-3 Patient performing sensory reeducation using a bracelet that she loved. (Photo by Cynthia Cooper. Used with permission.)

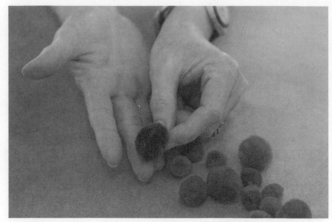

FIGURE 41-4 Many patients enjoy using soft pom-poms for soothing and pleasant sensory stimulation. (Photo by Cynthia Cooper. Used with permission.)

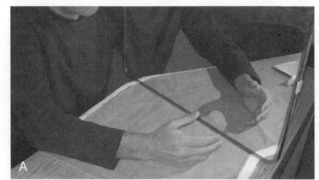

FIGURE 41-5 Mirror box therapy. (From Skirven T, Osterman AL, Fedorczyk JM, et al.: *Rehabilitation of the hand and upper extremity*, ed 6, Philadelphia, 2011, Mosby.)

Depending on the patient's needs, perform desensitization and sensory reeducation based on hand therapy's traditional body of knowledge in these areas.[10] Perform these interventions proximal to distal. Include the non-involved areas peripheral to the involved areas and treat bilaterally. Find desensitization materials that are meaningful to the patient (Figs. 41-3 and 41-4). Try vibration if it is not aversive to the patient.

Use laterality, graded motor imagery, and mirror box interventions (Fig. 41-5).[11,12] Try intentional confounding, such as having the patient wear an exam glove to perform dexterity tasks, then removing the glove and performing the same tasks again (Fig. 41-6). This form of sensory training seems to help the patient perceive or appreciate the available (albeit impaired) sensation, thereby promoting a sense of improved function; and it is based on exciting research by experts on the peripheral nervous system.[13]

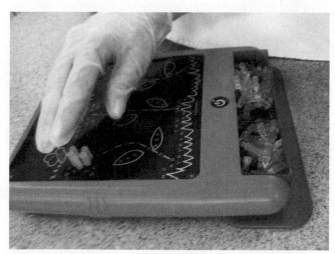

FIGURE 41-6 Patient performing pinch task with exam glove on; then patient will perform the same task with the glove off. (Photo by Cynthia Cooper. Used with permission.)

? *Questions to Discuss with the Physician*

- Has the patient had surgical disruption of the lymphatic system?
- What is the projected timeline of drug administration?

Diagnosis-Specific Information that Affects Clinical Reasoning

Patients with CIPN are different clinically from our traditional hand therapy patients with peripheral nerve trauma or repair. CIPN patients tend to present with sensory symptoms that do not follow the distribution of a particular peripheral nerve. This is because the pathology of chemotherapy toxicity is different from that of a peripheral nerve injury or repair.

The fatigue factor for patients with CIPN may necessitate shorter therapy sessions. Monitor their tolerances to the visit, and be prepared for them to need to shorten or cancel the visit possibly without notice if they are not feeling well enough to participate that day.

♡ *Tips from the Field*

- Light manual therapy can be very powerful for this patient population. Be prepared for the possibility of a moving emotional response from the patient or a family member.
- Use your training in joint protection and energy conservation to maximize the function of patients with CIPN.
- Focus on ADLs. Something as simple as an assistive device that improves patients' function will be well-appreciated by the patient and their family.

Marketing Dilemmas/Strategies

Patients with CIPN tell me that when they have complained to their doctors' offices about their neuropathy symptoms, they have been told there is no non-medicinal rehabilitation for this problem. My efforts to get referrals to hand therapy from oncologists have been frustrating with slow and only minimal

---

BOX 41-1   Sample Marketing Letter

To Whom It May Concern:

I am an occupational therapist/certified hand therapist at _____. I have a passion to work with oncology patients with upper extremity neuropathy. Although hand therapists routinely treat patients with other neuropathies, the oncology patients seem to have been overlooked by my profession, and this concerns me. I feel that patients with any subjective complaints of sensory changes or any signs of hand weakness/atrophy are good candidates for hand therapy. So far I have found that gentle soft tissue work, nerve gliding, and sensory reeducation techniques appear to be helpful, in addition to desensitization and other compensatory strategies, including adapted implements that maximize function. Most patients would probably not need more than a few therapy visits.

I would be very interested in communicating with you further regarding any opportunities to treat your patients. If you would be available for a phone call or a meeting in person, I would look forward to that.

Sincerely,

BOX 41-2   Sample Screening Tool

Hand Therapy Referral Screening Questions
- Do you have any numbness or tingling in your hands or fingers?
- Do you experience weakness in your arms or hands?

Referral Process
- Write a prescription for the patient to have hand therapy with _____(name of therapist)_____.
- Patient calls _____(phone number)_____ to schedule an appointment as a new patient.

Documentation
You will receive reports regarding the patient's clinical status and progress.

---

response. One reason for this is the physician's office's perception that these patients are already overloaded with medical appointments and do not really have time or interest in yet another appointment. My personal experience with these patients indicates otherwise. Many have asked me why they were not referred earlier. Some have cried when they experienced relief at their first therapy visit. It seems to me that there is a profound and as yet unarticulated importance of sensory function to these patients. Hand therapists are in a perfect position to explore this new territory. See Box 41-1 for a sample marketing letter to oncologists. See Box 41-2 for a sample screening tool that referrers might find useful.

Conclusion

Hand therapists who are interested in sensory problems have much to offer this population of potential patients who have not been identified in the hand therapy or oncology literature. Recognizing this population and providing hand therapy services to them can improve their quality of life, assist in their medical management, and provide hand therapists with personally rewarding work and new program growth and development.

References

1. Windebank AJ, Grisold W: Chemotherapy-induced neuropathy, *J Peripher Nerv Syst* 13:27–46, 2008.
2. Gutiérrez-Gutiérrez G, Sereno M, Miralles A, et al: chemotherapy-induced peripheral neuropathy: clinical features, diagnosis, prevention and treatment strategies, *Clin Transl Oncol* 12:81–91, 2010.
3. Sioka C, Kyritsis A: Central and peripheral nervous system toxicity of common chemotherapeutic agents, *Cancer Chemother Pharmacol* 63:761–767, 2009.
4. Wolf S, Barton D, Kottschade L, et al: Chemotherapy-induced peripheral neuropathy: prevention and treatment strategies, *Eur J Cancer* 44:1507–1515, 2008.
5. Kaley TJ, DeAngelis LM: Therapy of chemotherapy-induced peripheral neuropathy, *Br J Haematol* 145(3):14, 2009.
6. Barbour SY: Caring for the treatment-experienced breast cancer patient: the pharmacist's role, *Am J Health Syst Pharm* 65(10 Suppl 3):S16–S22, 2008.
7. Calford MB: Mechanisms for acute changes in sensory maps, *Adv Exp Med Biol* 508:451–460, 2002.
8. Malaviya GN: Sensory perception in leprosy-neurophysiological correlates, *Int J Lepr Other Mycobact Dis* 71(2):119–124, 2003.
9. Rosen B, Balkenius C, Lundborg G: Sensory re-education today and tomorrow: a review of evolving concepts, *Br J Hand Ther* 8(2):48–56, 2003.
10. Cooper C, Canyock JD: Evaluation of sensation and intervention for sensory dysfunction. In Pendleton HM, Schultz-Krohn W, editors: *Pedretti's occupational therapy: practice skills for physical dysfunction*, ed 7, St Louis, 2013, Mosby, pp 575–589.
11. Rosen B, Lundborg G: Training with a mirror in rehabilitation of the hand, *Scand J Plast Reconstr Surg Hand Surg* 39:104–108, 2005.
12. Rosen B, Lundborg G: Sensory reeducation. In Skirven TM, Osterman AL, Fedorczyk JM, et al, editors: *Rehabilitation of the hand and upper extremity*, ed 6, Philadelphia, 2011, Mosby, pp 634–645.
13. Rosén B, Bjorkman A, Lundborg G: Improved sensory relearning after nerve repair induced by selective temporary anaesthesia—a new concept in hand rehabilitation, *J Hand Surg Br* 31(2):126–132, 2006.

Index

Page numbers followed by *t* indicate tables; *f* indicate figures; *b* indicate boxes.